Nephrology

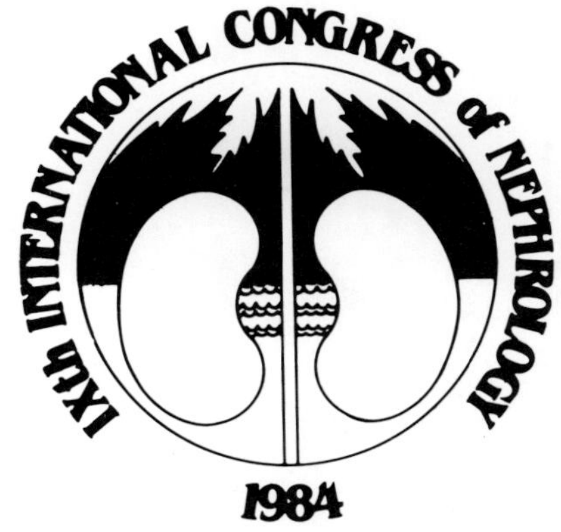

Nephrology VOLUME I

PROCEEDINGS OF THE
IXth INTERNATIONAL CONGRESS OF NEPHROLOGY

Editor

Roscoe R. Robinson

Associate Editors

Vincent W. Dennis · Thomas F. Ferris
Richard J. Glassock · Juha P. Kokko
C. Craig Tisher

With 220 Figures

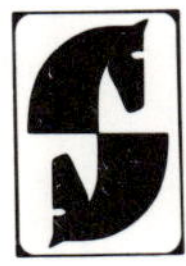

Springer-Verlag
New York Berlin Heidelberg Tokyo

Roscoe R. Robinson
Vanderbilt University Medical Center
Nashville, Tennessee, USA

Vincent W. Dennis, Duke University Medical Center, Durham, North
Carolina, USA

Thomas F. Ferris, University of Minnesota Medical Center, Minneapolis,
Minnesota, USA

Richard J. Glassock, Harbor-UCLA Medical Center, Torrance, California,
USA

Juha P. Kokko, Southwestern Medical School, University of Texas Health
Science Center, Dallas, Texas, USA

C. Craig Tisher, J. Hillis Miller Health Center, University of Florida, Gainesville, Florida, USA

Library of Congress Cataloging in Publication Data
International Congress of Nephrology (9th : 1984 : Los Angeles, Calif.)
   Nephrology : proceedings of the IXth International Congress of Nephrology.
   Includes bibliographies and index.
   Based on the proceedings of the IXth International Congress of Nephrology held in
Los Angeles, Calif., June 11–16, 1984.
   1. Kidneys—Diseases—Congresses. 2. Nephrology—Congresses. I. Robinson,
Roscoe R. II. Title.
[DNLM: 1. Nephrology—congresses. W3 IN446 9th 1984n / WJ 300 I59 1984n]
RC902.A2I56 1984   616.6′1   84–22136

The use of general descriptive names, trade names, trademarks, etc. in this publication, even
if the former are not especially identified, is not to be taken as a sign that such names, as
understood by the Trade Marks and Merchandise Marks Act, may accordingly be used freely
by anyone.

While the advice and information in this book are believed to be true and accurate at the
date of going to press, neither the authors nor the editors nor the publisher can accept any
legal responsibility for any errors or omissions that may be made. The publisher makes no
warranty, express or implied, with respect to the material contained herein.

Typeset by Kingsport Press, Kingsport, Tennessee.
Printed and bound by Halliday Lithograph, West Hanover, Massachusetts.
Printed in the United States of America.

9 8 7 6 5 4 3 2 1

ISBN 0–387–96072–4 Springer-Verlag New York Berlin Heidelberg Tokyo
ISBN 3–540–96072–4 Springer-Verlag Berlin Heidelberg New York Tokyo

Foreword

For many reasons, as President of the International Society of Nephrology, I am happy and honored to write a brief introduction to *Nephrology,* the Proceedings of the IXth International Congress of Nephrology. One of these reasons is specially treasured: I edited the two books published after our first Congress (Geneva-Evian 1960).

The 1984 vintage will certainly be as good as the preceding ones. And, for any nephrologist, whatever his or her field of interest, many observations will be found in the Proceedings that will enhance their personal work. It is characteristic for our Congresses to be the converging point upon which many different orientations join together and form the nephrology that is researched and practiced throughout the world.

What could replace a State-of-the-Art lecture delivered by a selected nephrologist whose work is of the highest quality? At times, even more revealing are those presentations made by non-nephrologists, the basic scientists who bring us fresh data and new concepts far removed from the reader's daily world. But attending such a lecture is never enough. Their texts should be read and reread. Symposia and workshops, as sources of precise and updated knowledge espoused by experts, are often heart-breaking as they shake established dogma. Therefore, they should be neither neglected nor forgotten but scrutinized carefully. The evidence which could eventually lead to new concepts or hypotheses has to be weighed accurately and then either rejected, discarded temporarily, or accepted, even if the latter implies dramatic change. These Proceedings provide the necessary means by which such decisions can be made wisely. *La règle du jeu, ce n'est pas la mode, mais l'imagination controlée par la raison:* The rule of the game is not the mode but imagination controlled by reason.

Dig into that heap of genuine facts that awaits you and you might find a nugget that could intellectually enlighten and boost your research program.

What a hope for a miraculous draught of fishes! I wish you good fortune and remember to prepare your best results for presentation at the Xth Congress of Nephrology to be held in London in 1987.

Gabriel Richet
President
International Society of Nephrology
(1981–1984)

Preface

Nephrology represents a unique venture. It is based on the Proceedings of the IXth International Congress of Nephrology held in Los Angeles, California, June 11–16, 1984. However, it differs from the proceedings of almost all previous congresses, international or national.

When policy was established for the Congress two years ago, a commitment was made to achieve a level of scientific excellence that had never before been achieved in an International Congress. The Program Committee worked diligently for 18 months in this pursuit. Simultaneously, steps were taken to assure the transmission of the information to a worldwide audience in written form using the most authoritative and comprehensive presentations.

To accomplish the latter, it was essential that Dr. Roscoe R. Robinson serve as the Editor-in-Chief; for he is the member of our society who has a proven track record of dealing with large numbers of papers, of transforming them (when necessary) into a form consistent with his own high values, of creating the required degree of flow and transition, and finally, of never sacrificing quality for other considerations. The book would be not only contemporary but meritorious, and the substantive points made by the essayists would not be modified.

Dr. Robinson accepted the challenge and immediately appointed a distinguished board of associate editors: Vincent W. Dennis, Thomas F. Ferris, Richard J. Glassock, Juha P. Kokko, and C. Craig Tisher.

Working as a team, Dr. Robinson and his associate editors subjected submitted manuscripts not only to editorial scrutiny but to peer review by independent referees. Many were returned to the authors for substantive revisions; almost all of the manuscripts were subjected to editorial modification. The resultant synthesis has, I believe, set yet another record for editorial accomplishment by Dr. Robinson, father and editor of *Kidney International* for its first 13 years.

Renal disease is a new and rapidly growing area of medical science and practice. It has, in fact, undergone the transition from a "footnote in some textbooks of urology" to one of the most rapidly advancing and extensive areas of biomedical science and practice; and all of this has happened within 25 years. This is due, in no small way, to Dr. Robinson's impact on the field in his capacity as Editor of *Kidney International.* He is now about to step aside from that position. It thus seems fitting that he should end that portion of an exciting and innovative career with an award-winning presentation of the state-of-the-nephrologic-art in *Nephrology.* Thank you, Ike.

Neal S. Bricker
President
IXth International Congress of Nephrology
Los Angeles, 1984

Officers and Committees
IXth International Congress of Nephrology
Los Angeles, California, U.S.A.
June 11–16, 1984

OFFICERS

President	Neal S. Bricker
Vice-President	Shaul G. Massry
Secretary General	Richard J. Glassock
Treasurer	Michael A. Kirschenbaum

ORGANIZING COMMITTEE

Donald A. Adams   Harvey C. Gonick   Nachman Brautbar
Charles R. Kleeman   Jack W. Coburn   Joel D. Kopple
Leon G. Fine   Kiyoshi Kurokawa   Dominick E. Gentile
Donald J. Marsh   Morton H. Maxwell

SCIENTIFIC PROGRAM COMMITTEE

Neal S. Bricker, *Chairman*
Richard J. Glassock   Charles R. Kleeman   Rex L. Jamison
Donald J. Marsh   Michael A. Kirschenbaum   Shaul G. Massry

EDITORIAL COMMITTEE

Roscoe R. Robinson, *Chairman*
Vincent W. Dennis   Richard J. Glassock   Thomas F. Ferris
Juha P. Kokko   C. Craig Tisher

LIAISON COMMITTEE, INTERNATIONAL SOCIETY OF NEPHROLOGY

Gabriel Richet, *Chairman*
Vittorio Bonomini   Colin Johnston   Jugoro Takeuchi

ADVISORY COMMITTEE, INTERNATIONAL SOCIETY OF NEPHROLOGY

George E. Schreiner, *Chairman*
Michael J. Dunn   Gary E. Striker   Guy Lemieux
Robert L. Vernier   Robert T. McCluskey   Guillermo Whittembury
Victor E. Pollak   Curtis B. Wilson, Jr.

SOCIAL COMMITTEE

Donald A. Adams   Dominick E. Gentile

COUNSEL

Harvey Shapiro

ADMINISTRATIVE DIRECTOR

Mary Frances Armbruster

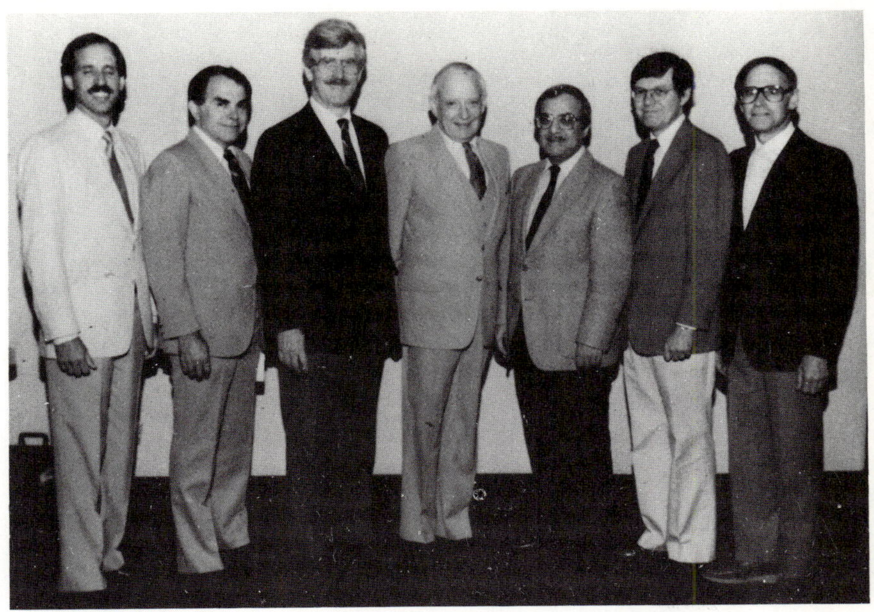

Scientific Program Committee (left to right): Michael A. Kirschenbaum, Donald J. Marsh, Richard J. Glassock, Neal S. Bricker (Chairperson), Shaul G. Massry, Rex L. Jamison, and Charles R. Kleeman.

Officers and Councillors
of the International Society of Nephrology
1981–1984

OFFICERS

President	Gabriel Richet, Paris
Immediate Past President	George E. Schreiner, Washington, D.C.
President-Elect	Donald W. Seldin, Dallas
Vice-President	Robert H. Heptinstall, Baltimore
Secretary General	John H. Moorhead, London
Treasurer	Robert W. Schrier, Denver
Editor, *Kidney International*	Roscoe R. Robinson, Nashville

COUNCILLORS

Stefan Angielski, Gdansk	Carl W. Gottschalk, Chapel Hill
Knut Aukland, Bergen	Renée Habib, Paris
A. William Asscher, Cardiff	Jean Hamburger, Paris
Jonas Bergstrom, Stockholm	Klaus Hierholzer, Berlin
Vittorio Bonomini, Bologna	Colin Johnston, Melbourne
J. Stewart Cameron, London	Guy Lemieux, Montreal
David P. Earle, Winnetka	Robert T. McCluskey, Boston
Laurence E. Earley, Philadelphia	E. J. Dorhout Mees, Utrecht
Carmelo Giordano, Naples	Floyd C. Rector, Jr., San Francisco
Richard J. Glassock, Torrance	Jugoro Takeuchi, Tokyo
Martin Goldberg, Cincinnati	Guillermo Whittembury, Caracas

Contents I

Two tables of contents have been provided. Contents I organizes the papers in a manner that provides the best sequential flow of content, irrespective of the order in which they were presented at the Congress or the type of presentation: State-of-the-Art lecture, Symposium manuscript, or Workshop summary. Contents II (see p. xxvii) is organized by the type of presentation.

Control of Acid and Electrolyte Excretion

Renal Metabolism, Prostaglandins, and Renin

The Endocrine System and the Kidney

Alterations of Extracellular Fluid Volume

Edema

Causes and Mechanisms of Renal Injury

Diseases of the Kidneys

Primary Glomerular Diseases

Acute Renal Failure

Volume II

Kidney Diseases in the Tropics

Diabetes Mellitus and the Kidney

Hypertension

Phosphate Depletion

Pathogenesis and Consequences of Chronic Renal Failure

Endocrine and Metabolic Abnormalities

Osteodystrophy

Hematopoietic System

Gastrointestinal

Evaluation and Management of Kidney Diseases and Renal Failure

Infections

Treatment of Glomerular Diseases

Contents II

Brush Border Transport Mechanisms

Regulation of Medullary Circulation

Intrarenal Control of Glomerular Filtration Rate

Transport Mechanisms in the Loop of Henle

Aldosterone and the Kidney

Mechanisms of Immune Complex Formation and Deposition in Glomeruli

Pathogenesis of Edema in Cirrhosis and Nephrotic Syndrome

IgA Nephropathy

Acute Renal Failure: Structure-Function Relationships

New Frontiers in the Prevention of Acute Renal Failure

Reflux Nephropathy: Current Status

Pathogenesis and Treatment of Calcium Nephrolithiasis

Tropical Nephrology

The Kidney and Malignant Disease

Nephrotoxicity and Drugs

Diabetic Nephropathy: Concepts of Pathogenesis and Treatment

Controversies in the Therapy of Hypertension

Endocrine and Metabolic Abnormalities in Renal Diseases

Parathyroid Hormone and Vitamin D in Uremia

Renal Osteodystrophy: Recent Advances

Renal and Vascular Consequences of Phosphate Depletion

Nutritional Aspects of Renal Disease

The Treatment of Glomerulonephritis

Continuous Ambulatory Peritoneal Dialysis

Immunomodulation for Transplantation: New Approaches

Workshops

Contributors

ABBUD-FILHO, MARIO. Department of Medicine, Beth Israel Hospital, Boston, Massachusetts, USA

ABE, KEISHI. Department of Internal Medicine, Tohoku University School of Medicine, Sendai, Japan

ABRAHAM, PAUL A. Regional Kidney Disease Program, Department of Medicine, Hennepin County Medical Center, Minneapolis, Minnesota, USA

ABRAHAMS, JOSEPHINE M. Department of Medicine, Monash University, Prince Henry's Hospital, Melbourne, Victoria, Australia

ACKERMANN, UWE. Department of Physiology, University of Toronto, Toronto, Ontario, Canada

ADLER, STEPHEN. Division of Nephrology, Department of Medicine, University of Washington, Seattle, Washington, USA

AGUS, ZALMAN S. Renal Section, Department of Medicine, University of Pennsylvania School of Medicine, Philadelphia, Pennsylvania, USA

ALFREY, ALLEN C. Medical and Research Services, Veterans Administration Medical Center, Denver, Colorado, USA

ALLAJANI, MOHAMMAD. Division of Renal Transplantation, Department of Surgery, Georgetown University Hospital, Washington, D.C., USA

ALPERN, ROBERT J. Department of Medicine, School of Medicine, University of California, San Francisco, California, USA

ALVESTRAND, ANDERS. Department of Renal Medicine, Karolinska Institute, Huddinge University Hospital, Stockholm, Sweden

AMIEL, CLAUDE. INSERM U 251, Département de Physiologie, Faculté de Médecine Xavier Bichat, Paris, France

AMSTUTZ, MARTIN. Department of Physiology, University of Zurich-Irchel, Zurich, Switzerland

ANDERSON, ROBERT J. Department of Medicine, University of Colorado Medical Center, Denver, Colorado, USA

ANDRESS, DENNIS L. Department of Medicine, University of Oklahoma Health Sciences Center, Oklahoma City, Oklahoma, USA

ANDREWS, PETER M. Department of Anatomy, School of Medicine, Georgetown University, Washington, D.C., USA

ARAKI, MASASUKE. Department of Anatomy, Jichi Medical School, Tochigi, Japan

ARANT, BILLY S., JR. Department of Pediatrics, Southwestern Medical School, University of Texas Health Science Center, Dallas, Texas, USA

ARDAILLOU, RAYMOND. Service d'Explorations Fonctionelles, Hôpital Tenon, Paris, France

ARNOLD, PATRICIA E. Department of Medicine, University of Colorado Medical School, Denver, Colorado, USA

ASSCHER, A. WILLIAM. Department of Renal Medicine, Welsh National School of Medicine, Royal Infirmary, Cardiff, Wales, UK

ATKINS, ROBERT C. Department of Nephrology, Prince Henry's Hospital, Monash University, Melbourne, Australia

AUKLAND, KNUT. Department of Physiology, University of Bergen, Bergen, Norway

BACKMAN, ULLA. Department of Internal Medicine, University Hospital, Uppsala, Sweden

BÁEZ-DÍAZ, LUIS. Departments of Medicine and Physiology, University of Puerto Rico School of Medicine, San Juan, Puerto Rico

BAILLY, CLAIRE. INSERM U 251, Département de Physiologie, Faculté de Médecine Xavier Bichat, Paris, France

BAKER, PATRICIA J. Division of Nephrology, Department of Medicine, University of Washington, Seattle, Washington, USA

BANKIR, LISE. INSERM U 90, Hôpital Necker, Paris, France

BANNISTER, KYM M. Department of Immunology, Research Institute of Scripps Clinic, La Jolla, California, USA

BARAJAS, LUCIANO. Department of Pathology, Los Angeles County Harbor-UCLA Medical Center, Torrance, California, USA

BARBARIC, ZORAN L. Department of Radiology, University of California at Los Angeles, Los Angeles, California, USA

BARBER, BARBARA. University Laboratory of Physiology, University of Oxford, Oxford, England, UK

BARFUSS, DALON W. Division of Nephrology, Department of Medicine, University of Alabama Medical Center, Birmingham, Alabama, USA

BAUD, LAURENT. Service de Néphrologie, Hôpital Tenon, Paris, France

BELL, P. DARWIN. Department of Physiology and Biophysics, University of Alabama Medical Center, Birmingham, Alabama, USA

BELLO-REUSS, ELSA. Department of Physiology, Washington University School of Medicine, St. Louis, Missouri, USA

BENIGNI, ARIELA. "Mario Negri" Institute for Pharmacological Research, Bergamo, Italy

BENNETT, WILLIAM M. Division of Nephrology, Department of Medicine, Oregon Health Sciences University, Portland, Oregon, USA

BERGERON, MICHEL. Department of Physiology, University of Montreal, Montreal, Quebec, Canada

BERGSTRÖM, JONAS. Department of Renal Medicine, Karolinska Institute, Huddinge University Hospital, Stockholm, Sweden

BERKSETH, ROBERT O. Regional Kidney Disease Program, Department of Medicine, Hennepin County Medical Center, Minneapolis, Minnesota, USA

BERNARD, DAVID B. Evans Memorial Department of Clinical Research, University Hospital and Renal Section, Department of Medicine, Boston University Medical Center, Boston, Massachusetts, USA

BERNSTEIN, JAY. Department of Anatomic Pathology, William Beaumont Hospital, Royal Oak, Michigan, USA

BERRY, CHRISTINE A. Division of Nephrology, Department of Medicine, University of California, San Francisco, California, USA

BETTER, ORI S. Department of Medicine, Rambam Hospital and Technion School of Medicine, Haifa, Israel

BIBER, JÜRG. Department of Physiology, University of Zurich-Irchel, Zurich, Switzerland

BINSWANGER, ULRICH. Section of Nephrology, Department of Internal Medicine, University of Zurich, Zurich, Switzerland

BLAINE, EDWARD H. Department of Renal Pharmacology, Merck Research Laboratories, West Point, Pennsylvania, USA

BLANTZ, ROLAND C. Division of Nephrology, Department of Medicine, Veterans Administration Medical Center, San Diego, California, USA

BLASCO, R. Servicio de Nefrología, Fundación Jiménez Díaz, Madrid, Spain

BOLTON, W. KLINE. Department of Internal Medicine, University of Virginia School of Medicine, Charlottesville, Virginia, USA

BOMSZTYK, KAROL. Department of Medicine, University of Washington School of Medicine, Seattle, Washington, USA

BONOMINI, VITTORIO. Department of Nephrology and Dialysis, St. Orsola University Hospital, Bologna, Italy

BONUCCI, ERMANNO. Dipartimento di Biopatologia Umana, Università di Roma, Rome, Italy

BONVALET, JEAN-PIERRE. INSERM U 246, Department of Biology, CEN/Saclay, Gif-sur-Yvette, France

BORDER, WAYNE A. Division of Nephrology, University of Utah Medical Center, Salt Lake City, Utah, USA

BORHANI, NEMAT O. Department of Community Health, School of Medicine, University of California, Davis, California, USA

BORN, WALTER. Research Laboratory for Calcium Metabolism, Balgrist Department of Orthopedic Surgery, University of Zurich, Zurich, Switzerland

BOUBY, NADINE. INSERM U 90, Hôpital Necker, Paris, France

BOUDAILLIEZ, B. Service de Néphrologie, Hôpital Nord, Amiens, France

BOUDJEMAA, AMAR. Department of Nephrology, Hôpital de la Pitie, Paris, France

BRAUN, WILLIAM E. Histocompatibility and Immunogenetics Laboratory, Cleveland Clinic Foundation, Cleveland, Ohio, USA

BRAUTBAR, NACHMAN. Division of Nephrology, Department of Medicine, University of Southern California, Los Angeles, California, USA

BRENNER, BARRY M. Renal Division, Department of Medicine, Brigham and Women's Hospital, Boston, Massachusetts, USA

BRIGGS, JOSEPHINE P. Physiology Institute, University of Munich, Munich, Federal Republic of Germany

BROWN, DAVID M. Division of Pediatric Nephrology, University of Minnesota Medical School, Minneapolis, Minnesota, USA

BROWN, DENNIS. Department of Morphology, Institute of Histology and Embryology, University of Geneva, Geneva, Switzerland

BUCKALEW, VARDAMAN M., JR. Departments of Medicine and Physiology and Pharmacology, Bowman Gray School of Medicine, Wake Forest University, Winston-Salem, North Carolina, USA

BULGER, RUTH E. Department of Pathology, University of Texas Medical School, Houston, Texas, USA

BURG, MAURICE. Laboratory of Kidney and Electrolyte Metabolism, National Heart, Lung, and Blood Institute, National Institutes of Health, Bethesda, Maryland, USA

BURKE, THOMAS J. Department of Medicine, University of Colorado Medical School, Denver, Colorado, USA

BUSHINSKY, DAVID. Division of Nephrology, Department of Medicine, University of Chicago Pritzker School of Medicine, Chicago, Illinois, USA

CAMERON, J. STEWART. Clinical Science Laboratories, Guy's Hospital Medical School, London, England, UK

CAMPESE, VITO. Division of Nephrology, University of Southern California, Los Angeles, California, USA

CAPASSO, GIOVAMBATTISTA. Department of Physiology, Albert Einstein College of Medicine, Bronx, New York, USA

CARDINAL, JEAN. Department of Physiology, University of Montreal, Montreal, Quebec, Canada

CARPI-MEDINA, PAOLA. Instituto Venezolano de Investigaciones Científicas, Caracas, Venezuela

CASE, DAVID B. Cardiovascular Center, Department of Medicine, Cornell University Medical College, New York, New York, USA

CATTRAN, DANIEL C. University of Toronto, Toronto General Hospital, Toronto, Ontario, Canada

CEREIJIDO, MARCELINO M. Centro de Investigación y Estudios Avanzados, Mexico City, Mexico

CHAIMOVITZ, CIDIO. Department of Nephrology, Soroka Medical Center and the Faculty of Health Sciences, Ben-Gurion University of the Negev, Beersheva, Israel

CHAN, JAMES C. M. Department of Pediatrics, Medical College of Virginia, Richmond, Virginia, USA

CHEKAL, MARCIA A. Department of Medicine, University of Chicago Pritzker School of Medicine, Chicago, Illinois, USA

CHESNEY, RUSSELL W. Department of Pediatrics, University of Wisconsin Hospitals, Madison, Wisconsin, USA

CHEVALIER, ROBERT L. Department of Pediatrics, University of Virginia Medical Center, Charlottesville, Virginia, USA

CHURG, JACOB. Department of Pathology, Mount Sinai Medical Center, New York, New York, USA

CLARK, MARY J. Department of Medicine, Veterans Administration Medical Center, Ann Arbor, Michigan, USA

CLEMENS, DANIEL L. Department of Biochemistry, Vanderbilt University School of Medicine, Nashville, Tennessee, USA

COBURN, JACK W. Research and Medical Services, Veterans Administration Medical Center, Wadsworth Division, Los Angeles, California, USA

COE, FREDRIC L. Renal Section, Department of Medicine, University of Chicago Pritzker School of Medicine, Chicago, Illinois, USA

COGGINS, CECIL H. Department of Medicine, Massachusetts General Hospital, Boston, Massachusetts, USA

COHEN, ARTHUR H. Department of Pathology, Harbor-UCLA Medical Center, Los Angeles, California, USA

COLE, BARBARA R. Department of Pediatrics, Washington University School of Medicine, St. Louis, Missouri, USA

COLEMAN, MICHAEL D. Holt-Krock Clinic, Fort Smith, Arkansas, USA

COLINDRES, ROMULO E. Department of Medicine, School of Medicine, University of North Carolina, Chapel Hill, North Carolina, USA

COLLINS, ALLAN J. Regional Kidney Disease Program, Hennepin County Medical Center, Minneapolis, Minnesota, USA

CORMAN, BRUNO. Department of Biology, INSERM U 246, CEN/Saclay, Gif-sur-Yvette, France

CORTES, PEDRO. Nephrology and Hypertension Division, Department of Medicine, Henry Ford Hospital, Detroit, Michigan, USA

CORVOL, PIERRE. INSERM U 36, Hôpital Broussais, Paris, France

COSIMI, A. BENEDICT. Department of Surgery, Massachusetts General Hospital, Boston, Massachusetts, USA

COSSETTE, PIERRE-YVES. Department of Nephrology, Hôpital de la Pitie, Paris, France

COUSER, WILLIAM G. Division of Nephrology, Department of Medicine, University of Washington, Seattle, Washington, USA

CRUTCH, BETH. University Laboratory of Physiology, University of Oxford, Oxford, England, UK

DABBS, DAVID. Department of Pathology, University of Washington, Seattle, Washington, USA

DAMBACHER, MAXIMILIAN A. Research Laboratory for Calcium Metabolism, Balgrist Department of Orthopedic Surgery, University of Zurich, Zurich, Switzerland

D'AMICO, GIUSEPPE. Division of Nephrology, San Carlo Borromeo Hospital, Milan, Italy

D'ANGELO, ANGELA. Department of Internal Medicine, University of Padova, Padova, Italy

DE BOLD, ADOLFO J. Department of Pathology, Queen's University, Kingston, Ontario, Canada

DEFRONZO, RALPH A. Department of Medicine, Yale University School of Medicine, New Haven, Connecticut, USA

DE ROUFFIGNAC, CHRISTIAN. Department of Biology, CEN/Saclay, Gif-sur-Yvette, France

DE SOUSA, RUI C. Departments of Physiology and Medicine, School of Medicine, University of Geneva, Geneva, Switzerland

DE ZEEUW, RICHARD. Section of Nephrology, Department of Internal Medicine, University of Groningen, Groningen, The Netherlands

DIBONA, DONALD R. Department of Physiology and Biophysics, University of Alabama Medical Center, Birmingham, Alabama, USA

DIBONA, GERALD F. Department of Internal Medicine, University of Iowa College of Medicine, Iowa City, Iowa, USA

DI STEFANO, ANTONIO. Max Planck Institute for Biophysics, Frankfurt, Federal Republic of Germany

DOBYAN, DENNIS C. Department of Pathology, University of Texas Medical School, Houston, Texas, USA

DONADIO, JAMES V., JR. Division of Nephrology, Department of Internal Medicine, Mayo Clinic and Mayo Foundation, Rochester, Minnesota, USA

DOYLE, AUSTIN E. Department of Medicine, University of Melbourne, Austin Hospital, Heidelberg, Victoria, Australia

DUBOSE, THOMAS D., JR. Division of Nephrology, Department of Medicine, University of Texas Medical Branch, Galveston, Texas, USA

DUMLER, FRANCIS. Nephrology and Hypertension Division, Department of Medicine, Henry Ford Hospital, Detroit, Michigan, USA

DUNN, MICHAEL J. Division of Nephrology, Department of Medicine, Case Western Reserve University School of Medicine, Cleveland, Ohio, USA

EGIDO, JESUS. Servicio de Nefrología, Fundación Jiménez Díaz, Madrid, Spain

EKNOYAN, GARABED. Renal Section, Department of Medicine, Baylor College of Medicine, Houston, Texas, USA

ELALOUF, JEAN-MARC. L.P.P.C., Department of Biology, CEN/Saclay, Gif-sur-Yvette, France

ELLIS, EILEEN N. Division of Pediatric Nephrology, University of Minnesota Medical School, Minneapolis, Minnesota, USA

EPSTEIN, MURRAY. Nephrology Section, Veterans Administration Medical Center, Miami, Florida, USA

FAIRLEY, KENNETH F. The Royal Melbourne Hospital, Parkville, Melbourne, Australia

FARMAN, NICOLETTE. INSERM U 246, Department of Biology, CEN/Saclay, Gif-sur-Yvette, France

FARQUHAR, MARILYN GIST. Department of Cell Biology, Yale University School of Medicine, New Haven, Connecticut, USA

FELSENFELD, ARNOLD J. Nephrology Section, College of Medicine, University of Oklahoma Health Sciences Center, Oklahoma City, Oklahoma, USA

FISCHER, JAN A. Research Laboratory for Calcium Metabolism, Balgrist Department of Orthopedic Surgery, University of Zurich, Zurich, Switzerland

FISCHER, SVEN. Department of Internal Medicine, University of Munich, Munich, Federal Republic of Germany

FLEUREN, GERT J. Department of Pathology, State University of Leiden, Leiden, The Netherlands

FOURNIER, ALBERT. Service de Néphrologie, Hôpital Nord, Amiens, France

FRIED, TERRANCE A. Division of Renal Diseases, Department of Medicine, University of Texas Health Science Center, San Antonio, Texas, USA

FRIEDENBERG, RICHARD M. Department of Radiology, University of California, Irvine, California, USA

FRIEDMAN, ELI A. Department of Medicine, State University of New York-Downstate Medical Center, Brooklyn, New York, USA

FRINDT, GUSTAVO. Department of Physiology, Cornell University Medical College, New York, New York, USA

FRÖMTER, EBERHARD. Max Planck Institute for Biophysics, Frankfurt, Federal Republic of Germany

GAGNADOUX, MARIE-FRANCE. Hôpital Necker Enfants-Malades, Paris, France

GARABÉDIAN, M. Hôpital Necker Enfants-Malades, Paris, France

GAROVOY, MARVIN R. Immunogenetics and Transplantation Laboratory, University of California School of Medicine, San Francisco, California, USA

GARRICK, RENÉE E. Renal Section, Department of Medicine, University of Pennsylvania School of Medicine, Philadelphia, Pennsylvania, USA

GAUDIO, KAREN M. Division of Nephrology, Department of Medicine, Yale University School of Medicine, New Haven, Connecticut, USA

GAUTHIER, V. JOYCE. Division of Rheumatology, Department of Medicine, University of Washington, Seattle, Washington, USA

GEBLER, BRIGITTE. Max Planck Institute for Biophysics, Frankfurt, Federal Republic of Germany

GEERING, KÄTHI. Pharmacology Institute, University of Lausanne, Lausanne, Switzerland

GENNARI, CARLO. Istituto di Semiotica Medica, Università di Siena, Siena, Italy

GIEBISCH, GERHARD. Department of Physiology, Yale University School of Medicine, New Haven, Connecticut, USA

GILL, WILLIAM B. Department of Urology, University of Chicago Pritzker School of Medicine, Chicago, Illinois, USA

GLAUSER, M. P. Division of Infectious Diseases, Department of Internal Medicine, CHU Vaudois, Lausanne, Switzerland

GMAJ, PIOTR. Department of Physiology, University of Zurich-Irchel, Zurich, Switzerland

GONZALEZ, ERNESTO. Instituto Venezolano de Investigaciones Cientificas, Caracas, Venezuela

GOOD, DAVID W. Laboratory of Kidney and Electrolyte Metabolism, National Heart,

Lung, and Blood Institute, National Institutes of Health, Bethesda, Maryland, USA

GRANTHAM, JARED J. Department of Medicine, University of Kansas Medical Center, Kansas City, Kansas, USA

GRAY, RICHARD W. Clinical Research Center, Froedtert Memorial Lutheran Hospital, Milwaukee, Wisconsin, USA

GREEN, JACOB. Department of Nephrology, Rambam Hospital and Technion School of Medicine, Haifa, Israel

GREGER, RAINER. Max Planck Institute for Biophysics, Frankfurt, Federal Republic of Germany

GRÉGOIRE, I. Service de Néphrologie, Hôpital Nord, Amiens, France

GUÉRIS, J. Laboratory of Radio-immunology, Hôpital Lariboisiere, Paris, France

GUGGINO, WILLIAM B. Department of Physiology, Johns Hopkins University, Baltimore, Maryland, USA

GUTTMANN, RONALD D. Royal Victoria Hospital, Montreal, Quebec, Canada

HABENER, JOEL F. Laboratory of Molecular Endocrinology, Massachusetts General Hospital and Howard Hughes Medical Research Institute, Harvard Medical School, Boston, Massachusetts, USA

HABER, EDGAR. Cardiac Unit, Massachusetts General Hospital and Department of Medicine, Harvard Medical School, Boston, Massachusetts, USA

HABIB, RENÉE. Hôpital Necker Enfants-Malades, Paris, France

HANCOCK, WAYNE. Department of Nephrology, Prince Henry's Hospital, Monash University, Melbourne, Victoria, Australia

HANDLER, JOSEPH S. Laboratory of Kidney and Electrolyte Metabolism, National Heart, Lung, and Blood Institute, National Institutes of Health, Bethesda, Maryland, USA

HAYASHI, MATUHIKO. Department of Pharmacology, Jichi Medical School, Tochigi, Japan

HEATON, ALEX. Department of Nephrology, Royal Victoria Hospital, Newcastle-upon-Tyne, England, UK

HEBERT, STEPHEN C. Department of Medicine, University of Texas Medical School, Houston, Texas, USA

HEIDLAND, AUGUST. Division of Nephrology, Department of Medicine, University of Würzburg, Würzburg, Federal Republic of Germany

HENRICH, WILLIAM L. Department of Internal Medicine, Southwestern Medical School, University of Texas Health Science Center, Dallas, Texas, USA

HERCZ, GAVRIL. Research and Medical Services, Veterans Administration Medical Center, Wadsworth Division, Los Angeles, California, USA

HERNANDO, LUIS. Servicio de Nefrología, Fundación Jiménez Díaz, Madrid, Spain

HILLMAN, BRUCE. Department of Radiology, University of Arizona, Tucson, Arizona, USA

HIWATARI, MASAO. Department of Medicine, Monash University, Prince Henry's Hospital, Melbourne, Victoria, Australia

HODSON, C. JOHN. Department of Diagnostic Radiology, Yale University School of Medicine, New Haven, Connecticut, USA

HOEDEMAEKER, PHILIP J. Department of Pathology, State University of Leiden, Leiden, The Netherlands

HOLDSWORTH, STEVEN R. Department of Medicine, Monash University, Prince Henry's Hospital, Melbourne, Victoria, Australia

HOPPE, RICHARD T. Department of Radiology, Stanford University Medical Center, Stanford, California, USA

HÖRL, WALTER H. Division of Nephrology, Department of Medicine, University of Freiburg, Freiburg, Federal Republic of Germany

HORSTER, MICHAEL F. Physiology Institute, University of Munich, Munich, Federal Republic of Germany

HRICAK, HEDVIG. Department of Radiology, University of California, San Francisco, California, USA

HRUSKA, KEITH A. Renal Division, Department of Internal Medicine, Washington University School of Medicine, St. Louis, Missouri, USA

HUMES, H. DAVID. Department of Medicine, Veterans Administration Medical Center, Ann Arbor, Michigan, USA

HUMPHREYS, MICHAEL H. Division of Nephrology, University of California School of Medicine, San Francisco General Hospital, San Francisco, California, USA

HUNT, DEBORAH A. Veterans Administration Medical Center, Ann Arbor, Michigan, USA

HUNT, JOHN. Department of Pathology. University of Otheo, Christchurch Clinical School of Medicine, Christchurch, New Zealand

ICHIKAWA, IEKUNI. Laboratory of Renal Physiology, The Children's Hospital, Boston, Massachusetts, USA

IMAI, MASASHI. Department of Pharmacology, National Cardiovascular Center, Research Institute, Osaka, Japan

INAGAMI, TADASHI. Department of Biochemistry, Vanderbilt University School of Medicine, Nashville, Tennessee, USA

ISSAD, BELKACEM. Department of Nephrology, Hôpital de la Pitie, Paris, France

IVANOVICH, PETER. Department of Medicine, Northwestern University School of Medicine, Chicago, Illinois, USA

IVES, HARLAN E. Nephrology Section, Department of Medicine, Veterans Administration Medical Center and Cardiovascular Research Institute and Department of Medicine, University of California, San Francisco, California, USA

JACOBSON, HARRY R. Department of Internal Medicine, Southwestern Medical School, University of Texas Health Science Center, Dallas, Texas, USA

JOHNSON, RICHARD J. Division of Nephrology, Department of Medicine, University of Washington, Seattle, Washington, USA

JOHNSTON, COLIN I. Department of Medicine, Monash University, Prince Henry's Hospital, Melbourne, Victoria, Australia

JONES, HENRY W., III. Department of Internal Medicine, Kaiser-Permanente Medical Center, Santa Clara, California, USA

KAISSLING, BRIGITTE. Anatomy Institute, University of Basel, Basel, Switzerland

KANGARLOO, HOOSHANG. Department of Radiology, University of California, Los Angeles, California, USA

KAPLAN, BERNARD S. Department of Pediatrics, McGill University, Montreal Children's Hospital, Montreal, Quebec, Canada

KAPLAN, NORMAN M. Department of Internal Medicine, Southwestern Medical School, University of Texas Health Science Center, Dallas, Texas, USA

KASHGARIAN, MICHAEL. Department of Pathology, Yale University School of Medicine, New Haven, Connecticut, USA

KATHOLI, RICHARD E. Department of Medicine, University of Alabama Medical Center, Birmingham, Alabama, USA

KATZ, ADRIAN I. Department of Medicine, University of Chicago Pritzker School of Medicine, Chicago, Illinois, USA

KEELER, RALPH. Department of Physiology, University of British Columbia, Vancouver, British Columbia, Canada

KERJASCHKI, DONTSCHO. Department of Pathological Anatomy, University of Vienna, Vienna, Austria

KIM, DONALD. Department of Medicine, Toronto Western Hospital and University of Toronto, Toronto, Ontario, Canada

KINCAID-SMITH, PRISCILLA S. Division of Nephrology, The Royal Melbourne Hospital, Parkville, Victoria, Australia

KINNE, ROLF. Max-Planck-Institut fur Systemphysiologie, Dortmund, Federal Republic of Germany

KIRK, KEVIN L. Department of Physiology and Biophysics, University of Alabama Medical Center, Birmingham, Alabama, USA

KJELLSTRAND, CARL M. Regional Kidney Disease Program, Department of Medicine, Hennepin County Medical Center, Minneapolis, Minnesota, USA

KLAHR, SAULO. Renal Division, Department of Medicine, Washington University School of Medicine, St. Louis, Missouri, USA

KLINKMANN, HORST. Department of Internal Medicine, Wilhelm-Pieck-University, Rostock, German Democratic Republic

KOEPPEN, BRUCE. Department of Medicine, University of Connecticut School of Medicine, Farmington, Connecticut, USA

KOKKO, JUHA P. Department of Internal Medicine, Southwestern Medical School, University of Texas Health Science Center, Dallas, Texas, USA

KON, VALENTINA. Laboratory of Renal Physiology, The Children's Hospital, Boston, Massachusetts, USA

KOPP, ULLA C. Department of Internal Medicine, University of Iowa School of Medicine, Iowa City, Iowa, USA

KOPPLE, JOEL D. Division of Nephrology and Hypertension, Harbor-UCLA Medical Center, Los Angeles, California, USA

KORKOR, ADEL B. Department of Medicine, Medical College of Wisconsin, Milwaukee, Wisconsin, USA

KRAEHENBUHL, JEAN-PIERRE. Biochemistry Institute, University of Lausanne, Lausanne, and Swiss Institute of Experimental Cancer Research, Epalinges, Switzerland

KU, GORDON. Department of Clinical Medicine, National University of Singapore, Singapore General Hospital, Singapore

KUROKAWA, KIYOSHI. Fourth Department of Medicine, Faculty of Medicine, University of Tokyo, Tokyo, Japan, and Department of Medicine, University of California, Los Angeles, California, USA

KUYTENS, RENÉE. Wilhelmina Kinderziekenhuis, Utrecht, The Netherlands

LACHIN, JOHN. Bio-statistics Center, Bethesda, Maryland, USA

LANGFORD, HERBERT G. Department of Medicine, University of Mississippi Medical Center, Jackson, Mississippi, USA

LANIER, LOUIS. Monoclonal Antibody Center, Becton Dickinson Company, Mountain View, California, USA

LAPOINTE, JACQUES. Department of Biochemistry, Laval University, Quebec City, Quebec, Canada

LAU, KAI. Renal Division, Michael Reese Hospital and University of Chicago, Chicago, Illinois, USA

LEE, DAVID B. N. Division of Nephrology, Sepulveda Veterans Administration Medical Center, Sepulveda, California, USA

LEGRAIN, MARCEL C. Department of Nephrology, Hôpital de la Pitie, Paris, France

LEMANN, JACOB, JR. Department of Medicine, Medical College of Wisconsin, Milwaukee, Wisconsin, USA

LEMKIN, MARGARET C. Department of Cell Biology, Yale University School of Medicine, New Haven, Connecticut, USA

LETTERI, JOSEPH M. Division of Nephrology, Department of Medicine, Nassau City Medical Center, East Meadow, New York, USA

LEVIN, BARRY. Renal Transplantation Service, Pacific Medical Center, San Francisco, California, USA

LEVIN, NATHAN W. Nephrology and Hypertension Division, Department of Medicine, Henry Ford Hospital, Detroit, Michigan, USA

LEWIS, EDMUND J. Department of Medicine, Rush-Presbyterian-St. Luke's Medical Center, Chicago, Illinois, USA

LIANOS, ELIAS A. Division of Nephrology, Department of Medicine, Medical College of Wisconsin, Milwaukee, Wisconsin, USA

LINARES, HENRY. Instituto Venezolano de Investigaciones Cientificas, Caracas, Venezuela

LINDHOLM, BENGT. Department of Renal Medicine, Karolinska Institute, Huddinge University Hospital, Stockholm, Sweden

LINSHAW, MICHAEL A. Department of Pediatrics, University of Kansas School of Medicine, Kansas City, Kansas, USA

LIVIO, MANUELA. "Mario Negri" Institute for Pharmacological Research, Bergamo, Italy

LLACH, FRANCISCO. Nephrology Section, Department of Medicine, College of Medicine, University of Oklahoma Health Science Center, Oklahoma City, Oklahoma, USA

LOCKWOOD, C. MARTIN. MRC Clinical Immunology Research Group, Department of Medicine, Royal Postgraduate Medical School, Hammersmith Hospital, London, England, UK

LOERTSCHER, ROLF. Department of Medicine, Beth Israel Hospital, Boston, Massachusetts, USA

LOMAX-SMITH, JANE D. Renal Unit, Royal Adelaide Hospital, Adelaide, South Australia, Australia

LORENZ, REINHARD. Department of Internal Medicine, University of Munich, Munich, Federal Republic of Germany

LOSCHIAVO, CARMELO. Division of Nephrology, University of Verona, Verona, Italy

LOZANO, L. Servicio de Nefrología, Fundación Jiménez Díaz, Madrid, Spain

LUND, BIRGER. Department of Orthopaedic Surgery, Rigshospital, Copenhagen, Denmark

LUND, BJARNE. Department of Orthopaedic Surgery, Rigshospital, Copenhagen, Denmark

MAACK, THOMAS. Department of Physiology, Cornell University Medical College, New York, New York, USA

MADSEN, KIRSTEN M. Division of Nephrology, Department of Medicine, J. Hillis Miller Health Center, University of Florida, Gainesville, Florida, USA

MALMSTRÖM, KERSTIN. Department of Physiology, University of Zurich-Irchel, Zurich, Switzerland

MANN, JOHANNES. Division of Nephrology, University of Heidelberg, Heidelberg, Federal Republic of Germany

MANNIK, MART. Division of Rheumatology, Department of Medicine, University of Washington, Seattle, Washington, USA

MANNING, MAURICE. Department of Biochemistry, Medical College of Ohio, Toledo, Ohio, USA

MARTIN, KEVIN J. Renal Division, Department of Internal Medicine, Washington University School of Medicine, St. Louis, Missouri, USA

MARTÍNEZ-MALDONADO, MANUEL. Medical Service, Veterans Administration Medical Center, San Juan, Puerto Rico

MASCHIO, GIUSEPPE. Istituto di Nefrologia Medica, Università di Verona, Verona, Italy

MASON, JUNE. Physiology Institute, University of Munich, Munich, Federal Republic of Germany

MAUER, S. MICHAEL. Department of Pediatrics, University of Minnesota Medical School, Minneapolis, Minnesota, USA

MCCARRON, DAVID A. Division of Nephrology and Hypertension, Department of Medicine, Oregon Health Sciences University School of Medicine, Portland, Oregon, USA

MCCLENNAN, BRUCE L. Department of Radiology, Washington University School of Medicine, St. Louis, Missouri, USA

MCKENZIE, JAMES C. Department of Biochemistry, Vanderbilt University School of Medicine, Nashville, Tennessee, USA

MENARD, JOËL. INSERM U 36, Hôpital Broussais, Paris, France

MENDRICK, DONNA L. Department of Pathology, Brigham and Women's Hospital, Boston, Massachusetts, USA

MEUNIER, P. INSERM U 234, University Alexis Carrel, Lyon, France

MEYER, JOHN L. Division of Research Grants, National Institutes of Health, Bethesda, Maryland, USA

MEYER, TIMOTHY W. Renal Division, Department of Medicine, Brigham and Women's Hospital, Boston, Massachusetts, USA

MICHAEL, ALFRED F. Departments of Pediatrics, Laboratory Medicine, and Pathology, University of Minnesota Medical School, Minneapolis, Minnesota, USA

MIGNON, FRANÇOISE. Service de Néphrologie, Hôpital Tenon, Paris, France

MILLINER, DAWN S. Division of Nephrology, Mayo Clinic, Rochester, Minnesota, USA

MITCH, WILLIAM E. Department of Medicine, The Brigham and Women's Hospital, Boston, Massachusetts, USA

MOGENSEN, CARL ERIK. Second University Clinic of Internal Medicine, Århus Kommunehospital, Århus, Denmark

MÖLLBY, ROLAND. National Bacteriological Laboratories, Stockholm, Sweden

MOORE, LEON C. Department of Physiology and Biophysics, Health Science Center, State University of New York, Stony Brook, New York, USA

MORGAN, TREFOR O. Department of Physiology, University of Melbourne, Parkville, Victoria, Australia

MORINIÈRE, PHILIPPE. Department of Nephrology, Hôpital Nord, Amiens, France

MORRIS, PETER J. Nuffield Department of Surgery, John Radcliffe Hospital, University of Oxford, Oxford, England, UK

MORRISON, AUBREY R. Department of Medicine and Pharmacology, Washington University School of Medicine, St. Louis, Missouri, USA

MORRISSEY, JEREMIAH J. Renal Division, Department of Internal Medicine, Washington University School of Medicine, St. Louis, Missouri, USA

MOSS, NICHOLAS G. Department of Physiology, School of Medicine, University of North Carolina, Chapel Hill, North Carolina, USA

MUJAIS, SALIM K. Department of Medicine, University of Chicago Pritzker School of Medicine, Chicago, Illinois, USA

MURER, HEINI. Department of Physiology, University of Zurich-Irchel, Zurich, Switzerland

MYERS, BRYAN D. Division of Nephrology, Department of Medicine, Stanford University School of Medicine, Stanford, California, USA

NAKAMARU, MITSUAKI. Department of Biochemistry, Vanderbilt University School of Medicine, Nashville, Tennessee, USA

NARINS, ROBERT G. Department of Medicine, Temple University Health Science Center, Philadelphia, Pennsylvania, USA

NARUSE, KIYOKO. Department of Biochemistry, Vanderbilt University School of Medicine, Nashville, Tennessee, USA

NARUSE, MITSUHIDE. Department of Biochemistry, Vanderbilt University School of Medicine, Nashville, Tennessee, USA

NAVAR, L. GABRIEL. Department of Physiology and Biophysics, University of Alabama Medical Center, Birmingham, Alabama, USA

NEBEKER, HENRY G. Research and Medical Services, Veterans Administration Medical Center, Wadsworth Division, Los Angeles, California, USA

NICAR, MICHAEL J. Department of Mineral Metabolism, University of Texas Health Science Center, Dallas, Texas, USA

NISER, ROGER L. Division of Nephrology, Department of Medicine, Veterans Administration Hospital, Miami, Florida, USA

NOLPH, KARL D. Division of Nephrology, Department of Medicine, University of Missouri Health Sciences Center, Columbia, Missouri, USA

NORBECK, HANS ERIK. Department of Renal Medicine, Karolinska Institute, Huddinge University Hospital, Stockholm, Sweden

OKA, TAKAHIRO. Department of Surgery, Kyoto Prefectural University of Medicine, Kamikyo-ku, Kyoto, Japan

OKAMURA, TOMIO. Department of Biochemistry, Vanderbilt University School of Medicine, Nashville, Tennessee, USA

O'NEIL, ROGER G. Department of Physiology, University of Texas Medical School, Houston, Texas, USA

OREOPOULOS, DIMITRIOS G. Department of Medicine, Toronto Western Hospital, University of Toronto, Toronto, Ontario, Canada

ORŁOWSKI, TADEUSZ. Transplantation Institute, Warsaw, Poland

OTT, SUSAN M. Department of Medicine, Harborview Medical Center, University of Washington, Seattle, Washington, USA

PAILLARD, MICHEL. Hôpital Louis Mourier, Colombes, France

PAK, CHARLES Y. C. Department of Internal Medicine, Southwestern Medical School, University of Texas Health Science Center, Dallas, Texas, USA

PANDEY, KAILASH. Department of Biochemistry, Vanderbilt University School of Medicine, Nashville, Tennessee, USA

PAREKH, NIRANJAN. Department of Physiology and Biophysics, University of Louisville Health Sciences Center, Louisville, Kentucky, USA

PARKS, JOAN H. Renal Section, Department of Medicine, University of Chicago Pritzker School of Medicine, Chicago, Illinois, USA

PEARL, MIRILEE. University Laboratory of Physiology, University of Oxford, Oxford, England, UK

PEDERSON, JAMES A. Nephrology Section, Department of Medicine, College of Medicine, University of Oklahoma Health Science Center, Oklahoma City, Oklahoma, USA

PERDUE, SONDRA. Tissue Typing Laboratory, UCLA School of Medicine, Los Angeles, California, USA

PEREZ, GUIDO O. Department of Medicine, University of Miami, Miami, Florida, USA

PEREZ, JOELLE. INSERM U 64, Hôpital Tenon, Paris, France

PERKINSON, DIANA A. Division of Nephrology, Department of Medicine, University of Washington, Seattle, Washington, USA

PERSSON, A. ERIK G. Departments of Physiology and Biophysics, University of Uppsala, Uppsala, Sweden

PETERS, D. KEITH. Department of Medicine, Royal Postgraduate Medical School, University of London, Hammersmith Hospital, London, England, UK

PUJOL, DIEGO. INSERM U 246, CEN/Saclay, Gif-sur-Yvette, France

PUSEY, CHARLES D. MRC Clinical Immunology Research Group, Department of

Medicine, Royal Postgraduate Medical School, University of London, Hammersmith Hospital, London, England, UK

RABINOWITZ, LAWRENCE. Department of Human Physiology, University of California, Davis, California, USA

RACUSEN, LORRAINE C. Department of Pathology, Johns Hopkins University School of Medicine, Baltimore, Maryland, USA

RAPAPORT, J. Department of Nephrology, Soroka Medical Center and the Faculty of the Health Sciences, Ben-Gurion University of the Negev, Beersheva, Israel

RECTOR, FLOYD C., JR. Cardiovascular Research Institute and Departments of Medicine and Physiology, University of California, San Francisco, California, USA

REES, ANDREW J. Department of Medicine, Royal Postgraduate Medical School, University of London, Hammersmith Hospital, London, England, UK

REMUZZI, GIUSEPPE. "Mario Negri" Institute for Pharmacological Research, Bergamo, Italy

RESNICK, LAWRENCE. Hypertension Center, New York Hospital-Cornell University Medical Center, New York, New York, USA

RIESELBACH, RICHARD E. Department of Medicine, Medical College of Wisconsin, Milwaukee, Wisconsin, USA

RITZ, EBERHARD. Section of Nephrology, University Medical Clinic, Heidelberg, Federal Republic of Germany

ROBERTS, JAMES A. Delta Regional Primate Center, Covington, Louisiana, USA

RODRÍGUEZ-ITURBE, BERNARDO. Renal Service and Laboratory, Hospital Universitario de Maracaibo, Maracaibo, Zulia, Venezuela

RODRÍGUEZ-SORIANO, JUAN. Department of Pediatrics, Hospital Infantile de la Seguridad Social, University School of Medicine, Cruces Bibao, Spain

ROINEL, NICOLE. L.P.P.C., Department of Biology, CEN/Saclay, Gif-sur-Yvette, France

RONCO, PIERRE. Service de Néphrologie, Hôpital Tenon, Paris, France

ROSS, BRIAN A. University of Oxford, Oxford, England, UK

ROSSIER, BERNARD C. Pharmacology Institute, University of Lausanne, Lausanne, Switzerland

ROTTEMBOURG, JACQUES B. Department of Nephrology, Hôpital de la Pitie, Paris, France

SABATINI, SANDRA. Section of Nephrology, Department of Medicine, University of Illinois College of Medicine, Chicago, Illinois, USA

SALANT, DAVID J. Department of Medicine, Boston University Medical Center, Boston, Massachusetts, USA

SAMPSON, DEREK. Renal Transplantation Service, Pacific Medical Center, San Francisco, California, USA (deceased)

SANCHO, JAIME. Servicio de Nefrología, Fundación Jiménez Díaz, Madrid, Spain

SASAKI, SEI. Department of Medicine, School of Medicine, University of California, San Francisco, California, USA

SAWYER, WILBUR H. Department of Pharmacology, College of Physicians and Surgeons of Columbia University, New York, New York, USA

SCHAFER, JAMES A. Department of Physiology and Biophysics, University of Alabama Medical Center, Birmingham, Alabama, USA

SCHLATTER, EBERHARD. Max Planck Institute for Biophysics, Frankfurt, Federal Republic of Germany

SCHNERMANN, JÜRGEN. Physiology Institute, University of Munich, Munich, Federal Republic of Germany

SCHOOLWERTH, ANTON C. Renal and Electrolyte Division, Department of Medicine, Pennsylvania State University, College of Medicine, Hershey, Pennsylvania, USA

SCHREINER, GEORGE F. Department of Pathology, Harvard Medical School, Boston, Massachusetts, USA

SCHRIER, ROBERT W. Department of Medicine, University of Colorado Medical Center, Denver, Colorado, USA

SCHULTZ, STANLEY G. Department of Physiology and Cell Biology, University of Texas Medical School, Houston, Texas, USA

SEALEY, JEAN E. Cardiovascular Center, New York Hospital-Cornell Medical Center, New York, New York, USA

SEBERT, J. L. Service de Néphrologie, Hôpital Nord, Amiens, France

SEGGIE, JANET L. Division of Nephrology, Department of Medicine, University of the Witwatersrand, Johannesburg, South Africa

SEIFFER, JULIAN. Laboratory of Kidney and Electrolyte Physiology, Brigham and Women's Hospital, Boston, Massachusetts, USA

SHAPIRO, FRED L. Regional Kidney Disease Program, Hennepin County Medical Center, Minneapolis, Minnesota, USA

SHEMESH, OVADIA. Division of Nephrology, Department of Medicine, Stanford University School of Medicine, Stanford, California, USA

SHERRARD, DONALD J. Department of Medicine, University of Washington School of Medicine, Seattle, Washington, USA

SIEGEL, NORMAN J. Department of Pediatrics, Yale University School of Medicine, New Haven, Connecticut, USA

SIESS, WOLFGANG. Department of Internal Medicine, University of Munich, Munich, Federal Republic of Germany

SILBERMAN, HOWARD. Department of Surgery, UCLA School of Medicine, Los Angeles, California, USA

SINNIAH, RAJA. Department of Pathology, National University of Singapore, Singapore

SITPRIJA, VISITH. Department of Medicine, Faculty of Medicine, Chulalongkorn University, Bangkok, Thailand

SLATOPOLSKY, EDUARDO. Renal Division, Department of Internal Medicine, Washington University School of Medicine, St. Louis, Missouri, USA

SMITH, DOUGLAS J. Section of Nephrology, Department of Medicine, Yale University School of Medicine, New Haven, Connecticut, USA

SMITH, LYNWOOD H. Nephrology Research Unit, Mayo Clinic and Mayo Foundation, Rochester, Minnesota, USA

SOLEZ, KIM. Department of Pathology, Johns Hopkins University School of Medicine, Baltimore, Maryland, USA

SOLOMON, SIDNEY. Department of Physiology, University of New Mexico School of Medicine, Albuquerque, New Mexico, USA

SONNENBERG, HARALD. Department of Physiology, Toronto General Hospital, Toronto, Ontario, Canada

SOUBRIER, FLORENT. INSERM U 36, Hôpital Broussais, Paris, France

SPENCER, HERTA C. Hines Veterans Administration Hospital, Hines, Illinois, USA

SPINELLI, FRANK. Ciba-Geigy Ltd., Basel, Switzerland

SPITZER, ADRIAN. Division of Pediatric Nephrology, Department of Pediatrics, Albert Einstein College of Medicine, Bronx, New York, USA

SPRING, KENNETH R. Laboratory of Kidney and Electrolyte Metabolism, National Heart, Lung, and Blood Institute, National Institutes of Health, Bethesda, Maryland, USA

STANTON, BRUCE. Department of Physiology, Yale University School of Medicine, New Haven, Connecticut, USA

STEFFES, MICHAEL W. Department of Chemistry, University of Minnesota Medical School, Minneapolis, Minnesota, USA

STEIN, JAY H. Division of Renal Diseases, Department of Medicine, University of Texas Health Science Center, San Antonio, Texas, USA

STEINHAUSEN, MICHAEL. Institute for Physiology, University of Heidelberg, Heidelberg, Federal Republic of Germany

STERZL, R. BERND. Department of Medicine, Veterans Administration Medical Center, Yale University School of Medicine, West Haven, Connecticut, USA

STOKES, JOHN B., III. Department of Internal Medicine, University of Iowa, Iowa City, Iowa, USA

STONE, DENNIS K. Department of Internal Medicine, Southwestern Medical School, University of Texas Health Science Center, Dallas, Texas, USA

STORK, JOHN E. Department of Medicine, Case Western Reserve University School of Medicine, Cleveland, Ohio, USA

STOW, JENNIFER L. Department of Cell Biology, Yale University School of Medicine, New Haven, Connecticut, USA

STRASSER, THOMAS. Department of Internal Medicine, University of Munich, Munich, Federal Republic of Germany

STRIKER, GARY E. Department of Pathology, University of Washington, Seattle, Washington, USA

STRIKER, LILIANE MOREL-MAROGER. Department of Pathology, University of Washington, Seattle, Washington, USA

STROBER, SAMUEL. Division of Immunology, Department of Medicine, Stanford University Medical Center, Stanford, California, USA

STROM, TERRY B. Department of Medicine, Beth Israel Hospital, Boston, Massachusetts, USA

SUKI, WADI N. Renal Section, Departments of Medicine and Physiology, Baylor College of Medicine, Houston, Texas, USA

SUMMERS, ROGER J. Department of Medicine, University of Melbourne, Austin Hospital, Heidelberg, Victoria, Australia

SUTTON, ROGER A. L. Department of Medicine, University of British Columbia, Vancouver, British Columbia, Canada

TABEI, KAORU. Department of Cardiology, Jichi Medical School, Tochigi, Japan

TANNEN, RICHARD L. Division of Nephrology, Department of Internal Medicine, University of Michigan Medical Center, Ann Arbor, Michigan, USA

TANNER, GEORGE A. Department of Physiology, Indiana University School of Medicine, Indianapolis, Indiana, USA

TARAZI, ROBERT C. Department of Clinical Science, Cleveland Clinic, Cleveland, Ohio, USA

TAUB, MARY. Department of Biochemistry, School of Medicine, State University of New York at Buffalo, Buffalo, New York, USA

TAYLOR, ANN. University Laboratory of Physiology, University of Oxford, Oxford, England, UK

TERASAKI, PAUL I. Tissue Typing Laboratory, UCLA School of Medicine, Los Angeles, California, USA

TESSITORE, NICOLA. Division of Nephrology, University of Verona, Verona, Italy

THOMAS, WILLIAM C. Division of Urology, Department of Surgery, J. Hillis Miller Health Center, University of Florida, Gainesville, Florida, USA

TISHER, C. CRAIG. Division of Nephrology, Department of Medicine, J. Hillis Miller Health Center, University of Florida, Gainesville, Florida, USA

TOBACK, F. GARY. Section of Nephrology, Department of Medicine, University of Chicago Pritzker School of Medicine, Chicago, Illinois, USA

TRANAEUS, ANDERS. Department of Renal Medicine, Karolinska Institute, Huddinge University Hospital, Stockholm, Sweden

TRINH-TRANG-TAN, MARIE-MARCELLE. INSERM U 90, Hôpital Necker, Paris, France

TRIPPODO, NICK C. Ochsner Medical Foundation, New Orleans, Louisiana, USA

TSCHOPP, FRITZ A. Research Laboratory for Calcium Metabolism, Balgrist Department of Orthopedic Surgery, University of Zurich, Zurich, Switzerland

TURNER, R. JAMES. Membrane Biology Group, Department of Medicine, University of Toronto, Toronto, Ontario, Canada

ULDALL, ROBERT. Renal Unit, Toronto Western Hospital, Toronto, Ontario, Canada

VAAMONDE, CARLOS A. Medical and Research Services, Veterans Administration Medical Center, Miami, Florida, USA

VALDERROBANO, FERNANDO. Nephrology Service, Hospital Provincial of Madrid, Madrid, Spain

VALENTICH, JOHN D. Department of Physiology and Cell Biology, University of Texas Medical School, Houston, Texas, USA

VALTIN, HEINZ. Department of Physiology, Dartmouth Medical School, Hanover, New Hampshire, USA

VANHOLDER, RAYMOND. Department of Nephrology, University Hospital, Ghent, Belgium

VARGHESE, ZACHARIAH. Royal Free Hospital, London, England, UK

VERRIER-JONES, KATE. Department of Renal Medicine, Welsh National School of Medicine, Royal Infirmary, Cardiff, Wales, UK

VERROUST, PIERRE. Service de Néphrologie, Hôpital Tenon, Paris, France

VIBERTI, GIANCARLO. Unit for Metabolic Medicine, Guy's Hospital Medical School, London, England, UK

VON SCHACKY, CLEMENS. Department of Internal Medicine, University of Munich, Munich, Federal Republic of Germany

WAER, MARK. Division of Immunology, Stanford University Medical Center, Stanford, California, USA

WARNOCK, DAVID G. Nephrology Section, Department of Medicine, Veterans Administration Medical Center and Cardiovascular Research Institute and Department of Medicine, School of Medicine, University of California, San Francisco, California, USA

WEBER, MICHAEL. Department of Medicine, Veterans Administration Medical Center, Long Beach, California, USA

WEBER, PETER C. Department of Internal Medicine, University of Munich, Munich, Federal Republic of Germany

WEENING, JAN J. Department of Pathology, State University of Leiden, Leiden, The Netherlands

WEIDMANN, PETER. Department of Medicine, University of Berne, Berne, Switzerland

WEIDTKE, CLAUDIA. Max Planck Institute for Biophysics, Frankfurt, Federal Republic of Germany

WEINBERG, JOEL M. Department of Medicine, Veterans Administration Medical Center, Ann Arbor, Michigan, USA

WERNERS, PETER G. Clinical Chemistry Laboratory, Mayo Clinic, Rochester, Minnesota, USA

WEST, CLARK D. Division of Nephrology, Children's Hospital Research Foundation, University of Cincinnati, Cincinnati, Ohio, USA

WHELTON, ANDREW. Department of Medicine, Johns Hopkins University School of Medicine, Baltimore, Maryland, USA

WHITE, MICHAEL P. Veterans Administration Medical Center, Ann Arbor, Michigan, USA

WHITTEMBURY, GUILLERMO. Instituto Venezolano de Investigaciones Científicas, Caracas, Venezuela

WIGGINS, ROGER C. Department of Internal Medicine, University of Michigan School of Medicine, Ann Arbor, Michigan, USA

WILSON, CURTIS B. Department of Immunology, Research Institute of the Scripps Clinic, La Jolla, California, USA

WILSON, DOUGLAS R. Division of Nephrology, Toronto General Hospital, Toronto, Ontario, Canada

WINBERG, JAN. Department of Pediatrics, Karolinska Institute, Huddinge University Hospital, Stockholm, Sweden

WINDHAGER, ERICH E. Department of Physiology and Biophysics, Cornell University Medical College, New York, New York, USA

WINSLADE, WILLIAM. Program in Medicine, Law and Human Values, Neuropsychiatric Institute, School of Medicine, University of California, Los Angeles, California, USA

WISEMAN, MARTIN J. Unit for Metabolic Medicine, Guy's Hospital Medical School, London, England, UK

WITTNER, MONIKA. Max Planck Institute for Biophysics, Frankfurt, Federal Republic of Germany

WOODROFFE, ANDREW J. Renal Unit, Royal Adelaide Hospital, Adelaide, South Australia, Australia

WORK, JACK. Division of Nephrology, Department of Medicine, University of Alabama Medical Center, Birmingham, Alabama, USA

WRIGHT, FRED S. Department of Physiology, Yale University School of Medicine, New Haven, Connecticut, USA

WU, AKIRA Y. T. Department of Nephrology, National University of Singapore, Singapore General Hospital, Singapore

WU, GEORGE. Department of Medicine, Toronto Western Hospital and University of Toronto, Toronto, Ontario, Canada

YARGER, WILLIAM E. Department of Medicine, Duke University Medical Center and Veterans Administration Medical Center, Durham, North Carolina, USA

ZAGER, RICHARD A. Department of Medicine, Ohio State University Medical Center, Columbus, Ohio, USA

ZIMMERMAN, STEPHEN W. Division of Nephrology, University of Wisconsin Medical School, Madison, Wisconsin, USA

Acknowledgments

An International Congress of Nephrology is held triennially under the auspices of the International Society of Nephrology, and in accordance with its by-laws. The Officers and Organizing Committee of the IXth Congress acknowledge the support of the Officers and Councillors of the International Society of Nephrology and its Committees, as well as many other distinguished individuals who contributed so enormously of their time and energy to the organization of the Congress. Generous contributions were received from the following corporations: *Major Donors:* Boehringer-Ingelheim Ltd., Schering Laboratories, Travenol Laboratories, Inc.; *Additional Corporate Donors:* Abbott Laboratories, Beach Pharmaceuticals, Burroughs Wellcome Company, Pfizer Pharmaceuticals, E. R. Squibb and Sons, and USV Laboratories.

Normal Structure and Function

Transport Processes and Epithelia

Determinants of Growth, Form, and Function in Epithelia

Chairpersons: Joseph S. Handler and Marcelino M. Cereijido
Discussants: Maurice Burg, Mary Taub, Michael F. Horster, and John D. Valentich

The participants in this Workshop agreed that the terminology and definitions suggested by the Tissue Culture Association should be used in the development of new techniques utilizing kidney-derived epithelial cell lines, an area of great potential use.

The utility of having a large library of continuous cell lines that express differentiated functions is illustrated by studies over the past few years with just a few epithelial cell lines. Methods used to study naturally occurring epithelia have been adapted for studying epithelia in culture and include: measurement of tracer fluxes and short-circuit current in intact epithelia, the use of special electrodes to assess other electrical properties of epithelia and the individual cells and tight junctions, tracer fluxes in plasma membrane vesicles, ligand binding to transporters, single-channel measurements using vesicles fused into planar lipid bilayers or patch clamping of intact epithelia, and studies of the regulation of transport by hormones and other signals. In certain respects, cultured epithelia are better suited than naturally occurring epithelia for some of these techniques. Cultured epithelia offer special advantages as well, in that it may become possible to apply the techniques of somatic cell and molecular genetics. In addition, differences between cultured and naturally occurring epithelia may provide useful information.

Burg and Green have attempted to start continuous kidney-derived epithelial cell lines for several years. After much frustration, they succeeded in starting a few cell lines. Burg proposed that the secret of starting cell lines is to keep improving culture conditions until continuous growth occurs. Their approach was begun with a complex medium composed of a mixture of Coon's and Liebovitz' medium. High concentrations of serum are usually deleterious to primary cultures of epithelial cells. However, it has not been possible to eliminate serum from culture media completely. Other partially

---

This manuscript is a summary of a Workshop entitled *Determinants of Growth, Form, and Function in Epithelia.*

defined additives such as pituitary extract have been useful. Defined mixtures of hormones and growth factors have been particularly useful (defined media are discussed later in this Workshop by Taub and Horster). Trace elements may be important. Certainly, selenium is required by some cell lines. Although tissue culture plastic is readily available and works well for some primary cultures, collagen-coated plastic dishes, or collagen membranes, or membranes prepared from amnions have been particularly useful. The amnions are from sheep placentas. They are denuded of epithelial cells by treatment with triton X-100 or hypertonic urea, and then held in an arrangement like an embroidery hoop. Medium is placed above the cells on the amnion and below the amnion. Finally, experience and skill may be required to handle delicate cells. One of the important skills is finding a way to subculture each type of cell successfully.

A line of cells has been developed from the epithelium lining the papilla in the renal pelvis. The line was started by dissecting the epithelium and culturing it in small plastic petri dishes. Later passages would grow only on collagen or amnion membranes. Currently, the cells grow best on plastic. Generally, several strains are carried in parallel under different conditions. When cultures were heterogeneous, one could select a given area under the phase contrast microscope, scraped off and subcultured. The cells have developed a transepithelial voltage when grown on collagen membranes or amnions only twice. At all other times tested, there was no potential difference. The only differentiated property this line currently shows is survival in hypertonic medium and medium with a high concentration of urea.

Another line of continuous cells is derived from the medullary thick ascending limb of Henle. These cells have been in continuous culture for over 3 years. Amnions and collagen membranes were useful in early passages. The cells now grow well on collagen-coated petri dishes. Primary cultures and two subsequent passages displayed apical surface-negative transepithelial potentials. Other passages had no potential differences although domes were seen when the cells were grown on petri dishes. In earlier passages, adenylate cyclase was not stimulated by any of the hormones that affect that segment. Tamm-Horsfall protein is localized to medullary thick ascending limb cells in the kidney. Two lines derived from cells of the medullary thick ascending limb are negative for Tamm-Horsfall protein; one line is positive.

It is evident that differentiation varies from line to line and from passage to passage in the same line. Also, although likely, it is uncertain that the papillary cell and medullary thick ascending limb cell lines are continuous and will continue to grow. Therefore, strategies have been developed to produce more stable growth and differentiation.

Cloning a differentiated cell may be useful, but is not easy because first the differentiated cell must be identified. In addition, most continuous cell lines in culture tend to drift; that is, their differentiated characteristics change. One approach is to select for differentiation. Although such selective conditions are not apparent for the two lines considered thus far, they may be available for cells derived from the proximal tubule. Generally, cells in culture require glucose. Glucose is needed not only for energy, but for metabolism through the pentose phosphate shunt to form nucleotides. Differentiated liver cells can grow without glucose in the culture medium because they can make it from other substances. The proximal tubule also has the capacity for gluconeogenesis. In addition, the brush border has enzymes capable of splitting complex carbohydrates into simple sugars. It may be possible to exert selective pressure for differentiated function by growing proximal tubule cells in glucose-free media that contain substrates for gluconeogenesis (that is, alpha-keto glutarate), or substrates for polysaccharidases (that is, maltose, trehalose).

It may be possible to immortalize cells by transfecting them with the appropriate DNA that can also contain a gene for resistance to a toxin such as neomycin, so that transfected cells can be selected. Many cultured cells have been immortalized by a variety of techniques. Usually, differentiation is sacrificed. Perhaps the addition of selective conditions such as those outlined above for proximal tubules will yield continuous differentiated cell lines.

Taub has concentrated on developing defined media for preparing primary cultures of kidney epithelial cells. She has been most successful with a medium developed originally for a continuous cell line designated MDCK. The medium has been used to grow primary cultures of proximal tubule cells from kidneys of baby mice and adult rabbits. The technique for harvesting cells has been adapted so that a large quantity of cells can be harvested and grown. The cultures manifest sodium-coupled glucose transport, sodium-dependent phosphate transport, and cyclic AMP production sensitive to parathyroid hormone. It is clear that the appropriately defined media can perform selection for epithelial cell growth and discourage fibroblast growth. At some point it may be possible to select for cells of a particular segment of the nephron using the appropriately defined medium.

Horster uses monolayer cultures of segmental nephron cells to study the induction of differentiated functions by hormones. He starts cultures by dissecting segments of rabbit, mouse, or rat kidney without proteases or chelating agents. Individual segments are placed on collagen membranes arranged so that the medium has access to both surfaces of the culture. Cells migrate from injured basement membrane sites and proliferate on a fibronectic coat of the collagen. Defined media have been developed on the basis of their effects on thymidine incorporation that favor cell growth from cortical or medullary segment of TAL or cortical collecting tubules (CCT). Cultures of the rabbit CCT have been used extensively recently to study the induction by hormones of differentiated cell functions. Cultured CCT epithelia are sensitive to corticosteroids [aldosterone (ALD), 10^{-9} M; dexamethasone (DEX) 10^{-8} M] and to thyroid hormone (T_3, 10^{-11} M). The magnitude of the transepithelial voltage (-28 to -12 mv) depends on the selective incubation with either ALD or DEX or T_3. Na-K-activated ATPase activity (fmoles/min · cell) is induced by aldosterone and to a smaller extent by T_3 and DEX. Enzyme activity decreases in CCT cultures after corticosteroid depletion of the medium and is restored by a specific ALD effect and a synergistic thyroid/glucocorticoid action after long-term incubation. There is preliminary evidence that these hormones also determine the level of ultrastructural differentiation in cultured CCT. These studies demonstrate that in vivo properties of renal epithelia are maintained in primary culture given an adequate environment. The differential inductive capacity of hormones might be utilized to select cell strains. Horster proposes that factors regulating epithelial transport functions, for example, may operate as epigenetic factors in the expression of differentiated epithelial functions.

Valentich described a cell line (M-mTAL-1C) established from identified, microdissected segments of the mouse medullary thick ascending limb (mTAL). Using a type I collagen gel as a substratum, he has been able to maintain these cells in culture for over 2 years without adherence to a plastic surface and without exposure to proteolytic enzymes and consequent disruption of intercellular contacts. These unique culture conditions permitted the development of a continuous cell line derived from a defined nephron segment that was capable of expressing the specific transport functions of that segment when transplanted to the subcutaneous environment of a mouse.

M-mTAL-1C cells in vitro exhibit a basal-positive transepithelial potential difference (V_{TE}) of 1.9 ± 1.6 mv, a transepithelial resistance (R_c) of $527 \pm 527 \ \Omega cm^2$ and a short-circuit current (I_{sc}) of $4.4 \pm 2.2 \ \mu A \ cm^{-2}$. None of these electrical parameters correspond to those reported for the isolated perfused mouse mTAL, which exhibits a basal-negative V_{TE}. The V_{TE} of M-mTAL-1C cells is also insensitive to furosemide or chloride-free bathing solutions, both of which abolish the V_{TE} of the intact mTAL. However, the V_{TE} of M-mTAL-1C cells is sensitive to micromolar concentrations of apically applied amiloride, a diuretic that has no known effect on the transport properties of the mTAL. Clearly, the transport phenotype of M-mTAL-1C cells in vitro fails to duplicate that of the freshly isolated mTAL. To determine if the humoral environment of the mouse could elicit re-expression of mTAL transport functions in M-mTAL-1C cells, a diffusion chamber was constructed that allows transplantation of M-mTAL-1C cultures subcutaneously into mice (the animal passage technique) and subsequent recovery for electrophysiology. When this procedure was carried out, about 20% of the successfully recovered animal passage M-mTAL-1C cultures exhibited reversion to the mTAL phenotype. This included a basal-negative V_{TE} (-3.7 ± -4.0 mv), which could be completely abolished by the addition of furosemide to the apical bathing solution or symmetrical removal of chloride. The ability of amiloride to modify the V_{TE} persisted. However, now its effects were to drive the spontaneous V_{TE} to a more negative voltage.

Valentich believes these results indicate that a continuous renal cell line when maintained under unique in vitro conditions does not necessarily lose its ability to re-express the phenotypic properties characteristic of its cells of origin. He suggests that defining the factors in the mouse subcutaneous environment responsible for the animal passage effect should significantly aid in the design of culture conditions for maintaining functional renal epithelium in long-term tissue culture.

Basolateral Membrane Properties of Sodium-absorbing Epithelia

Stanley G. Schultz

In the 25 years that have elapsed since the introduction of the Koefoed-Johnsen-Ussing (KJU) *double membrane* model for sodium absorption by isolated frog skin [1], its fundamental features have been confirmed beyond reasonable doubt and have been extended to a wide variety of sodium-absorbing epithelia [2]. In some epithelia, often classified as *tight* or *moderately tight* (for example, amphibian urinary bladder, mammalian colon, and urinary bladder), the original KJU notion that sodium enters the absorptive cells across the apical membrane by electrodiffusion through pores or channels has been amply validated by the results of current-voltage (I-V) studies [3–7] and fluctuation (noise) analyses [5, 8–10]. In other epithelia, often classified as *leaky* (for example, small intestine, gallbladder, renal proximal tubule), the entry of this cation is mediated by *carriers* that bring about its cotransport with a variety of organic solutes [11], its cotransport with chloride [12] and/or its countertransport to hydrogen ions [13].

But, regardless of the mechanisms by which sodium enters the absorptive cells, it is the function of the basolateral sodium-potassium pump to extrude it from those cells at a rate equal to the rate of entry and to maintain the low intracellular sodium activity and high intracellular potassium activity characteristic of virtually all cells of higher animals. At the same time, the potassium pumped into the cells across the basolateral membrane in exchange for sodium must exit, largely across that barrier,[1] at a rate equal to the pump rate. It follows that the pump-leak properties of the basolateral membrane must be responsive to the rate of sodium entry across the apical membrane or else the cell will be threatened with major swings in ionic composition and volume; in other words, in the final analysis, the pump-leak properties

---

This manuscript was presented as part of a Symposium on *Second Messengers and Epithelial Transport.*

[1] The apical membranes of some tight and leaky epithelia possess potassium-channels so that some of the potassium pumped into the cell diffuses out across that barrier. In general, however, the rate of potassium excretion by this mechanism is a small fraction of the potassium pumped into the cell.

of the basolateral membrane are responsible for intracellular ionic homeostasis and must be capable of coping with large and often rapid changes in the rate of transcellular sodium transport [14].

For several reasons, the small intestine of the amphibian *Necturus maculosus* has proved to be an ideal epithelium for studying how the pump-leak properties of the basolateral membrane respond to an increase in the rate of sodium entry across the apical membrane. First, the rate of sodium entry can be rapidly and physiologically increased 4-fold simply by adding a sugar or amino acid in low concentration (10 mM) to the mucosal bathing solution. Thus, one need not resort to changing the sodium activity in the mucosal solution or adding pharmacologic agents (for example, amiloride) or hormones (for example, antidiuretic hormone, aldosterone), which may have multiple effects, to bring about a change in the rate of sodium entry. Second, the villus cells are large and electrically coupled, forming a virtual syncytium, so that they can be readily impaled simultaneously with conventional, potassium-chloride-filled, and ion-selective microelectrodes for prolonged periods.

In this communication, we shall summarize the recent studies in which the *Necturus* small intestine was used. The results indicate that, in response to an increase in the rate of sodium entry across the apical membrane, there is an increase in the potassium conductance of the basolateral membrane ($g_{K^+}^S$) and a similar increase in the *capacity* of the sodium-potassium pump to extrude sodium. In addition, we shall cite evidence from studies on other epithelia suggesting that these are general phenomena. We shall conclude with some speculations regarding possible underlying mechanisms.

Relation Between the Rate of Sodium Entry and Basolateral Potassium Conductance

The effects of adding 10 mM galactose to the solution bathing the mucosal surface of *Necturus* small intestine are illustrated in Figure 1a.[2] Initially, there is a rapid depolarization of ψ^{MC} (the electrical potential difference across the apical membrane), often of sufficient magnitude to reverse the original polarity. This depolarization is accompanied by a significant decline in r^M/r^S (the ratio of the resistance of the apical membrane to that of the basolateral membrane). These phenomena are due to the activation of rheogenic *and* conductive carrier processes that mediate the coupled entry of sodium and the sugar.[3] This initial, rapid response is followed by a slower repolarization

---

[2] Identical results are observed when alanine is added to the mucosal bathing solution.

[3] The term *rheogenic* is used to indicate that these carrier processes mediate the transfer or flow of charge and thus generate a current. That they are also *conductive* processes means that they are not operating as constant current generators (i.e., current sources with infinite internal resistances or zero conductances); the activation of a constant current generator would change ψ^{MC}, but would not, in itself, reduce the apical membrane resistance (r^M). The important consequence of the finding that these sodium-coupled sugar and amino acid entry processes are *both* rheogenic and conductive is that the entry rate must be affected by ψ^{MC}.

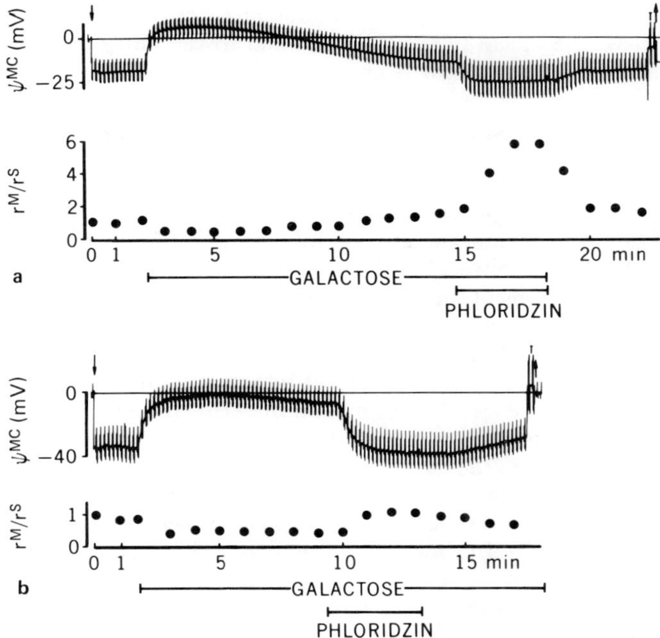

Fig. 1. a Effect of galactose on ψ^{MC} (the electrical PD across apical membrane) and r^M/r^S (ratio of apical-membrane resistance to basolateral-membrane resistance). Galactose was added to the solution bathing the mucosal surface of *Necturus* small intestine. Also shown are the effects of the subsequent addition of phloridzin to the mucosal solution. b Results of an identical experiment on tissue samples exposed to 1 mM cyanide plus 1 mM iodoacetamide for 1 hr.

of ψ^{MC} and an increase in r^M/r^S, with the latter often reaching steady-state values that exceed the ones observed in the absence of the sugar. Evidence that the increase in r^M/r^S is the result, at least in part, of a decrease in the basolateral membrane resistance (r^S) is also shown in Figure 1a; namely, the addition of phloridzin, a potent inhibitor of the sodium-sugar-coupled entry mechanism, to the mucosal solution results in a rapid repolarization of ψ^{MC} and a transient increase in r^M/r^S to levels much greater than that observed in the absence of the sugar. In other words, by suddenly aborting the sodium-sugar-coupled entry process, we were able to transiently catch the basolateral membrane with "its resistance down." Finally, as shown in Figure 1b, when the identical experiment is carried out on tissue samples exposed to metabolic inhibitors for 1 hr prior to study, the addition of galactose to the mucosal solution results in a prompt depolarization of ψ^{MC} and a decrease in r^M/r^S, but the slow repolarization and increase in r^M/r^S are not observed; under these conditions, the addition of phloridzin to the mucosal solution simply restores ψ^{MC} and r^M/r^S to control values [15].

Thus, we conclude that a sudden increase in the rate of sodium entry across the apical membrane, coupled to the entry of sugar (or amino acid), is followed by a slow decrease in r^S and that this response can be blocked by metabolic inhibitors.

There are several lines of evidence indicating, conclusively, that the decrease in r^S is due to an increase in the potassium conductance of the basolateral membrane, $g_{K^+}^S$. First, the repolarization of the cell interior is precisely the response one would predict if the total electromotive force across the basolateral membrane moves closer to that of potassium; that is, that barrier more closely approaches the behavior of a "potassium electrode" [15]. Second, determinations of intracellular potassium activities K_C^+, done with potassium-selective microelectrodes, indicate that the addition of sugars or amino acids to the mucosal solution results in a significant *decline* in K_C^+ despite the 3- to 4-fold increase in the rate at which sodium is being pumped out of the cell across the basolateral membrane [16]. If sodium extrusion by the pump is tightly coupled to potassium uptake, as is generally the case, then a 4-fold increase in the rate of sodium extrusion across the basolateral membrane should be accompanied by a 4-fold increase in the rate of potassium uptake across that barrier, and, all other things being equal, one would expect an *increase* in K_C^+. In short, assuming reasonably tight coupling of the basolateral sodium-potassium exchange pump, the observed decline in K_C in the face of a marked increase in pump activity can only be explained by an increase in $g_{K^+}^S$ [16].

Finally, perhaps the most direct evidence that the increase in r^M/r^S and the concomitant repolarization of ψ^{MC} are due to an increase in $g_{K^+}^S$ is illustrated in Figure 2. Thus, when the serosal solution contains 1 mM barium, the values of r^M/r^S in the absence of sugar are very low. The addition of galactose to the mucosal solution results in a depolarization of ψ^{MC}, but the normal repolarization and increase in r^M/r^S are not observed until barium is removed from the serosal solution [17]. It is well established that barium blocks potassium channels in a number of nonepithelial cells [18], and, recently, it has been shown to block the potassium conductance of the basolateral membranes of several epithelia [19–24]. The ability of this cation to block the decrease in r^S following the addition of galactose to the mucosal solution is compelling evidence that this decrease is due to an increase in the conductance of barium-inhibitable potassium channels in the basolateral membrane.

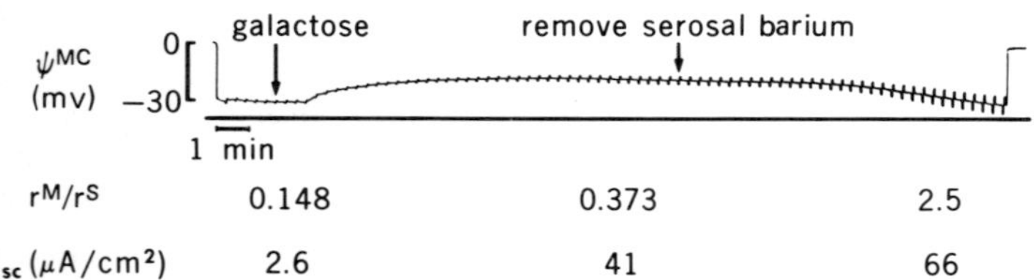

Fig. 2. Effect of galactose on ψ^{MC} and r^M/r^S when the serosal solution contains 5 mM barium and after removing barium from the serosal perfusate.

Transcellular Solute Transport and Volume Regulatory Responses

In recent years, it has become clear that a number of epithelial and nonepithelial cells possess mechanisms that tend to restore initial volume after these cells or tissues are exposed to anisotonic media [25]. In particular, exposure of renal tubules [26], frog urinary bladder [27], and *Necturus* gallbladder [28] to a hypotonic solution results in initial, rapid swelling followed by a slower shrinkage toward the original volume. This volume regulatory decrease (VRD) appears to be due to an increase in the permeability of the basolateral membrane to potassium (and, perhaps, chloride as well) leading to the efflux of potassium, chloride, and water from the cell. Further, evidence has been presented that this VRD can be blocked by metabolic inhibition [26].

It has long been known that sugars and amino acids are accumulated in osmotically active forms within small intestinal cells and, thus, are accompanied by an increase in cell water content and cell swelling [29–31].

Could cell swelling be the *signal* for the increase in g_K^S+ observed in *Necturus* small intestine following the addition of sugars or amino acids to the mucosal solution?

To explore this possibility, we examined the responses of *Necturus* small intestine to three conditions: (1) exposing it to a moderately (12%) hypotonic solution; (2) exposing it to the same hypotonic solution containing 1mM barium; and, (3) exposing it to the same hypotonic solution after exposing it to metabolic inhibitors for 1 hr [17]. The results, stated briefly, are that exposure of this epithelium to a 12% hypotonic solution brings about a slow hyperpolarization of ψ^{MC} and an increase in r^M/r^S and that both of these responses are blocked by barium or conditions of metabolic inhibition.

In short, exposure of the tissue to a moderately hypotonic solution leads to an increase in a barium-inhibitable, potassium conductance of the basolateral membrane, and this response is blocked by metabolic inhibitors. Thus, there is a one-for-one correspondence between the effect of sugars or amino acids and the effect of exposure to a hypotonic solution on g_K^S+. This close correspondence strongly suggests that the slow increase in g_K^S+ observed following the addition of sugars or amino acids to the solution bathing the mucosal surface of *Necturus* small intestine is a response to the accumulation of these solutes within the cell in osmotically active forms and, consequently, a response to cell swelling.

Relation of These Findings to Other Epithelia and Their Physiologic Importance

Parallelisms between sodium-potassium pump activity (that is, the rate of active transcellular sodium transport) and the conductance of the basolateral membrane have been reported for, or can be deduced from the results of studies on, a number of sodium-absorbing epithelia [7, 14, 27, 32–35] and, in some instances, reasonable evidence has been presented that the changes in r^S are at least in part attributable to changes in $g_{K^+}^S$ [27, 35]. In addition, compelling evidence has been presented for an increase in $g_{K^+}^S$ in canine tracheal mucosa under conditions where an acceleration of sodium-potassium pump activity is associated with the stimulation of active chloride secretion [24, 36]. Thus, it seems that the findings on *Necturus* small intestine may be reasonably general.

Further, since cell swelling appears to accompany increases in transcellular active sodium transport in several of these epithelia [25, 37–39], it may very well be that the increase in $g_{K^+}^S$ is part of a volume-regulatory mechanism. Indeed, inasmuch as volume regulation in response to exposure to anisotonic media has been observed in cells and tissues that are never likely to be exposed to an anisotonic extracellular milieu under physiologic conditions, it may very well be that the *physiologic functions* of these volume-regulatory processes are *to preserve cell volume in the face of changes in intracellular solute content rather than changes in extracellular osmolarity.*

There are at least three, immediately obvious, physiologically important consequences of this parallelism between sodium-potassium pump rate and $g_{K^+}^S$.

First, as discussed above, the increase in $g_{K^+}^S$ with increased pump rate (and vice versa) serves to preserve intracellular K_C^+ within reasonably narrow limits.

Second, in leaky epithelia, where the low-resistance paracellular shunt pathway electrically couples the apical and basolateral membranes [40], an increase in $g_{K^+}^S$ will hyperpolarize both the basolateral and the apical membranes (Fig. 1a). The hyperpolarization of the apical membrane will increase the driving force for all rheogenic and conductive sodium-entry processes [14, 15] (see footnote 3). In canine tracheal mucosa, it increases the driving force for the diffusional exit of chloride across the apical membrane [24, 36].[4]

Finally, the increase in $g_{K^+}^S$ not only facilitates the exit of potassium across the basolateral membrane but also increases the electrical driving force for the exit of chloride across that barrier; the efflux of potassium chloride accompanied by water appears to be the essence of the VRD [25–28].

Given the obvious importance of these three consequences of a parallelism between sodium-potassium pump activity and $g_{K^+}^S$, it would be surprising indeed if this phenomenon did not prove to be a ubiquitous property of sodium-absorbing epithelia.

---

[4] Thus, in leaky and moderately leaky epithelia, the effects of an increase in $g_{K^+}^S$ exert a "positive electrical feedback" on rheogenic and conductive cation-entry and anion-exit processes across the apical membrane (see footnote 3). In the absence of this increase in $g_{K^+}^S$, the effect of the activation of sodium-coupled entry processes for sugars or amino acids on ψ^{MC} would be "self-defeating" (Fig. 1a) [15].

Sodium Entry, the "Sodium Transport Pool," and Pump Activity

During the years that followed the introduction of the KJU model, the following scenario for the regulation of active sodium absorption evolved: (1) Sodium entry across the apical membrane is rate-limiting for overall transcellular transport; that is, changes in the rate of transcellular sodium transport are due primarily to changes in the permeability of the apical membrane to sodium. (2) Changes in the rate of sodium entry lead to changes in the size of an intracellular "sodium transport pool" (which may or may not be synonymous with the intracellular sodium activity; Na_C^+). (3) Changes in the size of this transport pool are responsible for changes in the rate of the sodium-potassium pump [2, 41]. In short, the activity of the basolateral pump emerged as a rather passive follower of events taking place at the apical membrane. Although some dissenting views were expressed [42, 43], the predominant notion was that the so-called sodium transport pool determined the rate of (or "drove") the sodium-potassium pump.

In recentyears, studies using microelectrophysiologic techniques and, in particular, sodium-selective microelectrodes have yielded results that challenge this notion.

For example, Table 1 summarizes the results of a study [44] in which galactose was added to the solution bathing the mucosal surface of *Necturus* small intestine to examine its effects on Na_C^+ and on the rate of active sodium transport, given by the short-circuit current (I_{sc}). In the absence of the sugar (control), Na_C^+ averaged 12 mM. Within 1 to 2 min after galactose was added to the mucosal bathing solution, Na_C^+ increased almost 2-fold. But, it then declined, and when a new steady-state was achieved (approximately 10 min) Na_C^+ did not differ significantly from the control value. During the course of these 10 min, the rate of active sodium transport increased 4-fold!

Table 1. Effect of galactose on electrical parameters and intracellular sodium activity in *Necturus* small intestine[a]

	ψ^{MC} (mv)	r^M/r^S	I_{SC} ($\mu A/cm^2$)	Na_C^+ (mM)
Control ($N = 12$)	-27 ± 3	0.82 ± 0.16	13.4 ± 2.0	12.1 ± 1.1
Galactose "peak" (1 to 2 min; $N = 5$)	-5 ± 5^b	0.18 ± 0.12^b	17.7 ± 2.3^b	20.7 ± 3.4^b
Galactose "steady-state" (10 min; $N = 7$)	-19 ± 5^b	1.04 ± 0.24^c	50.7 ± 2.5^b	14.1 ± 2.5^c

[a] Abbreviations: ψ^{MC}, the electrical potential difference across the apical membrane; r^M/r^S, the ratio of the resistance of the apical membrane to that of the basolateral membrane; I_{SC}, short-circuit current measuring rate of active sodium transport; and Na_C^+, intracellular sodium activity; N, the number of tissue samples studied.

[b] $P < 0.05$, vs. control.

[c] Not significantly different from control.

The initial increase in Na_C^+ is certainly consistent with an increase in the rate of sodium entry into the cell, coupled to the entry of galactose. Two factors may contribute to the subsequent decline in Na_C^+: namely, (1) an increase in basolateral sodium pump activity; and (2) an increase in cell water content secondary to the intracellular accumulation of galactose in an osmotically active form. But, the finding that the steady-state pump rate in the presence of the sugar is approximately four times greater than that under control conditions in the absence of a significant increase in Na_C^+ currently defies adequate explanation.

These findings do not stand alone. Lee and Armstrong [45] earlier found that the addition of 3-0-methylglucose to the solution bathing the mucosal surface of bullfrog small intestine resulted, if anything, in a small *decrease* in Na_C^+; although the effect of this sugar analog on the rate of active sodium absorption was not reported in this study, it is not unreasonable to infer from the results of earlier studies [46] that it was increased. Thomas et al [7] found that increasing the concentration of sodium in the solution bathing the apical surface of *Necturus* urinary bladder from 5 to 45 mM resulted in a 4-fold increase in the rate of active sodium absorption but no significant change in Na_C^+. Wills and Lewis [47] have reported that urinary bladders from rabbits maintained on a low-sodium diet for 13 to 15 days actively absorbed sodium at a rate twice that of bladders from rabbits fed a normal diet but that the Na_C^+ (and the K_C^+) of these bladders did not differ significantly.

In short, while we certainly do not doubt that changes in Na_C^+ can directly effect changes in pump rate, there is also no doubt that large increases in pump rate can occur in the absence of significant changes in Na_C^+. Indeed, we are unaware of any convincing demonstration in *intact epithelia* that a *physiologically induced* increase in the rate of active sodium absorption is associated with a significant increase in Na_C^+.

Speculations Regarding the Regulatory Mechanisms for Homocellular Sodium, Potassium (and Volume)

The findings just cited indicate conclusively that in response to an increase in sodium entry across the apical membrane of *Necturus* small intestine, resulting from the addition of a sugar or an amino acid to the mucosal bathing solution, there are parallel increases in (1) the ability of the basolateral sodium-potassium pump to extrude sodium actively across that barrier in the absence of a significant increase in Na_C^+; and, (2) the potassium conductance of the basolateral membrane.

In short, there is a concerted response on the part of the basolateral "pump-leak" system designed to prevent major changes in Na_C^+ and K_C^+ (and volume) in response to large changes in the rate of transcellular sodium transport. These changes in basolateral membrane properties may be due to one or more of the following: (1) an increase in the activity of a fixed number of functioning pumps or leaks already present in the basolateral membrane; (2) the activation of quiescent (nonfunctional) pumps or leaks already present in the basolateral membrane; and (3) the recruitment of "new" pumps or leaks into that barrier from intracellular sources. Clearly these possibilities are subject to many permutations and combinations.

In considering these possibilities, refer to Figure 3, which summarizes the emerging picture regarding the cytokinetics of basolateral membrane Na-K-ATPase activity. In this figure, the focus is on an element termed the *sodium-potassium pump, potassium-leak unit.* By this term I do not wish to imply, necessarily, that the pump and the leak are parts of the same molecule. Instead, I only suggest that there is a relatively constant proportionality between the number of operating sodium-potassium-pump molecules and the number of operating potassium-channel molecules. This notion is suggested by the linear relation between the basolateral membrane conductance and the rate of pump activity observed in *Necturus* urinary bladder [7] and several other epithelia [14, 24] and the relative constancy of K_C^+ (and, more important, the relative constancy of the electrochemical PD for potassium across the basolateral membrane) of several epithelia in the face of widely different pump rates [16, 24].

Given this assumption, consider Figure 3 in the light of what is currently known regarding Na-K-ATPase synthesis, its insertion into the basolateral membrane, and its subsequent internalization ("turnover"). The reader is referred to the excellent, recent review by Karin and Cook [48] for references to the primary literature on this relatively new but blossoming area of study.

Briefly, the scenario appears to be as follows: (1) The "pump" is synthesized in the rough endoplasmic reticulum and, like many other membrane-bound proteins, after initial processing it is inserted into vesicles that are then transferred to the Golgi apparatus for further processing. These fully processed vesicles are then, somehow, directed specifically toward the basolateral membrane and are inserted into that barrier. The transit time between the onset of synthesis of new pump molecules and their insertion into the basolateral membrane is estimated to be 2 to 3 hr. (2) However, like all membrane

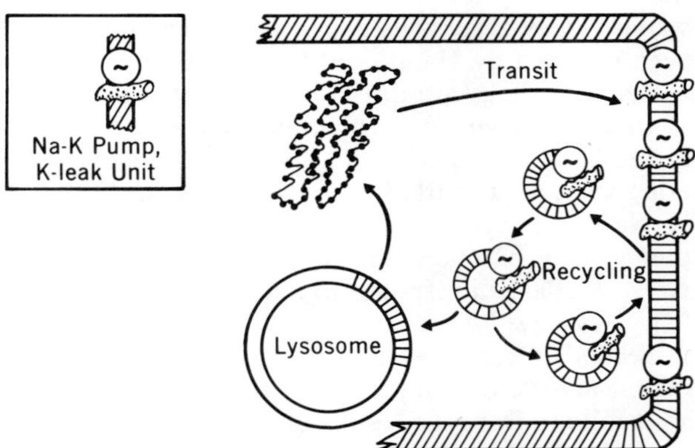

Fig. 3. Model illustrating cytokinetics of "pump-leak" units in basolateral membrane.

components, the residency of the pump in the basolateral membrane is transient, and, in time, it is internalized by an energy-dependent endocytotic process. These vesicles (endosomes) then travel to lysosomes for degradation.

If this scenario is correct, it seems reasonable that there is an intracytoplasmic endosomal compartment containing pump (and perhaps, leak) units that are in transit between the basolateral membranes and the lysosomes. Early attempts to identify such a compartment have not been successful, but Fishman and Cook [49] have shown that internalized (endocytosed) membrane sialoglycoconjugates (of HeLa and HTC cells) are recycled from the endosomal compartment and are reinserted into the plasma membrane; the endosomal compartment was estimated to be *twice* the size of the surface compartment.

It follows that the overall activity of the basolateral sodium-potassium pump is determined by the *activity* (turnover rate) of individual pump molecules in the membrane and the *number* of such molecules. The former is subject to regulation by extracellular and intracellular factors such as cellular calcium, cell pH, K_C^+, and so on. The latter is determined by the balance between the rates of insertion and internalization. It is generally felt that rapid changes in active transcellular sodium transport are accomplished by regulation of the activity (turnover rate) of a fixed number of pumps ("short-term" regulation); whereas long-term regulation may involve changes in the number of pump units as well [48].

However, if there is an endosomal pool of pump molecules that can be recruited into the membrane, changes in the number of active pump units could be effected rapidly.

In this regard, it is of interest to examine some recent findings on the effect of aldosterone on Na-K-ATPase activity. Petty, Kokko, and Marver [50] have reported that adrenalectomy markedly reduces the Na-K-ATPase activity of isolated segments of rabbit cortical collecting tubules (CCT) and that administration of physiologic doses of aldosterone to the adrenalectomized rabbits restores the control levels of Na-K-ATPase within 3 hr; a partial restoration was observed as early as 1.5 hr. However, this restoration was completely blocked by treating the rabbits with amiloride, which blocks sodium entry across the apical membrane of the CCT; similar findings have been reported by Handler et al [51] for cultured A6 cells.

These findings are intriguing from at least two points of view.

First, the *complete restoration* of Na-K-ATPase activity within 3 hr observed by Kokko, Petty, and Marver [50] seems to be very rapid when considering what is currently known regarding the time lag between the stimulation of Na-K-ATPase synthesis by aldosterone and the appearance of de novo pumps in the basolateral membrane; in toad urinary bladder newly synthesized Na-K-ATPase in response to aldosterone is *not detectable* prior to 3 hr [48, 52].

Second, Geering et al [52] have demonstrated that amiloride does not inhibit aldosterone-induced Na-K-ATPase synthesis.

It follows from the results of Petty, Kokko, and Marver [50] and Handler et al [51] that amiloride, by blocking sodium entry, prevents the *expression* or *insertion* of the Na-K-ATPase activity in the basolateral membrane; in other words, sodium entry into the cell appears to be a necessary stimulus for the insertion of already synthesized Na-K-ATPase into the basolateral membrane.

Clearly, there are many seminal questions that remain to be resolved regarding the cytokinetics and regulation of basolateral membrane Na-K-ATPase activity. Of paramount importance are: Is there a cytoplasmic compartment of sodium-potassium pumps (and perhaps potassium leaks)? And, if so, can an increase in Na_C^+ as a result of an increase in the rate of sodium entry across the apical membrane serve as a signal (direct or indirect) for the insertion of these pump (and perhaps, leak) units into the basolateral membrane? In short, can short-term regulation of overall pump (and leak) activity be the result of an increase in the number of pumps (and leaks) as well as an increase in the activity of individual pumps?

Summary

The results of recent studies on *Necturus* small intestine indicate that the pump-leak properties of the basolateral membrane respond rapidly to an increase in the rate of sodium entry across the apical membrane, coupled to the entry of sugar or amino acid, with (1) an increase in pump activity in the face of little or no increase in Na_C^+ and (2) a *parallel* increase in a barium-sensitive, K-conductance of the basolateral membrane. These responses serve to maintain intracellular ionic composition and volume. Seminal questions that remain to be resolved are whether these responses are the results of (1) an increase in the activity of a fixed number of functioning pump-leak units already present in the basolateral membrane; (2) the activation of previously quiescent pump-leak units already present in the basolateral membrane; and/or (3) the recruitment of new pump-leak units into that barrier. The *direct* signals for any and all of these possibilities are not known.

Acknowledgment. The research reported from our laboratories was supported by a grant from the NIH-NIA.

References

1. KOEFOED-JOHNSEN V, USSING HH: The nature of the frog skin potential. *Acta Physiol Scand* 42:298–308, 1958
2. MACKNIGHT ADC, DiBONA DR, LEAF A: Sodium transport across toad urinary bladder: A model tight epithelium. *Physiol Rev* 60:615–715, 1980
3. FUCHS W, LARSEN EH, LINDEMANN B: Current-voltage curve of sodium channels and concentration dependence of sodium permeability in frog skin. *J Physiol (Lond)* 267:137–166, 1977
4. PALMER LG, EDELMAN IS, LINDEMANN B: Current-voltage analysis of apical sodium transport in toad urinary bladder: Effects of inhibitors of transport and metabolism. *J Membr Biol* 57:59–71, 1980

5. LI JH-Y, PALMER LG, EDELMAN IS, LINDEMANN B: The role of sodium-channel density in the natriferic response of the toad urinary bladder to an antidiuretic hormone. *J Membr Biol* 64:77–89, 1982
6. THOMPSON SM, SUZUKI Y, SCHULTZ SG: The electrophysiology of rabbit descending colon: I. Instantaneous transepithelial current-voltage relations and the current-voltage relation of the Na-entry mechanism. *J Membr Biol* 66:41–54, 1982
7. THOMAS SR, SUZUKI Y, THOMPSON SM, SCHULTZ SG: The electrophysiology of *Necturus* urinary bladder: I. "Instantaneous" current-voltage relations in the presence of varying mucosal sodium concentrations. *J Membr Biol* 73:157–175, 1983
8. LINDEMANN B, VAN DRIESSCHE W: Sodium-specific membrane channels of frog skin are pores: Current fluctuations reveal high turnover. *Science* 195:292–294, 1977
9. PALMER LG, LI JH-Y, LINDEMANN B, EDELMAN I: Aldosterone control of the density of sodium channels in the toad urinary bladder. *J Membr Biol* 64:91–102, 1982
10. HELMAN SI, COX TC, VAN DRIESSCHE W: Hormonal control of apical membrane Na transport in epithelia: Studies with fluctuation analysis. *J Gen Physiol* 82:201–220, 1983
11. SCHULTZ SG: Sodium-coupled solute transport by small intestine: A status report. *Am J Physiol* 233:E249-E254, 1977
12. FRIZZELL RA, FIELD M, SCHULTZ SG: Sodium-coupled chloride transport by epithelial tissues. *Am J Physiol* 236:F1-F8, 1979
13. ARONSON PS: Identifying secondary active solute transport in epithelia. *Am J Physiol* 240:F1-F11, 1981
14. SCHULTZ SG: Homocellular regulatory mechanisms in sodium-transporting epithelia: Avoidance of extinction by "flush-through." *Am J Physiol* 241:F579-F590, 1981
15. GUNTHER-SMITH P, GRASSET E, SCHULTZ SG: Sodium-coupled amino acid and sugar transport by *Necturus* small intestine: An equivalent electrical circuit analysis of a rheogenic co-transport system. *J Membr Biol* 66:25–39, 1982
16. GRASSET E, GUNTER-SMITH P, SCHULTZ SG: Effects of Na-coupled alanine transport on intracellular K activities and the K conductance of the basolateral membranes of *Necturus* small intestine. *J Membr Biol* 71:89–94, 1983
17. LAU K, HUDSON RL, SCHULTZ SG: Cell swelling increases a barium-inhibitable energy dependent potassium conductance in the basolateral membrane of *Necturus* small intestine. *Proc Natl Acad Sci,* in press
18. LATORRE R, MILLER C: Conduction and selectivity in potassium channels. *J Membr Biol* 71:11–30, 1983
19. NAGEL W: Inhibition of potassium conductance by barium in frog skin epithelium. *Biochim Biophys Acta* 552:346–357, 1979
20. NIELSEN R: A 3 to 2 coupling of the Na-K pump responsible for the transepithelial Na transport in frog skin as disclosed by the effect of Ba. *Acta Physiol Scand* 107:189–191, 1979
21. KIRK KL, HALM DR, DAWSON DC: Active sodium transport by turtle colon via an electrogenic Na-K exchange pump. *Nature (Lond)* 287:237–239, 1980
22. BELLO-REUSS E: Electrical properties of the basolateral membrane of the straight portion of the rabbit proximal renal tubule. *J Physiol (Lond)* 326:49–63, 1982
23. WELSH MJ: Barium inhibition of basolateral membrane potassium conductance in tracheal epithelium. *Am J Physiol* 244:F639-F645, 1983
24. SMITH PL, FRIZZELL RA: Chloride secretion by canine tracheal epithelium: IV.

Basolateral membrane K permeability parallels secretion rate. *J Membr Biol* 77:187–199, 1984

25. MACKNIGHT ADC, LEAF A: Regulation of cell volume. *Physiol Rev* 57:510–573, 1977
26. DELLASEGA M, GRANTHAM JJ: Regulation of renal tubule cell volume in hypotonic media. *Am J Physiol* 224:1288–1294, 1973
27. DAVIS CW, FINN AL: Sodium transport inhibition by amiloride reduces basolateral membrane potassium conductance in tight epithelia. *Science* 216:525–527, 1982
28. FOSKETT JK, SPRING KR: Control of epithelial cell volume regulation (*abstract*). *J Gen Physiol* 82:21a, 1983
29. SCHULTZ SG, FUISZ RE, CURRAN PF: Amino acid and sugar transport in rabbit ileum. *J Gen Physiol* 49:849–866, 1966
30. CSAKY TZ, ESPOSITO G: Osmotic swelling of intestinal epithelial cells during active transport of sugars. *Am J Physiol* 217:753–755, 1969
31. ARMSTRONG WMD, MUSSELMAN DL, REITZUG HC: Sodium, potassium and water content of isolated bullfrog small intestinal epithelium. *Am J Physiol* 219:1023–1026, 1970
32. HIGGINS JT, GEBLER B, FRÖMTER E: Electrical properties of amphibian urinary bladder: II. The cell potential profile in *Necturus maculosa*. *Pflügers Arch* 371:87–97, 1977
33. NAGEL W, CRABBE J: Mechanism of action of aldosterone on active sodium transport across toad skin. *Pflügers Arch* 385:181–187, 1980
34. DAVIS CW, FINN AL: Sodium transport effects on the basolateral membrane in toad urinary bladder. *J Gen Phsiol* 80:733–751, 1982
35. MATSUMURA Y, COHEN B, GUGGINO WB, GIEBISCH G: Regulation of the basolateral potassium conductance of the *Necturus* proximal tubule. *J Membr Biol,* in press
36. WELSH MJ: Intracellular potassium activities in canine tracheal epithelium. *Am J Physiol* 245:C248-C254, 1983
37. VOUTE CL, USSING HH: Some morphologic aspects of active sodium transport: The epithelium of the frog skin. *J Cell Biol* 36:625–638, 1968
38. BROBRYCKI VA, MILLS JW, MACKNIGHT ADC, DiBONA DR: Structural responses to voltage-clamping in the toad urinary bladder: I. The principle role of granular cells in the active transport of sodium. *J Membr Biol* 60:21–35, 1981
39. DiBONA DR, SHERMAN B, BROBRYCKI VA, MILLS JW, MACKNIGHT ACD: Structural responses to voltage-clamping in the toad urinary bladder: II. Granular cells and the natriferic action of vasopressin. *J Membr Biol* 60:35–44, 1981
40. SCHULTZ SG: Electrical potential differences and electromotive forces in epithelial tissues. *J Gen Physiol* 59:794–798, 1972
41. MACKNIGHT ADC, LEAF A: The sodium transport pool. *Am J Physiol* 234:F1-F9, 1978
42. FINN AL: The kinetics of sodium transport in the toad urinary bladder: II. Dual effects of vasopressin. *J Gen Physiol* 57:349–362, 1971
43. FINN AL: Changing concepts of transepithelial sodium transport. *Physiol Rev* 56:453–464, 1976
44. HUDSON RL, SCHULTZ SG: Effects of sodium-coupled sugar transport on intracellular sodium activities and sodium-pump activity in *Necturus* small intestine. *Science,* in press
45. LEE CO, ARMSTRONG WM: Activities of sodium and potassium ions in epithelial cells of small intestine. *Science* 175:1261–1264, 1972
46. QUAY JF, ARMSTRONG WM: Enhancement of net sodium transport in isolated

bullfrog intestine by sugars and amino acids. *Proc Soc Exp Biol Med* 131:46–51, 1969
47. WILLS NK, LEWIS SA: Intracellular Na activity as a function of Na transport rate across a tight epithelium. *Biophys J* 30:181–186, 1980
48. KARIN NJ, COOK JS: Regulation of Na-K-ATPase by its biosynthesis and turnover, in *Current Topics in Membranes and Transport,* edited by HOFFMAN JF, FORBUSH B III, New York, Academic Press, 1983, pp 713–751
49. FISHMAN JB, COOK JS: Recycling of surface sialoglycoconjugates in HTC and HeLa cells. *J Biol Chem* 257:8122–8129, 1982
50. PETTY KJ, KOKKO JP, MARVER D: Secondary effect of aldosterone on Na-K-ATPase activity in the rabbit cortical collecting tubule. *J Clin Invest* 68:1514–1521, 1981
51. HANDLER JS, PRESTON AS, PERKINS FM, MATSUMURA M, JOHNSON JP, WATLINGTON CO: The effect of adrenal steroid hormones on epithelia formed in culture by A6 cells. *Ann NY Acad Sci* 372:442–454, 1981
52. GEERING K, GIRARDET M, BRON C, KRAEHENBUHL J-P, ROSSIER BC: Hormonal regulation of (Na,K)-ATPase biosynthesis in the toad bladder. *J Biol Chem* 257:10338–10343, 1982

Sodium-Glucose Cotransport Mechanisms

R. James Turner

Early studies of the active renal reabsorption of D-glucose established that
the uphill step in this process occurred at the brushborder membrane of
the proximal tubule via a highly selective, saturable, and sodium (Na)-depen-
dent transport mechanism [1, 2]. As the experimental evidence accumulated,
it became increasingly clear that this reabsorptive system was a further example of the scheme originally proposed by Crane et al [3, 4] for sugar absorption
in the intestine—and later extended by others to a variety of other solutes
and systems (for a list of recent reviews see [5]).

According to Crane's *gradient hypothesis,* the active accumulation of
D-glucose in the proximal tubular cell is accomplished by the coordinated action
of two transport systems: (1) a Na-coupled transporter for D-glucose localized
in the brushborder membrane, which drives glucose from the lumen into
the cell against a concentration gradient as a result of the electrochemical
gradient for Na across this membrane, and (2) the Na pump (Na$^+$, K$^+$)-
ATPase, localized in the basolateral membrane, which maintains the extracellular-to-intracellular Na electrochemical gradient at the expense of adenosine
triphosphate (ATP); thus, it provides the link to metabolic energy that ultimately drives the coupled luminal transport system. The final step in the
reabsorptive process occurs via a facilitative diffusion-type transporter for
glucose localized in the basolateral membrane. This transporter allows glucose
to diffuse out of the cell, down its own concentration gradient, and into
the blood. It is now known that the renal reabsorption of a number of ions
and metabolites follows this general scheme.

The Thermodynamics of Coupled Transport

The handling of D-glucose by the proximal tubular cell provides an excellent
model system for examining the thermodynamic principles behind coupled

---

This manuscript was presented as part of a Symposium on *Brushborder Transport Mechanisms.*

reabsorptive transport processes. From thermodynamic considerations, it can be shown [6] that the ratio of intracellular-to-extracellular glucose concentrations, $[G_{in}]/[G_{out}]$, in the proximal tubular cell must obey the following inequality:

$$\frac{[G_{in}]}{[G_{out}]} \leq \left[\frac{[Na_{out}]}{[Na_{in}]} \exp \frac{F\Delta\psi}{RT} \right]^n \qquad (1)$$

Where F, R, and T have their usual thermodynamic interpretations, $\Delta\psi = \psi_{out} - \psi_{in}$ is the transmembrane electrical potential, and n is the Na:glucose coupling stoichiometry; that is, the number of Na ions translocated by the brushborder membrane transporter per glucose molecule. The $\leq$ sign in Eq. 1 becomes an equality in the absence of glucose leak pathways. These leak pathways may be divided into two distinct classes: those that occur via the Na-dependent transporter (internal leaks) and those that do not (external leaks). External leaks include the basolateral glucose carrier, as well as the passive diffusion of D-glucose across the brushborder and basolateral membranes. Internal leaks arise when the flux of Na and glucose via the luminal carrier is not tightly coupled; or, more specifically, when glucose translocation is able to occur via the carrier with less than n (possibly zero) cotransported Na ions. In the presence of internal leaks, the actual number of moles of Na translocated per mole of glucose may vary with glucose and Na concentrations as well as with membrane potential. Thus n in Eq. 1 is better defined as the *maximum* number of Na ions translocated per glucose molecule. The existence of significant internal leak pathways in coupled transport systems would seem to be undesirable, since these would result in unproductive dissipation of substrate and/or Na gradients. There is now good evidence that renal Na-glucose cotransport is relatively tightly coupled, at least in the early proximal tubule (see below).

Several general points are worth emphasizing with regard to Na-coupled reabsorptive processes. First, note that the concentrating capacity of the cell for substrate (Eq. 1)—and hence its ability to effectively drive substrate reabsorption—varies as the power of the coupling stoichiometry, n. Thus, other factors being equal, one would expect a dramatic dependence of substrate reabsorption on n.

In this regard, it is interesting to consider how the energetic cost of substrate reabsorption varies with n. We neglect the energy expended by the cell in maintaining the Na electrochemical gradient in the presence of membrane processes that are unrelated to the reabsorptive system of interest. In this case, the energy expended in transporting a substrate molecule from lumen to cytosol via the Na-coupled carrier is simply the energy required to pump the cotransported Na ions back out of the cell. Provided that this substrate molecule does not return to the lumen via a dissipative pathway, this will be the total energetic cost for its reabsorption, since it will eventually diffuse from the cytosol into the blood down its own chemical gradient. The relevant dissipative pathways are simple diffusion across the brushborder membrane, internal leaks of the brushborder transporter, and diffusion from blood to lumen via the tight junctions between cells. Loss of substrate via all of these routes is expected to increase with increasing intracellular (and hence intercellular) substrate concentration; hence, with increasing n. Thus, as one might expect, the advantage of increased reabsorptive capacity resulting from higher Na:substrate coupling ratios will be offset, to some degree, by higher energetic costs and larger dissipative losses.

D-Glucose Transport in Brushborder Membrane Vesicles

The most convincing confirmation of the gradient hypothesis for renal D-glucose transport has been provided by experiments with brushborder membrane vesicles [7–17]. These systems allow the study of brushborder membrane transport phenomena in the absence of nonmembrane-related events. Both Na-dependent glucose transport [7–17] and glucose-dependent Na transport [14, 15] have been demonstrated in these systems. In addition, it has been shown that a Na gradient can drive the concentrative uptake of D-glucose [7–13]. The results of such an experiment are shown in Figure 1. In this

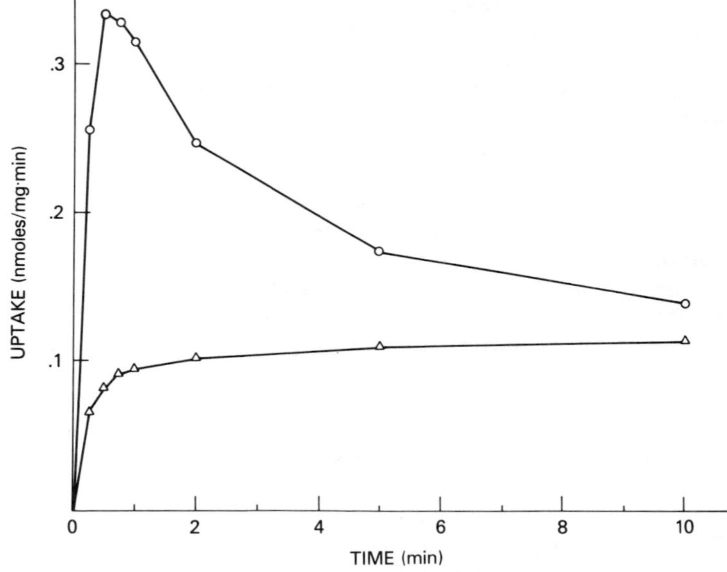

Fig. 1. Demonstration of the "overshoot" phenomenon for D-glucose in rabbit outer cortical brushborder membrane vesicles. Vesicles were prepared in 10 mM Tris-HEPES (pH 7.4) buffer containing 100 mM mannitol, 12.5 μg valinomycin/mg protein, and 100 mM KSCN, along with 90 mM choline chloride (*upper curve*) or 60 mM NaCl plus 30 mM choline chloride (*lower curve*). In each case, the composition of the incubation medium was such that the final extravesicular solution was 10 mM Tris-HEPES, 100 mM mannitol, 100 mM KSCN, 30 mM choline chloride, and 60 mM NaCl. Symbols are: O, Na gradient; △, Na equilibrium. (Reproduced with permission from [5])

figure, D-glucose uptake into brushborder membrane vesicles that are prepared from the outer cortex of rabbit kidney is studied in the presence and absence of an extravesicular-to-intravesicular Na gradient. In the presence of a Na gradient (upper curve), the intravesicular glucose concentration transiently rises above ("overshoots") its equilibrium value; then, it falls back toward equilibrium as the Na gradient dissipates. Thus, the concentrative uptake of D-glucose that is characteristic of the intact proximal tubular cell can be duplicated by the brushborder membrane alone in conjunction with a suitably oriented Na gradient. In the absence of a Na gradient (lower curve), no concentrative uptake is observed. This latter behavior is not surprising in view of the fact that no energy source is available under these experimental conditions. These overshoot experiments, carried out under the well-controlled conditions possible in vesicle systems, provide strong evidence for the direct coupling of Na and glucose fluxes across the brushborder membrane. Experiments described later in this chapter confirm these results in a quantitative way.

In addition to providing evidence supporting the gradient hypothesis, early studies of Na-dependent D-glucose transport in brushborder membrane vesicles showed a somewhat complex kinetic behavior. Curvilinear uptake/[glucose] versus uptake (Eadie-Hofstee) plots were observed in experiments with brushborder membrane vesicles that were prepared from the whole cortex of the dog [16] and human kidney [10]. These curvilinear Eadie-Hofstee plots cannot be accounted for by a single transporter that obeys Michaelis-Menten kinetics. Although more complex coupled transport models are capable of explaining the observed deviations from linearity [18], Turner and Silverman provided experimental evidence in the dog indicating that this effect may be due to the presence of two (or more) Na-dependent glucose transporters in renal brushborder membrane vesicle preparations [16]. These authors further suggested that the existence of multiple glucose carriers in the renal brushborder membrane may reflect heterogeneity of transport sites along the length of the proximal tubule. This conjecture later received support from the work of Barfuss and Schafer [19], who studied the glucose transport properties of various segments of the proximal tubule by using the isolated perfused tubule technique. Their studies demonstrated that the Michaelis constant (K_m) and V_{max} for active D-glucose reabsorption decreased progressively as a function of length along the proximal nephron.

Turner and Moran [13] were subsequently able to directly establish the existence of proximal tubular brushborder D-glucose transport heterogeneity. These authors compared the D-glucose transport properties of brushborder membrane vesicles prepared from two regions of the rabbit kidney: the outer cortex and the outer medulla. Owing to the structural organization of nephrons in the kidney [20, 21], the outer cortical preparation is expected to contain predominantly brushborder membranes from proximal convoluted tubules of superficial nephrons (early proximal tubule from S_1 and some S_2 cell types); the outer medullary preparation is expected to contain predominantly brushborder membranes from the late proximal straight tubule (from S_3 cell types). D-glucose transport was characterized by distinctly different Na-dependent transport systems in each of these preparations. These experiments and the physiologic rationale for this transport heterogeneity are described in detail later in this chapter.

Transport Studies—Methods

The methods used in the transport studies presented here have been described in detail elsewhere [13, 14, 17, 22]. A brief discussion emphasizing several important technical points is given below.

Transport measurements were made by using the "rapid filtration" technique. The basic procedure is as follows: At time zero, suitably prepared vesicles are combined with an incubation medium containing radioactively labeled ligands and other constituents as required. After an appropriate incubation period, a "stop solution" is added and the vesicles are collected on a filter that is subsequently washed and counted for radioactivity.

Most kinetic studies were carried out under zero trans conditions (at time zero, $[G_{in}] = [Na_{in}] = 0$). In all kinetic experiments, care was taken to measure initial transport rates. This precaution is essential for the quantitative interpretation of flux data in vesicle systems (or for that matter in any system), since intravesicular concentrations can change dramatically over relatively short time periods. Also, since Na-coupled D-glucose transport is rheogenic, D-glucose flux can influence and be influenced by the transmembrane potential. Accordingly, membrane potentials were controlled in all experiments by means of a K/valinomycin voltage clamp. Technically, this means that K was present in both the intravesicular and extravesicular solutions and that the K ionophore, valinomycin, was added to the vesicle preparation at a sufficient concentration so that the transmembrane potential was fixed at the K diffusion potential.

The quantitative interpretation of data obtained by using the rapid filtration technique also depends critically on the ability of the stop solution to prevent any further flux of labeled substrate into or out of the vesicles. Errors arising from the use of an inadequate stop solution can be large [5]. Methods for evaluating the effectiveness of the stop solution and tests of the stop solution used in the studies presented here (10 mM Tris-HEPES, pH 7.4, containing 300 mM NaCl, 1 mM phlorizin, and sufficient mannitol to compensate for intravesicular osmolarity) have been presented elsewhere [5, 13, 23].

Transport Studies—Results

Brushborder membrane vesicles were prepared from rabbit renal outer cortical or outer medullary tissue by the same divalent cation precipitation procedure [13]. Relative to the respective starting homogenates, each preparation was enriched by approximately 12-fold in the brushborder membrane marker maltase; and, they showed small-to-negligible contamination with nonbrushborder membrane material [13]. The flux of D-glucose into both preparations was markedly stimulated by Na ($\sim$ 20-fold at 1 mM D-glucose and 60 mM NaCl), was enhanced by negative intravesicular potentials, and was inhibited by phlorizin at concentrations in the micromolar range. Furthermore, both preparations exhibited the classic overshoot of intravesicular D-glucose concentration (Fig. 1) in the presence of an inwardly directed Na gradient [13]. Thus, both enzymatically and functionally, each preparation had many of the classic properties usually associated with brushborder membrane vesicle systems.

However, although the qualitative characteristics of D-glucose transport that were mentioned above were quite similar in the two vesicle preparations, marked quantitative differences were observed. The first of these is illustrated in Figure 2. In this case, we have measured the initial rate of Na-dependent D-glucose flux as a function of D-glucose concentration under zero transvoltage-clamped conditions. The data are illustrated as Eadie-Hofstee plots. In contrast to the curvilinear Eadie-Hofstee plots observed in earlier studies with whole cortical preparations [10, 16], linear plots with dramatically different slopes for outer cortical and outer medullary vesicles are observed here. The linearity of these plots indicates that the data fit the Michaelis-Menten equation; thus, they are consistent with the existence of a single transport site in each preparation. Fitting these data to the Michaelis-Menten equation, we find $K_m \cong 6$ mM in the outer cortex and $K_m \cong 0.4$ mM in the outer medulla. Thus, D-glucose reabsorption apparently is mediated by a low-affinity system in the early proximal tubule and by a high-affinity system in the late proximal tubule. We have also demonstrated that these two transporters show different specificity properties for glucose analogs and different sensitivity to inhibition by phlorizin [13]. For example, relative to D-glucose, α-methyl-D-glucoside is a better substrate for the outer cortical site than for the outer medullary one; whereas, the opposite holds true for D-galactose. Also, the outer medullary transporter is almost two orders of magnitude less sensitive to inhibition by phlorizin than the outer cortical site [17]. Furthermore, we have shown [14, 17] that it is the outer cortical transporter and not the outer medullary one that is associated with the high-affinity Na-dependent phlorizin binding site that is commonly found in renal brushborder membrane preparations [2].

Why then are there two D-glucose transporters arranged as a function of length along the renal proximal tubule? Initially, we thought that there might be some kinetic advantage to preceding a high-affinity system with a low-affinity one; however, we were unable to come up with a plausible rationale for this possibility. It seemed to us that if a high-affinity system were available, it would be more advantageous to use it to absorb the entire glucose load.

Our eventual understanding of the physiologic rationale for this transport heterogeneity came from studies of the Na dependence of the two transporters [14, 17]. The first experiments we attempted were measurements of glucose flux as a function of Na concentration. In the outer cortex, we found that our results indicated a hyperbolic dependence of flux on [Na] and yielded an excellent fit ($r = 0.99$) to the equation:

$$\text{Flux} = \frac{V_{max}[\text{Na}]}{K_{0.5} + [\text{Na}]} \tag{2}$$

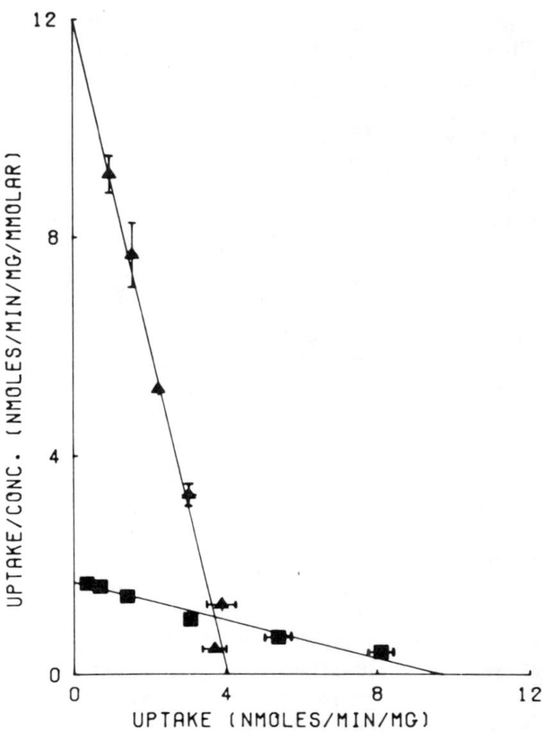

Fig. 2. Kinetics of the Na-dependent stereo-specific component of initial D-glucose flux into outer cortical and outer medullary brushborder membrane vesicles. Vesicles were prepared in 10 mM Tris-HEPES (pH 7.4) buffer containing 300 mM mannitol, 12.5 μg valinomycin/mg protein, and 100 mM KSCN. The incubation medium was 10 mM Tris-HEPES, 100 mM mannitol, 100 mM KSCN, 40 mM NaCl, or choline chloride (final concentrations), and various concentrations of labeled D- and L-glucose. Uptakes observed in the presence of choline were subtracted from those found in the presence of Na to obtain the Na-dependent component of D-glucose flux. Symbols are: ■, outer cortex; ▲, outer medulla. (Reproduced with permission from [13])

where V_{max} and $K_{0.5}$ are constants. This is exactly the functional relationship expected for a system with a Na:glucose stoichiometry of 1:1 [24, 25]. In contrast, plots of glucose flux versus [Na] for the outer medullary system were sigmoidal. This type of behavior is indicative of the involvement of more than one Na ion in the D-glucose transport event [5, 17, 24]. A lower limit on the number of Na ions involved, n, can be obtained by fitting the results to the Hill equation:

$$\text{Flux} = \frac{V_{max}[\text{Na}]^{n}}{K_{0.5}^{n} + [\text{Na}]^{n}} \tag{3}$$

A fit of the outer medullary data to this equation via nonlinear regression analysis typically yielded $n \cong 1.8$. Similar fits to the outer cortical data typically yielded $n = 1.0$, with an uncertainty of a few percentage points. These experiments suggested to us that the important physiologic difference between the outer cortical and outer medullary transporters might be their coupling stoichiometries, rather than their affinities for D-glucose. However, we knew that the above method for determining stoichiometric ratios does not distinguish between energetically and catalytically coupled Na; that is, between stimulation of glucose flux due to Na-glucose cotransport (energetic coupling) and Na-induced facilitation of glucose entry without concomitant Na transport (catalytic coupling). To determine the number of Na ions actually cotransported with glucose, another type of experiment is required. The experimental protocol typically used for this purpose in transport studies involves measuring and comparing the Na-dependent substrate flux and the substrate-dependent Na flux in the same preparation under the same experimental conditions. When this experiment was carried out for the outer cortical preparation, a $1:1$ correspondence between Na and glucose fluxes was observed, which again indicates a $1:1$ coupling ratio [14]. However, attempts to measure the Na:glucose coupling ratio in the outer medullary system by the same method were unsuccessful, owing to the small size of glucose-dependent Na fluxes relative to glucose-independent Na fluxes in this membrane. Thus, the crucial flux experiment could not be done.

We were aware that investigators working with bacterial and other systems that were capable of generating and maintaining Na (or proton) gradients over time used another method for measuring couplingratios [26–31]. In these experiments, the steady-state substrate gradient generated by the system in the presence of a known (measured) Na (or proton) electrochemical gradient is measured, and n (or more correctly a lower limit on n) is calculated from Eq. 1. However, this method was impractical for our purposes for two reasons. First, we had no means of estimating the relative importance of external leaks in our vesicle preparations, and thus had no way of determining the degree to which we were underestimating n by using Eq. 1. Second, a Na gradient cannot be maintained in brushborder membrane vesicle preparations, owing to significant Na leak pathways. Thus, the sustained steady-state substrate gradient required for this method never occurs. The additional error introduced into the determination of n by this problem is difficult, if not impossible, to determine.

The following technique for determining Na:substrate coupling ratios, which we refer to as the "static head method," provided a means around the two difficulties just discussed [5, 14, 17]. A similar procedure has been reported by Kinsella and Aronson [32]. Consider a tightly coupled cotransport system in which n Na ions are transported per glucose molecule. The thermodynamic condition—that there is no net flux of either substance via the transporter, or equivalently, that the thermodynamic driving forces for Na and glucose fluxes are balanced—is given by:

$$\frac{[G_{in}]}{[G_{out}]} = \left[\frac{[Na_{out}]}{[Na_{in}]} \right]^n \tag{4}$$

In this case, the effects of membrane potentials (compare Eq. 1) have been omitted, since it is assumed that $\Delta\psi$ can be set to zero by an appropriate voltage clamping procedure. We refer to the situation in which Eq. 2 holds as a static head condition. This equation is a thermodynamic relationship that involves only cotransported Na and glucose. The principle of the static head experiment is to search for experimental conditions under which Eq. 2 holds. In practical terms (see below), we search for a Na gradient that exactly balances a known glucose gradient. Once these static head conditions have been determined, the coupling stoichiometry can be calculated directly from Eq. 2 by using the known values of the Na and glucose gradients.

An example of a static head experiment for the renal outer cortical brush-border membrane D-glucose transporter is shown in Figure 3a. In this experi-

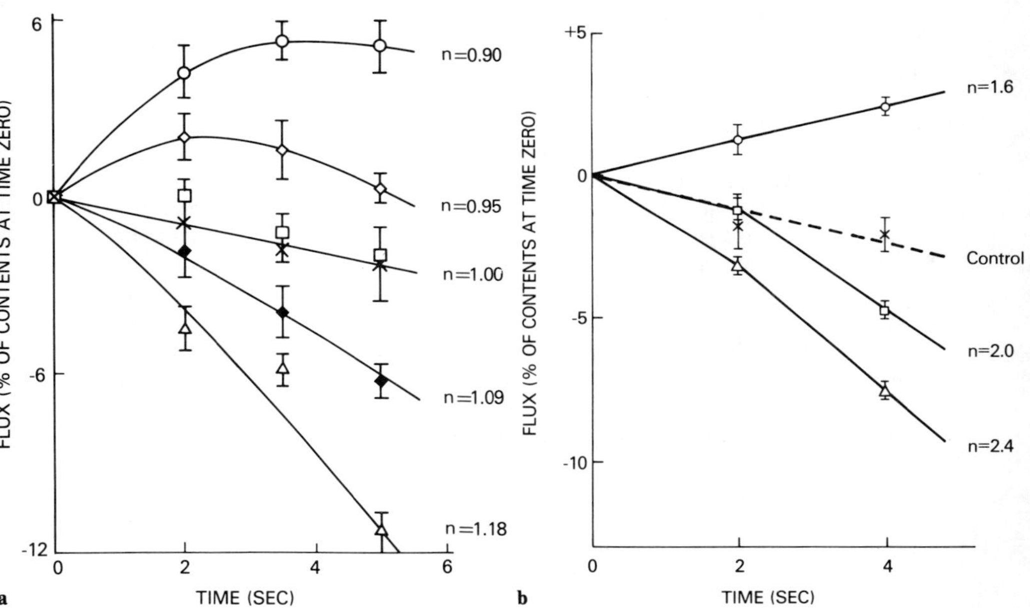

Fig. 3. The results of static head experiments for the outer cortical (**a**) and outer medullary (**b**) brushborder membrane D-glucose transporters. Vesicles were loaded with 20 mM NaCl, 180 mM choline chloride, and 0.5 mM labeled glucose (outer cortex) or 20 mM NaCl, 50 mM choline chloride, and 0.25 mM labeled glucose (outer medulla). Vesicles were diluted 1:5 into iso-osmotic media containing various concentrations of Na. The values of n indicated on the figures are the Na/glucose stoichiometries, which would be predicted if they were to result in static head conditions. A control run (x) was carried out in the absence of Na to measure efflux via unrelated sodium-independent pathways. The static head condition is characterized by that external sodium concentration which causes the test points to lie on the control. Membrane potentials were clamped at 0 by including 100 mM KSCN in all solutions and by adding the K^+ ionophore valinomycin at a concentration of 12.5 μg/mg membrane protein. (**a** redrawn with permission from [14]; **b** redrawn with permission from [17])

ment, vesicles were preloaded with known concentrations of Na and labeled D-glucose and then diluted $1:5$ into appropriate glucose-free media, thus establishing an intravesicular-to-extravesicular glucose gradient of $6:1$. The glucose retained in these vesicles then was measured as a function of time at various extravesicular Na concentrations. A control run, carried out in the absence of Na, was used to measure efflux via unrelated Na-independent pathways (external leaks). The static head condition (no net flux via the Na-dependent transporter) was characterized by that external Na concentration, which causes the test run to superimpose on the control. The values of n indicated on the figure are the Na:glucose stoichiometries, which would be predicted by Eq. 2 if that extravesicular Na concentration resulted in static head conditions. This experiment illustrates that the Na:glucose coupling ratio of the outer cortical transporter is $1:1$ with an uncertainty of less than 5%. The results of a similar experiment for the outer medullary transporter are shown in Figure 3b. Here a stoichiometry of slightly less than 2 (approximately 1.8) is predicted. This result is consistent with the stoichiometry predicted by the Hill analysis for the outer medullary transporter mentioned above.

Since the static head method involves a comparison of net influx or efflux rates under various initial conditions, the sustained steady-state substrate gradient used for stoichiometric determinations in bacterial systems (see above) is not required here. Also, external leaks are considered explicitly by the control run inthe static head experiment.

We recently have extended the static head method from the determination of the Na:substrate stoichiometry to the determination of charge:substrate stoichiometry [22]; that is, the determination of the number of electric charges transferred per substrate molecule. This parameter obviously is equal to the sum of the charges on all translocated species; thus, it provides a means of verifying other stoichiometric determinations, as well as indicating the possible involvement of previously overlooked ions (H^+) in the transport event. The principle of the charge stoichiometry experiment is similar to the one just discussed, except that instead of attempting to balance a glucose gradient with a Na gradient, we balance it with a valinomycin-induced K diffusion potential. The static head condition in this case is:

$$\frac{[G_{in}]}{[G_{out}]} = \exp\left(qF\Delta\psi/RT\right) \tag{5}$$

where q is the charge:substrate stoichiometry. Since $\Delta\psi = (RT/F)\,1n\,([K_{in}]/K_{out}])$, the K diffusion potential, the above equation reduces to:

$$\frac{[G_{in}]}{[G_{out}]} = \left[\frac{[K_{in}]}{[K_{out}]}\right]^q \tag{6}$$

In practical terms, the procedure for the charge stoichiometry experiment is very similar to that described for Figure 3. Now, however, vesicles are pre-equilibrated with K, labeled glucose, and valinomycin and are diluted into media containing various K concentrations. The charge stoichiometry experiment is carried out at Na equilibrium.

The values of q given by the charge stoichiometry experiments—0.9 for the outer cortical preparation and 1.5 for the outer medulla—agree well with the corresponding Na:glucose coupling ratios for these systems. Thus, these experiments are consistent with the hypothesis that Na is the only ion involved in renal brushborder membrane D-glucose transport.

Physiologic Rationale

The experiments described above show that D-glucose reabsorption across the brushborder membrane of the proximal tubule is mediated by at least two Na-coupled transport systems with differing Na:glucose coupling stoichiometries: (1) a low-affinity system, apparently localized to the early proximal tubule with a Na:glucose coupling ratio of $1:1$, and (2) a high-affinity system, apparently localized to the late proximal tubule with a Na:glucose coupling ratio of approximately $2:1$. The value of 1.8 obtained for the stoichiometry of the latter system could be indicative of a $2:1$ transporter with internal leaks; however, we favor the explanation that this deviation from a $2:1$ coupling ratio is due to the presence of a small, but significant, number of $1:1$ transporters in the outer medullary vesicle preparation.

As a result of these stoichiometric measurements, we have suggested the following physiologic rationale for the heterogeneity of D-glucose transport observed in the proximal tubule [17]. Most of the glucose load is reabsorbed early in the tubule by the outer cortical transporter at an energetic cost of one Na ion per glucose molecule. The driving force for this process includes both the chemical and electrical components of the Na electrochemical gradient. As glucose is reabsorbed along the length of the tubule, the intracellular glucose concentration falls along with the urinary concentration. Eventually, a point will be reached where the electrochemical gradient for Na is too low for a $1:1$ system to drive the intracellular glucose concentration to a value higher than that found in the blood. At this point, glucose reabsorption would cease. However, before this occurs, the $2:1$ system is already present in the apical membrane. Since the concentrating capacity of a coupled transporter increases as the power of the coupling stoichiometry (compare Eq. 1), this transporter can use the same driving force to produce substantially higher intracellular glucose concentrations than the $1:1$ system; thus, it can continue to drive D-glucose reabsorption in the late proximal tubule. These lasttraces of glucose are pumped from the urine at the higher energetic cost of two Na ions per glucose molecule. This arrangement of transporters in series along the proximal tubule leads to a more energy-efficient reabsorptive mechanism for D-glucose than could be achieved by either of the transporters acting alone.

Summary

The renal brushborder membrane transport system for D-glucose often has been used as a model system for Na-coupled reabsorptive mechanisms in the proximal tubule, as well as for Na-coupled transport mechanisms in general. Using brushborder membrane vesicle preparations from the outer cortex (early proximal tubule) and outer medulla (late proximal tubule) of rabbit kidney, we have demonstrated that the reabsorption of D-glucose across the brushborder membrane is, in fact, mediated by two distinct Na-dependent transporters arranged in a series along the proximal nephron. The first of these is a low-affinity system localized in the early proximal tubule, which cotransports one Na^+ per glucose molecule. The second is a high-affinity system localized in the late proximal tubule, which cotransports two Na^+ per glucose. In each case, the net charge that is translocated is equal to that on the cotransported Na ions, indicating that no other ions are involved in these contransport events. We have provided a physiologic rationale for this transport heterogeneity by indicating how this arrangement of carriers, in series along the proximal nephron, allows the kidney to reabsorb D-glucose in an energy-efficient fashion.

Acknowledgment. This review was prepared while the author was the holder of grant MA-8028 from the Medical Research Council of Canada.

References

1. MUDGE GH, BERNDT WO, VALTIN H: Tubular transport or urea, glucose, phosphate, uric acid, sulfate, and thiosulfate, in *Handbook of Physiology. Renal Physiology,* edited by ORLOFF J, BERLINER RW, Washington D.C., American Physiology Society, 1973, pp 587–652
2. SILVERMAN M: Glucose transport in the kidney. *Biochim Biophys Acta* 457:303–351, 1976
3. CRANE RK, MILLER D, BIHLER I: The restrictions on possible mechanisms of intestinal active transport of sugars, in *Membrane Transport and Metabolism,* edited by KLEINZELLER A, KOTYK K, New York, Academic Press, 1961, pp 439–449
4. CRANE RK: Hypothesis for mechanism of intestinal active transport of sugars. *Fed Proc* 21:891–895, 1962
5. TURNER RJ: Quantitative studies of co-transport systems: models and vesicles. *J Membr Biol* 76:1–15, 1983
6. ARONSON PS: Identifying secondary active transport in epithelia. *Am J Physiol* 240:F1–F11, 1981
7. ARONSON P, SACKTOR B: The Na^+ gradient-dependent transport of D-glucose in renal brush border membranes. *J Biol Chem* 250:6032–6039, 1975
8. BECK JC, SACKTOR B: Energetics of the Na^+-dependent transport of D-glucose in renal brush border membranes. *J Biol Chem* 250:8647–8680, 1975
9. KINNE R, MURER H, KINNE-SAFFRAN E, THEES M, SACHS G: Sugar transport by renal plasma membrane vesicles. *J Membr Biol* 21:375–395, 1975
10. TURNER RJ, SILVERMAN M: Sugar uptake into brush border vesicles from normal human kidney. *Proc Natl Acad Sci USA* 74:2825–2829, 1977
11. BECK J, SACKTOR B: The sodium electrochemical potential mediated transport of D-glucose in renal brush border membrane vesicles. *J Biol Chem* 253:5531–5535, 1978
12. TURNER RJ, SILVERMAN M: Sugar uptake into brush border vesicles from dog kidney. I. Specificity. *Biochim Biophys Acta* 507:305–321, 1978

13. TURNER RJ, MORAN A: Heterogeneity of sodium dependent D-glucose transport sites along the proximal tubule: Evidence from vesicle studies. *Am J Physiol* 242:F406–F414, 1982

14. TURNER RJ, MORAN A: Stoichiometric studies of the renal outer cortical brush border membrane D-glucose transporter. *J Membr Biol* 67:73–80, 1982

15. HILDEN SA, SACKTOR B: D-glucose-dependent sodium transport in renal brush border membrane vesicles. *J Biol Chem* 254:7090–7096, 1979

16. TURNER RJ, SILVERMAN M: Sugar uptake into brush border vesicles from dog kidney. II. Kinetics. *Biochim Biophys Acta* 511:470–486, 1978

17. TURNER RJ, MORAN A: Further studies of proximal tubular brush border membrane D-glucose transport heterogeneity. *J Membr Biol* 70:37–45, 1982

18. CRANE RK, DORANDO FC: On the mechanism of Na^+-dependent glucose transport, in *Function and Molecular Aspects of Biomembrane Transport,* edited by QUAGLIARIELLO E, Amsterdam, Elsevier/North Holland, 1979, pp 271–278

19. BARFUSS DW, SCHAFER JA: Differences in active and passive glucose transport along the proximal nephron. *Am J Physiol* 240:F322–F332, 1981

20. KAISSLING B, KRIZ W: *Structural Analysis of the Rabbit Kidney.* Berlin, Springer-Verlag, 1979, pp 42–59

21. MAUNSBACH AB: Ultrastructure of the proximal tubule, in *Handbook of Physiology. Renal Physiology,* edited by ORLOFF J, BERLINER RW, Washington D.C., American Physiology Society, 1973, pp 31–79

22. FUKUHARA Y, TURNER RJ: The static head method for determining the charge stoichiometry of coupled transport systems: applications to the sodium-coupled D-glucose transporters of the renal proximal tubule. *Biochim Biophys Acta* 770:73–78, 1984

23. FUKUHARA Y, TURNER RJ: Na-dependent succinate transport in renal outer cortical brush border membrane vesicles. *Am J Physiol* 245:F374–F381, 1983

24. SEGEL IH: *Enzyme Kinetics.* New York, John Wiley & Sons, 1975

25. TURNER RJ: Kinetic analysis of a family of cotransport models. *Biochim Biophys Acta* 649:269–280, 1981

26. RAMOS S, KABACK HR: pH-dependent changes in proton:substrate stoichiometries during active transport in *Escherichia coli* membrane vesicles. *Biochemistry* 16:4271–4275, 1977

27. LANYI JK: Coupling of aspartate and serine transport to the transmembrane electrochemical gradient for sodium ions in *Halobacterium halobium.* Translocation stoichiometries and apparent cooperativity. *Biochemistry* 17:3011–3018, 1978

28. JOHNSON RG, CARTY SE, SCARPA A: Proton:substrate stoichiometries during active transport of biogenic amines in chromaffin ghosts. *J Biol Chem* 256:5773–5780, 1981

29. KNOTH J, ZALLAKIAN M, NJUS D: Stoichiometry of H^+-linked dopamine transport in chromaffin granule ghosts. *Biochemistry* 20:6625–6629, 1981

30. BROEK PJA VAN DEN, CHRISTIANSE K, STEVENINCK J VAN: The energetics of D-fructose transport in *Saccharomyces fragilis.* The influence of the protonmotive force on sugar accumulation. *Biochim Biophys Acta* 692:231–237, 1982

31. PASTUSZKO A, WILSON DF, ERECINSKA M: Energetics of γ-aminobutyrate transport in rat brain synaptosomes. *J Biol Chem* 257:7514–7519, 1982

32. KINSELLA JL, ARONSON PS: Determination of the coupling ratio for Na^+-H^+ exchange in renal microvillus membrane vesicles. *Biochim Biophys Acta* 689:161–164, 1982

Cell Volume Regulation in Epithelia

Chairpersons: Jared J. Grantham and Kenneth R. Spring
Discussants: Michael A. Linshaw, Guillermo Whittembury,
Paola Carpi-Medina, Ernesto Gonzalez, Henry Linares,
William B. Guggino, Kevin L. Kirk, James A. Schafer,
Donald R. DiBona, and Peter M. Andrews

The Workshop began with a discussion of the mechanism of volume regulatory decrease in the proximal tubule. The acute stress of immersion in hypotonic medium causes renal proximal straight tubules (PST) to swell quickly to a peak volume within 1 min and then recover close to control size over the next several minutes as the tubules extrude solute and water. This volume regulatory decrease occurs presumably as potassium, sodium, anion, and water are extruded from the cells. Linshaw has studied some effects of altering cation and anion content in the bathing medium on the volume regulatory decrease of PST in dilute medium. He mounted rabbit PST with collapsed lumens between two micropipets and assessed tubule volume by measuring tubule diameter with an image-splitting eyepiece. Tubule size was stable in an isotonic medium. Tubules incubated for 20 min in 10^{-3} M $BaCl_2$ swelled in a manner similar to control tubules to a peak 55% above the baseline when immersed in dilute medium, but took more than twice as long to regulate to an apparent steady state close to control size. Barium reduces the potassium conductance of the basolateral membrane of epithelial cells and may be useful for studying cation extrusion. In further experiments, he loaded PST cells with sodium chloride and substantially depleted them of potassium by incubating the tubules in 10^{-4} M ouabain and isotonic Ringer solution without potassium (280 mOsm/liter) until the tubules swelled to an apparent steady state. When placed in hypotonic medium (170 mOsm/liter), control tubules swelled further and then decreased their size gradually over the next 10 to 20 min. Ouabain-treated tubules that were also incubated in 10^{-3} M $BaCl_2$ for 20 min showed volume regulation indistinguishable from control tubules.

In his anion exchange studies, PST were incubated initially in isotonic medium in a control (122 mM Cl) or zero chloride Ringer solution for 20 to 30 min. Upon immersion in dilute medium, the tubules swelled to a peak volume that was 50 to 60% above baseline; he could alter the volume regula-

---

This manuscript is a summary of a Workshop entitled *Cell Volume Regulation in Epithelia.*

tory decrease by varying the anion. Control tubules ($N = 6$) regulated 81% below the peak swelling, but tubules depleted of chloride by incubation in a chloride-free gluconate medium regulated only 33% ($N = 6$). Removing bicarbonate from the bathing medium had no apparent effect on hypotonic volume regulation. Linshaw concluded that (1) barium interferes with volume regulation in hypotonic medium probably by impairing potassium efflux, and (2) Cl, rather than bicarbonate, is the principal anion extruded with cation during hypotonic volume recovery in rabbit PST.

Next, Whittembury and his colleagues led a discussion of the osmometric behavior and cell volume regulation in the proximal kidney tubule. Cell volume (V) changes can be studied as changes in diameter of the tubule with a time resolution of less than 1 sec and a spatial resolution $< \pm 0.2$ μm ($\pm 2\sigma$) in PST isolated from the rabbit kidney mounted between crimping pipettes so that the lumen is occluded and water and ion movements mainly occur across the basolateral cell surface. Osmotic gradients across the peritubular cell membrane induce within 10 sec the V changes expected from a perfect osmometer (V/V_{iso}) $= 0.27$ (± 0.70) $+ 0.76$ (± 0.07) $\times C_{iso}/C_b$ where the ordinate is the ratio of V observed at the peak of the osmotic response (obtained with a bath concentration [C_b] to the control V observed at equilibrium with a bath concentration C_{iso}. The intercept is not different from the cell solid content of 0.30 ± 0.01 measured directly (*Am J Physiol* 242:F321, 1982). The slope is the ratio of cell water volume to V. Thus, all cell water is osmotically active. Bath potassium affected the magnitude of the osmotic response to swelling leading to responses smaller than (low potassium) and larger than (high potassium) those expected for a perfect osmometer. The water movements involved in this osmotic response can be either diffusive through the membrane lipids (involving strong interactions between water and the membrane) or viscous through aqueous pathways piercing the membrane. To differentiate between these possibilities, we have measured P^c_{os}, the water osmotic permeability coefficient, and its energy of activation, E_a (kcal/mole) under control conditions and after the addition of the highly specific, nonpenetrating sulfhydryl reagent, *p*CMBS (*p*-chloromercuribenzenesulfonic acid). We found that *p*CMBS did not markedly affect the magnitude of the osmometric response, but reduced P^c_{os} to 0.26 ± 0.17 of its control value and increased E_a from 3.2 ± 1.4 to 9.2 ± 2.2. This effect of *p*CMBS reverses with dithiothreitol. E_a for viscous flow is 4.2; therefore, water equilibration must occur through water-filled pathways that allow viscous flow. Sulfhydryl groups must be involved in determining the conformation of these pathways. If the change produced by *p*CMBS were in the pathway diameters, an alteration of only 30% would explain these observations. Finally, volume regulation was demonstrated when the bath tonicity was lowered in nonperfused tubules, and when the lumen osmolality was reduced while the tubules were bathed in mineral oil.

Next, Guggino initiated a discussion of those factors that control cell volume in the Amphiuma diluting segment. The diluting segment of the Amphiuma kidney (similar to the rabbit cortical thick ascending limb) maintains a lumen-positive transepithelial potential, and thus reabsorbs chloride against a transepithelial gradient. Both the positive transepithelial potential and chloride reabsorption are inhibited by the loop diuretic furosemide. There is evidence that the uphill entry of chloride into these cells across the apical cell membrane is a secondarily active process involving a single cotransport system transporting sodium, potassium, and chloride (*Pflügers Arch* 396:27–33, 1983). This apical cotransport system exists in parallel with a potassium conductance. The volume of a diluting segment cell depends on the entry and exit of solutes during net transport. This phenomenon can be exploited to study the processes involved in solute transport. Concerning apical solute entry mechanisms, cell volume measurements with a video optical system show that basolateral application of ouabain results in significant cell swelling at a rate of approximately 11 ± 3 μm^3/sec. This points out that inhibiting solute exit with continued entry results in cell swelling. This swelling is inhibited by prior application of furosemide to the luminal solution. Since furosemide inhibits solute entry via the sodium/potassium/chloride cotransport system, it follows that the apical cotransport system must be the major site of solute entry into these cells. Concerning solute entry mechanisms, simultaneous measurements of cell volume and basolateral cell membrane potential (V_{bl}) with conventional microelectrodes show that diluting segment cells are heterogeneous in regard to the mechanism of potassium and chloride transport across the basolateral cell membrane. The evidence is as follows: (1) increasing potassium to 98 mM or decreasing chloride to 16 mM in the basolateral solution depolarizes V_{bl} only by 58 ± 4 mv and 33 ± 4 mv, respectively, in one cell type (group 1) and by only 6 ± 2 mv and 4 ± 3 mv, respectively, in another cell type (group 2); (2) raising basolateral potassium to 98 mM in chloride-free solutions increases the depolarization of V_{bl} by 84 ± 8 mv in group 1 cells, but does not increase it significantly in group 2 cells, 6 ± 2 mv; and (3) the ratio of apical to basolateral resistances is greater than 10 ± 3 in group 1 cells and 1.3 ± 0.3 in group 2 cells. Thus, two cell types are present in the same Amphiuma diluting segment, a group 1 cell with a high potassium- and chloride-conductive basolateral cell membrane and a group 2 cell with low basolateral conductances for these ions. The cell volume increases in group 1 cells at a rate of 195 μm^3/sec in response to an increase in basolateral potassium to 98 mM at constant chloride. This swelling is inhibited by removing chloride from the solutions. Both responses are expected from a cell which is conductive to both potassium and chloride. Surprising, however, is the observation that potassium-induced swelling also occurs in group 2 cells, but at a rate significantly lower than in group 1 cells, 111 μm^3/sec. This suggests that although the conductance for potassium is virtually undetectable, rather large fluxes of this ion can occur via neutral mechanisms. This swelling is also inhibited by chloride removal, indicating that the electroneutral mechanism for potassium movement across the basolateral cell membrane of group 2 cells may involve potassium and chloride cotransport. Thus, combined cell volume and electrical measurements in the same cell have been important in showing that: (1) the sodium/potassium/chloride cotransport system on the apical cell membrane of the diluting segment is the major pathway for ions to move into the cells, and (2) the mechanisms of potassium and chloride movement out of the cell across the basolateral cell membrane appears to be heterogeneous with one cell type exhibiting primarily conductive transport, while the movement ina second cell type is electroneutral.

When perfused tubules were exposed to hypotonic bathing medium, the cells swelled, but there was no volume regulatory decrease.

Kirk et al then directed their attention to the cellular consequences of volume reabsorption in the mammalian collecting duct. The description that followed characterized the changes in cell volume and epithelial morphology associated with the onset of antidiuretic hormone (ADH)-stimulated, volume reabsorption in the mammalian collecting duct. Computer-assisted morphometric procedures were developed to provide estimates of cell volume and the geometry of the lateral intercellular spaces from Nomarski interference-contrast-microscopic images of isolated and perfused rabbit cortical collecting tubules. No structural changes were observed following the addition of ADH in the absence of a transepithelial osmotic gradient. However, in the presence of a lumen-to-bath osmotic gradient (130 mOsm perfusate/290 mOsm bath), the addition of a maximal dose of ADH (250 μU/ml) resulted in a nearly 10-fold stimulation in transepithelial volume flow (J_v) and the following structural changes: (1) bulging of the cells into the lumen; (2) dilation of the lateral intercellular spaces; and (3) the appearance of large intracellular vacuoles. Morphometric analyses revealed that the volume of the lateral intercellular spaces increased dramatically (+ 78%), whereas cell volume increased more modestly (+ 25%) during the onset of ADH-stimulated volume reabsorption. Cell and lateral space volume increased coincidentally with J_v and reached new steady-state values within 10 to 15 min that were maintained for at least another 30 min. Vacuolation was a secondary event that was not observed until the changes in water permeability and cell volume were nearly complete and vacuole formation continued for 45 to 60 min after these parameters had reached new steady-state values. Their results support the following conclusions. First, the pathway for ADH-stimulated volume reabsorption involves water entry into collecting tubular cells across the hormone-responsive luminal membrane and water exit via, in part, the lateral intercellular spaces. Second, vacuole formation is a secondary response to water reabsorption and does not represent the expansion of a preferential route for transcytoplasmic volume flow. Third, from the magnitude of the cell volume increase associated with the onset of volume reabsorption, they estimate that the luminal membrane is the rate-determining barrier to water flow in the presence of physiologic levels of ADH. Thus, changes in cell volume during enhanced volume reabsorption in the collecting duct are minimized due to the relatively large hydraulic conductivities of those barriers that exist in series with the hormone-responsive luminal membrane.

Proximal straight tubules were studied in a similar fashion. When tubules were perfused with isotonic fluid, substitution of hypotonic external bathing fluid caused the cells to swell, and to regulate volume back to baseline in a few minutes.

The final segment of the Workshop dealt with the control of cell volume during ischemic insult to the kidney. In vitro and in vivo studies of Andrews indicate that controlling cell swelling during ischemia is essential to protecting kidneys from postischemic acute renal failure. Light and electron microscopy of kidneys flushed with cold storage preservation solutions demonstrate progressive swelling of tubule cells as the length of storage time is increased. This swelling is especially damaging to the convoluted and straight segments of the proximal tubules, which eventually rupture and fill the tubule lumens with cytoplasmic debris. Swelling of cells can be controlled by adding the proper amounts of impermeant osmotic agents to the flushing solution. It was found that mannitol is more effective than dextrose and sucrose is more effective than mannitol in preventing cell swelling during cold storage, which agrees with their respective permeability coefficients. Based on these observations an isotonic, phosphate-buffered, cold flushing solution was developed which has proven to be consistently successful in the cold storage of dog kidney for 72 hr. Recently, the ability of the widely used Euro-Collins flushing solution to protect rat kidneys from 1 hr or normothermic ischemic insult was tested. Flushing kidneys with Euro-Collins containing dextrose and then clamping the renal vessels of the flushed kidneys for 1 hr in situ resulted in severe postischemic acute renal failure and usually death within 72 hr following the ischemic insult. When, however, the dextrose in Euro-Collins flushing solution was replaced with an equivalent osmolal contribution of mannitol or sucrose, all the animals exhibited only mild elevations in serum creatinine levels and most returned to normal within 72 hr following ischemic insult. In view of the above observations, it is strongly recommended that flushing solutions contain the proper amounts of effective impermeant osmotic agents (that is, sucrose, mannitol) in place of other commonly used osmotic agents (that is, dextrose).

Role of Cytosolic Calcium in Vasopressin-sensitive Epithelia

Ann Taylor, Mirilee Pearl, Barbara Barber, and Beth Crutch

Vasopressin promotes the absorption of water and sodium (Na) the amphibian urinary bladder and the mammalian collecting tubule. While the hormone initially binds to receptors in the basolateral membrane of its target epithelial cells, its stimulatory effects on water and Na transport ultimately depend on alterations in the water and Na permeability of the plasma membrane at the apical surface of the cells [1]. Many different elements of the cellular machinery evidently participate in the translation of the hormonal signal from one cell surface to the other. The changes in apical membrane function induced by vasopressin are mediated by cyclic AMP, but cytosolic calcium (Ca) ions also appear to play a rolein the response to the hormone.

The cellular action of vasopressin has been most extensively studied in the toad urinary bladder. In this tissue, the hormone-induced changes in water and Na permeability appear to be confined to the granular epithelial cells [2]. The vasopressin receptors at the basolateral cell surface are coupled to adenylate cyclase (they are of the V2 type) [3]. Hormone-receptor interaction leads to activation of the cyclase and to the generation of cyclic AMP. The second messenger role of cyclic AMP was established some 20 years ago, when Orloff, Handler, and Preston [4] demonstrated that exogenous cyclic AMP mimics the action of the hormone on transepithelial water and Na movement in the toad bladder and that vasopressin increases the cyclic AMP content of the bladder epithelial cells [5, 6]. The increase in cyclic AMP content has been shown to precede the stimulation of Na transport elicited by vasopressin [7] consistent with the postulate that the nucleotide serves as an intracellular mediator of the natriferic and hydrosmotic actions of the hormone [4]. Cyclic AMP is believed to bind to and to activate type II protein kinases (located in the cell cytosol) [1] that, in turn, regulate the level of phosphorylation of specific target proteins. However, the precise sub-

This manuscript was presented as part of a Symposium on *Second Messengers and Epithelial Transport*.

cellular distribution of the kinases and the identity and function of the phosphoprotein substrates are unknown.

Vasopressin increases the water and Na permeability of the rate-limiting barrier at the apical surface of the cell by two discrete mechanisms. The hormone increases apical membrane permeability to Na by activating a pre-existing population of Na channels (these channels are converted from a closed state to an open fully conducting state [8]). In contrast, the hormone-induced increase in water permeability involves the insertion of new membrane components into the apical membrane. This process is accompanied by specific changes in fine structure at the apical surface of the cell, including the appearance of particle aggregates in the apical membrane [9] and transformation of the microvilli from a ridge-like to a finger-like configuration [10]. The particle aggregates are believed to contain the channels through which water crosses the apical barrier. The aggregates exist preformed in a helical array in membrane vesicles in the subapical cytoplasm [11]. These vesicles are translocated toward the apical surface by a process that involves microtubules and microfilaments [12], and they are incorporated into the apical membrane by an exocytotic-like fusion event [13] under the influence of the hormone.

Cytoplasmic microtubules [14] and actin-containing microfilaments [15] have been identified as components of the cytoskeletal lattice in the apical region of toad bladder granular epithelial cells. Pharmacologic evidence indicates that the cytoskeletal organelles play a specific role in the hormone-induced increase in water permeability [14, 15] and in the associated structural changes at the apical cell surface [16, 17], including both the insertion of the particle aggregates [12] and the microvillus transformation [18]. Studies with heavy meromyosin have revealed that the microvillus cores and the cortical cytoplasm (terminal web) are composed, in large part, of actin filaments and that such filaments are intimately associated with the plasma and cytoplasmic organelle membranes [15]. While the granular cell microvilli are superficially similar to brushborder microvilli in that both contain actin filament cores, there are clear differences in their structural organization. The absence of conspicuous microfilament bundles in granular cell microvilli may be a reflection of the ability of these microvilli to undergo rapid transformation in response to hormonal stimulation.

While the cellular mechanisms underlying the changes in apical membrane permeability are beginning to be understood, the sequence of intracellular events—whereby vasopressin and cyclic AMP induce these changes—is still essentially unknown. Since cyclic AMP-dependent protein kinases have been described in association with cytoskeletal proteins in other tissues [19, 20], it seems likely that microtubule- and microfilament-associated proteins are target sites for such kinases in vasopressin-sensitive epithelial cells and that cyclic AMP directly regulates cytoskeletal activity. Vasopressin and cyclic AMP induce a modest increase ($\sim$30%, $P < 0.02$) in the content of cytoplasmic microtubules in toad bladder granular epithelial cells [14], which is consistent with the view that cyclic AMP is involved in some way in the regulation of microtubule assembly and/or function in these cells. Likewise, cyclic AMP might influence microfilament activity in vasopressin target cells, but there currently is no experimental evidence for this.

Calcium ions have been implicated in the control of a variety of cellular events in nonmuscle cells, including microtubule- and microfilament-dependent processes. Calcium ions are believed to regulate the state of assembly and organization of the cytoskeleton; low levels of Ca ($< 10^{-7}$ M) favor microtubule assembly and actin filament stabilization and bundling, while high Ca ($> 10^{-7}$ M) favors the disassembly of microtubules and the severing of actin filaments [21, 22]. In general, Ca ions play a complementary role to that of cyclic AMP, in that the two agents exert reciprocal effects on cytoskeletal organization and activity.

In view of the potential link between Ca ions and the cytoskeleton, we have explored the role of cytosolic Ca in the action of vasopressin. The role of Ca ions was first evaluated indirectly in a series of studies on the toad urinary bladder that used procedures designed to interfere with cellular Ca homeostasis. All functional studies were conducted on isolated toad bladder preparations. Transepithelial osmotic water movement was estimated gravimetrically [15]; net Na transport was measured by means of the short-circuit current technique [15].

In our initial experiments, we examined the effects of quinidine. Quinidine was tested because of its reputed ability to block Ca uptake by intracellular organelles [23]. (Recent measurements with Ca^{++}-selective microelectrodes in epithelial cells of *Necturus* kidney have shown that quinidine increases cytosolic Ca ion activity by some 10-fold [24].) In functional studies on the toad bladder, we demonstrated that quinidine inhibits both vasopressin- and cyclic AMP-induced water movement (Fig. 1). The inhibition was dose-dependent and readily reversible [25]. In separate experiments, quinidine was found to inhibit the basal short-circuit current, but not the natriferic response to vasopressin. At a concentration of 4×10^{-4} M, the drug induced a fall in net Na transport to $43 \pm 4\%$ of the paired controls over 45 min ($N = 19$, $P < 0.001$). In these experiments, the addition of vasopressin, 20 mU/ml, to the quinidine-treated hemibladders elicited an increase in short-circuit current to levels observed in the controls. Thus, vasopressin apparently reversed the effect of the drug [25].

To determine the effect of quinidine on epithelial cell morphology, we recently examined thick sections through the apical surface of the granular cells in the high-voltage electron microscope [26]. This technique permits the three-dimensional visualization of events occurring at the cell surface. Figure 2 is a series of micrographs that compares the microvillus architecture of resting bladders with that of bladders receiving vasopressin or quinidine plus vasopressin. A comparison of the upper and middle panels demonstrates the normal transformation from ridge- to finger-like microvilli that is elicited by vasopressin or cyclic AMP. The lower panel shows the effect of exposing the tissue to quinidine (3×10^{-4} M) prior to stimulation with vasopressin. In this micrograph, the apical surface is flattened and the microvilli appear to have collapsed.

The disruption of normal microvillus architecture by quinidine may be due to solation of the microvillus core actin filaments by high Ca. This effect could be mediated by a Ca-activated actin filament-severing protein similar to those that have been described in many nonmuscle cell types [22]. This

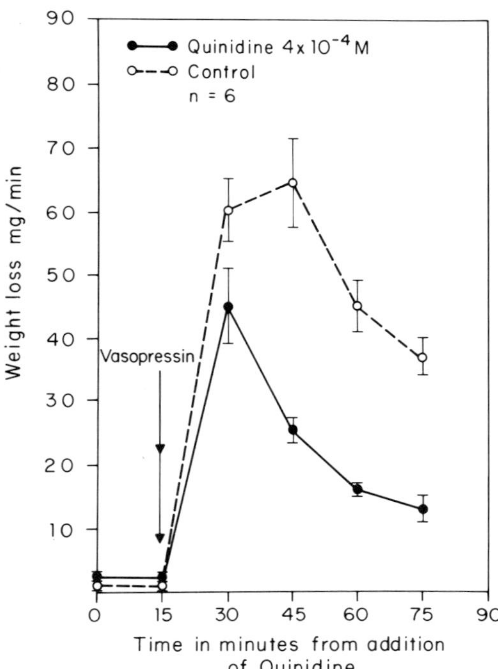

Fig. 1. Inhibition of the hydrosmotic response to vasopressin in isolated toad bladders by quinidine. One member of each pair of hemibladders was exposed to quinidine 4×10^{-4} M for 15 min prior to hormone stimulation. (Reproduced from [30])

type of protein has recently been identified in vitro in studies on toad bladder homogenates [27]. Our electron microscopic findings support the view that the organization of cytoskeletal elements in the microvilli is sensitive to changes in cytosolic Ca in vivo. Thus, quinidine may inhibit the hydrosmotic response to vasopressin and cyclic AMP partly by interfering with Ca-sensitive cytoskeletal-dependent events that underlie the change in apical membrane water permeability.

Additional evidence of a role for cytosolic Ca in vasopressin-sensitive epithelia has been obtained in studies with the Ca ionophores, A23187 and X537A. Like quinidine, these agents inhibit vasopressin- and cyclic AMP-induced water flow. They also inhibit the basal rate of net Na transport across the toad bladder, but this effect is at least partially reversed by vasopressin [25]. In a recent study, A23187 was shown to interfere with the increase in apical membrane area (estimated as membrane capacitance) that is induced by vasopressin [28]. This finding is consistent with the view that elevated cytosolic Ca interferes with the structural changes at the apical cell surface elicited by the hormone.

Manipulation of the Na-Ca exchanger that is now known to operate across the basolateral membrane of toad bladder epithelial cells [29] provides another means of increasing the level of free Ca in the epithelial cell cytosol. If the concentration of Na in the medium bathing the serosal surface of the epithelium is reduced, the driving force for Na-Ca exchange is decreased; this

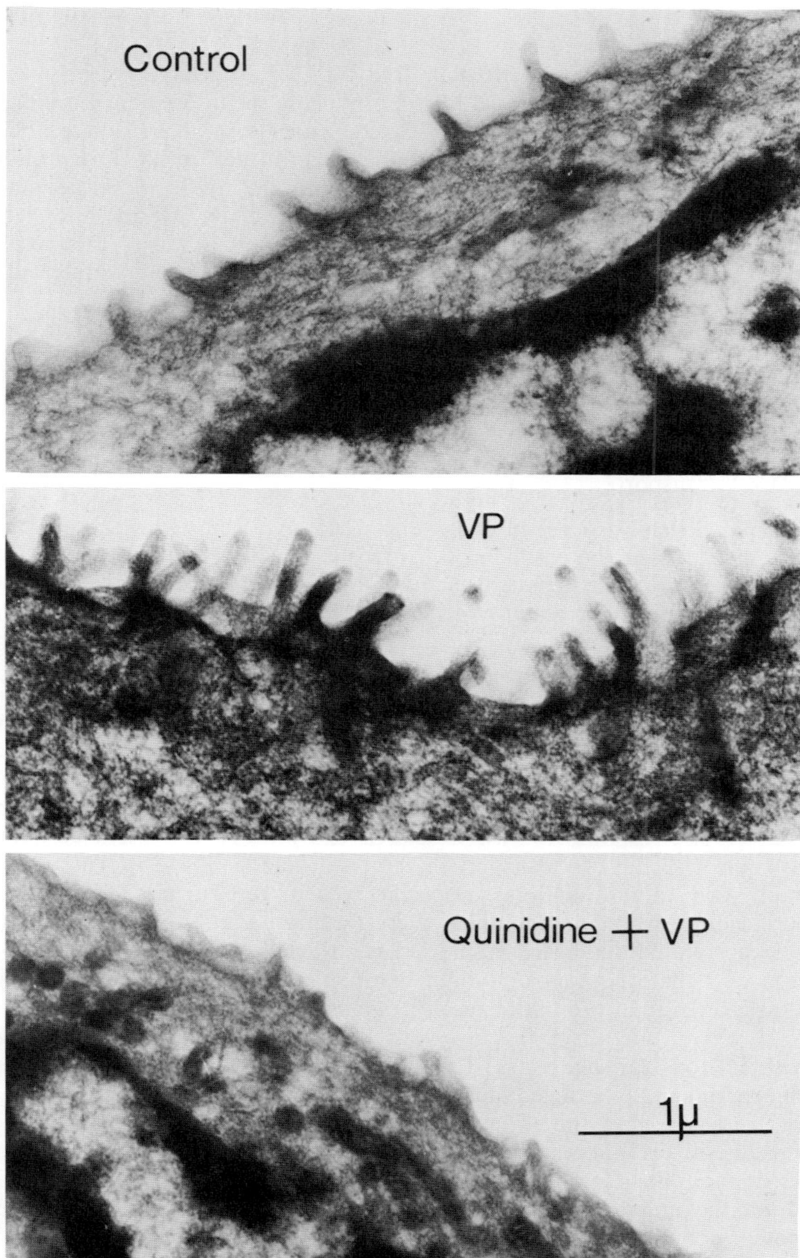

Fig. 2. Bladders were incubated as sacs in Ringer's solution (*top*); or vasopressin (20 mU/ml) in Ringer's solution for 5 min (*middle*); or quinidine (3×10^{-4} M) in Ringer's for 15 min, followed by vasopressin (VP) for 5 min (*bottom*). Samples were fixed in 2% glutaraldehyde and embedded in epoxy resin. Sections (~ 0.3 μm) were stained with uranyl acetate and lead citrate and examined in the AEI HVEM at 1000 KeV. ($\times$37,000)

results in an increase in cytosolic-free Ca [30]. We have recently verified this experimentally in the toad bladder by using the fluorescent Ca indicator, Quin 2, to measure cytosolic-free Ca ion concentration in isolated bladder epithelial cells [31]. In functional studies, exposure of isolated toad bladders to low-serosal Na was shown to inhibit both the hydrosmotic response to hormonal stimulation and the basal rate of net Na transport; however, the effect on the latter was again reversed by vasopressin [25]. Thus, exposure to low serosal Na resulted in a pattern of transport events similar to that observed with quinidine and the Ca ionophores.

Our functional studies provided indirect evidence that cytosolic Ca ions play a role in the regulation of apical membrane water permeability and also modulate a rate-limiting step (presumed to be the apical entry step) in the Na transport process [25]. (Since our studies were commenced, other investigators have shown that micromolar levels of Ca decrease apical membrane permeability to Na [29].) Based on the finding that vasopressin selectively reverses the effect of high cytosolic Ca on net Na transport, we have speculated that vasopressin and cyclic AMP may transiently lower the level of ionized Ca in the epithelial cell cytosol. We have suggested that such a decrease in cytosolic Ca might mediate the stimulatory action of the hormone on both transcellular water and Na movement [25, 30].

In recent years, other investigators have explored the potential messenger role of Ca in vasopressin-sensitive epithelial cells by examining the role of calmodulin. This high-affinity Ca-binding protein has been implicated as a mediator of many Ca-activated cellular events. It is thought to function as an intracellular Ca receptor and also to be involved in Ca-signal transduction when cytosolic Ca is elevated above 10^{-7} M [32]. Several laboratories have reported that calmodulin-binding agents, such as trifluoperazine, inhibit the hydrosmotic response to vasopressin or to cyclic AMP, but have no effect on transepithelial Na transport in the toad bladder [33–36]. These findings imply that calmodulin plays aspecific role in the hormone-induced water permeability response. Based on these findings, some investigators [33, 34] have postulated that vasopressin increases the level of free Ca in the epithelial cells and that the Ca-calmodulin complex that is formed plays a second messenger role in the hydrosmotic response to the hormone.

However, not all of the functions of calmodulin involve its interaction with Ca ions (or vice versa) [27, 32]. To determine whether the effects of an experimentally induced increase in cytosolic Ca are mediated by calmodulin, we have tested the effects of trifluoperazine on bladders exposed to low serosal Na. Trifluoperazine does not block the inhibition of hormone-stimulated water flow (or net Na transport) that is induced by low serosal Na; rather, the inhibitory effects of the two experimental procedures on the hydrosmotic response are additive [36]. These results suggest that Ca and calmodulin play independent roles in the sequence of cellular events that underlies the action of the hormone. It is relevant to note that the Ca-dependent actin-modulating protein implicated in the control of microfilament organization in the toad bladder (as discussed above) is calmodulin-independent [27].

From this survey of the literature, it is apparent that based on indirect evidence, two opposing views of the role of cytosolic Ca ions in the cellular action of vasopressin have been postulated by different investigators. To directly assess the role of Ca ions in the hormonal response, we have used the Quin 2 method [31] to determine the effect of vasopressin on the level of cytosolic-free Ca in toad bladder epithelial cells. This method, which was recently developed by Tsien, Pozzan and Rink [37], permits the estimation of the average free Ca ion concentration in isolated cell suspensions.

In these experiments, isolated epithelial cells were loaded with the acetoxymethyl ester of Quin 2 (5 to 10 μM) at a cell density of 5×10^7 cells/ml. The lipid-soluble ester rapidly enters the cells, where it is hydrolyzed to the impermeant free acid; intracellular Quin 2 concentrations ranged from 0.2 to 2.0 mM. The fluorescent signal from freshly washed Quin 2-loaded cells was monitored at 492 nm (emission) and 339 nm (excitation). Figure 3 shows the response of the fluorescent signal to a change in extracellular Ca concentration and to addition of the Ca-specific ionophore, ionomycin. This trace indicates that the Quin 2 signal is reporting changes in free Ca within the epithelial cells in a predictable manner. In a representative sample of 100 measurements obtained under resting conditions in cells suspended in normal amphibian Ringer's solution (Ca 0.89 mM, pH 7.4), cytosolic free Ca ion concentration averaged 91 $\pm$ 3 nM (SEM). Thus, the resting level of ionized Ca in toad bladder epithelial cells is very similar to that in excitable cells.

We have recently determined the effects of vasopressin and other agonists on both cytosolic Ca ion concentration and cellular cyclic AMP content of Quin 2-loaded epithelial cells. The results are illustrated in Figure 4. When precautions are taken to avoid quenching artifacts, vasopressin stimulation has no detectable effect on the fluorescent Quin 2 signal; that is, on the level of cytosolic-free Ca. (The commercial vasopressin preparations that we have tested may be contaminated with heavy metals; their addition leads

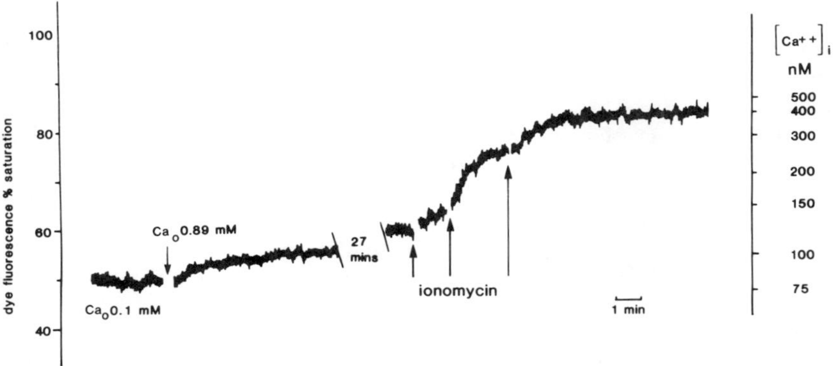

Fig. 3. Quin 2-loaded cells were initially suspended in a solution containing Ca 0.1 mM. On restoration of normal extracellular Ca (0.89 mM), cytosolic Ca ion concentration rose from 75 to 110 nM over 30 min. The addition of ionomycin led to sequential, dose-dependent increases in cytosolic Ca.

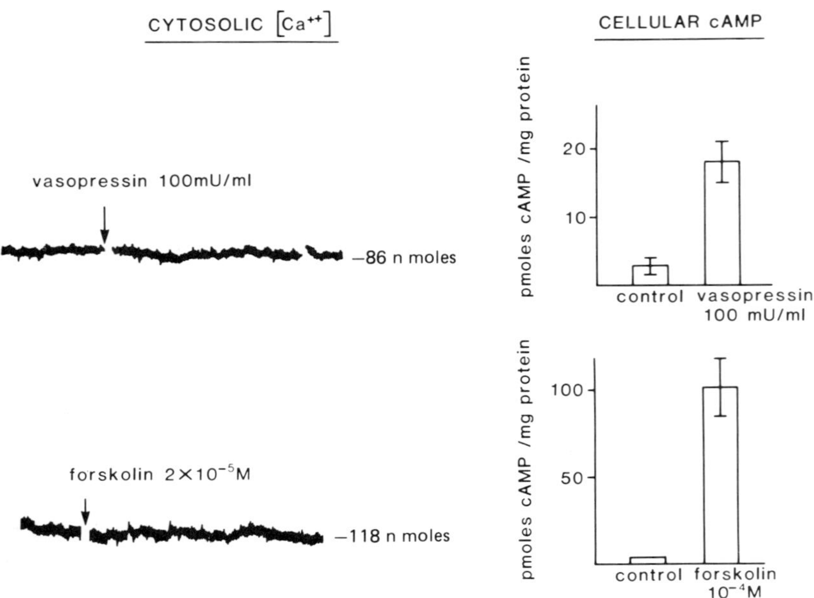

Fig. 4. Effects of vasopressin and forskolin on cytosolic Ca ion concentration and cellular cyclic AMP content of Quin 2-loaded cells. Intracellular (Quin 2) was ~1.5 mM. Measurements of cyclic AMP were made in the presence of theophylline, 10 mM.

to the quenching of the fluorescence of Quin 2 in solution. However, this can be prevented or reversed by means of heavy metal-chelating agents.)

Forskolin is a potent activator of adenylate cyclase; at a concentration of 2×10^{-5} M, this agent mimics the vasopressin response in the toad bladder (unpublished observations of the authors). Like vasopressin, forskolin had no effect on cytosolic Ca. Similar results were obtained in experiments with exogenous cyclic AMP.

Measurements of cellular cyclic AMP content were made parallel with the estimations of cytosolic Ca to ascertain whether isolated epithelial cells, loaded with millimolar concentrations of Quin 2, were still capable of responding to both vasopressin and forskolin. These measurements were made on aliquots of the same cell suspensions that were used for the cytosolic Ca estimates. As shown in Figure 4, both vasopressin and forskolin elicited marked increases in cellular cyclic AMP content in the Quin 2-loaded cells, although they had no apparent effect on cytosolic Ca.

Thus, according to these data, vasopressin neither increases nor decreases cytosolic free Ca levels in toad bladder epithelial cells. This conclusion must necessarily be qualified, since the Quin 2 method only reports the average value of cytosolic free Ca in the epithelial cell suspension, which contains several cell types. Thus, it is conceivable that vasopressin lowers cytosolic

Ca in one cell type, while increasing it in another. It is also possible that localized changes in the level of free Ca may occur in restricted domains within the epithelial cell cytosol, which we cannot detect with the Quin 2 method. More sophisticated techniques undoubtedly will be required to establish whether or not localized differences in free Ca ion concentration exist within the cytoplasmic compartment of individual granular epithelial cells.

Since the available evidence indicates that cytosolic Ca does not change in response to vasopressin, Ca cannot be classified as a second messenger in vasopressin-sensitive epithelial cells. Nevertheless, Ca ions clearly play adecisive regulatory role in transepithelial water and Na transport; they are important components of the overall control system in these cells [38]. It is now recognized that Ca-dependent regulation may be effected in at least two distinct ways: (1) by alteration of the level of cytosolic free Ca, and/or (2) by modulation of the Ca-sensitivity of Ca-dependent processes through cyclic AMP-dependent phosphorylation events. Such a sensitivity modulation mechanism is known to be involved in the control of contractility in smooth muscle [20].

We conclude that cytosolic Ca ions may act as regulators of specific rate-limiting steps that determine apical membrane permeability to water and Na in the toad bladder. We suggest that the hormonal second messenger, cyclic AMP, may selectively lower the sensitivity to Ca at predetermined sites in the cellular machinery. Cyclic AMP and Ca ions, thus, may act in concert (for example, at the level of microtubules and/or microfilaments or the apical Na channels) to elicit the cascade of events that culminates in specific increases in apical membrane permeability. Such a mechanism would have the advantage of allowing maximum selectivity and, hence, versatility of the overall control system.

Summary

Both cyclic AMP and cytosolic calcium ions appear to be involved in the control of membrane permeability by vasopressin. In the toad urinary bladder, procedures that increase cytosolic calcium inhibit both the hydrosmotic response to vasopressin or cyclic AMP and the basal rate of sodium transport, and also disrupt microvillus architecture in the granular epithelial cells. These effects are independent of calmodulin; however, this protein apparently plays a specific role in the water permeability response to the hormone. Direct measurements of cytosolic calcium ion concentration have been obtained in isolated bladder epithelial cells. Our findings indicate that vasopressin does not itself influence the level of cytosolic calcium. Instead, the hormone may alter the sensitivity to calcium of cellular mechanisms that determine apical membrane water and sodium permeability.

Acknowledgments. These investigations have been supported by the United States Public Health Service Grants AM19022 and AM28409.

References

1. AUSIELLO DA, ROBINSON RR: Regulation by vasopressin and cyclic nucleotides of water and electrolyte movement in the kidney, in *Handbook of Experimental Pharmacology* (vol 58 [II]), edited by KEBABIAN WJ, NATHANSON JA, Heidelberg, Springer-Verlag, 1982, pp 271–303
2. DIBONA DR, CIVAN MM, LEAF A: The cellular specificity of the effect of vasopressin on toad urinary bladder. *J Membr Biol* 1:79–91, 1969
3. MICHELL RH: Inositol phospholipids and cell surface receptor function. *Biochim Biophys Acta* 415:81–147, 1975
4. ORLOFF J, HANDLER JS, PRESTON AS: The similarity of effects of vasopressin, adenosine-3', 5'-monophosphate (cyclic AMP) and theophylline on the toad bladder. *J Clin Invest* 41:702–709, 1962
5. HANDLER JS, BUTCHER RW, SUTHERLAND EW, ORLOFF J: The effect of vasopressin and of theophylline on the concentration of adenosine 3',5'-phosphate in the urinary bladder of the toad. *J Biol Chem* 240:4524–4526, 1965
6. OMACHI RS, ROBBIE DE, HANDLER JS, ORLOFF J: Effects of ADH and other agents on cyclic AMP accumulation in toad bladder epithelium. *Am J Physiol* 226:1152–1157, 1974
7. SAPIRSTEIN VS, SCOTT WN: Cyclic AMP and sodium transport. Quantitative and temporal relationships in toad urinary bladder. *J Clin Invest* 52:2379, 1973
8. LI JH-Y, PALMER LG, EDELMAN IS, LINDEMANN B: The role of sodium-channel density in the natriferic response of the toad urinary bladder to an antidiuretic hormone. *J Membr Biol* 64:77–89, 1982
9. CHEVALIER J, BOURGUET J, HUGON JS: Membrane associated particles: Distribution in frog urinary bladder epithelium at rest and after oxytocin treatment. *Cell Tiss Res* 152:129–140, 1974
10. LEFURGEY A, TISHER CC: Time course of vasopressin-induced formation of microvilli in granular cells of toad urinary bladder. *J Membr Biol* 61:13–19, 1981
11. WADE JB: Modulation of membrane structure in the toad urinary bladder by vasopressin, in *Water Transport Across Epithelia,* edited by USSING HH, BINDSLEV N, LASSEN NA, STEN-KNUDSEN O, Copenhagen, Munksgard, 1981
12. KACHADORIAN WA, ELLIS SJ, MULLER J: Possible roles for microtubules and microfilaments in ADH action on toad urinary bladder. *Am J Physiol* 236: (suppl I): F14–F20, 1979
13. MULLER J, KACHADORIAN WA, DISCALA VA: Evidence that ADH-stimulated intramembrane particle aggregates are transferred from cytoplasmic to luminal membranes in toad bladder epithelial cells. *J Cell Biol* 85:83–95, 1980
14. REAVEN E, MAFFLY R, TAYLOR A: Evidence for involvement of microtubules in the action of vasopressin in toad urinary bladder. III. Morphological studies on the content and distribution of microtubules in bladder epithelial cells. *J Membr Biol* 40:251–267, 1978
15. PEARL ML, TAYLOR A: Actin filaments and vasopressin-stimulated water flow in toad urinary bladder. *Am J Physiol* 245:C28–C39, 1983
16. GRONOWICZ G, MASUR SK, HOLTZMAN E: Quantitative analysis of exocytosis and endocytosis in the hydroosmotic response of toad bladder. *J Membr Biol* 52:221–235, 1980
17. PALMER LG, LORENZEN M: Antidiuretic hormone-dependent membrane capacitance and water permeability in the toad urinary bladder. *Am J Physiol* 244:F195–F204, 1983

18. GROSSO A, SPINELLI F, DESOUSA RC: Cytochalasin B and water transport. A scanning electron microscope study of the toad urinary bladder. *Cell Tiss Res* 188:375–388, 1978

19. VALLEE RB, DIBARTOLOMEIS MJ, THEURKAUF WD: A protein kinase bound to the projection portion of MAP 2 (microtubule-associated protein 2). *J Cell Biol* 90:568–576, 1981

20. ADELSTEIN RS, CONTI MA, HATHAWAY DR, KLEE CB: Phosphorylation of smooth muscle myosin light chain kinase by the catalytic subunit of adenosine 3':5'-monophosphate-dependent protein kinase. *J Biol Chem* 253:8347–8358, 1978

21. GOLDMAN R, POLLARD T, ROSENBAUM J: *Cell Motility,* Cold Spring Harbor, New York, Cold Spring Harbor Laboratory, 1976

22. CRAIG SW, POLLARD TD: Actin-binding proteins. *Trends Biochem Sci* 7:88–92, 1982

23. FUCHS G, GERTZ EW, BRIGGS FDN: The effects of quinidine on calcium accumulation by isolated sarcoplasmic reticulum of skeletal and cardiac muscle. *J Gen Physiol* 52:955–968, 1968

24. LORENZEN M, LEE CO, WINDHAGER EE: Effect of quinidine and ouabain on intracellular calcium (a^iCa) and sodium (a^iNa) ion activities in isolated perfused proximal tubules of *Necturus* Kidney (*abstract*). *Kidney Int* 21:281, 1982

25. TAYLOR A, EICH E, PEARL M, BREM A: Role of cytosolic calcium and Na-Ca exchange in the action of vasopressin, in *Hormonal Control of Epithelial Transport,* edited by BOURGUET J, CHEVALIER J, PARISI M, RIPOCHE P, Paris, Inserm, 1979, pp 167–174

26. PEARL M, TAYLOR A: High voltage electron microscopy (HVEM) of toad urinary bladder (*abstract*). *J Cell Biol* 97:312a, 1983

27. AUSIELLO DA, CORWIN HL, HARTWIG JH: Identification of actin-binding protein and villin in toad bladder epithelia. *Am J Physiol* 246:F101–F104, 1984

28. PALMER LG, SPEEZ N: Modulation of antidiuretic hormone-dependent capacitance and water flow in toad urinary bladder. *Am J Physiol* 246:F501–F508, 1984

29. CHASE H JR, AL-AWQATI Q: Submicromolar calcium regulates Na permeability of luminal membrane vesicles from toad bladder as measured by fast reaction methods (*abstract*). *Kidney Int* 21:270, 1981

30. TAYLOR A: Role of cytosolic calcium and sodium-calcium exchange in regulation of transepithelial sodium and water absorption, in *Ion Transport by Epithelia,* edited by SCHULTZ SG, New York, Raven Press, 1981, pp 233–259

31. CRUTCH B, TAYLOR A: Measurement of cytosolic free Ca^{2+} concentration in epithelial cells of toad urinary bladder (*abstract*). *J Physiol (Lond)* 345:109P, 1983

32. CHEUNG WY: Calmodulin plays a pivotal role in cellular regulation. *Science* 207:19–27, 1980

33. LEVINE SD, KACHADORIAN WA, LEVIN DN, SCHLONDORFF D: Effects of trifluoperazine on function and structure of toad urinary bladder. *J Clin Invest* 67:662–672, 1981

34. GROSSO A, COX JA, MALNOE A, DESOUSA RC: Evidence for a role of calmodulin in the hydrosmotic action of vasopressin in toad bladder. *J Physiol (Paris)* 78:270–278, 1982

35. BEAUWENS R, RENTMEESTERS M: Role of calmodulin in antidiuretic hormone mediated water transport. *Biochem Biophys Res Commun* 99:491–495, 1981

36. BARBER B, TAYLOR A: Calmodulin antagonists block vasopressin-stimulated water flow, but not the inhibitory effects of raised cytosolic Ca^{2+} in toad urinary bladder (*abstract*). *J Physiol (Lond)*, 354:47P, 1984

37. TSIEN RY, POZZAN T, RINK TJ: Calcium homeostasis in intact lymphocytes: cytoplasmic free calcium monitored with a new intracellularly trapped fluorescent indicator. *J Cell Biol* 94:325–334, 1982
38. TAYLOR A, WINDHAGER EE: Cytosolic calcium and its role in the regulation of transepithelial ion and water transport, in *Physiology and Pathophysiology of Electrolyte Metabolism,* edited by SELDIN D, GIEBISCH G, New York, Raven Press, in press

Role of Cytosolic Calcium in Renal Tubular Transport

Erich E. Windhager and Gustavo Frindt

It has been known for many years that changes in extracellular calcium (Ca) concentration can influence renal tubular transport of sodium (Na). However, only with the introduction of techniques for directly measuring intracellular Ca^{++} activities has it become apparent that changes in cytosolic Ca^{++} play an important role in regulating tubular reabsorption of Na. The first suggestive evidence for this view had been Taylor's observation [1] that quinidine, which is a drug known to increase intracellular Ca concentration in other tissues, inhibits the net transport of Na in the urinary bladder of the toad. Subsequently, Grinstein and Erlij [2] found that a reduction in Na concentration of the solution bathing the inside of isolated frog skins inhibits the short-circuit current in a Ca-dependent manner. They interpreted their findings to be evidence of an inhibitory action of intracellular Ca^{++} on the Na permeability of the apical cell membrane. This view was based on the previous proposal of Blaustein [3] that a Na-Ca exchange process operates in the basolateral cell membrane of renal tubular cells. Direct evidence for the existence of a Na-Ca exchange mechanism, in addition to an ATP-driven Ca pump in the basolateral membrane of renal tubular epithelium, was then provided by Gmaj, Murer, and Kinne [4] in studies on inside-out vesicles of peritubular cell membranes that were prepared from the rat kidney cortex. All of these and other studies [5, 6] have led to a hypothesis [7] that cytosolic Ca^{++} is involved in a negative feedback mechanism that regulates Na transport in Na-absorbing epithelia, as shown in Figure 1.

According to this hypothesis, a primary change in active Na extrusion from the cell would alter the intracellular Na^+ concentration and, consequently, also the electrochemical driving force for passive Na backflux into the cell across the basolateral cell membrane. In the presence of a Na-Ca exchange process operating in this cell membrane, changes in intracellular Na^+ concentration will alter the rate of Ca^{++} extrusion so that cytosolic

This manuscript was presented as part of a Symposium on *Second Messengers and Epithelial Transport.*

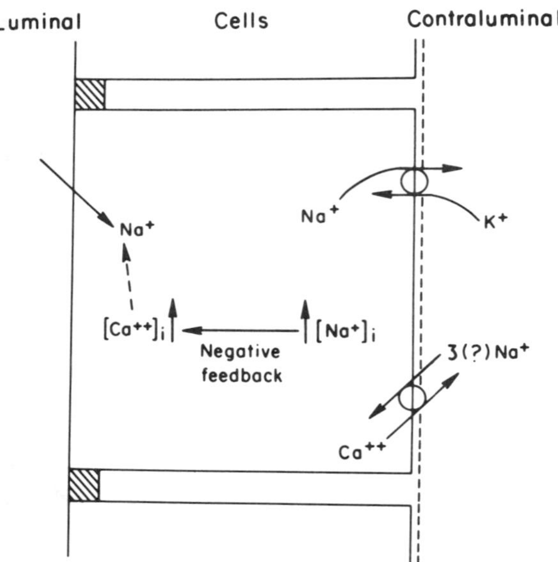

Fig. 1. Model of feedback mechanism. (Modified from [7])

Ca^{++} will parallel intracellular Na$^+$ activity; as Na$^+$ activity rises, Ca^{++} activity will also increase. The change in cytosolic Ca^{++} activity is then believed to modify the Na permeability of the apical cell membrane in such a way that the rate of Na entry across the apical membrane is kept in step with the rate of Na extrusion across the basolateral cell membrane. For example, if the Na pump is inhibited by a cardiac glycoside, the intracellular concentration of Na$^+$ will rise and less Na$^+$ would be driven into—and less Ca^{++} would be extruded out of—the cell via the Na-Ca exchanger. The resulting increase in cytosolic Ca^{++} levels would then inhibit the rate of Na$^+$ entry across the luminal cell membrane.

To test the relevance of this model for renal tubular epithelia, we have performed several studies on isolated, perfused renal tubules—some of them on amphibian nephrons in which cytosolic Ca- and Na- ion activities could be measured directly by using ion-selective microelectrodes.

The first experiments were carried out on isolated, perfused proximal convoluted tubules of rabbit kidneys [8] by using the method of Burg et al [9]. In these studies, tubules were perfused with solutions containing 145 mM Na at all times. The same concentration of Na was present in the peritubular bathing solution during control and recovery periods. Only during the experimental periods was the peritubular Na concentration reduced to 40 mM by substitution of Na with lithium, choline, or tetraethylammonium. During the experimental periods when bath Na concentration was reduced, fluid reabsorption was only 0.45 nl · min^{-1} · mm^{-1}; that is, some 46% of the control level. Fluid reabsorption was recovered when the peritubular Na concentration was restored to physiologic levels.

To test whether the inhibition of fluid reabsorption was caused by a decrease in Na efflux from lumen to bath, ^{22}Na was added to the luminal perfusion fluid. During the experimental periods when bath Na was partially replaced by lithium, Na efflux dropped to 72% of the control value. This corresponded with 51% of the simultaneously measured decrease in fluid reabsorption. These findings demonstrate that the reduction in water reabsorption that is brought about by the low peritubular Na concentration is largely the consequence of an inhibition of unidirectional efflux of Na from lumen to bath; lithium backflux and the resulting small drop in luminal Na concentration could not account for the full magnitude of the inhibition of water reabsorption. The inhibition of Na efflux took place despite an Na concentration gradient of 105 mM that favored Na efflux from lumen to bath. Experiments using choline or tetraethylammonium instead of lithium gave similar results.

In separate experiments, the degree of inhibition of fluid reabsorption at a given reduction in peritubular Na concentration was examined as a function of the concentration of ultrafilterable Ca in the extracellular fluid. Within the range of 0.2 to 1.0 mM-ultrafilterable Ca in external medium, the degree of inhibition of fluid reabsorption was proportional to the extracellular Ca concentration. Thus, low external Ca resulted in the least inhibition of fluid transport at a low peritubular Na concentration that presumably was due to a lesser degree of elevation of cytosolic Ca^{++} activity.

Further support for the view that increased intracellular Ca ion levels inhibit proximal tubular Na reabsorption was obtained in experiments with quinidine and the Ca ionophore, A23187. Both compounds are thought to increase cytosolic Ca^{++} concentrations. When added to the peritubular bathing solution, they significantly reduced proximal tubular fluid reabsorption and ^{22}Na efflux [8].

In isolated, perfused cortical collecting tubules (CCTs) of rabbits, the same experimental maneuvers, which were thought to elevate cytosolic Ca^{++} concentration, also reduced Na reabsorption [10]. Tubules were obtained from rabbits pretreated with DOCA for 2 weeks to obtain maximal values of Na efflux. When tubules were exposed to 145 mM Na in luminal and peritubular fluid, the Na efflux was 22 pmoles $\cdot$ cm^{-1} $\cdot$ sec^{-1}. Sodium efflux was diminished to 17 pmoles $\cdot$ cm^{-1} $\cdot$ sec^{-1} when the peritubular Na concentration was reduced to 5 mM by choline substitution. This reduction in Na efflux occurred while Na backflux was also reduced due to the low peritubular Na concentration. However, efflux was reduced more than backflux, which resulted in a significant inhibition of net reabsorption of Na. In other experiments, the effect of quinidine on Na transport was tested. At a concentration of 2 $\times$ 10^{-4} M (equal to k_i) in the peritubular bath, the drug caused a reversible inhibition of 40% of Na efflux. Sodium backflux was not changed by quinidine, indicating that it is the transcellular route, rather than the paracellular pathway of Na transport, that is inhibited by this drug. Thus, both of the maneuvers that are believed to increase intracellular Ca^{++} activity—low peritubular Na concentration and quinidine administration—led to an inhibition of Na reabsorption by CCTs of the rabbit kidney.

It is clear that the interpretation of these experiments is limited by the fact that there are no methods available for measuring cytosolic Ca^{++} activity in the perfused mammalian tubules. However, we were able to obtain this information in perfused proximal tubules of the *Necturus* kidney by using Ca^{++}-selective microelectrodes [11]. These electrodes were prepared by using the neutral ligand described and supplied by Simon, Ammann, and Morf [12]. Under control conditions, the cytosolic Ca^{++} activity averaged 71 nM, which is comparable to values observed in other tissues.

To test whether intracellular Ca^{++} activity changes in a manner predicted by the operation of a Na-Ca exchanger process in the basolateral cell membrane, cytosolic Ca^{++} and Na^+ activities were measured during a reduction of the Na concentration in the peritubular fluid. When the bath Na concentration was reduced from 100 to 10 mM via choline substitution, the intracellular Ca^{++} activity increased from 73 to 382 mM, while cytosolic Na^+ activity decreased from 13 to 8 mM. In other experiments, the addition of 10^{-4} M ouabain to the peritubular bathing solution led to an increase of 71 to 546 nM in cytosolic Ca^{++} activity and caused a rise in intracellular Na^+ activity of 15 to 70 mM. These results are consistent with the existence of the operation of a Na-Ca counterpart within the peritubular cell membrane.

The addition of 10^{-4} M quinidine to the fluid bathing isolated, perfused proximal tubules of *Necturus* kidneys also increased intracellular Ca^{++} activity from 87 to 556 nM. The mechanism by which the compound increases cellular levels of Ca^{++} in renal epithelia is presently unknown to our knowledge. However, this drug can be used to distinguish whether cytosolic Ca^{++} inhibits net Na transport by reducing the rate of luminal Na entry or by inhibiting the activity of the Na-K pump. This distinction is made possible by evaluating the changes in cytosolic Na^+ and Ca^{++} activities that are produced by quinidine, and then by relating these changes with the observed inhibition of transepithelial Na efflux from lumen to bath. Quinidine (10^{-4} M) caused a decrease of 15 to 12 mM in cytosolic Na^+ activity. The fact that the intracellular Na concentration was not elevated argues against a primary inhibition of the Na pump as an explanation of the reduction in Na reabsorption. The observation that intracellular Na concentration was actually diminished significantly is best explained by a Ca-induced inhibition of the rate of entry of Na^+ across the luminal cell membrane.

Strong support for the view that high cytosolic Ca^{++} levels inhibit the Na permeability of the luminal cell membrane have been obtained in studies with amphotericin B on isolated, perfused CCTs of rabbits pretreated for 3 weeks with DOCA [10]. This regimen of mineralocorticoid administration stimulates Na efflux approximately 3-fold. In these and subsequently discussed experiments, the same Na concentration of 145 mM was used in luminal and peritubular fluids. When amphotericin B, which is a drug known to increase membrane permeability to Na^+, was added to the luminal perfusate (at 5×10^{-6} M), Na efflux did not increase above the control value of 23 pmoles $\cdot$ cm^{-1} $\cdot$ sec^{-1}. Sodium backflux was not changed significantly by amphotericin B. These findings indicate that Na reabsorption in these tubules operated at the apparent saturation level of the Na pump. In the absence of amphotericin B, the addition of 2×10^{-4} M quinidine to the bathing fluid reduced the Na efflux from 24 to 12 pmoles $\cdot$ cm^{-1} $\cdot$ sec^{-1}. This inhibition of Na efflux could be fully reversed when amphotericin B was added to the luminal perfusate—in the presence of quinidine and amphotericin B, Na efflux averaged 24 pmoles $\cdot$ cm^{-1} $\cdot$ sec^{-1}, which is not different from the control levels. The fact that amphotericin B increased Na efflux to its apparent pump maximum in the presence of quinidine demonstrates that the drug-induced increase in cytosolic Ca^{++} activity did not inhibit the Na pump, but it must have reduced the rate of Na entry across the luminal cell membrane.

Recent electrophysiologic studies on CCTs [13, 14] showed a marked increase in transepithelial electrical resistance during reductions of the peritubular Na concentration or during addition of quinidine to the bathing solution. When a 5-mM Na bathing solution was applied, the electrical resistance rose from 17 to 22 K$\Omega \cdot$ cm. Quinidine (2×10^{-4} M), in separate experiments, increased the resistance from 15 to 19 K$\Omega \cdot$ cm. The effect of both experimental maneuvers was abolished by the addition of 5×10^{-5} M amiloride to the luminal perfusate. In contrast, the addition of 2 mM barium to the luminal fluid failed to prevent the rise in transepithelial resistance. These results support the view that increased levels of cytosolic Ca^{++} inhibit an amiloride-sensitive Na conductance in the luminal cell membrane.

In summation, results obtained in proximal tubules and CCTs of rabbit kidneys and in proximal tubules of *Necturus* are consistent with the existence of a Na-Ca exchanger-process in the peritubular cell membrane and with the view that high cytosolic Ca inhibits tubular Na reabsorption by decreasing the rate of Na entry into the cell across the luminal cell boundary.

References

1. TAYLOR A: Effect of quinidine in the action of vasopressin (*abstract*). *Fed Proc* 34:185, 1975
2. GRINSTEIN S, ERLIJ D: Intracellular calcium and the regulation of sodium transport in the frog skin. *Proc R Soc London (Biol Sec)* 202:353–360, 1978
3. BLAUSTEIN MP: The interrelationship between sodium and calcium fluxes across cell membranes. *Rev Physiol Biochem Pharmacol* 70:33–82, 1974
4. GMAJ P, MURER H, KINNE R: Calcium ion transport across plasma membranes isolated from rat kidney cortex. *Biochem J* 178:549–557, 1979
5. ULLRICH KJ, RUMRICH G, KLOSS S: Active Ca^{2+} reabsorption in the proximal tubule of rat kidney. Dependence on sodium and buffer transport. *Pflügers Arch* 364:223-228, 1976
6. WIESMANN W, SINHA S, KLAHR S: Effects of ionophore A23187 on base-line and vasopressin-stimulated sodium transport in the toad bladder. *J Clin Invest* 59:418–425, 1977
7. TAYLOR A, WINDHAGER EE: Possible role of cytosolic calcium and Na-Ca exchange in regulation of transepithelial sodium transport. *Am J Physiol* 236:F505–F512, 1979
8. FRIEDMAN PA, FIGUEIREDO JF, MAACK T, WINDHAGER EE: Sodium-calcium interactions in the renal proximal convoluted tubule of the rabbit. *Am J Physiol* 240:F558–F568, 1981
9. BURG M, GRANTHAM J, ABRANOW M, ORLOFF J: Preparation and study of fragments of single rabbit nephrons. *Am J Physiol* 210:1293–1298, 1966
10. FRINDT G, WINDHAGER EE: Effect of quinidine, low peritubular [Na] or [Ca]

on Na transport in isolated perfused rabbit cortical collecting tubules (*abstract*). *Fed Proc* 42:305, 1983

11. LORENZEN M, LEE CO, WINDHAGER EE: Cytosolic Ca^{2+} and Na^+ activities in perfused proximal tubules of Necturus kidney. *Am J Physiol,* in press
12. SIMON W, AMMANN D, MORF WE: Calcium-selective electrodes. *Am NY Acad Sci* 307:52–70, 1978
13. FRINDT G, WINDHAGER EE: Effect of quinidine on low peritubular Na concentration on rabbit cortical collecting tubule transepithelial electrical resistance (*abstract*). *Fed Proc* 43:303, 1984
14. FRINDT G, WINDHAGER EE: Transepithelial electrical resistance (R_t) of cortical collecting tubules at reduced peritubular Na concentration (*abstract*). *IXth Int Congr Nephrol,* Los Angeles, 1984, p 413A

Sodium Phosphate Cotransport: Studies with Vesicles and LLC-PK$_1$ Cells

Heini Murer, Martin Amstutz, Jürg Biber, Piotr Gmaj, and Kerstin Malmström

In this brief review we will discuss three different aspects of the cotransport of sodium and phosphate: (1) the effect of sodium and pH, (2) the evidence for and against involvement of phosphorylation and ribosylation reactions in the regulation, and (3) sodium phosphate cotransport and its regulation to LLC-PK$_1$ cells and apical vesicles isolated therefrom.

Effect of Sodium and pH on Phosphate Transport Across the Brushborder Membrane

It has been shown in microperfusion experiments and studies with isolated perfused nephron segments that transepithelial transport in the renal proximal tubule is sodium-dependent and sensitive to ouabain [1–3]. The observed sodium dependence led to the formulation of the concept of a secondary active transcellular transport of inorganic phosphate energized by the sodium gradient across the brushborder membrane. This concept includes sodium phosphate cotransport across the brushborder membrane as the mechanism for the uphill movement of phosphate from the tubule into the cell. Transcellular transport is completed by a transport mechanism in the basolateral membrane allowing quilibration between cell and interstitium (for review, see [4]).

The properties of the sodium phosphate cotransport mechanism have been analyzed in several studies with isolated brushborder membrane vesicles (for review, see [4]). The increased sodium-dependent phosphate transport rate by increasing pH led to the conclusion that the divalent phosphate ion is the preferred substrate [5–10]. The evidence for a preferential transport of divalent phosphate is supported by two recent observations: (1) In rabbit

This manuscript was presented as part of a Symposium on *Regulation of Potassium Excretion*.

renal brushborder vesicles, sodium phosphate cotransport was stimulated by an outwardly directed proton gradient [7]. (2) In studies with rabbit and renal brushborder vesicles [7, 9, 10], an apparent insensitivity to medium pH was found when the transport was calculated on the basis of divalent phosphate concentrations.

In our studies with rat renal brushborder vesicles, evidence has been obtained that suggests strongly that the pH effect is mainly related to altered carrier properties, rather than to preferential transport of divalent phosphate ions [8] (Amstutz and Murer, manuscript in preparation). Phosphate transport is influenced strongly by pH at physiologic sodium concentrations, but is only marginally dependent on pH at high sodium concentrations. This suggests that the pH effect is not primarily a function of the monovalent-to-divalent phosphate concentration ratio [8]. These observations have now been extended by a kinetic analysis of initial linear flux measurements (Amstutz and Murer, manuscript in preparation). As shown in Table 1, an increased proton concentration leads to a decrease in the affinity of the transport system for sodium (experiment 1). Sodium increases the affinity of the transport system for phosphate (experiment 2), and phosphate itself has no influence on the interaction of the transport system with sodium (experiment 3). Thus, at nonsaturating sodium concentrations, an increase of proton concentration leads to a decreased affinity of the transport system for sodium and secondarily to a decreased affinity for phosphate. These findings explain the previous observations that the pH dependence of phosphate transport is different at different sodium concentrations [8]. However, the pH dependence of sodium phosphate cotransport cannot be completely abolished by increasing sodium [8] (Amstutz and Murer, manuscript in preparation). Even at saturating sodium concentrations, there is a small increase in the transport rate upon increasing the pH. However, it must be emphasized that—in the presence of pH effects on the affinity of the carrier for sodium and indirectly for phosphate—it is most difficult to conclude from pH-dependence studies whether monovalent or divalent phosphate is transported preferentially.

On the basis of the results presented above, we postulate the following model for sodium phosphate cotransport. Sodium interacts first with the transport system and facilitates its interaction with phosphate. Protons interfere with the sodium-binding site and reduce its affinity for sodium. Thus, lowering the pH at nonsaturating sodium concentrations indirectly alters the affinity of the transport system for phosphate. The potential dependence of sodium phosphate cotransport at low but not at high pH [8, 11], as well as a 2:1 stoichiometry between sodium and phosphate flux, implies that both monovalent and divalent phosphate can be transported.

Little is known about the exit mechanism in the basolateral membranes. The early work of Hoffmann, Thees, and Kinne [6] on isolated rat renal basolateral membrane vesicles provided evidence that the membrane contains no sodium-dependent transport system. More recently, an anion-exchange mechanism has been described in basolateral membranes of rat proximal tubule [12–14]. This mechanism can operate in the complete absence of sodium and also interacts with phosphate [13, 14]. The anion exchange was found to be electroneutral [13]. Recently, Hammerman and Schwab [15] reported

Table 1. Kinetic parameters of sodium-phosphate cotransport[a]

		Concentration		Apparent K_m		Apparent N	
	pH	P_i (mmoles/liter)	Sodium (mmoles/liter)	Phosphate (mmoles/liter)	Sodium (mmoles/liter)	Phosphate	Sodium
Exp. 1	7.4	0.1	40 to 300	—	103	—	2.0
	6.4	0.1	40 to 300	—	192	—	2.2
Exp. 2	7.4	0.05 to 1.0	60	0.423	—	1.0	—
		0.05 to 1.0	120	0.188	—	1.0	—
	6.4	0.05 to 1.0	130	0.878	—	1.0	—
		0.05 to 1.0	250	0.324	—	1.0	—
Exp. 3	7.4	5.0	40 to 300	—	72	—	2.0
		0.2	40 to 300	—	74	—	1.9

[a] The kinetic parameters were obtained from initial linear influx values (corrected for sodium-independent uptake). The K_m values were obtained from linear regression analysis of the Hanes-Woolf equation. The appropriate N values were obtained from the linear regression analysis of the Hill equation. The values presented are from three independent experiments performed in quadruplicate (within 5%). The r^2 values were between 0.98 and 1.0. The vesicles were preloaded with 600 mmoles/liter choline chloride, 20 mmoles/liter potassium chloride, and 20 mmoles/liter HEPES-Tris (pH, 7.4) or MES-Tris (pH, 6.4). The incubation medium had the same composition except for partial replacements of choline chloride with sodium chloride and the addition of $KH_2^{32}PO_4$ at different concentrations. The membrane potential was clamped by the addition of valinomycin (10 μg/100 μl). The data are from recent experiments in our laboratory (Amstutz and Murer, manuscript in preparation).

on the existence of a sodium-independent transport system in the basolateral membranes isolated from dog kidney proximal tubule. In contrast to the findings on rat kidney, this system involves the transfer of negative charges; that is, there is a movement of the phosphate anion that is not electrically compensated within the transport processes. In addition to the sodium-independent mechanism, evidence for a sodium-dependent high-affinity, low-capacity system for inorganic phosphate was obtained [15] in a study with dog basolateral membranes. Such a system might be involved in the uptake of phosphate from the interstitium into the cell in situations where luminal transport of phosphate was insufficient to cover the needs of the cellular metabolism.

Evidence for and Against the Involvement of Phosphorylation and Ribosylation Reactions in the Regulation of Sodium Phosphate Cotransport

Over the last few years, the attention of several laboratories has been focused on the regulation of the sodium phosphate cotransport mechanism. Different physiologic conditions are known to be associated with altered tubular handling of phosphate and with alterations of the sodium phosphate cotransport at the membrane level (for review, see [4, 16]). Specifically, two types of regulatory processes have been postulated to represent the final event in the regulation of the sodium phosphate cotransport mechanism: (1) membrane phosphorylation [16–20], and (2) membrane ADP-ribosylation [21–26]. Parathyroid hormone (PTH) increases cellular cyclic AMP by interaction with vesicles in the basolateral membranes [27, 28]. The increase in cellular cyclic AMP levels leads via a stimulation of gluconeogenesis to an increase in the NAD/NADH ratio [16, 21, 22, 29].

The brushborder membranes contain cyclic AMP-dependent protein phosphorylation mechanisms [17–20, 30, 31]. In addition, evidence for ADP-ribosylation reactions and calcium-protein kinase C-dependent phosphorylation has recently been obtained [23, 32, 33]. Thus, it is feasible to speculate that phosphorylation and ADP-ribosylation reactions are directly involved in the regulation of sodium phosphate cotransport. However, it is very difficult to correlate biochemical modifications in studies with vesicles. Three major difficulties should be mentioned: (1) Brushborder membrane vesicles represent a closed and right-side-out-oriented membrane population; that is, the membrane-bound regulatory phenomena are cryptic, as they are mainly located on the cytoplasmic membrane surface only [18]. (2) NAD^+ and ATP are rapidly hydrolyzed by the brushborder enzymes [26, 34–36]. (3) Membrane isolation requires several hours and leads to a separation of cytosolic components from the membrane; that is, the regulatory phenomena might be inactivated or lost during isolation [37]. Different approaches have been adapted to overcome these difficulties (for example, an osmotic shock procedure, which allows for a transient permeabilization of the vesicles) [17, 18, 26]. However, in view of the clearly defined orientation of brushborder vesicles, the extent of transient permeabilization must be documented, for example by (1) showing a clear difference in the phosphorylation pattern under isotonic or hypotonic phosphorylation or ribosylation conditions [18, 26]; (2) quantifying the vesicular space accessible during osmotic shock [18, 26]; (3) documenting the resealing of the vesicles after opening [18, 26]; (4) identifying the intravesicular substance after osmotic shock [26].

In a study on membrane phosphorylation with γ-^{32}P-ATP, it could be shown that phosphorylation sites (except alkaline phosphatase) are predominantly located on the cytoplasmic membrane surface (Fig. 1) [18]. The addition of γ-^{32}P-ATP after osmotic shock produced the same phosphorylation pattern as did the phosphorylation under isotonic conditions (phosphorylation of external membrane proteins only), indicating that vesicles reclose after the shock with the original orientation. A quantification showed that at least 70% of the vesicles were transiently opened under osmotic shock conditions [18, 26]. In studies where no quantification of the transient opening of the vesicles was made, it is difficult to conclude that the observed biochemical modifications of the membrane components occur in a representative fraction

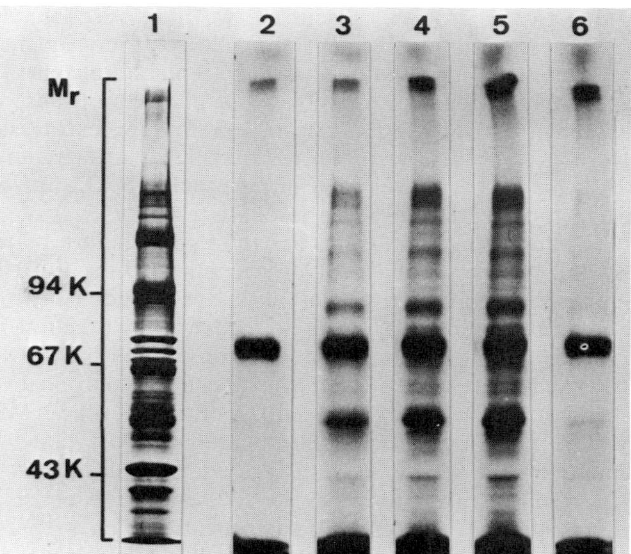

Fig. 1. Phosphorylation of rat kidney brushborder membrane vesicles by γ-^{32}P-ATP under isotonic and hypotonic conditions. Membrane protein phosphorylation was performed by 20 μmoles of γ^{32}P-ATP (per liter) and analyzed by SDS-gel-electrophoresis. *Lane 1* was made visual by Coomassie Blue staining; *lanes 2 to 6*, by autoradiographies. Phosphorylation was performed under isotonic conditions (*lane 2*) or under hypotonic conditions at the dilution ratios of 1:4 (*lane 3*), 1:8 (*lane 4*), or 1:16 (*lane 5*). *Lane 6* represents the phosphoprotein pattern obtained when γ-^{32}P-ATP was added to preshocked vesicles (1 min after osmotic shock). (Reprinted with permission from [18])

of the vesicle population (for examples, see [17, 23]). It has been documented that different nucleotides—or their hydrolysis products—are inhibitors of sodium-dependent phosphate transport [34]. This interaction with the phosphate transport system represents actually the most serious difficulty in analyzing the regulatory phenomena in isolated vesicles. Anyspecific effects of phosphorylation or ribosylation reactions on phosphate transport are always overlapped by the effects not related to regulation, but *only* to interaction with the transport system (for example, competition, isotope dilution). Thus, it is a requirement that the regulatory phenomena be analyzed by either of the two following procedures: (1) removal of the extravesicular nucleotides and identification of the intravesicular nucleotides before analysis of phosphate transport at the brushborder membrane level [26]; (2) an analysis of the kinetic parameters of phosphate transport without removal of the nucleotides and their hydrolysis products [34] (Malmström and Murer, manuscript in preparation). The first approach has the limitation that the introduced modification might be lost during the time required for a removal of extravesicular products. In the second approach, it is assumed that the regulatory phenomena are expressed as changes in V_{max}, whereas the direct interactions with the transport system would probably show up as competitive inhibition [34]. Owing to the problems discussed, we have been unable in our laboratory to document the involvement of cyclic AMP-dependent phosphorylation in the inhibition of sodium-dependent phosphate transport [18, 33]. In our laboratory, NAD-dependent inhibition of phosphate transport under conditions favorable for ribosylation was observed when extravesicular NAD and its hydrolysis products were not removed [26]. After removal of extravesicular NAD but in the presence of intravesicular NAD (including its breakdown products), no inhibition of phosphate transport was obtained [26].

The foregoing discussion, as well as the failure of our experiments [18, 26, 33], on the involvement of phosphorylation and ribosylation reactions in phosphate transport regulation do not exclude its existence [17, 23]. However, in our opinion, there is no evidence for a causal link between altered transport and biochemical modification of the brushborder membrane. Thus, the evidence for these mechanisms to occur in phosphate transport regulation is indirect and related to correlations of tissue cyclic AMP levels and $NAD^+/NADH$ ratios and altered phosphate transport under various physiologic conditions (for review, see [16]). An additional evidence for the phosphorylation mechanism is the induction of membrane phosphorylation events in rabbit kidney slice incubation experiments, which are paralleled by the altered transport at the vesicular level [38, 39]. However, these experiments also failed in our laboratory with rat kidney cortex slices (Biber, Scalera, and Murer, submitted for publication).

Sodium Phosphate Cotransport and Its Regulation in LLC-PK$_1$ Cells

Over the last 10 years, epithelial cell lines derived from various transporting epithelia have gained wide acceptance as useful models for the study of the mechanisms of transepithelial ion and solute fluxes [40, 41]. LLC-PK$_1$, a renal epithelial cell line derived from pig kidney, has been used extensively in the study of transport events normally associated with renal proximal tubule, such as sodium-dependent hexose transport [42–44] and amino acid transport [45–47]. In recent publications, a sodium phosphate cotransport mechanism in the intact LLC-PK$_1$ cells as well as in the apical membrane vesicles isolated from LLC-PK$_1$ has been described [48–50]. Similar to the studies in rat kidney proximal tubule, our studies found evidence for a 2:1 stoichiometry between sodium and phosphate flux [49, 50]. Also in close similarity to rat renal proximal tubular membrane vesicles, an increased sodium concentration increased the apparent affinity of the transport system for phosphate [49, 50]. This latter observation is in contrast to the observation on rabbit duodenal sodium phosphate cotransport, where increasing sodium concentrations augmented the V$_{max}$ [51]. Thus, LLC-PK$_1$ cells can represent a useful model to study the mechanism and regulation of sodium phosphate cotransport, which in some aspects can be similar to renal proximal tubule.

But in contrast to renal proximal tubule, LLC-PK$_1$ cells are sensitive to vasopressin and calcitonin but apparently not to PTH [28, 40, 52, 53]. To simulate the effects of PTH, we increased cellular cyclic AMP levels by the addition of forskolin, a potent stimulator of adenylate cyclase [54]. When the cells were preincubated for 20 min with 10 μmoles of forskolin per liter, cellular cyclic AMP increased more than 20-fold (Malmström and Murer, manuscript in preparation). This increase in cellular cyclic AMP was without effect on sodium-dependent phosphate uptake by LLC-PK$_1$ cells grown to different degrees of confluency and for different time periods after reaching a confluent monolayer (Malmström and Murer). Thus, in LLC-PK$_1$ cells, an increased cellular cyclic AMP level does not seem to be associated with the inhibition of phosphate transport, although it cannot be excluded that the cells have lost the PTH- or cyclic AMP-dependent regulatory mechanism along with their PTH receptors. Studies on a renal cell line containing sodium phosphate cotransport and PTH receptors are required to clarify this possibility. However, the studies with LLC-PK$_1$ might suggest that the increase in cellular cyclic AMP alone is insufficient to trigger the inhibition of sodium phosphate cotransport.

The increase in the proximal tubular sodium phosphate cotransport after dietary phosphate deprivation is an event independent of the PTH system [55, 56]. In LLC-PK$_1$ cells, phosphate deprivation for 15 to 17 hr in subconfluent or confluent monolayers leads to a marked increase in sodium phosphate cotransport [57] (Fig. 2 and Table 2). The increase in phosphate transport after phosphate deprivation in the absence of protein synthesis (that is, in the presence of cycloheximide) is only about 20% (Table 2) and similar to the increase observed already after 15 min of deprivation in the presence and absence of cycloheximide. These adaptive alterations in phosphate transport are also expressed at the level of the brushborder membrane [57] (Table 2); that is to say, they are not related to alterations in the cellular driving forces, but rather reflect a change at the level of the brushborder membrane. These observations suggest the existence of two different mechanisms in response to phosphate deprivation (adaptation): a fast component not involving de novo protein synthesis and a slow component involving protein synthesis.

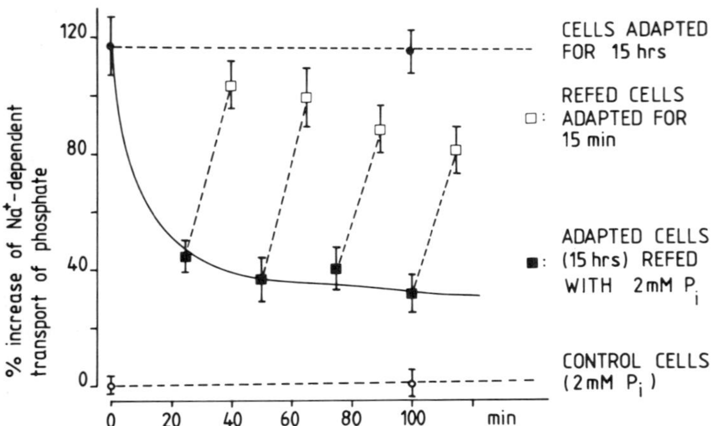

Fig. 2. Rapid alteration of phosphate transport in LLC-PK$_1$ cells. Initial linear rate of sodium-dependent phosphate uptake by LLC-PK$_1$ cells was first increased by about 120% by exposing LLC-PK$_1$ monolayers for 15 hr to a growth medium containing less than 10 μmoles of inorganic phosphate per liter (●). Then the medium was replaced by a medium containing 1.0 mmoles of inorganic phosphate per liter. After various time intervals, phosphate uptake was analyzed (■). The cells were again exposed to low-phosphate medium for 15 min, and phosphate transport was analyzed (□). The basic methods are described in [49].

The fast component—which does not depend on de novo protein synthesis— can be analyzed also in cells that have first been phosphate-deprived for 15 hr (Biber and Murer, manuscript in preparation) (Fig. 2). Refeeding of the cells leads to a fast decrease in the transport capacity and within 3 hr reaches the level of nondeprived cells (Fig. 2 and Table 2). This *down-regulation* is not influenced by cycloheximide (Table 2). An exposure of the refed cells for 15 min to phosphate-deprived medium leads to a fast readaptation, which again is not influenced by cycloheximide; in other words, the fast adaptation process is independent of protein synthesis.

The described study shows that it is possible to use LLC-PK$_1$ cells to analyze cellular mechanisms involved in the regulation of renal phosphate transport. Further studies are now required to analyze the cellular mechanism involved in the adaption of the sodium phosphate cotransport in the apical membrane of LLC-PK$_1$ cells.

Conclusions

On the basis of studies on intact epithelia and with isolated membrane vesicles, we obtained a detailed knowledge of sodium phosphate cotransport located in the luminal membrane of proximal tubular epithelial cells. The transport system in the basolateral membrane has not been well defined as yet. In

Table 2. Regulation of sodium-dependent transport of phosphate in LLC-PK$_1$ cells

	Percent of altered sodium-dependent transport of phosphate[a]	
Conditions	Cellular uptake	Vesicular uptake
Control cells (2 mmoles/liter P$_i$)	100	100
P$_i$ deprivation, (10 μmoles/liter P$_i$)		
For 17 hr	180 to 200	200
For 17 hr + cycloheximide[b]	120	ND
For 15 min	120 to 130	125
For 15 min + cycloheximide[b]	120 to 130	ND
P$_i$ deprived cells (17 hr):	(180 to 200)	
Refed with 1 mmole/liter P$_i$ for 3 hr	100	ND
Refed for 3 hr + cycloheximide[b]	100	ND
Refed for 90 min and readapted for 15 min	140	ND
Refed for 90 min and readapted for 15 min + cycloheximide[b]	140	ND
Forskolin (10 μmoles/liter)[c]	100	ND

[a] Cellular uptake was determined after 5 min [49]. Uptake in isolated apical membrane vesicles was determined after 30 sec under the inwardly directed gradient of sodium (sodium chloride, 100 mmoles/liter) [50].

[b] Cells were preincubated with 20 μmoles of cycloheximide (per liter) for 1 hr before a change of the media. The incorporation of ^{35}S-methionine into cell protein was prevented completely under these conditions (Biber and Murer, manuscript in preparation).

[c] Preincubation time was 20 min at 37°C. Forskolin concentration was 10 μmoles/liter; the cellular cyclic AMP level after 20 min of preincubation was increased about 20-fold (Malmström and Murer, manuscript in preparation).

rat basolateral membranes, a sodium-independent anion-exchange mechanism has been shown [12–14]. The finding in dog basolateral membranes of a sodium-independent high-capacity low-affinity transport system involving the transfer of net negative charges and of a sodium-dependent high-affinity low-capacity system is difficult to interpret [15]. In the intact cell, the high capacity system would be involved in exit and also determine the intracellular inorganic phosphate concentrations in situations where luminal phosphate entry is limiting. A feeding of the cell metabolism with inorganic phosphate from the interstitium via the sodium-dependent transport system would require some compartmentalization, that is, the separation of a transport pool and of a metabolic pool.

Concerning the regulation of proximal tubular phosphate transport, it is certainly most interesting that for different physiologic situations the final event is expressed at the level of the brushborder membrane's sodium phosphate cotransport system [16]. Although different mechanisms for post-translational modifications of protein function are present in the brushborder membrane, until now it has not been possible to convincingly document their involvement in the regulation of phosphate transport (see above). Future studies will have to consider the intact cell again. It is hoped that the combination of experiments on the intact tissue (including cell culture) and on different subcellular structures also including cytosolic fractions will allow us to define the cellular mechanisms leading to altered sodium-dependent influx of phosphate across the luminal membrane.

Finally, different laboratories concentrate their efforts on the identification of the molecular units involved in phosphate transport across the luminal membrane and contraluminal membrane. Sodium phosphate cotransport system was solubilized from rat proximal tubular brushborder membranes and reconstituted into liposomes [58]. More recently, the isolation of a phosphate-binding proteolipid from rabbit brushborder membranes has been reported; it has been suggested that this proteolipid is involved in phosphate transport [59]. The molecule probably involved in sodium-independent anion exchange in rat basolateral membranes has recently been identified by affinity labeling experiments [60]. Such experiments certainly represent the first important steps in the purification of the transport systems from the brushborder membrane and the basolateral membrane.

References

1. BAUMANN K, DE ROUFFIGNAC C, ROINEL N, RUMRICH G, ULLRICH KJ: Renal phosphate transport: Inhomogeneity of local proximal transport rates and sodium dependence. *Pflügers Arch* 356:287–297, 1975
2. DENNIS VW, WOODHALL PB, ROBINSON RR: Characteristics of phosphate transport in isolated proximal tubule. *Am J Physiol* 231:979–985, 1976
3. DENNIS VW, BRAZY PC: Divalent anion transport in isolated renal tubules. *Kidney Int* 22:498–506, 1982
4. MURER H, BURCKHARDT G: Membrane transport of anions across epithelia of mammalian small intestine and kidney proximal tubule. *Rev Physiol Biochem Pharmacol* 96:1–51, 1983
5. CHENG L, SACKTOR B: Sodium gradient dependent phosphate transport in renal brush border membrane vesicles. *J Biol Chem* 256:1556–1564, 1981
6. HOFFMANN N, THEES M, KINNE R: Phosphate transport by isolated brush border membrane vesicles. *Pflügers Arch* 362:147–156, 1976
7. SACKTOR B, CHENG L: Sodium gradient-dependent phosphate transport in renal brush border membrane vesicles: Effect of an intravesicular > extravesicular proton gradient. *J Biol Chem* 256:8080–8084, 1981
8. BURCKHARDT G, STERN H, MURER H: The influence of pH on phosphate transport into rat renal brush border membrane vesicles. *Pflügers Arch* 340:191–197, 1981
9. CHENG L, LIANG T, SACKTOR B: Phosphate uptake by renal membrane vesicles of rabbits adapted to high and low phosphorus diets. *Am J Physiol* 245:F175–F180, 1983
10. BRUNETTE MG, BELIVEAU R, CHAN M: Effect of temperature and pH on phosphate transport through brush border membrane vesicles in rat. *Can J Physiol Pharmacol,* in press
11. FROEMTER E, SAMARZIJA J, GESSNER K: Electrical analysis of Na$^+$-dependent cotransport systems in the rat kidney proximal tubule, in *Abs Proc II Eur Colloq Renal Physiol,* Balatonfüred, 1977, no 28
12. PRICHARD JB, RENFRO JL: Renal sulfate transport at the basolateral membrane is mediated by anion exchange. *Proc Natl Acad Sci USA* 80:2603–2607, 1983
13. LOEW J, FRIEDRICH T, BURCKHARDT G: Properties of anion exchanger in the contraluminal membrane of rat proximal tubular epithelial cells: Studies with sulfate uptake into basolateral membrane vesicles. *Am J Physiol,* in press

14. HAGENBUCH B, STANGE G, MURER H: Transport of inorganic anions in rat small intestinal and renal proximal tubular basolateral membrane vesicles (*abstract*). *Experientia,* in press
15. HAMMERMAN MR, SCHWAB SJ: Phosphate transport in the kidney, studies with isolated membrane vesicles (*abstract*). *Second Int Workshop on Calcium and Phosphate Transport across Biomembranes,* Vienna, 1984
16. DOUSA JP, KEMPSON SA: Regulation of renal brush border membrane transport of phosphate. *Mineral Electrolyte Metab* 7:113–121, 1982
17. HAMMERMAN MR, HRUSKA KA: Cyclic AMP-dependent protein phosphorylation in canine renal brush-border membrane vesicles is associated with decreased phosphate transport. *J Biol Chem* 257:992–999, 1982
18. BIBER J, MALMSTROEM K, SCALERA V, MURER H: Phosphorylation of rat kidney proximal tubular brush border membranes: A role of cAMP dependent protein phosphorylation in the regulation of phosphate transport. *Pflügers Arch* 398:221–226, 1983
19. HAMMERMAN MR, HANSEN VA, MORRISSEY JJ: Cyclic AMP-dependent protein phosphorylation and dephosphorylation alter phosphate transport in canine renal brush border vesicles. *Biochim Biophys Acta* 755:10–16, 1983
20. HAMMERMAN MR, COHN DE, TAMAYO J, MARTIN KJ: Effect of parathyroid hormone on Na⁺-dependent phosphate transport and cAMP-dependent ³²P phosphorylation in brush border vesicles from isolated perfused canine kidney. *Arch Biochem Biophys* 227:91–97, 1983
21. BERNDT TJ, KNOX FG, KEMPSON SA, DOUSA TP: Nicotinamide adenine dinucleotide and renal response to parathyroid hormone. *Endocrinology* 108:2005–2007, 1981
22. KEMPSON SA, COLON-OTERO G, LISE OU S-Y, TURNER ST, DOUSA TP: Possible role of nicotinamide adenine dinucleotide as an intracellular regulator of renal transport of phosphate transport. *J Clin Invest* 67:1347–1360, 1981
23. HAMMERMAN MR, HANSEN VA, MORRISSEY JJ: ADP ribosylation of canine renal brush border membrane vesicle proteins is associated with decreased phosphate transport. *J Biol Chem* 257:12380–12386, 1982
24. HAMMERMAN MR, CORPUS VM, MORRISSEY JJ: NAD⁺-induced inhibition of phosphate transport in canine renal brush-border membranes: Mediation through a process other than or in addition to NAD⁺ hydrolysis. *Biochem Biophys Acta* 732:110–116, 1983
25. BRAUN-WERNESS JL, JACKSON BA, WERNESS PG, DOUSA TP: Binding of nicotinamide adenine dinucleotide by the renal brush-border membrane from rat kidney cortex. *Biochim Biophys Acta* 732:553–561, 1983
26. GMAJ P, BIBER J, ANGIELSKI S, STANGE G, MURER H: Intravesicular NAD has no effect on sodium-dependent phosphate transport in isolated renal brush border vesicles. *Pflügers Arch* 400:60–65, 1984
27. SCHLATZ LJ, SCHWARTZ JL, KINNE-SAFFRAN E, KINNE R: Distribution of parathyroid hormone-stimulated adenylate cyclase in plasma membranes of cells of the kidney cortex. *J Membr Biol* 24:145–159, 1975
28. MOREL F: Sites of hormone action in the mammalian nephron. *Am J Physiol* 240:F159–F164, 1981
29. KEMPSON SA, KOWALSKI JC, PUSCHETT JB: Inhibition of renal brush border phosphate transport and stimulation of renal gluconeogenesis by cAMP and parathyroid hormone. *Biochem Pharmacol* 32:1533–1537, 1983
30. HRUSKA KA, MILLS SC, KHALIFA S, HAMMERMAN MR: Phosphorylation of renal brush-border membrane vesicles: Effect on calcium uptake and membrane content of polyphosphoionositides. *J Biol Chem* 258:2501–2507, 1983
31. KINNE R, SCHLATZ LJ, KINNE-SAFFRAN E, SCHWARTZ JL: Distribution of

membrane bound cyclic AMP-dependent protein kinase in plasma membranes of cells of the kidney cortex. *J Membr Biol* 24:145–159, 1975

32. KEMPSON SA, CURTHOYS NP: NAD⁺-dependent ADP-ribosyltransferase in renal brush border membrane. *Am J Physiol* 245:C449–C456, 1983

33. MALMSTRÖM K, MURER H: Calcium-dependent phosphorylation in rat renal brush border vesicles (*abstract*). *Fed Proc,* in press

34. LANG RP, YANAGAWA N, NORD EP, SAKHRANI L, LEE S-H, FINE LG: Nucleotide inhibition of phosphate transport in the renal proximal tubule. *Am J Physiol* 245:F263–F271, 1983

35. TENENHOUSE HS, CHU YL: Hydrolysis of nicotinamide-adenine dinucleotide by purified renal brush-border membrane. *Biochem J* 204:635–638, 1982

36. ANGIELSKI S, ZIELKIEWICZ J, DZIEZKO G: Metabolism of NAD by isolated rat renal brush border membranes. *Pflügers Arch* 395:159–161, 1982

37. MURER H, KINNE R: The use of isolated membrane vesicles to study epithelial transport processes. *J Membr Biol* 55:81–95, 1980

38. AUSIELLO D, HANDLER J, ORLOFF J: Effect of parathyroid hormone and cyclic AMP in protein phosphorylation in rabbit kidney cortex. *Biochim Biophys Acta* 451:372–381, 1976

39. TAKENAWA T, WADA E, TSUMITA T, MASAKI T, FILBURN CR, SACKTOR B: Effect of parathyroid hormone, cyclic AMP and Ca⁺⁺ on the phosphorylation of brush border membranes in rabbit kidney. *Mineral Electrolyte Metab* 10:103–112, 1984

40. HANDLER JS, PERKINS FM, JOHNSON JP: Studies of renal cell function using cell culture techniques. *Am J Physiol* 238:F1–F9, 1980

41. WRIGHT EM: Transepithelial transport in cell culture. *Am J Physiol* 240:C91, 1981

42. MULLINS JM, DIAMOND JL, KLEINZELLER A: Uptake of alpha-methyl-D-glucoside and 3-0-methyl-D-glucose by an established pig renal epithelial line (*abstract*). *Fed Proc* 38:1058, 1979

43. RABITO CA, AUSIELLO DA: Na⁺ dependent sugar transport in a cultured epithelial pig kidney cell line. *J Membr Biol* 54:31–38, 1980

44. SANDERS MJ, SIMON M, MISFELD DS: Transepithelial transport in cell culture: Bioenergetics of Na,D-glucose coupled transport. *J Gen Physiol* 114:263–266, 1982

45. RABITO CA, KARISH MV: Polarized amino acid transport by an epithelial cell line of renal origin (LLC-PK₁). *J Biol Chem* 257:6802–6808, 1982

46. RABITO CA, KARISH MV: Polarized amino acid transport by an epithelial cell line of renal origin (LLC-PK₁): The basolateral system. *J Biol Chem* 258:2543–2547, 1983

47. SEPULVEDA FV, PEARSON JD: Characterization of neutral amino acid uptake by cultured epithelial cells from pig kidney. *J Cell Physiol* 112:182–188, 1982

48. RABITO CA: Phosphate uptake by a kidney epithelial cell line (LLC-PK₁). *Am J Physiol* 245:F22–F31, 1983

49. BIBER J, BROWN CDA, MURER H: Sodium dependent transport of phosphate in LLC-PK₁ cells. *Biochim Biophys Acta* 735:325–330, 1983

50. BROWN CDA, BODMER M, BIBER J, MURER H: Sodium dependent phosphate transport by apical membrane vesicles from a cultured renal epithelial cell line (LLC-PK₁). *Biochim Biophys Acta* 769:471–478, 1984

51. DANISI G, MURER H, STRAUB RW: The effect of pH on phosphate transport into intestinal brush border vesicles. *Am J Physiol,* in press

52. SAKHRANI LM, FINE GL: Renal tubular cells in culture. *Mineral Electrolyte Metab* 9:276–281, 1983

53. HERON FJ, DAYER JM, GOLDRING SR, KRANE SM: Factors modulating the

response of a porcine renal tubular cell line to calcitonin and antidiuretic hormone. *Calcif Tissue Int* 33:41–50, 1981

54. HUDSON TN, FAIN JN: Forskolin-activated adenylate cyclase. *J Biol Chem* 258:9755–9761, 1983

55. BONJOUR J-P, TROEHLER U, PRESTON C, FLEISCH H: Parathyroid hormone and renal handling of P$_1$: Effect of dietary P$_1$ and diphosphonates. *Am J Physiol* 234:F497–F505, 1978

56. STOLL R, MURER H, FLEISCH H, BONJOUR J-P: Effect of diphosphonate treatment on phosphate transport by renal brush border vesicles. *Am J Physiol* 239:F13–F16, 1980

57. BIBER J, BROWN CDA, MURER H, CAVERZASIO J, BONJOUR J-P: Characterization and adaptation to low inorganic phosphate of phosphate transport system in LLC-PK$_1$ cells (*abstract*). *Fed Proc,* in press

58. KINNE R, FAUST RG: Incorporation of D-glucose, L-alanine and phosphate transport systems from rat renal brush border membranes into liposomes. *Biochem J* 168:311–314, 1977

59. KESSLER RJ, VAUGHAN DA, FANESTIL DD: Phosphate binding proteolipid from brush border. *J Biol Chem* 257:14311–14317, 1982

60. FRIEDRICH T, BURCKHARDT G, FASOLD H: Identification of a polypeptide in rat renal basolateral membrane vesicles possibly involved in sulfate transport (*abstract*). *Hoppe Seyler's Z Physiol Chem,* in press

Regulation of the Na$^+$/H$^+$ Antiporter in Cells of the Proximal Tubule

David G. Warnock and Harlan E. Ives

Asymmetric Distribution of the Na$^+$/H$^+$ Antiporter

The hypothesis that the Na$^+$/H$^+$ antiporter causes net H$^+$ movement rests on the assumption that it is present on the brushborder and reduced or absent on the basolateral membrane, since if it were equally active on both membranes, net proton movement would not occur as a result of its action. This assumption has been shown to be false in the tiger salamander where Boron and Boulpaep [3] showed that the Na$^+$/H$^+$ antiporter is present in both apical and basolateral membranes of the proximal tubule cell. These workers believe that in the salamander proximal tubule (which does not acidify its fluid), the Na$^+$/H$^+$ antiporter has a more important role in intracellular pH regulation than in the vectorial transport of H$^+$. Na$^+$/H$^+$ antiporters also appear to be involved in intracellular pH regulation in many nonepithelial cells [4]. Thus, it was not certain whether the Na$^+$/H$^+$ antiporter, which has been demonstrated in brushborder membranes from the mammalian proximal tubule [2, 5, 6], was truly responsible for the net transfer of H$^+$ across the proximal tubule epithelium.

We have examined this issue by subcellular fractionation of proximal tubule cells from the rabbit renal cortex [4]. A crude membrane preparation containing both brush border and basolateral membranes was subjected to sucrose density gradient fractionation (Fig. 1). The location of brushborder membranes in the gradient was ascertained by maltase activity and the location of basolateral membranes by Na$^+$/K$^+$-ATPase activity. Brushborder and basolateral membranes were separated into two distinct peaks by this techniques. We assayed the fractions for Na$^+$-H$^+$ antiporter using the acridine orange method [6]. Na$^+$/H$^+$ antiporter activity paralleled the maltase activity and was absent in the basolateral fractions (Na$^+$-K$^+$-ATPase activity). As a control, we have shown that acridine orange is quenched by basolateral

This manuscript was presented as part of a Symposium on *Brushborder Transport Mechanisms.*

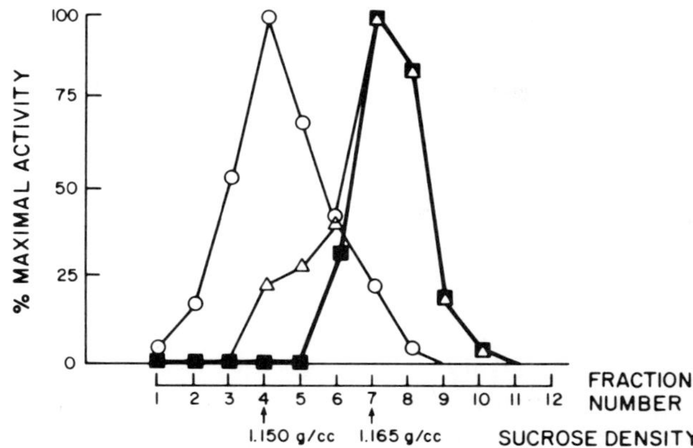

Fig. 1. Separation of basolateral from apical membranes by sucrose density gradient fractionation. Na^+/H^+ antiporter activity was detected in the apical fractions (maltase activity) and not in the basolateral fractions (Na-K-ATPase activity). O—O, Na^+/K^+ ATPase; △—△, maltase; ■—■, Na^+/H^+ antiporter.

membranes and that the assay works well if an exogenous antiporter (nigericin) is added to these membranes. Thus, the lack of activity observed in the basolateral fractions is due to the absence of the Na^+/H^+ antiporter from the basolateral membrane. These findings demonstrate that the Na^+/H^+ antiporter is asymmetrically distributed in the rabbit proximal tubule, and thus fulfill an important criteria for defining the role of the Na^+/H^+ antiporter in net H^+ transport.

While these sucrose gradients clearly separated brushborder and basolateral membranes, the separation between brushborder and intracellular membranes was not as sharp [4]. To improve upon this resolution, we have done preliminary experiments [7] using aqueous phase separation (with dextran and polyethylene glycol) to subfractionate brushborder membranes prepared by divalent cation precipitation.

Use of this two-phase system in a countercurrent distribution device gave rise to four populations of membranes. Only one of these appears to be true brushborder membrane, in that it contains 95% of the maltase and 60% of the Na^+/H^+ antiporter. Two other populations are most likely of endoplasmic reticulum and Golgi origin. The fourth contains no maltase, but does contain 20% of the Na^+/H^+ antiporter activity and 40% of the acid phosphatase. If it is assumed that maltase is found on all brush-border membranes, this result suggests that the Na^+/H^+ antiporter is found on membranes other than the brushborder. Since the antiporter is absent from the basolateral membrane (Fig. 1), it is possible that this fourth membrane population consists of intracellular membranes. Alternatively, the fourth population may consist of brushborders that lack maltase activity in situ or that lost maltase activity during the preparation. However, because of the potential significance of intracellular Na^+/H^+ antiporter activity (see below), it will be important to further characterize these populations and establish their true cellular origin.

Regulation of the Na^+/H^+ Antiporter

There are several lines of physiologic evidence that indicate that the rate of proximal acidification can be altered. Alpern, Cogan, and Rector [8] have shown that, at constant luminal bicarbonate concentration, the proximal reabsorption of bicarbonate is stimulated by metabolic acidosis and inhibited by metabolic alkalosis. There are also now a number of preliminary reports that Na^+/H^+ antiporter activity itself can be regulated. Three different groups (9–11) have reported increased antiporter activity in brushborder vesicles from animals with metabolic acidosis; one [9] has shown that this response is dependent on glucocorticoids. Our own studies [11] have shown that antiporter activity increases in a graded fashion, in direct relation to the degree of in vivo acidosis in rabbits gavaged with ammonium chloride. Figure 2 demonstrates this relationship.

Taken together, these studies provide compelling evidence that Na^+/H^+ antiporter activity in the brushborder can be altered, raising the intriguing possibility that the proximal tubule can vary its capacity to reabsorb bicarbonate by changing the activity of the Na^+/H^+ antiporter.

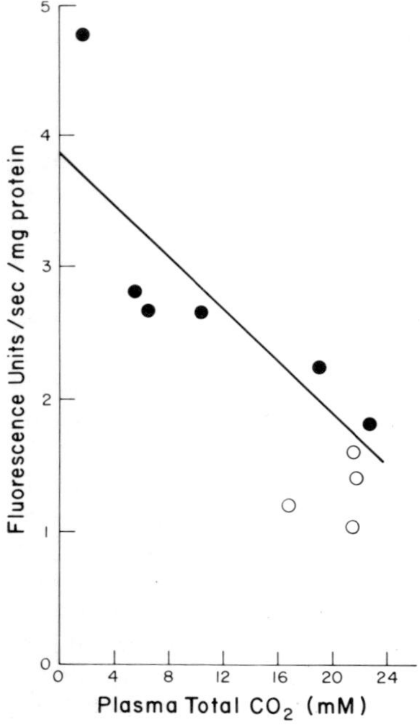

Fig. 2. Effect of metabolic acidosis on Na^+/H^+ antiporter activity. The V_{max} (fluorescence U/sec/mg) in each experiment was determined by Eadie-Hofstee analysis, and plasma total CO_2 measurement by microcalorimetry. The *open circles* (○) represent results obtained with brushborder membranes prepared from individual control animals, and the *closed circles* (●) represent results obtained for individual rabbits that had been gavaged with NH_4Cl for 3 days. (Reprinted with permission from [11])

Cellular and Biochemical Mechanisms of Regulation

We have been interested in establishing the mechanisms whereby regulation of the Na^+/H^+ antiporter may take place. In theory, regulation could occur through either synthesis of new antiporters, or modification of existing antiporters.

There is now a large body of evidence that plasma membrane constituents are constantly recycled via coated vesicles, endosomes, lysosomes, and Golgi [12]. Considerable precedent exists for the contribution of these processes in controlling the levels of membrane transport systems. For example, the H^+-ATPase in turtle bladder [13] and the glucose transport systems from the adipocyte [14] both exhibit "up regulation" in response to physiologic stimuli by fusion of intracellular vesicles with the plasma membrane. Therefore, the establishment of Na^+/H^+ antiporters (either active or inactive) on intracellular membranes would be potentially very important. It is of interest to note that endosomes isolated from rabbit renal cortex have an H^+-translocating ATPase, but do not appear to have Na^+/H^+ antiporter activity [15]. This finding implies that Na^+/H^+ antiporter may not undergo membrane recycling via endosomes, or else that the antiporter is rapidly inactivated following endocytosis.

A second type of regulation that has been explored in more depth is the possibility of a direct chemical interaction between a messenger molecule and the Na^+/H^+ antiporter.

We first became interested in this possibility when we noticed an unexpected interaction between sodium and lithium on the antiporter. It has been shown [5] that lithium can exchange for hydrogen via the antiporter and that lithium is a competitive inhibitor of the antiporter with the acridine orange assay [16]. Lithium caused proton efflux at lower concentrations than sodium (K_m for $Li^+ = 1.2$ mM; K_m for $Na^+ = 14.3$ mM) and exhibited a lower V_{max} (2.40 fluorescence U/sec/mg protein for Li^+; 7.10 U/sec/mg protein for Na^+). It appeared that sodium and lithium were simply two different substrates for the same transport system (Fig. 3).

However, when Na^+/H^+ exchange over a range of sodium concentrations (1.0 to 90 mM) was measured in the presence of a small amount of lithium (1.0 mM), a noncompetitive interaction was observed. Surprisingly, at high sodium concentrations, 1.0 mM lithium had a 30% inhibitory effect rather than the 5% that would be predicted from simple competition. Thus, lithium appeared to be binding to a modifier site separate from the site at which sodium was binding.

To determine the concentration range for this noncompetitive inhibition of the antiporter by Li^+-Na^+/H^+, exchange due to 90 mM sodium was measured with from 25 μM to 1.0 mM lithium (Fig. 4). A significant competitive interaction of lithium with the transport site was not expected under these conditions. What was revealed is a remarkably low inhibitory $K_{1/2}$ of 50 to 100 μM. This $K_{1/2}$ when compared to the agonist K_m for lithium of 1.2 mM, is further evidence that lithium has two separate binding sites on the antiporter. However, it is worth emphasizing that noncompetitive inhibition

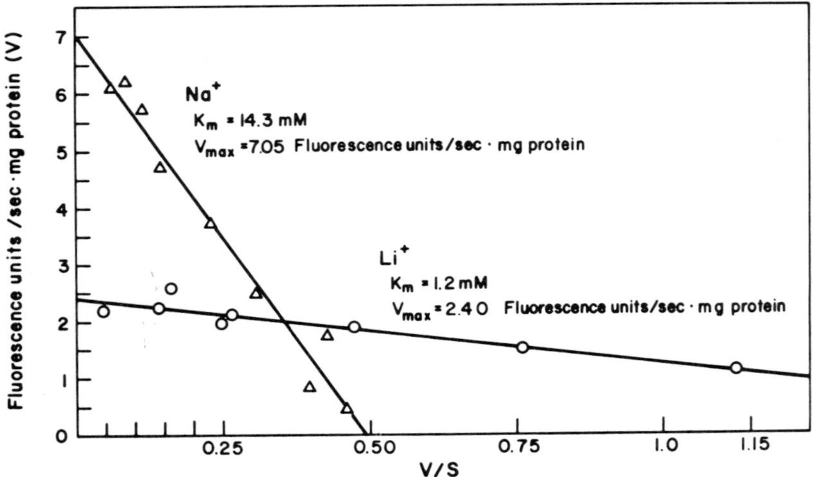

Fig. 3. Eadie-Hofstee plot of concentration response curves for Na⁺ and Li⁺. Brush-border membrane vesicles (pH 6.0) were suspended in external buffer at pH 7.5, and cations subsequently added to the external buffer. Initial rates of pH gradient collapse (fluorescence U/sec/mg protein) were measured with the acridine orange technique. (Reprinted with permission from [6])

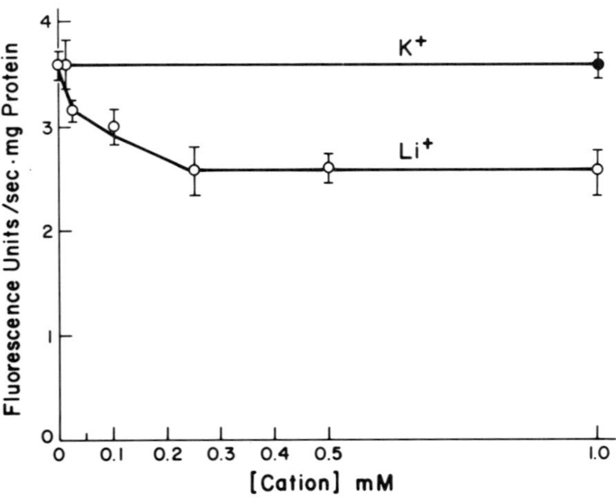

Fig. 4. Inhibition of Na⁺/H⁺ exchange by Li⁺. Initial rates of pH gradient collapse were measured with brushborder membrane vesicles following addition of 90 mM Na⁺ and the indicated concentrations of Li⁺ or K⁺.

does not, per se, require two separate binding sites. Amiloride and lithium may each bind to a single site that is not simply competitive with the sodium binding site.

A modifier site for hydrogen has been found on the inside renal brush-border membranes by Aronson, Nee and Suhm [17]. Of note, this same group has been unable to detect an interaction between hydrogen and the external modifier site described in our work [18]. Whether these two modifier sites are truly different has not been firmly established. Aronson's group has described a noncompetitive inhibition of the Na^+/H^+ antiporter by quinidine [19], a finding that is consistent with an external modifier site.

To explore the interaction of known inhibitors of the Na^+/H^+ antiporter with the modifier site, we studied the inhibition by amiloride of Na^+/H^+ exchange (Fig. 5). Eadie-Hofstee plots of Na^+/H^+ exchange rates at concentrations of amiloride from 0 to 100 μM (concentrations greater than 100 μM could not be examined because of an artificial interference by amiloride with the assay) revealed a decreasing V_{max} and increasing K_m with increasing amiloride concentration. This is characteristic of mixed-type inhibition. Dixon plots revealed a K_i (the binding constant in the absence of sodium) for amiloride of 30 μM, and Cornish Bowden plots revealed a K_i (the binding constant at infinite sodium) of 90 μM.

The finding of mixed-type inhibition of Na^+/H^+ exchange by amiloride supported our hypothesis of a modifier site on the antiporter, since amiloride also required a second binding site beside the sodium transport site. We therefore asked whether the modifier site we had found for Li^+ and amiloride were in fact the same site. This was studied by examining the kinetics of

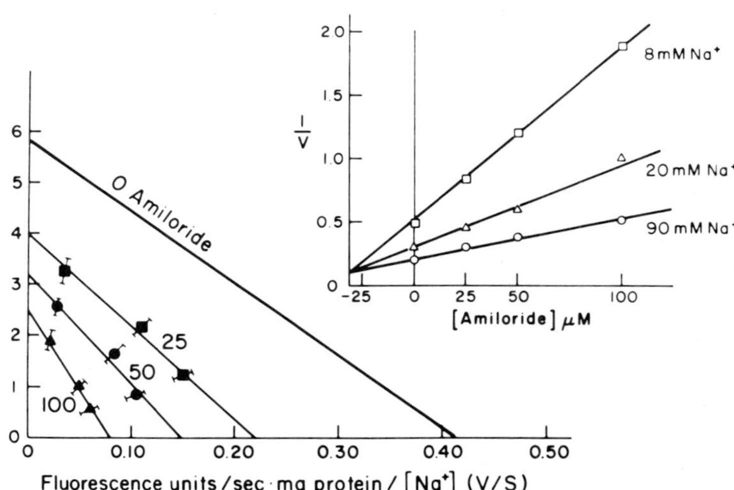

Fig. 5. Inhibition of Na^+/H^+ exchange by amiloride. Concentration response curves for Na^+ were obtained in the presence of the indicated concentrations of amiloride. *Inset:* Dixon plot to determine K_i.

inhibition of Li$^+$/H$^+$ exchange by amiloride. Since we knew that lithium could occupy the modifier site at extremely low concentrations (K$_{1/2}$ = 50 to 100 μM), we were curious to see if amiloride would inhibit Li$^+$/H$^+$ exchange. Amiloride did inhibit Li$^+$/H$^+$ exchange (Fig. 6), but Eadie-Hofstee plots of Li$^+$/H$^+$ exchange in the presence of 0 to 100 μM amiloride, in marked contrast to those of Na$^+$/H$^+$ exchange, intersected at the same V$_{max}$, which is evidence for pure competitive inhibition. The simplest explanation for this finding is that under the conditions of this experiment (lithium greater than 1.0 mM), the modifier site was occupied by lithium. Amiloride and lithium then interact only by simple competition at the transport site. A model that incorporates the features of an external modifier site and an external transport site is presented in Figure 7.

It is worth noting that the results obtained with lithium and amiloride utilized the AO fluorescence quenching technique. Similar studies have been done by Kinsella and Aronson [5] utilizing ^{22}Na uptake, and only simple competitive inhibition could be observed. It is unknown at present if this represents a fundamental difference in the two techniques or a limitation of one technique compared to the other in the description of the kinetics of the Na$^+$/H$^+$ antiporter.

In summary, the Na$^+$/H$^+$ antiporter is absent from the basolateral membrane in the mammalian proximal tubule and thus participates in vectorial transport of hydrogen across the epithelium. Since the rate of proton secretion is almost certainly regulated, we hypothesize that the Na$^+$/H$^+$ antiporter participates in this regulation. Much indirect evidence exists for such participation. Preliminary experiments aimed at delineating potential mechanisms for regulation raise the possibility of an intracellular pool of Na$^+$/H$^+$ anti-

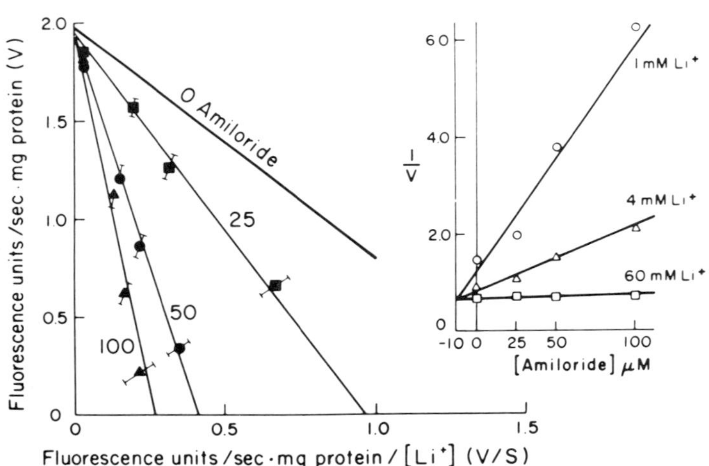

Fig. 6. Inhibition of Li$^+$/H$^+$ exchange by amiloride. Concentration response curves for Li$^+$ were obtained in the presence of the indicated concentrations of amiloride. *Inset:* Dixon plot to determine K.

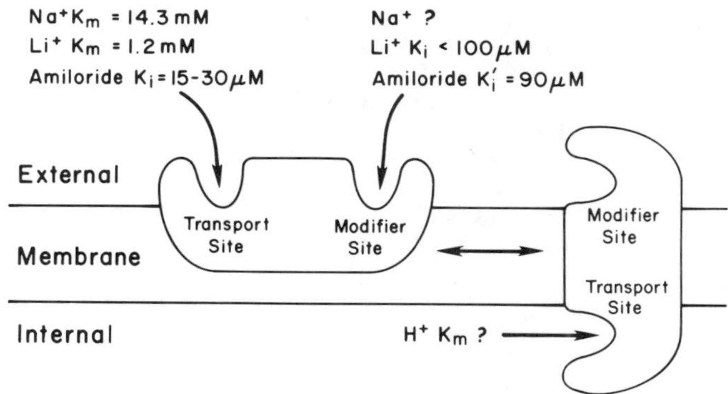

Fig. 7. Model of the external aspect of Na$^+$/H$^+$ antiporter.

porter activity and have identified modifier sites on the antiporter, which could be loci for direct kinetic regulation. The nature of endogenous substances that may regulate the activity of the antiporter remains to be determined. It seems certain from studies by Aronson and his colleagues [17, 18] that pH, especially intracellular acidity, plays an important role in regulation of the antiporter. It is also conceivable that substances in the luminal fluid may have a direct effect on the antiporter through an interaction at the external modifier site. Studies from Satta et al [20] and Blumenthal, Ware, and Kleinman [21] have recently demonstrated a stimulatory effect of alpha$_1$ catecholamines on Na$^+$/H$^+$ antiporter activity in brushborder membranes and cells from the proximal tubule. Further studies are required to define the role of luminal factors, both inhibitory like lithium and amiloride and stimulatory like norepinephrine, on the activity of the Na$^+$/H$^+$ antiporter.

References

1. WARNOCK DG, RECTOR FC JR: Renal acidification mechanisms, in *The Kidney,* 2nd edition, edited by BRENNER BM, RECTOR FC JR, Philadelphia, Saunders, 1981, pp 440–449
2. MURER H, HOPFER U, KINNE R: Sodium/proton antiporter in brush-border membrane vesicles isolated from rat small intestine and kidney. *Biochem J* 154:597–604, 1976
3. BORON WF, BOULPAEP EL: Intracellular pH regulation in the renal proximal tubule of the salamander. *J Gen Physiol* 81:29–52, 1983
4. IVES HE, YEE VJ, WARNOCK DG: Assymetric distribution of the Na$^+$/H$^+$ antiporter in the renal proximal tubule epithelial cell. *J Biol Chem* 258:13513–13516, 1983
5. KINSELLA JL, ARONSON PS: Properties of the Na$^+$/H$^+$ exchanger in renal microvillus membrane vesicles. *Am J Physiol* 238:F461–F469, 1980
6. WARNOCK DG, REENSTRA WW, YEE VJ: Na$^+$/H$^+$ antiporter of brush-border vesicles: Studies with acridine orange uptake. *Am J Physiol* 238:F733–F739, 1982
7. MIRCHEFF AK, IVES HE, YEE VJ, WARNOCK DG: Na$^+$/H$^+$ antiporter in mem-

brane populations resolved from a renal brush-border vesicle preparation. *Am J Physiol* 246:F853–F858, 1984

8. ALPERN RJ, COGAN MG, RECTOR FC JR: Effects of extracellular fluid volume and plasma bicarbonate concentration on proximal acidification in the rat. *J Clin Invest* 71:736–746, 1983

9. KINSELLA JL, SACKTOR B: Role of glucocorticoids in the response to chronic metabolic acidosis (*abstract*). *Fed Proc* 42:989, 1983

10. COHN DE, KLAHR S, HAMMERMAN MR: Metabolic acidosis and parathyroidectomy increase Na^+/H^+ exchange in brush border vesicles. *Am J Physiol* 245:F217–F222, 1983

11. TSAI C-J, IVES HE, ALPERN RJ, YEE VJ, WARNOCK DG, RECTOR FC JR: Increased V_{max} for Na^+/H^+ antiporter activity in proximal tubule brush border vesicles from rabbits with metabolic acidosis. *Am J Physiol,* in press

12. BROWN MS, ANDERSON RGW, GOLDSTEIN JL: Recycling receptors: the round-trip itinerary of migrant membrane proteins. *Cell* 32:663–667, 1983

13. GLUCK S, CANNON C, AL-AWQATI Q: Exocytosis regulates urinary acidification by rapid insertion of H^+ pumps into the luminal membrane. *Proc Natl Acad Sci USA* 79:4327–4331, 1982

14. KONO T, ROBINSON FW, BLEVINS TL, EZAKI O: Evidence that translocation of the glucose transport activity is the major mechanism of insulin action on glucose transport in fat cells. *J Biol Chem* 257:10942–10947, 1982

15. GURICH RW, YEE VJ, WARNOCK DG: H^+ transport systems in apical and intracellular membrane vesicles from rabbit renal cortex (*abstract*). *Proc Int Cong Nephrol* 9:382, 1984

16. IVES HE, YEE VJ, WARNOCK DG: Mixed type inhibition of the renal Na^+/H^+ antiporter by Li^+ and amiloride: evidence for a modifier site. *J Biol Chem* 258:9710–9716, 1983

17. ARONSON PS, NEE J, SUHM MA: Modifier role of internal H^+ in activating the Na^+-H^+ exchanger in renal microvillus membrane vesicles. *Nature* 299:161–163, 1982

18. ARONSON PS, SUHM MA, NEE J: Interaction of external H^+ with the Na^+-H^+ exchanger in renal microvillus membrane vesicles. *J Biol Chem* 258:6767–6771, 1983

19. MAHNENSMITH RL, LOULAKIS P, ARONSON PS: Quinidine inhibition of the Na-H exchanger in renal microvillus membrane vesicles (*abstract*). *Kidney Int* 25:309, 1984

20. SATTA A, CONTU B, FAEDDA R, BRANCA GF, BARTOLI E: In vitro effects of catecholamine on Na efflux across proximal brush border vesicles (*abstract*). *Proc Int Cong Nephrol* 9:374A, 1984

21. BLUMENTHAL S, WARE R, KLEINMAN J: $Alpha_1$ adrenergic agonist stimulation of Na^+-H^+ exchange in proximal tubule cells (*abstract*). *Proc Int Cong Nephrol* 10:379, 1984

Renal Nerves

Functions of the Renal Nerves

Chairpersons: Gerald F. DiBona and Romulo E. Colindres
Discussants: Luciano Barajas, Roger J. Summers, Nicholas G. Moss,
Ulla C. Kopp, and Richard E. Katholi

Light microscopy and ultrastructural examination of kidneys from rats given tritiated norepinephrine consistently disclose nerves at the sites where autoradiographic grains (AAGs) accumulate. Neurotubular contact or close proximity can also be reasonably predicted when AAGs overlap a tubular profile in the autoradiograms. With this approach, neurotubular contact has been shown ultrastructurally in the proximal tubule (PT), the ascending thick limb of Henle (ATLH), the collecting duct (CD), and the connecting tubule (CNT). It has also allowed a quantitative assessment of the innervation of the different portions of the cortical nephron to be carried out. The results indicate that although the PT showed the largest number of innervated profiles, the highest frequency of innervation (defined by the ratio of the number of innervated profiles to the total number of profiles surveyed) occurred in the ATLH, followed by the distal convoluted tubule (including the CNT) and the PT. The CD was also found to be innervated; however, it showed the lowest number of innervated profiles. These findings suggest that all portions of the nephron are under some degree of neural influence.

Summers stated that renal adrenoceptors can be labeled in vitro with high-affinity radioligands, and their distribution then examined by light microscopic autoradiography. ^{125}Icyanopindolol (cyp) and tritiated-rauwolscine were used accordingly to examine the distribution of sites with the biochemical characteristics of β-adrenoceptors and α_2-adrenoceptors. Highly localized populations of β-adrenoceptors were found in rat, dog, and guinea pig kidney. The β_1- and β_2-adrenoceptor subtypes were resolved by using the selective antagonists betaxolol and ICI 118,551.

The glomeruli of all three species contained high concentrations of β_1-adrenoceptors, which covered the entire area of these structures. In the rat, β_1-adrenoceptors were also found on distal and cortical collecting tubules; β_2-adrenoceptors were more widespread and less localized. High concentra-

This manuscript is a summary of a Workshop entitled *The Function of the Renal Nerves*.

tions of β_2-adrenoceptors were associated with the straight portion of the proximal tubule (alkaline phosphatase-positive) in guinea pig and with medullary rays in the dog.

In the rat kidney, α_2-adrenoceptors were confined to the proximal tubules, whereas in the dog, high concentrations were localized to glomeruli, blood vessels, and areas in the medulla.

These results indicate that adrenoceptor subtypes are highly localized to structures in the kidney, with particularly high concentrations in glomeruli. The distribution and concentration of adrenoceptors in other nephron segments varies markedly with species.

DiBona noted that, in a previous study, he and his colleagues had found that conscious rats, in the absence of anesthetic and surgical stress, require intact renal innervation for normal renal sodium conservation and maintenance of body sodium balance during dietary sodium restriction. The role of the renal nerves in the renal responses to acute and chronic changes in total body sodium was further studied by using measurements of renal nerve activity in conscious rats in balance on low, normal, or high dietary sodium intake and subjected to acute intravenous saline volume expansion. In the control period, right atrial pressure and urinary sodium excretion ($U_{Na}V$) were directly related and renal nerve activity was inversely related to the dietary sodium intake. During volume expansion, right atrial pressure and $U_{Na}V$ increased and renal nerve activity decreased in all three dietary groups; however, the increase in $U_{Na}V$ was greater in the low-sodium rats than in the normal or high-sodium rats. A decrease in renal nerve activity was associated with a greater natriuresis in the low-sodium rats than in the normal or high-sodium rats. The greater contribution of inhibition of renal nerve activity to the increased natriuretic response to volume expansion in low-compared with normal-sodium rats was further examined in renal denervated animals. Bilateral renal denervation substantially reduced the natriuretic response to volume expansion in the low-sodium rats but had no significant effect in the normal-sodium rats. Thus, when basal levels of renal nerve activity are elevated, the natriuretic response to acute intravenous saline volume expansion includes a component related to withdrawal of renal nerve activity with decreased renal tubular sodium reabsorption. Similar findings are observed in spontaneously hypertensive rats (SHR), which have elevated basal renal nerve activity and an exaggerated natriuresis associated with an exaggerated inhibition of renal nerve activity during intravenous saline volume expansion compared to normotensive Wistar-Kyoto rats (WKY). Bilateral renal denervation attenuates the exaggerated natriuresis in SHR, but has no effect in WKY.

Colindres considered chronic renal denervation in conscious rats and its effects on sodium balance, blood pressure (BP), and the renin-angiotensin-aldosterone system. He noted first that there is some controversy regarding the contribution of the renal nerves to the maintenance of sodium balance in conscious animals. Furthermore, the influence of the renal nerves on the responses of the renin-angiotensin-aldosterone system in such animals has not been evaluated. Studies were done in unrestrained conscious rats on varying sodium intake before and after bilateral renal denervation or sham denervation. Functional and chemical evidence of denervation was obtained in all denervated rats at the end of these long-term experiments. The results show that chronic bilateral renal denervation in conscious, unstressed rats leads to a reproducible fall in mean arterial blood pressure and to partial suppression of the renin-angiotensin-aldosterone system in rats on a normal sodium diet. Denervated rats subjected to sodium restriction for 10 days maintained a blood pressure that was lower than that seen in sham-denervated rats and were able to maintain sodium balance as well as they did before denervation. Plasma renin concentration during sodium deprivation did not increase to the degree seen before denervation or to that seen in sham-denervated rats. Plasma aldosterone concentration increased normally during sodium deprivation, both in innervated and denervated animals. Glomerular filtration rate, as measured by creatinine clearance, was unchanged after renal denervation or sham denervation. The results of this study demonstrate that the renal nerves influence the function of the juxtaglomerular apparatus in unrestrained conscious rats. These results do not exclude an effect of renal denervation on proximal sodium reabsorption with compensation in more distal nephron segments.

Moss addressed the neurophysiology of renal afferent nerves. He stated that the afferent innervation of the kidney is composed of chemoreceptive and mechanoreceptive nerves that enter the spinal cord in the dorsal roots of the late thoracic segments (T11, T12, and T13). The most numerous type of afferent fibers innervating the kidney are R2-chemoreceptive. These receptors have a basal discharge that is excited to high levels of activity during reflux of urine into the renal pelvis or during complete renal ischemia. Recent studies have revealed that a reduction in renal perfusion pressure to between 70 and 80 mm Hg also leads to excitation of R2 chemoreceptors. The chemical nature of the stimulus for these receptors is still unclear. Potassium chloride solutions introduced into the renal pelvis are excitatory and mimic the effects of reflux of urine. However, the effect of other chemical stimuli such as the release of kinins within the kidney is supported by the finding that renal artery injections of bradykinin also excite R2 chemoreceptors. The threshold dose for this response was determined for 14 single R2 units in the rat and found to be 104 ± 57 ng in bolus injections of 50 μl into the renal artery.

Kopp focused on the neural and functional responses of renorenal reflexes. In the rat, she noted that renal mechanoreceptors can be stimulated by increasing the ureteral pressure (UP), and that renal chemoreceptors can be stimulated by retrograde ureteropelvic perfusion with 0.9 M sodium chloride. These maneuvers cause an increase in ipsilateral afferent renal nerve activity (ARNA), a decrease in contralateral efferent RNA (ERNA) and an increase in contralateral urinary flow rate (V) and urinary sodium excretion ($U_{Na}V$), that is, a contralateral inhibitory renorenal reflex response. Stimulation of the renal mechanoreceptors by increasing the UP 31 mm Hg or increasing the renal venous pressure (RVP) 23 mm Hg resulted in similar increases in contralateral V, 53 ± 13 and $40 \pm 9\%$ ($P < 0.01$, $N = 8$). When RVP was increased 22 mm Hg, the ipsilateral ARNA increased from 11 ± 2 to 40 ± 7 counts/sec ($P < 0.05$), and the contralateral ERNA decreased from 51 ± 5 to 9 ± 3 counts/sec ($P < 0.05$, $N = 6$). Renal pelvic administration of lidocaine (5 μg/ml) abolished the contralateral inhibitory renorenal reflex responses to the increase in UP and the retrograde ureteropelvic perfusion with 0.9 M sodium chloride. However, the renorenal reflex response to the increase in RVP was not affected by renal pelvic administration of lidocaine. Spinal cord section at T6 18 hr before the experiment abolished the renorenal reflex responses to the increase in UP and RVP and the retrograde ureteropelvic perfusion with 0.9 M sodium chloride. Furthermore, T6 spinal cord section abolished the ipsilateral ARNA responses to renal mechanoreceptor and chemoreceptor stimulation, suggesting a trophic influence of ERNA on ARNA. In preliminary studies, this was confirmed by experiments using ganglionic blockade, which also abolished the ipsilateral ARNA response to mechanoreceptor stimulation. These results demonstrate that renal mechanoreceptor stimulation by either an increase in UP or RVP results in a contralateral inhibitory renorenal reflex response with contralateral diuresis and natriuresis. The renorenal reflex response to an increase in UP and to retrograde ureteropelvic perfusion with 0.9 M sodium chloride is elicited by activation of neuroreceptor complexes in the region of the renal pelvis. The renorenal reflex response to an increase in RVP is elicited by neuroreceptor complexes in the renal interstitium beyond the renal pelvis. The level of integration of the renorenal reflex response to mechanoreceptor and chemoreceptor stimulation is supra spinal.

Katholi stated that studies of the renal nerves in experimental hypertension suggested that the afferent renal nerves from the clipped kidney enhance the activity of the sympathetic nervous sytem in established one-kidney one-clip and two-kidney one-clip Goldblatt hypertension. Recent experiments have been performed to determine the relative contribution of the sympathetic fibers and the adrenal medullae in these models. Adrenal demedullation lowered arterial pressure and decreased sympathetic activity (assessed by ganglionic blockade) to the same degree as occurred with renal denervation or combined adrenal demedullation and renal denervation. Thus, the adrenal medullae contribute importantly to the maintenance of hypertension in the conscious one-kidney one-clip and two-kidney one-clip Goldblatt hypertensive rat. These data also suggest that the afferent renal nerves activate the adrenal medulla in these models.

Recent studies have shown that there are adenosine-sensitive nerve endings located within or near the renal pelvis and that, when stimulated, they activate the sympathetic nervous system producing moderate hypertension. This intrarenal adenosine-induced sympathetic response is characterized by an increased cardiac output, an increased contralateral renal vascular resistance, no change in resistance of the splanchnic or hindlimb vascular beds, and enhanced norepinephrine (but not epinephrine) release from the adrenal medullae. Intrarenal adenosine administration in an adrenal-demedullated animal results in little or no hypertension. These results suggest that the adrenal medullae contribute importantly to the intrarenal adenosine-induced sympathetic response through selective release of norepinephrine.

In summary, the renal nephron receives noradrenergic innervation along its entire length, with a greater density in the thick ascending limb of Henle's loop than in the distal convoluted tubule, proximal convoluted tubule, or collecting duct. In vitro labeling and autoradiographic techniques using selective ligands allow a more precise anatomic localization and biochemical characterization of adrenoceptors. β_1- and β_2-adrenoceptors are found in the kidneys of the rat, guinea pig, and dog. In the rat, β_1-adrenoceptors were found in the glomeruli and distal and cortical collecting tubules, whereas β_2-adrenoceptors were more widespread and less localized; α_2-adrenoceptors were confined to the proximal tubules. The proportion and distribution of renal adrenoceptors vary markedly between species. To avoid the potentially confounding influences of anesthetic and surgical stress, studies of renal denervation and renal nerve activity have been performed in conscious rats. There is disagreement as to whether intact renal innervation is required for normal renal sodium conservation and maintenance of body sodium balance during dietary sodium restriction. Renal nerve activity recordings in conscious rats indicate a relationship between changes in renal nerve activity and urinary sodium excretion during both acute and chronic alteration in sodium balance. Plasma renin and aldosterone concentrations are subnormal in conscious rats with bilateral renal denervation during basal conditions, and plasma renin (but not aldosterone) concentration fails to increase normally during dietary sodium deprivation. Renal R2 chemoreceptors show a previously unrecognized excitation by reductions in renal perfusion pressure to 70 to 80 mm Hg. Furthermore, R2 chemoreceptors are also excited by renal artery injections of bradykinin. The interaction between the excitation produced by these two stimuli requires further definition. When specific stimuli for activation of both renal mechanoreceptors and chemoreceptors are used in combination with measurements of renal function and nerve activity, contralateral inhibitory renorenal reflexes integrated at the supraspinal level can be identified. Decreases in efferent renal nerve activity produced by spinal cord section or ganglionic blockade modulate the response of afferent renal nerves to renal mechanoreceptor stimulation. In certain models of experimental hypertension, the afferent renal nerves carry information to central nervous system autonomic centers. This causes an increase in the level of systemic sympathetic neurohumoral activity, which contributes to the hypertension via an increase in systemic vascular resistance. Recent evidence indicates that the adrenal medulla is importantly involved in this process. It releases norepinephrine in response to a reflex initiated by increased afferent renal nerve activity, which is stimulated by adenosine or other stimuli.

Renal Circulation

Organization of the Medullary Circulation: Functional Implications

Lise Bankir, Nadine Bouby, and Marie-Marcelle Trinh-Trang-Tan

It is the renal medulla that enables the kidney to concentrate urine above plasma osmolality. With equivalent nephron segments (that is, the proximal tubule, short "intermediate" tubule, "diluting segment," and distal tubule, but not folded into a "U" shape), the amphibian and reptile kidneys can adequately maintain the composition of their "milieu intérieur" and can excrete their nitrogen end-products, but they cannot produce hypertonic urine [1]. On the other extreme, kidneys of desert-adapted rodents exhibit the main structural features permitting the elaboration of a highly concentrated urine.

The medullary circulation is not uniformly organized from the cortico-medullary border to papillary tip, but it comprises three concentric zones containing different tubular segments: the outer and the inner stripes of the outer medulla and the inner medulla. A glance at a sagittal section of a kidney whose vessels have been filled with a silicone rubber (Fig. 1) reveals that each of these three medullary zones has its own vascular pattern. The mammalian renal medulla, therefore, must be considered as a *multicompartmental structure*. The scope of this chapter is to describe the medullary vessels, their relationships with the tubules in each renal zone, and the functional consequences of this organization. This description is based not only on a survey of the literature, but also on personal observations of kidneys of more than 20 mammals. Detailed descriptions of the medullary vessels have been previously published [2–7], as have anatomic-functional and vasculotubular relationships [8–20].

Vascular Organization of the Medulla

The blood supply to the medulla is derived almost exclusively from the efferent arterioles of a small percentage of the glomeruli, which are located in the

---

This manuscript was presented as part of a Symposium on *Medullary Circulation.*

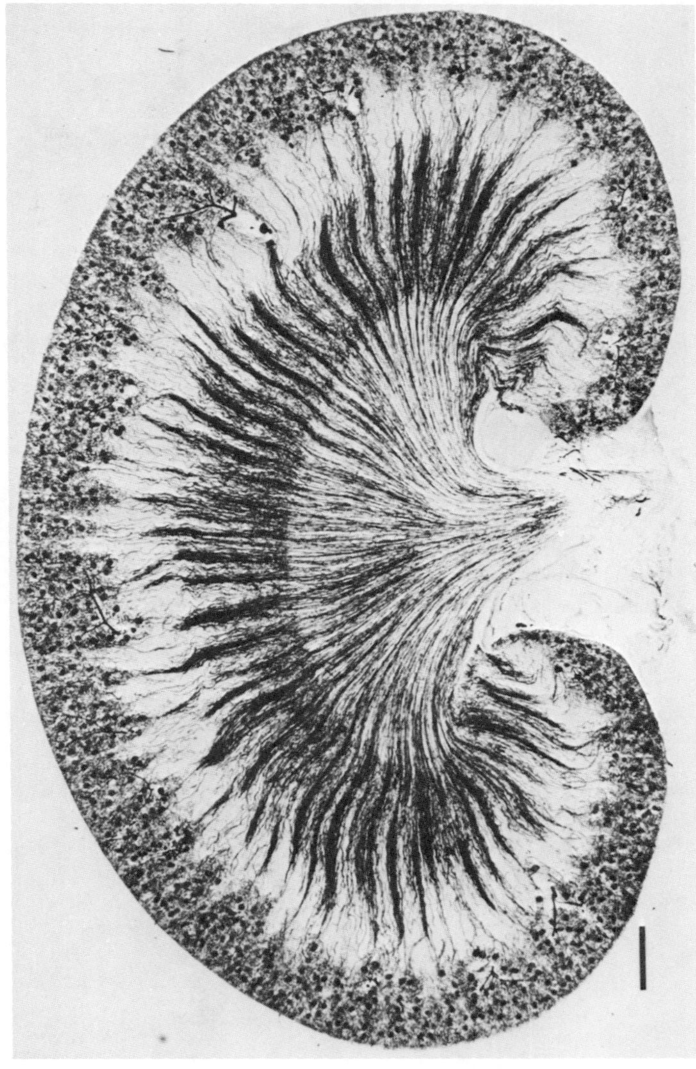

Fig. 1. Longitudinal section of rat kidney following arterial injection with Microfil silicone rubber. Each of the four concentric zones, cortex, and outer and inner stripes of the outer medulla and inner medulla has its own vascular pattern and is easily recognized. Note the paucity of capillaries in the *outer stripe,* the radial vascular bundles of the *inner stripe,* and the abrupt transition from the inner stripe capillary plexus to the inner medulla. (Bar, $\cong$ 1.2 mm; picture by Wilhelm Kriz, Heidelberg, Federal Republic of Germany)

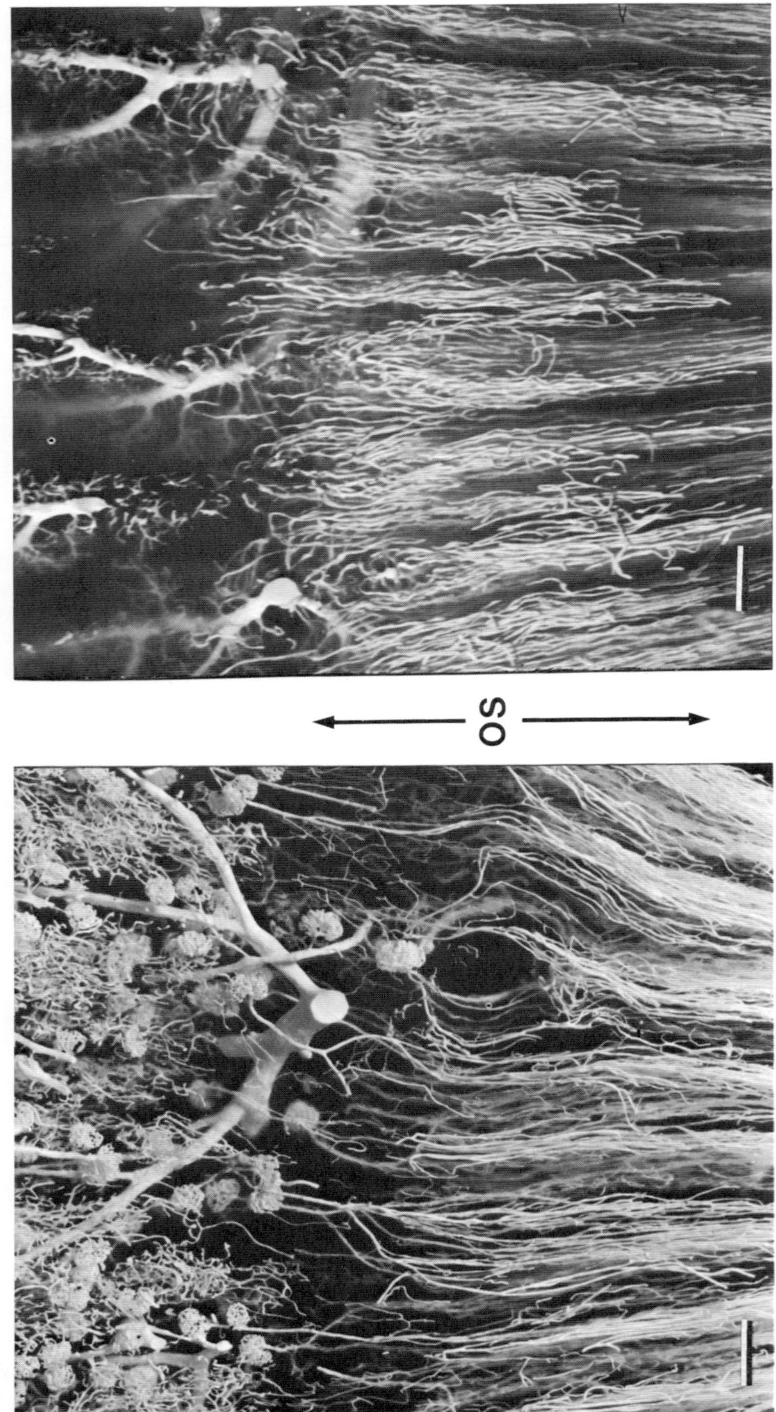

Fig. 2

deep cortex. Other pathways, which represent only an insignificant contribution to medullary blood flow, may come either from arterioles arising directly from the arcuate arteries or from afferent-efferent shunts remaining after glomeruli degeneration [4, 7, 21, 22]. Thus, the medullary blood supply can be considered to be almost entirely postglomerular. The percentage of "juxtamedullary glomeruli" (those giving rise to vasa recta supplying the medulla) varies from 7 to 20% [7, 18, 23], but the percentage of "long-looped nephrons" varies from 0 (beaver) to 100% (carnivores such as the cat and the dog), with values of 60% in the rabbit [24] and 35 to 45% in most rodents (rat, mouse, and *Psammomys*) [7, 25]. Thus, except for the few species that have no long loops, juxtamedullary glomeruli are associated with long-looped nephrons.

Let us first follow the medullary vessels from their origin (the efferent arterioles of juxtamedullary glomeruli) to their end-point (their junction with the arcuate vein system). During their descent through the outer stripe, efferent arterioles—after a relatively long unbranched course—divide repeatedly over a short distance to form numerous parallel vasa recta that give off very few side branches to the surrounding region (Fig. 2, bottom) [26, 27]. The vasa recta from a few adjacent glomeruli gather to form bundles of descending vessels in the inner stripe that run in close apposition to the vessels ascending from the inner medulla. These groups of vessels are called vascular bundles and are observed in the inner stripe of the outer medulla in all mammals. The descending vasa recta at the periphery of the bundles in both the deep outer stripe and the inner stripe break off into capillaries to form a rich plexus between the vascular bundles (Fig. 3). This capillary network resolves into numerous wide venous vessels that do not re-enter the vascular bundles, but ascend directly to rejoin the arcuate veins at the corticomedullary border (Fig. 2, top). The descending vasa recta at the center of each vascular bundle descend into the inner medulla, between the tubules, and divide (at various levels) into a few branches that then turn and become ascending vasa recta without giving a real mesh of capillaries (except at the very tip of the papilla). These vasa recta ascend individually up to the border between the inner and outer medulla. There, vasa recta ascending from the inner medulla join the vascular bundles and cross the inner stripe (Fig. 4, bottom) without merging with the capillary network in the inner stripe. In the outer stripe, the ascending vasa recta from the inner medulla (which have crossed the inner stripe within the vascular bundles) and the ascending vasa recta from the inner stripe capillary network (which as-

---

Fig. 2. Deep cortex and outer stripe (*OS*) of rabbit kidney following arterial (*bottom*) or venous (*top*) injection with Microfil silicone rubber. Efferent arterioles of deep glomeruli give rise to numerous arterial vasa recta that form vascular bundles as they descend toward the inner stripe (*bottom*). Numerous, wide venous vasa recta ascend towards the corticomedullary border and empty into arcuate or interlobular veins (*top*). Note the paucity of arterially filled capillaries in the *outer stripe* and (in contrast) the richness in the venous vessels at the same level. Compare with cross-section shown in Figure 6. (Bar, $\cong$ 300 μm)

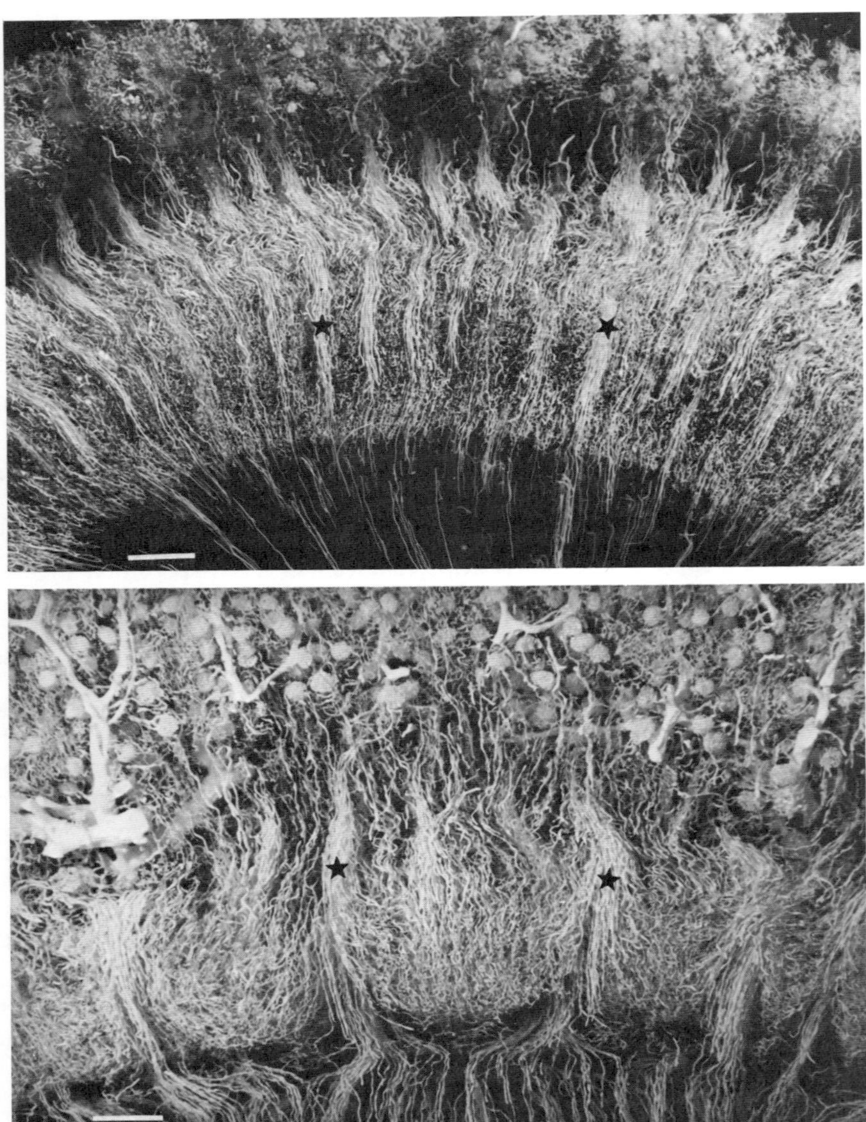

Fig. 3. Sagittal sections of rat (*top*) and Mongolian gerbil (*Meriones shawii*) (*bottom*) kidneys following arterial injection with Microfil silicone rubber, showing deep cortex, outer and inner stripes of the outer medulla, and the early inner medulla. In the inner stripe, vascular bundles (*stars*) alternate with interbundle capillary plexus. The functional separation of the two adjacent compartments exists in both species, but is amplified in the desert-adapted Mongolian gerbil. [Bar, $\cong$ 600 μm (*top*) and $\cong$ 350 μm (*bottom*)]

cend between the bundles) both continue as single, wide venous channels and empty into the arcuate veins or into the interlobular veins in the medullary rays of the cortex (Fig. 2, top, Fig. 4, bottom).

If we now consider each medullary zone successively (Fig. 5), it can be seen that the *outer stripe* (Fig. 2) receives only very few capillaries from the efferent arterioles of the juxtamedullary glomeruli and their branches. The majority of the vessels observed in the outer stripe are ascending venous vasa recta that come from the inner medulla via the vascular bundles, and also from the inner stripe capillary plexus. The *inner stripe* (Fig. 3) contains two distinct vascular territories: (1) the vascular bundles containing vessels going down to or coming up from the inner medulla, and (2) the interbundle capillary plexus that originates from branches of the bundles and then makes no further contact with them. The *inner medulla* mainly contains descending and ascending vasa recta with few capillaries. These inner medullary vessels have passed through the inner stripe in the vascular bundles. This special vascular organization gives each medullary zone (and its characteristic nephron segments) a specific blood supply, and it establishes between adjacent zones definite relationships or separations that will be described below.

In species such as beaver [28, 29], hippopotamus, or pig [28], the inner medulla is virtually absent, and there are no or very few long-looped nephrons. This is considered to be an adaptation to life in a water-rich environment and it does not correspond to a primitive form of mammalian kidney, since nearly all Eutherians (mammals in the strictest sense) [28]—but also Protherians (marsupials) [30]—have both short- and long-looped nephrons; hence, they have an inner medulla. In the medulla of these kidneys that lack long loops, the medullary vessels show a less strict organization than in other mammals [31]; however, numerous narrow vascular bundles are present (Kriz, personal communication). Even in species where it is normally developed, the inner medulla—because of its conical shape—represents a very small fraction of the total kidney volume (2 to 4% in the rat, rabbit, hamster, and humans) [7].

Vascular-Tubular Relationships in the Medulla

The kidney includes two systems of fluids that circulate in different structures: urinary fluid in the tubules and blood in the blood vessels. Exchanges between or within juxtaposed elements of these two systems may be influenced by the wall properties of each structure, the area of contact between them, their relative flow rates, and the presence of an interstitium between them. The permeability and transport properties of the various nephron segments have been reviewed [32, 33] and the ultrastructure of the medullary vessels has been described in detail elsewhere [3, 6, 7, 34, 35]. Regarding the interstitium, the volume occupied by the interstitial space and cells in the different zones of the rat kidney has been determined recently [36, 37]. The outer stripe is the region with the least interstitium; hence, it is the region where tubules and vessels make the closest contacts. The inner stripe has a

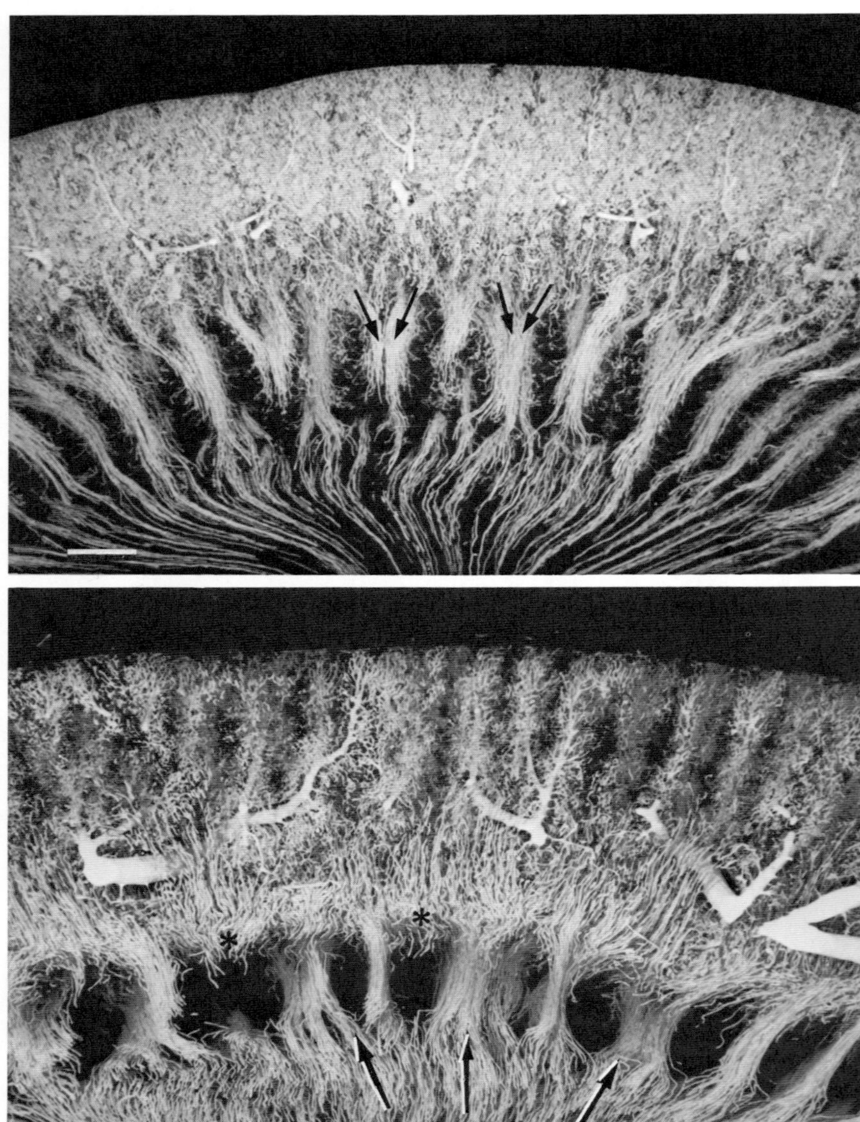

Fig. 4. Sagittal sections of gerboa (*Jaculus orientalis*) kidneys following arterial (*top*) or venous (*bottom*) injection with Microfil silicone rubber. The arterial filling adequately shows the fusion of primary vascular bundles into larger units in the lower outer stripe (*arrows*). The venous filling shows how vasa recta ascending from the inner medulla (*arrows*) rejoin the bundles to cross the inner stripe. The vascular bundles dissipate in the outer stripe and their vessels merge with those ascending from the interbundle region of the inner stripe (*asterisks*). (Bar, $\cong$ 800 μm)

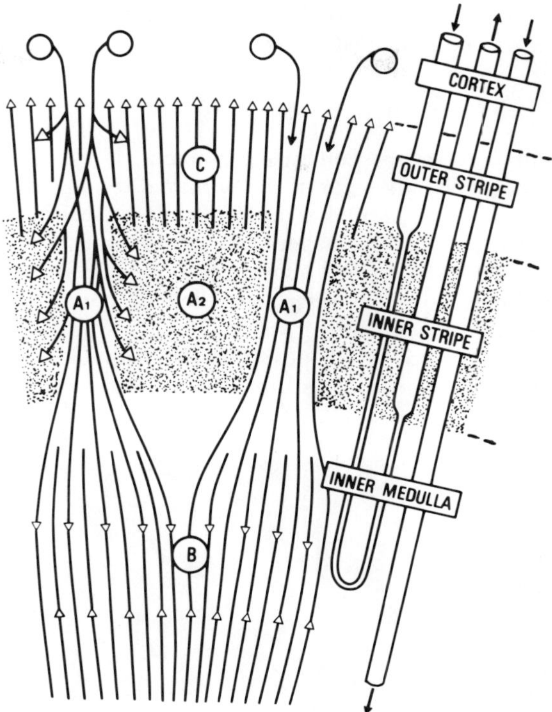

Fig. 5. Schematic representation of the medullary circulation. Efferent arterioles of juxtamedullary glomeruli (*circles*) give rise to the descending vasa recta, some of which descend to the inner medulla (*B*), while others supply the inner stripe capillary plexus (A_2). Vessels supplying or returning from the inner medulla cross the inner stripe in the vascular bundles (A_1). (The vascular bundles always contain both descending and ascending vessels. Some vessels have been omitted here for clarity.) The outer stripe (*C*) receives its main blood supply from the venous vasa recta that ascend from both the inner stripe and the inner medulla. At the corticomedullary border, these venous vasa recta empty into the arcuate veins or the late interlobular veins (not shown). In summary, each medullary zone (outer stripe, inner stripe, and inner medulla) has its own unique vascular organization (*C, A,* and *B,* respectively) and tubular composition (see schematic nephron on the right). In addition, the inner stripe includes, at the same level, two spatially separated compartments (A_1 and A_2).

moderately developed interstitium that increases in relative volume from the outer-inner medullary border to the papillary tip. The interstitium is unequally distributed in the inner stripe. Relatively abundant in the interbundle region, it is virtually absent in the vascular bundles (Kriz, personal communication), thus allowing very intimate contact between vascular and possibly tubular (short-looped thin limb, see below) structures running in the bundles.

The relationships between vessels and tubules vary in the different zones of the medulla, and they favor different types of exchanges between them, as will be described below.

The Outer Stripe

The outer stripe contains pars recta, thick ascending limbs, and collecting ducts. The pars recta of the proximal tubules is the most prominent segment of this zone; it makes up 80% of the epithelial tissue [37], with a large contribution of the longer and more tortuous pars "recta" of the deep nephrons [9, 11]. As described above, there is little arterial blood supply in this zone and the "nutrient" vessels are the vasa recta that ascend from both the inner medulla and the inner stripe (Fig. 2). Since ascending vasa recta are wide channels whose walls adjust to the available space between the tubules (Fig. 6) with very little interstitium, there is a large area of contact between descend-

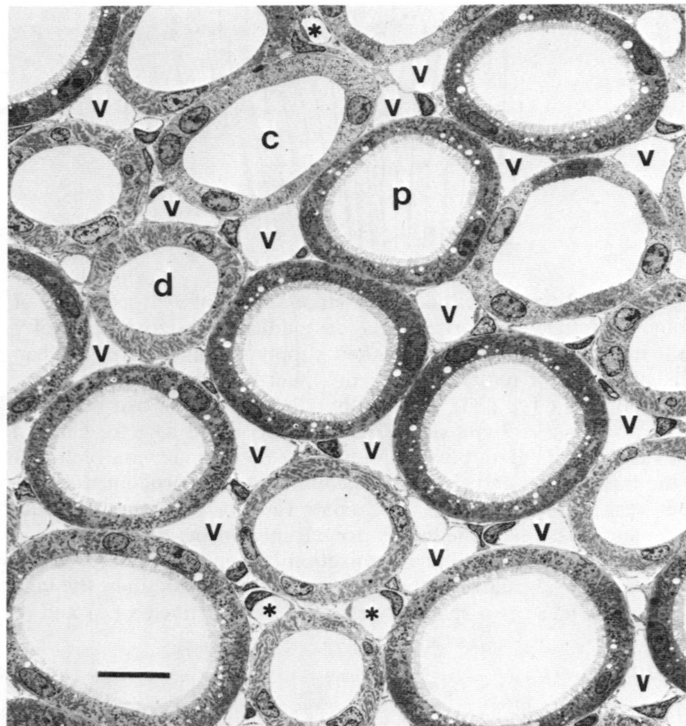

Fig. 6. Electron micrograph of the outer stripe of the rat kidney in a cross-section showing pars recta of proximal and distal (that is, thick ascending limb) tubules (*p* and *d,* respectively), collecting ducts (*c*), and arterial and venous vasa recta (*asterisk and V*). Note the virtual absence of interstitium, the high density of venous vasa recta, and their large area of contact with the proximal straight tubules. Compare with Figure 2. (Bar $\cong$ 15 μm; picture by Wilhelm Kriz, Heidelberg, Federal Republic of Germany)

ing pars recta and ascending vasa recta. The vasa recta wall consists of a thin, fenestrated endothelium, like that of capillaries [5–7]. The blood velocity in these vessels is probably low, since their total cross-sectional area is extremely large (there is a great number of wide vessels, 20 to 40 μm in diameter [7]). These factors will favor the re-entry into the descending tubules—just at the entrance of the medullary osmotic gradient—of solutes coming up from the deeper medullary regions that are about to escape from the kidney in the venous blood [9, 11]. Urea, which can be secreted by the pars recta [38], probably is recycled by this route.

There are only slight species differences regarding the organization of the outer stripe. They include a certain variation in the relative thickness of this zone and a variable penetration of the ascending vasa recta into the deep cortex. Both of these factors affect the total tubular length along which those exchanges and transports (characteristic for the outer stripe) are possible. The outer stripe is very narrow in dogs, cats, and humans and is well developed in rats [10]. In most mammals (including the rat, rabbit, mouse, dog, and humans), ascending vasa recta empty into arcuate veins or into the deep interlobular arteries, penetrating only for a short distance into the medullary rays. Consequently, the medullary rays of the cortex—although having the same tubular composition as the outer stripe (with no or little contribution of deep nephron segments)—have a different blood supply, since they receive their blood from the cortical capillary plexus that originates from efferent arterioles of superficial and midcortical glomeruli. In a few desert-adapted rodents (such as *Psammomys*), ascending vasa recta rise high into the medullary rays and penetrate nearly three-quarters of the total thickness of the cortex [18]. This extends the vascular environment of the outer stripe and, hence, the possibility of solute recycling into the medullary rays.

The Inner Stripe

The inner stripe contains two adjacent compartments, as is clearly visible in Figures 3 and 7 (top). The vascular bundles can be compared to a highway that supplies and drains the inner medulla. The interbundle capillary plexus supplies the thin descending limbs, thick ascending limbs, and collecting ducts. Departing from this general pattern, fundamental species differences exist in the organization of the inner stripe in some rodents [7, 10, 11, 39]. They involve: (1) the position of the thin descending limbs of short-looped nephrons with respect to the bundles, and (2) the size of the vascular bundles.

In the basic pattern observed in most mammals (including the cat, dog, monkey, humans, pig, rabbit, guinea pig, and golden hamster [7, 10, 12, 17, 24, 40]), vascular bundles are numerous, relatively small, and exclusively comprise descending and ascending vessels. In the interbundle region, short-looped nephrons lie closer to the collecting ducts and long-looped nephrons lie closer to the vascular bundles; this can be expected from the ontogenic development of the successive nephron populations. In some rodents, the thin descending branches of short-looped nephrons deviate slightly from their normal course in the deep outer stripe and early inner stripe, and they come closer to the vascular bundles (as in the rat [39]), or even penetrate the

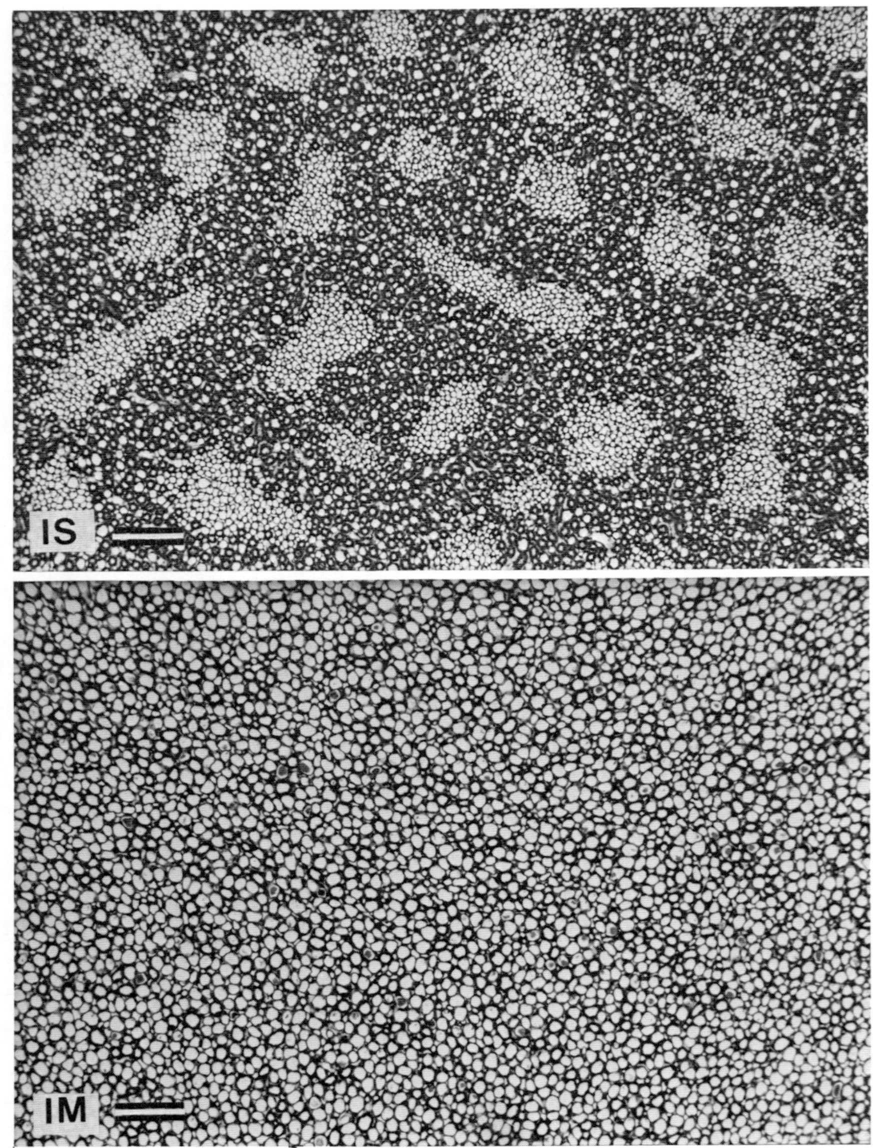

Fig. 7. Cross-sections of rat kidney through the mid-inner stripe (*IS, top*) and early inner medulla (*IM, bottom*). The inner stripe includes two distinct compartments: the vascular bundles (*light*) and the interbundle regions (*dark*). In contrast, the inner medulla displays a homogeneous structure, with vascular and tubular elements evenly distributed in a single compartment. [Bar, $\cong$ 200 μm (*IS*) and $\cong$ 100 μm (*IM*)]

vascular bundles (as in the mouse [41] and several desert-adapted rodents such as the Mongolian gerbil, gerboa [10], *Psammomys* [25], or the pocket mouse [42]). The result of this is that in the inner stripe, the thin descending limbs of short loops lie at the periphery of or even within the vascular bundles, among the descending and ascending vessels. This reorganization is depicted schematically in Figure 8. When they turn close to the inner stripe-inner medulla transition, the short loops leave the bundles and ascend in the inter-bundle region. This structural modification never involves the long loops, whose descending and ascending limbs always lie in the interbundle region. Vascular bundles containing only vasa recta are called "simple-type bundles," whereas those also containing thin limbs of short loops are called "complex-type bundles" [10].

A second species difference is the size of the bundles. In a few rodents, several "primary" vascular bundles converge early in their course through the inner stripe to form fewer "secondary" (mouse) or even fewer "giant" vascular bundles (Mongolian gerbil, gerboa, *Psammomys*) (Fig. 3, bottom, and Fig. 4, top) [7, 10, 11, 18, 43].

These two adaptations of the inner stripe organization are found only in rodents, and they are best developed in desert-inhabiting species. Both adaptations often are associated, but the incorporation of short-looped thin limbs into the bundles can be observed in the absence of vascular bundle fusion in the pocket mouse [42]. Both may be absent in some desert-inhabiting species, such as the gundi [43] and the chinchilla [16]. These adaptations might influence the maximum concentrating ability of the kidney, but also the time required to establish the medullary osmotic gradient (Bankir and de Rouffignac, in preparation).

Another species difference is the thickness of the inner stripe. The thickness of a given zone determines, for "straight" nephron segments, the length along which they will be in a characteristic environment. The inner stripe is relatively thin in *Psammomys* [18, 25] and much thicker in the pocket mouse [44]—two species that have a long papilla and a high urine concentrating ability. However, *Psammomys* has few giant vascular bundles, while the pocket mouse has numerous narrow bundles, although the bundles include short-looped thin limbs in both cases [25, 42].

What are the functional consequences of the particular organization of the inner stripe vessels? How do the modifications displayed by some rodents affect the concentrating mechanism?

Vascular Bundles

The fact that the vessels going to or coming from the inner medulla run in bundles separated from the tubules of the inner stripe hinders exchanges with the tubules and promotes exchange between the ascending and descending vessels in the bundles. As clearly explained by Kriz in many articles [5, 7–11, 18], "blood flowing to the inner medulla has not previously been exposed to tubules of the outer and inner stripes. Blood that has perfused tubules of the inner medulla does not then perfuse tubules of the inner stripe"

[7]. In the bundles, both the parallel arrangement of descending and ascending vessels and the virtual absence of interstitium between them favor countercurrent exchanges of water and solutes (Fig. 8A). Water can be short-circuited from descending to the ascending vessels, while solutes coming from the solute-rich inner medullary interstitium may be added to descending vessels, thereby preventing their loss in the venous blood. The fusion of primary bundles into larger groups of vessels improves the efficiency of this exchange, and it better isolates the inner medulla from the outer medulla [7, 10, 18].

The incorporation of the thin limbs of short loops into the vascular bundles (Fig. 8 B and C) creates new possibilities for solute recycling; and, it probably enhances solute recovery from the inner medulla and its selective addition to the short loops. What are the solute-recycling possibilities in the simple-

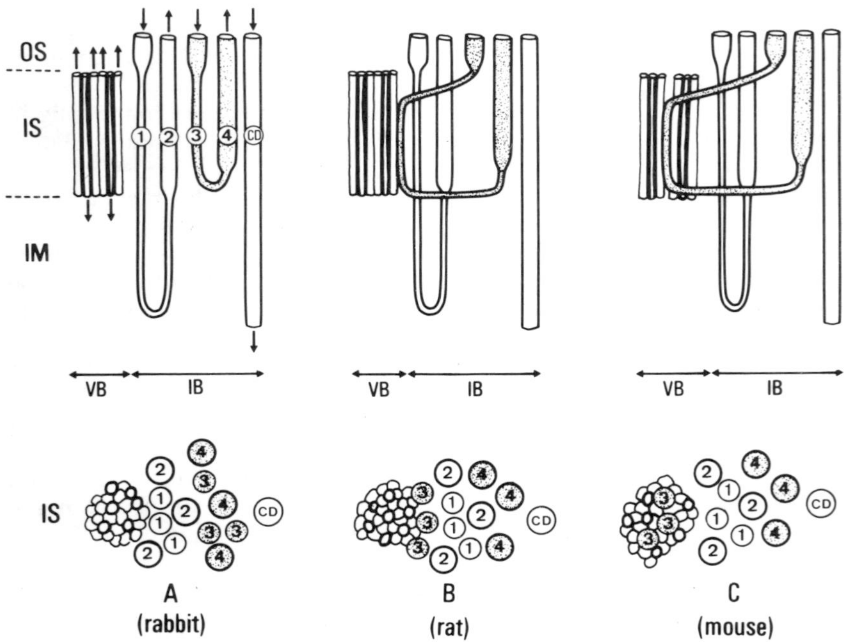

Fig. 8. Organization of the inner stripe schematically shown longitudinally (*top*) and cross-sectionally (*bottom*). The location of the tubular segments with respect to the vascular bundles, as it appears in a typical mammalian kidney, is depicted on the left (**A**). Varying degrees of modifications are observed in some rodents. Thin descending limbs of short-looped nephrons are incorporated at the periphery of (**B**) or into the vascular bundles (**C**). In addition (not shown here), several vascular bundles may fuse to form larger, but fewer, units (see Fig. 4). Abbreviations are: *OS, IS,* and *IM,* outer stripe, inner stripe, and inner medulla, respectively; *VB* and *IB,* vascular bundles and interbundle region, respectively; *1* to *4,* loops of Henle, that is, thin descending (*1*) and thick ascending (*2*) limbs of long-looped nephrons, and thin descending (*3*) and thick ascending (*4*) limbs of short-looped nephrons; *CD,* collecting ducts.

type kidney (rabbit, humans)? To establish and maintain a high osmotic gradient in the inner medulla, it is essential to minimize the escape of solutes from this zone. Solute escape from the inner medulla in an upward direction can occur through three possible ways: (1) through ascending vessels, (2) through ascending tubules, and (3) through axial diffusion in the interstitium. The escape of medullary solutes via the renal lymph does not seem possible, since there are no lymphatics in the medulla [45]. Axial diffusion is reduced by the ladder arrangement of the interstitial cells. Regarding the first two routes: (1) Solutes leaving the inner medulla *via the tubules* (thick ascending limbs) are partly returned to the inner medulla by two routes: in the inner stripe, sodium chloride is reabsorbed by the thick ascending limbs, and may be reintroduced from the solute-rich interstitium of the interbundle region into the descending thin limbs lying nearby. Urea is little reabsorbed in the ascending thick limb, distal tubule, and early collecting duct; thus, it is carried to the more urea-permeable inner medullary collecting ducts [46] from where it may diffuse into the inner medullary interstitium. (2) Solutes leaving the inner medulla *via the ascending vessels* can be recaptured in the descending vasa recta running in parallel in the vascular bundles. If the thin descending limbs of short loops are also incorporated at the periphery of—or into— the bundles (as in the rat, mouse, and some desert rodents), the close contact between thin limbs and ascending vasa recta will favor the recapture of solutes ascending from the inner medulla into the short loops of Henle. Subsequently, sodium chloride can be reabsorbed by the thick ascending limbs, and urea that is not reabsorbed in the distal nephron can diffuse across the medullary collecting duct, as already described. The importance of short loops in both urea recycling and efficiency of the urine concentrating mechanism is empha- sized both in comparative anatomy (Table 1 in [47]) and computer simulation studies [48].

Since such structural modifications to the vascular bundles certainly affect the composition of the fluid entering the medullary thick ascending limbs of short loops (and hence the workload delivered to this segment), they should be considered when comparing data obtained from different species with different degrees of vascular bundle modification; or, when comparing data obtained in vivo with that obtained in vitro.

Interbundle Regions

In these regions, the existence of a dense capillary plexus—representing the largest relative vascular volume in the kidney—and the presence of a relatively well-developed interstitium create a totally different situation than in the nearby bundles. The vessels form a random capillary plexus, suggesting a nutrient role without direct countercurrent exchanges between vessels and tubules in this compartment. In all species, the capillary plexus of the inner stripe stops at the inner stripe-inner medullary border (Fig. 3) [2, 5, 12, 16, 18, 44]. This transition coincides exactly with the equally abrupt transition of thin-into-thick ascending limbs (Fig. 5). The latter segment (or straight part of the distal tubule), which makes up 60% of the epithelium volume in the inner stripe [36, 37], has a high metabolic rate [49, 50], is rich in mitochondria [37, 51], and displays a high Na/K-ATPase activity [52, 53] in accordance with its intensely active sodium chloride transport. This nephron segment is the first to suffer from anoxic damage in the isolated perfused kidney [54], and the inner stripe is the first medullary region in which blood flow is impaired in ischemic renal failure [55].

Due to the vigorous reabsorption of sodium chloride by the medullary thick ascending limb, the interstitial sodium chloride concentration should be relatively high in the interbundle compartment, thus favoring salt entry there into the thin descending limbs. In most mammals and in the rabbit, all thin descending limbs are found in the interbundle region. However, in the rat and even more so in the mouse and in some desert rodents (*Psammomys*, Mongolian gerbil, gerboa, but not in the hamster), the thin descending limbs of short loops are removed from this environment because they are included into the vascular bundles. Thus, in these species, only the thin descending limbs of long loops cross the salt-rich interbundle interstitium. The early part of the thin limbs in long loops have a more complex epithelial structure than that of short loops [7, 10, 56] (for detailed description and interspecies differences). The extremely developed intercellular infoldings and the amplification of the tight junctional belt (except in the rabbit) are suggestive of an important paracellular pathway. In agreement with this morphology, a high permeability to sodium was recently demonstrated in this segment (except in the rabbit) [57]; therefore, it seems that sodium may be added to the tubular fluid and, thus, may be returned to the inner medulla via the thin descending limbs of long loops. In addition, a significant Na/K-ATPase activity, which is also found in this segment, could be involved in potassium recycling [58]. (The main species differences with regard to the inner stripe organization [namely the incorporation of thin limbs of short loops into the vascular bundles, the fusion of bundles, and the development of a special type of epithelium in the early thin descending limbs of long loops] may be present and/or variably developed *independently* of each other in the different rodent species.)

The Inner Medulla

The vascular and tubular structures in the inner medulla form a homogeneous compartment without any apparent regular pattern (Fig. 7, bottom). In the early inner medulla, vascular bundles may still be present, but their vessels progressively disperse among thin limbs and collecting ducts. Descending and ascending vasa recta can be distinguished according to the ultrastructure of their wall. Descending vessels display a continuous endothelium, whereas ascending ones are fenestrated [35]. The abundant interstitium around tubules and vessels creates a homogeneous environment at any level of the inner medulla. Lateral diffusion is certainly favored and axial diffusion is restricted by numerous interstitial cells that are arranged horizontally like the rungs of a ladder between tubules and vessels [7].

Several studies have revealed that ascending vessels outnumber descending ones in the inner medulla [59–61]. Because of the well-developed interstitium in this zone, the functionally important consequence of the more numerous ascending vasa recta is not the increase in the area of contact with descending vessels and loops, but the reduction in vascular resistance and flow velocity in ascending vessels. As confirmed experimentally, flow is slower in ascending than in descending vasa recta [59, 60, 62]. This improves the diffusion of solutes out of the vessels as blood ascends through the decreasing osmotic gradient; thus it reduces the loss of solute from the inner medulla to the venous blood. As described above, the anatomic vascular-tubular relationships suggest an additional recovery of solutes from ascending vasa recta in the next two medullary regions that they cross; that is, the inner and the outer stripes, but by different routes at each level in accordance with their specific vascular and interstitial patterns. In the outer stripe, solutes can be reintroduced preferentially into the pars recta of mainly the long loops. In the inner stripe, they can be reintroduced along the vascular bundles into the vasa recta descending to the inner medulla; and, in some species, possibly into the thin limbs of short loops. In the inner medulla, solutes can be reintroduced into both descending vasa recta and descending thin limbs of long loops via the interstitium.

No major species differences exist in the organization of the inner medulla. However, the length of the papilla [7, 10, 28, 63, 64] and the relative number of loops and collecting ducts [36] vary from one species to another. A longer papilla supplies a greater distance for the operation of the countercurrent multiplication system. A relatively high collecting duct-to-loop ratio in the rat, as opposed to the rabbit [36], probably favors the influence of inner medullary collecting ducts on the final composition of the urine.

Regulation of the Medullary Blood Supply

Possible Sites and Modes of Regulation

Because of the topographic organization of the medullary vessels, two successive steps must be considered regarding the regulation of the medullary circulation. First, is the total blood flow to the medulla from the efferent arterioles of juxtamedullary glomeruli regulated? Second, within the medulla itself, is the blood flow to the inner stripe and that to the inner medulla controlled independently? In other words, is there a regulation of the "intramedullary distribution of blood flow?" Several anatomic features are relevant to these two points.

First, the efferent arterioles of the juxtamedullary glomeruli are much wider than the afferents, in contrast to the situation in other glomeruli; and, their muscular wall is much better developed, with up to three layers of smooth muscle cells in their early course and their first branches in the outer stripe [2, 4, 7, 12, 23, 27]. The number of muscle cells decreases as the vessels penetrate the deeper regions of the medulla, where they are progressively replaced by pericytes. The innervation of the juxtaglomerular apparatus is highly developed in juxtamedullary nephrons [65, 66]; also, adrenergic axons run along the efferent arterioles and vasa recta for a relatively long distance within the outer medulla [67, 68]. This muscular and nervous equipment suggests that the medullary circulation may well be controlled by circulating vasoactive substances and by neuroadrenergic stimuli.

Concerning the independent control of blood flow to the inner stripe capillary plexus and to the inner medulla, two possible sites of regulation may be considered. The blood flow to each territory may be controlled at an early site. A selective constriction of some descending vasa recta, and not of others, in the outer and/or inner stripe is conceivable. This seems possible, since two types of descending vasa recta have been identified [6]. In all species, a few vessels located centrally in each vascular bundle, which probably reach the deepest levels in the inner medulla, have a larger caliber and a thicker wall than other arterial vasa recta. Their endothelium resembles that of early juxtamedullary efferent arterioles with numerous cells and nuclei protruding into the lumen. These features may be retained in some vessels down to the inner medulla [6, 7].

The blood flow to each territory also may be controlled more distally by alterations in vascular resistance in later portions of the vasculature. Changes in interstitial pressure in the interbundle region of the inner stripe may affect vascular resistances in the inner stripe capillary plexus, without affecting blood supply to the inner medulla. This type of situation is seen in postischemic renal failure, when blood stasis is observed in the inner stripe even though inner medullary perfusion is well preserved [55]. Alternatively, the high inner medullary osmotic pressure in the concentrating kidney could reduce vascular bundle [69] and inner medullary blood flow by increasing blood viscosity [70]. Indeed, papillary plasma flow is low in rats that produce a maximally concentrated urine after 48 hr of water deprivation [71]. However, captopril (blocking angiotensin II formation), given before and during water deprivation, increases papillary plasma flow to very high values without impairing urinary concentration [71]; this suggests that papillary blood supply is controlled by hormonally mediated vasoconstriction, rather than by osmotically mediated changes in vascular resistance. One further factor could possibly affect inner medullary blood flow without exerting much effect on outer medullary flow. Peristaltic contractions of the pelvic wall make papillary vasa recta flow discontinuous [72]. The frequency and duration of these contractions may influence time-averaged papillary blood flow.

From the large number of ascending vessels and from their increasing cross-sectional area (7 to 15 μm in the inner medulla and inner stripe, 20 to 40 μm in the outer stripe) [7], one can expect: (1) blood to decrease in velocity as it moves toward the corticomedullary border, and (2) the vascular resistance in the outer stripe to be minimized. In most capillary beds, capillaries converge progressively to form venules and veins. In the medulla, ascending vessels converge not at all or only at the very last moment, just before reaching the arcuate veins; thereby, they delay their reduction in the total cross-sectional area.

Measurement of Medullary Blood Flow

Because of the organization of the medullary circulation into compartments, evaluation of the medullary blood flow is difficult. The concept itself is ambiguous, as already underlined [73]. Theoretically, "medullary blood flow" should include the total flow entering the medulla, which is a flow very close to the sum of blood flow in all efferent arterioles of juxtamedullary glomeruli. Then, this flow functionally divides into one part supplying the inner stripe and another part supplying the inner medulla. The concept of blood flow per gram of tissue in the medulla is meaningless, except in the interbundle capillary plexus of the inner stripe. However, due to the juxtaposition of vascular bundles and interbundle region, it is technically not feasible to assess separately blood flow *to* the inner stripe and blood flow *through* the inner stripe to supply the inner medulla. Furthermore, the short-circuiting of water between descending and ascending vasa recta decreases descending flow; the addition of water reabsorbed from collecting ducts increases the ascending flow.

In addition, plasma and red blood cell flows are not similar in all compartments of the medulla. The hematocrit is lower in the inner than in the outer medulla [74, 75]. This diminishes the exposure of erythrocytes to the high osmotic pressures of the inner medulla and extends their lifespan [76]. However, the short-circuiting of water between descending and ascending vasa recta in the vascular bundles and in the inner medulla should increase the hematocrit progressively as blood proceeds in the medulla and papilla. Therefore, the low papillary hematocrit implies that some plasma-red blood cell separation occurs at a postglomerular level, so that red blood cell-enriched blood is directed to the inner stripe and plasma-enriched blood is directed to the inner medulla. Curiously, "arterial cushions" generally are observed at the origin of the afferent arterioles of juxtamedullary glomeruli [77, 78]. They might induce the formation of streamlines that are differently enriched in plasma or red blood cells. However, it is difficult to conceive that these lines could be maintained through the glomerular tufts and efferent arterioles. The mechanism that is responsible for the low inner medullary hematocrit remains unclear.

In works aimed at studying the regulation of the medullary blood flow, either in the entire medulla or in certain regions of the medulla, the consequences of the structural organization of the medullary vascular beds should be discussed, in addition to the specific technical or theoretic limitations inherent to each of the presently available methods.

Summary

Each of the three medullary zones (the outer stripe and inner stripe of the outer medulla, and the inner medulla) has its own vascular pattern. This creates a specific vascular environment for the nephron segments found in each zone. In the *outer stripe,* the efferent arterioles of the juxtamedullary glomeruli divide into bundles of parallel vessels that give only a few side branches to supply the outer stripe tubules. The real "nutrient" blood supply of the outer stripe is provided by the numerous capillary-like vasa recta ascending from the inner stripe and the inner medulla. These vessels show a large area of direct contact (no interstitium) with the pars recta of proximal tubules, thus offering an ultimate recycling possibility for solutes that are about to escape from the medulla in the venous blood. The *inner stripe* contains two distinct vascular territories: (1) the "vascular bundles," containing the vessels going to or coming from the inner medulla, and (2) the "interbundle regions," where the tubules are surrounded by a rich capillary plexus originating from the most external branches of the vascular bundles. This plexus supplies the metabolically very active thick ascending limbs. It makes no contact with the inner medulla and stops abruptly at the outer-inner medullary border (also the limit of the thick ascending limbs), thus isolating the inner medulla from the inner stripe. The *inner medulla* itself receives blood from the most central branches of the bundles. Descending and ascending vasa recta run parallel with loops and collecting tubules and are surrounded by an abundant interstitium. Vasa recta ascending from the inner medulla join the vascular bundle to cross the inner stripe, making no contact in this zone with the capillary plexus and tubules. However, in a few rodents, thin limbs of short-looped nephrons deviate from their normal course and run within the vascular bundles, thereby making intimate contact with the vessels descending to and ascending from the inner medulla, creating a possible route for solute (mainly urea) recycling, thus improving urine concentrating ability. The vascular organization of the medulla isolates different medullary compartments and creates in each of them several possible routes for reintroducing, in descending tubules, solutes that would otherwise escape from the medulla.

References

1. DANTZLER WH, BRAUN EJ: Comparative nephron function in reptiles, birds and mammals. *Am J Physiol* 239(*Reg Integr Comp Physiol* 8): R197–R213, 1980
2. MOFFAT DB, FOURMAN J: The vascular pattern of the rat kidney. *J Anat* 97:543–553, 1963
3. MOFFAT DB: The fine structure of the blood vessels of the renal medulla with particular reference to the control of the medullary circulation. *J Ultrastruct Res* 19:532–545, 1967
4. FOURMAN J, MOFFAT DB: *The Blood Vessels of the Kidney.* Oxford and Edinburgh, Blackwell Scientific Publications, 1971
5. ROLLHÄUSER H, KRIZ W, HEINKE W: Das Gefäßsystem der Rattenniere. *Z Zellforsch Mikrosk Anat* 64:381–403, 1964
6. KRIZ W, DIETERICH HJ: The supplying and draining vessels of the renal medulla in mammals, in *Proc 4th Int Cong Nephrol, Stockholm 1969,* Basel, Karger, 1970, vol 1, pp 138–144
7. JAMISON RL, KRIZ W: *Urinary Concentrating Mechanism: Structure and Function.* New York and Oxford, Oxford University Press, 1982
8. KRIZ W, BARRETT JM, PETER S: The renal vasculature: anatomical-functional aspects, in *Kidney and Urinary Tract Physiology II,* edited by THURAU K, Baltimore, University Park Press, 1976, vol II, pp 1–21
9. KRIZ W: Structural organization of renal medullary circulation. *Nephron* 31:290–295, 1982
10. KRIZ W: Structural organization of the renal medulla: comparative and functional aspects. *Am J Physiol* 241(*Reg Integr Comp Physiol* 10):R3–R16, 1981

11. KRIZ W: Structural organization of the renal medullary counterflow system. *Fed Proc* 42:2379–2385, 1983
12. BEEUWKES R III: Efferent vascular patterns and early vascular-tubular relations in the dog kidney. *Am J Physiol* 221:1361–1374, 1971
13. BEEUWKES R III, BONVENTRE JV: Tubular organization and vascular-tubular relations in the dog kidney. *Am J Physiol* 229:695–713, 1975
14. BEEUWKES R III: The vascular organization of the kidney. *Ann Rev Physiol* 42:531–542, 1980
15. BEEUWKES R III: Vascular-tubular relationships in the human kidney, in *Renal Pathophysiology,* edited by LEAF A, COTRAN RS, New York, Raven Press, 1980, pp 155–163
16. PRONG LA, BJORAKER DG, HARVEY RB: Comparison of the renal medullary vascular systems of dog and chinchilla. *Microvasc Res* 1:275–286, 1969
17. BULGER RE, CRONIN RE, DOBYAN DC: Survey of the morphology of the dog kidney. *Anat Rec* 194:41–66, 1979
18. BANKIR L, KAISSLING B, DE ROUFFIGNAC C, KRIZ W: The vascular organization of the kidney of Psammomys obesus. *Anat Embryol* 155:149–160, 1979
19. SPELLER AM, MOFFAT DB: Tubulo-vascular relationships in the developing kidney. *J Anat* 123:487–500, 1977
20. KNEPPER M, BURG M: Organization of nephron function. *Am J Physiol* 244(*Renal Fluid Electrolyte Physiol* 13):F579–589, 1983
21. TAKAZAKURA E, SAWABU N, HANDA A, TAKADA A, SHINODA A, TAKEUCHI J: Intrarenal vascular changes with age and disease. *Kidney Int* 2:224–230, 1972
22. CASELLAS D, MIMRAN A: Shunting in renal microvasculature of the rat: a scanning electron microscopic study of corrosion casts. *Anat Rec* 201:237–248, 1981
23. BANKIR L, FARMAN N: Hétérogénéité des glomérules chez le lapin. *Arch Anat Microsc Morphol Exp* 62:281–291, 1973
24. KAISSLING B, KRIZ W: Structural analysis of the rabbit kidney. *Adv Anat Embryol Cell Biol* 56:1–123, 1979
25. KAISSLING B, DE ROUFFIGNAC C, BARRETT JM, KRIZ W: The structural organization of the kidney of the desert rodent *Psammomys obesus. Anat Embryol* 148:121–143, 1975
26. EVAN AP, DAIL WG: Efferent arterioles in the cortex of the rat kidney. *Anat Rec* 187:135–145, 1977
27. EDWARDS JG: Efferent arterioles of glomeruli in the juxtamedullary zone of the human kidney. *Anat Rec* 125:521–529, 1956
28. SPERBER I: Studies on the mammalian kidney. *Zool Bidr Uppsala* 22:249–432, 1944
29. PFEIFFER EW, NUNGESSER WC, IVERSON DA, WALLERIUS JF: The renal anatomy of the primitive rodent, *Aplodontia rufa,* and a consideration of its functional significance. *Anat Rec* 137:227–232, 1960
30. BURGER CH, CROSS RB: Aspects of renal vascular organization and early vascular tubular relations of the marsupial *Isoodon obesulus. Anat Rec* 203:47–54, 1982
31. PLAKKE RK, PFEIFFER EW: Blood vessels of the mammalian renal medulla. *Science* 146:1683–1685, 1964
32. BERRY CA: Heterogeneity of tubular transport processes in the nephron. *Ann Rev Physiol* 44:181–201, 1982
33. JACOBSON HR, KOKKO JP: Isolated perfused tubules. *Kidney Int* 22:415–570, 1982
34. DIETERICH HJ, SCHÜRHOLZ KH: Die Ultrastruktur der Gefäße im Mark der Rattenniere. *Verh Anat Ges* 67:S47–58, 1973
35. SCHWARTZ IL, KARNOVSKY MA, VENKATACHALAM MA: Ultrastructural differ-

ences between rat inner medullary descending and ascending vasa recta. *Lab Invest* 35:161–170, 1976

36. KNEPPER MA, DANIELSON RA, SAIDEL GM, POST RS: Quantitative analysis of renal medullary anatomy in rats and rabbits. *Kidney Int* 12:313–323, 1977

37. PFALLER W: Structure-function correlation on rat kidney: Quantitative correlation of structure and function in the normal and injured rat kidney. *Adv Anat Embryol Cell Biol* 70:1–106, 1982

38. KAWAMURA S, KOKKO JP: Urea secretion by the straight segment of the proximal tubule. *J Clin Invest* 58:604–612, 1976

39. KRIZ W, SCHNERMANN J, KOEPSELL H: The position of short and long loops of Henle in the rat kidney. *Z Anat Entwickl Gesch* 138:301–319, 1972

40. TISHER CC, SCHRIER RW, MCNEIL JS: Nature of urine concentrating mechanism in the macaque monkey. *Am J Physiol* 223:1128–1137, 1972

41. KRIZ W, KOEPSELL H: The structural organization of the mouse kidney. *Z Anat Entwickl Gesch* 144:137–163, 1974

42. NAGEL RB, ALTSCHULER EM, DOBYAN DC, DONG S, BULGER RE: The ultrastructure of the thin limbs of Henle in kidneys of the desert heteromyid (*Perognathus penicillatus*). *Am J Anat* 161:33–47, 1981

43. DE ROUFFIGNAC C, BANKIR L, ROINEL N: Renal function and concentrating ability in a desert rodent: the gundi (*Ctenodactylus vali*). *Pflügers Arch* 390:138–144, 1981

44. ALTSCHULER EM, NAGLE RB, BRAUN EJ, LINDSTEDT SL, KRUTZSCH PH: Morphological study of the desert heteromyid kidney with emphasis on the Genus perognathus. *Anat Rec* 194:461–468, 1979

45. KRIZ W, DIETERICH HJ: Das Lymphgefäßsystem der Niere bei einigen Säugetieren. Licht- und Elektronenmikroskopische Untersuchungen. *Z Anat Entwickl Gesch* 131:111–147, 1970

46. ROCHA AS, KOKKO JP: Permeability of medullary nephron segments to urea and water: Effect of vasopressin. *Kidney Int* 6:379–387, 1974

47. VALTIN H: Structural and functional heterogeneity of mammalian nephrons. *Am J Physiol* 233(*Renal Fluid Electrolyte Physiol* 2):F491–F501, 1977

48. STEPHENSON JL, MEJIA R: Theoretical bounds on the passive concentrating mechanism, in *Abs Proc Int Union Physiol Sci 29th Congr,* Sidney, Australia, 1983, p 419

49. KIIL F, JOHANNESEN J, AUKLAND K: Metabolic rate in renal cortex and medulla during mannitol and saline infusion. *Am J Physiol* 220:565–570, 1971

50. SEJERSTED OM, LIE M, KIIL F: Effect of ouabain on metabolic rate in renal cortex and medulla. *Am J Physiol* 220:1488–1493, 1971

51. PFALLER W, RITTINGER M: Quantitative morphology of the rat kidney. *Int J Biochem* 12:17–22, 1980

52. SCHMIDT U, DUBACH UC: Activity of (Na^+K^+)-stimulated adenosine triphosphatase in the rat nephron. *Pflügers Arch* 306:219–226, 1969

53. KATZ AI, DOUCET A, MOREL F: Na-K-ATPase activity along the rabbit, rat and mouse nephron. *Am J Physiol* 237(*Renal Fluid Electrolyte Physiol* 6):F114–F120, 1979

54. BREZIS M, ROSEN S, SILVA P, EPSTEIN F: Selective vulnerability of the medullary thick ascending limb to anoxia in the isolated perfused rat kidney. *J Clin Invest* 73:182–190, 1984

55. TORHORST J, DE ROUGEMONT D, BRUNNER FP, THIEL G: Morphology of the renal medulla in ischemic acute renal failure in the rat. *Nephron* 31:296–300, 1982

56. SCHWARTZ MM, VENKATACHALAM MA: Structural differences in thin limbs of Henle: Physiological implications. *Kidney Int* 6:193–208, 1974

57. IMAI M, ARAKI M: Internephron heterogeneity and interspecies differences in the function of the descending limbs of Henle's loop, in *Abs Proc Int Union Physiol Sci 29th Cong,* Sidney, Australia, 1983, p 418, no 489.07

58. GARG LC, TISHER CC: Na-K-ATPase activity in thin limbs of rat nephron (*abstract*). *Kidney Int* 23:255, 1983

59. MARSH DJ, SEGEL LA: Analysis of countercurrent diffusion exchange in blood vessels of the renal medulla. *Am J Physiol* 221:817–828, 1971

60. HOLLIGER C, LEMLEY KV, SCHMITT SL, THOMAS FC, ROBERTSON CR, JAMISON RL: Direct determination of vasa recta blood flow in the rat renal papilla. *Circ Res* 53:401–413, 1983

61. BÖTTCHER W, STEINHAUSEN M: Microcirculation of the renal papilla of rats under control conditions and after temporary ischemia. *Kidney Int* 10(suppl):S74–S80, 1976

62. GUSSIS GL, ROBERTSON CR, JAMISON RL: Erythrocyte velocity in vasa recta: effect of antidiuretic hormone and saline loading. *Am J Physiol* 237(*Renal Fluid Electrolyte Physiol* 6):F326–F332, 1979

63. SCHMIDT-NIELSEN B, O'DELL R: Structure and concentrating mechanism in the mammalian kidney. *Am J Physiol* 200:1119–1124, 1961

64. BROWNFIELD MS, WUNDER BA: Relative medullary area: A new structural index for estimating urinary concentrating capacity of mammals. *Comp Biochem Physiol* 55A:69–75, 1976

65. BARAJAS L: Anatomy of the juxtaglomerular apparatus. *Am J Physiol* 237(*Renal Fluid Electrolyte Physiol* 6):F333–F343, 1979

66. GORGAS K: Structure and innervation of the juxtaglomerular apparatus of the rat. *Adv Anat Embryol* 54:5–84, 1978

67. DIETERICH HJ: Electron microscopic studies of the innervation of the rat kidney. *Z Anat Entwickl Gesch* 145:169–186, 1974

68. NEWSTEAD J, MUNKACSI I: Electron microscopic observations on the juxtamedullary efferent arterioles and Arteriolae rectae in kidneys of rats. *Z Zellforsch* 97:465–490, 1969

69. FOURMAN J, KENNEDY GC: An effect of antidiuretic hormone on the flow of blood through the vasa recta of the rat kidney. *J Endocrinol* 35:173–176, 1966

70. SCHMID-SCHÖNBEIN H, WELLS RE, GOLDSTONE J: Effect of ultrafiltration and plasma osmolarity upon the flow properties of blood: A possible mechanism for control of blood flow in the renal medullary vasa recta. *Pflügers Arch* 338:93–114, 1973

71. ELOY L, GRÜNFELD JP, BAYLE F, BANKIR L, RAMOS-FRENDO B, TRINH-TRANG-TAN MM: Papillary plasma flow in rats. II. Hormonal control. *Pflügers Arch* 398:253–258, 1983

72. REINKING LN, SCHMIDT-NIELSEN B: Peristaltic flow of urine in the renal papillary collecting ducts of hamsters. *Kidney Int* 20:55–60, 1981

73. RASMUSSEN SN: Red cell and plasma volume flows to the inner medulla of the rat kidney. Determinations by means of a step function input indicator technique. *Pflügers Arch* 373:153–159, 1978

74. RASMUSSEN SN: Intrarenal red cell and plasma volumes in the non-diuretic rat. *Pflügers Arch* 342:61–72, 1973

75. PINTER GG, O'MORCHOE CCC, BLAUMANIS OR, ZISOW DL: Functional implications of differences in red cell and plasma transit through the renal medulla, in *Int Symp Renal Handling Sodium, Brestenberg 1971,* Basel, Karger, 1972, pp 190–197

76. ALEXANDER CS, SWAIM WR, GARCIA MC: Urine concentration and dilution: Effect on red cell survival. *Proc Soc Exp Biol Med* 150:295–298, 1975

77. MOFFAT DB, CREASEY M: The fine structure of the intra-arterial cushions at the origins of the juxtamedullary afferent arterioles in the rat kidney. *J Anat* 110:409–419, 1971
78. CASELLAS D, DUPONT M, JOVER B, MIMRAN A: Scanning electron microscopic study of arterial cushions in rats: A novel application of the corrosion-replication technique. *Anat Rec* 203:419–428, 1982

Pathophysiology of the Medullary Circulation

June Mason

In the mammalian organism, the circulation of the renal medulla is unique, differing markedly in its arrangement and in its function from that of other vascular beds. The renal medulla alone is entrusted with the task of concentrating or diluting the urine, of conserving or excreting the water necessary to preserve the internal ionic concentrations, and the medullary circulation plays a central role in this activity.

The contribution of the medullary circulation toward this achievement can be divided into three components. First, it supplies the metabolic substrates to fuel the active transport of sodium chloride out of the tubules and into the interstitium. Second, through the countercurrent exchange between ascending and descending vasa recta in the vascular bundles, it traps urea reabsorbed from the collecting ducts and sodium chloride transported out of the tubule lumen and establishes the medullary hypertonicity that is necessary for urinary concentration. Third, during the process of urinary concentration, it reabsorbs and removes from the medulla the water extracted from the collecting ducts and descending thin loops of Henle as they penetrate the hypertonic medulla and preserves this hypertonicity.

These different activities place different and, to some extent, opposing demands on the medullary circulation. Medullary blood flow must be *sufficient* to supply the substrates needed for active tubular transport, it must be *low* enough to permit equilibration between ascending and descending vasa recta to ensure adequate trapping of solutes, and it must be *high* enough to effect water removal and prevent dilution of the medullary interstitium. It is the conflicting nature of these individual demands on the medullary circulation that forms the basis of its pathophysiology. Any increase or decrease in medullary blood flow that disturbs the delicate balance between the metabolic, solute-trapping, and water-removing requirements of the circulation, all of which are essential for urinary concentration, will lead to a reduction of urinary concentrating power. Alterations in medullary blood flow, however,

This manuscript was presented as part of a Symposium on *Regulation of Medullary Circulation.*

will have less influence on urinary diluting ability, for this activity depends on the medullary circulation only for the supply of metabolic substrates needed to fuel tubular reabsorption in the thick ascending loops of Henle.

The exact amount of blood supplying the renal medulla is difficult to determine for methodologic reasons, but it is generally agreed that the outer medulla receives 5 to 13% of the total blood flow to the kidney [1–6], whereas the inner medulla does not receive more than 3% of that supplying the whole kidney [1, 3–9]. These seemingly small fractions should not be interpreted as indicating that medullary blood flow is low in absolute terms, for in the outer medulla it is greater per gram of tissue than it is in either brain or cardiac muscle; and in the inner medulla, where it is comparable to that in brain and cardiac muscle, it is still several times higher than that of resting skeletal muscle.

Despite the apparent adequacy of medullary blood flow, it seems that the oxygen supply to the medullary tissues may indeed by very low. First, because of the efficient countercurrent exchange for small molecules in the vascular bundles, oxygen diffuses out of the descending (arterial) vasa recta and into the ascending (venous) vessels, causing the oxygen tension of blood and tissue to fall with increasing depth into the medulla. This has been demonstrated by inserting oxygen electrodes through the cortex and into the medulla [10–12] and by measuring the oxygen tension in renal pelvic urine, which is considered to reflect that of papillary tissue [13–17]. Second, the hematocrit of the inner medullary blood in the papillary vasa recta is only one-half of that found systemically [18, 19], which is due both to erythrocyte shrinkage in the hypertonic papilla and to a decrease in erythrocyte number and hemoglobin concentration [19] and, therefore, in oxygen transporting capacity. Third, much of the blood supply to the outer stripe of the outer medulla comes from those ascending vasa recta that are not organized into vascular bundles but are interspersed among the tubules like true capillaries [20]. These "venous" vessels contain blood that has already perfused either the inner medulla or the inner stripe of the outer medulla. Whereas the vessels originating in the inner medulla, which have traversed the inner stripe in vascular bundles, may have been enriched with oxygen through countercurrent exchange there, those that drain the inner stripe and that have never been organized into bundles may be seriously deficient in oxygen.

Such a poor oxygen supply to the renal medulla would be of little consequence if the medullary tissue were to derive most of its metabolic energy from anaerobic processes, as has been previously supposed from studies on isolated tissue slices [21]. This conclusion seems justified for the inner medulla but is not applicable to the outer medulla, as indicated by several experimental observations. First, there is a sudden and marked drop in tissue oxygen tension immediately beyond the corticomedullary junction [10, 11], suggesting that the outer medullary tissue consumes considerable amounts of oxygen. Second, oxygen utilization rises with increasing medullary work, which is illustrated by the increase in oxygen consumption in slices of outer medullary tissue exposed to increasing sodium concentrations [22] and by the decrease in urinary oxygen tension in kidneys undergoing osmotic diuresis, which increases solute delivery to the distal nephron [16]. Third, oxygen utilization is decreased by loop diuretics, which decrease medullary work, as witnessed by the increased oxygen tension in the urine [16, 23] and by the enhanced oxidation of cytochrome oxidase in the isolated, perfused kidney [24]. Thus, the oxygen supply to the medulla may well be of critical importance in determining what happens to the concentrating and diluting processes during alterations in medullary blood flow.

Conditions under which medullary blood flow is increased are relatively seldom seen and are only well-documented during the application of vasodilatory substances and in the early phase of ureteral obstruction. It is known that acetylcholine [25, 26], bradykinin [26], dopamine [27], and ureteral obstruction [28, 29] all raise renal blood flow by increasing blood flow to the inner cortical regions more than to the superficial ones. Since it is the efferent arterioles of the juxtamedullary glomeruli that supply the medulla with blood, an increase in deep cortical perfusion seems most likely to increase blood flow to the medulla. The influence that an increase in blood flow will exert on urinary concentrating ability is perhaps to favor tubular transport by increasing oxygen delivery and reducing the axial fall in oxygen tension caused by countercurrent oxygen exchange, to enhance water removal from the interstitium, but also to lower medullary hypertonicity by reducing solute trapping. The resulting net decrease in concentrating ability has been observed during acetylcholine administration [30] and following release of ureteral obstruction [31, 32], and found to accompany a decrease in papillary solute concentration [30, 31]. An increase in medullary blood flow would be expected to influence urinary diluting ability little, because tubular transport out of the thick ascending limb of Henle's loop is not compromised under these circumstances.

In contrast, conditions under which medullary blood flow is decreased are many and varied. A common situation is one in which blood flow to the inner medulla is predominantly affected. A reduction in medullary blood flow seems possible during chronic ureteral obstruction, since deep cortical blood flow is already depressed at 18 hr [33] and renal blood flow has yet to fall further [34]. The expected decrease in urinary concentrating ability has been observed [35, 36], and diluting ability has been shown to be little affected [35]. A decrease in papillary perfusion is thought also to accompany analgesic nephropathy [37, 38], in which urinary concentrating ability is known to be reduced [39]. Clinically, in both of these conditions and also in diabetic nephropathy, obliteration of the vasa recta is common, and papillary necrosis may result [40], which must certainly cause some loss of concentrating power.

One condition in which the reduction in papillary flow is not primarily due to vascular damage but to an increase in blood viscosity is sickle cell nephropathy. In this disease, deformability of nonsickled erythrocytes is reduced, owing both to an increase in membrane rigidity and a decrease in internal fluidity; and sickling upon exposure to hypoxic and hypertonic conditions, such as prevail in the medulla, increases viscosity even further [41]. Morphologically, a reduction in the number of vasa recta has been demonstrated using microangiographic techniques [42]; vasa recta congestion and obliteration typify the histologic findings [43, 44], and papillary necrosis may develop [40]. Thus, even though medullary blood flow determinations have not been reported either for sickle cell nephropathy or for the animal model of sicklemia [41], it seems clear from the morphologic findings that it could be reduced. Consequently, it can be concluded that solute trapping will be enhanced since vasa recta flow is slowed, but that the removal of water reabsorbed from the collecting ducts will be limited. In addition, congestion of the glomeruli [44, 45] may lead to a decrease in filtration rate with increasing age [46], thus reducing the availability of solutes with which to generate medullary hypertonicity [47]. The net effect of all these factors is a decrease in concentrating ability [48–52], which becomes more pronounced with increasing age and increasing vascular derangement [49, 52]. In young children who do not have irreversible ischemic tissue damage, transfusions of normal blood promptly restore concentrating ability [50, 51], presumably because the reduction in blood viscosity [53] reestablishes vasa recta flow. As anticipated, the ability to dilute the urine is unimpaired [48–50] because the papillary circulation plays no part in this process.

Another condition on which medullary blood flow is diminished, but in which the perfusion of the outer medulla is predominantly affected, is seen following renal ischemia. Blood flow to the inner cortex is substantially reduced after ischemia [33, 54], so that medullary perfusion is almost certainly affected, even though blood flow to the papilla seems unimpaired [55, 56]. Morphologically, these kidneys are characterized by a redness or "hyperemia" of the inner stripe region of the outer medulla (Fig. 1). This results from a capillary congestion with densely packed erythrocytes (Fig. 2) [56, 57] that

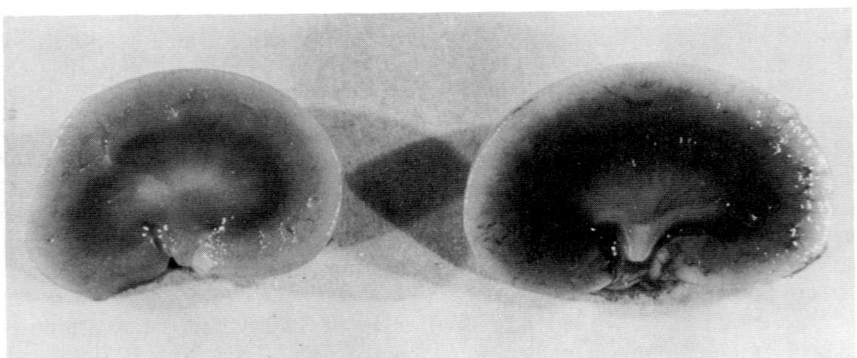

Fig. 1. The cut surfaces of the freshly removed, unfixed kidneys of one animal. The left kidney, which was subjected to 45 min of warm ischemia followed by 2 hr of reperfusion, is shown on the *right*, next to the untouched contralateral kidney (*left*), which was removed at the same time. The ischemically damaged kidney shows a red "hyperemic" zone, confined mainly to the inner stripe of the outer medulla, which is characteristic for the early phase of ischemic renal failure and is always absent from control kidneys. (Reproduced from [56])

is so severe that vascular filling of this region by arterial injection is no longer possible (Fig. 3) [56]. The functional significance of this perfusion deficit is illustrated by the correlation between the degree of vascular congestion and the loss of concentrating ability and renal function after ischemia. In the early maintenance and recovery phases of ischemic renal failure, the kidneys showing the most congestion display the worst function, whereas those with the least congestion show relatively little functional impairment [56]. Removal of the aggregated blood by acutely elevating perfusion pressure immediately after ischemia leads to a rapid and substantial improvement in urinary concentrating ability and renal function [58]. Similarly, prevention of erythrocyte accumulation by lowering arterial hematocrit to 30% immediately prior to ischemia also improves concentrating ability and renal function (unpublished observations). The exquisite sensitivity of the outer medulla to oxygen deprivation is known from studies on the isolated, perfused kidney preparation. Perfusion with isoncotic, erythrocyte-free solutions rapidly leads to anoxic damage of those thick ascending limbs in the outer medulla that lie farthest away from the vascular bundles (Fig. 4) [59–61]. The addition of erythrocytes to the perfusion medium to enhance oxygen transporting capacity prevents these lesions [61]. Thus, in the ischemically damaged kidney, where vascular congestion most certainly limits the oxygen supply to the thick ascending limbs of Henle, diminished diluting power is to be expected. Such a decrease in diluting ability after ischemia has been demonstrated in superficial nephrons [62] and isolated thick ascending limbs [63], and the Na-K-ATPase activity in the outer medulla has been shown to be reduced by ischemia [64]. As the inner medullary circulation seems little affected, it must be assumed that water removal is possible and that solute trapping could proceed normally, if only the severe reduction both in filtration rate and thick ascending limb transport were not to limit solute delivery and diminish medullary hypertonicity. Such a reduction in papillary solute concentration in ischemic renal failure has indeed been identified as the cause of the restriction in concentrating power observed [65].

In summary, pathophysiologic alterations to the medullary circulation become apparent as alterations in urinary concentrating and diluting power. The contribution that the medullary circulation makes toward the concentrating process is manyfold. It must supply the metabolic substrates for tubular transport, generate medullary hypertonicity by trapping solutes, and preserve this hypertonicity by removing water. Changes in blood flow in either direction will lead to a loss of concentrating power by favoring one activity at the expense of another. The contribution the circulation makes toward the diluting process, however, is only to supply the thick ascending loop of Henle ("diluting segment") with metabolic substrates. Only decreases in blood flow to the outer medulla will therefore affect urinary dilution. Thus, the processes of concentration and dilution can be separately and differently influenced by changes in medullary blood flow. Increases in blood flow, as during vasodilation or early after ureteral occlusion, lead to a loss of concentrating power through diminished solute trapping ("solute washout") but should have little influence on dilution. Decreases in blood flow affecting mostly the inner medulla, such as during chronic ureteral obstruction, analgesic, diabetic, or

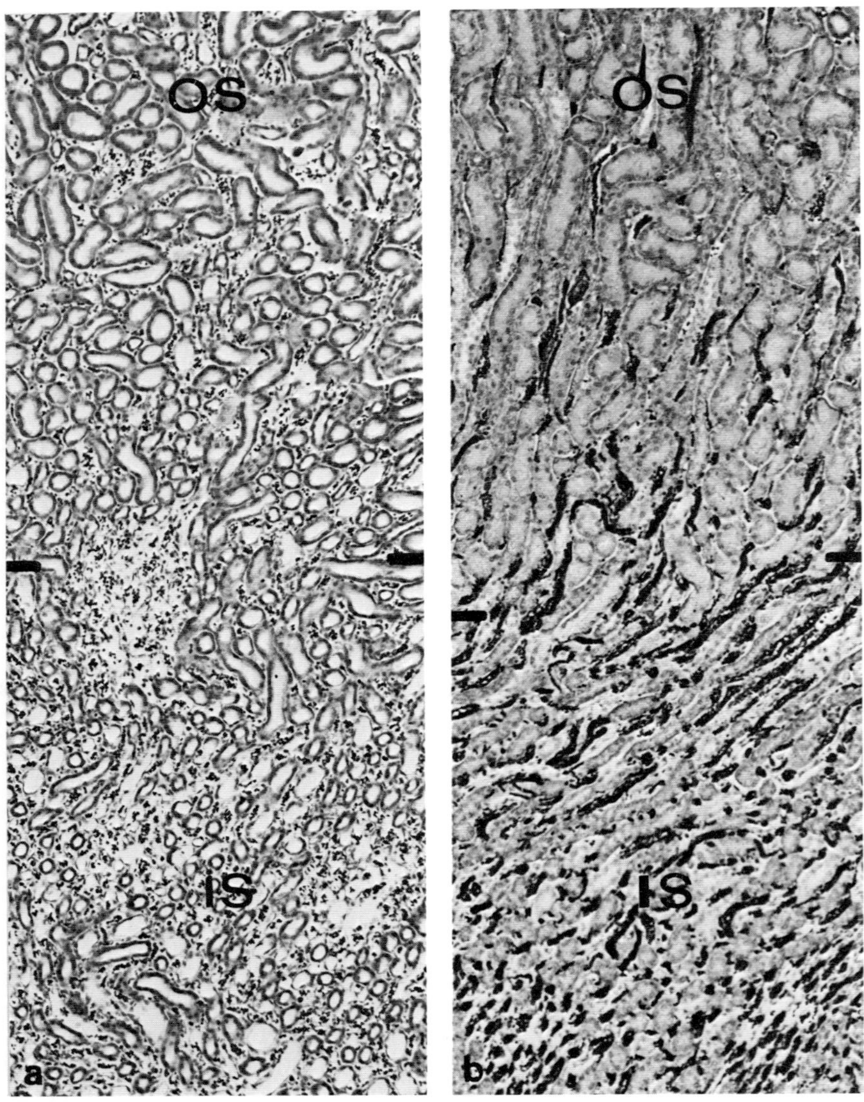

Fig. 2 a and **b.**

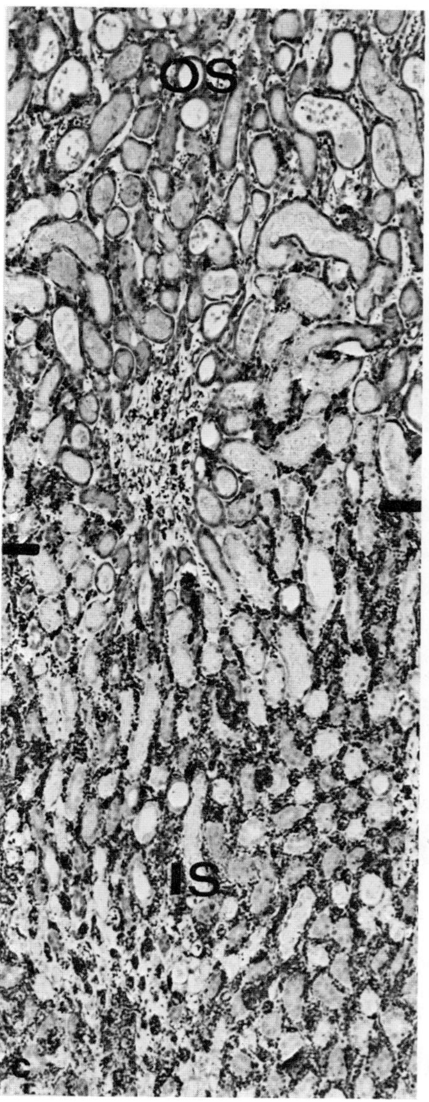

Fig. 2. Sections across the outer stripe (*OS*), inner stripe (*IS*) border of the outer medulla in a control kidney (**b**) and in two kidneys subjected to 45 min of warm ischemia, one without reflow (**a**) and one after 1 hr of reperfusion (**c**). The kidneys were shock-frozen at −180°C and freeze-dried, before conventional preparation, to preserve the in vivo structural relationships. In both ischemic kidneys, a massive interbundle capillary congestion is seen, which predominates in the *inner stripe* and is little evident in the *outer stripe* (Kriz, Joeris, and Mason, unpublished observations).

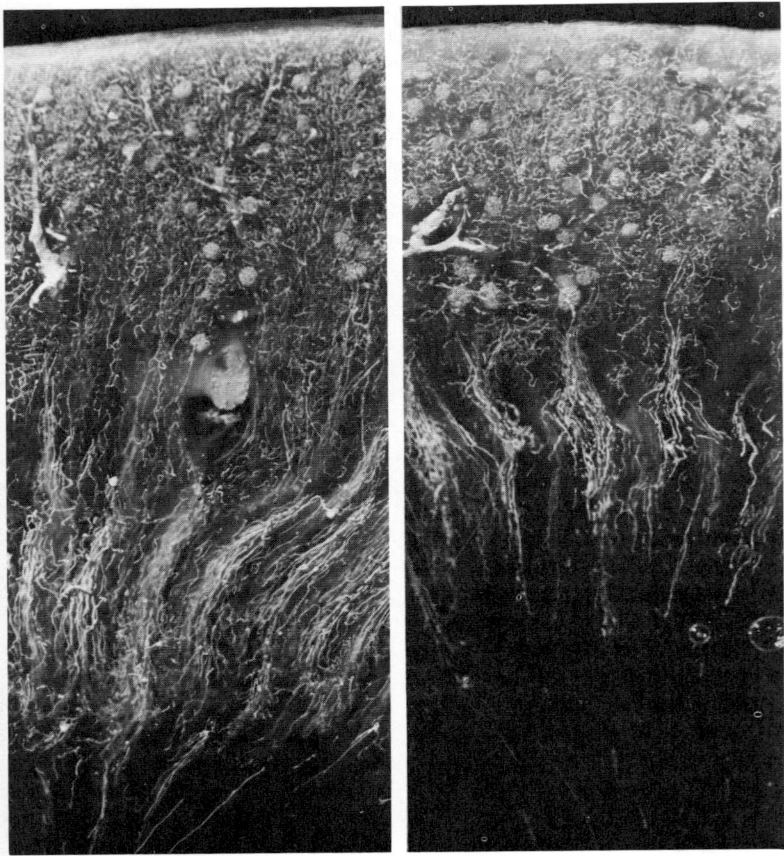

Fig. 3. Sections from both kidneys of one animal obtained after synchronous arterial filling from the carotid artery, fixation in alcohol, and clearing in methyl salicylate. The left kidney, which was subjected to 45 min of warm ischemia, followed by 1 hr of reperfusion, is shown on the *right,* next to the untouched contralateral kidney (*left*). Compared to the control kidney, the ischemically damaged kidney displays good filling of the cortical capillaries and descending vasa recta, but poor filling of the capillary plexus of the inner stripe. (Reproduced from [56])

Fig. 4. Transverse sections obtained from a kidney isolated and perfused with erthrocyte-free colloids for several hours. The sections were stained with methylene blue and azure II, which preferentially colors those thick ascending limbs that are not necrotic. Taken at a lower magnification (**a**), the regular appearance of darkly stained, thick ascending limbs in the immediate vicinity of the vascular bundles is apparent. At a higher magnification (**b**), the presence of darkly stained, non-necrotic tubules close to the vessels and lightly stained necrotic ones farther away is more evident. Some tubules display both necrotic and nonnecrotic cells; the non-necrotic cells are always directed toward the vascular bundle and the necrotic cells always face away from the vessels. (Reproduced from [62])

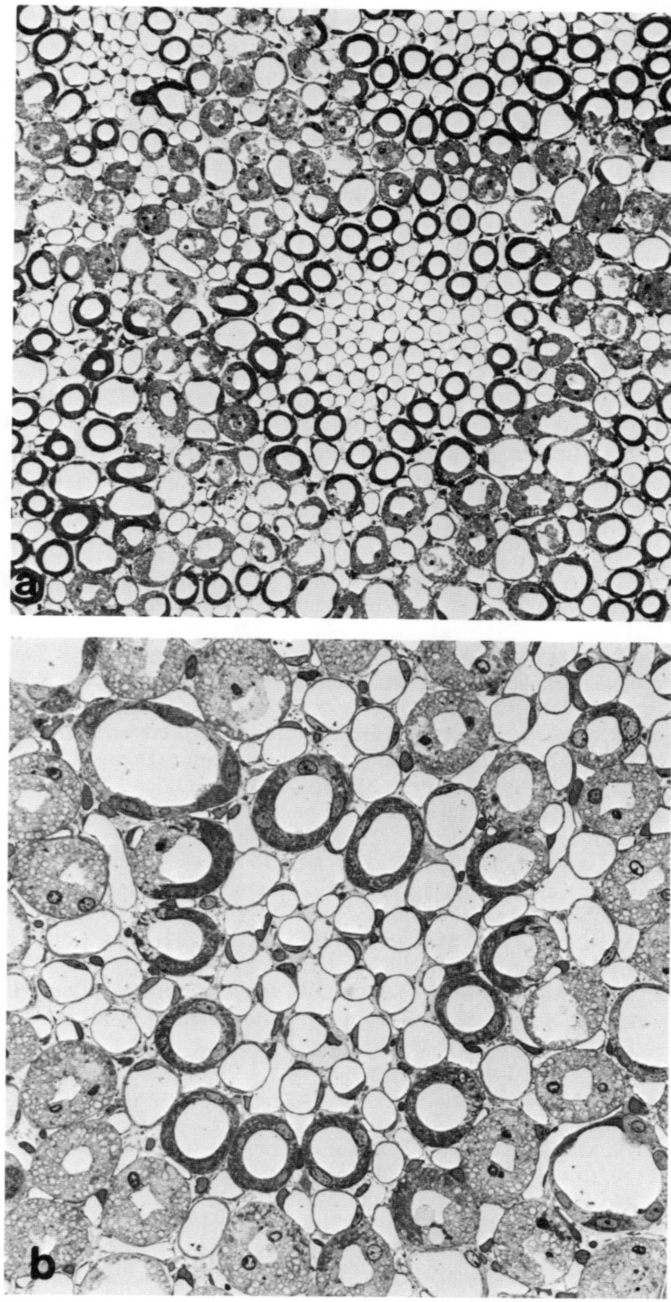

Fig. 4 a and b.

sickle cell nephropathies, decrease concentrating power while influencing dilution little; and relief of the inner medullary vascular obstruction in young sicklemia patients by transfusion restores the concentrating ability. Decreases in blood flow affecting mostly the outer medulla, such as occur after renal ischemia, lead to a loss of thick ascending limb transport, so that both diluting ability and concentrating power are reduced, and prevention or relief of the outer medullary congestion greatly improves concentrating ability.

References

1. THORNBURN GD, KOPALD HH, HERD JA, HOLLENBERG M, O'MORCHOE CCC, BARGER AC: Intrarenal distribution of nutrient blood flow determined with Krypton[85] in the unanesthetized dog. *Circ Res* 13:290–307, 1963
2. DEETJEN P, BRECHTELSBAUER H, KRAMER K: Hämodynamik des Nierenmarks: III. Mitteilung: Farbstoffpassagezeiten in äusserer Markzone und V. renalis. Die Durchblutungsverteilung der Niere. *Pflügers Arch* 279:281–293, 1964
3. HARSING L, PELLEY K: Die Bestimmung der Nierenmarkdurchblutung auf Grund der Ablagerung und Verteilung von [86]Rb. *Pflügers Arch* 285:302–312, 1965
4. CARRIÈRE S, THORNBURN GD, O'MORCHOE CCC, BARGER AC: Intrarenal distribution of blood flow in dogs during hemorrhagic hypotension. *Circ Res* 19:167–179, 1966
5. WOLGAST M: Studies on the regional blood flow with P[32]-labelled red cells and small beta-sensitive semiconductor detectors. *Acta Physiol Scand* 73(Suppl 313):1–109, 1968
6. GIRNDT J, OCHWADT B: Durchblutung des Nierenmarks, Gesamtnierendurchblutung und corticomedulläre Gradienten beim experimentellen renalen Hochdruck der Ratte. *Pflügers Arch* 313:30–42, 1969
7. RASMUSSEN SN: Red cell and plasma volume flows to the inner medulla of the rat kidney. *Pflügers Arch* 373:153–159, 1978
8. KRAMER K, THURAU K, DEETJEN P: Hämodynamic des Nierenmarks: I. Mitteilung: Kapilläre Passagezeit, Durchblutung, Gewebshämatokrit und O_2-Verbrauch des Nierenmarks in situ. *Pflügers Arch* 270:251–269, 1960
9. LILIENFELD LS, MAGANZINI HC, BAUER MH: Blood flow in the renal medulla. *Circ Res* 9:614–617, 1961
10. LEICHTWEISS HP, LÜBBERS DW, WEISS C, BAUMGÄRTL H, RESCHKE W: The oxygen supply of the rat kidney: measurements of intrarenal pO_2. *Pflügers Arch* 309:328–349, 1969
11. BAUMBÜRTL H, LEICHTWEISS HP, LÜBBERS DW, WEISS C, HULAND H: The oxygen supply of the dog kidney: measurements of intrarenal pO_2. *Microvasc Res* 4:247–257, 1972
12. AUKLAND K, KROG J: Renal oxygen tension. *Nature* 188:671, 1960
13. AUKLAND K, KROG J: Influence of various factors on urine oxygen tension in the dog. *Acta Physiol Scand* 52:350–365, 1961
14. LEONHARDT KO, LANDES RR: Oxygen tensions of the urine and renal structures, preliminary report of clinical findings. *N Engl J Med* 269:115–121, 1963
15. APERIA AC, LIEBOW AA: Implications of urine pO_2 for renal medullary blood flow. *Am J Physiol* 206:499–504, 1964
16. WASHINGTON JA, HOLLAND JH: Urine oxygen tension: Effect of osmotic and saline diuresis and of ethacrynic acid. *Am J Physiol* 210:243–250, 1966

17. RENNIE DW, REEVES RB, PAPPENHEIMER JR: Oxygen pressure in urine and its relation to intrarenal blood flow. *Am J Physiol* 195:120–132, 1958

18. RASMUSSEN SN: Effect of osmotic diuresis and water diuresis on intrarenal red cell and plasma volumes in the rat. Determination by means of ^{51}Cr labelled red cells and ^{125}I-γ-M immunoglobulin. *Pflügers Arch* 348:1–11, 1974

19. ULLRICH KJ, PEHLING G, STÖCKLE H: Hämoglobinkonzentration, Erythrozytenzahl und Hämatokrit im vasa recta Blut. *Pflügers Arch* 273:573–578, 1961

20. KRIZ W: Structural organisation of renal medullary circulation. *Nephron* 31:289–323, 1982

21. LEE JB, VANCE VK, CAHILL GF: Metabolism of ^{14}C-labelled substrates by rabbit kidney cortex and medulla. *Am J Physiol* 203:27–36, 1962

22. ULLRICH KJ, PEHLING G: Aktiver Natriumtransport und Sauerstoffverbrauch in der äußeren Markzone der Niere. *Pflügers Arch* 267:207–217, 1958

23. AUKLAND K, JOHANNESEN J, KIIL F: In vivo measurements of local metabolic rate in dog kidney: Effect of mersalyl, chlorothiazide, ethacrynic acid and furosemide. *Scand J Clin Lab Invest* 23:317–323, 1969

24. EPSTEIN FH, BALABAN RS, ROSS BD: Redox state of cytochrome aa$_3$ in isolated perfused rat kidney. *Am J Physiol* 243:F356–F363, 1982

25. McNAY JL, ABE Y: Distribution of blood flow during renal vasodilation in dogs. *Circ Res* 27:1023–1032, 1970

26. STEIN JH, FERRIS TF, HAPRICH JE, SMITH TC, OSGOOD RW: Effect of renal vasodilatation on the distribution of cortical blood flow in the kidney of the dog. *J Clin Invest* 50:1429–1438, 1971

27. HARDAKER WT, WECHSLER AS: Redistribution of renal intracortical blood flow during dopamine infusion in dogs. *Circ Res* 33:437–444, 1973

28. BAY WH, STEIN JH, RECTOR JB, OSGOOD RW, FERRIS TF: Redistribution of renal cortical blood flow during elevated ureteral pressure. *Am J Physiol* 222:33–37, 1972

29. ABE Y, KISHIMOTO T, YAMAMOTO K, UEDA J: Intrarenal distribution of blood flow during ureteral and venous pressure elevations. *Am J Physiol* 224:746–751, 1973

30. VANDER AJ: Effects of acetyl choline, atropine and physostigmine on renal function in the dog. *Am J Physiol* 206:492–498, 1964

31. JAENIKE JR, BRAY GA: Effects of acute transitory urinary obstruction in the dog. *Am J Physiol* 199:1219–1222, 1960

32. SELKURT EE: Effect of ureteral blockade on renal blood flow and urinary concentrating ability. *Am J Physiol* 205:286–292, 1963

33. MASON J, WELSCH J, TAKABATAKE T: The disparity between surface and deep nephron function early afterrenal ischemia. *Kidney Int* 24:27–36, 1983

34. VAUGHAN ED, SORENSEN EJ, GILLENWATER JM: The renal hemodynamic response to chronic unilateral complete ureteral occlusion. *Invest Urol* 8:78–90, 1970

35. EKNOYAN G, SUKI WN, MARTINEZ-MALDONADA M, ANHALT MA: Chronic hydronephrosis: Observations on the mechanism of the defect in urine concentration. *Proc Soc Exp Biol Med* 134:634–642, 1970

36. HARRIS RH, YARGER WE: Renal function after release of unilateral renal obstruction in rats. *Am J Physiol* 227:806–815, 1974

37. MOLLAND EA: Experimental renal papillary necrosis. *Kidney Int* 13:5–14, 1978

38. NANRA RS, CHIRAWONG P, KINCAID-SMITH P: Medullary ischaemia in experimental analgesic nephropathy: The pathogenesis of renal papillary necrosis. *Aust NZ J Med* 3:580–583, 1973

39. STEELE TW, GYÖRY AZ, EDWARDS KDG: Renal function in analgesic nephropathy. *Br Med J* 2:213–216, 1969

40. EKNOYAN G, QUNIBI WY, GRISSOM RT, TUMA SN, AYUS JC: Renal papillary necrosis: An update. *Medicine* 61:55–73, 1982
41. KLUG PP, LESSIN LS, RADICE P: Rheological aspects of sickle cell disease. *Arch Intern Med* 133:577–590, 1969
42. STATIUS VAN EPS LW, PINEDO-VEELS C, DE VRIES GH, DE KONING J: Nature of concentrating defect in sickle cell nephropathy. *Lancet* 1:450–452, 1970
43. MOSTOFI FK, VORDERBRUEGGE CF, DIGGS LW: Lesions in kidneys removed for unilateral hematuria in sickle-cell disease. *Arch Pathol* 63:336–351, 1957
44. BERNSTEIN J, WHITTEN CF: Histological appraisal of the kidney in sickle cell anemia. *Arch Pathol* 70:407–418, 1960
45. PITCOCK JA, MUIRHEAD EE, HATCH FE, JOHNSON JG, KELLY BJ: Early renal changes in sickle cell anemia. *Arch Pathol* 90:403–410, 1970
46. ETTELDORF JN, SMITH JD, TUTTLE AH, DIGGS LW: Renal hemodynamic studies in adults with sickle cell anemia. *Am J Med* 18:243–248, 1955
47. LEVINSKY NG, DAVIDSON DG, BERLINER RW: Effects of reduced glomerular filtration on urine concentration in the presence of antidiuretic hormone. *J Clin Invest* 38:730–740, 1959
48. HATCH FE, CULBERTSON JW, DIGGS LW: Nature of the renal concentration defect in sickle cell disease. *J Clin Invest* 46:336–345, 1967
49. SCHLITT L, KEITEL HG: Pathogenesis of hyposthenuria in persons with sickle cell anemia or the sickle cell trait. *Pediatrics* 26:249–254, 1960
50. KEITEL HG, THOMPSON D, ITANO HA: Hyposthenuria in sickle cell anemia: A reversible renal defect. *J Clin Invest* 35:998–1007, 1956
51. STATIUS VAN EPS LW, SCHOUTEN H, LA PORTE-WIJSMAN H, STRUYKER-BOUDIER AM: The influence of red blood cell transfusions on the hyposthenuria and renal hemodynamics of sickle cell anemia. *Clin Chim Acta* 17:449–461, 1967
52. STATIUS VAN EPS LW, SCHOUTEN H, VER HAAR ROMENY-WACHTER CC, LA PORTE-WIJSMAN H: The relation between age and renal concentrating capacity in sickle cell disease and haemoglobin C disease. *Clin Chim Acta* 27:501–511, 1970
53. HARRIS JW, BREWSTER HH, HARN TH, CASTLE WB: Studies on the destruction of red blood cells: X. The biophysics and biology of sickle cell disease. *Arch Intern Med* 97:145–168, 1956
54. NORLEN J, ENGBERG A, KÄLLSKÖG Ö, WOLGAST M: Intrarenal hemodynamics in the transplanted rat kidney. *Kidney Int* 14:1–9, 1978
55. BÖTTCHER W, STEINHAUSEN M: Microcirculation of rats under control conditions and after temporary ischemia. *Kidney Int* 10(Suppl 6):574–580, 1976
56. MASON J, TORHORST J, WELSCH J: The role of the medullary perfusion defect in the pathogenesis of ischemic renal failure. *Kidney Int* 26:283–293, 1984
57. TORHORST J, DE ROUGEMENT D, BRUNNER FP, THIEL G: Morphology of the renal medulla in ischemic acute renal failure in the rat. *Nephron* 31:296–300, 1982
58. MASON J, WELSCH J, TORHORST J: The functional significance of medullary congestion in acute renal failure, in *Abs Proc IXth Int Congr Nephrol,* Los Angeles, 1984, p 330A
59. KRIZ W: Discussion comment and figure, in "Workshop on the Role of Renal Medullary Circulation in the Pathogenesis of Acute Renal Failure," edited by MASON J, THIEL G *Nephron* 31:199–230, 1982
60. ALCORN D, EMSLIE KR, ROSS BD, RYAN GB, TANGE, JD: Selective distal nephron damage during isolated kidney perfusion. *Kidney Int* 19:638–647, 1981
61. BREZIS M, ROSEN S, SILVA P, EPSTEIN FH: Selective vulnerability of the medullary thick ascending limb to anoxia in the isolated perfused rat kidney. *J Clin Invest* 73:182–190, 1984

62. MASON J, GUTSCHE H-U, MÜLLER-SUUR R, MOORE L: The early phase of experimental acute renal failure: IV. The diluting ability of the short loops of Henle. *Pflügers Arch* 379:11–18, 1979

63. HANLEY MJ: Isolated nephron segments in a rabbit model of ischemic acute renal failure. *Am J Physiol* 239:F17–F23, 1980

64. KRAMER HJ, KLINGMÜLLER D, GLÄNZER K: Protection from ischemic acute renal failure (iARF) by mannitol (M) and verapamil (V) in conscious rats (*abstract*). *Kidney Int* 25:233, 1984

65. ANDERSON RJ, GORDON JA, KIM J, PETERSON LM, GROSS PA, VAN PATTEN V, ELLIS M: Renal concentrating defect following non-oliguric acute renal failure in the rat. *Kidney Int* 21:583–591, 1982

Intrarenal Control of Medullary Blood Flow and the Urinary Concentrating Mechanism

Leon C. Moore

The concentration of excreted urine in hydropenia is determined by the dynamic balance between two primary factors. First, the generation of high medullary osmolarity depends on the relative rates of water and solute reabsorption into the medullary interstitium from the collecting ducts and Henle's loop. The primary source of sodium chloride (NaCl) in the medullary interstitium is NaCl reabsorption from the ascending limb of Henle's loop, which is a process that is driven by active transport in the outer medulla and by a passive mechanism in the inner medulla. In both parts of the medulla, the rate of ascending limb NaCl reabsorption is a key determinant of concentrating ability. The major source of urea is passive reabsorption from the inner medullary collecting ducts, which is a process that is indirectly dependent on active NaCl transport in the medullary thick ascending limb. The second major factor is the rate by which the accumulated solutes are dissipated by diffusion into the cortex and by convection into the renal venous system; for example, vasa recta "washout." Much research on the regulation of the countercurrent system has dealt with control of distal nephron water permeability by vasopressin, which is the principal extrarenal hormonal effector controlling urine concentration. In this chapter, the focus will be on intrarenal mechanisms and will include: (1) the relationship between the rate of medullary blood flow and urine concentrating ability, (2) how tubuloglomerular feedback in juxtamedullary nephrons may act as a key intrarenal regulator of the urine concentrating mechanism by directly stabilizing the degree of tubular fluid dilution in the ascending limbs and, concurrently, by regulating medullary blood flow, and (3) how the unique characteristics of tubuloglomerular feedback in juxtamedullary nephrons might provide a partial explanation of the effects of arterial pressure on urine concentrating ability.

This manuscript was presented as part of a Symposium on *Medullary Circulation*.

Method of Analysis: Countercurrent System Model

Given that urine concentrating ability depends on a delicate dynamic balance between many factors, prediction of the effects of primary changes in key variables (such as the rate of medullary blood flow and nephron filtration rate) requires a systematic analysis of a multitude of direct and indirect effects. To this end, a mathematic model of the renal countercurrent system was used to investigate these questions and to obtain quantitative estimates of the predicted effects. This model has been used in previous studies of the concentrating mechanism [1, 2] and is based on the same physical principles as the models developed by others [3, 4]. It consists of a set of partial differential equations that express conservation of mass within the tubular structures and vessels of the medulla. When solved numerically, these equations—along with appropriate auxiliary expressions describing tubular and vascular transport and the anatomy of the medulla—yield a prediction of the steady-state concentrating ability of the kidney. For a detailed description of the model and a complete list of all parameters, the original work should be consulted [1]. In this chapter, only those features and limitations of the model that are relevant to the issues in question will be discussed.

First, the model is configured to simulate the medulla of a rat, and it considers only the transport of NaCl, urea, and water. Mass transport along the corticopapillary axis is by convection within the nephrons and vasa recta and by diffusion within the interstitium. Transepithelial transport is by passive diffusion, osmosis, or active transport that incorporates Michaelis-Menton kinetics. Second, the model includes a population of short (75%) and long (25%) Henle's loops and distal tubules, as well as collecting ducts that progressively merge in the inner medulla. Two percent of the loops of Henle descend to the tip of the papilla. The short loops of Henle, which are assumed to arise from superficial or midcortical nephrons, turn at the junction between the inner and outer medulla. Third, transport parameters for the nephron were taken from the literature where possible [1]. The descending limbs are identical except for their length, while the thick ascending limbs from short- and long-looped nephrons have somewhat different active transport rates. These rates were selected to be consistent with in vivo micropuncture measurements made in rats [5] and the results of in vitro perfusion studies of rat and rabbit nephron fragments, as summarized in the comprehensive review of the urine concentrating mechanism by Jamison and Kriz [6].

The features of the medullary vasculature included in the model are a population of ascending and descending vasa recta that are configured to represent vascular bundles. Ten percent of the total descending blood flow, which is assumed to consist solely of postglomerular blood from juxtamedullary nephrons, enters the inner medulla. The number of ascending vasa recta exceeds the number of descending vessels; their radii are larger in accordance with experimental observations [7]. The functional effects of the grouping of vasa recta into vascular bundles is represented by permitting direct diffusion of solute between ascending and descending vessels.

Although this model has been shown to simulate adequately the countercurrent system in several complex situations [2], there are three inherent limitations that should be considered. First, the mechanism of tubular fluid dilution by the thin ascending limbs in this model is via active NaCl transport. This feature was included to produce a significant concentrating effect in the inner medulla, although studies by Imai and Kokko [8] clearly show that thin ascending limbs perfused in vitro lack any significant ability to actively transport NaCl. Kokko and Rector [9] and Stephenson [3] independently proposed models of inner medullary urine concentration that do not require active NaCl transport in the thin ascending limb. Both hypotheses assume that inner medullary thin descending limbs have very low NaCl and urea permeabilities and high osmotic water permeability. However, a recent in vitro perfusion study by Imai and Araki [10] provides evidence that long-looped thin descending limbs have high NaCl permeability in rats and hamsters. As discussed at length in a previous analysis of the countercurrent system [1], solute entry into inner medullary thin descending limbs significantly compromises the ability of these passive models to explain urinary concentration in the inner medulla. Hence, to generate a significant axial osmotic gradient along the inner medulla with this model of a rat kidney, an active sodium (Na) transport capability was incorporated into the thin ascending limbs. The inner medullary descending limb permeabilities used in the simulation studies are consistent with the findings of Imai and Araki [10].

Second, the vascular elements included in the model are merely a first-order approximation of the complex circulation of the medulla. As discussed at length by Jamison and Kriz [6] and by Bankir in this volume, the medullary vasculature is composed of several components that may be regulated differently, and it may be of fundamental importance to the urinary concentrating mechanism.

Third, any model that describes only NaCl and urea cannot simulate the full range of transport mechanisms that are present in the renal tubule. In this particular model, this is especially true of the collecting ducts, where it is assumed that no NaCl is reabsorbed, but where important final adjustments in urine composition are known to occur.

These limitations notwithstanding, the results described below arise mainly from the flow-dependent characteristics of nephron solute and water reabsorption, as well as the flow dependency of passive countercurrent exchange in the vasa recta. Due to this phenomena, it is unlikely that elimination of the limitations listed above would have a major effect on the general nature of the responses, although some quantitative differences would be expected.

Coupling of the Medullary Circulation and the Countercurrent System

All of the major determinants of urine concentrating ability described above, with the exception of vasopressin levels in plasma, are influenced either directly or indirectly by changes in medullary blood flow. One direct linkage is due to the effect of vasa recta solute washout on urine concentrating ability, which is a process that strongly depends on the rate of vasa recta blood flow. A second direct effect arises from coupling of the juxtamedullary nephron filtration rate to medullary blood flow, since virtually all of the blood perfusing the medulla consists of postglomerular blood from juxtamedullary nephrons. More indirect, but important, effects arise because of the general flow-dependent nature of reabsorption in the loop of Henle and the distal nephron. This phenomenon, which has been discussed at length by Wright [11], manifests itself as a rise in absolute reabsorption and a fall in fractional reabsorption as tubular fluid flow increases [5]. Hence, any increase in delivery of tubular fluid into Henle's loop will propagate along the distal nephron, thereby influencing the flow and composition of the final urine. The following examples illustrate the possible quantitative significance of these concepts.

Increases in medullary blood flow enhance the convective dissipation of the axial medullary concentration gradient, thereby reducing the final urine concentration. This effect was the subject of an earlier analysis by Marsh and Segel [7]. The predicted consequences on urine osmolarity and flow of changes in the rate of blood flow into descending vasa recta are illustrated in Figure 1. In this figure, the rates of tubular fluid flow into the short- and long-looped descending limbs were held constant at values of 10 and 15 nl/min, respectively. The control (100%) value of descending vasa recta blood flow was calculated by assuming both a 30% filtration fraction and a filtration rate of 45 nl/min in each of the juxtamedullary nephrons. The marked effect on urine osmolarity of low blood flow into the descending vasa recta arises, because the loss of solutes from the medulla via vasa recta washout decreases exponentially as descending blood flow falls [1]. The exponential nature of this curve agrees with experimental measurements of the relationship between medullary blood flow and urine osmolarity made by Thurau and Deetjen in 1962 [12].

The effect of the flow dependence of nephron reabsorption on urine concentrating ability was simulated by varying the flow rate into descending Henle's loops in juxtamedullary nephrons while holding medullary blood flow constant. The results are shown in Figure 2. In this figure, the normal rate of

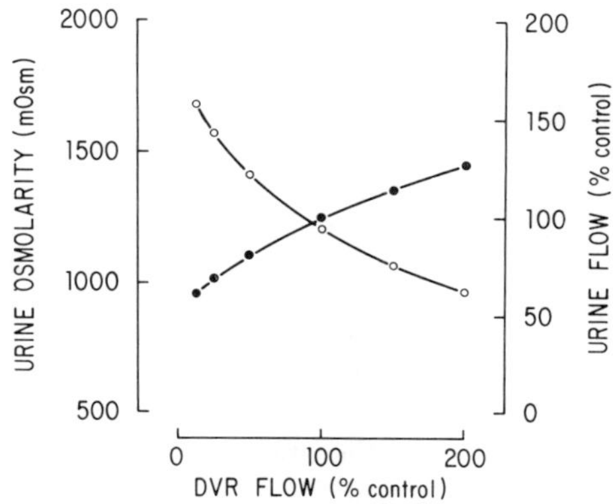

Fig. 1. The predicted effects of increased blood flow into the descending vasa recta (DVR) on urine osmolarity (*open circles*) and flow (*closed circles*). The *circles* indicate the values of the vasa recta inflow at which simulation studies were performed. Since all other variables were held constant, these responses are due to the strong flow dependency of solute loss from the medulla via the vasa recta.

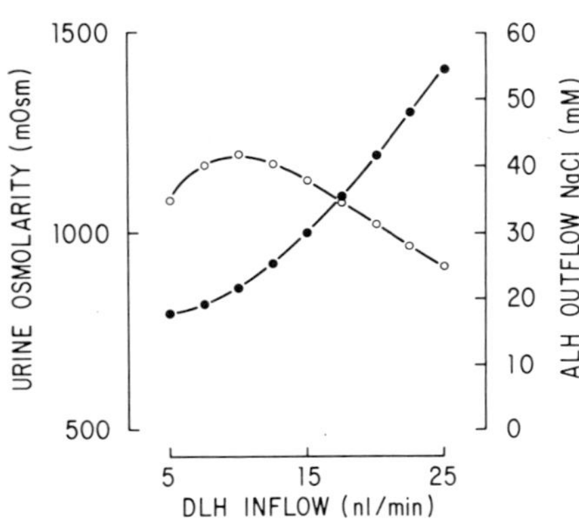

Fig. 2. The predicted effects of increased flow into juxtamedullary descending limbs (DLH) on urine osmolarity (*open circles*) and the NaCl concentration of the ascending limb (ALH) effluent (*closed circles*). All other variables were held constant. The fall in urine osmolarity is due to a decrease in the ratio of the rate of NaCl reabsorption from the ascending limb to the rate of water reabsorption from the descending limbs and collecting ducts. The rise in NaCl concentration in the ascending limb effluent is thought to be the signal for excitation of tubuloglomerular feedback.

juxtamedullary descending limb flow was assumed to be 15 nl/min. The effect on urine osmolarity is primarily due to alterations in the state of the urine concentrating mechanism in the inner medulla. The biphasic nature of the curve results from the interaction of several factors. First, as flow into the juxtamedullary descending limbs decreases below normal, NaCl transport out of the ascending limbs also falls due to the reduced delivery of NaCl. This is especially true for the inner medullary thin ascending limbs, which arise entirely from juxtamedullary nephrons. Urine osmolarity drops, because the absolute rate of solute reabsorption from the thin ascending limbs decreases to a greater extent than does the load of tubular fluid entering the inner medullary collecting ducts—a variable that is an important determinant of the absolute rate of collecting duct water reabsorption. The relative constancy of tubular fluid flow into the inner medullary collecting ducts reflects the fact that most of the fluid entering the collecting duct system in the cortex arises from superficial nephrons. First, these disproportionate changes in the rates of water and solute reabsorption into the inner medullary interstitium depress interstitial NaCl concentration and osmolarity. As interstitial osmolarity falls, the rate of water reabsorption from the collecting ducts will also decrease until a new steady state is established in which the reduced rate of NaCl reabsorption into the medullary interstitium is in dynamic balance with the rate of collecting duct water reabsorption.

Second, as shown in Figure 2, urine osmolarity drops as flow into the juxtamedullary descending limb rises because of a decrease in the dilution of tubular fluid in the ascending limbs. This is a result of the flow dependency of NaCl reabsorption in this segment [11]. This effect is reflected in experimental studies by a rise in the NaCl concentration of the ascending limb effluent [5]; the prediction of the model of this experimental observation is also shown in Figure 2. In the distal tubule, the higher osmotic and water loads result in elevated absolute, but lower fractional solute, reabsorption. As a result, the fluid load entering the collecting duct system is elevated, which causes an increase in the absolute amount of water reabsorbed into the medulla. This depresses interstitial NaCl concentration and osmolarity, particularly in the inner medulla. As inner medullary osmolarity falls, fractional water reabsorption from the collecting ducts subsides, although absolute water reabsorption remains elevated. Eventually, a new steady state is established. Hence, an uncontrolled rise in juxtamedullary nephron filtration will produce a fall in urine osmolarity. If blood flow into the descending vasa recta also increases, the net effect on urine concentrating ability will be more pronounced as the responses shown in Figures 1 and 2 occur simultaneously. It should be noted that these conclusions generally agree with the results of an elegant analysis of a central core model of the medullary countercurrent system by Stephenson [3].

Tubuloglomerular Feedback in Juxtamedullary Nephrons

The results discussed above illustrate how changes in the rates of both medullary blood flow and tubular fluid flow into descending limbs of juxtamedullary nephrons can have important effects on urine flow and osmolarity. Clearly, stability of the concentrating mechanism requires some intrarenal mechanism to regulate these key variables. Given the unique structure and function of the medullary countercurrent system, the most important intrarenal regulatory mechanism is probably tubuloglomerular feedback. This assertion is based on the fact that tubuloglomerular feedback in both superficial and juxtamedullary nephrons appears to monitor and to regulate the NaCl concentration of the ascending limb effluent as it passes the macula densa [13, 14]. As discussed above, this is an important determinant of urine concentrating ability, since it reflects the extent of tubular fluid dilution by the medullary thick ascending limb. In addition, if tubuloglomerular feedback in juxtamedullary nephrons controls filtration rate by modulating arteriolar resistance, then tubuloglomerular feedback in deep nephrons will also stabilize medullary blood flow. Thus, all of the flow-dependent determinants of the urine concentrating mechanism might be regulated in parallel by tubuloglomerular feedback.

Analysis of the possible significance of tubuloglomerular feedback as a regulator of the urine concentrating mechanism requires consideration of its functional characteristics. The existence of tubuloglomerular feedback in juxtamedullary nephrons has been demonstrated by two independent studies [13, 15]. However, three features are of interest to this discussion. First, experimental results are consistent with the assumption that the basic functional organization of tubuloglomerular feedback in juxtamedullary nephrons is similar to that in superficial nephrons [13]. Second, available evidence indicates that tubuloglomerular feedback in deep nephrons can produce a significantly greater decrease in the nephron filtration rate than in superficial nephrons [13, 15]. This suggests that the efficacy of tubuloglomerular feedback as a regulator of deep-nephron function may be greater than in superficial nephrons. Third, available evidence indicates that at normal levels of arterial pressure, tubuloglomerular feedback in deep nephrons operates very near saturation [13, 15]. This finding implies that tubuloglomerular feedback has a limited ability to prevent increases in the deep-nephron filtration rate and blood flow, but it has a substantial capacity to maintain these variables as arterial pressure falls below normal levels.

Renal Autoregulation and the Urine Concentrating Mechanism

Given the sensitivity of urine flow and osmolarity to changes in both medullary blood flow and tubular fluid load, it is interesting to consider how well the urine concentrating mechanism is insulated from changes in arterial pressure via renal autoregulation. Recent work clarifies many issues related to the mechanisms underlying renal autoregulation of blood flow and filtration rate. Both micropuncture measurements of superficial nephrons [16] and a recent study of the frequency of renal blood flow [17] have supported the hypothesis that at least two mechanisms are involved in renal autoregulation: tubuloglomerular feedback and a myogenic reflex in the afferent vasculature. Theoretic objections to a myogenic mechanism that regulates vessel wall tension have been largely answered in a recent analysis by Øien and Aukland [18].

The development of the dual-slit video technique for measuring erythrocyte velocity in vasa recta has provided an interesting picture of the autoregulatory ability of juxtamedullary nephrons [19]. The principal advantage of this method is that measurements at different levels of arterial pressure can be made in the same animal, thereby eliminating much of the variability and lack of precision associated with some of the more traditional methods of measuring medullary blood flow [6]. While some problems remain concerning the quantitative conversion of erythrocyte velocity into estimates of blood flow [19, 20], the changes in erythrocyte velocity provide an important qualitative estimate of the autoregulatory behavior of juxtamedullary nephrons. In general, the results indicate that autoregulation of vasa recta flow is similar to that in more superficial nephrons, except that the autoregulatory range is somewhat lower. A substantial loss of autoregulatory ability is seen at arterial pressures just slightly higher than normal. It is interesting to note that these experimental results are consistent with predictions of deep-nephron autoregulation that can be drawn from the measured characteristics of tubuloglomerular feedback in juxtamedullary nephrons.

Given this difference in autoregulatory behavior between deep and superficial nephrons, it is to be expected that changes in arterial pressure will influence the urine concentrating mechanism. To estimate the magnitude of this effect, the renal countercurrent model was used in a series of studies in which the rates of flow into descending Henle's limbs and vasa recta were selected to simulate the autoregulatory patterns found with the dual-slit video method by Cohen, Marsh, and Kayer [19]. An essential assumption was that flow into the descending limbs and descending vasa recta paralleled the measured changes in erythrocyte velocity; additional assumptions were the constant glomerular filtration fraction and proximal tubular fractional reabsorption, which was assumed to be 67% in all nephrons. Autoregulation of filtration rate in superficial nephrons was patterned after the results of micropuncture studies. No attempt was made to include the effects of the sympathetic nervous and renin-angiotensin systems on tubular reabsorption or glomerular dynamics. In this case, our focus is limited to the acute effects of physical mechanisms related to the flow dependency of solute and water transport in the vasa recta and renal tubules.

The simulation study of renal autoregulation is summarized in Figure 3. The filtration rate in superficial nephrons is constant between 100 and 150 mm Hg, while the filtration rate in juxtamedullary nephrons is constant between 70 and 120 mm Hg. As shown, the resulting autoregulatory pattern for whole kidney glomerular filtration rate (KGFR) follows that of the superficial nephrons because of their greater number. Given this autoregulatory pattern, the model predicts that changes in arterial pressure will have a substantial effect on urine concentrating ability. As arterial pressure falls below normal, urine osmolarity rises and urine flow falls; also, there is a fractional redistribution of blood flow and filtration rate toward the deep nephrons. As arterial pressure rises above the autoregulatory range of the juxtamedullary nephrons, urine flow rises and urine osmolarity falls; and, there is again a redistribution of blood flow and filtration rate toward the deep nephrons. Both urine flow and osmolarity curves show a plateau region that results from the constancy of all variables between 100 and 120 mm Hg, which is

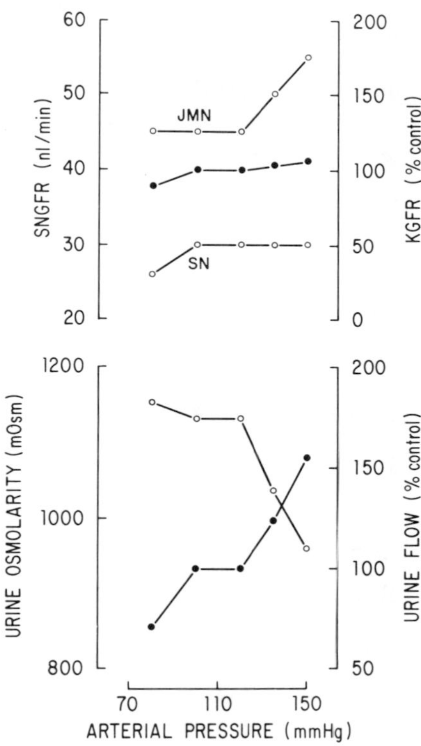

Fig. 3. The effect of differential autoregulation ranges in juxtamedullary (*JMN*) and superficial (*SN*) nephrons on urine flow and osmolarity. The *upper panel* shows the assumed autoregulatory pattern for SNGFR (*open circles*) and the resulting changes in kidney GFR (KGFR) (*closed circles*). Flow into the descending vasa recta (not shown) was assumed to parallel the autoregulatory pattern of the juxtamedullary nephron filtration rate. The *lower panel* shows the predicted changes in urine osmolarity (*open circles*) and flow (*closed circles*).

a feature that would be much less evident in vivo because of the smoothing effect of the variability of the autoregulatory response between individual nephrons.

The relationships between arterial pressure and urine flow and osmolarity are a clear prediction of the development of a pressure diuresis, which is a phenomenon that has been observed in intact and isolated perfused kidneys [12, 21–24] and is thought to play a pivotal role in the regulation of extracellular volume and arterial pressure [25]. In quantitative terms, the magnitude of the predicted pressure diuresis is somewhat smaller than that measured in whole kidney studies; however, in this case, only those changes related to the flow dependency of nephron and vasa recta transport were considered. However, these results do suggest that at least part of the pressure diuresis response may arise from differences in autoregulation between superficial and deep nephrons, which is a mechanism proposed in 1962 by Thurau and Deetjen [12].

Summary

The strong coupling between medullary blood flow and the intrarenal determinants of urine concentrating ability demonstrate the importance of effective regulation of medullary blood flow. Tubuloglomerular feedback may be an important intrarenal regulator of the renal countercurrent system, since it directly senses and stabilizes tubular fluid dilution in the ascending limbs and controls medullary blood flow, which are two important determinants of urine concentrating ability. Full evaluation of this hypothesis will require a great deal of imaginative experimental work.

Acknowledgment. Portions of this work were supported by NIADDKD Grant AM26341.

References

1. MOORE LC, MARSH DJ: How descending limb of Henle's loop permeability affects hypertonic urine formation. *Am J Physiol* 239:F57–F71, 1980
2. MOORE LC, MARSH DJ, MARTIN CM: Loop of Henle during the water-to-antidiuresis transition. *Am J Physiol* 239:F72–F83, 1980
3. STEPHENSON JL: Concentration of urine in central core model of the renal countercurrent system. *Kidney Int* 2:85–94, 1972
4. LORY P, GILIG A, HORSTER M: Renal countercurrent system: role of collecting duct convergence and pelvic urea predicted from a mathematical model. *J Math Biol* 16:281–304, 1983
5. MASON J, GUTSCHE H, MOORE L, MÜLLER-SUUR R: The early phase of acute renal failure: IV. The diluting ability of the short loops of Henle. *Pflügers Arch* 379:11–18, 1979
6. JAMISON RL, KRIZ W: *Urinary Concentrating Mechanism.* New York, Oxford University Press, 1982

 7. MARSH DJ, SEGEL LA: Analysis of countercurrent diffusion exchange in blood vessels of the renal medulla. *Am J Physiol* 221:817–828, 1971
 8. IMAI M, KOKKO JP: Mechanism of sodium and chloride transport in the thin ascending limb of Henle. *J Clin Invest* 58:1054–1060, 1976
 9. KOKKO JP, RECTOR FC: Countercurrent multiplication without active transport in the inner medulla. *Kidney Int* 2:214–223, 1972
10. IMAI M, ARAKI M: Internephron heterogeneity and interspecies differences in the function of the descending limb of Henle's loop (*abstract*). *Proc XXth Congr Int Union of Physiol Sciences,* Sydney, 1983, p 418
11. WRIGHT FS: Flow-dependent transport processes: filtration, absorption, secretion. *Am J Physiol* 243:F1–F11, 1982
12. THURAU K, DEETJEN P (mit einem Beitrag VON GÜNZLER H): Die Diurese bei arteriellen Drucksteigerungen. *Pflügers Arch* 274:567–580, 1962
13. MÜLLER-SUUR R, ULFENDAHL HR, PERSSON AEG: Evidence for tubuloglomerular feedback in juxtamedullary nephrons of young rats. *Am J Physiol* 244:F425–F431, 1983
14. SCHNERMANN J, BRIGGS JP: Concentration-dependent sodium chloride transport as the signal in feedback control of glomerular filtration rate. *Kidney Int* 22(Suppl 12):S82–S89, 1982
15. MOORE LC: Tubuloglomerular feedback in hamster superficial and juxtamedullary nephrons (*abstract*). *Fed Proc* 41:1257, 1982
16. MOORE LC, SCHNERMANN J, YARIMIZU S: Feedback mediation of SNGFR autoregulation in hydropenic and DOCA- and salt-loaded rats. *Am J Physiol* 237:F63–F74, 1979
17. SAKAI T, MARSH DJ: Analysis of frequency response of renal blood flow autoregulation in rats (*abstract*). *Fed Proc* 42:1090, 1983
18. ØIEN AH, AUKLAND K: A mathematical model of the myogenic hypothesis with special reference to autoregulation of renal blood flow. *Circ Res* 52:241–252, 1983
19. COHEN HJ, MARSH DJ, KAYSER B: Autoregulation in vasa recta of the rat kidney. *Am J Physiol* 245:F32–F40, 1983
20. GUSSIS GL, ROBERTSON CR, JAMISON RL: Erythrocyte velocity in vasa recta: effect of antidiuretic hormone and saline diuresis. *Am J Physiol* 237:F326–F332, 1979
21. SHIPLEY RE, STUDY RS: Changes in renal blood flow, extraction of inulin, GFR, tissue pressure and urine flow with acute alterations of renal artery blood pressure. *Am J Physiol* 167:676–688, 1951
22. SELKURT EE, WOMACK I, DAILEY WN: Mechanism of naturesis and diuresis during elevated renal arterial pressure. *Am J Physiol* 209:95–99, 1965
23. KALOYANIDES GJ, DiBONA GF, RASKIN P: Pressure naturesis in the isolated kidney. *Am J Physiol* 220:1660–1666, 1971
24. NAVAR LG, BELL PD, BURKE TJ. Autoregulatory responses of superficial nephrons and their association with sodium excretion during arterial pressure alterations in the dog. *Circ Res* 41:487–496, 1977
25. GUYTON AC: *Arterial Pressure and Hypertension.* Philadelphia, W.B. Saunders Co., 1980, p 87

Glomerular Filtration

Intrarenal Control of Glomerular Filtration: Cellular Mechanisms of Tubuloglomerular Feedback

P. Darwin Bell and L. Gabriel Navar

The maintenance of an optimum balance between the metabolically dependent reabsorptive functions of the tubules and the hemodynamically determined filtered volume at the glomerulus requires the existence of effective mechanisms for the regulation of GFR. Because of this notion, the intimate association between the macula densa cells of the distal tubule and the vascular pole of its own nephron unit has been an intriguing morphologic characteristic, and even early investigators were prompted to suggest that the macula densa region might serve as an important site of communication between the tubular structures and the glomerular blood vessels [1]. The fundamental hypothesis states that changes that occur in the luminal composition of the tubular fluid at the level of the macula densa in response to alterations in flow of fluid into the loop of Henle are perceived by the macula densa cells, which then initiate a sequence of cellular events culminating in a change in vascular tone of the glomerular blood vessels and an adjustment of GFR [2]. During this last decade, this important concept has received widespread recognition and support. With the establishment of this general phenomenon, the investigational issues have become much more specific, with one major thrust focusing on the process by which macula densa cells receive and transmit information. This chapter will discuss our current level of understanding regarding this aspect of the tubuloglomerular feedback mechanism.

General Characteristics of the Tubuloglomerular Feedback Pathway

The characteristics of the distal tubule-to-glomerular feedback mechanism, or simply tubuloglomerular feedback (TGF), have been studied in several

This manuscript was presented as part of a Symposium on *Intrarenal Control of Glomerular Filtration Rate.*

species and in both superficial and deep nephrons [3–8]. One means of assessing tubuloglomerular feedback responses is to block a proximal tubular segment with oil or wax and measure either the single nephron glomerular filtration rate (SNGFR) or the stop-flow pressure (SFP), an index of glomerular capillary pressure, while perfusing the segment of the nephron beyond the block at different flow rates. The highest values are observed in the absence of perfusion. When an isotonic Ringer's solution is used and the late proximal tubule is perfused at flow rates varying from 5 to 40 nl/min, the values decrease. At low perfusion rates of 8 to 12 nl/min, SNGFR and SFP are only slightly reduced; sodium chloride concentration in the early distal tubular fluid is between 40 and 60 mM, and osmolality is below 200 mOsm/kg owing to continued transport of sodium chloride out of the lumen of the water-impermeable thick ascending limb of the loop of Henle. With increases in the perfusion rate to 30 to 40 nl/min, there are further progressive decreases in SNGFR (30 to 50%) and SFP (20 to 30%), whereas there are increases in the distal tubular fluid sodium chloride concentrations and osmolality owing to corresponding flow-related decreases in the fractional reabsorption of sodium chloride by the thick ascending limb. Absolute sodium chloride reabsorption by this segment may actually increase [8]. The values shown in Figure 1 are representative of those obtained in superficial nephrons of the rat; however, it should be mentioned that SFP and SNGFR show substantial decreases in the range of 15 to 25 nl/min when a larger number of measurements are made in each nephron. Studies performed in dogs [5] and in deep juxtamedullary nephrons of the rat [7] indicate that, under some conditions, feedback-mediated reductions in SNGFR can be even greater. Indeed, very high perfusion for several minutes can elicit complete cessation of filtration in some circumstances (personal observations).

The decreases in SNGFR and SFP elicited in response to an increased orthograde perfusion are generally attributed to feedback-mediated increases in afferent arteriole resistance [1, 9, 10]. This conclusion is based, in part, on the assumption that alterations in SFP reflect changes in glomerular capillary pressure. This point of view, however, has been challenged in a recent study [11], which found that directly measured glomerular capillary pressure in the nonobstructed nephron of the Munich-Wistar rat was not responsive to increases in late proximal perfusion but that SNGFR still decreased as it does in other rat strains. This finding has not been substantiated by other recent studies [12, 13], which demonstrate that glomerular capillary pressure does decrease during increases in perfusion rate, even in nephrons in which proximal tubule fluid flow is not interrupted and proximal tubule pressure is unaltered. Also, the magnitude of the response of glomerular capillary pressure is remarkably similar to previously reported decreases in SFP. Indeed, data from our laboratory presented in Figure 1 show decreases in glomerular pressure averaging 12 mm Hg in response to an increased flow rate out of the proximal tubule. Taken together, the data indicate that feedback-mediated decreases in SNGFR result predominantly as a consequence of preglomerular vasoconstriction, which reduces glomerular capillary pressure, effective filtration pressure, and glomerular plasma flow.

Our recent investigations focus on the delineation of the sequence of events

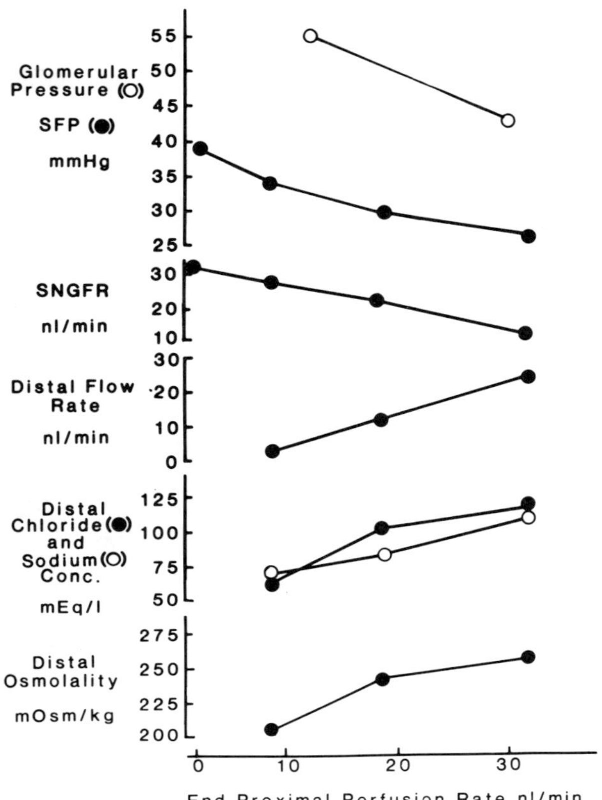

Fig. 1. Changes in glomerular function and distal tubular flow and composition occurring in response to variations in the perfusion rate from a late proximal tubule site in normal Sprague-Dawley rats. All data except for directly measured glomerular capillary pressures, which were measured in Munich-Wistar rats, were obtained in wax-blocked nephrons. In the glomerular capillary pressure series, the perfusion solution was added to the normal tubular flow, and late proximal tubule flow rates are estimated. (Data were taken from [3, 4, 8, 10, 12, 13, 17])

that are involved in the processing and transmission of feedback signals [2]. The first event in the transmission of feedback signals is a change in the composition of the distal tubular fluid, which is brought about by a change in the tubular fluid flow rate through the thick ascending limb. The second step involves a mechanism located in the macula densa cells, the putative "sensing cells" that detect changes in luminal composition. These sensing cells must then activate a cellular mechanism that eventually leads to their communication with extraglomerular mesangial cells and the contractile cells of the glomerular vasculature. This intermediate step may involve complex intracellular biochemical events. (An understanding of this process is fundamental to a complete analysis of the tubuloglomerular feedback mechanism.)

The final step in the feedback pathway is the excitation-contraction event at the smooth muscle cells.

It must be recognized that the macula densa cells are not definitively established as the sensing cells for the transmission of feedback signals. However, their unique morphologic and enzymologic characteristics [14], as compared with surrounding cells of the ascending loop of Henle and their intricate association with the extraglomerular mesangial and smooth muscle cells of the vascular tuft, make them the most likely candidate. Recent morphologic studies by Kaissling and Kriz [15] indicate that, in contrast to the closed intercellular spaces of the thick ascending limb cells, the intercellular spaces between macula densa cells are dilated. Kaissling and Kriz suggest that the macula densa cell segment has a greater water permeability than the surrounding thick ascending limb of the loop of Henle.

Tubular Fluid Compositional Changes Associated with Feedback Signals

Microperfusion studies have shown that feedback-mediated changes in SNGFR and SFP are associated with changes in distal tubular fluid composition, which, in turn, normally result from altered volume flow rate into the thick ascending limb. Compositional changes can thus be expressed in terms of factors that influence this flow rate into the thick ascending limb (such as changes in GFR or tubular reabsorption rate) [9]. Under physiologic conditions, changes in tubular fluid osmolality and sodium chloride concentration occur concurrently. One current issue of uncertainty is related to the precise mechanism by which the macula densa cells detect the changes in concentration. In an effort to gain insight regarding the mechanism by which changes in tubular fluid composition are sensed, several studies have examined the effects of changes in luminal fluid composition, in particular, the substitution of sodium and chloride ions.

Studies designed to evaluate the degree of specificity of the sensing step, for any of the constituents of tubular fluid, have used either the orthograde microperfusion technique, involving perfusion from a late proximal tubule site, or the retrograde microperfusion technique, which involves perfusion from the earliest accessible distal tubule segment backwards toward the macula densa. The orthograde microperfusion studies generally demonstrate that substitution of either sodium or chloride with other electrolytes such as potassium, choline, acetate, isethionate, or bicarbonate does not alter the magnitude of the SFP or SNGFR feedback responses compared to those obtained with an isotonic sodium chloride containing artificial tubular fluid [5, 8, 16–18]. In addition, we have reported that when most of the sodium chloride is replaced with a nonelectrolyte solute such as mannitol, the feedback mechanism maintains its responsiveness to tubular perfusion [8, 16]. In studies involving concomitant analysis of distal tubular fluid, we demonstrated that there is no correlation between changes in distal tubular fluid chloride concentration and feedback-mediated decreases in SNGFR and SFP when most of the sodium chloride was replaced with sodium isethionate [17]. These and related studies led to the proposal that the macula densa cells are probably not sensitive to one specific constituent, but rather are responsive to the overall osmolality of distal tubular fluid.

Studies using the retrograde microperfusion procedure have allowed a more detailed assessment of the initial sensing step. The major advantage of the retrograde microperfusion technique is the close proximity of the early distal tubular perfusion site to the macula densa segment. Therefore, only minor changes in the composition of the perfusate are to be expected between the point of perfusion and the sensing site. The maximum decreases in SFP or SNGFR during retrograde perfusion are not different from those obtained with orthograde microperfusion; however, the magnitude of the feedback responses is independent of flow and primarily dependent on the concentration of the perfusate over a relatively narrow range from 40 to 120 mOsm. The SFP feedback responses obtained during retrograde perfusion with a variety of solutions are shown in Figure 2.

Using the retrograde microperfusion technique, Schnermann, Ploth, and Hermle [19] reported that feedback responses were obtained most consistently with solutions of sodium chloride and other chloride-containing single-salt solutions. Substitution of chloride with other anions reduced the consistency of the feedback responses. Also, mannitol or urea did not significantly enhance the feedback responses found with hypotonic sodium chloride solutions [20]. They suggested that the sensing step might be chloride specific, involving either changes in chloride concentration or chloride transport, or both. Using a slightly different approach involving retrograde microperfusion of more

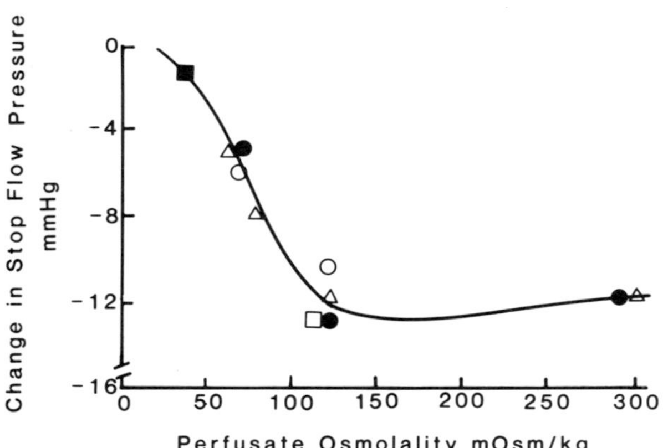

Fig. 2. Influence of the perfusate osmolality on the change in SFP obtained in response to retrograde perfusion at 15 nl/min. The matrix solution contained normal tubular concentrations of monovalent and divalent electrolytes and a chloride concentration of 7 mEq/liter. Increases in perfusate osmolality were achieved by adding specific salts as indicated. Symbols are: ■, matrix solution; ●, sodium chloride; △, sodium isethionate; ○, sodium bicarbonate; □, choline chloride. (Data were taken from [21])

complete solutions, studies from our laboratory [21] indicate that other electrolytes such as isethionate, choline, and bicarbonate can be substituted for almost all of the sodium or chloride without an apparent effect on the magnitude of the feedback responses when compared with a Ringer's solution of similar osmolality (Fig. 2). In our experiments, emphasis was placed on the use of more complex perfusates that contain many of the constituents normally found in tubular fluid and low concentrations of sodium and chloride. Using this approach, we observed a consistent inverse relationship between the magnitude of the SFP feedback response and the perfusate osmolality over a range of 40 to 120 mOsm/kg. These studies support the premise that the detection process is responsive to an overall change in tubular fluid osmolality.

Although our studies dissociated the magnitude of the feedback responses from changes in distal sodium chloride concentration, other studies indicate that complete removal of chloride from the perfusion solution can result in diminished or abolished feedback responses [19]. It is possible, however, that certain constituents, such as sodium chloride, must be present, at least in small quantities, to maintain the integrity of the feedback mechanism. This interpretation suggests that the capability of the macula densa cells to detect changes in luminal fluid osmolality and transmit feedback signals may require an intact electrolyte transport step such as the Na:Cl:K transporter known to exist in the cortical thick ascending limb [22]. Evidence that such a transport mechanism influences feedback responses is the finding that loop diuretics, such as furosemide, that are known to block this cotransport step can completely inhibit feedback responses [10, 23]. However, furosemide induces several cellular electrolyte disturbances, including decreases in intracellular sodium and chloride concentrations, abolished transepithelial potential difference, hyperpolarization of the basolateral membrane, and reduced energy consumption [22]. If these alterations also occur in the macula densa cells, they could render the "sensing cells" unable to detect luminal osmolality changes and to transmit signals. It is thus possible that the deletion of all chloride from the perfusate [19] could have produced a "furosemide-like" effect in that the complete absence of chloride effectively inhibited the Na:Cl:K entry step. In our experiments, sodium chloride was never completely removed, and it is possible that the amount remaining at the macula densa was sufficient to maintain the requisite cellular transport and to preserve the functional integrity of the macula densa cells.

Role of Calcium in the Mediation of Feedback Responses

The cellular mechanism responsible for detecting changes in luminal fluid composition presents an intriguing problem, because it requires a system that is highly sensitive to small changes in tubular fluid composition, has a fast response time, and is capable of transmitting signals to the contractile cells. Recent experimental findings suggest an important role for intracellular calcium in the transmission of feedback signals [24]. In other tissues, a variety of extracellular events, such as hormone binding, membrane electrical potential changes, and alterations in electrolyte concentrations, lead to increases in cytosolic calcium concentration, which in turn elicit specific alterations in cell function [25]. Since the feedback process requires the detection of an extracellular event and the subsequent transmission or communication with other cell types, we were attracted to the idea that a macula densa intracellular calcium system might serve such a role [2], and we performed studies to examine this proposal. To increase cytosolic calcium concentration, we used the calcium ionophore, A23187, to increase the permeability of luminal cell membranes to calcium. Since intracellular calcium is maintained at very low levels in many cell systems (10^{-7} M), the normal tubular fluid calcium concentrations represent a substantial calcium gradient, which should result in calcium entry and elevations in cytosolic calcium concentration [25]. As shown in Figure 3, the addition of A23187 to a hypotonic solution, which normally elicits only a small feedback response when perfused retrograde,

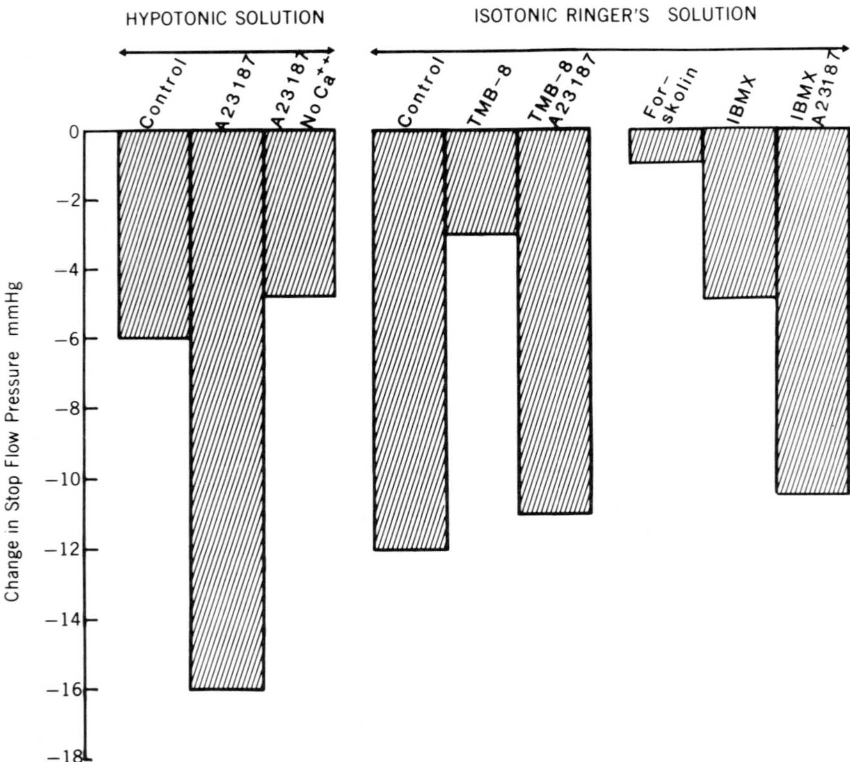

Fig. 3. Average SFP feedback responses obtained during retrograde microperfusion with solutions containing various agents that influence cytosolic calcium concentration or elevate cyclic AMP levels. The control solution in the hypotonic group was 70 mOsm/kg. Refer to the text for information concerning the actions of the various drugs. (Data were taken from [24, 27, 33])

resulted in markedly augmented feedback responses. In fact, the feedback responses obtained with A23187 were even greater than the feedback responses obtained with an isotonic solution. This effect of A23187 appeared to be calcium specific, since removal of calcium from the perfusate blunted the enhanced responses obtained with A23187.

The addition of A23187 presumably increased luminal membrane permeability to calcium and allowed influx from the tubular fluid. For several reasons, however, it is unlikely that the normal activation step involves calcium translocation from the tubular fluid into the cells. Other studies have reported that changes in perfusate calcium concentration do not alter the magnitude of feedback responses obtained with retrograde microperfusion [26]. We have confirmed that feedback responses obtained during retrograde perfusion are not perceptibly altered by varying the calcium concentration or eliminating calcium from the perfusate [27]. Also, the addition of a calcium chelator or a calcium channel blocker to the isotonic perfusion solution does not influence the feedback responsiveness during retrograde perfusion.

Because it appeared that the feedback mechanism did not require a calcium entry step from the luminal fluid into the macula densa cells, yet appeared to be activated by increased cellular calcium concentrations, further studies were conducted to determine if feedback responses could be influenced by procedures that affect intracellular calcium mobilization. Such reasoning is consistent with the concept that the level of cytosolic calcium is controlled, to a large extent, by calcium storage sites such as mitochondria, endoplasmic reticulum, and cellular membranes, and that extracellular events can elicit increases in cytosolic calcium through calcium mobilization from these storage sites into the cytosol [25]. To assess this possibility, we performed retrograde microperfusion studies using 8-(N,N-diethyl-amino)-octyl 3,4,5-trimethoxy-benzoate (TMB-8), which stabilizes cellular calcium and prevents or attenuates calcium movement from storage sites into the cytosol [28]. We observed that the addition of TMB-8 at concentrations of 100 to 500 μM to an isotonic Ringer's solution (having a calcium concentration of 1 mEq/liter) resulted in a dose-dependent inhibition of SFP feedback responses [27]. Importantly, the inhibitory effects of TMB-8 were completely reversed by the addition of A23187 to the perfusion solution. This action was consistent with the presumed ability of TMB-8 to influence calcium mobilization from storage sites and not directly antagonize the actions of free cytosolic calcium. These results suggest that the TMB-8 entered the sensing cells and prevented the increases in cytosolic calcium concentration that presumably would have occurred during increases in luminal fluid osmolality.

In other tissues in which cytosolic calcium participates as an intracellular mediator, other intracellular messengers and cellular proteins often contribute either directly or indirectly to calcium-mediated events. As pointed out by Rasmussen [29], there is a complex interaction between cytosolic calcium and other intracellular messenger systems, an interaction that is highly dependent on the particular tissue and system under investigation. This interaction can be either synergistic or inhibitory. Accordingly, we attempted to evaluate the influence of other intracellular messenger systems on calcium-mediated feedback responses.

One system closely linked to the actions of calcium is the calcium-binding protein calmodulin. Calmodulin has been found in all systems examined to date, and its effects on a wide variety of cellular functions have been characterized [30]. Activation of calmodulin may directly mediate the effects of an increase in cytosolic calcium concentration. Alternatively, it may indirectly influence calcium-mediated responses by regulating cytosolic calcium concentration through an energy-linked calcium transport mechanism that promotes the lowering of cytosolic calcium concentration. To evaluate this issue, we added trifluroperazine (TFP), a potent inhibitor of calmodulin activity, to the isotonic perfusion solution. We were unable to establish that TFP altered the magnitude or the onset characteristics of SFP feedback responses obtained during retrograde microperfusion [31]. These results suggest that calmodulin does not participate directly in the mediation of feedback responses. We noticed, however, that in the tubules perfused with the TFP containing isotonic solution, the recovery patterns were delayed. The time required for SFP to return to control values following cessation of perfusion was doubled from that normally measured when an isotonic Ringer's solution is used alone (69 to 160 sec). The finding that TFP significantly prolonged the time required for SFP to return to preperfusion levels suggests an impaired ability of the macula densa cells to restore cytosolic calcium concentration to a normal level when calmodulin activity is inhibited. One interpretation of these results is that calmodulin, while not directly participating in the transmission of feedback signals, could contribute to the regulation of cytosolic calcium concentration by enhancing either calcium extrusion from the cell or calcium uptake into intracellular storage sites, or both [30]. Thus, calmodulin could contribute to the rapidity of the restoration in glomerular pressure that occurs when perfusion to the macula densa segment is stopped.

Influence of Cyclic Nucleotide and Calcium Interactions on the Feedback Mechanism

The relationship between the cytosolic calcium system and cyclic AMP has been examined in several different systems. Depending on the system under investigation, cyclic AMP has been shown to either enhance calcium-mediated responses or to inhibit calcium-mediated events. The reason for the directionally different types of interaction between these two systems is not clear, but one suggestion is that cyclic AMP can either raise or lower cytosolic calcium concentration depending on which intracellular calcium storage site is susceptible to its control [29].

In previous studies, it was reported that the methylxanthines, isobutyl methylxanthine (IBMX) and theophylline, inhibit feedback responses when perfused from either a late proximal tubule segment or an early distal tubular site [32]. One action of these methylxanthines is to elevate cellular cyclic AMP by inhibition of phosphodiesterase activity, the enzyme that is responsible for the degradation of cyclic AMP. In recent studies [33], we confirmed the finding that IBMX attenuates SFP feedback responses obtained during retrograde microperfusion with an isotonic Ringer's solution. Although IBMX causes inhibition of phosphodiesterase activity, it also has additional actions, such as adenosine receptor antagonism. Thus, additional maneuvers were used for evaluating the possibility of a specific cyclic AMP action. When dibutyryl cyclic AMP was added to the perfusate in the presence of a low concentration of IBMX, we again found marked attenuation of feedback responses. In further studies, forskolin, a diterpene agent that stimulates adenylate cyclase activity [34] and thereby elevates endogenous intracellular cyclic AMP concentrations, was added to the perfusate. This agent almost completely eliminated SFP feedback responses during retrograde microperfusion with an isotonic Ringer's solution. To determine if the inhibition of feedback responses resulting from elevations in cellular cyclic AMP levels was related to the cytosolic calcium system, the calcium ionophore A23187 was added to the Ringer's solution containing a concentration of IBMX sufficient to significantly inhibit feedback responses. Perfusion with A23187 restored SFP feedback responses to normal levels even when IBMX was present. These results suggest that cyclic AMP interrupts transmission of feedback signals by preventing increases in cytosolic calcium concentration. This effect may occur through an enhanced sequestering of calcium into intracellular storage sites or calcium extrusion from the macula densa cells.

Alterations in feedback responsiveness or sensitivity are known to occur in response to a number of different maneuvers [1, 2]. The mechanism by which feedback responses are altered or "reset" has not been completely characterized. Although it has been suggested that changes in interstitial fluid pressure or volume are capable of altering feedback sensitivity [35], it is also possible that cellular cyclic AMP levels could serve to modulate feedback sensitivity. Thus, conditions or circumstances that result in an enhanced adenylate cyclase activity could elevate cyclic AMP concentrations within the macula densa cells, which, in turn, would decrease the cellular responsiveness to changes in tubular fluid osmolality.

Possible Role of Arachidonic Acid Metabolites in Mediating Feedback Signals

Recent work indicates that cellular prostaglandins participate in a variety of stimulus-secretion coupling mechanisms [25]. In fact, products of arachidonic acid metabolism can, in some systems, directly stimulate secretion, whereas there are other examples in which prostaglandins inhibit secretion. In addition, there is a complex interaction between prostaglandin production and cytosolic calcium. Increases in cytosolic calcium concentration can activate certain phospholipases, which increase the availability of free arachidonic acid and lead to the production of various metabolites through the cyclooxygenase and lipoxygenase pathways. Furthermore, certain metabolites of arachidonate metabolism, as well as phosphatidic acid, which is generated by phospholipase C, may serve as calcium ionophores. Thus, elevations in cytosolic calcium concentration can stimulate prostaglandin production, and intracellular production of prostaglandins may result in mobilization of cellular calcium [25].

In agreement with previous studies [36], our experiments assessing the possible involvement of prostaglandins in the tubuloglomerular feedback mechanism demonstrated that cyclooxygenase inhibitors, such as indomethacin, prevented the manifestation of tubuloglomerular feedback responses to increases in flow rate to the distal nephron [37]. Such studies implicate a prostaglandin contribution to the mediation of TGF signals. To determine if there is an interaction between cellular prostaglandins and the cytosolic calcium system, studies were performed in which arachidonic acid was added to a hypotonic solution, which normally elicits small responses during retrograde microperfusion. With the addition of arachidonic acid (160 μM), there was a marked enhancement of tubuloglomerular feedback responses. This finding suggests the interesting possibility that the feedback pathway includes an arachidonic acid metabolite that may either directly elicit contraction of the smooth muscle effector cells or at least indirectly influence cytosolic calcium concentraion, perhaps through enhanced calcium mobilization. The exact nature of this interaction awaits additional studies.

The specific mechanism responsible for the transmission of feedback signals from the macula densa cells to the vascular elements remains unknown. Low-resistance gap junctions have been found to connect extraglomerular and intraglomerular mesangial cells, granular cells, and vascular smooth muscle cells [38]. Thus, once the signal has been transmitted to the extraglomerular mesangial cells, it may be propagated to the smooth muscle cells through the low-resistance pathways. However, gap junctions have not been found between the macula densa cells and extraglomerular mesangial cells, and it would appear that a chemical mediator is necessary for this communication step. The arachidonic acid perfusion studies raise the interesting possibility that the macula densa cells may release a metabolite of arachidonic acid that elicits vasoconstriction.

Acknowledgments. Our experimental work has been supported by research grants from the National Heart, Lung and Blood Institute and the American Heart Association.

References

1. WRIGHT FS, BRIGGS JP: Feedback control of glomerular blood flow, pressure, and filtration rate. *Physiol Rev* 59:958–1006, 1979
2. BELL PD, NAVAR LG: Macula densa feedback control of glomerular filtration: Role of cytosolic calcium. *Mineral Electrolyte Metab* 8:61–77, 1982
3. SCHNERMANN J, WRIGHT FS, DAVIS JM, STACKELBERG WV, GRILL G: Regulation of superficial nephron filtration rate by tubulo-glomerular feedback. *Pflügers Arch* 318:147–175, 1970
4. SCHNERMANN J, PERSSON AEG, AGERUP B: Tubuloglomerular feedback: Nonlinear relation between glomerular hydrostatic pressure and loop of Henle perfusion rate. *J Clin Invest* 52:862–869, 1973

5. BELL PD, THOMAS C, WILLIAM RH, NAVAR LG: Filtration rate and stop-flow pressure feedback responses to nephron perfusion in the dog. *Am J Physiol* 234 (*Renal Fluid Electrolyte Physiol 3*):F154–F165, 1978

6. PERSSON BF, PERSSON AEG: The existence of a tubulo-glomerular feedback mechanism in the Amphiuma nephron. *Pflügers Arch* 391:129–134, 1981

7. MULLER-SUUR R, ULFENDAHL HR, PERSSON EG: Evidence for tubuloglomerular feedback in juxtamedullary nephrons of young rats. *Am J Physiol* 244(*Renal Fluid Electrolyte Physiol 13*):F425–F431, 1983

8. BELL PD, NAVAR LG, PLOTH DW, MCLEAN CB: Tubuloglomerular feedback responses during perfusion with nonelectrolyte solutions in the rat. *Kidney Int* 18:460–471, 1980

9. NAVAR LG: Renal autoregulation: perspectives from whole kidney and single nephron studies. *Am J Physiol* 234(*Renal Fluid Electrolyte Physiol 3*):F357–F370, 1978

10. BRIGGS JP, WRIGHT FS: Feedback control of glomerular filtration rate: site of the effector mechanism. *Am J Physiol* 236(*Renal Fluid Electrolyte Physiol 5*):F40–F47, 1979

11. ICHIKAWA I: Direct analysis of the effector mechanism of the tubuloglomerular feedback system. *Am J Physiol* 243(*Renal Fluid Electrolyte Physiol 12*):F447–F455, 1982

12. NAVAR LG, REDDINGTON M, BELL PD, PLOTH DW: Tubuloglomerular feedback mediated reductions in directly measured glomerular capillary pressure in response to increased distal volume delivery (*abstract*). *Physiologist* 26:A127, 1983

13. BLANTZ RC, GUSHWA LC, PERSSON AEG: Tubuloglomerular feedback (TGF) released response in glomerular capillary hydrostatic pressure (P_G) and nephron filtration rate (SNGFR) in hydropenic (H) and in angiotensin (AII) and prostaglandin (PG) blocked rats (B) (*abstract*). *Kidney Int* 25:286, 1984

14. BARAJAS L: The juxtaglomerular apparatus: Anatomical considerations in the feedback control of glomerular filtration rate. *Fed Proc* 40:78–86, 1981

15. KAISSLING B, KRIZ W: Variability of intercellular spaces between macula densa cells: a transmission electron microscopic study in rabbits and rats. *Kidney Int* 22(Suppl 12):S-9–S-17, 1982

16. NAVAR LG, BELL PD, THOMAS CE, PLOTH DW: Influence of perfusate osmolality on stop pressure feedback responses in the dog. *Am J Physiol* 235(*Renal Fluid Electrolyte Physiol 4*):F352–F358, 1978

17. BELL PD, MCLEAN CB, NAVAR LG: Dissociation of tubulo-glomerular feedback responses from distal tubular chloride concentration in the rat. *Am J Physiol* 240(*Renal Fluid Electrolyte Physiol 9*):F111–F119, 1981

18. MULLER-SUUR R, GUTSCHE H-U: Effect of intratubular substitution of Na$^+$ and Cl$^-$ ions on the operation of the tubuloglomerular feedback. *Acta Physiol Scand* 103:353–362, 1978

19. SCHNERMANN J, PLOTH DW, HERMLE M: Activation of tubulo-glomerular feedback by chloride transport. *Pflügers Arch* 362:229–240, 1976

20. BRIGGS JP, SCHNERMANN J, WRIGHT FS: Failure of tubule fluid osmolality to affect feedback regulation of glomerular filtration. *Am J Physiol* 239(*Renal Fluid Electrolyte Physiol 8*):F427–F432, 1980

21. BELL PD, NAVAR LG: Relationship between tubulo-glomerular feedback responses and perfusate hypotonicity. *Kidney Int* 22:234–239, 1982

22. GREGER R, SCHLATTER E: Cellular mechanism of the action of loop diuretics on the thick ascending limb of Henle's loop. *Klin Wochenschr* 61:1019–1027, 1983

23. WRIGHT FS, SCHNERMANN J: Interference with feedback control of glomerular filtration rate by furosemide, triflocin, and cyanide. *J Clin Invest* 53(6):1695–1708, 1974

24. BELL PD, NAVAR LG: Cytoplasmic calcium in the mediation of macula densa tubulo-glomerular feedback responses. *Science* 215:670–673, 1982
25. RUBIN RP: *Calcium and Cellular Secretion.* New York, Plenum Press, 1982, pp 1–43, 192–215
26. SCHNERMANN J, HERMLE M: Maintenance of feedback regulation of filtration dynamics in the absence of divalent cations in the lumen of the distal tubule. *Pflügers Arch* 358:311–323, 1975
27. BELL PD, REDDINGTON M: Intracellular calcium in the transmission of tubulo-glomerular feedback signals. *Am J Physiol* 245(*Renal Fluid Electrolyte Physiol 14*):F295–F302, 1983
28. SHAW JO: Effects of extracellular Ca^{++} and the intracellular Ca^{++} antagonist 8-(N,N-diethylamino)octyl-3,4-5-trimethoxybenzoate on rabbit platelet conversion of arachidonic acid to thromboxane. *Prostaglandins* 21:571–579, 1981
29. RASMUSSEN H: *Calcium and cAMP as Synarchic Messengers.* New York, John Wiley & Sons, 1981, pp 1–59
30. MEANS AR, TASH JS, CHAFOULEAS JG: Physiological implications of the presence, distribution, and regulation of calmodulin in eukaryotic cells. *Physiol Rev* 62:1–37, 1982
31. BELL PD, REDDINGTON M: Tubuloglomerular feedback responses during calmodulin inhibition with trifluoperazine in the rat (*abstract*). *Physiologist* 26:A127, 1983
32. SCHNERMANN J, OSSWALD H, HERMLE M: Inhibitory effect of methylxanthines on feedback control of glomerular filtration rate in the rat kidney. *Pflügers Arch* 369(1):39–48, 1977
33. BELL PD, REDDINGTON M: Cyclic nucleotide-calcium interaction in the mediation of macula densa tubuloglomerular feedback signals (*abstract*). *Fed Proc* 42:298, 1983
34. SEAMON KB, DALEY JW: Forskolin: a unique diterpene activator of cyclic AMP-generating systems. *J Cyclic Nucleotide Res* 224:201–224, 1981
35. PERSSON AEG, BOBERG U, HAHNE B, MULLER-SUUR R, NORLEN B-J, SELEN G: Interstitial pressure as a modulator of tubuloglomerular feedback control. *Kidney Int* 22(Suppl 12):S122–S128, 1982
36. SCHNERMANN J, BRIGGS JP: Participation of renal cortical prostaglandins in the regulation of glomerular filtration rate. *Kidney Int* 19:802–815, 1981
37. BELL PD: Participation of prostaglandins in the mediation of tubuloglomerular feedback responses (*abstract*). *Fed Proc* 43:409, 1984
38. FORSSMANN WG, TAUGNER R: Studies on the juxtaglomerular apparatus: V. The juxtaglomerular apparatus in tupania with special reference to intercellular contacts. *Cell Tissue Res* 177:291–295, 1977

Regulatory Role of the Tubuloglomerular Feedback Mechanism

Josephine P. Briggs and Jürgen Schnermann

There is accumulating evidence that the juxtaglomerular apparatus (JGA)—the anatomic curiosity that links the microvascular pole of every glomerulus with its own distal tubule—plays an important functional role in the control of filtration rate. It is well established that an elevation of flow into the loop of Henle leads to a prompt reduction in the single nephron glomerular filtration rate (SNGFR) of the same nephron, a phenomenon commonly called tubuloglomerular feedback (TGF). It is likely that this response is a reflection of backtalk between the macula densa and its parent glomerulus, communicated via the extraglomerular mesangial cells of the JGA. A substantial body of experimental work has explored the mechanism of this response. This work, which has been reviewed elsewhere [1], will not be discussed here. This report will concentrate on recent studies that address the question of the regulatory role of this mechanism. The question we pose is: Is it possible to extrapolate from the response of the single nephron, studied under the somewhat artificial conditions of in situ microperfusion, to the response of the whole kidney? We will review evidence suggesting that the answer to this question in a number of circumstances is a qualified yes.

The Macula Densa Signal

The thick ascending limb performs a critical function in the operation of the TGF mechanism; by virtue of its capacity to transport sodium chloride without water, it converts changes in tubular flow rate into changes in sodium chloride concentration. The macula densa is located at the distal-most end of the thick ascending limb, right before the transition to the distal convoluted tubule [2]. Although macula densa of most nephrons is inaccessible to micro-

---

This manuscript was presented as part of a Symposium on *Intrarenal Control of Glomerular Filtration Rate*.

puncture, there is good indirect evidence that sodium and chloride concentrations at this site are a direct function of tubular flow rate [3, 4]; at low flow rates, minimum values in the range of 15 to 20 mEq/liter are achieved, with progressively higher values at higher flow rates.

In studies in which tubular fluid composition in the macula densa segment is experimentally manipulated by single nephron perfusion, filtration rate is an inverse function of sodium chloride concentration ($[NaCl]_{MD}$). The response range, approximately 20 to 60 mEq/liter [5], corresponds with the probable free-flow range. Our studies suggest that the important ion for the response is chloride [5]; sodium plays no regulatory role, probably because its concentration is always supramaximal. Bell, McLean, and Navar [6] have advanced the hypothesis that tubular fluid osmolarity may be the regulated quantity. We have been unable to demonstrate any influence of noncharged solutes (urea or mannitol) on responses [7], but agree with their observation that isethionate, an impermeant anion, enhances responses [8]. Although uncharged solutes and cations are apparently without important physiologic influence, the effect of chloride appears to be modified to a substantial degree by the presence of impermeant anions [9]. The JGA mechanism can be viewed as a regulatory response linking distal sodium chloride concentration and filtration rate. Distal sodium chloride concentration is, in turn, a function of flow into the loop of Henle.

The Feedback Loop

When two quantities (A and B) are interrelated such that an increase in A leads to an increase in B, but an increase in B yields a decrease in A, a potential negative or homeostatic feedback loop results. When the two relationships can be defined quantitatively, A as a function of B and B as a function of A, the steady-state values of A and B are required to lie at the point yielded by simultaneous solution of the two equations. The TGF loop is shown in Figure 1. An elevation of filtration rate results in an increase in tubular flow rate. This is the feed*forward* function, shown as f_1. An elevation in tubular flow results, via the TGF mechanism, in a suppression in filtration rate; this relationship can be defined by a feed*back* function, f_2. Quantitative estimates of this relationship, derived from single nephron microperfusion experiments are presented below. Because the macula densa is inaccessible to micropuncture, our quantitative analysis uses the flow into the loop of Henle ($\dot{V}_{LP}$) as the second quantity in the homeostatic loop rather than the macula densa sodium chloride concentration. $\dot{V}_{LP}$ is defined from the viewpoint of the micropuncturist; it is the flow rate at the end of the most superficial convolution of the proximal tubule. $\dot{V}_{LP}$ is a quantity that can be manipulated experimentally. The standard technique for study of the TGF mechanism is to perfuse the loop of Henle of a single nephron from the last segment of the proximal tubule with a microperfusion pump that allows flow to be varied from 0 to 50 nl/min. Usually the tubule is blocked, just upstream from the perfusion pipette, with an immobile wax block. Filtration rate, flow rate, or intratubular pressure is then measured in an early proximal site.

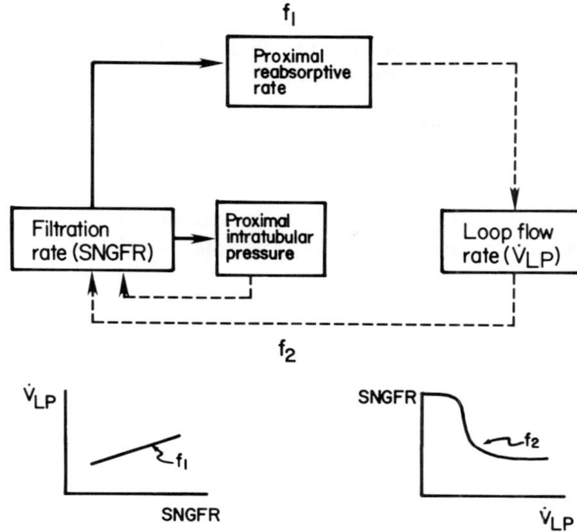

Fig. 1. Schematic depiction of interrelationships between glomerular and tubular function. A *solid arrow* depicts a relationship in which increases in the first variable lead to increases in the second variable; a *broken arrow,* one in which the two quantities change in opposite directions.

The TGF loop is not the only potential intrinsic homeostatic regulator of SNGFR and $\dot{V}_{LP}$. There are two other interrelationships between tubular and glomerular function that may have homeostatic function. When filtration rate rises, intratubular pressure rises. Because the resulting diminished transcapillary pressure gradient tends to reduce filtration rate, this response creates a potential feedback loop. The quantitative importance of this response has been the subject of controversy. Single nephron microperfusion studies suggest that the tubule is compliant enough to accommodate moderate increases in flow with only very minimal elevations in intratubular pressure [10, 11]. In one study increments or decrements of flow of 5 nl/min produced no measurable change in intratubular pressure [11]. Where loop flow rises very substantially, however, as, for example, during furosemide or mannitol diuresis, elevation in intratubular pressure may exert a significant suppressing effect on filtration rate.

Glomerulotubular balance is another intrinsic regulator of $\dot{V}_{LP}$. Proximal tubular transport rises and falls with increases and decreases in GFR. These changes in proximal transport tend to blunt the change in flow into the loop of Henle that results from a change in GFR. They are thus an important determinant of the signal that reaches the macula densa. To determine the effectiveness (or, in engineering terminology, the open loop gain) of the TGF loop from loop perfusion results, it is necessary to know what proportion of a change in filtration rate will be transmitted to the loop of Henle. In other words, it is necessary to define the slope of f_1, the feed*forward* function.

A precise experimental assessment of this slope is not a straightforward problem. Nevertheless, it is possible to set limits. In the absence of any proximal tubule adjustments, a change in filtration rate would result in an equal change in loop flow rate. In this case (the *absent* glomerulotubular balance assumption), f_1 would have a slope of 1, and the signal to the TGF mechanism would be maximum. A reasonable minimum value is calculated by assuming that a constant fraction of the filtrate is reabsorbed along the proximal tubule (the *perfect* glomerulotubular balance assumption). With this assumption, if the TF/P_{inulin} ratio in the late proximal tubule were 2, the slope of f_1 would be one-half, which is to say half of a change in filtration rate would be transmitted to the loop. Most available measurements would suggest that the adjustments in proximal transport with changing GFR are not sufficient to maintain a constant late proximal TF/P_{inulin} ratio. Therefore, the reality probably lies between these two estimates.

The Feedback Function

We recently performed a series of experiments designed to describe the feedback function [12]. For these studies we used rats of three sizes. The smallest

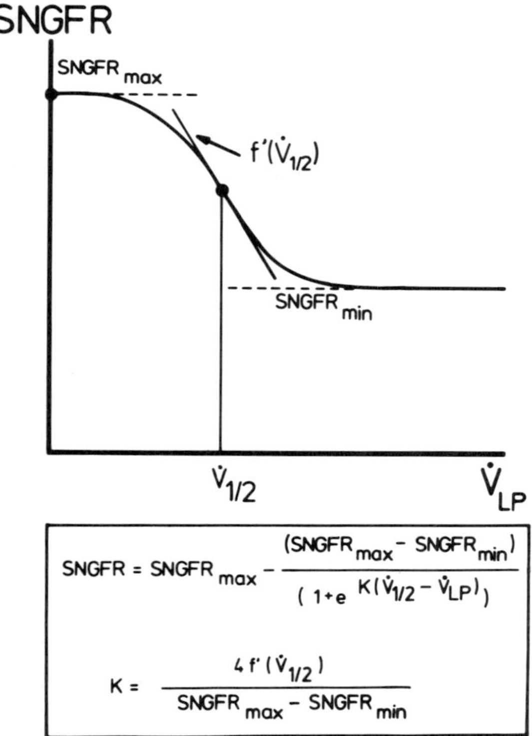

$$SNGFR = SNGFR_{max} - \frac{(SNGFR_{max} - SNGFR_{min})}{(1 + e^{K(\dot{V}_{1/2} - \dot{V}_{LP})})}$$

$$K = \frac{4 f'(\dot{V}_{1/2})}{SNGFR_{max} - SNGFR_{min}}$$

Fig. 2. Equation used to describe observed sigmoidal relationship between $\dot{V}_{LP}$ and SNGFR.

group weighed 100 g and were approximately 30 days old, a size and age at which renal function is essentially mature. The intermediate group, 220 g, corresponded to the standard micropuncture rat in our laboratory. A group of large animals, weighing an average of 350 g, were also studied. Surgical protein losses were replaced to maintain arterial hematocrit approximately constant and thus, at least by this parameter, euvolemia. We found that when flow into the loop of Henle was progressively increased, SNGFR, measured in the proximal tubule, fell in a sigmoidal fashion. It was insensitive at high and low flows, but fell steeply in an intermediate flow range. A sigmoidal equation of the form shown in Figure 2 was found to provide a good fit to the data. We therefore used this function to provide a simple quantitative description of the observed relationship. This function describes the dependence of SNGFR on $\dot{V}_{LP}$ in terms of four parameters: $SNGFR_{Max}$ and $SNGFR_{Min}$, the maximum and minimum values of SNGFR; $\dot{V}_{1/2}$, the flow rate at which the response is half-maximum; and $f'(V_{1/2})$, the slope at the midpoint.

The feedback curves in the three size groups are shown in Figure 3. Curves plotted are based on the overall averages of parameters determined separately for each perfused nephron. In the intermediate weight group, SNGFR fell from 46.5 ± 1.5 to 27.3 ± 1.3 nl/min, a decrease of 41%, when loop flow was elevated from 0 to 40 nl/min. The response was half maximal at a tubular flow rate of 15.4 ± 0.8 nl/min, and the midpoint slope was 1.7 ± 0.2. In the smaller and larger rats, the curve was shifted to the left and right, respectively; the curve shift was essentially proportionate. The maximum depression of filtration rate averaged between 40 and 50% in all three groups. The value of filtration rate measured when loop flow was zero rose

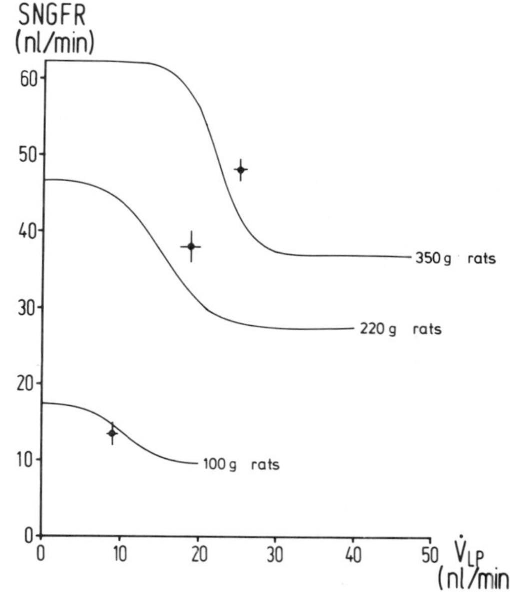

Fig. 3. Feedback function in rats of three sizes. Function is derived from measurements of SNGFR made during microperfusion of the loop of Henle. Shown for comparison by the *closed circles* are free-flow measurements of SNGFR and $\dot{V}_{LP}$ made with minimal perturbation of loop of Henle flow.

progressively, as did $\dot{V}_{1/2}$, the flow at which 50% of the response occurred. The maximum slope also increased with growth; however, expressed as a fractional change, sensitivity did not increase. The data suggest that in all three groups a 10% increase in loop flow at the midpoint would produce a 5 to 10% decrease in SNGFR.

Tubuloglomerular Feedback in the Subnormal Flow Range

The microperfusion measurements just discussed would suggest that when the loop of Henle flow is reduced from normal to zero, SNGFR should rise. Sensitivity in the subnormal flow range can also be assessed by comparing proximal and distal measurements of SNGFR (see Fig. 3). When SNGFR is measured in the distal tubule, flow past the macula densa is not disturbed. Measurement of SNGFR in the proximal tubule, however, involves blockade of the tubule and therefore interruption of the TGF loop. A large number of laboratories have confirmed the original observation of Schnermann et al [13], that SNGFR is systematically higher when measured in the proximal than in the distal tubule (Fig. 4) [14–17]. In a number of studies, no difference was detected, however [18, 19]. The reasons for this discrepancy are not entirely clear. There are a number of potential experimental differences that can influence a comparison of filtration rate at the two sites. With appropriate care, however, these differences can be excluded.

In the microperfusion studies just discussed, we also measured SNGFR in the distal tubule. In all three groups, this value was found to lie approxi-

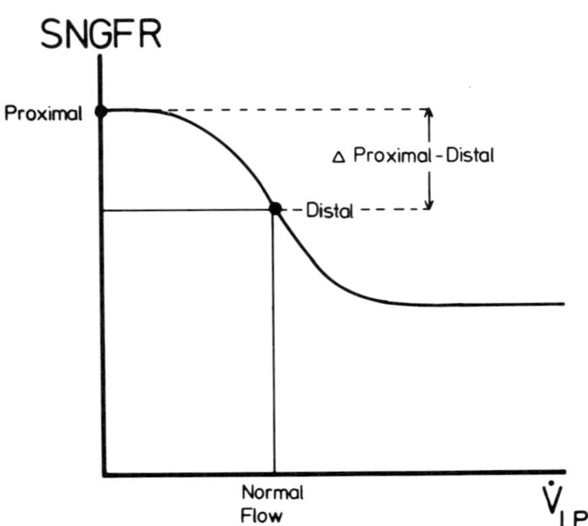

Fig. 4. Prediction of the proximal-distal SNGFR difference from microperfusion curves.

mately half-way between the maximum and minimum SNGFR values measured during microperfusion. The free-flow value of $\dot{V}_{LP}$, estimated by *stealing* fluid from the late proximal tubule at a low collection rate, was found to be close to the microperfusion estimate of $\dot{V}_{1/2}$. These studies provide evidence that under the conditions of these studies a substantial portion of the TGF response occurs in the subnormal flow range and indicate that in the basal state TGF (or distal flow) is exerting a tonic effect on vascular tone.

The magnitude of this basal tone seems to be quite variable, more so than the magnitude of the maximum responses. There is evidence that it depends on rat size [12], sodium chloride balance [20], dietary protein content, and arterial pressure [21]. Such factors may have contributed to the failure of certain studies to detect a significant difference between SNGFR measured in the proximal and distal tubules.

The Intact Feedback Loop

External Forcing—Autoregulation

The open-loop characteristics of the tubuloglomerular feedback loop outlined so far permit predictions about its regulatory role under normal closed-loop operating conditions. It is to be realized that the system is constructed to keep distal delivery of sodium chloride within narrow limits. Therefore, the response to an external forcing imposed on filtrate formation will be to alter vascular resistance and thus blunt the impact of the changed forces. In the new steady state, GFR and distal sodium chloride concentration will be relatively well maintained, but vascular resistances will be readjusted.

A change in arterial pressure has been the most widely studied model for external forcing of the feedback loop. In a number of studies, it has been found that virtual constancy of GFR is achieved only when the flow perturbation is permitted to reach the macula densa sensor [21–23]. In agreement with the position of the operating point within the steep portion of the feedback function, a regulatory response is obtained during both increases and decreases in pressure. Thus, as suggested by the microperfusion results, in the control state, the feedback mechanism has both vasodilatory and vasoconstrictive capacity. The nature of the signal maintaining the adjusted resistance, even though GFR has been returned to its original level, is unclear. It has been pointed out that relatively small, pressure-dependent alterations in tubular absorption may be sufficient to supply the error signal [24]. While most results support a role of TGF in the resistance adjustments in response to an arterial pressure change, it appears that autoregulatory precision is the result of an interplay between several control systems. Prostaglandins, the renin-angiotensin system, and the intrinsic myogenic capacity of the renal vasculature all appear to also contribute [21]. Our estimate is that in the subnormal flow range, one-third to one-half of the autoregulatory resistance changes are feedback-mediated.

In contrast to the GFR stabilizing effect of TGF in response to an external forcing, the system will destabilize filtration rate when either the feedforward or feedback function is altered.

Effect of an Altered Feedforward Function

An alteration in the feedforward function results when there is a change in sodium chloride transport along the proximal tubule. As shown schematically in Figure 5a, a decrease in transport will induce a shift of the feedforward function to the right, and an increase in transport a shift to the left. In confirmation of these predictions, it has been found that the decrease in GFR produced by infusion of hypertonic sodium chloride is blocked by blocking the loop of Henle [25]. Proximal fluid transport is reduced, which has the effect of perturbing the macula densa signal. In the steady state, GFR is moderately decreased and $\dot{V}_{LP}$ moderately increased. There is evidence that the same mechanism may be the cause for the decrease in GFR during inhibition of carbonic anhydrase [26, 27], during maleate-induced reduction in proximal fluid transport, and possibly in chloride-depletion alkalosis [28]. In all these circumstances, tubuloglomerular feedback subserves the function of preventing the distal sodium chloride overload that would occur without the GFR adjustment.

Effect of an Altered Feedback Function

As has already been pointed out, the feedback function cannot be considered a fixed relationship. In fact, as summarized in Table 1, numerous conditions have been defined in which the feedback function is altered. The consequences of such an alteration are schematically depicted in Figure 5b. As long as the feedforward function is constant, a left shift of the feedback function will lead to a decrease of both GFR and $\dot{V}_{LP}$. A right shift in the feedback function will cause a parallel increase in GFR and $\dot{V}_{LP}$. By and large, the experimental findings agree with these predictions; the conditions listed on the left of Table 1 are generally associated with an increase in GFR and

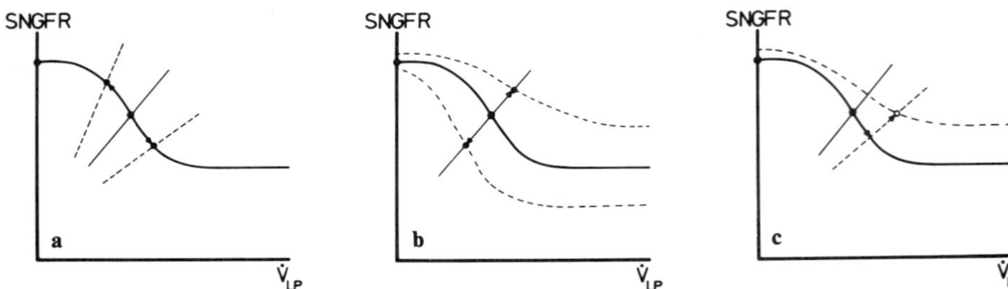

Fig. 5. a Effect of change in the transport function; **b** effect of change in the feedback function; and **c** effect of change in both functions.

Table 1. Conditions associated with an altered feedback function.[a]

Decreased sensitivity	Increased sensitivity
Acute NaCl infusion	Dietary NaCl restriction
Acute plasma infusion	Hemorrhage
Chronic dietary NaCl loading	Dehydration
Chronic dietary NaCl loading + DOCA	Reduction of arterial pressure to 70 mm Hg for >20 min
High-protein diet	Renal artery stenosis
Acute hyperglycemia	Transplanted kidney
Contralateral nephrectomy	Adrenalectomy + dexamethasone
Contralateral renal artery stenosis	Release of ureteral obstruction
Acute unilateral ureteral obstruction	Chloride depletion alkalosis (?)

[a] Decreased or increased sensitivity refers to a right or a left shift in the feedback function. In most cases, a decreased sensitivity is characterized by a decrease in the maximum response, a decrease in slope, and an increase in $\dot{V}_{1/2}$; the converse is in general associated with increased sensitivity.

those listed on the right with a decrease. Deviations from these predictions occur during simultaneous changes in both feedforward and feedback functions. Figure 5c is a schematic illustration of the consequence of a decreased transport function with simultaneous resetting of the feedback function to the right. In this circumstance, feedback desensitization is only capable of compensating for the GFR lowering effect of the shift in the transport function. In the new steady state, GFR is unchanged, although $\dot{V}_{LP}$ is elevated.

Conclusions

Tubuloglomerular feedback has been recognized as a control mechanism that regulates sodium chloride delivery into the more distal portions of the nephron by adjustments in glomerular filtration rate. A number of details in signal generation and transmission at the cellular level are still unclear and remain under intense investigation. Because of these uncertainties, we have used a phenomenologic approach to describe the mutual interdependence between a signal correlate, $\dot{V}_{LP}$, and SNGFR. This approach avoids the necessity of making assumptions about the precise nature of either the signal or the mechanism of its effect on filtration rate; however, it permits one to make testable predictions as to the role that TGF plays in setting GFR under various experimental conditions. The assumption we do make is that the feedback curve, derived from microperfusion of single superficial nephrons with artificial solutions, is representative of the function of all nephrons in situ. This is clearly only a first approximation. Future investigation of the physiologic role of TGF will need to consider other factors, such as the feedback function of deep nephrons [29] and the possible role of alterations in tubular fluid composition.

Acknowledgment. Dr. J. P. Briggs is an Established Investigator of the American Heart Association.

References

1. WRIGHT FS, BRIGGS JP: Feedback control of glomerular blood flow, pressure and filtration rate. *Physiol Rev* 59:958–1006, 1979
2. KAISSLING B, PETER S, KRIZ W: The transition of the thick ascending limb of Henle's loop into the distal convoluted tubule in the nephron of the rat kidney. *Cell Tissue Res* 182:111–118, 1977
3. SCHNERMANN J, SCHUBERT G, BRIGGS JP: In situ studies of the distal convoluted tubule in the rat: I. Evidence for NaCl secretion. *Am J Physiol* 243:F160–F166, 1982
4. GUTSCHE H-U, MÜLLER-SUUR R, HEGEL U, HIERHOLZER K: Electrical conductivity of tubular fluid of the rat nephron. Micropuncture study of the diluting segment in situ. *Pflügers Arch* 383:113–122, 1980
5. SCHNERMANN J, PLOTH DW, HERMLE M: Activation of tubulo-glomerular feedback by chloride transport. *Pflügers Arch* 362:229–240, 1976
6. BELL PD, MCLEAN CB, NAVAR LG: Dissociation of tubuloglomerular feedback responses from distal tubular chloride concentration in the rat. *Am J Physiol* 240:F111–F119, 1981
7. BRIGGS JP, SCHNERMANN J, WRIGHT FS: Failure of tubule fluid osmolarity to affect feedback regulation of glomerular filtration. *Am J Physiol* 239:F427–F432, 1980
8. BELL PD, NAVAR LG, PLOTH DW, MCLEAN CB: Tubuloglomerular feedback responses during perfusion with nonelectrolyte solutions in the rat. *Kidney Int* 18:460–471, 1980
9. SCHNERMANN J, SCHUBERT G, BRIGGS JP: In situ studies of the distal convoluted tubule in the rat: I. Evidence for NaCl secretion. *Am J Physiol* 243:F160–F166, 1982
10. MOORE LC, MASON J: Perturbation analysis of tubuloglomerular feedback in hydropenic and hemorrhaged rats. *Am J Physiol* 245:F554–F563, 1983
11. HÄBERLE DA, DAVIS JM: Interrelationship between proximal tubular hydrodiuremia and tubuloglomerular feedback in the rat kidney. *Kidney Int* 22(Suppl): S-193–S-197, 1982
12. BRIGGS JP, SCHUBERT G, SCHNERMANN J: Quantitative characterization of the tubuloglomerular feedback response: effect of growth. *Am J Physiol,* in press
13. SCHNERMANN J, DAVIS JM, WUNDERLICH P, LEVINE DZ, HORSTER M: Technical problems in the micropuncture determination of nephron filtration rate and their functional implications. *Pflügers Arch* 329:307–320, 1971
14. KAUFMAN JS, HAMBURGER RJ, FLAMERBAUM W: Tubuloglomerular feedback: Effect of dietary NaCl intake. *Am J Physiol* 231:1744–1749, 1976
15. PLOTH DW, RUDULPH J, THOMAS C, NAVAR LG: Renal and tubuloglomerular feedback response to plasma expansion in the rat. *Am J Physiol* 235:F156–F162, 1978
16. MASON J, KAIN H, SHIIGAI T, WELSCH J: The early phase of experimental acute renal failure: V. The influence of suppressing the renin angiotensin system. *Pflügers Arch* 380:233–258, 1979
17. MÜLLER-SUUR R, NORLEN B-J, PERSSON AEG: Resetting of tubuloglomerular feedback in rat kidneys after unilateral nephrectomy. *Kidney Int* 18:48–57, 1980
18. BARTOLI E, EARLEY LE: Measurement of nephron filtration rate in the rat with and without occlusion of the proximal tubule. *Kidney Int* 3:372–380, 1973
19. MADDOX DA, TROY JL, BRENNER BM: Autoregulation of filtration rate in the absence of macula densa-glomerulus feedback. *Am J Physiol* 227:123–131, 1974
20. DEV B, DRESCHER C, SCHNERMANN J: Resetting of tubuloglomerular feedback sensitivity by dietary salt intake. *Pflügers Arch* 346:262–277, 1974

21. Schnermann J, Briggs JP, Weber PC: Tubuloglomerular feedback, prostaglandins and angiotensin in the autoregulation of glomerular filtration rate. *Kidney Int* 25:53–64, 1984
22. Moore LC, Schnermann J, Yarimizu S: Feedback mediation of SNGFR autoregulation in hydropenic and DOCA- and salt-loaded rats. *Am J Physiol* 236:F63–F74, 1979
23. Navar LG, Burke TJ, Robinson RR, Clapp JR: Distal tubular feedback in the autoregulation of single nephron glomerular filtration rate. *J Clin Invest* 53:516–525, 1974
24. Moore LC: Interaction of tubuloglomerular feedback and proximal nephron reabsorption in autoregulation. *Kidney Int* 12(Suppl):S-173–S-178, 1982
25. Schnermann J, Briggs JP, Wright FS: Feedback-mediated reduction of GFR during infusion of hypertonic saline. *Kidney Int* 20:462–468, 1981
26. Persson AEG, Wright FS: Evidence for feedback mediated reduction glomerular filtration rate during infusion of acetazolamide. *Acta Physiol Scand* 114:1–7, 1982
27. Tucker BJ, Steiner WR, Gushwa LC, Blantz RC: Studies of tubuloglomerular feedback system in rat: Mechanism of reduction in filtration rate with benzolamide. *J Clin Invest* 62:993–1004, 1978
28. Galla JH, Bonduris DN, Luke RG: Reduction in SNGFR in chloride depletion alkalosis unexplained by volume contraction (*abstract*). *Kidney Int* 25:230, 1984
29. Müller-Suur R, Ufendahl HR, Persson AEG: Evidence for tubuloglomerular feedback in juxtamedullary nephrons of young rats. *Am J Physiol* 244:F425–F431, 1983

Influence of Renal Nerves on the Glomerular Microcirculation

Valentina Kon and Iekuni Ichikawa

It has been known for a long time that the renal vasculature is not only a target for a variety of circulating vasoactive substances but also a locus for regulation by the sympathetic nervous system. Stimulation of the renal nerves causes renal vasoconstriction, conservation of fluid, and renin release [1–6]. Immunohistochemical and electron microscopic studies have demonstrated direct adrenergic innervation of a variety of renal structures, including epithelia of proximal and distal tubules, the loop of Henle, as well as afferent and efferent arterioles and the glomerular mesangium [7–9]. In particular, the study by Barajas and Muller [7] has demonstrated direct contact of axons with the bodies of mesangial cells.

Our previous understanding of adrenergic effects on renal hemodynamics had been limited to the level of whole kidney GFR and blood flow rate. Hermansonn et al [4] were the first to examine the effects of renal nerve stimulation of preglomerular, glomerular, and postglomerular pressures and flows in cortical microcirculation of mammalian kidney. In this early study, single nephron glomerular filtration rate (SNGFR) fell by 15% in response to direct electrical stimulation of the renal nerves at 2 Hz and by more than 50% in response to 5 Hz. Single nephron glomerular plasma flow rate (Q_A) estimated from the whole kidney clearance of para-aminohippurate (PAH) was also found to fall in a dose-dependent manner during stimulation of the renal nerves. Q_A fell by about 15 and 50% in response to stimulation at 2 and 5 Hz, respectively. Glomerular capillary pressure, estimated by the stop-flow method, was shown to be essentially unaffected during mild stimulation, but decreased slightly at higher frequencies. These findings of glomerular capillary pressures led these investigators to conclude that the renal vasoconstriction induced by activation of the renal nerves involved the afferent and efferent arterioles. At a higher sympathetic discharge, there appeared to be a somewhat more pronounced tone in the afferent arterioles.

This manuscript was presented as part of a Symposium on *Intrarenal Control of Glomerular Filtration Rate.*

Thus, progressive arteriolar constriction accounted for the reduction in glomerular plasma flow, glomerular capillary pressure, and glomerular filtration.

It should be recognized that glomerular pressure and plasma flow are but two of several factors potentially capable of regulating the rate of single

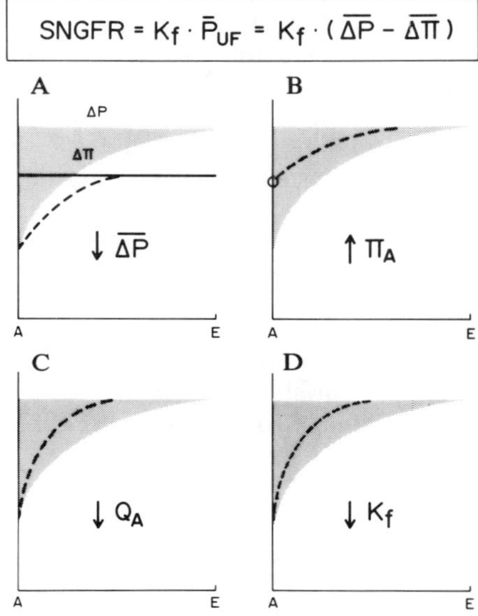

Fig. 1. Determinants of single nephron glomerular filtration rate (SNGFR) and effects of individual perturbation. The Starling equation describes the determinants of SNGFR. In each panel, pressure profiles are schematically portrayed along the unitless glomerular capillary length from afferent to efferent ends (left and right). The effects of selective perturbation of each of the determinants of SNGFR are depicted in each of the four panels. The *shaded areas* represent normal mean net ultrafiltration pressure ($\bar{P}_{UF}$) as defined by the mean difference between hydraulic ($\overline{\Delta P}$) and colloid osmotic ($\Delta\Pi$) pressures. *Panel A* shows a reduced mean glomerular transcapillary hydraulic pressure difference ($\overline{\Delta P}$). Since $\overline{\Delta P} = P_{GC} - P_T$, a change in either mean glomerular capillary hydraulic pressure ($\bar{P}_{GC}$) or Bowman's space hydraulic pressure (P_T) will affect $\overline{\Delta P}$, hence $\bar{P}_{UF}$ and SNGFR. *Panel B* shows increased systematic colloid osmotic pressure (Π_A). The level of systemic protein, hence Π_A, is important, for it determines the inlet value of $\Delta\Pi$ and therefore $\bar{P}_{UF}$ and SNGFR. $\overline{\Delta\Pi}$ is also modulated by glomerular plasma flow rate (Q_A). *Panel C* shows the effects of changes in Q_A on SNGFR. When Q_A is decreased, a given amount of colloid-free solution filtered into Bowman's space results in higher intracapillary protein concentration; hence, the rise in $\Delta\Pi$ along the capillary is accelerated so that $\bar{P}_{UF}$ and SNGFR are expected to fall. In addition to these three determinants that directly affect $\bar{P}_{UF}$, SNGFR also depends on the glomerular capillary ultrafiltration coefficient (K_f) (*panel D*). Changes in K_f accompany directionally reciprocal changes in $\bar{P}_{UF}$ by modulating the $\Delta\Pi$ profile. This tendency is most prominent when K_f is increased from normal values (*dotted line*), whereas a reduction in K_f below the normal level brings a relatively small fall in $\Delta\Pi$ and $\bar{P}_{UF}$ (not shown) so that a marked reduction in K_f is capable of reducing SNGFR. (Reprinted with permission from [19])

nephron GFR. The summary of all the determinants of SNGFR and the effects of perturbation of each one are given in Figure 1. A more recent study by Kon and Ichikawa [10] measured the hydraulic pressure difference across the glomerular capillary directly, which permitted a detailed description of all the determinants of SNGFR and allowed a more precise description of the mechanisms of adrenergic influence on glomerular filtration. In their study, micropuncture measurements were made during direct renal nerve stimulation, and the results were compared with values obtained before or after stimulation in the same animal. Stimulation of the renal nerves at low frequency (0.5 to 1.5 Hz; LFS) or high frequency (3 to 5 Hz; HFS) increased the resistances in afferent and efferent arterioles. Again, the magnitude of renal vasoconstriction was proportional to the strength of stimulation. The effects of the high renal nerve stimulation on the individual determinants of SNGFR are shown in Figure 2. Single nephron GFR fell, on the average by 60%, from 24 ± 4 to 10 ± 2 nl/min. Direct measurement of glomerular capillary hydraulic pressure ($\overline{P}_{GC}$) revealed a uniform decrease, on the average, from 48 ± 1 to 43 ± 1 mm Hg. Proximal tubule hydraulic pressure (P_T) also decreased from 15 ± 1 to 11 ± 1 mm Hg. The comparable fall in these two variables contributed to the virtually unchanged mean glomerular transcapillary hydraulic pressure difference ($\overline{\Delta P}$), which remained at 33 mm

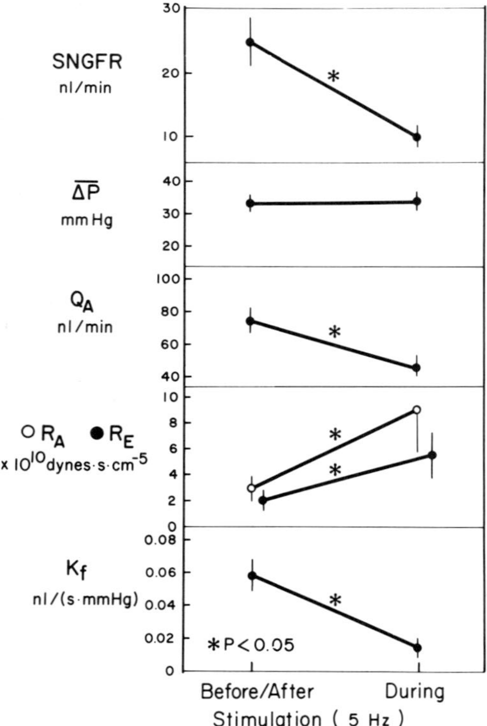

Fig. 2. Summary of SNGFR and various determinants of SNGFR in the absence of and during high frequency renal nerve stimulation ($N = 7$ rats). (Reprinted with permission from [17])

Hg during HFS. Thus, this determinant was not responsible for the fall in SNGFR with HFS. Although not shown in this figure, protein concentration in the systemic plasma, hence the calculated systemic colloid osmotic pressure (Π_A), was also unaffected. By contrast, the glomerular plasma flow rate (Q_A) fell by almost 40%, from 71 ± 11 to 44 ± 10 nl/min. This reduction in Q_A was the result of the marked increase in the afferent and efferent arteriolar resistances, particularly the former, during renal nerve stimulation. The direct measurement of glomerular capillary pressure also permitted assessment of the glomerular capillary ultrafiltration coefficient (K_f). K_f fell by more than 70% during HFS, from 0.055 ± 0.014 to 0.015 ± 0.002 nl/(sec $\cdot$ mm Hg). Thus, the profound fall in SNGFR during HFS was due to a reduction in Q_A, a result of constriction of both afferent and efferent arterioles, and a reduction in K_f. The changes in Q_A and K_f were found to contribute comparably to the observed fall in SNGFR.

At a lower level of renal nervestimulation, the degree of vasoconstriction was qualitatively similar, but quantitatively much less than it was with HFS. The mild constriction of the afferent and efferent arterioles was reflected in the tendency toward a decrease in Q_A. The vasoconstriction was also evidenced by a decrease in hydraulic pressure in the downstream postglomerular circulation. Thus, the inlet peritubular capillary hydraulic pressure was found to be lower during LFS, on the average by 4 mm Hg. The ultrafiltration coefficient, K_f, also decreased in response to the lower frequency stimulation, on the average by some 30%, from 0.091 ± 0.016 to 0.064 ± 0.011 nl/(sec $\cdot$ mm Hg). These studies show that the effector loci of the sympathetic nervous system include afferent and efferent arterioles and the glomerulus itself. Thus, by varying the tone within the arterioles and glomerulus, renal nerves influence the rate of glomerular plasma flow and the ultrafiltration coefficient.

In keeping with these findings in vivo are the results of a recent study by Edwards [11] using isolated rabbit arterioles. He examined the contractile response of isolated afferent and efferent arterioles treated with norepinephrine at concentrations of 10^{-9} to 10^{-5} M and found significant reductions in the luminal diameter of both these arterioles.

The adrenergically induced glomerular effect of decreased K_f was observed during HFS as well as during LFS. Since K_f is the product of the effective hydraulic permeability of the glomerular capillary wall and total capillary surface area available for filtration, either component may be influenced by activation of renal nerves. Of note in this regard, the glomerular capillary wall is in direct contact with mesangial cells, which possess numerous intracellular contractile myofilaments [12, 13]. Studies of isolated mesangial cells in culture have demonstrated that these cells contract in response to angiotensin II (AII), antidiuretic hormone, and norepinephrine [14, 15]. Furthermore, Ichikawa, Miele, and Brenner found that the AII-induced increase in afferent and efferent resistances and decrease in glomerular capillary ultrafiltration coefficient were completely reversed by verapamil and manganese, inhibitors of excitation-contraction coupling in smooth muscle cells [16]. These data support the notion that a decrease in area available for filtration, induced by mesangial contraction, hence K_f, may account for the decreased SNGFR found with increased adrenergic activity.

Further support for the functional changes in cortical microcirculation induced by adrenergic stimulation comes from experiments by Ichikawa and Kon. They investigated the arteriolar and glomerular morphologic changes in response to adrenergic stimulation [17]. Figure 3 shows silicone-injected glomeruli from the left (top) and right (bottom) kidneys of the same rat. The kidneys were perfusion-fixed, whereas the right renal nerves were stimu-

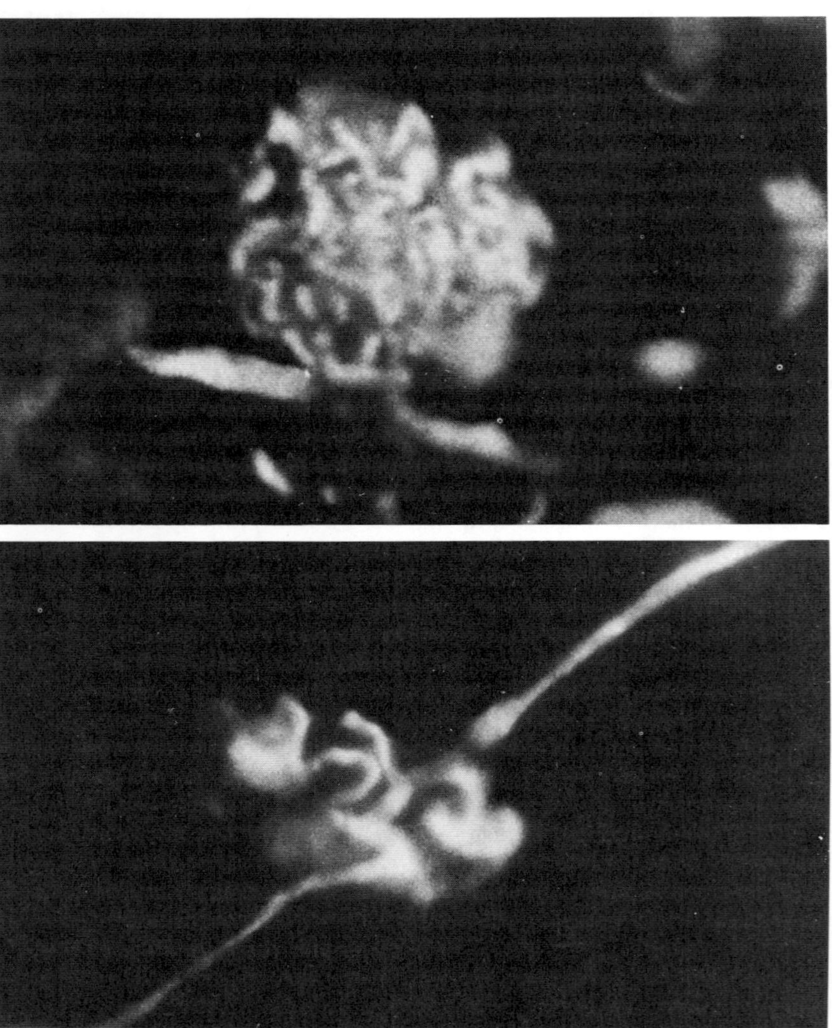

Fig. 3. Silicone-injected glomeruli from left (*top*) and right (*bottom*) kidneys of the same rat. The kidneys were perfusion-fixed, whereas the right renal nerves were stimulated at high frequency. (Reprinted with permission from [17])

lated selectively. After fixation, the kidneys were injected with silicone rubber. This approach permitted evaluation of increased adrenergic activity in one kidney, using the contralateral kidney of the same animal as the control. The glomerulus from the nonstimulated kidney showed many fine capillary tufts, which were open, whereas the stimulated glomerulus showed an opening of only relatively large-diameter channels consistent with a dramatic reduction in the filtering surface area. Also noted were marked narrowings of afferent and efferent arterioles in the glomerulus from stimulated kidneys.

In addition to vasoconstriction, stimulation of renal nerves is known to elicit renal release of renin and therefore increase the generation of AII [5, 6]. It is possible, therefore, that the renal hemodynamic changes following sympathetic activation are mediated by AII, or that this hormone enhances any direct adrenergic effects. This issue was addressed in a recent study by Pelayo and Blantz [18], who evaluated glomerular hemodynamics during renal nerve stimulation (3 Hz) before and after pharmacologic inhibition of AII. They found that administration of an AII antagonist attenuated the fall in the rate of glomerular plasma flow and SNGFR. Whereas renal nerve stimulation alone decreased SNGFR from 50 ± 2 to 38 ± 1 nl/min and Q_A from 187 ± 9 to 144 ± 11 nl/min, stimulation of renal nerves during AII inhibition decreased SNGFR and Q_A to only 45 ± 2 and 175 ± 11 nl/min, respectively. Thus, the magnitude of decrease in both of these parameters in response to adrenergic stimulation was lessened by 50% following AII inhibition. This was due, at least in part, to amelioration of vasoconstriction in afferent and efferent arterioles. On the other hand, in this study, a fall in glomerular capillary ultrafiltration coefficient was not evident during renal nerve stimulation. In conclusion, the available evidence suggests that neural regulation of glomerular ultrafiltration appears to be channeled through the vasomotor tone of the afferent and efferent arterioles and contractility of the glomerular mesangium, which affects the surface area. These adrenergic effects seem, at least in part, to be mediated through AII.

Acknowledgment. This work is supported by Public Health Grant 32160. Dr. V. Kon is a recipient of a Clinician-Scientist Award from the American Heart Association.

References

1. BLOCK M, WAKIM KG, MANN FC: Renal function during stimulation of renal nerves. *Am J Physiol* 169:670–677, 1952
2. DiSALVO J, FELL C: Changes in blood flow during renal nerve stimulation. *Proc Soc Exp Biol Med* 136:150–153, 1971
3. KATZ MA, SHEAR L: Effect of renal nerves of renal hemodynamics: I. Direct stimulation and carotid occlusion. *Nephron* 14:246–256, 1975
4. HERMANSSON K, LARSON M, KALLSKOG O, WOLGAST M: Influence of renal nerve activity on arteriolar resistance, ultrafiltration dynamics and fluid reabsorption. *Pflügers Arch* 389:85–90, 1981
5. SCHRIER RW: Effects of adrenergic nervous system and catecholamines on systemic and renal hemodynamics, sodium and water excretion and renin secretion. *Kidney Int* 6:291–306, 1974

6. VANDER AJ: Effect of catecholamines and the renal nerves on renin secretion in anesthetized dogs. *Am J Physiol* 209:659–662, 1965

7. BARAJAS L, MULLER J: The innervation of the juxtaglomerular apparatus and surrounding tubules: A quantitative analysis of serial section electron microscopy. *J Ultrastruct Res* 43:107–132, 1973

8. LJUNGQVIST A, WAGERMARK J: The adrenergic innervation of intrarenal glomerular and extraglomerular circulatory routes. *Nephron* 7:218–229, 1970

9. MULLER J, BARAJAS L: Electron microscopic and histochemical evidence of tubular innervation in the renal cortex of the monkey. *J Ultrastruct Res* 41:533–549, 1972

10. KON V, ICHIKAWA I: Effector loci for renal nerve control of cortical microcirculation. *Am J Physiol* 245(*Renal Fluid Electrolyte Physiol 14*):F545–F553, 1983

11. EDWARDS RM: Segmental effects of norepinephrine and angiotensin on isolated renal microvessels. *Am J Physiol* 244(*Renal Fluid Electrolyte Physiol 13*):F526–F534, 1983

12. KREISBERG JI, KARNOVSKY MJ: Characterization of rat glomerular cells in vitro, in *Immune Mechanisms in Renal Disease,* edited by CUMMINGS MB, MICHAEL AF, WILSON CB, New York, Plenum, 1982, pp 189–248

13. PEASE DC: Myoid features of renal corpuscles and tubules. *J Ultrastruct Res* 23:304–320, 1968

14. AUSIELLO DA, KREISBERG JI, ROY C, KARNOVSKY MJ: Contraction of cultured rat glomerular mesangial cells after stimulation with angiotensin II and arginine vasopressin. *J Clin Invest* 65:754–760, 1980

15. MAHIEU PR, FOIDART JB, DUBOIS CH, DECHENNE CA, DEHENEFFE J: Tissue culture of normal rat glomeruli: contractile activity of the cultured mesangial cells. *Invest Cell Pathol* 3:121–128, 1980

16. ICHIKAWA I, MIELE JF, BRENNER BM: Reversal of renal cortical actions of angiotensin II by verapamil and manganese. *Kidney Int* 16:137–147, 1979

17. ICHIKAWA I, KON V: Glomerular mesangium as an effector locus for the tubuloglomerular feedback system and renal sympathetic innervation. *Fed Proc* 42:3075–3079, 1983

18. PELAYO JC, BLANTZ RC: Glomerular hemodynamic alterations during renal nerve stimulation: effects of Angiotensin II inhibition (*abstract*). *Clin Res* 31(2):517A, 1983

19. YARED A, ICHIKAWA I: Renal blood flow and glomerular filtration rate: Function and development, in *Pediatric Nephrology,* edited by HOLLIDAY MA, BARRATT TM, VERNIER RL, Baltimore, Williams & Wilkins, 1984, in press

Structure and Transport Along the Nephron

Hydrogen Ion Transport Along the Nephron

Floyd C. Rector, Jr.

The renal tubule participates in acid-base homeostasis by conserving filtered base (primarily bicarbonate) and excreting protons bound to either filtered buffers (as titratable acid) or ammonia (as ammonium ions). The tubule is subject to precise physiologic control and is capable of augmenting the excretion of titratable acid and ammonium when the intake or production of nonvolatile acids is increased and is capable of augmenting the excretion of bicarbonate if alkali is ingested. Most segments of the nephron participate in this process of acid-base regulation, although the mechanisms involved differ in the individual segments. In general, most segments participate primarily by secreting hydrogen ions, although some of the more distal segments are capable of secreting either hydrogen ions or bicarbonate, depending on the acid-base status of the animal.

Proximal Segments

The proximal convoluted tubule (PCT) reabsorbs 80 to 90% of the filtered bicarbonate and reduces the tubular fluid pH 0.6 to 1.0 U below that of blood. The PCT exhibits considerable axial heterogeneity in its capacity to reabsorb bicarbonate. Studies by Liu and Cogan (submitted for publication), in which the PCT of Munich-Wistar rats was sequentially micropunctured from the last accessible loop to the glomerulus, revealed that the rate of bicarbonate reabsorption was approximately 350 pmoles/mm/min in the first loop and only 80 pmoles/mm/min in the later loops. In addition to the reabsorption of bicarbonate, filtered buffers are titrated to form titratable acid, and ammonia is added to proximal tubule fluid in an amount equal to 80 to 100% of that appearing in final urine.

This manuscript was presented as a State-of-the-Art lecture.

In both PCT and proximal straight tubule (PST), hydrogen ions are transported from cell to lumen across the apical membrane, and hydroxyl ions are liberated within the cytoplasm. The hydroxyl ions combine with carbon dioxide to form bicarbonate ions, which are then transported across the basolateral membrane into peritubular fluid. The electrochemical gradients across the apical and basolateral cell membranes can be estimated from measurements of cell pH and basolateral membrane potential difference (PD). Cell pH is approximately 7.4 to 7.5 measured with DMO in suspensions of PCT [1–3] and is approximately 7.1 to 7.2 measured with pH-sensitive microelectrodes [4]. Basolateral membrane PD is approximately 40 to 70 mV (cell interior is negative) in PCT [5, 6] and PST [6, 7]. Thus, hydrogen ions must be transported up an electrochemical gradient across the apical membrane, while bicarbonate (or its base equivalent hydroxyl ion) moves down its electrochemical gradient across the basolateral membrane. The movement of hydrogen ions across the apical membrane, therefore, must involve some type of active transport process.

A variety of mechanisms for hydrogen transport have been identified in different tissues and subcellular organelles, but in the kidney interest has been focused primarily on two models (Fig. 1). The first mechanism is a form of secondary active transport in which the uphill transport of hydrogen ions is coupled to the downhill movement of sodium ions via a sodium/hydrogen antiporter in the luminal membrane. The process is electroneutral and is driven by the sodium concentration gradient across the apical membrane. Consequently, it depends on the presence of sodium and an intact Na-K-ATPase system. Murer, Hopfer, and Kinne [8] were the first to demonstrate the existence of a neutral sodium/hydrogen antiporter in brushborder membrane vesicles prepared from kidney cortex. Subsequent studies have extensively characterized this antiporter [9]. The antiporter is electroneutral with 1:1 coupling between sodium and hydrogen ions. In addition to sodium/hydrogen exchange, the antiporter is capable of Na/Na, Li/H, Li/Na, and Na/NH_4 exchange. The antiporter is selectively inhibited by amiloride with an apparent K_i of 7 to 30 × 10^{-6} M. The concentration of amiloride required to inhibit the antiporter is approximately two orders of magnitude higher than that required to inhibit the sodium channels in tight epithelia. The mechanism by which amiloride inhibits the antiporter is controversial. Kinsella and Aronson [10] have obtained kinetics consistent with simple competitive inhibition, whereas Ives, Yee, and Warnock [11] have obtained kinetics indicative of a mixed type of inhibition. A similar discrepancy has been observed with the effects of lithium. Kinsella and Aronson [12] have found that lithium can serve as substrate for Li/H exchange and competitively inhibit Na/H exchange. Ives, Yee, and Warnock [11], on the other hand, have found that lithium can serve as substrate for Li/H exchange but gives a mixed type of inhibition of Na/H exchange. They have proposed that both amiloride and lithium can compete with sodium at the active transport site, and can also bind to a modifier site to produce noncompetitive inhibition. Aronson, Nee, and Suhm [13] have found that raising internal hydrogen ion concentration stimulates both Na/H and Na/Na exchange in a manner that cannot be explained by a simple substrate effect and have proposed

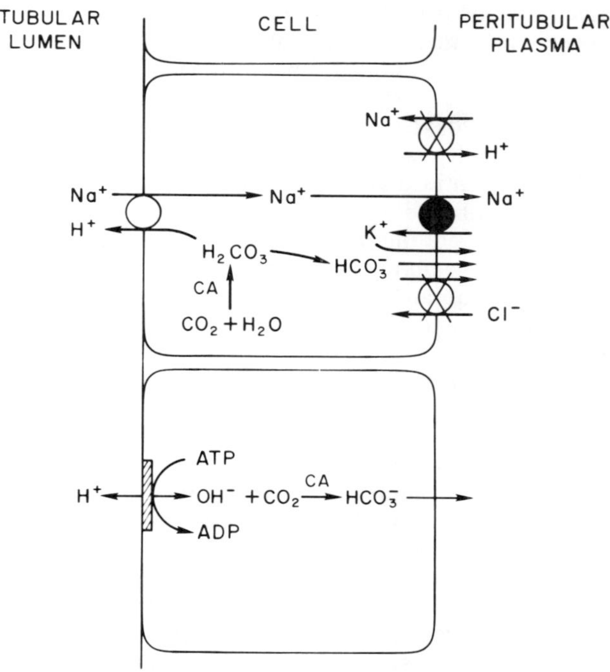

Fig. 1. Hydrogen ion transport in the proximal tubule. A Na/H antiporter in the luminal membrane in a series with a conductive bicarbonate exit pathway in the basolateral accounts for most of the acidification. A proton-translocating ATPase may account for a smaller fraction. Basolateral Na/H and Cl/HCO₃ exchangers do not appear to be present.

that internal hydrogen interacts with a modifier site to allosterically increase activity of the antiporter. Whether hydrogen, lithium, and amiloride are reacting at the same or different modifier sites is not known.

The Na/H antiporter in renal brushborder membrane vesicles appears to be similar to that present in the plasma membrane of many different cell types; in these other tissues, it plays a key role in the regulation of cell pH. Boron and Boulpaep [14] have found that in the salamander proximal tubule, the Na/H antiporter is present in both the luminal and antiluminal membranes. These investigators have raised the suggestion that its primary role may be the regulation of cell pH rather than vectoral transport of bicarbonate. In that tissue, the vectoral transport of bicarbonate is the consequence of the exit mechanism for bicarbonate across the basolateral membrane. In contrast, Ives, Yee, and Warnock [15] have found that in the rabbit kidney the Na/H antiporter is located in the luminal, but not in the basolateral membrane. Thus, in the mammalian PCT the Na/H antiporter is well suited to mediate vectoral transport of bicarbonate.

Other forms of sodium-coupled secondary active transport have been identified in renal brushborder membrane vesicles, and these may also play some role in proximal acidification [9]. Phosphate appears to be reabsorbed as the dibasic or alkaline member of the conjugate base pair, and as such would generate a hydrogen ion in the lumen and a hydroxyl ion in the cell. The contribution of this process, however, would be small and would be limited by the quantity of dibasic phosphate in the filtrate. Blomstedt and Aronson [16] have identified an organic anion/hydroxyl (OA/OH) antiporter in brushborder membrane vesicles from rat, but not rabbit, kidneys. This OA/OH antiporter operatingsynchronously with either the Na/OA symporter in the basolateral membrane (for secreted anions) or the Na/OA symporter in the luminal membrane (for reabsorbed anions) could effect net acidification of proximal tubular fluid. The quantitative significance of this process is unknown.

A second major possibility for hydrogen ion transport across the apical membrane of the proximal tubule is some form of primary active transport. Such a process would notbe coupled to sodium and thus would continue in the absence of sodium or sodium transport, would be electrogenic, and would thus generate a lumen-positive PD. Such a process might be mediated by a proton-translocating ATPase in the membrane and would derive its energy from the splitting of ATP (Fig. 1); or it might be mediated by a redox system in the membrane and would derive its energy from the oxidation of NADH or some other suitable substrate.

Kinne-Saffran, Beauwens, and Kinne [17, 18] have obtained evidence for a proton-translocating ATPase in brushborder membrane vesicles prepared from rat renal cortex. Vesicles loaded with an ATP-generating system will extrude hydrogen ions from the vesicles and alkalinize the vesicle interior. The steady-state intravesicular ATP concentration represents a balance between the rates of ATP generation and ATP splitting; the latter rate is controlled by the pH gradient between the inside and outside of the vesicle. If the interior alkalinity is dissipated by adding a protonophore to the vesicle preparation, the rate of splitting is accelerated and the intravesicular concentration of ATP falls. This proton-translocating ATPase activity can be demonstrated in the presence of sufficient oligomycin to inhibit mitochondrial ATPase and is inhibited by high concentrations of dicyclohexylcarbodiimide (DCCD; 0.1 mM). Since oligomycin-insensitive proton-translocating ATPases are present in many intracellular organelles (lysosomes, Golgi, and so forth) it is not yet certain whether ATPase activity of the brushborder membrane preparation is truly resident in the brushborder membrane or whether it represents contamination with intracellular organelles. Recently, Rodman et al [19] have demonstrated extensive coating of the intervillous area of the brushborder microvilli with clathrin, suggesting the presence of clathrin-coated pits performing the same endocytic function as in other tissues. Vesicles prepared from clathrin-coated pits from nonrenal tissue contain an oligomycin-insensitive proton-translocating ATPase [20] similar to that reported by Kinne-Saffran, Beauwens, and Kinne [17]. When proteins, hormones, viruses, or other substances bind to receptors on plasma membranes, the bound material and its receptor are internalized by the formation of an endocytotic vesicle at the clathrin-coated pit. The proton-translocating ATPase serves to acidify the interior of the endosome and cause dissociation of the bound substance and its receptor, allowing recycling of the receptor back to the cell surface. In view of the extensive absorption of small proteins and hormones by the proximal tubule, it is highly likely that there is a high density of clathrin-coated pits with their intrinsic proton-translocating ATPase resident in the brushborder membrane. It is not clear, however, whether the proton pump functions on the cell surface extruding hydrogen ions into the lumen or whether it functions only after the clathrin-coated pit is internalized as an endosome.

Another possibility for primary active transport of hydrogen ions across the luminal membrane is some type of redox system, such as the cytochrome electron transport chain that is responsible for generating pH gradients in mitochondria. Garcia et al [21, 22] have reported that preparations of rat renal brushborder membrane vesicles contain NADH oxidase activity that is linked to a cytochrome system and that is capable of generating electrical and pH gradients across the vesicle membrane with the interior negatively charged and alkaline relative to the exterior fluid. Again, however, it is not clear whether this activity is intrinsic to the brushborder membrane or represents contaminants from mitochondria.

The use of brushborder membrane vesicles prepared from renal cortex has been extremely useful for identifying and characterizing potential transport systems. However, there are potential problems arising from contamination by intracellular organelles, membranes, or enzymes and from heterogeneity of nephron segments. Moreover, they do not answer the important physiologic question concerning the relative contribution of the various transport systems to the in vivo tubule function, particularly for a complex function such as acidification. This question requires more physiologic approaches, such as micropuncture and in vivo or in vitro microperfusion of well-defined tubule segments.

Burg and Green [23] and McKinney and Burg [24] were the first to demonstrate that removal of sodium or inhibition of sodium transport would reduce the rate of bicarbonate absorption in isolated rabbit PCT and PST by 60 to 80%. More recent studies by Sasaki, Berry, and myself [25] examine the question of whether or not there is any residual acidification independent of sodium transport. In their studies in the isolated rabbit PCT, Na-K-ATPase was inhibited by removal of potassium from ambient fluids. At zero bath, potassium bicarbonate absorption was reduced to 6% of the control rate. This rate of bicarbonate absorption, however, was not different from that measured when the luminal perfusate was passed directly into the collecting pipette without passing through the tubule. These studies suggest, therefore, that all acidification in the rabbit PCT is in some way coupled to active sodium transport, presumably via a Na/H antiporter in the luminal membrane.

The role of sodium transport inproximal acidification has been less clearcut in other species. In hamsters, Ullrich et al [26] used glycodiazine absorption from stationary droplets as an indirect assessment of the rate of acidification and found that adding ouabain to the peritubular perfusate inhibited volume and sodium-coupled glucose absorption, but had no effect on the rate of glycodiazine absorption. De Mello-Aires and Malnic [27] measured the rate of bicarbonate absorption from stationary droplets of fluid containing very high concentrations of bicarbonate in rat PCT and found it to be very insensitive to either removal of ambient sodium or inhibition of sodium transport. More recent studies, however, have shown that in the rat removal of sodium from ambient fluids or inhibition of sodium transport by removal of potassium from peritubular perfusates inhibited bicarbonate absorption by 80 to 90% [28, 29]. In rats, as in rabbits, the rate of acidification strongly depends on active sodium transport, but there may be an additional component, amounting to 10 to 20% of the total, of primary active proton transport that is independent of sodium transport and is electrogenic.

Direct evidence for any component of electrogenic proton transport is not compelling. Frompter and Sato [30] perfused lumens and peritubular capillaries of rat PCT with a solution of sodium chloride and sodium bicarbonate that was free of organic solutes. They found a lumen-positive PD of +1 mv which was partially inhibited by acetazolamide. Although this finding is consistent with electrogenic proton secretion, it is also consistent with an electroneutral Na/H antiporter operating synchronously with conductive bicarbonate exit in the basolateral membrane and a potassium conductance in the luminal membrane [9]. In the rabbit, Berry [31] has failed to find any evidence for a lumen-positive acidification PD, a finding that would suggest that luminal potassium conductance is smaller in the rabbit than in the rat and is consistent with the almost total dependence of acidification on sodium transport in that species.

Recently, Bank, Aynedjian, and Mutz [32] used the inhibitor dicyclohexyl-carbodiimide (DCCD) to evaluate the possible contribution of a luminal membrane proton-translocating ATPase to proximal acidification. Addition of 1 mM DCCD to luminal perfusate had noeffect on sodium chloride or glucose absorption, but inhibited bicarbonate absorption by 20%. These results indicate that this very high concentration of DCCD was not nonspecifically inhibiting cellular metabolism, sodium transport, or sodium-coupled transport; DCCD has no effect on Na/H antiporter activity in brushborder membrane vesicles in vitro. Although DCCD in high concentrations is known to inhibit a variety of proton-translocating ATPases, including that present in brushborder membrane preparations, it is a nonspecific inhibitor that will inactivate any carrier with a carboxyl group in a key position. In addition to proton-translocating ATPases, DCCD inhibits proton transport via the cytochrome system and the K/H exchanger in mitochondria. Thus, these results are consistent with a small (20%) component of proximal acidification in the rat being mediated by primary active transport via either a proton-translocating ATPase or a NADH oxidase cytochrome-coupled system in the luminal membrane.

The largest component of proximal acidification in both rabbit and rat is mediated by secondary active transport coupled to active sodium transport. The Na/H antiporter in the luminal membrane is the most obvious candidate for this role. Amiloride is an effective inhibitor of this transporter and thus should provide a means of evaluating its contribution. If amiloride inhibits the antiporter competitively with a K_i of 10^{-6}M and the K_m for sodium is

15 mM [10], then 1 mM amiloride in the presence of 150 mM sodium should inhibit the antiporter by approximately 85%. If the mode of inhibition is mixed as found by Ives, Yee, and Warnock [11], then the percent inhibition should be even greater. Howlin, Alpern, and I [33] performed such studies and found the percent inhibition to be only 25%, a value much less than predicted. The reason for this discrepancy is not clear. Possibilities, however, include inaccessibility of inhibitor to the antiporter in vivo, changes in intracellular pH and sodium which secondarily blunt the inhibitory effect, or a significant contribution of some sodium-coupled transport process other than Na/H exchange to overall acidification.

Secretion of hydrogen ions into the luminal fluid liberates hydroxyl ions in the cell cytoplasm, which react with carbon dioxide to form bicarbonate ions that must exit the cell across the basolateral membrane. Since the intracellular pH and bicarbonate concentration are similar to those of peritubular blood, and basolateral membrane PD is approximately 60 mV (cell interior negative), there is a large electrochemical gradient available for driving bicarbonate out of the cell. To harness this electrochemical energy effectively, however, the basolateral membrane must be conductive to bicarbonate ions. The conductive properties of the basolateral membrane have been examined by measuring the change in basolateral membrane PD in response to rapid and selective changes in ionic composition of the peritubular fluid. All studies in rat [5] and rabbit PCT [34] and rabbit PST [6, 7] have shown the basolateral membrane to be highly conductive to potassium, but not to sodium or chloride. Assessment of bicarbonate conductance has been complicated by the fact that the potassium conductance is very pH-sensitive; lowering pH reduces potassium conductance whereas raising pH increases potassium conductance. In early studies [6, 7] in rabbit PST, lowering peritubular bicarbonate concentration shifted the PD in a positive direction, consistent with a bicarbonate conductance; however, this effect was not observed if potassium conductance was first blocked by barium. Thus, it was concluded that there was no bicarbonate conductance in rabbit PST. In more recent studies in both rat PCT [30] and rabbit PCT and PST [34], the membrane depolarization produced by lowering peritubular bicarbonate concentration is not blocked by barium, and in fact, actually is amplified, as would be predicted if there were both potassium and bicarbonate conductances in the basolateral membrane.

A different approach to determining the mechanism of bicarbonate exit has been taken by Sasaki and Berry [35]. In their studies, the rate of bicarbonate absorption was measured in rabbit PCT, and the effects of either removing chloride from ambient fluids or depolarizing the basolateral membrane PD with 2 mM barium were examined. Replacing all chloride in luminal perfusate and bath solutions had no effect on bicarbonate absorption, thus excluding Cl/HCO$_3$ exchange as the mechanism of bicarbonate exit. The addition of 2 mM barium to the bath solution, which has been shown to reduce the basolateral membrane PD by approximately 50%, also reduced bicarbonate absorption by 50%. These results, therefore, suggest that bicarbonate exits the cell by a voltage-dependent process. This process could be by either simple conductance or the more complex process of coupled Na/CO$_3$ symport proposed by Boron and Boulpaep [36] for the salamander proximal tubule. This latter mechanism was detected by depolarization of the basolateral membrane, when peritubular sodium concentration was reduced. However, electrophysiologic studies in the rat [5] have failed to show such an effect. Thus, simple bicarbonate (or OH) conductance is the most likely mechanism for bicarbonate exit in the mammalian tubule.

In addition to the transport processes just described, there may be some passive diffusion of H/OH and bicarbonate. In brushborder membrane vesicles, Reenstra et al [37] have shown significant voltage-dependent transport of hydrogen ions. Similar findings have been reported by Seifter, Knickelbein, and Aronson [38]. Thus, the luminal membrane has a significant conductance to protons. However, it is highly unlikely that this has any quantitative significance for overall acidification. Schwartz [39] and Hamm et al [40] have measured the transepithelial permeability to hydrogen in the rabbit PCT and have found it to be very high (0.10 to 0.3 cm/sec). Despite the very high permeability coefficient, when multiplied by the very small concentrations of hydrogen ions in the ambient fluids, the absolute rate of hydrogen ion diffusion is extremely small. Of much more quantitative significance is the passive diffusion of bicarbonate. The measured bicarbonate permeability is 3.5×10^{-5} cm/sec in the rat [41] and 1.5×10^{-5} cm/sec in the rabbit [42]. This permeation probably represents movement of bicarbonate through the paracellular pathway and can give rise to significant back diffusion when the luminal concentration of bicarbonate falls below that of plasma.

In summary, acidification in the proximal tubule is coupled to active transport through a Na/H antiporter in the luminal membrane and a voltage-dependent bicarbonate (or hydroxyl) exit mechanism in the basolateral membrane. Other sodium-coupled processes, such as phosphate and organic anion (OA) transport plus OA/OH exchange, may contribute to a smaller degree. There may also be a small component of primary active proton transport, most likely mediated by the proton-translocating ATPase associated with the clathrin-coated pits in the microvillous spaces. In parallel with these transcellular processes is passive bicarbonate permeation, most likely through the paracellular pathway.

The rate at which this overall process operates is controlled in part by the acid-base composition of the luminal and peritubular fluids. In rabbit PCT [42], raising the concentration of bicarbonate in luminal perfusate from 24 to 40 mM at a constant P_{CO_2} of 40 mm Hg increased bicarbonate absorption from 95 to 135 pmoles/mm/min. Increasing bicarbonate to 40 mM in both luminal and bathing fluids at a constant P_{CO_2} of 40 mm Hg raised the pH to 7.6 and reduced the absorptive rate to 70 pmoles/mm/min. If P_{CO_2} was raised to 70 mm Hg while keeping bicarbonate concentration in bath and perfusate at 40 mM, the pH of the ambient fluids was restored to 7.4 and the rate of bicarbonate absorption (95 pmoles/mm/min) was the same as in the first period, in which pH was also 7.4 but P_{CO_2} was 40 mm Hg and bicarbonate concentration was 24 mM. This finding suggests that pH of luminal and peritubular fluid is the critical determinant and that the chemical or electrochemical gradients for H/OH across each cell membrane regulate, at least in part, the overall rate of acidification.

Similar results have been obtained in rat proximal tubules perfused in situ [41, 43]. Raising the concentration of bicarbonate in the luminal fluid, while keeping the acid-base composition of blood constant, progressively increases net bicarbonate absorption. Absorption begins to saturate only after the concentration exceeds 45 mM. The greater net absorption is due in part to greater diffusion of bicarbonate out of the lumen down the increased concentration gradient and in part to the stimulation of proton secretion. The passive component of bicarbonate transport, calculated from the bicarbonate permeability and the concentration gradient, was in the secretory direction when luminal concentration was below the plasma concentration and was in the absorptive direction when the concentration of bicarbonate was greater in lumen than in plasma. The residual component accounts for most of the bicarbonate transport and represents proton secretion. The rate of proton secretion increases progressively as luminal bicarbonate concentration is raised and then plateaus above a mean luminal concentration of 45 mM at a maximal rate of approximately 200 pmoles/mm/min.

Accelerating the flow of luminal fluid stimulates the rate of bicarbonate absorption [44]. In part, this is due to delivering more bicarbonate into the tubule and minimizing the fall of luminal concentration. However, only a small portion of the stimulation can be attributed to an increase in mean luminal concentration, and the remainder appears to be due to a flow-dependent diffusion barrier in the microvillous space. This flow dependence is observed only at lower mean luminal concentrations and disappears at a higher concentration in which the proton secretory system has reached its maximal capacity. The flow-dependent changes in mean luminal concentration and alterations in the luminal diffusion barrier combine to give the well-known glomerulotubular balance for bicarbonate reabsorption when GFR is increased.

The maximal proton secretory rate can be influenced by the acid-base status of the animal. Acute metabolic alkalosis, produced by infusing sodium bicarbonate into rats reduces the maximal proton secretory rate to 75 pmoles/mm/min [43]. Acute metabolic acidosis has the reverse effect and stimulates the maximal secretory rate. These changes can be explained, in part, by alterations in the proton gradients acting across the Na/H antiporter (and any other proton secretory mechanism). However, the intrinsic activity of the transporters might be changed. As proposed by Aronson, Nee, and Suhm [13], alterations in intracellular pH might modify the activity of the Na/H antiporter by allosteric effects. In addition, chronic acid-base changes can produce adaptive changes in Na/H antiporter activity assayed in brushborder membrane vesicles [45–47].

Distal Segments

Thick Ascending Limb

Micropuncture studies in rats have shown disappearance of bicarbonate between the end of the superficial PCT and the beginning of the distal convoluted tubule. It is known that the PST absorbs bicarbonate and could account for part, if not all, of this bicarbonate absorption. The contribution of other segments in the loop of Henle has remained conjectural until recently. Good, Knepper, and Burg [48] have perfused cortical and medullary thick ascending limbs (TAL) of the rat and have found very low rates of bicarbonate absorption, ranging from 5 to 9 pmoles/mm/min. Inhibition of carbonic anhydrase reduces these rates by approximately 80% [49]. These rates are only 3 to 5% of the rates found in rat PCT. To demonstrate these very low rates experimentally, it was necessary to perfuse the tubules very slowly (1.5 nl/min), which may explain why in earlier studies in which mouse cortical TAL were perfused at higher rates (10 nl/min), Friedman and Andreoli [50] failed to find any bicarbonate absorption. Earlier, Ino and Burg [51] could not demonstrate any bicarbonate absorption in TAL of rabbits, but this species, in contrast to rats and mice, does not have any carbonic anhydrase in the TAL. More recently, Good [49] has shown that the acidification process in the rat TAL is inhibited by removingsodium from the luminal perfusate and potassium from the serosal fluid (to inhibit sodium transport). Thus, Na/H exchange in the luminal membrane is the most likely process mediating bicarbonate absorption in this nephron segment.

Cortical Collecting Tubule (CCT)

The contribution of the CCT to tubular acidification is complex [52–54]. The CCT obtained from either rats or rabbits pretreated with alkali secrete bicarbonate into luminal fluid against concentration gradients (Fig. 2). The CCT obtained from animals pretreated with acid loads absorb bicarbonate against concentration gradients (Fig. 2).

One possible mechanism by which CCT might secrete bicarbonate is illustrated in the upper panel of Fig. 2. According to this model, a Na/H antiporter located in the basolateral membrane extrudes protons from the cell liberating hydroxyl ions, which subsequently react with carbon dioxide to form bicarbonate ions. The bicarbonate ions exit the cell into the lumen by a chloride-independent process [53, 55], presumably via conductive pathways driven by the favorable electrochemical gradient. In support of this model is the finding by McKinney and Burg [53] that removal of sodium from the ambient fluids inhibits bicarbonate secretion, but removal of chloride has no effect [53, 55]. More recently, Chaillet and Boron [56] demonstrated that regulation of cell pH in the CCT depends on bath, but not luminal sodium, and can be blocked completely by bath amiloride. These findings provide strong evidence for the existence of a Na/H antiporter in the basolateral membrane. The sodium that enters the cell via the Na/H antiporter can be pumped out of the cell by means of a basolateral Na/K ATPase system; alternatively, the sodium could be pumped out of the cell by a luminal Na/K ATPase. Which of these two possibilities is responsible for sodium removal is not clear. The addition of ouabain to the bathing fluid inhibits bicarbonate secretion slightly, but not completely; the effect of ouabain added to the luminal fluid has not been adequately tested.

Absorption of bicarbonate by the CCT is probably mediated by a proton-

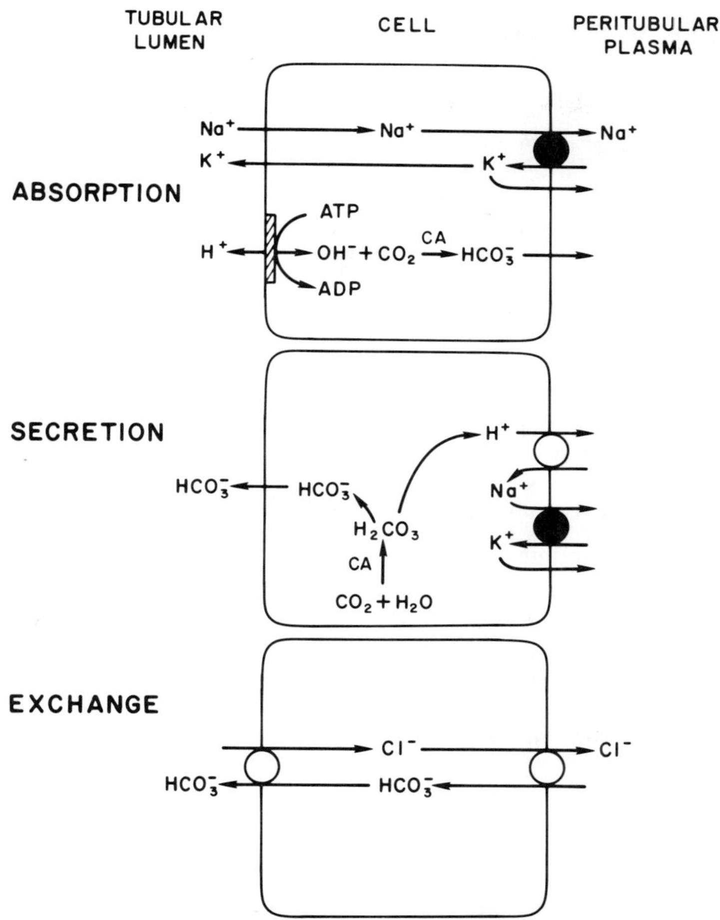

Fig. 2. Hydrogen transport in the cortical collecting tubule. Bicarbonate ions can be either absorbed or secreted. There may also be some Cl/HCO$_3$ exchange.

translocating ATPase in the luminal membrane, similar to that present in turtle bladder and the medullary collecting duct (MCD), where it has been more completely characterized. The proton pump in the CCT is probably electrogenic, generating a lumen-positive PD, but its true electrical properties are partially obscured by simultaneous electrogenic sodium transport. However, when sodium transport is inhibited, an acetazolamide-sensitive lumen-positive PD has been observed [57]. The rate of hydrogen ion secretion by an electrogenic proton-translocating ATPase should be sensitive to transepithelial electrical gradients and, thus, should be secondarily influenced by sodium transport. Earlier studies by McKinney and Burg [54] did not completely confirm this prediction; luminal amiloride obliterated the sodium transport PD and partially inhibited bicarbonate absorption, whereas inhibition of sodium transport by bath ouabain reduced the PD but had no effect on the rate of bicarbonate absorption. More recent studies by Laski and Kurtzman [58], however, show that inhibition of sodium transport by ouabain or a variety of other means produces a reproducible reduction in the rate of bicarbonate absorption. Thus, the proton pump in the CCT is similar to that in the turtle bladder; it is electrogenic and sensitive to pH and electrical gradients; it can operate in the absence of sodium transport but is secondarily influenced by sodium transport PDs.

Laski, Warnock, and I [55] have shown that superimposition of chloride concentration gradients across the CCT can drive either bicarbonate secretion or absorption, depending on the orientation of the chloride gradient. We proposed the existence of a parallel Cl/OH exchanger; however, our studies did not exclude electrical coupling as an explanation for the findings.

In summary, the CCT is a complex transporting epithelium that can absorb sodium and potassium and can secrete potassium, protons, or bicarbonate ions. The CCT is also an important target organ for aldosterone. Aldosterone stimulates sodium transport by an effect on the metabolic control of the sodium channels in the apical membrane and thereby increases the lumen-negative sodium transport PD. As a consequence, aldosterone can indirectly influence the rate of proton transport. However, in the absenceof active sodium transport, aldosterone stimulates proton secretion and increases the lumen-positive PD [57]. Thus, aldosterone appears to act directly on the proton pump, as it does in the turtle bladder and the MCT. Rather surprisingly, mineralocorticoid hormone (DOC) has also been shown to stimulate bicarbonate secretion in alkalotic rats and rabbits [59].

Outer Medullary Collecting Tubule (MCD)

The MCD is an unusual nephron segment that neither absorbs sodium nor secretes potassium actively [60], but does absorb bicarbonate [61–63], presumably by active proton transport across the luminal membrane (Fig. 3). The

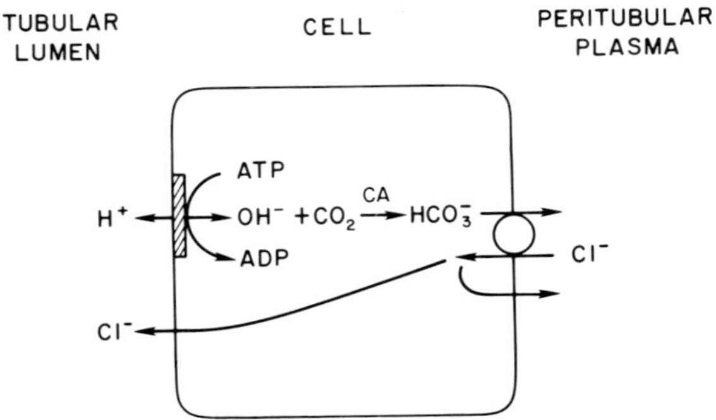

Fig. 3. Hydrogen ion transport in the medullary collecting duct.

proton transport system is independent of sodium transport and is electrogenic, generating an acetazolamide-sensitive lumen-positive PD. Bicarbonate absorption (or proton secretion) is matched by equivalent secretion of chloride. Bicarbonate that is generated in the cell as a consequence of proton secretion leaves the cell by a SITS-sensitive Cl/HCO_3 exchange in the basolateral membrane. Removal of chloride from or addition of SITS to the bath solution completely blocks proton secretion. In contrast, the addition of SITS to the luminal fluid has no effect, whereas removal of luminal chloride actually stimulates proton secretion. It is not clear whether stimulation of proton secretion by removal of luminal chloride is due to electrical coupling or is by a more direct effect; removal of chloride did reduce the lumen-positive PD, which opposes proton secretion, but the reduction was not statistically significant.

The mechanism by which the chloride that enters the cell via the Cl/HCO_3 exchange exits the cell is controversial. Two possibilities, however, can be considered. First, the chloride could move through a conductive pathway in the luminal membrane driven by its favorable electrochemical gradient. Equivalent transport of protons and chloride across the luminal membrane would give rise to apparent electrogenic proton transport only if the luminal membrane were much more conductive than the paracellular pathway. An alternative possibility is that chloride leaves the cell via a conductive pathway in the basolateral membrane and is secreted into the lumen by passive movement through the paracellular pathway driven by the lumen-positive proton secretory PD. Either of these two models could explain the inhibition of proton secretion by removal of bath chloride and stimulation of secretion by removal of luminal chloride. In the first case, the electrical coupling would occur across the luminal membrane, whereas in the second case, the electrical coupling would be between chloride movement through the paracellular pathway and proton movement through the apical membrane. There is experimental evidence to support each of these two possibilities.

Stone, Xie, and Racker [64] have isolated from the renal medulla membrane vesicles that contain an oligomycin-insensitive and vanadate-insensitive proton-translocating ATPase. This ATPase is inhibited by high concentrations of DCCD and is very similar to the proton-translocating ATPase in clathrin-coated vesicles isolated from brain and other tissues. The net movement of protons into these vesicles is stimulated by the addition of ATP to the outside fluid and requires the presence of chloride or bromide. Thus, an intrinsic chloride-conductive pathway is present in the same membrane that contains the proton pump. However, it has not been proven that the vesicles prepared from the renal medulla represent luminal membranes.

In contrast, electrophysiologic studies by Koeppen [65] have failed to find any evidence of chloride conductance in the apical membrane of the MCD. The MCD is a high-resistance tissue with a transepithelial resistance of 747 $\Omega \cdot cm^2$. The apical membrane is less than 1% as conductive as the basolateral membrane and has no chloride conductance, but the basolateral membrane is highly conductive to chloride. Thus, the membrane vesicle studies support the first possibility, whereas the electrophysiologic studies refute the first and support only the second possibility.

The MCD is also a target tissue for aldosterone [62]. Aldosterone stimulates proton secretion and increases the lumen positivity, presumably by a direct effect on the pump. The papillary collecting duct in rats also secretes hydrogen ion by a sodium-independent mechanism that is inhibited by SITS applied to the basolateral membrane [66]. In addition, recent evidence indicates that proton secretion in this segment is also stimulated by aldosterone [67].

Acknowledgment. This study was supported in part by grant AM27045 from the National Institutes of Health.

References

1. STRUYVENBERG A, MORRISON RB, RELMAN AS: Acid-base behavior of separated canine renal tubule cells. *Am J Physiol* 214:1155–1162, 1968
2. BICHARA M, PAILLARD M, LEVIEL F, GARDIN JP: Hydrogen transport in rabbit kidney proximal tubules—Na:H exchange. *Am J Physiol* 238(*Renal Fluid Electrolyte Physiol* 7):F445–F451, 1980
3. KLEINMAN JG, BROWN WW, WARE RA, SCHWARTZ JH: Cell pH and acid transport in renal cortical tissue. *Am J Physiol* 239(*Renal Fluid Electrolyte Physiol* 8):F440–F444, 1980
4. SASAKI S, IINO Y, SHIIGAI T, TAKEUCHI J: Intracellular pH of isolated perfused rabbit proximal tubule: Effects of luminal Na and Cl (*abstract*). *Kidney Int* 25:282, 1984
5. FROMTER E, MULLER CW, WICK T: Permeability properties of the proximal tubular epithelium of the rat kidney studied with electrophysiological methods, in *Electrophysiology of Epithelial Cells* (Symposia Medica Hochst), edited by GIEBISCH G, New York, F.K. Schatlauer, 1971, pp 119–146
6. BIAGI B, KUBOTA T, SOHTELL M, GIEBISCH G: Intracellular potentials in rabbit proximal tubules perfused in vitro. *Am J Physiol* 240(*Renal Fluid Electrolyte Physiol* 9):F200–F210, 1981
7. BELLO-REUSS E: Electrical properties of the basolateral membrane of the straight portion of the rabbit proximal renal tubule. *J Physiol* (*Lond*) 326:49–63, 1982
8. MURER H, HOPFER U, KINNE R: Sodium/proton antiport in brush-border membrane vesicles isolated from rat small intestine and kidney (*abstract*). *Biochem J* 154:597, 1976
9. ARONSON PS: Mechanisms of active H^+ secretion in the proximal tubule. *Am J Physiol* 245(*Renal Fluid Electrolyte Physiol* 14):F647–F659, 1983
10. KINSELLA JL, ARONSON PS: Amiloride inhibition of the Na^+-H^+ exchanger in renal microvillus membrane vesicles. *Am J Physiol* 241(*Renal Fluid Electrolyte Physiol* 10):F374–F379, 1981
11. IVES HE, YEE VJ, WARNOCK DG: Mixed type inhibition of the renal Na^+/H^+ antiporter by Li^+ and amiloride: Evidence for a modifier site. *J Biol Chem* 258:9710–9716, 1983
12. KINSELLA JL, ARONSON PS: Interaction of NH_4^+ and Li^+ with the renal microvillus membrane Na^+-H^+ exchanger. *Am J Physiol* 241(*Cell Physiol* 10):C220–C226, 1981
13. ARONSON PS, NEE J, SUHM MA: Modifier role of internal H^+ in activating the Na^+-H^+ exchanger in renal microvillus membrane vesicles. *Nature* 299:161–163, 1982
14. BORON WF, BOULPAEP EL: Intracellular pH regulation in the renal proximal tubule of the salamander: Na-H exchange. *J Gen Physiol* 81:29–52, 1983

15. IVES HE, YEE VJ, WARNOCK DG: Asymmetric distribution of the Na^+/H^+ antiporter in the renal proximal tubule epithelial cell. *J Biol Chem* 257:13513–13516, 1983
16. BLOMSTEDT JW, ARONSON PS: pH gradient-stimulated transport of urate and p-aminohippurate in dog renal microvillus membrane vesicles. *J Clin Invest* 65:931–934, 1980
17. KINNE-SAFFRAN E, BEAUWENS R, KINNE R: An ATP-driven proton pump in brush-border membranes from rat renal cortex. *J Membr Biol* 64:67–76, 1982
18. KINNE-SAFFRAN E, KINNE R: ATP-driven proton transport systems in renal proximal tubule and collecting duct plasma membranes, in *Hydrogen Ion Transport in Epithelia,* edited by FORTE JG, WARNOCK DG, RECTOR FC JR, John Wiley & Sons (in press, 1984)
19. RODMAN JS, KERJASCHKI D, MERISKO EM, FARQUHAR MG: Extensive clathrin coating on the apical membrane of the kidney proximal tubule (*abstract*). *J Cell Biol* (in press, 1984)
20. FORGAC M, CNATLEY L, WIEDENMANN B, ALTSTIEL L, BRANTON D: Clathrin-coated vesicles contain an ATP-dependent proton pump. *Proc Natl Acad Sci USA* 80:1300–1303, 1983
21. GARCIA ML, BENAVIDES J, GIMENEZ-GALLEGO G, VALDIVIESO F: Coupling between reduced nictinamide adenine di-nucleotide oxidation and metabolite transport in renal brush border membrane vesicles. *Biochemistry* 19:4840–4843, 1980
22. GARCIA ML, BENAVIDES J, VALDIVIESO F, MAYOR F: Cytochromes in the rat kidney brush border membrane. *Biochem Biophys Res Commun* 82:738–744, 1978
23. BURG M, GREEN N: Bicarbonate transport by isolated perfused rabbit proximal convoluted tubules. *Am J Physiol* 233(*Renal Fluid Electrolyte Physiol* 2):F307–F314, 1977
24. MCKINNEY TD, BURG MB: Bicarbonate and fluid absorption by renal proximal straight tubules. *Kidney Int* 12:1–8, 1977
25. SASAKI S, BERRY CA, RECTOR FC JR: Effect of potassium concentration on bicarbonate reabsorption in the rabbit proximal convoluted tubule. *Am J Physiol* 244(*Renal Fluid Electrolyte Physiol* 13):F122–F128, 1983
26. ULLRICH KJ, CAPASSO G, RUMRICH G, PAPAVASSILIOU F, KLOSS S: Coupling between proximal tubular transport processes: Studies with ouabain, SITS and HCO_3^- free solutions. *Pflügers Arch* 368:246, 1977
27. DEMELLO AIRES M, MALNIC G: Sodium in renal tubular acidification kinetics. *Am J Physiol* 236(*Renal Fluid Electrolyte Physiol* 5):F434–F441, 1979
28. CHAN YL, GIEBISCH G: Relationship between sodium and bicarbonate transport in the rat proximal convoluted tubule. *Am J Physiol* 240(*Renal Fluid Electrolyte Physiol* 9):F222–F230, 1981
29. CHANTRELLE B, COGAN MG, RECTOR FC JR: Evidence for coupled sodium/hydrogen exchange in the rat superficial proximal convoluted tubule. *Pflügers Arch* 395:186–189, 1982
30. FROMTER E, SATO K: Electrical events in active H^+/HCO_3^- transport across rat proximal tubular epithelium, in *Gastric Hydrogen Ion Secretion,* edited by KASBEKER D, SACHS G, REHM W, New York, Marcel Dekker, 1976, p 382
31. BERRY CA: Electrical effects of acidification in the rabbit proximal convoluted tubule. *Am J Physiol* 240(*Renal Fluid Electrolyte Physiol* 9):F459–F470, 1981
32. BANK N, AYNEDJIAN HS, MUTZ BF: Quantitative contribution of H^+ ATPase to proximal HCO_3^- reabsorption in normal rats (*abstract*). *Kidney Int* 25:271, 1984
33. HOWLIN KJ, ALPERN RJ, RECTOR FC JR: Sodium bicarbonate and sodium absorption in the proximal convoluted tubule (PCT): Effect of amiloride (*abstract*). *Kidney Int* 25:277, 1984

34. BIAGI B, SOHTELL M: Bicarbonate voltage transients in the rabbit proximal tubule (*abstract*). *Kidney Int* 25:271, 1984
35. SASAKI S, BERRY CA: The mechanism of bicarbonate exit across the basolateral membrane of the rabbit proximal tubule. *Am J Physiol* (in press, 1984)
36. BORON WF, BOULPAEP EL: Intracellular pH regulation in the renal proximal tubule of the salamander: Basolateral HCO_3^- transport. *J Gen Physiol* 81:53–94, 1983
37. REENSTRA WW, WARNOCK DG, YEE VJ, FORTE JG: Proton gradients in renal cortex brush-border membrane vesicles. *J Biol Chem* 256:11663–11666, 1981
38. SEIFTER J, KNICKELBEIN R, ARONSON PS: Cl transport in rabbit renal microvillus membrane vesicles: Evidence against Cl-OH exchange. *Kidney Int* 23:266, 1983
39. SCHWARTZ GJ: Na^+-dependent H^+ efflux from proximal tubule: Evidence for reversible Na^+-H^+ exchange. *Am J Physiol* 241(*Renal Fluid Electrolyte Physiol* 10):F380–F385, 1981
40. HAMM LL, PUCACCO LR, KOKKO JP, JACOBSON HR: Hydrogen ion permeability of the rabbit proximal convoluted tubule. *Am J Physiol* 246(*Renal Fluid Electrolyte Physiol* 15):F3–F11, 1984
41. ALPERN RJ, COGAN MG, RECTOR FC JR: Effect of luminal bicarbonate concentration on proximal acidification in the rat. *Am J Physiol* 243(*Renal Fluid Electrolyte Physiol* 12):F53–F59, 1982
42. SASAKI S, BERRY CA, RECTOR FC JR: Effect of luminal and peritubular HCO_3^- concentrations and P_{CO_2} on HCO_3^- reabsorption in rabbit proximal convoluted tubules perfused in vitro. *J Clin Invest* 70:639–649, 1982
43. ALPERN RJ, COGAN MG, RECTOR FC JR: Effects of extracellular fluid volume and plasma bicarbonate concentration on proximal acidification in the rat. *J Clin Invest* 71:736–746, 1983
44. ALPERN RJ, COGAN MG, RECTOR FC JR: Flow dependence of proximal tubular bicarbonate absorption. *Am J Physiol* 245(*Renal Fluid Electrolyte Physiol* 14):F478–F484, 1983
45. COHN DE, KLAHR S, HAMMERMAN MR: Metabolic acidosis and parathyroidectomy increase Na^+-H^+ exchange in brush border vesicles. *Am J Physiol* 245(*Renal Fluid Electrolyte Physiol* 14):F217–F222, 1983
46. TSAI C-J, IVES HE, ALPERN RJ, YEE VJ, WARNOCK DG, RECTOR FC JR: Increased V_{max} for Na^+/H^+ antiporter activity in proximal tubule brush border vesicles from rabbits with metabolic acidosis. *Am J Physiol* (*Renal Fluid Electrolyte Physiol*) (in press, 1984)
47. KINSELLA J, CUJDIK T, SACKTOR B: Na^+-H^+ exchange activity in renal brush border membrane vesicles in response to metabolic acidosis: The role of glucocorticoids. *Proc Natl Acad Sci USA* 81:630–634, 1984
48. GOOD DW, KNEPPER MA, BURG MB: Ammonia and bicarbonate transport by thick ascending limb of rat kidney (*abstract*). *Kidney Int* 25:275, 1984
49. GOOD DW: Sodium dependent bicarbonate absorption by rat cortical thick ascending limb (*abstract*). *Clin Res* 32:448A, 1984
50. FRIEDMAN PA, ANDREOLI TE: CO_2-stimulated NaCl absorption in the mouse renal cortical thick ascending limb of Henle: Evidence for synchronous Na^+/H^+ and Cl^-/HCO_3^- exchange in apical plasma membranes. *J Gen Physiol* 80:683–711, 1982
51. IINO Y, BURG MB: Effect of acid-base status in vivo on bicarbonate transport by rabbit renal tubules in vitro. *Jpn J Physiol* 31:99–107, 1981
52. MCKINNEY TD, BURG MB: Bicarbonate transport by rabbit cortical collecting tubules: Effect of acid and alkali loads in vivo on transport in vitro. *J Clin Invest* 60:766–768, 1977

53. MCKINNEY TD, BURG MB: Bicarbonate secretion by rabbit cortical collecting tubules in vitro (*abstract*). *J Clin Invest* 61:1421, 1978
54. MCKINNEY TD, BURG MB: Bicarbonate absorption by rabbit cortical collecting tubules in vitro. *Am J Physiol* 234(*Renal Fluid Electrolyte Physiol* 3):F141, 1978
55. LASKI ME, WARNOCK DG, RECTOR FC JR: Effects of chloride gradients on total CO_2 flux in the rabbit cortical collecting tubule. *Am J Physiol* 244(*Renal Fluid Electrolyte Physiol* 13):F112–F121, 1983
56. CHAILLET JR, BORON WF: Basolateral Na-H exchange in the rabbit cortical collecting tubule (*abstract*). *Fed Proc* 43:1089, 1984
57. KOEPPEN BM, HELMAN SI: Acidification of luminal fluid by the rabbit cortical collecting tubule perfused in vitro. *Am J Physiol* 242(*Renal Fluid Electrolyte Physiol* 11):F521–F531, 1982
58. LASKI ME, KURTZMAN NA: Characterization of acidification in the cortical and medullary collecting tubule of the rabbit. *J Clin Invest* 72:2050–2059, 1983
59. KNEPPER M, GOOD D, GARCIA-AUSTT J, BURG M: Deoxycorticosterone-stimulated bicarbonate secretion in cortical collecting ducts from rabbits and rats (*abstract*). *Kidney Int* 25:278, 1984
60. STOKES JB: Na and K transport across the cortical and outer medullary collecting tubule of the rabbit: Evidence for diffusion across the outer medullary portion. *Am J Physiol* 242(*Renal Fluid Electrolyte Physiol* 11):F514–F520, 1982
61. LOMBARD WE, KOKKO JP, JACOBSON HR: Bicarbonate transport in cortical and outer medullary collecting tubules. *Am J Physiol* 244(*Renal Fluid Electrolyte Physiol* 13):F289–F296, 1983
62. STONE DK, SELDIN DW, KOKKO JP, JACOBSON HR: Mineralocorticoid modulation of rabbit medullary collecting duct acidification. *J Clin Invest* 72:77–83, 1983
63. STONE DK, SELDIN DW, KOKKO JP, JACOBSON HR: Anion dependence of rabbit medullary collecting duct acidification. *J Clin Invest* 71:1505–1508, 1983
64. STONE DK, XIE X-S, RACKER E: Comparison of the protonATPase and chloride transporter from bovine clathrin-coated vesicles and renal medullary vesicles (*abstract*). *Kidney Int* 25:283, 1984
65. KOEPPEN BM: Conductive properties of rabbit outer medullary collecting duct (*abstract*). *Kidney Int* 25:278, 1984
66. ULLRICH KJ, PAPAVASSILIOU F: Bicarbonate reabsorption in the papillary collecting duct of rats. *Pflügers Arch* 389:271–275, 1981
67. HIGASHARA E, CARTER NW, PUCACCO L, KOKKO JP: The effect of aldosterone on papillary collecting duct pH profile of normal and adrenalectomized rat (*abstract*). *Kidney Int* 25:276, 1984

Proximal Tubule Transport

Chairpersons: Harry R. Jacobson and Jean Cardinal
Discussants: Christine A. Berry, Bruno Corman, Dalon W. Barfuss, Jacques Lapointe, Elsa Bello-Reuss, Sei Sasaki, Keith A. Hruska, and Julian Seifter

Three major topics were discussed in the Workshop on proximal tubule transport. The first topic related to the controversy as to which pathways (transcellular or paracellular) are taken by solute and water as they traverse the intact epithelium. The other two topics were designed to disseminate updated information on the application of newer experimental techniques to the study of proximal tubule transport: the application of cell puncture for electrophysiologic measurements on both apical and basolateral cell membranes and the use of cell membrane vesicles to study regulation and adaptation of proximal tubule transport.

Berry initiated the discussion on the first topic by presenting studies designed to elucidate whether water molecules cross the proximal convoluted tubule via mostly transcellular or paracellular routes. Using the disappearance of [^{3}H] water from luminal perfusate in proximal convoluted tubule perfused in vitro, Berry calculated a diffusive water permeability coefficient (P_{DW}) of 5×10^{-3} cm/sec. Unstirred (luminal and peritubular) water layer effects were corrected by the simultaneous measurement of the lumen-to-bath permeability coefficient for the highly permeant organic solute [^{14}C]n-butanol (P_{DNB}). P_{DNB} was 3.6×10^{-3} cm/sec. The very high P_{DW} provides substantial proof that water diffuses through predominantly a cellular and not a paracellular pathway. Because neither P_{DW} nor P_{DNB} was affected by increasing bath fluid viscosity 10-fold, it was calculated that in the isolated perfused proximal convoluted tubule peritubular unstirred water layers must be less than 1 μ thick and thus physiologically insignificant.

To gain further insight into the mechanism of water permeation, activation energies (E_A) of P_{DNB} were calculated by multiple measurements of the permeability coefficient at several temperatures (range, 20 to 40°C). Of interest, E_A ranged between 3.4 to 5.5 kcal/mole with a mean of 4.3 kcal/mole. The value for E_A of P_{DNB} is very close to the activation energy of water diffusion

---

This manuscript is a summary of a Workshop entitled *Reabsorption in the Proximal Tubule.*

in water (E_A 4.6 kcal/mole), suggesting that water traverses proximal tubule cells through aqueous pathways that do not involve significant interactions with the cell membranes.

The organic mercurial, sulfhydral reagent p-chloromercuribenzene sulfonate (PCMBS), is known to reduce the osmotic water permeability of the red blood cell and rabbit proximal tubule peritubular cell membrane by almost 90%. In studies with PCMBS present in the bath, P_{DW} was reduced by 30% while P_{DNB} was unaffected. These results suggest that the water permeability of luminal and peritubular membranes are comparable. The PCMBS studies, in concert with the activation energy measurements and the high P_{DW}, under normal circumstances are consistent with a model of proximal tubule water transport where the water molecules diffuse through small gramicidin-like channels in a transcellular pathway. The data are inconsistent with solubility diffusion of water through lipid-protein matrix of lumen and peritubular cell membranes. In addition, it is likely that lumen and peritubular cell membranes exhibit similar water permeabilities.

Corman addressed the issue of proximal tubule reflection coefficient for sodium chloride and the implication of this reflection coefficient for the coupling of solute and water movement. Previously determined values for the proximal tubule reflection coefficient for sodium chloride range from 0.7 to 0.89, possibly predicting that a measurable amount of solute would be dragged across the proximal convoluted tubule by an osmotically induced transepithelial water flux. Attempts to measure such solvent drag have raised significant questions regarding the accuracy of the reflection coefficient; that is, measurements of almost no solvent drag for sodium chloride suggest that the reflection coefficient for this solute does not differ from 1.0. It is thus possible that results obtained by different investigators for the sodium chloride reflection coefficient may suffer from problems with the actual measurements, or from a problem equating the reflection coefficient for osmosis to that obtained from solvent drag experiments. In other words, do measurements of reflection coefficient obtained by measuring the osmotic pressure generated by sodium chloride compared to that generated by a solute that has a reflection coefficient of 1.0 (raffinose) assess the same epithelial characteristics as estimates of reflection coefficients from measurement of solvent drag? To address these questions, Corman considered two experimental features: (1) Measurements of streaming and diffusion potentials in proximal tubules perfused in vitro suggested that a sweeping away of solutes in the lateral intercellular spaces as a result of osmotic water flow would reduce the effect of osmotic pressure of raffinose across the tubule. The same process would apply to sodium chloride placed in the peritubular environment, but to a lesser extent, because the sodium chloride diffusion in water is faster than that of raffinose and would theoretically persist in higher concentrations in the lateral intercellular space. Such a process would overestimate the ratio of sodium chloride reflection coefficient to that of raffinose. (2) Because sodium chloride is more permeant than raffinose, an equiosmolar transepithelial gradient of sodium chloride will be dissipated faster than that of raffinose along the perfused tubule. Thus, the resulting water flow with the sodium chloride addition to peritubular fluid would be reduced relative to that seen with an equivalent osmolar addition of raffinose. Thus, a true reflection coefficient for sodium chloride would be underestimated.

Corman, in an attempt to clarify the question of solute-solvent interactions, estimated a new reflection coefficient for sodium chloride which considered the above two points. The results of these estimations suggest that the reflection coefficient of proximal tubule for sodium chloride is 0.95 and thus consistent with the lack of significant solvent drag for this salt.

Barfuss addressed the mechanism whereby alterations in tubular flow rate affect solute transport in proximal tubules perfused in vitro. Previous studies both in vivo and in vitro in proximal convoluted tubules have demonstrated the flow-rate dependence of reabsorption of a number of solutes. Classically, it is considered that the flow-rate dependence of these solutes was critically a function of the affect that flow rate had on the axial concentration profile of the solute in question. In other words, the higher the flow rate, the higher the mean luminal concentration of the solute and the more favorable are conditions for its entry into the cell or its exchange for an intracellular solute. Previous measurements by Barfuss and his colleagues with proximal tubule glucose transport showed that by using glucose concentrations in the lumen that are above the K_m of the apical glucose transporter (1.6 mM), flow-rate dependence of glucose absorption existed and could be accounted for by changes in the mean luminal concentration profile for glucose. However, these and other studies examining flow dependence have not been able to determine whether there are independent effects of flow rate and flow rate-induced changes in the concentration profile of the solute in question. Studies presented here attempt to address this issue by measuring the effects of flow rate on glucose absorption with low luminal concentrations of glucose (0.6 mM). The results of these studies could be used to develop a model for flow-rate dependence of transport that contains a component of flow dependence that is not due to changes in the luminal concentration profile for glucose. This derives from the results of studies in which flow rate was increased while attempts were made to keep mean luminal fluid glucose concentration constant. Under these circumstances there was a significant increase in net glucose absorption that correlated with flow rate. However, there was also a flow rate-dependent increase in mean luminal glucose concentration. Thus, in vitro studies of this transport process fail to disclose evidence for a luminal diffusion barrier to glucose.

This Workshop next considered the application of cell puncture technique to in vitro microperfusion. The first discussion was presented by Lapointe. These studies utilized rabbit proximal convoluted tubules perfused in vitro and punctured from the peritubular side with standard Ling-Gerard microelectrodes. Basolateral (V_{BL}) potential differences, transepithelial potential (V_T) and the ratio of apical to basolateral membrane resistances (R_A/R_{BL}) were measured with different artificial perfusates. Control perfusate was a standard bicarbonate Ringer's solution containing glucose and alanine. Perfusate substitutions were of five types.

Because the apical membrane potential difference is related to the sum of an electromotive force (E_A) and an ohmic voltage drop across the apical resistance (R_A), alterations in V_A can be attributed to variations in I, R_A, and E_A, since E_A is equal to

$$\Sigma_i \cdot \frac{G_i}{G_{total}} \cdot E_1$$

where G_i/G_{total} represents partial conductance for the solute in question. The absolute value of E_A can be obtained for each perfusate by subtracting the term $R_A \times I$ from the measured value of V_A. Utilizing the first perfusate, P1, which is a bicarbonate Ringer's lacking amino acids or glucose and producing a transepithelial voltage very close to zero, the transepithelial current is relatively small and E_A should approximate V_A. For the other perfusates where ion substitutions were made, transepithelial diffusion potentials were generated and the epithelial current could not be evaluated from the measurements of V_T. For these perfusates the term $R_A I$ can be calculated from the value of R_A/R_{BL} and the change in V_{BL} compared to V_{BL} with perfusate P1 where the epithelial current is close to zero. Therefore, $R_A \times I = R_A \times \triangle V_{BL}/R_{BL}$.

Transport numbers for ions are obtained by dividing the variation of E_A during a particular ionic substitution by the calculated variation of the reversal potential (using the Nernst equation) for this ion. However, when a concentration of an ion is changed by substitution, the conductance made by this ion is also expected to change, which must be considered in the analysis. If the ionic flux mechanism is not saturated, the change in specific ion conductance can be evaluated using the Goldman equation. For example, in the case of sodium in the presence of cotransport (results with solution P2 vs. P2 choline solution), the Goldman equation predicts that sodium conductance decreases by as much as 69% when the sodium is partially replaced by choline. Similar analysis can be applied to the case of potassium replacing choline in P2 perfusate (P2/choline vs. P2/potassium). Such an analysis demonstrates that the potassium conductance could increase by a factor of 7.1 when potassium is added to the perfusate.

Utilizing this approach for individual ionic conductances, the sodium conductance can be calculated to represent 33% of the total apical membrane conductance when proximal convoluted tubules are perfused with the P2 perfusate. The potassium conductance using P2/choline perfusate would represent only 6% of the apical conductance. These values agree with the partial conductances calculated using the measured change in the ratio R_A/R_{BL} during the same experiments, but contradict the values that would be obtained without correction for variations in individual ionic conductances. These intracellular potential analyses demonstrate the importance of cell membrane resistance measurements in the proximal convoluted tubule and stress the need for further kinetic details on different membrane permeation pathways.

Sasaki discussed intracellular pH measurements in isolated perfused rabbit proximal straight tubules. Measurements of intracellular pH in mammalian renal tubule cells have been difficult to achieve, because the available electrodes contained too large a tip diameter. Therefore, utilizing a pH microelectrode with a small enough tip constructed with the use of a liquid ion exchange resin using a proton ligand, Sasaki and his colleagues examined proximal straight tubule intracellular pH and alterations in pH with luminal substitution of sodium with choline.

Segments of rabbit proximal tubules were perfused in vitro according to standard methods. Perfusion and bath fluids under control conditions were artificial solutions mimicking plasma ultrafiltrate. Basolateral membrane potential was measured with standard Ling-Gerard electrodes filled with either 3 or 1 mM KCl and exhibiting resistances of 20 to 50 MΩ. Using salinized Ling-Gerard microelectrodes, pH electrodes were constructed by placing a small droplet of proton ligand (a mixture of 10% tri-N-dodeclamine, 89.3% O-nitro-pheny-N-octyl-ether, and 0.7% sodium tetra-phenylborate) into the tip. The remainder of the pH electrode was filled with buffer solution (0.04 M KH_2PO_4, 0.023 M sodium hydroxide, and 0.015 M NaCl, pH 7.0). The resistance of these pH electrodes were 1 to 6 $\times$ 10^{11} Ω and the response times were about 10 sec.

Calibration studies with these electrodes demonstrated that with 20 mM Tris buffer the potential measured was linear between pH 6.6 and 8.0 with a mean slope of 48.8 $\pm$ 2.9 mv per pH unit. The addition of 100 mM KCl or NaCl to the 20 mM Tris buffer did not affect the slope of the electrode significantly, demonstrating that the cation interference in this pH range was minimal.

The investigators also looked for interaction of this electrode with other ions which are present in the physiologic solutions used in the experiments. Thus, the slopes are compared in phosphate-buffered and bicarbonate-buffered solutions. For 11 pH microelectrodes the slope was 45.5 $\pm$ 1.7 mv in phosphate buffer and 47.2 $\pm$ 1.6 mv per pH unit in bicarbonate buffer fluids. Intracellular pH was calculated from the following equation: pHi = pH bath + 1/S (V_{pH} − V_{BL}) where pH bath is the bath pH, S is the slope of the pH microelectrode, V_{pH} is the voltage measured by the pH electrode, and V_{BL} is the basolateral cell membrane voltage. It is preferred that the V_{pH} and V_{BL} are measured in the same cell simultaneously, but this could not be accomplished in the present studies due to the utilization of a single-barrel pH microelectrode.

In 57 tubules, 65 measurements of V_{BL} and 58 measurements of V_{pH} were performed under control conditions. The mean values for V_{BL} and V_{pH} were −48.5 $\pm$ 1.1 and −33.8 $\pm$ 1.1 mv, respectively, P <0.001. Calculated pHi ranged from 6.74 to 7.65 with a mean of 7.11 $\pm$ 0.03. This pHi is significantly lower than the bath pH of 7.42 $\pm$ 0.01, P <0.001. However, this pHi is higher than the calculated equilibrium pHi of 6.64 $\pm$ 0.01 predicted from passive proton distribution.

Since V_{pH} was lower than V_{BL}, it was possible that the pH microelectrode impalement was leaky. To assess for this, the response of V_{BL} and V_{pH} to luminal glucose addition was tested in 10 tubules. The luminal glucose addition depolarized V_{BL} by a mean of 4.6 mv and V_{pH} by a mean of 4.3 mv. The equality of these depolarizations suggested that the pH microelectrodes were properly sealed inside the cell.

When luminal sodium was replaced with choline, V_{BL} hyperpolarized quickly (90% change within 30 sec) from -46.6 ± 2.1 to -63.2 ± 1.5 mv, $P <0.001$. V_{pH} also hyperpolarized at essentially the same rate from -33.2 ± 3.4 to -38.5 ± 3.7 mv, $P <0.005$. Both these changes were reversible. The resultant pHi change calculated in the sodium replacement experiments was from 7.14 ± 0.06 to 6.91 ± 0.07 ($P <0.001$). Recovery upon reintroduction of sodium into the lumen was complete.

These studies of Sasaki represent the first measurements of intracellular pH of mammalian renal proximal tubule cells utilizing microelectrodes. The results obtained in these experiments are in keeping with its low intracellular pH values obtained by previous studies using the pH-sensitive distribution of the 5,5-dimethyloxazoline-2,4-dione. This more acidic intracellular pH measurement by the electrode could be due to the possibility that proximal straight tubules have a more acid pH because of lower rates of proton secretion or because of the microelectrode measures cytoplasmic pH, whereas the dye distribution technique measures total intracellular pH including that observed in intracellular compartments including the alkaline compartments represented by mitochondria.

The decline in intracellular pH after sodium removal is consistent with the presence of a luminal sodium proton exchanger. Of note is that the intracellular pH after luminal sodium removal was still above equilibrium. If the sodium proton exchanger at the luminal membrane is the only mechanism for proton secretion, then the intracellular pH value might be expected to approach that of the equilibrium pH when luminal sodium is withdrawn. The fact that intracellular pH was higher than equilibrium could be accounted for by any of the following: (1) presence of sodium proton exchanger at the basolateral cell membrane; (2) a sodium-independent mechanism for proton exit from the cell; (3) the persistence of some luminal sodium to allow for the sodium proton exchanger to continue operation. Further studies will be necessary to clarify the residual of the equilibrium distribution of protons.

Bello-Reuss addressed measurements of transepithelial as well as apical and basolateral cell membrane resistances utilizing intracellular electrodes. Transepithelial-specific resistance (R_E) was measured in isolated perfused proximal convoluted tubules using cable analysis and intracellular microelectrode measurements. R_E in 29 tubules was measured to be 15.5 ± 2.0 $\Omega \cdot cm^2$. The measurements of tubule diameter using electrical measurements were compared to those measured optically. The optical diameter was 22 ± 1 μ and was not significantly different from the electrical diameter of 24 ± 3 μ. Measurement of R_E was further validated by examining the changes in R_E resulting from removal of peritubular calcium and decreasing bath temperature, maneuvers which should decrease and increase R_E respectively. Removal of bath calcium resulted in R_E falling to a value not different from 0, while decreasing temperature from $37^\circ C$ to $10^\circ C$ resulted in a significant increase in R_E from 15.5 ± 2.0 to 31 ± 9 $\Omega \cdot cm^2$.

Measurements of the resistance ratio of apical to basolateral cell membrane, R_a/R_b, was 3.1 ± 0.3. The values of the specific membrane resistances R_a and R_b were calculated from the transepithelial resistance, the ratio of R_a

to R_b, and the effects of three different maneuvers on basolateral and apical membrane voltages. These three maneuvers included peritubular barium (1 mM), peritubular nystatin, and the addition of 8 mM glucose to the luminal perfusate. Calculations were made assuming that the initial effects of barium, nystatin, and glucose were restricted to the ipsilateral membrane. Utilizing these techniques, R_a was found to be 248 ± 68 $\Omega \cdot cm^2$ with the barium studies, 120 ± 59 $\Omega \cdot cm^2$ with the nystatin studies, and 227 ± 42 $\Omega \cdot cm^2$ with the glucose studies. The respective values of R_e were 70 ± 11, 76 ± 48, and 66 ± 13. Simultaneous measurement of the paracellular or transepithelial resistance with these three maneuvers was, respectively, 17 ± 5, 22 ± 1, and 15 ± 0.1.

The calculated values of R_a and R_e agree well with the luminal glucose and peritubular barium experiments; however, the values obtained with peritubular nystatin appear to be low, specifically with the apical cell membrane resistance measurement. The reason for this underestimate with the nystatin technique is unclear. The measurements do show, however, that the proximal tubule has a paracellular pathway resistance that is approximately 20 times more conductive than the cellular pathway. They also demonstrate that addition of glucose to perfusate or barium to the bath are good alternative methods for the measurement of cell membrane resistances.

The relatively new area of application of vesicle techniques to the study of adaptation of proximal tubule transport was first discussed by Hruska. By way of introduction Hruska outlined the transport processes that have been shown to retain adaptive function when vesicles are studied in vitro. With respect to brushborder membrane transport processes that retain adaptive function, sodium-hydrogen antiporter, sodium-dependent phosphate transport, and calcium transport all have been demonstrated to retain adaptive function. With respect to the basolateral cell membrane of proximal tubules, sodium-calcium exchange, Ca-Mg-ATPase, and Na-K-ATPase are transport processes that have been shown to retain adaptive function when studied in vitro. Hruska then concentrated on studies of sodium-dependent phosphate transport in the brushborder membrane vesicles. Studies of this transport process in brushborder membrane vesicles have demonstrated adaptation in response to in vivo changes in parathyroid hormone, growth hormone, phosphorus load, and vitamin D deficiency.

To help address the studies of adaptation with respect to understanding the mechanism, the sodium-dependent phosphate transport was characterized with respect to its sodium dependency, its kinetics, the ratio of sodium to phosphorus coupling, and the effects of pH on the transport. Subsequently, the effects of parathyroid hormone on this transport process were discussed, including hypothetical presentation of the mechanism of the parathyroid response and the likelihood that membrane phosphorylation was involved. Next, the effects of vitamin D were discussed, including various possible mechanisms such as the lipinomic effects of vitamin D and the genomic effects of vitamin D. Also presented was evidence for effects of annular lipid on phosphate transport.

Seifter then discussed the adaptation of the luminal cell membrane sodium-hydrogen antiporter. Three general areas were covered. First a listing of the physiologic functions of the sodium-hydrogen antiporter in proximal tubular acidification, sodium reabsorption, the regulation of intracellular pH, the regulation of cell volume, and in processes of cell growth and mitogenesis. These functions attest to the physiologic importance of the antiporter in proximal tubules.

Seifter then discussed the chronic rat models in which proximal tubule sodium-bicarbonate is thought to increase. These include models of renal ablation, acid-base disturbances, and potassium depletion. The response of proximal tubule brushborder membrane vesicle sodium-hydrogen exchange to these maneuvers was analyzed. Seifter presented data from his laboratory, in which the antiporter function was studied in vesicles harvested from animals with metabolic acidosis, metabolic alkalosis, respiratory acidosis, and potassium depletion; in animals ingesting high-protein diets; and in animals with a remnant kidney. The sodium-hydrogen antiporter activity was correlated with changes in the glomerular filtration rate, renal mass, and presumed intracellular pH. Chronic potassium depletion increased sodium-dependent changes in vesicle H^+ transport via an increase in V_{max}. Interestingly, metabolic alkalosis induced by furosemide, chloride depletion, and potassium bicarbonate feeding was associated with no change in brushborder vesicle sodium-dependent proton transport. Respiratory acidosis also produced no change in vesicle transport.

Metabolic acidosis in BB/W diabetic rats untreated with insulin was associated with increased brushborder vesicle sodium-hydrogen exchange that was normalized with insulin treatment of the animals, but was also normalized by sodium bicarbonate treatment of the animals (hyperglycemia persisted).

Finally, urinephrectomy was associated with increased sodium-hydrogen exchange in vesicles prepared from the remnant kidney when compared to control. High-protein (40%) diet increased sodium-hydrogen exchange even more in vesicles from the remnant kidney. There was a significant correlation between brushborder membrane vesicle sodium-hydrogen exchange and renal size as well as glomerular filtration in the remnant kidney model.

Transport Properties of the Pars Recta

James A. Schafer and Jack Work

Although often neglected in discussions of the function of the loop of Henle, the medullary portion of the pars recta or proximal straight tubule is the initial segment of the loop and should be considered when examining the transport events leading to the delivery of a relatively concentrated tubular fluid to the tip of the loop of Henle. In both superficial and juxtamedullary nephrons, the medullary region of the proximal straight tubule extends from the corticomedullary junction to the border of the outer and inner stripes of the outer medulla and consists exclusively of the S_3 (or P_3) cell type [1, 2]. Whereas the medullary segment is a relatively straight extension of the superficial proximal straight tubule from the medullary ray, that of the juxtamedullary nephron extends from the late convoluted tubule near the corticomedullary junction outside of the medullary rays and is more tortuous than its superficial counterpart [1].

The S_3 segment of the proximal tubule can be examined directly only by using the technique of isolated tubule perfusion; however, relatively few studies have been conducted with this segment, probably because of its relatively short length and the greater difficulty of dissection compared with the superficial S_2 segment. Nevertheless, it is known that the rate of volume absorption in this segment is comparable to that in the S_2 segment, at least when bathed in isosmotic media resembling rabbit serum [3–5]. On the other hand, the spontaneous lumen-negative transepithelial voltage is greater than in the corresponding S_2 segment, which may be indicative of a lower shunt conductivity [3, 4]. The only other reports directly related to the S_3 segment concern the relative ion selectivity of the shunt pathway [5], bicarbonate transport [6], and para-aminohippurate (PAH) secretion [7]. With regard to the latter, the S_3 segment has a lower PAH secretory rate than does S_2, and thus resembles the early convoluted segment more closely.

This presentation considers the potential role of the medullary portion

This manuscript was presented as part of a Symposium on *Transport Mechanisms in Henle's Loop.*

of superficial and juxtamedullary proximal straight tubules in the postulated medullary recycling of potassium and the relation of this process to volume absorption in the outer medulla. Jamison et al [8] and Battilana [9] observed that the potassium load delivered to the tip of the loop of Henle of juxtamedullary nephrons in the rat was comparable to the filtered load of potassium in normal animals and that it was approximately two times greater than the filtered load in potassium-loaded animals. On the other hand, in potassium-depleted animals, only 30 to 40% of the filtered load was delivered to the tip of the loop, that is, approximately the amount expected to be delivered from the cortical portion of the proximal nephron [10]. Based on further evidence that furosemide and amiloride decreased delivery to the tip of the loop [11] and the fact that the load to the tip of the loop showed a direct correlation with the rate of potassium excretion [9], Jamison et al [8], Battilana et al [9], Dobyan, Lacy, and Jamison [10], Dobyan et al [11], Sufit and Jamison [12], along with Jamison and ourselves [13] proposed that potassium may be recycled within the medulla in a manner similar to urea. However, this hypothesis requires that potassium be secreted into the descending limb of the loop of Henle. As shown by Jamison et al [8], given previously measured values of the potassium permeability of the descending limb [14], the mechanism of entry may be passive in the descending limb of the loop of Henle if the potassium concentration in the medullary interstitium is sufficiently higher than that in the lumen. The results from our laboratory [3], which are reviewed below, as well as those of Wasserstein and Agus [15], indicate that the proximal straight tubule is capable of net active potassium secretion as had been previously suggested by the results of Grantham, Qualizza, and Irwin [16]. However, the magnitude of this secretion is negligible in comparison with the rate of potassium delivery observed at the tip of the loop of Henle in the rat. Work, Troutman, and Schafer [3] also noted that the permeability of the juxtamedullary pars recta to potassium was significantly higher than that of the early or late regions of the superficial pars recta. This higher permeability would allow significant passive potassium secretion if there was an elevated potassium concentration in the medullary interstitium of the outer stripe. However, the magnitude of the inward potassium gradient would also depend on the extent of osmotic water abstraction in the same region. These interrelated processes are considered below.

Methods

The segments of interest were dissected from rabbit kidney slices. Superficial S_3 segments were identified as the medullary portion of proximal straight tubules that extended to the cortical surface. Juxtamedullary segments were identified by their attachment to a long thin descending limb. (In this context, we refer to long-looped nephrons as "juxtamedullary," while recognizing that most actually derive from midcortical nephrons [2].) Both types of segments averaged 1.0 mm in length before attachment to the perfusion pipets. All tubules were studied at 38°C. The artificial bathing solution resembled rabbit serum, whereas the perfusate was essentially an ultrafiltrate of the bathing solution. Both perfusate and bath had an osmolality of 290 mOsm/ kg H_2O.

Unidirectional fluxes of both potassium 42 and rubidium 86 were measured in both the lumen-to-bath ($J^{l\text{-}b}$) and bath-to-lumen ($J^{b\text{-}l}$) directions using standard methods [3]. We confirmed that both potassium-42 and rubidium-86 fluxes were not statistically different under identical conditions in the same segment, and both were equally effective in supporting volume absorption [3], as expected from their similar renal clearances observed in other studies [17, 18]. Flux coefficients (or apparent permeabilities) were calculated from these unidirectional fluxes as the quotient of the flux divided by the potassium or rubidium concentration on the side of the epithelium containing the isotope, or calculated from the slope of the linear regression line relating the measured flux to concentration. These flux coefficients were expressed in units of pmoles $\cdot$ min^{-1} $\cdot$ mm^{-1} $\cdot$ mM^{-1} for convenience in other calculations, but were also converted to the more usual permeability units of micrometers per second by division by πd (using the apparent inside diameter of the tubule) and conversion of units.

Results and Discussion

Unidirectional lumen-to-bath ($J^{l\text{-}b}$) fluxes of both isotopes were measured in early superficial and juxtamedullary proximal straight tubules with 5 mM of either potassium or rubidium in both the perfusate and the bathing solution; and no significant difference was found between the fluxes as measured by the two isotopes. Both isotopes were also used to measure bath-to-lumen ($J^{b\text{-}l}$) fluxes in the juxtamedullary segment, and again there was no significant difference. Consequently, data from both isotopes were pooled to obtain the unidirectional flux estimates presented in Figure 1. It can be seen from the figure that both $J^{l\text{-}b}$ and $J^{b\text{-}l}$ were higher in the juxtamedullary than in the superficial S_3 segments ($P < 0.001$). The mean $J^{l\text{-}b}$ in S_2 segments from the superficial proximal straight tubule was slightly higher than that in the S_3 segment ($P < 0.025$), but $J^{b\text{-}l}$ fluxes were identical, indicating that there were no substantial differences in potassium transport in the cortical and medullary regions of the superficial proximal tubule (data not shown; see [3]).

As shown in Figure 1, $J^{b\text{-}l}$ significantly exceeded $J^{l\text{-}b}$ in the superficial S_3 segment ($P < 0.001$). The unpaired difference between the two unidirectional fluxes gave a net secretion rate of 3.18 $\pm$ 0.83 pmoles $\cdot$ min^{-1} $\cdot$ mm^{-1}, which was significantly different from zero ($P < 0.001$). The same flux asymmetry was observed in the juxtamedullary segment, indicating a net secretory flux of 4.8 $\pm$ 2.19 pmoles $\cdot$ min^{-1} $\cdot$ mm^{-1} ($P < 0.025$). In both segments, the inequality in unidirectional fluxes indicated active secretion, since the transepithelial voltage was far from sufficient to account for the observed flux ratio, and any flux resulting from solvent drag would have opposed the secretory flux. It might seem reasonable that the secretory flux was occur-

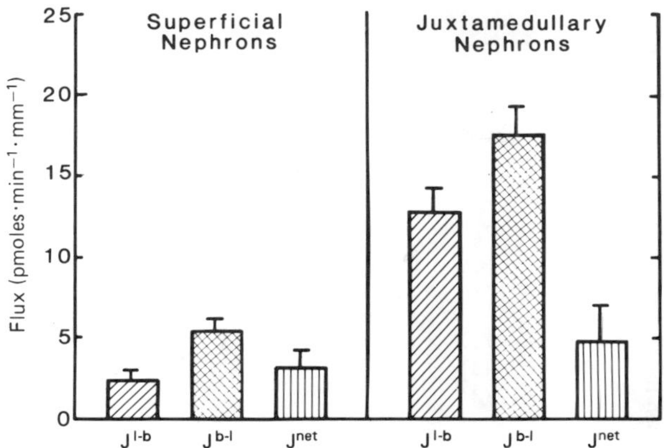

Fig. 1. Unidirectional fluxes of potassium 42 and rubidium 86 in isolated medullary proximal straight tubules from superficial and juxtamedullary nephrons. Lumen-to-bath ($J^{l\text{-}b}$) and bath-to-lumen ($J^{b\text{-}l}$) fluxes were measured in separate groups of tubules, and results using both isotopes were combined. Net fluxes were computed as the unpaired difference in the unidirectional fluxes. SEMs are indicated.

ring as a consequence of active potassium transport across the basolateral membranes by the Na-K-ATPase activity, with passive leak from the cell into the lumen. If this were the case, then we would have expected that ouabain would abolish the secretory flux. However, in the presence of 0.1 mM ouabain, there was no significant change in any fluxes measured in either segment.

Wasserstein and Agus [15] have recently confirmed the existence of net potassium secretion in both the S_2 and S_3 regions of superficial nephrons and in the juxtamedullary proximal straight tubule by the direct measurement of net fluxes using electron microprobe methodology. Their results agree with ours in the magnitude of the active secretory flux (their values were in the range of 1.4 to 2.8 pmoles · min^{-1} · mm^{-1}); however, in their experiments either ouabain in the bathing solution or, surprisingly, 1 mM amiloride in the luminal perfusate was found to eliminate the net secretion. The difference between the studies of Wasserstein and Agus [15] and ours [3] with regard to the effect of ouabain is unexplained, except that in our studies it may have been difficult to see a small change in the rather large unidirectional fluxes in the presence of the inhibitor.

In other experiments we measured unidirectional rubidium-86 fluxes at concentrations of 2, 5, and 10 mM. In all cases for both unidirectional fluxes, and in the absence and presence of ouabain, there was a linear relationship between flux and concentration. The results for $J^{b\text{-}l}$ in the juxtamedullary straight tubule are shown in Figure 2. The results reinforce the lack of any effect of ouabain on $J^{b\text{-}l}$ and also indicate the relatively high rubidium-86 permeability of this segment. The linearity of the flux also suggests that the flux is occurring by a nonsaturable pathway, although a negative finding

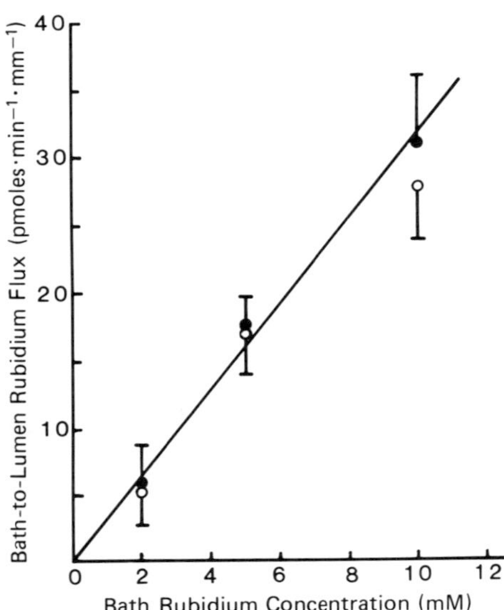

Fig. 2. Concentration dependence of bath-to-lumen rubidium-86 fluxes ($J^{b\text{-}l}$) in juxtamedullary proximal straight tubules in the presence (○) and absence (●) of 0.1 mM ouabain in the bathing solution. The *line* is drawn by linear regression of the control data. SEM are indicated.

in this regard cannot be regarded as proof, since saturation might have occurred if it had been possible to use yet higher rubidium concentrations without damage to the epithelium. The fact that ouabain had no effect on the fluxes also suggests that rubidium is moving primarily by a paracellular route. Because ouabain would be expected to decrease intracellular potassium and to depolarize the cells, it would be expected to alter transcellular flux even if the flux were occurring by purely passive mechanisms. The flux coefficient estimated from the slope of the line in Figure 2 was 3.28 ± 0.28 pmoles $\cdot$ min^{-1} $\cdot$ mm^{-1} $\cdot$ mM^{-1}, which corresponds to an apparent permeability of 0.68 μm/sec. For comparison, the flux coefficients for the superficial straight segments are listed in Table 1. The considerably higher apparent permeability of the juxtamedullary segments to potassium may be a reflection of their relatively high cation selectivity. The sodium-to-chloride permeability

Table 1. Comparison of apparent potassium permeability coefficients in proximal straight tubules[a]

	Potassium permeability	
Segment	pmoles $\cdot$ min^{-1} $\cdot$ mm^{-1}	μm/sec
Superficial S$_2$	0.70 ± 0.04	0.14 ± 0.02
Superficial S$_3$	0.45 ± 0.11	0.10 ± 0.02
Juxtamedullary S$_3$	2.56 ± 0.27[b]	0.52 ± 0.07[b]

[a] Flux coefficients were calculated from average $J^{l\text{-}b}$ fluxes with 5 mM ^{42}K$^+$ or ^{86}Rb$^+$ present in the lumen and assuming a linear dependence of flux on concentration with a zero intercept.

[b] Significantly greater than either superficial segment, $P < 0.001$.

ratio in the juxtamedullary straight segment was measured to be in excess of 2.0 [5], whereas the same ratio in early and late superficial segments was 0.3 to 0.5 [19].

The important question raised by these findings is whether the potassium transport properties, particularly of the juxtamedullary proximal straight tubule, could explain the high rate of potassium delivery to the tip of the loop of Henle. From the magnitude of the secretory fluxes observed by ourselves [3] and Wasserstein and Agus [15], it appears that an active potassium secretion in the medullary proximal straight tubule could contribute a potassium mass flow equivalent to, at most, 10% of the filtered load, which would explain only a minor fraction of the load observed at the tip of the loop. On the other hand, it is quite possible that the higher permeability of the juxtamedullary segment would favor a significant passive potassium secretion if there were a favorable electrical and concentration gradient for diffusion in this direction. In the juxtamedullary proximal straight tubule, the transepithelial voltage is normally lumen-negative, favoring potassium secretion. Unfortunately, there are no direct measurements of its concentration in the outer medulla; however, given the measured values of potassium in vasa recta blood in the papilla obtained by micropuncture [8, 20] and from electron microprobe analysis [21], it is likely that there is at least a 40-mM potassium gradient from the corticomedullary junction to the tip of the loop of Henle. To obtain an index of the importance of an elevated medullary interstitial potassium concentration on potassium secretion in the medullary regions of the proximal straight tubule, we [3] assumed that the potassium concentration in the outer stripe of the medulla rises linearly from 5 to 10 mM at the junction with the inner stripe. Assuming a constant volume absorption rate of 0.5 nl/min, a constant transepithelial voltage equivalent to that measured in each segment, the active secretion rates reported above, and the permeabilities reported in Table 1, we have modeled the change in potassium mass flow along the 1.0-mm length of both the superficial and juxtamedullary proximal straight tubule as shown in Figure 3 (see [3]). It can be seen that, owing to its higher permeability, there is significantly greater potassium secretion into the juxtamedullary segment, such that the load delivered to the descending limb of the loop of Henle is augmented by about 40% (20%, relative to the original filtered load of potassium [3, 13]). On the other hand, diffusional entry contributes significantly less to potassium secretion in the superficial proximal straight tubule owing to its considerably lower permeability. In the presence of active secretion alone, with no elevation in medullary potassium concentration (shown by the dashed line in Fig. 3), the augmentation of a potassium mass flow would be insignificant.

The calculations above, in their simplicity, assume that the volume absorption from the medullary proximal straight tubules is equivalent to that in the cortex where the interstitium is isosmotic to plasma. However, cryoscopic studies of the total solute content of the outer medulla indicate that it may be hyperosmotic to plasma and thus to the tubular fluid that enters it [22, 23]. Although the increase in osmolality occurs exponentially in the inner medulla [22, 23], the data suggest that the outer medulla may be slightly

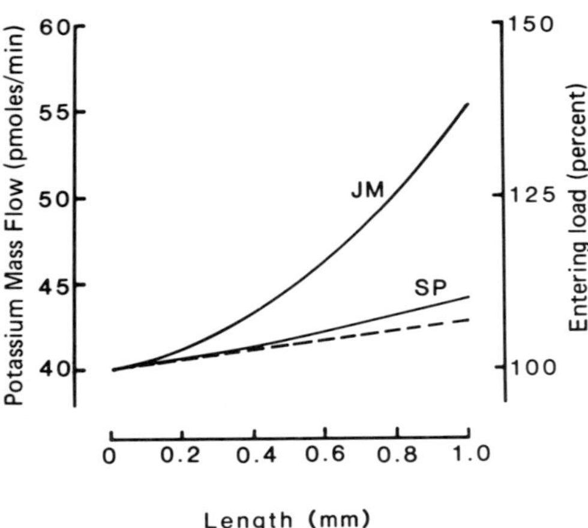

Fig. 3. Theoretical predictions of the effect of potassium permeability on the luminal potassium flow in superficial (*SP*) and juxtamedullary (*JM*) proximal straight tubules. The *solid lines* show the results predicted assuming that the potassium concentration of the interstitium of the outer stripe rises from 5 to 10 mM. The *dashed line* shows the predicted load with no transepithelial potassium concentration gradient and only active net potassium transport.

hyperosmotic to plasma, particularly after prolonged antidiuretic hormone administration [23]. In addition, the outer medullary sodium concentration is also shown to be slightly elevated [25]. Consequently, a small osmotic gradient could favor water abstraction from the medullary regions of the proximal straight tubule just as it does from the descending thin limb. This would result in a rise in the luminal potassium concentration and leave a less favorable gradient for passive potassium entry. To examine the effect of a hyperosmotic outer medullary interstitium on tubular fluid osmolality, we considered a "worst case" situation in which we assumed that interstitial osmolality increases by 2-fold (from 290 to 580 mOsm/kg H_2O) in the outer stripe of the outer medulla. We have modeled the change in tubular fluid osmolality along the length of the medullary proximal straight tubule assuming water permeabilities from 150 μm/sec to the minimum value measured in the superficial S_2 segment (2000 μm/sec [25]). It can be seen from the results presented in Figure 4 that the luminal osmolality nearly follows the interstitial osmolality, especially at the higher water permeability. In other words, the osmotic water permeability of the proximal straight tubule may be sufficiently high that the tubular fluid is always nearly in osmotic equilibrium with the interstitium. If this were the case, then there would be negligible passive potassium secretion. On the other hand, if the potassium concentration in the interstitium were elevated to a greater extent than the osmolality, then a passive potassium secretion would be favored. The answer to this question can only be resolved by a knowledge of the relation of the potassium concentration in the interstitium of the outer stripe to the osmolality.

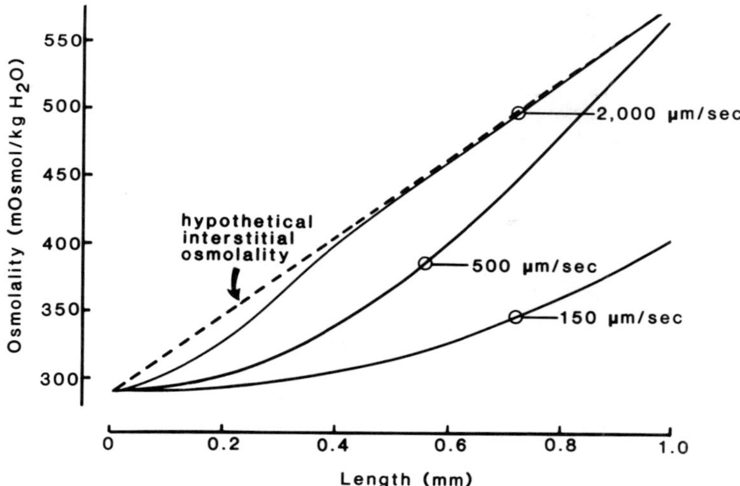

Fig. 4. Theoretical predictions of the osmotic equilibration of proximal fluid with medullary interstitial osmolality in the outer stripe. The *dashed line* indicates a hypothetical increase in the outer stripe interstitial osmolality from 290 to 580 mOsm/kg H_2O. The *solid lines* give the predicted rise in luminal osmolality assuming three different osmotic water permeabilities.

In summary, the results show that both superficial and juxtamedullary proximal straight tubules exhibit net active potassium secretion, but the relatively small magnitude of this secretion is unlikely to be a significant contributor to the large potassium delivery to the tip of the loop of Henle in juxtamedullary nephrons. On the other hand, the much higher passive potassium permeability of the juxtamedullary segment would favor significant passive secretion if there were a sufficient potassium concentration in the surrounding medullary interstitium relative to that in the lumen after osmotic equilibration. Obviously, the answers to these questions must await measurements of potassium concentrations in the tubular fluid of medullary proximal straight tubules and the surrounding interstitium. Given the considerable recent successes with electron microprobe analysis of thin sections, such measurements may soon be possible.

References

1. JAMISON RL, KRIZ W: *Urinary Concentrating Mechanism: Structure and Function.* New York, Oxford University Press, 1982, pp 113–132
2. KAISSLING B, KRIZ W: *Structural Analysis of the Rabbit Kidney.* Berlin, New York, Springer-Verlag, 1979, pp 13–59
3. WORK J, TROUTMAN SL, SCHAFER JA: Transport of potassium in the rabbit pars recta. *Am J Physiol* 242:F226–F237, 1982

4. BARFUSS DW, SCHAFER JA: Differences in active and passive glucose transport along the proximal nephron. *Am J Physiol* 240:F322–F332, 1981
5. KAWAMURA S, IMAI M, SELDIN DW, KOKKO JP: Characteristics of salt and water transport in superficial and juxtamedullary straight segments of proximal tubules. *J Clin Invest* 55:1269–1277, 1975
6. WARNOCK DG, BURG MB: Urinary acidification: CO_2 transport by the rabbit proximal straight tubule. *Am J Physiol* 232:F20–F25, 1977
7. WOODHALL PB, TISHER CC, SIMONTON CA, ROBINSON RR: Relationship between para-aminohippurate secretion and cellular morphology in rabbit proximal tubules. *J Clin Invest* 61:1320–1329, 1978
8. JAMISON RL, LACY FB, PENNELL JP, SANJANA VM: Potassium secretion by the descending limb of pars recta of juxtamedullary nephron in vivo. *Kidney Int* 9:323–332, 1976
9. BATTILANA CA, DOBYAN DC, LACY FB, BHATTACHARYA J, JOHNSTON PA, JAMISON RL: The effect of chronic potassium loading on potassium secretion by the pars recta or descending limb of the juxtamedullary nephron in the rat. *J Clin Invest* 62:1093–1103, 1978
10. DOBYAN DC, LACY FB, JAMISON RL: Suppression of potassium-recycling in the renal medulla by short-term potassium deprivation. *Kidney Int* 16:704–709, 1979
11. DOBYAN DC, ARRASCUE JF, DE ROUFFIGNAC C, ROINEL N, JAMISON RL: Effect of furosemide on sodium and potassium flow at the end of the juxtamedullary descending limb in *Psammomys obesus*. *Renal Physiol* 5:105–114, 1982
12. SUFIT CR, JAMISON RL: Effect of acute potassium load on reabsorption in Henle's loop in the rat. *Am J Physiol* 245:F569–F576, 1983
13. JAMISON RL, WORK JW, SCHAFER JA: New pathways for potassium transport in the kidney. *Am J Physiol* 242:F297–F312, 1982
14. ROCHA AS, KOKKO JP: Membrane characteristics regulating potassium transport out of the isolated perfused descending limb of Henle. *Kidney Int* 4:326–330, 1973
15. WASSERSTEIN AG, AGUS ZS: Potassium secretion in the rabbit proximal straight tubule. *Am J Physiol* 245:F167–F174, 1983
16. GRANTHAM JJ, QUALIZZA PB, IRWIN RL: Net fluid secretion in proximal straight renal tubules in vitro: Role of PAH. *Am J Physiol* 226:191–197, 1974
17. KUNIN AS, DEARBORN EH, BURROWS BA, RELMAN AS: Comparison of renal excretion of rubidium and potassium. *Am J Physiol* 197:1297–1302, 1959
18. CORTNEY MA, MOREAU GP: Microinjections of [86]Rb: A study of reduced renal potassium absorption in the rat. *Am J Physiol* 225:1529–1534, 1973
19. SCHAFER JA, TROUTMAN SL, ANDREOLI TE: Volume reabsorption, transepithelial potential differences, and ionic permeability properties in mammalian superficial proximal straight tubules. *J Gen Physiol* 64:582–607, 1974
20. JOHNSTON PA, BATTILANA CA, LACY FB, JAMISON RL: Evidence for a concentration gradient favoring outward movement of sodium from the thin loop of Henle. *J Clin Invest* 59:234–240, 1977
21. BULGER RE, BEEUWKES R III, SAUBERMANN AJ: Application of scanning electron microscopy to analysis of frozen-hydrated sections: III. Elemental content of cells in the rat renal papillary tip. *J Cell Biol* 88:274–280, 1981
22. WIRZ H, HARGITAY B, KUHN W: Lokalisation des Konzentrierungsprozesses in der Niere durch direkte Kryoscopie. *Helv Physiol Pharmacol* 9:196–207, 1951
23. HAI MA, THOMAS S: The time-course of changes in renal tissue composition during lysine vasopressin infusion in the rat. *Pflügers Arch* 310:297–319, 1969
24. KOEPSELL H, NICHOLSON WAP, KRIZ W, HÖHLING HJ: Measurements of expo-

nential gradients of sodium and chlorine in the rat kidney medulla using electron microprobe. *Pflügers Arch* 350:167–184, 1974
25. SCHAFER JA, PATLAK CS, TROUTMAN SL, ANDREOLI TE: Volume absorption in the pars recta: II. Hydraulic conductivity coefficient. *Am J Physiol* 234:F340–F348, 1978

Function of the Thin Limb of Henle's Loop

Masashi Imai, Matuhiko Hayashi, Masasuke Araki, and Kaoru Tabei

It has been well established that the renal medulla plays a crucial role in the mechanisms of formation of concentrated urine [1]. The loop of Henle is assumed to play an integral part in the countercurrent multiplication system by generating a steep osmotic gradient of the renal medullary interstitium. The function of the thick ascending limb of Henle's loop has been settled [2]. This segment has characteristics of the diluting segment, in which sodium chloride is actively transported across the water-impermeable epithelia. On the other hand, the function of the thin limbs of Henle's loop is still in considerable dispute with many respects.

For example, it has not been established whether an active ion transport mechanism is playing an important part in the operation of the single effect for the countercurrent multiplier in the thin ascending limb of Henle's loop. Although it is well known that the function of the descending limb of Henle's loop is distinct from that of the thin ascending limb, there has been a considerable dispute as to whether the osmotic equilibration of the luminal fluid along this segment occurs mainly by the abstraction of water or the addition of solutes. These controversial issues might be, at least in part, accounted for by species differences. In addition, it is possible that internephron heterogeneity also contributes to the apparently discrepant results, since micropuncture techniques can approach only the long-loop nephron—whereas the in vitro microperfusion techniques can examine only upper portions of the thin-loop segments.

To solve these problems, it is necessary to compare function of the thin-loop segments between different nephrons, as well as among different mammalian species, by using the same technique. The purpose of this communication is to review the data on the function of thin-loop segments that are obtained via the technique of in vitro microperfusion. The topics will focus mainly on interspecies differences and on internephron heterogeneity of the thin

---

This manuscript was presented as part of a Symposium on *Transport Mechanisms in Henle's Loop.*

limbs of Henle's loop. Physiologic significance of nephron heterogeneity will be briefly discussed with respect to the mechanisms of the formation of concentrated urine.

Morphologic Heterogeneity

Heterogeneity of Epithelia and Tight Junctions

Anatomic studies have elucidated that the morphology of epithelia composing the thin limbs of Henle's loop are heterogeneous between the short- and long-loop nephron (internephron heterogeneity), as well as within the same nephron (intranephron heterogeneity). For example, in the rat, the descending

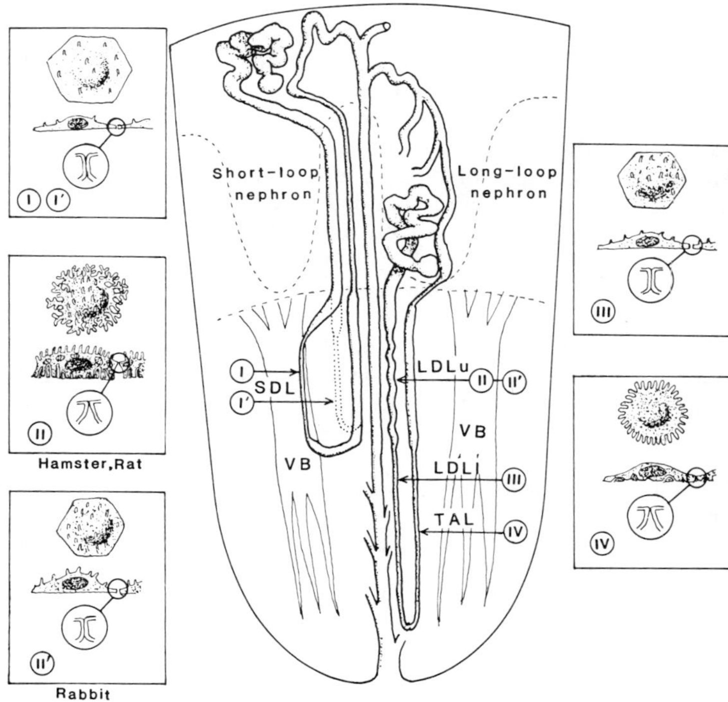

Fig. 1. Inter- and intranephron heterogeneity and species difference of the thin limbs of Henle's loop. The nephron architecture or epithelium marked by I′ and II′ are typical for rabbits. Figures in *circles* illustrate the morphology of tight junctions. Abbreviations: *SDL,* short descending limb (descending limb of the short-loop nephron); *LDL1,* lower portion of long descending limb (descending limb of long-loop nephron); *LDLu,* upper portion of the long descending limb; *VB,* vascular bundle; *TAL,* thin ascending limb.

limb of Henle's loop of the short-loop nephron (SDL) consists of relatively simple, flat epithelia with noninterdigitated intercellular junctions. This type of epithelia was named type I cells by Dietrich [3]. Although Schwartz and Venkatachalam [4] used different nomenclature, we selected the nomenclature of the former in this chapter to avoid confusion. In marked contrast, the upper portion of the descending limbs of the long-loop nephron (LDLu) consists of epithelium with complicated infolding of the basolateral membranes, with extensive interdigitation with neighboring cells, called type II cells. This type of epithelium has abundant microvilli at the luminal membrane; it contains numerous mitochondria in the cytoplasm. These differences are schematically illustrated in Figure 1.

In addition to the differences in the appearance of epithelium, morphology of the tight junction also is quite different between these cell types (5–8). The tight junction of the SDL has characteristics of the tight-junction, which consists of deep junctions with several ramified junctional strands as revealed by the freeze-fracture technique (Table 1). In contrast, the tight junction of the LDLu is very shallow, and it usually contains only one simple junctional strand.

Morphology of the lower portion of the descending limbs of Henle's loop of the long-loop nephron (LDL1) is very similar to that of the SDL, although this is called a type III cell. Thus, morphologic intranephron heterogeneity exists along the descending limbs of the LDL1. The thin ascending limb of Henle's loop consists of type IV epithelium, which is characterized by an absence of microvilli on the luminal membrane, but an abundance of lateral cell processes. The tight junctions are also shallow. In this regard, type IV epithelium resembles type II epithelium. However, the former is different from the latter in that cells generally are flat and contain relatively few organelles.

These unique differences in morphology of epithelia and tight junctions have been observed in many mammalian species, including the rat [3–5], mouse [6], *Psammomys* [7, 8], *Meriones* [9], *Perognathus penicellatus* [10],

Table 1. Heterogeneity and species difference of the tight junction of the thin-loop segments[a]

	Apical-basal depth, (nm)			Number of junctional strands	
	Rat	Rabbit	Hamster	Rat	Rabbit
SDL	46.6 ± 31.1(5)	142.5 ± 56.8(5)	160 ± 100(11)	2.3 ± 1.0(5) 3.8 ± 0.09(14)	5.9 ± 1.5(5)
LDLu	18.7 ± 7.6(5)	98.8 ± 48.8(5)	52 ± 24(11)	1.5 ± 0.5(5) 1.0 ± 0.0(14)	5.2 ± 1.0(5)
LDL1	39.2 ± 20.2(5)	132.1 ± 65.2(5)	82 ± 22(11)	4.2 ± 1.6(5) 3.1 ± 0.14(14)	3.1 ± 1.3(5)
TAL	23.9 ± 17.7(5)	27.6 ± 14.8(5)	25 ± 2(11)	2.1 ± 0.9(5) 1.3 ± 0.09(14)	1.6 ± 0.7(5)

Abbreviations: SDL, short descending limb; LDLu, upper portion of long descending limb; LDL1, lower portion of long descending limb; TAL, thin ascending limb.

[a] Numbers in parentheses indicate references cited. Values are means ± SD.

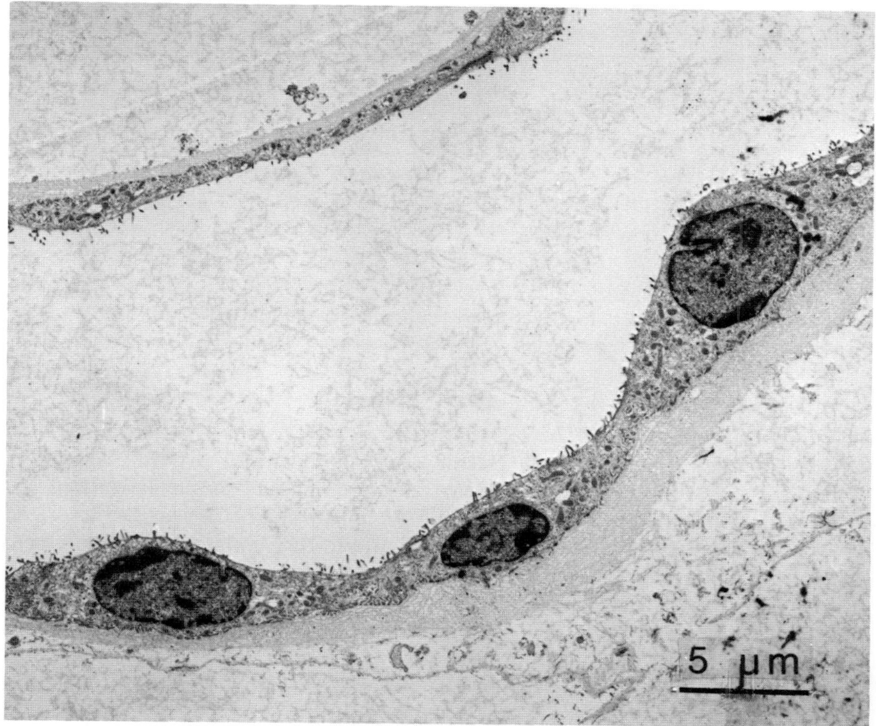

Fig. 2. Electron-microscopic feature of hamster LDLu. The isolated tubule during perfusion was fixed with 2% glutaraldehyde in 0.1 M cacodylate buffer (pH 7.4).

and hamster [11]. Although the thin limbs of hamster kidney have similar characteristics, some tubules of the LDLu consist of epithelia that are taller than those of the usual type II cells (Fig. 2). They have a more elaborate mode of cellular interdigitation. This type of epithelium is called type IIa. On the other hand, in the rabbit, the LDLu consists of epithelia with different morphology. Their morphology is very similar to that of epithelia in the LDL1; the epithelia are flat and noninterdigitated, containing sparse cell organelles. Thus, interspecies difference exists in the morphology of epithelia of the descending limb.

Heterogeneity of Membrane Particles

Freeze-fracture or freeze-replica techniques can visualize intramembrane particles that are assumed to represent functional proteins in the cell membrane. Distribution of membrane particles in the thin limbs of Henle's loop has been examined in the rabbit [12] and the rat [13, 14]. Table 2 summarizes the data obtained in the rabbit. It should be noted that both luminal and

Table 2. Numbers of intramembrane particles in the rabbit thin-loop segments[a]

	Luminal		Basolateral	
	PF	EF	PF	EF
SDL	396 ± 27(14)	95 ± 1.6(14)	407 ± 38(14)	154 ± 20(14)
LDLu	7213 ± 364(14)	487 ± 68(14)	6343 ± 364(14)	363 ± 34(14)
	4009 ± 55(13)	765 ± 88(13)	3921 ± 72(13)	581 ± 30(13)
LDL1	839 ± 81(14)	109 ± 14(14)	768 ± 51(14)	152 ± 22(14)
TAL	631 ± 38(14)	206 ± 38(14)	1662 ± 71(14)	405 ± 43(14)
	1006 ± 44(13)	44 ± 5(13)	1542 ± 48(13)	87 ± 11(13)

Abbreviations: PF, P face; EF, E face. Other abbreviations are the same as in Table 1.

[a] Numbers in parentheses indicate references cited. Values are means ± SD (for [14]) and means ± SEM (for [13]).

basolateral membranes of the LDLu are characterized by the extremely high density of membrane particles. Basolateral membrane of the thin ascending limbs are also rich in membrane particles, but not as much as that of the LDLu. In contrast, membranes of the SDL and the LDL1 are characterized by scarce membrane particles. Although quantitative data were not given, the similar heterogeneity of distribution of membrane particles was observed in the rabbit [12]. It is interesting to note that membranes of the rabbit LDLu are also rich in particles, although the structure of epithelium and the morphology of the tight junctions are different from those of the rat, as discussed previously. This suggests that the function of individual membranes of the LDLu is similar among different species.

Histotopographic Heterogeneity

In addition to these structural distinctions of epithelia, histotopographic distinctions also exist between the long- and the short-loop nephrons [1, 15]. In most species, the descending limbs of the long-loop nephrons are distributed in the regions that are apart from the vascular bundles. The descending limbs appear to be separated from the vascular bundles by the interposed, thick ascending limbs. On the other hand, the pattern of distribution of the SDL is different among species; it can be classified roughly into two groups, depending on the relation of the descending limbs with vascular bundles.

The first group consists of simple vascular bundles that do not contain any thin-loop segments. The descending limbs are distributed around the vascular bundles and do not make any direct contact with the vasa recta. This type of architectural organization has been found in the golden hamster, guinea pig, rabbit, prairie dog, opossum, muskrat, bat, cat, dog, pig, rhesus monkey, and humans [1].

The second group consists of complex vascular bundles that include the SDL. This type of architectural arrangement could allow countercurrent exchange not only between the descending and the ascending vasa recta, but also between the ascending vasa recta and the descending limbs. The vascular bundles tend to fuse to form larger bundles. The extent of the fusion of vascular bundles varies among species. In *Psammomys* and *Jerboa,* several vascular bundles fuse to form giant bundles, whereas in the mouse and *Meriones* (and to a certain extent in the rat), a couple of bundles tend to fuse together.

These architectural and species differences, along with structural differences in epithelia, provide a basis for the hypothesis that the function of the thin limbs of Henle's loop may be heterogeneous between nephrons and among species.

Functional Heterogeneity

Function of the Descending Limbs of Henle's Loop

Micropuncture studies in the renal papilla of rats, hamsters, and *Psammomys* have demonstrated that fluid in the descending limbs is concentrated as it flows down into the renal papilla. However, there is controversy as to whether the fluid in the descending limbs is concentrated mainly by abstraction water or by addition of solutes into the tubular lumen.

The studies of Gottschalk et al in the hamster [16] suggested that the fluid in the descending limbs is equilibrated with that of the interstitium mainly by abstraction of water. The TF/P inulin ratio at the tip of the thin loop ranged from 6 to 17, with a mean of 11. Marsh [17] performed a very difficult study by inserting two micropipettes into the same descending limb at the bend and 1 mm proximal to the bend of the loop. He found that at the terminal portion of the descending limbs, the TF/P ratios for inulin, osmolality, and sodium all increased by approximately 10%, which supports the view that osmotic equilibration occurs mainly by abstraction of water. However, at the same time, he showed unequivocal evidence that a certain amount of urea is added to the descending limbs. Sakai, Tadokoro, and Teraoka [18] performed in vivo microperfusion of the thin loop of the hamster; they found that the descending limbs are highly permeable to water as well as to sodium.

By using Brattleboro strain rats, Pennel, Lacy, and Jamison [19] demonstrated that 33 to 40% of the increase in osmolality of descending limb fluid in vivo is attributed to solute entry; the rest is attributed to water removal. By in vitro microperfusion of papillary slices of rat kidney, Morgan and Berliner [20] reported that the descending limbs are highly permeable to water. However, they also showed the data that suggests this segment is highly permeable to urea.

Microperfusion studies of the descending limb of *Psammomys obesus* performed by de Rouffignac et al [21, 22] demonstrated that 85% of the increase in osmolality of the descending limb fluid is due to the addition of sodium and that 15% is due to abstraction of water. By using in vitro microperfusion of isolated rabbit renal tubules, Kokko [23, 24] reported that the descending limbs are highly permeable to water, but less permeable to sodium and to urea. While the results of these studies were initially questioned [25], they have been confirmed by the recent studies of Miwa and Imai [26].

The data obtained from various mammalian species strongly suggest that there are species differences in the membrane characteristics of the descending limb. On the basis of morphologic heterogeneity, it is reasonable to assume that internephron heterogeneity also exists in the function of the descending limb. Recently, we have succeeded in perfusing the upper portion of the LDLu as well as the SDL isolated from kidneys of various mammals, including rabbits, rats, and hamsters [27].

The LDLu of rats and hamsters was easily identified by its large diameter, thickness of the cells, and tortuous appearance running through the outer medulla. The SDL was identified as the thinnest straight segments running in the outer medulla. Initially, we compared membrane characteristics of these two different segments that were obtained from hamster kidneys. Permeability properties of these segments are summarized in Table 3. Although both segments were highly permeable to water, the LDLu was more permeable to sodium and chloride, whereas the SDL was more permeable to urea. This would suggest that significant amounts of sodium can enter into the LDLu if the diffusional gradients are favorable. To estimate the contribution of solute entry for the increase in osmolality along the LDLu, we measured the reflection coefficient of the LDLu for sodium chloride (NaCl) as well as for urea. The reflection coefficient for NaCl was 0.83, whereas for urea, it was not different from unity. This would indicate that significant amounts of NaCl can enter into the LDLu in the presence of transepithelial concentration gradient.

Next, we compared permeability properties of the descending limb among rabbits, hamsters, and rats by measuring transepithelial voltage (V) under conditions in which osmolality or ionic composition of the bathing fluid was varied. Table 4 summarizes the permeability for sodium and potassium in relation to chloride calculated from the diffusion potential generated when ionic composition of the bathing fluid was varied. It is clear that the LDLu of both hamsters and rats are highly permeable to sodium as well as to potassium. In marked contrast, the segments of the SDL of both species are less permeable to sodium and potassium. These observations clearly indicate that internephron heterogeneity exists in the descending limb of these

Table 3. Permeability properties of the thin-loop segments of the hamster[a]

	Lp	Klb, $(10^{-7}$ cm^2 s$^{-1})$		
	$(10^{-8}$ cm^2 atm^{-1} s$^{-1})$	^{22}Na	^{36}Cl	^{14}C-urea
SDL	260.0	2.8	0.9	5.5
LDLu	139.0	41.0	3.8	1.4
TAL	1.3	55.0	123.1	11.6

Abbreviations: Lp, osmotic water permeability; Klb, flux coefficient from bath to lumen. Other abbreviations are the same as in Table 1.
[a] Data are from [34].

Table 4. Species difference of permeability of the descending limbs for sodium relative to chloride (P_{Na}/P_{Cl})

	SDL	LDLu
Rabbit	0.83	1.08
Rat	0.67	7.28
Hamster	0.75	5.55

Abbreviations are the same as in Table 1.

species. On the other hand, internephron heterogeneity is less remarkable in the rabbit. In the LDLu of both hamsters and rats, the lumen-negative voltage was generated when the transepithelial osmotic gradient was imposed by adding raffinose to the bath. This indicates that streaming potential can be generated in the LDLu of both species because of high water permeability combined with cation selectivity.

To obtain more detailed analysis of the LDLu ion selectivity of hamsters, Tabei and Imai [28] performed a series of studies in which deflection of voltage was observed by varying the ion composition of the bathing fluid. They found that the LDLu is selectively permeable to cations, with the order of permeability being as follows: $NH_4^+ > K^+ > Rb^+ > Na^+ = Cs^+ > Li^+$. Permeability to NO_3^-, I^-, Br^-, and acetate relative to chloride were less than unity. It is interesting to note that the membrane characteristics of the LDLu are analogous to the gramicidin channel, with respect to high permeability to water and cation selectivity.

Function of the Thin Ascending Limbs of Henle's Loop

There also is controversy concerning the function of the thin ascending limb. The most important problem concerns whether active NaCl transport exists in this segment. Marsh and Azen [29] demonstrated that sodium concentration in the fluid of the ascending limbs decreased by 50 mEq/liter below that of plasma in the adjacent vessels when the luminal flow was reduced by aspirating tubular fluid at the portion proximal to the collection site. They interpreted this to mean that an increase in contact time uncovered the existence of active NaCl transport, which otherwise was undetectable. Marsh and Martin [30] reported that transepithelial voltage of the thin ascending limbs of hamsters was 2 mV-oriented positive in the lumen, and that this voltage was abolished when ouabain or furosemide was added to the lumen. They argued that these observations suggest the existence of active chloride transport in this segment.

By in vivo microperfusion of thin ascending limb of hamster kidney, Sakai et al [18] reported that this segment was highly permeable to water as well as to sodium. By in vitro microperfusion of the thin ascending limb of rat

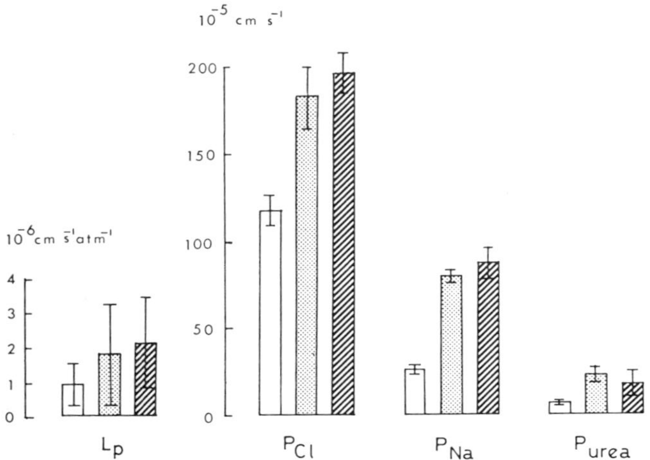

Fig. 3. Comparison of membrane characteristics of the thin ascending limbs of Henle's loop of rabbits, rats, and hamsters. Symbols are: □, rabbit; ▣, rat; ▨, hamster.

kidney slices, Morgan and Berliner [20] reported that this segment was less permeable to water, but was highly permeable to sodium as well as to urea. It is unclear whether these discrepancies represent species difference, since these results were derived by different techniques.

We have compared the function of the thin ascending limb of rabbits, rats, and hamsters by perfusing the isolated renal tubules in vitro [31–35]. As summarized in Figure 3, there is no qualitative difference in the membrane characteristics of the thin ascending limb among these mammals. The segment is impermeable to water, is highly permeable to NaCl, and is moderately permeable to urea. These characteristics are very similar to those predicted by models of countercurrent multiplication systems by passive diffusion of solutes [36, 37].

Physiologic Significance of Nephron Heterogeneity

Most of the models for countercurrent multiplication systems in the renal medulla are based on the assumption that there is no difference in the function of the descending limb. Since morphologic and functional differences exist in the descending limb of mammalian species with high urinary concentrating capacity, it is possible that these characteristics may have physiologic significance.

Since both the LDLu and the SDL are highly permeable to water, increases in osmolality of the luminal fluid in the descending limb may be caused primarily by water absorption. However, in the LDLu, sodium entry also might contribute to the increase in osmolality of the luminal fluid, since this segment is highly permeable to sodium. Since the LDLu makes close countercurrent contact with the thick ascending limb, it is possible that a favorable diffusion gradient exists from the thick ascending limb surroundings into the descending limb. This would fit exactly with the classic countercurrent multiplication model proposed by Kuhn and Ramel [38].

On the other hand, the membrane characteristics and histotopographic localization of the SDL cannot be incorporated into the classic model. It is tempting to speculate that the SDL is playing an important role as one of the sites of urea recycling. Since the SDL of some species is making close contact with the vascular bundles, urea carried via ascending vasa recta from the renal papilla and/or pelvis will be trapped by a countercurrent exchange mechanism into the SDL—which delivers urea to more distal nephron segments, thereby providing a source for accumulation of urea in the medullary interstitium.

The membrane characteristics of the thin ascending limb are favorable for operations of single effect by passive diffusion of solutes as proposed by Kokko and Rector [36] and Stephenson [37], although it is not clear whether active solute transport processes also contribute a component to the countercurrent multiplication system in the inner medulla. To the extent that NaCl diffuses into the descending limb of Henle, this would increase the favorable gradient for NaCl diffusion out of the thin ascending limb, and thus facilitate the operation of the *passive* countercurrent multiplication system.

Thus, the existence of morphologic and functional internephron heterogeneity in the thin descending limb agrees with the hypothesis that both active and passive models of countercurrent multiplication participate in the mechanism of formation of concentrated urine. However, this hypothesis is still highly speculative; more detailed computer simulation studies are necessary to provide quantitative bases for this model.

Acknowledgment. Some of the works quoted in this review were supported, in part, by a grant from the Ministry of Education, Science, and Culture of Japan (# 58480104).

References

1. JAMISON RL, KRIZ W: *Urinary Concentrating Mechanism. Structure and Function.* New York, Oxford Press, 1982
2. BURG M: Thick ascending limb of Henle's loop. *Kidney Int* 22:454–464, 1982
3. DIETRICH HJ: Die Ultrastruktur der Gefassbundel im Mark der Rattenniere. *Z Zellforsch* 84:350–371, 1968
4. SCHWARTZ NM, VENKATACHALAM MA: Structural differences in thin limbs of Henle: Physiological implications. *Kidney Int* 6:193–208, 1974
5. KRIZ W, SCHILLER A, KAISSLING B, TAUGNER R: Comparative and functional aspects of thin loop limb ultrastructure, in *Functional Ultrastructure of the Kidney,* edited by MAUNSBACH AB, OLSEN TS, CHRISTENSEN EI, London, Academic Press, 1980, pp 241–250
6. DIETRICH HJ, BARRETT JM, KRIZ W, BULHOFF JP: The ultrastructure of thin loop limbs of the mouse kidney. *Anat Embryol* 147:1–13, 1975

7. BARRETT JM, KRIZ W, KAISSLING B, DE ROUFFIGNAC C: The ultrastructure of the desert rodent (*Psammomys obesus*) kidney. I. Thin limb of Henle of short-looped nephrons. *Am J Anat* 151:487–498, 1978

8. BARRETT JM, KRIZ W, KAISSLING B, DE ROUFFIGNAC C: The ultrastructure of the desert rodent (*Psammomys obesus*) kidney. II. Thin limb of Henle of long-looped nephrons. *Am J Anat* 151:499–514, 1978

9. KRIZ W, KAISSLING B, PSCZOLLA M: Morphological characterization of the cell in Henle's loop and the distal tubule, in *New Aspects of Renal Function*, edited by VOGEL HG, ULLRICH K, Amsterdam, Excerpta Medica, 1978, pp 67–78

10. NAGLE RB, ALTSCHULER EM, DOBYAN DC, DONG S, BULGER RE: The ultrastructure of the thin limbs of Henle in kidneys of the heteromyid (*Perognathus penicillatus*). *Am J Anat* 161:34–47, 1981

11. BACHMAN S, KRIZ W: Histotopography and ultrastructure of the thin limbs of the loop of Henle in the hamster. *Cell Tissue Res* 225:111–127, 1982

12. SCHILLER A, TAUGNER R, KRIZ W: The thin limbs of Henle's loop in the rabbit: A freeze fracture study. *Cell Tissue Res* 207:247–265, 1980

13. HUMBERT F, PRICAM C, PERRELET A, ORCI L: Freeze-fracture differences between plasma membranes of descending and ascending branches of rat Henle's thin loop. *Lab Invest* 33:407–411, 1975

14. SCHWARTZ MM, KARNOVSKY MJ, VENKATACHALAM MA: Regional membrane specialization in the thin limbs of Henle's loop as seen by freeze-fracture electron microscopy. *Kidney Int* 16:577–589, 1979

15. KRIZ W: Structural organization of the renal medulla: comparative and functional aspects. *Am J Physiol* 241:R3–R16, 1981

16. GOTTSCHALK CW, LASSITER WE, MYLLE M, ULLRICH K, SCHMIDT-NIELSEN B, O'DELL R, PEHLING G: Micropuncture study of composition of loop of Henle fluid in desert rodents. *Am J Physiol* 204:532–535, 1963

17. MARSH DJ: Solute and water flows in thin limbs of Henle's loop in the hamster kidney. *Am J Physiol* 218:824–831, 1970

18. SAKAI F, TADOKORO M, TERAOKA M: Experimentelle Untersuchungen über die Funktion des Nierenmarkes mit der Mikropunktionsmethode. *Tokyo J Med Sci* 79:1–30, 1971

19. PENNEL JP, LACY FB, JAMISON RL: An *in vivo* study of the concentrating process in the descending limb of Henle's loop. *Kidney Int* 5:337–347, 1974

20. MORGAN T, BERLINER RW: Permeability of loop of Henle, vasa recta, and collecting duct to water, urea, and sodium. *Am J Physiol* 215:108–115, 1968

21. DE ROUFFIGNAC C, MOREL F: Micropuncture study of water, electrolyte and urea movements along the loop of Henle in Psammomys. *J Clin Invest* 48:474–486, 1969

22. JAMISON RL, ROINEL N, DE ROUFFIGNAC C: Urinary concentrating mechanism in the desert rodent *Psammomys obesus*. *Am J Physiol* 236:F448–F453, 1979

23. KOKKO JP: Sodium and water transport in the descending limb of Henle. *J Clin Invest* 49:1838–1846, 1970

24. KOKKO JP: Urea transport in the proximal tubule and the descending limb of Henle. *J Clin Invest* 51:1999–2009, 1972

25. STONER LC, ROCH-RAMEL F: The effects of pressure on the water permeability of the descending limb of Henle's loop of rabbit. *Pflügers Arch* 382:7–15, 1979

26. MIWA T, IMAI M: Flow-dependent water permeability of the rabbit descending limb of Henle's loop. *Am J Physiol* 245:F743–754, 1983

27. IMAI M, ARAKI M: Internephron heterogeneity and interspecies differences in

the function of the descending limbs of Henle's loop (DLH) (*abstract*). *Proc Int Union Physiol Sci* 15:418, 1983

28. TABEI K, IMAI M: Ion permselectivity of the descending limb of long loop nephron of the hamster, in *Abstr 26th Congr Jpn Soc Nephrol* (in Japanese), Kyoto, 1983, p 493

29. MARSH DJ, AZEN SP: Mechanism of NaCl absorption by hamster thin ascending limb of Henle's loop. *Am J Physiol* 228:71–79, 1975

30. MARSH DJ, MARTIN CM: Origin of electrical PDs in hamster thin ascending limbs of Henle's loop. *Am J Physiol* 232:F348–F357, 1977

31. IMAI M, KOKKO JP: Relative permeability of the thin ascending limb of Henle(tALH) to various ions, in *Abstr 6th Annu Mtg Am Soc Nephrol*, Washington D.C., 1973, p 52

32. IMAI M, KOKKO JP: NaCl, urea and water transport in the thin ascending limb of Henle: generation of osmotic gradients by passive diffusion of solutes. *J Clin Invest* 5:393–402, 1974

33. IMAI M, KOKKO JP: Mechanism of sodium and chloride transport in the thin ascending limb of Henle. *J Clin Invest* 58:1054–1060, 1976

34. IMAI M: Function of the thin ascending limb of Henle of rats and hamsters perfused in vitro. *Am J Physiol* 232:F201–F209, 1977

35. IMAI M: Transport properties of the thin ascending limb of Henle's loop, in *Edema: Recent Advances,* edited by SEKI K, CASLEY-SMITH JR, ANDREOLI TE, Proceedings of the International Conference on Edema in Tokyo, 1981, pp. 199–209

36. KOKKO JP, RECTOR FC JR: Countercurrent multiplication system without active transport in renal inner medulla. *Kidney Int* 2:214–223, 1972

37. STEPHENSON JL: Concentration of urine in a central core model of the counterflow system. *Kidney Int* 2:85–94, 1972

38. KUHN W, RAMEL L: Aktiver Salztransport als Möglicher (und warscheinlicher) Einzeleffekt bei der Harnkonzentrierung in der Niere. *Helv Chim Acta* 42:628–660, 1959

Regulation of Sodium Chloride Transport by the Loop of Henle

John B. Stokes III

The process of sodium chloride (NaCl) transport by the various segments of the loop of Henle varies considerably. Due to the strikingly different morphology of the pars recta, the thin limbs, and the thick-limb segments, it is not surprising that the mechanisms of transport are different. However, functional heterogeneity exists not only between these major segments, it also exists within each segment. It is now clear that the cortical portion of the thick ascending limb (cTALH) of the mouse [1] has (at least in part) a different mechanism for NaCl absorption than does the medullary portion (mTALH) [2, 3]. In the rabbit, there does not appear to be the same type of heterogeneity. However, the cTALH and the mTALH of the rabbit demonstrate considerable differences in hormonal sensitivities and rates of NaCl absorption. From these few examples, it should be obvious that generalizations regarding mechanisms of regulation of NaCl transport in the loop of Henle must be viewed with a great deal of circumspection. Species differences in mechanisms of transport, species and segmental heterogeneity of hormonal responses, and axial heterogeneity all make attempts in presenting an integrated rational approach to regulation rather difficult. However, there are certain themes that have surfaced recently that may have general applicability. The extent to which they operate in humans or even in the species studied remains somewhat speculative. However, there is a good probability that these regulatory processes contribute in some way to loop function in vivo.

The discussion of the regulation of NaCl absorption in Henle's loop must begin with the examination of factors that regulate NaCl transport in the thick ascending limb. There is now a considerable body of information regarding humoral effects on this segment. Both the biochemical responses and the functional responses to various hormones have provided a reasonably consistent framework from which to assess their role in loop function. In addition to the hormonal regulation of transport, it is becoming clear that

This manuscript was presented as part of a Symposium on *Transport Mechanisms in Henle's Loop.*

important physical aspects related to the special position of the mTALH within the renal medulla can play a major role in the regulation of NaCl absorption.

In contrast to regulatory aspects of NaCl absorption by the thick ascending limb, regulation of NaCl transport by the thin limbs is less well understood. There currently is no information, to our knowledge, regarding the possibility that passive permeabilities to these ions can be regulated. Furthermore, there appears to be substantial variation in permeability characteristics from species to species. In some species, NaCl enters the descending limb [4], while in other species, it appears unlikely that this phenomenon occurs to any great extent. Functional and morphologic heterogeneity along the length of the descending limb further complicates the analysis of NaCl transport and its regulation. Since there is no active transport in the thin ascending limb [5], the magnitude of NaCl absorption in the segment is a function of the concentration gradient. Therefore, the magnitude of NaCl absorption in the loop is a complex function of water absorption in the thin descending limb, passive NaCl transfer in the thin limbs, active NaCl absorption in the thick ascending limb, and (in addition) in the vasa recta blood flow [6, 7]. Given the complexities of these regulatory features regarding NaCl transport in the loop of Henle, it is little wonder that there currently is no generally accepted model for solute and water transport in the loop of Henle that can completely explain the solute concentration gradients measured along the axis of the papilla [8].

Flow Dependence in the Thick Ascending Limb

The initial studies of the isolated, perfused mTALH and cTALH of the rabbit demonstrated that chloride (Cl) and not sodium (Na) was absorbed against its electrochemical gradient [9, 10]. The mechanism of NaCl absorption in both the cTALH and the mTALH demonstrated considerable similarities; there also appeared to be some differences. One of the important differences was the extent to which these segments could lower the NaCl concentration of the luminal fluid. Burg and Green [10] noted that the lowest Na concentration that could be maintained in the lumen of the cTALH was $\sim$ 60 mM. By contrast, under similar conditions, Rocha and Kokko [9] reported that the lowest Na concentration that could be maintained at very low flow rates in the lumen of the mTALH was $\sim$ 100 mM. These results demonstrated important differences between each other despite the fact that both groups of investigators used isotonic bath concentrations.

Rocha and Kokko [9] also conducted experiments that examined the flow dependence of solute absorption. They determined that the magnitude of Cl absorption at flow rates less than 1 nl/min was approximately 4 pEq/cm/sec, while the rate of absorption in tubules perfused at greater than 10 nl/min was approximately 40 pEq/cm/sec. Greger [11], by using electrical estimates of Na absorption in the cTALH, has demonstrated a rate of Cl absorption that reaches approximately 11 pEq/cm/sec at high flow rates.

In a study conducted in this laboratory, the rates of Cl transport in the cTALH and mTALH were compared by using the same perfusion rate and the same length of tubule [12]. The mTALH was bathed in either isotonic fluid or rabbit serum, or it was perfused and bathed in hypertonic fluid. These different conditions had no effect on the magnitude of Cl absorption in the mTALH. In every case, Cl absorption in mTALH was approximately twice that of Cl absorption in the cTALH.

These observations, when taken together, indicate that the cTALH and the mTALH have different basal rates of NaCl absorption. The mTALH appears to be a high-capacity low-gradient system, while the cortical thick limb appears to be a lower capacity system with a greater ability to generate a concentration gradient. This general theme is characteristic of the respective proximal and distal segments of the nephron, the proximal convoluted tubule, and the collecting tubule representing the extreme examples of this phenomenon.

The notion that the rate of NaCl absorption by the loop of Henle depends on the delivery of NaCl to the ascending limb has been recognized for many years. Clearance studies have demonstrated that the generation of solute-free water depends on Cl delivery [13]. In vivo microperfusion of superficial loops has demonstrated that solute absorption is flow-dependent [14]. Thus, it seems completely consistent that the thick ascending limb of Henle's loop participates in the flow-dependent or load-dependent NaCl absorption by the loop of Henle.

Hormonal Regulation of NaCl Absorption

One of the earliest demonstrations that a humoral substance could act on the thick ascending limb to regulate NaCl absorption was the inhibitory effect of exogenous prostaglandin E_2 (PGE_2) on the isolated mTALH of the rabbit [12]. This inhibitory action was localized to the medullary segment, and the cTALH was not influenced by PGE_2. Assigning a role for PGE_2 for the regulation of NaCl absorption by the thick limb has several attractive features. First (and most obviously), the mTALH resides in a region of the kidney that is rich in prostaglandin production [15]. Second, the effect of prostaglandin on the rate of Cl absorption can be expressed either from the peritubular surface or from the luminal surface [12, 16]. Thus, it is conceivable that prostaglandin secretion by the pars recta and/or production by interstitial cells in the renal medulla could influence the magnitude of NaCl absorption by the thick ascending limb. Finally, the selective effect on the medullary portion regulates medullary solute content; thus, it can influence water excretion by limiting the maximum urinary osmolality. The absence of effects in the cTALH limits the renal prostaglandin system to the regulation of negative free-water excretion without limiting the ability of the kidney to generate or excrete a dilute urine.

The demonstration by Morel et al [17] that the adenylate cyclase of the mTALH was activated by vasopressin led several groups of investigators to examine its effect on NaCl transport in this segment. The biochemical and physiologic effects of vasopressin correlate well in the rabbit and mouse mTALH. In the mouse, vasopressin dramatically stimulates both adenylate cyclase activity and net NaCl absorption [2, 17–19]. In the rabbit mTALH, the effects are inconsistent, but in the aggregate, they are rather modest [2, 17, unpublished observations]. In the rat, there is brisk stimulation of adenylate cyclase, but little or no increase in NaCl transport [18]. The reasons for this discrepancy in the rat are not clear. As is the case for PGE_2, the effect of vasopressin appears to be localized to the mTALH with minimal or no effect on the cTALH [2].

In addition to the effects of vasopressin and prostaglandin, several other hormones have been implicated in the regulation of NaCl absorption via the loop of Henle. Glucagon has been shown to stimulate adenylate cyclase activity in the rat mTALH [17], and it has been reported to stimulate the transepithelial voltage in the mouse mTALH [20]. Likewise, isoproterenol has been shown to stimulate the transepithelial voltage of the mTALH of the mouse [20, 21]; although, in the rat and rabbit, isoproterenol has little or no effect on adenylate cyclase activity [17]. Calcitonin and parathyroid hormone (PTH) stimulate adenylate cyclase activity in the rat thick ascending limb; although, in contrast to glucagon and vasopressin, calcitonin and PTH have a more pronounced effect in the cTALH than in the mTALH [17].

There is accumulating evidence indicating that the hormone-stimulated adenylate cyclase activity described for the in vitro systems is closely associated with regulation of NaCl transport in vivo. Systemic infusion of vasopressin increases NaCl absorption by the superficial loop in the Brattleboro rat [22]. In this setting, Cl excretion also was reduced. These results complement the in vitro biochemical and functional effects of vasopressin, and they suggest that vasopressin can increase NaCl absorption by the thick limb in vivo. The effects of calcitonin and glucagon have also been examined in vivo by using the same experimental setting. Calcitonin has effects similar to vasopressin [23], but glucagon has no effect on NaCl transport [24]. The reasons for the differences may be related to species-dependent differences in sensitivities to these hormones. Despite the sometimes dramatic species differences regarding segmental response to a given hormone, there is a generally consistent theme relating the patterns of hormone-sensitive adenylate cyclase activity and the ability of the hormone to stimulate NaCl absorption by the appropriate segment in vivo.

An interesting discrepancy between biochemical hormone response and functional response is evident in the case of isoproterenol. There appears to be no increase in adenylate cyclase activity in the rat mTALH [17], yet there is a brisk functional response in the in vitro-perfused mouse mTALH [20, 21]. The demonstration that low-frequency renal nerve stimulation enhances NaCl absorption in the absence of water absorption is supportive evidence for an in vivo effect of adrenergic agents [25].

The molecular nature of the interaction between vasopressin, glucagon (and perhaps isoproterenol), and the mTALH appears to be coupled to activation of adenylate cyclase and the generation of intracellular cyclic AMP. Exogenous cyclic AMP can produce stimulation of NaCl transport [2], as can forskolin [20], which an agent that stimulates cyclic AMP production by bypassing the receptor and interacting with the catalytic protein. Thus, there is a reasonably consistent theme regarding the mechanisms by which NaCl absorption can be stimulated by hormones.

The mechanism by which PGE_2 inhibits NaCl absorption is less clear. In the mouse mTALH, PGE_2 inhibits transport only after stimulation [16]. In the rabbit mTALH, which is considerably less sensitive to stimulation by vasopressin, PGE_2 inhibits basal transport [12]. It is likely that the differences are owed to the nonstimulated levels of cyclic AMP in these species. Culpepper and Andreoli [16] have examined the interaction between vasopressin and PGE_2 in the mouse mTALH, and they have found an apparent competitive antagonism by PGE_2. A concentration of 1 μM PGE_2 shifts the vasopressin dose-response curve to the right, but it does not prevent a full response, provided that high enough concentrations of vasopressin are used. These investigators have further examined this interaction and have reported that PGE_2 inhibits the stimulatory effect of glucagon and isoproterenol as well. Prostaglandin E_2 had no effect on the response to exogenous cyclic AMP or forskolin. The site of the PGE_2-vasopressin interaction, thus, would be distal to the vasopressin receptor and proximal to the catalytic protein. It is possible that PGE_2 interacts with the guanine nucleotide regulatory subunit to prevent transmission of a variety of receptor-mediated signals [20].

In Vivo Evidence for Action of PGE_2 and Antidiuretic Hormone on NaCl Transport

There now is considerable evidence that both endogenously produced prostaglandins and vasopressin produce their effects on mTALH-NaCl transport in the intact kidney. The effects of stimulating or inhibiting NaCl absorption by the mTALH produce some important changes in the intrarenal distribution of NaCl absorption, which may or may not result in alteration of NaCl excretion. One of the most important effects of altering the rate of NaCl absorption in the mTALH is the alteration of the NaCl content of the medullary interstitium. (Increasing NaCl absorption by the mTALH will increase medullary NaCl content; the converse would be true for a decrease in the rate of NaCl absorption.) An increase in medullary NaCl content, by virtue of raising medullary tonicity, would cause an increase in water abstraction from the thin descending limb (tDLH). This effect would decrease axial volume flow through the loop and the distal tubule. The alteration in the NaCl gradients across the thin limbs would favor enhanced, passive NaCl absorption by the tALH. These changes would have a major effect on the ability of the kidney to produce a maximally concentrated urine.

A second major consequence of regulating NaCl absorption by the mTALH and not by the cTALH becomes apparent when one considers that the population of nephrons in the kidney can be divided into at least two groups. The extreme examples of this nephron heterogeneity are the superficial nephrons with short loops and the juxtamedullary nephrons with long loops. The superficial nephrons have short segments of thin limbs, but they have a long cTALH. By contrast, the deep nephrons have long segments of thin limbs, but little cTALH. From consideration of the consequences of medullary tonicity on passive NaCl absorption, one might predict that agents regulating NaCl absorption only in the mTALH would influence deep nephron function more dramatically than they would superficial nephron function. The *single effect* on deep nephron function, thus, would be magnified by the passive NaCl transport of the longer thin limbs.

In contrast to the long loops, the effect of altering NaCl transport by the mTALH of superficial loops would not be magnified. Instead, the thin limbs would not play a significant role in the amplification of mTALH-NaCl absorption. Furthermore, the cTALH—because of its immunity to the action of agents that modify mTALH function—would mitigate the alteration in mTALH transport. For example, during conditions under which mTALH absorption was avid and loop flow rates were low, absolute NaCl absorption by the cTALH would be low due to the (relatively) early attainment of the limiting NaCl concentration. On the other hand, when mTALH absorption is low and axial flow rate is high, cTALH absorption would be increased because of the more distal attainment of the limiting NaCl concentration. Thus, because of the selective alteration of NaCl absorption in the mTALH, the deep nephrons may play a particularly active role in regulating delivery of NaCl out of the loop.

Demonstrating that a substance modulates NaCl by the mTALH selectively is most readily accomplished by using isolated nephron segments perfused in vitro; demonstrating that such an effect occurs in vivo is more difficult. Because the mTALH is not accessible to micropuncture, the evaluation must rely on more indirect techniques. The most commonly used techniques in this regard are: (1) measurement of interstitial solute content, (2) changes in the maximum urine osmolality, (3) alteration of absorbed solute in perfused superficial loops, and (4) demonstration of discrepancies in Na delivery between the late distal tubule and the most proximal, accessible portion of the papillary collecting duct. Each of these determinations is subject to multiple interpretations, but they can provide useful evidence to evaluate the possibility of whether an effect that has been demonstrated in vitro might be operative in vivo.

One of the earliest clues that NaCl absorption by the mTALH might be regulated is contained in the measurements of papillary solute content by Bartelheimer and Senft [26]. They found that nonsteroidal anti-inflammatory drugs increased papillary solute content. The agents, which were subsequently shown to inhibit cyclo-oxygenase, might produce this effect either by increasing NaCl absorption by the mTALH or by decreasing vasa recta blood flow. The separation of these parameters was done by Ganguli et al [27], who measured papillary blood flow and medullary solutes in the rat after the administration of indomethacin. They found that solute content increased even when blood flow changed minimally. These results are consistent with those found by other investigators [28, 29], and they support the notion that endogenous prostaglandins inhibit NaCl absorption by the mTALH in vivo.

These in vivo data, addressing the notion that endogenous prostaglandins inhibit absorption by the mTALH, are complemented by two other types of results: (1) clearance data indicating that the maximum urine osmolality increases after the inhibition of prostaglandin synthesis, and (2) micropuncture data of the accessible portions of the nephron, following inhibition of prostaglandin synthesis.

The increase in urine osmolality following administration of cyclo-oxygenase inhibitors is one of the most consistently reported renal effects of these agents [30, 31]. Anderson et al [32] showed dramatic increases in U_{Osm} in water-loaded dogs following indomethacin. Similar effects have been reported in Brattleboro rats [29, 33], which indicates that this effect does not necessarily depend on the presence of circulating vasopressin. Furthermore, the effect occurs without a fall in glomerular filtration rate (GFR). These results clearly indicate that the increased medullary solute content caused by inhibition of prostaglandin production is functionally translated to the excretion of a more concentrated urine.

The localization of the major effect of endogenous prostaglandins to the mTALH is supported by studies that examine free water clearance following inhibition of prostaglandin production. These clearance studies demonstrate little or no effect on free water generation [34–36]. Thus, combined with the data on excretion of a concentrated urine, they are consistent with the localization of the site of action of renal prostaglandins to the mTALH.

There now is considerable evidence that the superficial nephrons and the juxtamedullary nephrons function differently. One of the ways they differ relates to their respective position in the kidney and to the extent to which the thin limbs descend into the medulla. The idea that the deep nephrons might play a role in the excretion of an acute NaCl load was advanced by Stein et al [37]. The important observation was that during volume expansion, sodium delivery to the most proximal accessible papillary collecting duct was greater than delivery out of the late distal nephron. Similar results have been obtained by Sonnenberg [38] by using the technique of collecting duct microcatheterization. The most attractive explanation for this phenomenon is that the deep nephrons reabsorb a significantly smaller fraction of the filtered NaCl than the superficial nephrons. Thus, they add their filtrate to the collecting duct in a region below the surface of the kidney that is not accessible to conventional micropuncture. Higashihara et al [28] have provided evidence that this effect depends on an intact renal prostaglandin system. Administration of indomethacin or meclofenamate eliminated the increase in the delivery of Cl to the base of the collecting duct that is evoked by volume expansion. These results provide good supporting evidence that endogenous prostaglandins can reduce NaCl absorption by the mTALH in vivo.

Solute Concentration Effects on NaCl Absorption

The fact that the mTALH is situated in an environment that is substantially different from that of most other cells in the body has prompted an investigation of the influence of some special environmental factors on NaCl absorption by this segment. The two conditions that have been most carefully examined are osmolality and potassium (K) concentration.

The effect of osmolality on NaCl absorption has been examined in the mouse mTALH under conditions in which Cl absorption has been stimulated with antidiuretic hormone (ADH). Hebert, Culpepper, and Andreoli [39] found that a rapid increase in the ambient osmotic pressure by using either urea, mannitol, or NaCl, produced a prompt and reversible reduction in NaCl absorption. Although the mechanism for this effect of osmolality on the ability to absorb NaCl is not clear, the results indicate that it is not simply an alteration in cell volume. Urea had no effect on cell volume, whereas the mannitol and NaCl conditions clearly reduced cell volume; yet, all three agents had similar effects. This effect could not be eliminated with supermaximal doses of vasopressin. Hypertonicity probably influences NaCl absorption in the mouse mTALH, even in the absence of vasopressin, since tubules dissected and studied in the hypertonic fluids had lower transepithelial voltage (V_T) than did tubules similarly handled—but examined in an isotonic solution [40]. In contrast to the mouse, hypertonic fluids apparently do not alter the net Cl absorption by the rabbit mTALH, nor does hypertonicity impair the inhibitory effect of PGE_2 [12].

The effect of K concentration on NaCl absorption has been examined in our laboratory. Potassium concentration, when increased from 5 to 25 mM inhibits within minutes the V_T in a reversible fashion. Potassium concentrations of 10 mM cause a small effect and concentrations of 25 mM reduce V_T by approximately 90%. In this setting (as is the case for most other situations in which mTALH V_T is altered), the direction and the magnitude of the change reflects changes in net Cl absorption. The K effects operate in both the mouse and rabbit mTALH, as well as under isotonic or hypertonic conditions [40].

The physiologic relevance of the effects of K concentration on NaCl absorption by the mTALH rests importantly on the observation that the K concentration in the loop fluid and in the interstitial fluid is substantially greater than that of the peripheral blood. The K concentration of vasa recta blood of the rat papilla ranges from 20 to 50 mM [41, 42]. Thus, while the ambient K concentration of the medullary thick limb is not known, it is reasonable to suspect that the concentration can range from 5 to 25 mM.

The mechanism whereby increased K concentration would lead to reduced net NaCl absorption by this segment becomes apparent when one considers the mechanism of NaCl absorption, as recently elucidated by Greger [11], Greger, Schlatter, and Lang [43], and Greger and Schlatter [44–46]. It is apparent that the entry of Na and Cl across the luminal membrane is coupled to K entry [43]. In addition, the extrusion of Na across the basolateral membrane via the Na-K pump obligates a large influx of K across the basolateral membrane. Potassium exits the cell via a conductive pathway on the apical membrane [46] and a Cl-coupled pathway on the basolateral membrane [46]. Thus, raising K concentrations either in the lumen or the bath reduces the driving force for Cl exit at the basolateral membrane. Raising lumen K by depolarizing the cell membrane voltage would reduce the electrical driving force for Cl exit. Raising basolateral K concentrations would reduce the chemical driving force for (electrically neutral) coupled KCl exit across the basolateral membrane. This type of an effect of K concentration on Cl transport has recently been demonstrated for the canine trachea, which possesses a similar array of transport processes [47]. In this tissue, raising K concentration reduces the short-circuit current (Cl transport) and depolarizes the cell. Thus, the observed effects of K concentration on mTALH are completely consistent with our understanding of the nature of the process by which NaCl is absorbed.

Integrated Aspects of the Regulation of NaCl Absorption

From a teleologic perspective, perhaps the most important function of the mTALH is to create a hypertonic medulla. According to our current understanding, this segment of the nephron provides virtually all of the energy for the operation of the countercurrent multiplier; therefore, it is either directly or indirectly responsible for the axial solute profile along the renal papilla. Alterations in the magnitude of salt addition to the renal medullary interstitium have a major influence on medullary tonicity. A detailed understanding of the mechanisms that are responsible for the solute content of the medulla is still elusive. Nevertheless, certain principles are known to be of major importance in the maintenance of a hypertonic medulla. They are: (1) net solute transport out of the ascending limb of Henle, (2) the *washout* due to medullary vasa recta blood flow, and (3) the addition of water to the medulla from the collecting duct.

We have, thus far, focused only on the portion of these parameters that deals with the absorption of NaCl from the ascending limb of Henle's loop. However, it is becoming clear that ADH and prostaglandins not only regulate NaCl absorption by the mTALH, but they also affect vasa recta blood flow in such a way as to produce opposite effects on medullary tonicity. A schematic illustration of the interactions of vasopressin and medullary prostaglandins on these parameters is illustrated in Figure 1. Importantly, vasopressin and medullary prostaglandins act in opposite ways to regulate the magnitude of NaCl absorption by the medullary thick limb. In addition, they have antagonistic effects on the hydraulic conductivity (P_f) of the collecting tubule [48]. Finally, they probably have opposite effects on vasa recta blood flow. The effect of vasopressin is to increase the medullary solute content, while the effect of the prostaglandin system is to reduce the medullary solute content. Acting in concert with their independent effects on the P_f on the collecting tubule, these agents antagonize each other's action with respect to U_{osm} and the magnitude of water excretion. The effects of the regulation of NaCl absorption in the mTALH are amplified by both the thin limbs and the addition of NaCl to the medulla by passive mechanisms. The NaCl content and osmolality of the papilla are major factors in determining the magnitude of water absorption from the thin descending limb, and—according to the principles involved in the passive countercurrent exchanger—they are important in de-

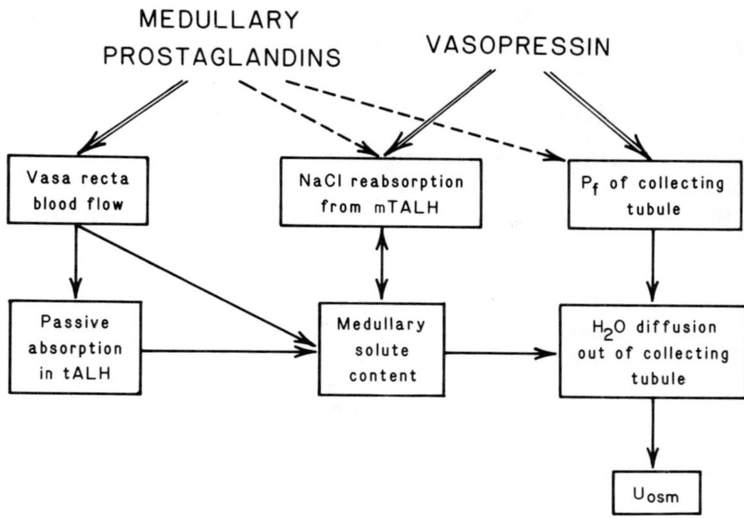

Fig. 1. Schema of counter-regulatory effects of renal medullary prostaglandins and vasopressin. *Double lines* indicate a direct stimulatory or enhancing effect of the prostaglandins or vasopressin, *single solid lines* indicate an indirect stimulatory effect, and *dashed lines* indicate an inhibitory effect. Vasopressin increases both NaCl reabsorption by the mTALH and by the hydraulic conductivity (P_F) of the collecting tubule. Vasopressin may also reduce vasa recta blood flow. Medullary prostaglandins enhance vasa recta blood flow. In addition, they diminish mTALH absorption and P_F of collecting tubule. In these ways, vasopressin and prostaglandins exert opposite effects on urine osmolality.

termining the actual NaCl gradients in the thin ascending limb. These gradients determine the magnitude of passive salt addition to the renal papilla [42, 49, 50].

Thus, the ADH prostaglandin system regulates NaCl absorption in the loop as one of several mechanisms used to alter papillary solute content and ultimately to regulate water excretion. In the process of regulating NaCl absorption in this segment, there may be effects on NaCl balance and, thus, on extracellular fluid volume. However, alterations in any one segment may not be necessarily translated into major effects on extracellular fluid volume regulation.

Potassium Recycling to the Medulla

The discovery that ambient K concentration exerts a potent regulatory effect on NaCl absorption by the mTALH answered, at least in part, the question regarding the effects of high K concentration on medullary function. However, the consequences of such an effect require a more concerted appraisal of both the mechanisms involved in medullary K accumulation and the integrated response to reduced NaCl absorption by the mTALH.

Interest in K transport within the medulla received renewed interest as a result of studies by Battilana et al [41], Jamison et al [51], Arrascue et al [52], and Dobyan, Lacy, and Jamison [53]. These investigators demonstrated that K was *recycled* to the renal medulla in a manner that was reminiscent of urea recycling. However, there are many important differences between urea recycling and K recycling—one of the most important of which is the ultimate effect on renal function. Urea accumulation is critically important in producing a maximally concentrated urine; K accumulation reduces the ability to excrete a maximally concentrated urine.

The pathways that result in medullary K accumulation are depicted in Figure 2. The initiating event is K secretion by the distal convoluted tubule (DCT) and the cortical collecting tubule (CCT). The mechanism of K secretion by these two segments differs in several important respects. The DCT is a high-capacity low-gradient system [54], while the CCT is a lower capacity system capable of generating large K concentration gradients [55]. Under

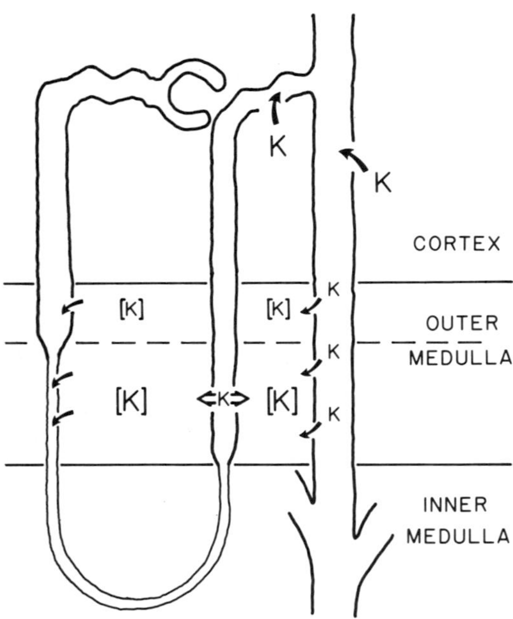

Fig. 2. Pathways of K transport along the nephron. Secretion of K occurs in the distal nephron (DCT and CCT). A small portion of the secreted K is reabsorbed by the medullary collecting tubule because of a favorable chemical gradient and a lack of an active transport mechanism. The increased K concentration in the medullary interstitium permits passive entry of K into the pars recta and thin descending limb. The cycle is completed when K is absorbed by the medullary thick ascending limb. The accumulation of K in the renal medulla can inhibit NaCl absorption in the thick limb. The functional significance of this recycling may have to do with the excretion of acute K loads. (Reproduced with permission from [40])

physiologic conditions, these properties of the DCT render the magnitude of K secretion as being primarily dependent on axial volume flow [56]. By contrast, K secretion by the CCT depends primarily on having an adequate concentration of Na in the lumen [57].

The secreted K can reach a lumen concentration of over 100 mM in the CCT [55]. As the luminal fluid enters the medullary collecting tubule, K secretion stops because the K secretory mechanisms are no longer present [58]. The high K concentration in the lumen provides sufficient driving force for a small amount of K to be reabsorbed passively down its concentration gradient [59]. In this way, the K concentration of the medullary interstitium is increased. The K concentration gradient from interstitium to the pars recta and tDLH is sufficient to cause net K secretion [51, 60, 61]. Under conditions of acute or chronic K loading, K secretion by the tDLH and/or pars recta can cause K delivery to the bend of the loop to exceed 100% of the filtered load [51, 52]. The final step in the sequence of K recycling occurs in the mTALH. In this segment, K is reabsorbed [40], thus completing the recycling process and effectively trapping K in the interstitium. The extent to which this final recycling step occurs is not clear. In the rabbit, K is absorbed by a process that cannot be explained by simple diffusion; that is, a cellular process favors absorption [40]. In the rat, K may be secreted [62]. The reasons for these species differences are not clear.

The effect of K recycling on overall renal function can be predicted, based on the inhibitory effect of K on NaCl absorption by the mTALH. The reduction of this *single effect* would be to reduce medullary solute content, reduce water absorption by the tDLH, and increase axial volume flow through the loop and the DCT. In addition, it would increase Na delivery to the CCT. Both of these alterations in delivery to the distal nephron create more favorable conditions for K secretion by the DCT and CCT. Via this scenario, K recycling is a mechanism by which acute K loads can be rapidly excreted. Reabsorbing a small amount of the secreted K would create conditions that would favor maximum K secretion by the distal nephron.

The extent to which K recycling produces these changes in vivo is not yet clear. The overall renal response to enhanced K recycling appears to be consistent with the predicted results: diuresis, natriuresis, kaliuresis, and a less than maximally concentrated urine. The extent to which these changes operate in the superficial loop following acute K loading appear to be modest [63, 64]. However, the interposition of the cTALH and the relatively short thin limbs may render the effects less pronounced than the effects of the deep nephrons. In this way, regulation of NaCl by the mTALH affects not only the solute content of the medulla, but it also accentuates differences between superficial and deep nephron populations.

Summary

Considerable information has recently become available regarding regulation of NaCl transport in the loop of Henle. Much of the information has its origins in the study of isolated nephron segments in vitro. The mechanism of NaCl absorption via the thick ascending limb of Henle's loop appears to be basically homogeneous along its length, but the basal transport rates and sensitivity to hormones are not homogeneous. The medullary portion is sensitive to regulation by prostaglandins and vasopressin, while the cortical portion is not. Furthermore, the medullary portion, by virtue of its position, is exposed to alterations in ambient osmolality and K concentration—both of which can alter NaCl absorption. Alterations in the rate of NaCl transport can produce changes in medullary solute content that can have significant effects on the patterns of solute and water delivery to different segments of the nephron. Finally, the selective regulation of transport by the medullary segment may accentuate differences between superficial and juxtamedullary nephrons.

Acknowledgment. The author's work was supported by National Institutes of Health grants AM 25231 and HL 14388.

References

1. FRIEDMAN PA, ANDREOLI TE: CO_2-stimulated NaCl absorption in the mouse renal cortical thick ascending limb of Henle. Evidence for synchronous Na^+/H^+ and Cl^-/HCO_3^- exchange in apical plasma membranes. *J Gen Physiol* 80:683–711, 1982

2. HEBERT SC, CULPEPPER RM, ANDREOLI TE: NaCl transport in mouse medullary thick ascending limbs. I. Functional nephron heterogeneity and ADH-stimulated NaCl cotransport. *Am J Physiol* 241(*Renal Fluid Electrolyte Physiol* 10):F412–F431, 1981

3. HEBERT SC, CULPEPPER RM, ANDREOLI TE: NaCl transport in mouse medullary thick ascending limbs. II. ADH enhancement of transcellular NaCl cotransport; origin of transepithelial voltage. *Am J Physiol* 241(*Renal Fluid Electrolyte Physiol* 10):F432–F442, 1981

4. IMBERT M, DE ROUFFIGNAC C: Role of sodium and urea in the renal concentrating mechanism in *Psammomys obesus*. *Pflügers Arch* 361:107–114, 1976

5. IMAI M, KOKKO JP: Mechanism of sodium and chloride transport in the thin ascending limb of Henle. *J Clin Invest* 58:1089–1097, 1976

6. KOKKO JP, RECTOR FC: Countercurrent multiplication system without active transport in inner medulla. *Kidney Int* 2:214–223, 1972

7. STEPHENSON JL: Concentration of urine in a central core model of the renal counterflow system. *Kidney Int* 2:85–94, 1972

8. MOORE LC, MARSH DJ: How descending limb of Henle's loop permeability affects hypertonic urine formation. *Am J Physiol* 239(*Renal Fluid Electrolyte Physiol* 8):F57–F71, 1980

9. ROCHA AS, KOKKO JP: Sodium chloride and water transport in the medullary thick ascending limb of Henle. Evidence for active chloride transport. *J Clin Invest* 52:612–623, 1973

10. BURG MB, GREEN N: Function of the thick ascending limb of Henle's loop. *Am J Physiol* 224:659–668, 1973

11. GREGER R: Chloride reabsorption in the rabbit cortical thick ascending limb of the loop of Henle: a sodium dependent process. *Pflügers Arch* 390:38–43, 1981

12. STOKES JB: Effect of prostaglandin E_2 on chloride transport across the rabbit thick ascending limb of Henle. Selective inhibition of the medullary portion. *J Clin Invest* 64:495–502, 1979

13. DANOVITCH GM, BRICKER NS: Influence of volume expansion on NaCl reabsorption in the diluting segments of the nephron: a study using clearance methods. *Kidney Int* 10:229–238, 1976

14. SCHNERMANN J: Microperfusion study of single short loops of Henle in rat kidney. *Pflügers Arch* 300:255–282, 1968

15. LARSSON C, Änggård E: Regional differences in the formation and metabolism of prostaglandins in the rabbit kidney. *Eur J Pharmacol* 21:30–36, 1973

16. CULPEPPER RM, ANDREOLI TE: Interactions among prostaglandin E_2 antidiuretic hormone, and cyclic adenosine monophosphate in modulating Cl-absorption in single mouse medullary thick limbs of Henle. *J Clin Invest* 71:1588–1601, 1983

17. MOREL F: Sites of hormone action in the mammalian nephron. *Am J Physiol* 240(*Renal Fluid Electrolyte Physiol* 9):F159–F164, 1981

18. SASAKI S, IMAI M: Effects of vasopressin on water and NaCl transport across the in vitro perfused medullary thick ascending limb of Henle's loop of mouse, rat and rabbit kidneys. *Pflügers Arch* 383:215–221, 1980

19. HALL DA, VARNEY DM: Effect of vasopressin on electrical potential difference and chloride transport in mouse medullary thick ascending limb of Henle's loop. *J Clin Invest* 66:792–802, 1980

20. CULPEPPER RM, ANDREOLI TE: Site of PGE_2 inhibition of ADH-mediated NaCl transport in mouse medullary thick ascending limb (mTAL) (*abstract*). *Kidney Int* 23:253, 1983

21. POLHEMUS RE, HALL DA: Effect of catecholamines on the potential difference and chloride efflux in the mouse thick ascending limb of Henle's loop (*abstract*). *Kidney Int* 19:253, 1981

22. DE ROUFFIGNAC C, CORMAN B, ROINEL N: Stimulation by antidiuretic hormone of electrolyte tubular reabsorption in rat kidney. *Am J Physiol* 244(*Renal Fluid Electrolyte Physiol* 13):F156–F164, 1983

23. ELALOUF JM, ROINEL N, DE ROUFFIGNAC C: ADH-like effects of calcitonin on electrolyte transport by Henle's loop of rat kidney. *Am J Physiol* 246(*Renal Fluid Electrolyte Physiol* 15):F213–F220, 1984

24. BAILLY C, ROINEL N, AMIEL C: PTH-like glucagon stimulation of Ca and Mg reabsorption in Henle's loop of the rat. *Am J Physiol* 246(*Renal Fluid Electrolyte Physiol* 15):F205–F212, 1984

25. DIBONA GF, SAWIN LL: Effect of renal nerve stimulation on NaCl and H_2O transport in Henle's loop of the rat. *Am J Physiol* 243(*Renal Fluid Electrolyte Physiol* 12):F576–F580, 1982

26. BARTELHEIMER VHK, SENFT G: Zur lokolisation der tubulären wirkung einiger antirheumatisch wirkender substanzen. *Arzneimittel-Forsch* 18:567–570, 1968

27. GANGULI M, TOBIAN L, AZAR S, O'DONNELL M: Evidence that prostaglandin synthesis inhibitors increase the concentration of sodium and chloride in rat renal medulla. *Circ Res* 40 (Suppl I): I-135–I-139, 1977

28. HIGASHIHARA E, STOKES JB, KOKKO JP, CAMPBELL WB, DuBOSE TD: Cortical and papillary micropuncture examination of chloride transport in segments of the rat kidney during inhibition of prostaglandin production: a possible role for prostaglandins in the chloruresis of acute volume expansion. *J Clin Invest* 64:1277–1287, 1979

29. STOFF JS, ROSA RM, SILVA P, EPSTEIN FH: Indomethacin impairs water diuresis in the DI rat: role of prostaglandins independent of ADH. *Am J Physiol* 241(*Renal Fluid Electrolyte Physiol* 10):F231–F237, 1981

30. ZAMBRASKI EJ, DUNN MJ: Renal effects of drugs that inhibit prostaglandin synthesis. *Kidney Int* 18:609–622, 1980

31. STOKES JB: Integrated actions of renal medullary prostaglandins in the control

of water excretion. *Am J Physiol* 240(*Renal Fluid Electrolyte Physiol* 9):F471–F480, 1981

32. ANDERSON RJ, BERL T, MCDONALD KM, SCHRIER RW: Evidence for an in vivo antagonism between vasopressin and prostaglandin in the mammalian kidney. *J Clin Invest* 56:420–426, 1975

33. DUNN MJ, KINTER LB, BEEUWKES R, SHIER D, GREELEY HP, VALTIN H: Interaction of vasopressin and renal prostaglandins in the homozygous diabetes insipidus rat, in *Advances in Prostaglandin and Thromboxane Research,* vol 7, edited by SAMUELSSON B, RAMWELL PW, PAOLETTI R, New York, Raven Press, 1980, pp 1009–1015

34. WORK J, BAEHLER RW, KOTCHEN TA, TALWALKER R, LUKE RG: Effect of prostaglandin inhibition on sodium chloride reabsorption in the diluting segment of the conscious dog. *Kidney Int* 17:24–30, 1980

35. Düsing R, Nicolas V, Glänzer K, Kipnowski J, Kramer HJ: Prostaglandins participate in the regulation of NaCl absorption in the diluting segment of the nephron in vivo: effects of furosemide. *Renal Physiol* [*Basel*] 5:115–123, 1982

36. KAOJARERN S, CHENNAVASIN P, ANDERSON S, BRATER DC: Nephron site of effect of nonsteroidal anti-inflammatory drugs on solute excretion in humans. *Am J Physiol* 244(*Renal Fluid Electrolyte Physiol* 13):F134–F139, 1983

37. STEIN JH, OSGOOD RW, KUNAU RT: Direct measurement of papillary collecting duct sodium transport in the rat. Evidence for heterogeneity of nephron function during Ringer loading. *J Clin Invest* 58:767–773, 1976

38. SONNENBERG H: Secretion of salt and water into medullary collecting duct of Ringer-infused rats. *Am J Physiol* 228:565–568, 1975

39. HEBERT SC, CULPEPPER RM, ANDREOLI TE: NaCl transport in mouse medullary thick ascending limbs. III. Modulation of the ADH effect by peritubular osmolality. *Am J Physiol* 241(*Renal Fluid Electrolyte Physiol* 10):F443–F451, 1981

40. STOKES JB: Consequences of potassium recycling in the renal medulla. Effects on ion transport by the medullary thick ascending limb of Henle's loop. *J Clin Invest* 70:219–229, 1982

41. BATTILANA CA, DOBYAN DC, LACY FB, BHATTACHARYA J, JOHNSTON PA, JAMISON RL: Effect of chronic potassium loading on potassium secretion by the pars recta or descending limb of the juxtamedullary nephron in the rat. *J Clin Invest* 62:1093–1103, 1978

42. JOHNSTON PA, BATTILANA CA, LACY FB, JAMISON RL: Evidence for a concentration gradient favoring outward movement of sodium from the thin loop of Henle. *J Clin Invest* 59:234–240, 1977

43. GREGER R, SCHLATTER E, LANG F: Evidence for electroneutral sodium chloride cotransport in the cortical thick ascending limb of Henle's loop of rabbit kidney. *Pflügers Arch* 396:308–314, 1983

44. GREGER R, SCHLATTER E: Presence of luminal K^+, a prerequisite for active NaCl transport in the cortical thick ascending limb of Henle's loop of rabbit kidney. *Pflügers Arch* 392:92–94, 1981

45. GREGER R, SCHLATTER E: Properties of the basolateral membrane of the cortical thick ascending limb of Henle's loop of rabbit kidney. A model for secondary active chloride transport. *Pflügers Arch* 396:325–334, 1983

46. GREGER R, SCHLATTER E: Properties of the lumen membrane of the cortical thick ascending limb of Henle's loop of rabbit kidney. *Pflügers Arch* 396:315–324, 1983

47. WELSH MJ: Evidence for basolateral membrane potassium conductance in canine tracheal epithelium. *Am J Physiol* 244(*Cell Physiol* 13):C377–C384, 1983

48. GRANTHAM JJ, ORLOFF J: Effect of prostaglandin E_1 on the permeability response

of the isolated collecting tubule to vasopressin, adenosine, 3',5'-monophosphate, and theophylline. *J Clin Invest* 47:1154–1161, 1968

49. REINECK JH, PARMA R: Effect of medullary tonicity on urinary sodium excretion in the rat. *J Clin Invest* 69:971–978, 1982
50. HOGG RJ, KOKKO JP: Comparison between the electrical potential profile and the chloride gradients in the thin limbs of Henle's loop in rats. *Kidney Int* 14:428–436, 1978
51. JAMISON RL, LACY FB, PENNELL JP, SANJANA VM: Potassium secretion by the descending limb or pars recta of the juxtamedullary nephron in vivo. *Kidney Int* 9:323–332, 1976
52. ARRASCUE JF, DOBYAN DC, JAMISON RL: Potassium recycling in the renal medulla: effects of acute potassium chloride administration to rats fed a potassium-free diet. *Kidney Int* 20:348–352, 1981
53. DOBYAN DC, LACY FB, JAMISON RL: Suppression of potassium recycling in the renal medulla by short term potassium deprivation. *Kidney Int* 16:704–709, 1979
54. MALNIC G, KLOSE RM, GIEBISCH G: Microperfusion study of distal tubular potassium and sodium transfer in rat kidney. *Am J Physiol* 211:548–559, 1966
55. GRANTHAM JJ, BURG MB, ORLOFF J: The nature of transtubular Na and K transport in isolated rabbit renal collecting tubules. *J Clin Invest* 49:1815–1825, 1970
56. GOOD DW, WRIGHT FS: Luminal influences on potassium secretion: sodium concentration and fluid flow rate. *Am J Physiol* 236:F192–F205, 1979
57. STOKES JB: Potassium secretion by the cortical collecting tubule: relation to sodium absorption, luminal sodium concentration, and transepithelial voltage. *Am J Physiol* 241(*Renal Fluid Electrolyte Physiol* 10):F395–F402, 1981
58. STOKES JB, INGRAM MJ, WILLIAMS AD, INGRAM D: Heterogeneity of the rabbit collecting tubule: localization of mineralocorticoid hormone action to the cortical portion. *Kidney Int* 20:340–347, 1981
59. STOKES JB: Sodium and potassium transport across the cortical and outer medullary collecting tubule of the rabbit: evidence for diffusion across the outer medullary portion. *Am J Physiol* 242(*Renal Fluid Electrolyte Physiol* 11):F514–F520, 1982
60. WORK J, TROUTMAN WL, SCHAFER JA: Transport of potassium in the rabbit pars recta. *Am J Physiol* 242(*Renal Fluid Electrolyte Physiol* 11):F226–F237, 1982
61. ROCHA AS, KOKKO JP: Membrane characteristics regulating potassium transport out of the isolated perfused descending limb of Henle. *Kidney Int* 4:326–330, 1973
62. WORK J, SCHAFER JA: Rubidium transport in rat medullary thick ascending limb (*abstract*). *Kidney Int* 23:271, 1983
63. KIRCHNER KA: Effect of acute potassium infusion on loop segment chloride reabsorption in the rat. *Am J Physiol* 244(*Renal Fluid Electrolyte Physiol* 13):F599–F606, 1983
64. SUFIT CR, JAMISON RL: Effect of acute potassium load on reabsorption in Henle's loop in the rat. *Am J Physiol* 245(*Renal Fluid Electrolyte Physiol* 14):F559–F576, 1983

Sodium Chloride Reabsorption in the Thick Ascending Limb of the Loop of Henle

Rainer Greger, Monika Wittner, Eberhard Schlatter, Brigitte Gebler, Claudia Weidtke, and Antonio Di Stefano

The early in vitro studies by Burg and Green [1] and by Rocha and Kokko [2] of the thick ascending limb (TAL) of the loop of Henle indicated that it was poorly permeable to water and that its mechanism for sodium chloride reabsorption generated a lumen-positive transepithelial potential difference (PD_{TE}). They claimed that the reabsorption of sodium ions was entirely passive while that of chloride ions was active. This issue was reexamined by Greger at our laboratory [3], who reported that the lumen-positive PD_{TE} was dependent on the active transport of sodium. He concluded that chloride reabsorption was secondarily active, linked to that of sodium, and that the primary active process was the pumping of sodium and potassium through the activity of sodium-potassium-adenosine triphosphatase (Na-K-ATPase). Greger's results have been confirmed by others [4].

The mechanism of sodium chloride reabsorption in the TAL has been the topic of several recent reviews [5–8]. Some of these reviews contain concise tables on the individual properties of the TAL (both medullary and cortical segments) of mouse, rat, and rabbit. To avoid repetition, we shall focus on some new aspects concerning (1) the conductive properties of the TAL, (2) the cotransport systems in the apical and basolateral membrane, (3) the role of Na-K-ATPase, (4) the different means by which sodium chloride reabsorption can be inhibited in the TAL, and (5) the mechanism of stimulation of sodium chloride reabsorption by antidiuretic hormone (ADH) in the mouse medullary TAL.

Conductive Properties of, and Diffusive Fluxes in, the TAL Cell

Studies utilizing transepithelial diffusion potentials [1, 4, 9] and transmembrane diffusion potentials [10–12] have characterized the conductive properties

This manuscript was presented as part of a Symposium on *Transport Mechanisms in Henle's Loop.*

of the individual barriers. The conclusions arrived at (see below) have generally agreed with observations made in the amphibian diluting segment [13, 14] and the flounder intestine [15]. The paracellular pathway is cation-selective; the luminal (apical) cell membrane is conductive to potassium, and the basolateral cell membrane is conductive to chloride. It is interesting that the conductive properties of the cell membranes of chloride-secreting epithelia are reversed, with the basolateral membrane being potassium-conductive [16] and the luminal cell membrane being chloride-conductive [17, 18]. As will be shown, this polarity of the cell is responsible for the lumen-positive PD_{TE} in the TAL and for the lumen-negative PD_{TE} in the secretory epithelia [12]. The cation selectivity of the shunt pathway (see Fig. 1) allows for the passive transport of sodium; the lumen-positive PD_{TE} acts as a driving force for the passive reabsorption of sodium (TAL), and the lumen-negative PD_{TE} acts as a driving force for the passive secretion of sodium (secretory epithelia).

The Paracellular Pathway

As denoted in Table 1, the transepithelial resistance is 34 Ωcm^2 in the cortical TAL segment of the rabbit [9]. The resistance of the paracellular pathway is approximately 47 Ωcm^2 [11]. That this resistance seems to reside almost exclusively in the tight junctions can be deduced from the observation that a marked narrowing of the lateral spaces (after ouabain) does not reduce the cation selectivity of the paracellular shunt pathway [9]. This argument rests on the fact that:

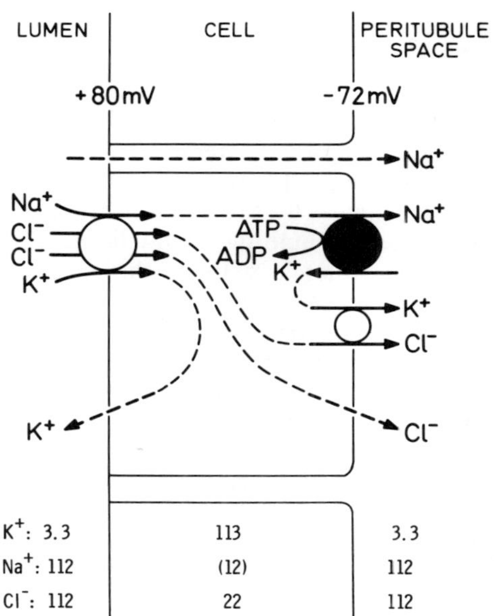

Fig. 1. Cell model for the thick ascending limb. Symbols denote diffusion ($-- \rightarrow$), carrier-mediated transport ($\bigcirc^\rightarrow$), and primary active pump ($\underline{\quad\bullet}^\rightarrow$). At the bottom, activities (mmoles·liter^{-1}) are given for sodium, potassium, and chloride. (Data are taken from [13, 32, 45].)

Table 1. Effect of inhibitors of sodium chloride reabsorption in the thick ascending limb on transepithelial and membrane resistances[a]

	R_{TE}			R_S	R_L	R_{BL}
	(Ωcm^2)	FR_{BL}	VDR		(Ωcm^2)	
Control	34	0.34	1.9	47	88	47
Barium[b]	46[f]	0.03[f]	36[f]	47	1700	47
DPC[c]	38[f]	0.53[f]	0.9[f]	47	88	98
Furosemide[d]	42[f]	0.70[f]	0.4[f]	47	88	220
Ouabain[e]	40[f]	0.03[f]	32[f]	47	>1000	<47

Abbreviations: R_{TE}, R_S, R_L, and R_{BL}, resistances across the epithelium, across the paracellular shunt, across the luminal membrane, and across the basolateral membrane; FR_{BL}, the fractional resistance of the basolateral membrane, that is, the current-pulse-induced voltage deflection across the basolateral membrane divided by that across the epithelium; VDR, the voltage divider ratio, that is, the current-pulse-induced voltage deflection across the lumen membrane divided by that across the basolateral membrane.

[a] R_S, R_L, and R_{BL} are calculated assuming that the inhibitors act mainly on one individual conductance. Data are taken from [6, 11, 43, and from unpublished observations from our laboratory].

[b] Barium was added to lumen at 3 mmoles $\cdot$ liter^{-1}.

[c] Diphenylcarboxylate (DPC) was added to bath at 10^{-4} moles $\cdot$ liter^{-1}.

[d] Furosemide was added to lumen at $5 \cdot 10^{-5}$ moles $\cdot$ liter^{-1}.

[e] Ouabain was added to bath at 10^{-5} moles $\cdot$ liter^{-1}.

[f] The value shown is significantly different from the control value.

$$g^S = \frac{g^{TJ} \cdot g^{LIS}}{g^{TJ} + g^{LIS}} \tag{1}$$

$$g^{LIS} = g^{LIS}_{Na} + g^{LIS}_{\alpha} \tag{2}$$

$$g^{LIS}_{Na}/g^{LIS}_{\alpha} = 0.7 \tag{3}$$

where g^S, g^{TJ}, and g^{LIS} are the conductances of the paracellular pathway, of the tight junctions, and of the lateral interstitial space, respectively. The conductance of the lateral interstitial space, g^{LIS}, is composed essentially of a sodium- and chloride-conductive pathway, and the ratio of these conductances is given by the mobility ratio of 0.7 for Na^+/Cl^- in free solution. If g^{LIS} were the limiting conductance, a reduction of the space width should shift the permselectivity of the entire paracellular pathway (g^S) toward the value of the mobility ratio for Na^+/Cl^- in free solution. This is not the case. Instead, the permeability ratio of sodium to chloride (P_{Na}/P_{Cl}) of the shunt pathway remains between 2 and 3 after ouabain, indicating that the limiting conductance is that of the tight junctions and that the tight junctions are cation-selective.

The permselectivity of the tight junctions is modulated by calcium and magnesium [19]. Increases in the luminal or peritubular calcium or magnesium concentration to 2.5 mmoles$\cdot$liter^{-1} (maximum effect, $\approx$ 5 mmoles$\cdot$liter^{-1}) decrease the P_{NA^+}/P_{Cl^-} from 3.0 to values $\cong$ 2.0; that is, a permselectivity ratio close to the ratio predicted by the free solution mobility is achieved.

Since the transepithelial resistance increases by approximately 20% under these conditions, it appears that calcium or magnesium reduces the sodium conductance of the tight junctions. A very similar finding has been reported for the tight junctions of the gallbladder [20].

As to the integrated function of the TAL segment, the cation selectivity of the shunt, predominant under control conditions, serves to drive sodium across this pathway in the reabsorptive direction. This flux of sodium amounts to some 40% of the total unidirectional sodium flux from lumen to bath [12]. A marked reduction of the passive sodium flux will occur when the permselectivity of the tight junctions is reduced to $\approx$ 2.0. This may, in fact, occur in hypercalcemia and may explain why the reabsorption of sodium chloride in the TAL segment is impaired under these conditions [21].

The Luminal Cell Membrane

The luminal membrane has a resistance on the order of 88 Ωcm^2 [11] (see Table 1), corresponding to a conductance of 11 mS cm^{-2}. The main, if not the only, conducting ion across this membrane seems to be potassium [11]. The potassium conductance can be blocked by barium (see below), which increases the resistance of this membrane by a factor of $\approx$10. A high potassium conductance of the luminal membrane has also been confirmed recently for the mouse medullary TAL [22]. Measurements of the cellular potassium activity in rabbit cortical TAL segments revealed that the activity was approximately 110 mmoles·liter^{-1}, which is some 50 mmoles·liter^{-1} higher than predicted for passive distribution (compare Table 2). From the electrochemical PD for potassium across the luminal membrane of approximately 15 mV and from the potassium conductance of this membrane, a potassium current from cell to lumen of 160 μA cm^{-2} can be calculated. This current is equivalent to a flux of 7 pmoles·cm^{-1}·sec^{-1}, which is about 60% of the rate of net reabsorption of sodium or chloride [5]. As depicted in Figure 1, this ratio is expected for a complete recycling of potassium across the luminal cell membrane, and for a 1Na$^+$:1K$^+$ stoichiometry of the luminal carrier. An almost complete recycling of potassium across the luminal cell membrane

Table 2. Effect of furosemide in isolated perfused cortical thick ascending limb[a]

	PD$_L$	PD$_{BL}$	a_K^{cell}	$a_{K,pass}^{cell}$	a_{Cl}^{cell}	$a_{Cl,pass}^{cell}$
	mV			mmoles · liter^{-1}		
Control	+80	−72	113	58	22	7
Furosemide[b]	+90[c]	−90[c]	117	85	7[c]	5

Abbreviations: PD$_L$ and PD$_{BL}$, potential differences (PD) across the luminal and basolateral membrane, respectively; a^{cell}, measured cellular activity; a_{pass}^{cell}, activity calculated for passive distribution.

[a] For simplification only mean values are given. The data are taken from [32, 45].

[b] The furosemide concentration was 5 · 10^{-5} moles · liter^{-1} (lumen).

[c] The value is significantly different from the control value.

has to be postulated since (1) the lumen fluid contains only little potassium when compared with luminal concentrations of sodium and chloride, and (2) the net transport of potassium in the TAL segment is small when compared to that of sodium and chloride [23, 24]. In fact, inhibition of potassium recycling by barium impedes the reabsorption of sodium chloride [25]. Similar observations have meanwhile been reported for the mouse and rabbit medullary TAL [24, 26], as well as for the diluting segment of the amphibian kidney [27] and for the flounder intestine [28]. Also, the potassium-conductive pathway in the apical membrane seems to be downregulated when Na-K-ATPase is inhibited.

Apart from the potassium conductance, there appears to be no other quantitatively significant conductance in the apical membrane. Specifically, a chloride-conductive pathway [11] and a sodium-conductive pathway have been excluded [6, 29, 30].

The Basolateral Cell Membrane

An increase in the peritubular potassium concentration leads to a depolarization of the basolateral membrane PD (PD_{BL}) in the cortical TAL [10, 12] as well as in the amphibian diluting segment [14]. Similarly, a reduction in peritubular chloride concentration also leads to a depolarization; however, these effects are quite variable [10, 12]. It has been argued that these findings are compatible with one of three constellations: (1) a potassium- and a chloride-conductive pathway in parallel; (2) a potassium-conductive pathway in parallel with a potassium chloride symport; and (3) a chloride-conductive pathway in parallel with a potassium chloride symport. As will be shown in the section "Inhibitors of Sodium Chloride Reabsorption in the TAL," the changes in PD_{BL} induced by alterations of peritubular chloride concentration can be blocked by inhibitors of chloride channels; the changes in PD_{BL} induced by alterations of peritubular potassium concentration can be abolished by barium [12]. On the basolateral cell side, barium does not increase either the transepithelial resistance or the fractional resistance of the basolateral cell membrane. Blockers of the chloride channel, however, clearly increase both these resistances. These data suggest that the potassium pathway in the basolateral membrane, though blocked by barium, is nonconductive. Thus, a constellation of a chloride-conductive pathway in parallel with a potassium chloride symport was postulated for the basolateral membrane of the cortical TAL [12]. The existence of a potassium chloride symport at the basolateral cell side has been postulated recently for the amphibian diluting segment [14, 31]. This symport will be discussed further in the next section.

Recent measurements of intracellular chloride activity obtained in the rabbit cortical TAL (Fig. 1) have shown levels two to three times above passive equilibrium [32]. Thus, the driving force for chloride exit across the basolateral cell membrane is approximately 20 to 30 mV (Table 2). The absolute conductance of this membrane is around 20 mS·cm^{-2} (Table 1). If this conductance were entirely due to chloride, the chloride current leaving the cell ought to be 400 to 600 $\mu A \cdot cm^{-2}$. This value translates into a flux of some 20 pmoles$\cdot cm^{-1} \cdot sec^{-1}$, which is in the same order of magnitude as the rate of chloride absorption in the TAL [5]. This quantitative consideration is hampered by the fact that responses of PD_{BL} to changes in the basolateral chloride concentration are variable [12]. Recently, it has been speculated that this variability may be caused by variations in intracellular chloride [30]. The chloride conductance (g_{Cl}^{BL}) was strongly dependent on the cellular chloride activity; with a reduction of cell chloride, g_{Cl}^{BL} fell [6] and it rose with an increase in cell chloride (see also Table 1). The basolateral chloride conductance can be blocked by anthracene-9-COO^- and even more effectively by diphenylamine-2-COO^-. This blocking and the effects of hormonal stimulation on the chloride conductance will be discussed in later sections of this chapter.

Figure 1 indicates the conductive pathways that have been discussed thus far. The potassium flux from cell to lumen, the chloride flux from cell to peritubular space, and the sodium flux across the shunt pathway comprise a current loop. The transcellular path of this loop generates the transepithelial lumen-positive PD. The paracellular pathway dissipates this PD by moving sodium passively from the lumen to the peritubular side. The lumen-positive PD is sustained as long as potassium and chloride are kept above equilibrium by the inward movement of these ions via the $Na^+2Cl^-K^+$ carrier (see below). The advantage of this type of sodium chloride reabsorption over the previously postulated [33] mode via a Na^+Cl^- carrier (with a stoichiometry of 1:1) is obvious. The latter system operates at a $3Na^+/ATP$ stoichiometry; the former, however, reaches a stoichiometry of up to $6Na^+/ATP$, since up to 50% of total sodium can be reabsorbed passively.

Cotransport Systems in the TAL

Thus far, the following carrier systems have been claimed to exist in the TAL: (1) Na^+Cl^- cotransport [4], (2) $Na^+2Cl^-K^+$ cotransport [25], (3) Na^+H^+ countertransport [34], (4) OH^-Cl^- countertransport [34], (5) K^+Cl^- cotransport [12]. Other systems such as Na^+-glucose or Na^+-amino acid cotransport have been ruled out at least for the luminal membrane [35]. The Na^+Cl^- cotransport, originally postulated to explain the secondary active nature of chloride reabsorption in the TAL, has been abandoned, meanwhile, because it is generally accepted that potassium participates in the carrier-mediated uptake of Na^+ and $2Cl^-$ [22]. Also, the coexistence of the $Na^+2Cl^-K^+$ cotransport and of the Na^+/H^+ and Cl^-/OH^- antiporters in the luminal cell membrane seems to be a finding unique to the mouse cortical TAL [34]. In the rabbit cortical TAL, as well as the medullary portion of the mouse TAL, no evidence is available for the two antiporter systems [23, 30]. The evidence for the symport of Na^+, Cl^-, and K^+ in the luminal membrane of a diluting segment is compelling [11–13, 23, 26, 36–40]. The carrier in the secretory epithelia, localized there in the basolateral membrane, seems to have the $Na^+2Cl^-K^+$ stoichiometry [40]. The evidence for the potassium chloride symport on the basolateral cell side, however, is still indirect (see below).

$Na^+2Cl^-K^+$ Cotransport

The existence of the $Na^+2Cl^-K^+$ cotransport was originally suggested on the basis of transepithelial measurements of the equivalent short-circuit current (I_{SC}) as a function of sodium, potassium, and chloride concentrations [3, 25, 41] in the perfusates. These data are summarized in Figure 2. Three aspects are noteworthy: (1) The curves for sodium and potassium are steep in the low-concentration range and reach the maximum I_{SC} at relatively low concentrations. (2) The dependence of I_{SC} on the potassium concentration has an intercept, since the bath potassium was kept at 2 mmoles·liter^{-1} and potassium backleak is likely to occur when the lumen potassium concentration is reduced below 2 mmoles·liter^{-1}. Note that the luminal cell membrane will be hyperpolarized at low luminal potassium concentrations, and part of this hyperpolarization will be apparent as a lumen-positive PD$_{TE}$ generated by a circular current loop. In addition, a small lumen-positive PD$_{TE}$ will be generated because of the cation selectivity of the paracellular pathway. The correction for the latter two factors, at a lumen concentration of 0.5 mmoles·liter^{-1}, is on the order of 2 mV, that is, 70 μA cm^{-2} (unpublished observations). (3) Unlike the curves for sodium and probably potassium,

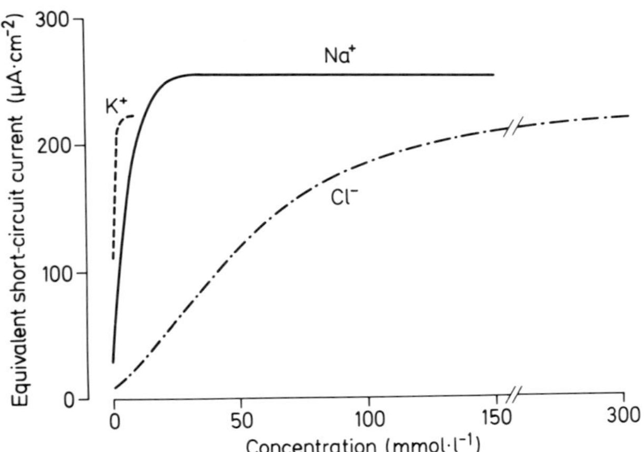

Fig. 2. Equivalent short-circuit current in the cortical thick ascending limb as a function of sodium, potassium, and chloride concentration. Each *curve* (mean values taken from [3, 41] and unpublished observations from our laboratory) was obtained by varying the concentration of one ion and keeping the two other ions at control values (sodium, 150; chloride, 150; potassium, 4.4 mmoles·liter^{-1}). For sodium and chloride, ion replacements were done symmetrically, that is, on both sides of the epithelium. Potassium was only reduced in the lumen perfusate, with the bath potassium concentration set at 2 mmoles·liter^{-1} (a value at which the sodium-potassium pump is not inhibited; unpublished observation from our laboratory).

the curve for chloride is sigmoid, revealing a Hill coefficient of 2. The apparent affinities to the three ions are: Na^+, 3 to 4; K^+, 1; and Cl^-, 50 mmoles·liter^{-1}. These values obviously describe only the case where one ion is varied and the others are at control levels. Very similar apparent affinities have been reported for the amphibian diluting segment [37]. Also, similar values for the apparent K_m's for sodium and chloride have been obtained in membrane vesicles prepared from medullary TAL cells [42]. These data are direct proof for the $Na^+2Cl^-K^+$ coupling inasmuch as they show that sodium uptake is both chloride- and potassium-dependent and that potassium uptake (measured as rubidium uptake) is chloride- and sodium-dependent. Both the uptake of sodium and rubidium are inhibited by furosemide. Furthermore, it has been shown in the cortical TAL segment that furosemide, by reducing cellular chloride, induces a hyperpolarization of PD_{BL} and that the same hyperpolarization is achieved when either luminal sodium or chloride are removed [43]. In the amphibian diluting segment, it was reported that either removal of luminal chloride, sodium, potassium or the addition of furosemide to the lumen perfusate reduces cellular sodium and chloride [13, 27, 44]. Therefore evidence is most consistent with the view that the carrier serves to transport all three ion species and that it has an absolute requirement for all three ions. With respect to the stoichiometry, firm conclusions are not possible at present. A $1Na^+:1K^+$ stoichiometry was suggested on the basis of a quantitative estimation of potassium recycling across the luminal cell membrane [11, 30]. A $2Cl^-:1Na^+$ stoichiometry is based on the transepithelial kinetics (see Fig. 2) [3, 37, 41] and on the Hill coefficients obtained in vesicle studies [38]. A more direct measurement of the stoichiometry was obtained recently in the rectal gland (Greger and Schlatter, submitted for publication). There it was shown that the initial rate at which cellular chloride declines after furosemide was twice as rapid as that for sodium. A $1Na^+:2Cl^-:1K^+$ stoichiometry was also postulated on the basis that this carrier is electrically silent [41]. From this stoichiometry and measurements of the cellular ion activity, a driving force for the carrier of some 50 to 70 mV can be calculated. It should be mentioned at this point that the participation of potassium in the carrier-mediated uptake of sodium and chloride serves to keep cellular potassium high [46]. The high cellular potassium hyperpolarizes the TAL cell and thus generates the lumen-positive PD_{TE} that is needed to move sodium passively across the shunt pathway. It is apparent from Figure 1 that the carrier is driven by the chemical potentials of chloride and sodium and that inhibition of the sodium-potassium pump will lead to an increase in cellular chloride and sodium (the increase in sodium may be smaller than that of chloride) until the carrier stops to operate (see below). The interaction of furosemide and related diuretics will be discussed under "Inhibitors of Sodium Chloride in the TAL."

Basolateral KCl Cotransport

In the preceding section on conductance properties, we briefly summarized the indirect evidence pointing toward the existence of this cotransport system in the basolateral membrane of the TAL. The key finding was a nonconductive movement of potassium associated with that of chloride [12]. A potassium chloride symport was also postulated from more recent data in the amphibian diluting segment, where it was shown that inhibition of the chloride exit by anthracene-9-COO$^-$ did not completely abolish the reabsorption of sodium chloride [31]. Furthermore, it was shown that at least in some of these diluting segment cells the basolateral conductances were far too small to explain the observed transepithelial reabsorptive flux on the basis of a conductive movement [14]. A basolateral potassium chloride symport has also been postulated recently for the gallbladder [46, 47] and for the amphibian proximal tubule [48]. It was shown that the movement of chloride across the basolateral cell membrane in these tissues was much larger than could be accounted for by the chloride conductance. Furthermore, it was shown that intracellular chloride increases when bath potassium is increased. A potassium chloride symport as a recycling pathway for the potassium taken up by the basolateral Na-K-ATPase activity has the advantage that the chemical potential of potassium is utilized *directly* to move chloride out of the cell against an unfavorable chemical potential for chloride. Two parallel conductive pathways for potassium and chloride can also lead to such coupling. The hyperpolarization caused by a cellular concentration of potassium above equilibrium would serve to drive out chloride; and conversely, the depolarization caused by a cell concentration of chloride above equilibrium would drive out potassium. However, in the special case of the TAL, any significant potassium conductance of the basolateral membrane would lead to an interruption of the circular current loop and thus compromise the lumen-positive transepithelial PD [12]. Therefore, for the TAL, the operation of a potassium chloride symport rather than two parallel conductances serves to sustain the most economical mode of sodium chloride reabsorption (see above). It has been shown that barium (1 to 3 mmoles·liter^{-1}) inhibits this symport in the TAL just as it inhibits the potassium conductance of the luminal cell membrane. Also, it has been reported that the potassium chloride symport can be blocked by high doses of furosemide [49]. Unfortunately, so specific inhibitor is known thus far for this pathway.

Other Carrier Systems

The mouse cortical TAL seems to be unique inasmuch as it has two means of entry into the cell for sodium chloride: (1) the $Na^+2Cl^-K^+$ cotransporter, and (2) a parallel arrangement of Na^+/H^+ and Cl^-/OH^- antiporters [34]. Little or no net transport of HCO_3^- is provided by this system, since the Na^+/H^+ and Cl^-/OH^- exchangers operate at similar rates. Still, all the sodium chloride reabsorption in the mouse TAL can be blocked by furosemide. High doses (10^{-4} moles·liter^{-1}) were used in this study, and thus it seems likely that furosemide did not block only the $Na^+2Cl^-K^+$ carrier but also the Cl^-/OH^- exchanger [50]. On the other hand, the Na^+/H^+ and Cl^-/OH^--mediated portion of sodium chloride reabsorption can be blocked by removal of bicarbonate from the perfusates or by addition of ethoxzolamide (a lipophilic carboanhydrase inhibitor) or the stilbene derivative SITS. It is tempting to speculate that the mouse cortical TAL resembles a nephron portion that combines properties of the diluting segment with that of the early distal tubule. A comparable observation, namely, that the diluting segment has an additional component of sodium entry, has been shown recently for the amphibian diluting segment [51]. When the animal was adapted to high potassium (and low sodium) concentrations, an amiloride-sensitive Na^+/H^+ exchanger was demonstrable that was absent in control animals.

The Sodium-Potassium Pump in the Basolateral Membrane and the Generation of ATP

The role of the sodium-potassium pump in the reabsorption of sodium chloride has already been discussed (see Fig. 1). Recent studies of the TAL have focused on two aspects: (1) How is the ATP generated to drive this pump? (2) How much of the ATP consumption of the pump is utilized for sodium chloride reabsorption via the pathways that are described above? First, it was found that removal of metabolic substrates led to a rapid decline of active sodium chloride reabsorption (Wittner, Weidtke, Schlatter, Di Stefano, and Greger, submitted). After only 10 min of substrate-free perfusion, the equivalent short-circuit current was reduced to 20 to 30%, and only a partial recovery was observed when the substrates were readmitted. This strong dependence on the presence of substrates is an expression of the high rates of sodium chloride reabsorption, corresponding to high rates of ATP consumption, and of small energy stores. Next, it was shown that substrate uptake occurs exclusively from the peritubular side and that the monocarboxylic acids, such as acetate, L-lactate, β-OH-butyrate, and pyruvate, as well as the sugars D-glucose and D-mannose, are good substrates. The metabolism is strictly aerobic. Finally, it was shown that substrate removal from, or ouabain addition to, the peritubular side led to cell swelling and a depolarization of PD_{BL} only if the $Na^+2Cl^-K^+$ cotransport system was operating. If the carrier were blocked by furosemide, substrate removal or ouabain addition were easily tolerated (Table 3) [30, 52]. These data indicate (1) that essentially

Table 3. Effect of furosemide on rabbit cortical thick ascending limb in the absence and in the presence of ouabain[a]

	Control	Furosemide[b]	Ouabain[c]	Ouabain + furosemide
PD_{TE}, (mV)	+8	$\approx 0^d$	$\approx +1^d$	$\approx 0^d$
PD_{BL}, (mV)	−72	$−90^d$	$−23^d$	$−90^d$

Abbreviations: PD_{TE}, transepithelial potential difference; PD_{BL}, PD across the basolateral membrane.
[a] For reasons of simplification, only mean values are reported. Data were taken from [6, 43].
[b] The furosemide concentration was $5 \cdot 10^{-5}$ moles $\cdot$ liter^{-1} (lumen).
[c] The ouabain concentration was 10^{-5} moles $\cdot$ liter^{-1} (bath).
[d] The value is significantly different from the control value.

the entire ATP consumption reflects active reabsorption of sodium chloride and (2) that furosemide reduces the turnover of the Na-K-ATPase to rates not distinguishable from zero. These data emphasize how loop diuretics like furosemide can be used to protect the TAL against the hazards of substrate shortage and hypoxia [6].

Inhibitors of Sodium Chloride Reabsorption in the TAL

The process of sodium chloride reabsorption in the TAL can be impeded or interrupted at several levels. In fact, it is possible to inhibit each of the individual components depicted in Figure 1. Already, we have described how substrate removal (or inhibition of substrate uptake) can inhibit sodium chloride reabsorption. At the level of Na-K-ATPase activity, inhibition is possible not only by ouabain but also by phloretin [53] (see below). The potassium chloride symport can be blocked by barium and the conductive chloride exit by anthracene-9-COO^- or even more effectively by diphenyla-mine-2-COO^- (see below). On the luminal cell side, the $Na^+2Cl^-K^+$ cotransport system can be blocked completely by diuretics related to furosemide (see below). The potassium recycling pathway of this membrane is blocked by barium (see below). And, finally, even the sodium conductance of the tight junctions can be blocked by the addition of the divalent cations, calium or magnesium (see the preceding section on "Conductive Properties," under "Paracellular Pathways").

Barium Inhibition of the Luminal Potassium Conductance

We have already stated that barium can block the potassium-recycling pathway in the TAL [11, 26] and in the amphibian diluting segment [27]. The results of this inhibition are (1) a reduction in the active transport PD across the epithelium, (2) an increase in transepithelial resistance, and (3) an increase in the resistance of the apical membrane (see Table 1). Furthermore, as indicated in Figure 3a, barium depolarizes the luminal PD and abolishes the depolarization induced by a rapid increase in luminal potassium concentration. The explanation of these findings would be straightforward except for two observations: (1) Why was the collapse in transepithelial PD not complete? (2) Why did the luminal PD depolarize after barium? One would predict that a complete inhibition of the potassium conductance should abolish PD_{TE} completely. Since PD_{TE} decreased only to 50%, one might argue that barium inhibition was incomplete. However, the potassium recycling is defined by

$$I_{K^+}^{cell \rightarrow lumen} = g_{K^+}^L (\Delta \tilde{\mu}/F)_{K^+}^L$$

Even if barium reduced $g_{K^+}^L$ to only 10%, $I_{K^+}^{cell \rightarrow lumen}$ would not be reduced as much, since the electrochemical driving force, $(\Delta \tilde{\mu}/F)_{K^+}^L$, for potassium recycling increases after barium (the luminal membrane depolarizes by 27 mV). Thus, $(\Delta \tilde{\mu}/F)_{K^+}^L$ will be 42 instead of 15 mV, and $I_{K^+}^{cell \rightarrow lumen}$ will be reduced to only 30%. The increase in $(\Delta \tilde{\mu}/F)_{K^+}^L$ may even be more marked, since cell potassium is expected to rise after barium. This has recently been

Fig. 3. a Inhibition of the luminal potassium conductance by barium (3 mmoles·liter⁻¹) and **b** of the basolateral conductance by diphenylamine carboxylate (*DPC*), 10^{-4} mmoles·liter⁻¹. The luminal membrane PD (PD_L) is depolarized significantly by barium. A potassium concentration step in the lumen from 4.4 to 19 mmoles·liter⁻¹ leads to a marked depolarization under control conditions, but has no significant effect (*NS*) in the presence of barium. The basolateral membrane PD (PD_{BL}) is hyperpolarized significantly by DPC. A chloride concentration step in the bath perfusate from 150 to 50 mmoles⁻¹ leads to a marked depolarization under control conditions, but has no significant effect in the presence of DPC.

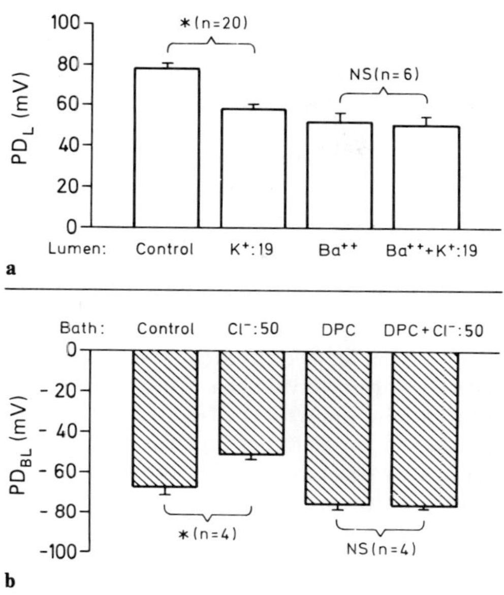

shown for the rectal gland (Greger and Schlatter, submitted). To conclude this consideration, an incomplete inhibition of PD$_{TE}$ is to be expected even though the examination of the potassium conductance reveals a $\approx$ 80 to 90% inhibition. The depolarization of the luminal PD after barium can be explained on the basis of the scheme shown in Figure 1. Blocking the potassium-conductive pathway by barium will drive PD$_{BL}$ toward the chemical PD of chloride and will also depolarize the luminal cell membrane, since the two cell membranes are partially short-circuited by the paracellular pathway. In fact, the depolarization is diminished or abolished if cellular chloride is first reduced by furosemide. Now the chemical PD for chloride is close to the chemical potential of potassium, and barium loses its depolarizing effect (Greger and Schlatter, submitted).

Inhibition of Chloride Conductance by Anthracene-9-COO⁻ (A9C) and by Diphenylamine-2-COO⁻ (DPC)

A9C has been described as an inhibitor of chloride conductance in neuromuscular membranes [54]. In the diluting segment of the amphibian kidney, it has a strong inhibitory effect [31]. The effect is less marked in the rabbit cortical TAL [43]. A recent systematic search of compounds related to A9C led to DPC, which is more effective in the rabbit cortical TAL [55]. DPC increases the transepithelial resistance, reduces the PD$_{TE}$ by 60 to 80%, and increases the resistance of the basolateral membrane (Table 1). In addition, the depolarization of PD$_{BL}$, observed after the reduction in bath chloride concentration, disappears in the presence of DPC (Fig. 3). The hyperpolarization of PD_{BL} after DPC can be explained by a shift of the cell PD toward the chemical PD of potassium. Again, inhibition of the chloride current from cell to peritubular space ($I_{Cl^-}^{cell \rightarrow bath}$) will be less, proportionally, than the inhibition of the chloride conductance, since the driving force for chloride exit increases after DPC (PD_{BL} hyperpolarizes). Also, an increase in cellular chloride has been shown in the amphibian diluting segment after A9C [31].

Inhibition of the $Na^+2Cl^-K^+$ Cotransporter by Furosemide

The molecular requirements for a diuretic to interact with the $Na^+2Cl^-K^+$ cotransporter have been studied recently [56]. The key findings were (1) that interaction with the $Na^+2Cl^-K^+$ carrier necessitates a molecular structure related to furosemide, and (2) that the side chain of the molecule reacting with the carrier is probably the anionic group of position 1. A similar conclusion was drawn recently from affinity binding studies in membranes prepared from the rectal gland [40] and from the renal medulla [57]. Also, it has been shown that the Tamm-Horsfall protein, lining the luminal membrane of the TAL [58], exhibits affinity binding to furosemide. This binding occurs only in the presence of sodium, chloride, and potassium with apparent $K_{1/2}$ values very similar to the ones reported in the section on "$Na^+2Cl^-K^+$ Cotransport." Still, however, evidence is lacking that the Tamm-Horsfall protein is present in all cells for which the furosemide-sensitive $Na^+2Cl^-K^+$ carrier has been demonstrated.

The observations made after the addition of furosemide to the lumen perfusate in the TAL are summarized in Tables 1, 2, and 3. The PD_{TE} collapses, both cell membranes hyperpolarize to the same value, cellular chloride falls to passive equilibrium values, and cellular potassium stays constant [10, 32, 41, 45]. The transepithelial resistance increases [5, 59] after furosemide, because the chloride conductance of the basolateral membrane decreases [6]. Identical observations have been made in the amphibian diluting segment [13, 36, 60]. All these effects of furosemide can be explained simply by an interference with the $Na^+2Cl^-K^+$ cotransporter. As a first step, the entry of Na^+, $2Cl^-$, and K^+ will be blocked. Chloride will continue to leak out of the cell until the electrochemical driving force for chloride exit becomes zero. Cellular sodium will fall [13] until a minimal value is achieved and the sodium-potassium pump is blocked by the high cellular potassium. During the period of falling cellular sodium, potassium will still be pumped into the cell. This flux balances the potassium diffusion from cell to lumen, thus maintaining cellular potassium fairly constant after furosemide. The PD of both cell membranes is pulled toward the chemical potential of potassium; that is, the cell hyperpolarizes. The fall in basolateral chloride conductance has been explained by the fall in cellular chloride [30]. All these events occur within seconds and probably even less than 1 sec after the addition of furosemide [41]. This extremely rapid response is possible because of the small volume of the cortical TAL cells and because these cells have such high rates of transepithelial sodium chloride transport.

Inhibition of Na-K-ATPase Activity by Ouabain and Phloretin

The effects of adding ouabain or phloretin to the peritubular perfusate are summarized in Tables 1 and 3. In the case of ouabain, an IC_{50} in the micromolar range is obtained for the rabbit cortical TAL segment. The effects are poorly reversible. The transepithelial PD collapses, and PD_{BL} depolarizes. The cells swell [6, 30]. Phloretin in doses greater than 50 μmoles·liter^{-1} probably also acts on Na-K-ATPase and not through inhibition of mitochondrial ATP production, since the phloretin effect is rapid and easily reversible (provided exposure lasted for less than 3 min). Transepithelial resistance increases because the apical membrane potassium conductance is reduced dramatically (see Table 1). A comparable observation has been made recently in the rectal gland (Greger and Schlatter, submitted). There it was shown that ouabain reduces the basolateral potassium conductance and thus results in an almost constant cellular potassium concentration. The depolarization was accounted for entirely by an increase in cellular chloride and a concomitant increase in the apical chloride conductance. These events in the TAL cell and in the rectal gland cell are examples of the postulated feedback between the sodium-potassium pump and the potassium conductance [59]. One advantage of this type of feedback has been pointed out recently (Greger and Schlatter, submitted). In a transient state of ATP shortage, cellular potassium is kept high because the conductance is shut down. During recovery, the channel will open and the high cellular potassium will hyperpolarize the cell instantaneously and thus drive out the chloride gained during the period of ATP shortage. In other words, chloride can be driven out without the need to increase cellular potassium first by active pumping.

Table 3 also contains PD_{TE} and PD_{BL} values for simultaneous application of ouabain and furosemide. The important finding is that the cell loses its sensitivity to ouabain completely when the $Na^+2Cl^-K^+$ cotransport is blocked by furosemide.

Stimulation of Sodium Chloride Reabsorption by Cyclic AMP

In mouse and rat medullary TAL, sodium chloride reabsorption is controlled by vasopressin [4, 63, 64]. This response is mediated by cyclic AMP and can also be elicited by isoproterenol, glucagon, and calcitonin [65]. The acute effects of *db*-cyclic AMP comprise an increase in the net reabsorption of sodium chloride and an increase in PD_{TE}. Recently, it has been shown that the transepithelial resistance falls after cyclic AMP [26, 64]. For chloride-transporting epithelia, it has been claimed that cyclic AMP stimulation acts through an increase in the chloride conductance [33]. Recently, it was found for the rectal gland that a cyclic AMP-induced increase in chloride conductance was in fact the primary event (Greger, Schlatter, Wang, and Forrest, submitted). In contrast, it was postulated that in the mouse medullary TAL

Table 4. Effect of stimulation on medullary thick ascending limb of mice[a]

	PD_{TE} (mV)	R_{TE} (Ωcm^2)	I_{SC} ($\mu A\ cm^{-2}$)	PD_{BL} (mV)
Nonstimulated	+6	24	290	−81
Stimulated[b]	+12[c]	20[c]	660[c]	−68[c]

Abbreviations: PD_{TE}, transepithelial potential difference; R_{TE}, transepithelial resistance; I_{SC}, equivalent short-circuit current; PD_{BL}, PD across the basolateral membrane.

[a] For reasons of simplification, only mean values are reported. Data were taken from [66].

[b] Stimulators were *db*-cyclic AMP ($4 \cdot 10^{-4}$), forskolin (10^{-6}), and ADH (10^{-9} moles $\cdot$ liter^{-1}) added to bath.

[c] The value is significantly different from the nonstimulated value.

the primary event should be an increase in the luminal potassium conductance [22, 26]. This question is currently under study, and preliminary data [66] are summarized in Table 4. It is evident that the fall in transepithelial resistance is accompanied by a depolarization luminal of PD and of PD_{BL}. This suggests that cyclic AMP leads to an increase in basolateral chloride conductance. In fact, paired measurements of the fractional resistance of this membrane [66] support this view. We conclude that in the TAL cell, as in other chloride-transporting epithelia, stimulation by cyclic AMP is expressed primarily as an increase in the chloride conductance.

Conclusion

This chapter was intended to supplement several excellent reviews already published [5, 7, 8] with recent findings on (1) the individual transport components in the TAL cell, (2) how they can be inhibited, and (3) possible modes of their regulation. The latter aspect is still very new and will be one area of further extensive research. Also, this chapter did not touch controversial points of the mechanisms of electrolyte transport in the TAL, namely (1) the mechanism of calcium and magnesium reabsorption, (2) the modulation of net potassium transport, (3) the mechanism of ammonium and bicarbonate transport. These three topics are currently under study and will certainly be the focus of later reviews.

Seen from the viewpoint of comparative biology, one of the most intriguing fields of research will be the purification of the $Na^+2Cl^-K^+$ carrier, which, now that one is searching for it, has appeared in many different tissues.

Acknowledgment. This work was supported by Deutsche Forschungsgemeinschaft Gr 480/4-8.

References

1. BURG M, GREEN N: Function of the thick ascending limb of Henle's loop. *Am J Physiol* 224:659–668, 1973
2. ROCHA AS, KOKKO JP: Sodium chloride and water transport in the medullary thick ascending limb of Henle. *J Clin Invest* 52:612–624, 1973
3. GREGER R: Chloride reabsorption in the rabbit cortical thick ascending limb of the loop of Henle. *Pflügers Arch* 390:38–43, 1981
4. HEBERT SC, CULPEPPER RM, ANDREOLI TE: NaCl transport in mouse medullary thick ascending limbs: I. Functional nephron heterogeneity and ADH-stimulated NaCl cotransport. *Am J Physiol* 241:F412–F431, 1981
5. BURG MB: Thick ascending limb of Henle's loop. *Kidney Int* 22:454–464, 1982
6. GREGER R, SCHLATTER E: Cellular mechanism of the action of loop diuretics on the thick ascending limb of Henle's loop. *Klin Wochenschr* 61:1019–1027, 1983
7. HEBERT SC, ANDREOLI TE: Salt and water transport in the mouse medullary thick ascending limb: Role of antidiuretic hormone, in *Membranes and Transport,* edited by MARTONOSI A. New York, London, Plenum Press, 1982, pp 187–196
8. BURG M, GOOD D: Sodium chloride coupled transport in mammalian nephrons. *Ann Rev Physiol* 45:533–547, 1983
9. GREGER R: Cation selectivity of the isolated perfused cortical thick ascending limb of Henle's loop of the rabbit kidney. *Pflügers Arch* 390:30–37, 1981
10. GREGER R: Coupled transport of Na^+ and Cl^- in the thick ascending limb of Henle's loop of rabbit nephron. *Scand Audiol (Suppl)* 14:1–15, 1981
11. GREGER R, SCHLATTER E: Properties of the lumen membrane of the cortical thick ascending limb of Henle's loop of rabbit kidney. *Pflügers Arch* 396:315–324, 1983
12. GREGER R, SCHLATTER E: Properties of the basolateral membrane of the cortical thick ascending limb of Henle's loop of rabbit kidney. *Pflügers Arch* 396:325–334, 1983
13. OBERLEITHNER H, GIEBISCH G, LANG F, WANG W: Cellular mechanism of the furosemide sensitive transport system in the kidney. *Klin Wochenschr* 60:1173–1179, 1982
14. GUGGINO WB: Hydraulic and electrical properties of the amphiuma diluting segment: Evidence for cellular heterogeneity (*abstract*). *Kidney Int* 25:301, 1984
15. MUSCH MW, ORELLANA SA, KIMBERG LS, FIELD M, HALM DR, KRASNY EJ JR, FRIZZELL RA: Na^+-K^+-Cl^- cotransport in the intestine of a marine teleost. *Nature* 300:351–353, 1982
16. WELSH MJ: Barium inhibition of basolateral membrane potassium conductance in tracheal epithelium. *Am J Physiol* 244:F639–F645, 1983
17. REUSS L, REINACH P, WEINMAN SA, GRADY TP: Intracellular ion activities and Cl^- transport mechanisms in bullfrog corneal epithelium. *Am J Physiol* 244:C336–C347, 1983
18. SHOROFSKY SR, FIELD M, FOZZARD HA: The cellular mechanism of active chloride secretion in vertebrate epithelia: Studies in intestine and trachea. *Philos Trans R Soc Lond [Biol]* 299:597–607, 1982
19. DI STEFANO A, WITTNER M, GEBLER B, GREGER R: Increased Ca^{++} or Mg^{++} reduces the Na^+ conductance of the paracellular pathway in isolated perfused cortical thick ascending limbs of Henle loops (cTAL) of rabbit kidney. *Pflügers Arch* (in press, 1984)
20. BARRY PH, DIAMOND JM, WRIGHT EM: The mechanism of cation permeation

in rabbit gallbladder, dilution potentials and bionic potentials. *J Membr Biol* 4:358–394, 1971

21. SUTTON RAL, WONG NLM, QUAMME GA, DIRKS JH: Renal tubular calcium transport: Effects of changes in filtered calcium load. *Am J Physiol* 245:F515–F520, 1983

22. HEBERT SC, ANDREOLI TE: The effects of antidiuretic hormone on cellular conductive pathways in mouse medullary thick ascending limbs of Henle: II. Determinants of the ADH-mediated increases in transepithelial voltage and in net Cl⁻ absorption. *J Membr Biol* (in press, 1984)

23. BURG MB, BOURDEAU JE: Function of the thick ascending limb of Henle's loop, in *New Aspects of Renal Function,* vol 6, edited by VOGEL HG, ULLRICH KJ, Amsterdam, Oxford, Excerpta Medica, 1978, pp 91–102

24. STOKES JB: Consequences of potassium recycling in the renal medulla: Effects on ion transport by the medullary thick ascending limb of Henle's loop. *J Clin Invest* 70:219–229, 1982

25. GREGER R, SCHLATTER E: Presence of luminal K^+, a prerequisite for active NaCl transport in the cortical thick ascending limb of Henle's loop of rabbit kidney. *Pflügers Arch* 392:92–94, 1981

26. HEBERT SC, FRIEDMAN PA, ANDREOLI TE: The effects of antidiuretic hormone on cellular conductive pathways in mouse medullary thick ascending limbs of Henle. I. ADH increases transcellular conductance pathways. *J Membr Biol* (in press, 1984)

27. OBERLEITHNER H, GREGER R, NEUMANN S, LANG F, GIEBISCH G, DEETJEN P: Omission of luminal potassium reduces cellular chloride in early distal tubule of amphibian kidney. *Pflügers Arch* 398:18–22, 1983

28. HALM DR, KRASNY EJ JR, FRIZZELL RA: Inhibition of K-independent Na/Cl uptake increases apical membrane K conductance in flounder intestine. *Bull Mount Des Isl Biol Lab* 22:80–82, 1982

29. GREGER R, SCHLATTER E, WEIDTKE C, WITTNER M: Active NaCl transport in the cortical thick ascending limb of Henle's loop (cTAL) of rabbit nephron does not require the presence of bicarbonate (*abstract*). *Pflügers Arch* 394:65, 1982

30. GREGER R, WITTNER M, SCHLATTER E, DI STEFANO A: $Na^+2Cl^-K^+$-cotransport in the thick ascending limb of Henle's loop and mechanism of action of loop diuretics, in *Coupled Transport in Nephron,* edited by HOSHI T, Tokyo, Miura Foundation (in press, 1984)

31. OBERLEITHNER H, RITTER M, LANG G, GUGGINO W: Antracene-9-carboxylic acid inhibits renal chloride reabsorption. *Pflügers Arch* 398:172–174, 1983

32. GREGER R, OBERLEITHNER H, SCHLATTER E, CASSOLA AC: Chloride activity in cells of isolated perfused cortical thick ascending limbs of rabbit kidney. *Pflügers Arch* 399:29–34, 1983

33. FRIZZELL RA, FIELD M, SCHULTZ SG: Sodium-coupled chloride transport by epithelial tissues. *Am J Physiol* 236:F1–F8, 1979

34. FRIEDMAN PA, ANDREOLI TE: CO_2-stimulated NaCl absorption in the mouse renal cortical thick ascending limb of Henle. Evidence for synchronous Na^+/H^+ and Cl^-/HCO^- exchange in apical plasma membranes. *J Gen Physiol* 80:683–711, 1982

35. SCHLATTER E, GREGER E: Metabolic substrates for maintaining active NaCl transport in the isolated cortical thick ascending limb (cTAL) of rabbit kidney (*abstract*). *Pflügers Arch* 394:64, 1982

36. OBERLEITHNER H, GUGGINO W, GIEBISCH G: Mechanism of distal tubular chloride transport in Amphiuma kidney. *Am J Physiol* 342:F331–F339, 1982

37. HOSHI T, KURAMOCHI G, YOSHITOMI K: Lumen-positive chloride transport potential in the early distal tubule of Triturus kidney: Its absolute dependence on the presence of Na$^+$ and K$^+$ in the luminal fluid. *Jpn J Physiol* 33:855–861, 1983

38. NISHIMURA H, IMAI M, OGAWA M: Transepithelial voltage in reptilian and mammalian-type nephrons from Japanese quail (*abstract*). *Fed Proc* 42:70, 1983

39. NISHIMURA H, IMAI M, OGAWA M: Sodium chloride and water transport in the renal distal tubule of the rainbow trout. *Am J Physiol* 244:F247–F254, 1983

40. HANNAFIN J, KINNE-SAFFRAN E, FRIEDMANN D, KINNE R: Presence of a sodium potassium chloride cotransport system in the rectal gland of *Squalus acanthias*. *J Membr Biol* 75:73–83, 1983

41. GREGER R, SCHLATTER E, LANG F: Evidence for electroneutral sodium chloride cotransport in the cortical thick ascending limb of Henle's loop of rabbit kidney. *Pflügers Arch* 396:308–314, 1983

42. KOENIG B, RICAPITO S, KINNE R: Chloride transport in the thick ascending limb of Henle's loop: potassium dependence and stoichiometry of the NaCl cotransport system in plasma membrane vesicles. *Pflügers Arch* 399:173–179, 1983

43. GREGER R, WARNOCK DG, GREGER R, DUNHAM PB, FRIZZELL RA, FIELD M, SPRING KR, IVES HE, ARONSON PS, SEIFTER J: Symposium: Ion transport processes in apical membranes of epithelia. *Fed Proc* (in press, 1984)

44. OBERLEITHNER H, GUGGINO W, GIEBISCH G: The effect of furosemide on luminal sodium, chloride and potassium transport in the early distal tubule of Amphiuma kidney. Effects of potassium adaptation. *Pflügers Arch* 396:27–33, 1983

45. GREGER R, WEIDTKE C, SCHLATTER E, WITTNER M, GEBLER B: Potassium activity in cells of isolated perfused cortical thick ascending limbs of rabbit kidney. *Pflügers Arch* (in press, 1984)

46. REUSS L: Basolateral KCl co-transport in a NaCl-absorbing epithelium. *Nature* 305:723–726, 1983

47. ARMSTRONG WM, CORCIA A, GARCIA-DIAZ JF, BAXENDALE LM: Use of ion-selective microelectrodes to study ion transport mechanisms in epithelial cells. *Proc XXIXth Int Congr Physiol Sci*, Sydney, Australia, 1983, p 174

48. SHINDO T, SPRING KR: Chloride movement across the basolateral membrane of proximal tubule cells. *J Membr Biol* 58:35–42, 1981

49. DUNHAM PB, WARNOCK DG, GREGER R, FRIZZELL RA, FIELD M, SPRING KR, IVES HE, ARONSON PS, SEIFTER J: Symposium: Ion transport processes in apical membranes of epithelia. *Fed Proc* (in press, 1984)

50. ARONSON PS, WARNOCK DG, GREGER R, DUNHAM PB, FRIZZELL RA, FIELD M, SPRING KR, IVES HE, ARONSON PS, SEIFTER J: Symposium: Ion transport processes in apical membranes of epithelia. *Fed Proc* (in press, 1984)

51. OBERLEITHNER H, LANG F, WANG W, MESSNER G, DEETJEN P: Evidence for an amiloride sensitive Na$^+$ pathway in the amphibian diluting segment induced by K$^+$ adaptation. *Pflügers Arch* 399:166–172, 1983

52. GREGER R, SCHLATTER E, WITTNER M: Cellular mechanism of action of furosemide-like diuretics in the thick ascending limb of the loop of Henle, in *1st Int Congr on Diuretics*, edited by PUSCHETT J, Amsterdam, New York, Elsevier Science Publishing Co., Inc. (in press, 1984)

53. SCHLATTER E: Phloretin (PTN) inhibits active NaCl reabsorption in the cortical thick ascending limb segment (cTAL) of rabbit nephron (*abstract*). *Naunyn Schmiedebergs Arch Pharmacol* 322:R18, 1983

54. PALADE PT, BARCHI RL: On the inhibition of muscle membrane chloride conductance by aromatic carboxylic acids. *J Gen Physiol* 69:879–896, 1977

55. WITTNER M, GREGER R, DI STEFANO A, GEBLER B, MEYER C: Inhibitors of

the basolateral Cl^--conductance in isolated perfused cortical thick ascending limbs of Henle loops (cTAL) of rabbit nephrons. *Pflügers Arch* (in press, 1984)

56. SCHLATTER E, GREGER R, WEIDTKE C: Effect of "high ceiling" diuretics on active salt transport in the cortical thick ascending limb of Henle's loop of rabbit kidney. Correlation of chemical structure and inhibitory potency. *Pflügers Arch* 396:210–217, 1983

57. FORBUSH B III, PALFREY HC: (H^3) Bumetanide binding to membranes isolated from dog kidney outer medulla. Relationship to the Na, K, Cl co-transport system. *J Biol Chem* 258:11787–11792, 1983

58. GREVEN J: Studies on the renal receptors of loop diuretics. *Clin Exper Hyper–Theory and Practice* A5(2):193–208, 1983

59. GREGER R, FRÖMTER E: Time course of ouabain and furosemide effects on transepithelial potential difference in cortical thick ascending limb of rabbit nephrons, in *Kidney and Body Fluids,* vol 11, edited by TAKACS L. Budapest, Adv Physiol Sci, Pergamon Press, 1981, pp 375–379

60. GUGGINO WB, STANTON BA, GIEBISCH G: Electrical properties of isolated early distal tubule of the Amphiuma kidney (*abstract*). *Fed Proc* 41:1597, 1982

61. SCHULTZ SG: Homocellular regulatory mechanisms in sodium-transporting epithelia: An extension of the Koefoed-Johnsen-Ussing model. *Semin Nephrol* 2:343–347, 1982

62. DIAMOND JM: Transcellular cross-talk between epithelial cell membranes. *Nature* 300:683–685, 1982

63. HALL DA, VARNEY DM: Effect of vasopressin on electrical potential difference and chloride transport in mouse medullary thick ascending limb of Henle's loop. *J Clin Invest* 66:792–802, 1980

64. SASAKI S, IMAI M: Effects of vasopressin on water and NaCl transport across the in vitro perfused medullary thick ascending limb of Henle's loop of mouse, rat, and rabbit kidneys. *Pflügers Arch* 383:215–221, 1980

65. IMAI M: Regulation of ion transport in the thick ascending limb of Henle's loop, in *Coupled Transport in Nephron,* edited by HOSHI T. Tokyo, Miura Foundation (in press, 1984)

66. SCHLATTER E, GREGER R: Mechanism of cAMP-stimulation of active NaCl reabsorption in the isolated perfused medullary thick ascending limb of Henle's loop (mTAL) of mouse nephron. *Pflügers Arch* (in press, 1984)

Structural Heterogeneity of the Distal Nephron

Chairpersons: C. Craig Tisher and Brigitte Kaissling
Discussants: Kirsten M. Madsen, Lise Bankir, Bruce Stanton,
Dennis Brown, and Michel Bergeron

The distal nephron encompasses the distal tubule, which is composed of the thick ascending limb of Henle (TALH), the macula densa and the distal convoluted tubule (DCT), the connecting tubule (CNT), and the collecting duct. The latter includes the initial collecting tubule (ICT), the cortical collecting duct (CCD), and the outer (OMCD) and the inner (IMCD) medullary collecting ducts. This Workshop was devoted to a discussion of the recent observations that have been made concerning the structure of these segments; such observations have been derived from the application of a host of morphologic and physiologic techniques in both rat and rabbit kidney.

The pars recta or TALH is the initial portion of the distal tubule and is divided into a medullary and a cortical segment. In long-looped nephrons, the TALH begins as an abrupt transition from the thin ascending limb, and this transition marks the boundary between the inner medulla and the inner stripe of the outer medulla. The transition to the TALH in short-looped nephrons usually occurs along the thin descending limb shortly before the hairpin turn. The medullary segment extends upward to the boundary between the outer stripe of the outer medulla and the inner cortex. In the rat kidney, the cells in the inner stripe of the outer medulla have an average cell height of approximately 7 μ, which decreases to approximately 5 μ in the outer stripe.

The cells of the medullary TALH contain numerous elongated mitochondria oriented perpendicularly to the membrane. The mitochondria are enclosed by plications or invaginations of the basal plasma membrane. These invaginations can extend two thirds or more into the cell toward the luminal border. In the rat, the junctional complex is formed by a tight junction or zonula occludens, which is 0.1 to 0.2 μ in depth. An intermediate junction or zonula adherens is also present, but desmosomes are lacking. Ultrastructural tracer studies with lanthanum have demonstrated the presence of a

---

This manuscript is a summary of a Workshop of the same title.

potential intercellular or paracellular shunt pathway for solute and fluid movement in this segment of the nephron.

Scanning electron microscopy in the TALH of both rat and rabbit kidney has revealed the existence of two distinctly different patterns of luminal surface structure among the cell population forming the epithelium of this segment of the nephron. One group of cells has a rough surface owing to the presence of extensive microvilli, while a second group has a smooth surface that is largely devoid of microvilli except along the lateral cell margins. Most cells possess one and occasionally two cilia. In both the medullary and cortical TALH, the rough-surfaced cells possess more extensive lateral processes that radiate from the main cell body. In comparison, lateral processes of smooth-surfaced cells are less common in the inner stripe of the outer medulla, but they do increase in number and complexity in the outer stripe of the outer medulla and throughout the cortical TALH. Smooth-surfaced cells predominate in the medullary segment, whereas those with a rough surface predominate in the cortical segment. Additional morphologic differences between the rough- and smooth-surfaced cells have not been described, and it is not clear at present whether these differences are indicative of the existence of two distinct cell types or whether they merely represent a variation in the structure of a single cell type in this region of the distal nephron.

The cortical TALH begins at the corticomedullary junction and extends to the glomerulus of the nephron of origin. At the point of contact with the extraglomerular mesangial region, the immediately contiguous portion of the tubule forms the macula densa. Recent studies in both the rat and rabbit have revealed that the macula densa is a specialized segment of the TALH since, in most instances, the TALH extends well beyond the vicinity of the macula densa to form a rather abrupt transition with the pars convoluta. Recent studies in the rat TALH reveal that major morphologic differences, both qualitatively and quantitatively, exist between the inner stripe segment and the remainder of the TALH.

The cells of the cortical TALH also possess numerous elongated mitochondria oriented perpendicular to the basement membrane. They are enclosed in plications or invaginations of the basal plasma membrane. In this region of the distal tubule, the lateral interdigitating processes in the apical portion of the cell are extensive, as are the number of rough-surfaced cells.

The pars convoluta portion of the distal tubule begins at a variable distance beyond the macula densa and extends to the region of transition with the connecting segment. In the rabbit kidney this segment of the nephron averages about 0.5 mm in length, but is slightly longer in the rat. The cells of the DCT are cuboidal and contain abundant quantities of elongated mitochondria that are oriented perpendicular to the basement membrane of the tubule. Individual cells often have a convex luminal surface that is covered by short, blunt microvilli. These microvilli are more extensive in the rabbit than the rat DCT.

Scanning electron microscopy has demonstrated that the luminal surface of the DCT differs rather substantially from that of the TALH. In contrast to the cortical TALH, there is a marked absence of lateral interdigitations in the apical region between adjacent cells. Prominent microvilli accentuate the rather straight lateral cell margins. The individual cells possess one and sometimes two centrally placed cilia. In contrast to the apical cell region, lateral interdigitations in the lower half of the cell of the DCT are extensive and resemble those in the TALH.

Transmission electron microscopy has demonstrated that the junctional complex in this region of the nephron is freely permeable to ultrastructural tracers such as lanthanum, suggesting the existence of a potential paracellular shunt pathway for solute and water movement in this segment of the nephron.

The participants in the Workshop directed their attention next to the application of morphometric procedures to the quantification of renal structure. A basic requirement for the conduct of a morphometric analysis is the use of a randomized sampling procedure. This requirement becomes extremely important when working with highly anisotropic structures such as kidney tubules and, especially, with those segments located in the renal medulla. However, for a variety of reasons it has been common to use only tubule cross-sections rather than randomly oriented sections for morphometric measurements.

A variety of problems can arise if a morphometric analysis is performed on renal tubules that have not been sampled and oriented at random. For the purposes of this discussion, an analysis is described that was performed on the rat TALH. The kidneys of four rats were preserved by an in vivo perfusion with glutaraldehyde. Tissue samples were taken from the inner stripe of the outer medulla for examination of the TALH and divided into three groups for analysis. In the first group, the tubules were cut perpendicular to the long axis of the tubule. In the second group, the tubules were cut parallel to the long axis. In the third group, the tissue samples were oriented and cut at random. Several tubule profiles are obtained with these different sectioning angles. For instance, a transverse section of a tubule will give rise to a donut-shaped profile, whereas a longitudinal section of a tubule can give rise to two rectangular profiles. With a randomly oriented section, virtually any profile between these two extremes will appear.

The morphometric analysis was carried out by point and intersect counting on transmission electron micrographs at a final magnification of $\times 20,000$. The surface density of the apical and basolateral membranes was determined, and the results were expressed in mm^2/mm^3. Significant differences were found between the three groups with respect to both parameters. The surface density of the apical plasma membrane was significantly greater when measured on longitudinal sections versus randomly oriented sections, while the surface density of the basolateral membrane was significantly smaller when determined on cross-sections versus longitudinal or randomly oriented sections.

In a transverse section of a medullary TALH, the basolateral invaginations appear irregular and are sometimes difficult to identify. In contrast, on a longitudinal section the invaginations of the basolateral plasma membrane are extensive. When this configuration is compared with that on a transverse section, it becomes obvious that the membranes must exhibit some preferential orientation. In a randomly oriented tubule, a section may include only the basal region of the cell, which is packed with invaginations of the plasma membrane. The section may not include the lumen and, therefore, will not contain any apical membrane.

Thus, in summary, the surface density of the apical membrane is overestimated when only sections including both apical and basal regions are used. On the other hand, the surface density of the basolateral membrane is significantly underestimated on transverse sections owing to the orientation of the basolateral invaginations.

The quantitative differences in the surface density of the basolateral membrane could have been predicted on the basis of an excellent study by Welling and his associates on the rabbit cortical TALH published in *Kidney International* in 1978. They pointed out that the typical cell of the TALH is oriented with its long axis extending around the tubule perpendicular to the long axis of the tubule. Thus, transverse sections of tubules will have fewer cross-sections, whereas longitudinal sections will have numerous cross-sections of the basolateral membrane. Whenever possible, morphometric analysis of kidney tubules should be performed on tubules that are sampled and oriented randomly.

Another segment of the Workshop was devoted to presentation of a morphometric study undertaken to quantify the morphologic changes induced by antidiuretic hormone (ADH) availability in the rat kidney. Homozygous Brattleboro rats with hereditary diabetes insipidus (DI) were compared with a control group of heterozygous Brattleboro rats (HZ) and with DI rats that received 6 weeks of continuous ADH infusion with Alzet osmotic minipumps (TDI). Urine osmolality in the three groups was 216, 1660, and 2770 mOsm/kg H_2O, respectively. ADH treatment was associated with a 37% increase in mass of kidney per unit of body weight; however, not all zones of the kidney nor all nephron segments were increased uniformly. With ADH, the inner stripe of the outer medulla was enlarged more than other renal zones and represented $22.2 \pm 1.5\%$ of the total kidney height along the corticopapillary axis in TDI rats and $15.5 \pm 0.7\%$ in DI animals ($P < 0.025$). Selective increases in epithelial thickness and tubular diameter were observed in the earliest part of the TALH in the inner stripe, resulting in a 2-fold increase in epithelial volume per unit of tubular length (1146 ± 35 μm^3 in TDI rats vs. 566 ± 15 μm^3 in DI rats; $P < 0.001$). HZ rats demonstrated intermediate values. As a result of the increase in epithelial volume per unit length and of the increase in the height of the inner stripe, the total volume of medullary TALH epithelium per kidney was more than tripled, thus increasing dramatically the mass of epithelium available for sodium chloride reabsorption in the inner stripe. Since hypertrophy of the TALH declined along the course of the segment, and since collecting ducts were not affected, a direct effect of ADH on its target cells does not appear to explain the observed changes. It is possible that the increased solute delivery to the medullary TALH that is likely to occur in the concentrating kidney could induce the hypertrophy of the TALH by increasing the work load in the early part of this segment. This work demonstrates that ADH, when present in amounts inducing a high urine concentration for several weeks, leads to profound morphologic changes in the kidney comprising a selective increase of the ADH target segments involved in the *single effect* of the concentrating process.

In addition to the axial heterogeneity of the TALH morphology, transport properties, and hormone sensitivity, the heterogeneity of its vascular environment should also be considered. The early TALH in the inner stripe is surrounded by the dense capillary plexus of the interbundle region. This plexus originates from branches of the efferent arteriole of deep glomeruli leaving the periphery of the vascular bundle to supply the inner stripe tubules. In the outer stripe, the direct blood supply by branches of the deep efferent arterioles is extremely scarce, and the real nutrient blood supply of the tubules there is provided by the very numerous venous vasa recta ascending from both the interbundle region of the inner stripe and from the inner medulla via the vascular bundles. Finally, in the cortex the vessels surrounding the cortical TALH belong to the medullary ray elongated capillary mesh originating from the efferent arterioles of midcortical and superficial glomeruli.

The second half of the Workshop concerned the issues relative to that portion of the nephron beyond the macula densa. The three cortical segments beyond the macula densa (DCT, CNT, and CCD) are composed of four different cell types. These include DCT cells, CNT cells, principal cells, and intercalated cells. Three (DCT, CNT, and principal cells) display a substantial increase in basolateral plasma membrane area. In DCT cells, this is achieved by the formation of large lateral interdigitating cell processes, and in CNT and principal cells by infoldings of the basal plasma membrane into the cell body. The fourth cell type, the intercalated cell, can display a substantial increase in luminal surface area.

Basolateral membrane amplification (basolateral plasma membrane area divided by the tubular basement membrane area) is highest in the DCT ($\sim$ 20 in the rat and rabbit and $\sim$ 40 in *Psammomys obesus*), decreases in the CNT cells along the connecting tubule, and is lowest in the principal cells (about 5 in rabbits). Basolateral membrane area and Na-K-ATPase activity vary proportionally. Axial changes are also apparent in the luminal surface of intercalated cells of the rabbit, with values being highest in the CNT at about 40% of the tubular luminal area and decreasing gradually along the collecting duct within the medullary ray to about 10%.

The basolateral membrane amplification changes with adaptation to altered electrolyte metabolism induced by means of dietary, hormonal, or diuretic treatment. The changes are assumed to reflect changes in transport capacity of the respective cells or nephron segments. In the cells of the DCT that functionally might be associated with sodium reabsorption, an increase in membrane area has been observed with a high sodium intake in the rabbit, and with inhibition of sodium chloride reabsorption in the TALH by furosemide treatment in rats. Apparently, the chronically high sodium load of the tubular fluid is the specific functional stimulus for this cell type.

Cells of the CNT are associated with sodium reabsorption and potassium secretion. They increase their basolateral membrane area with a high potassium intake and high plasma mineralocorticoid levels. The axial decrease in membrane area of CNT cells becomes conspicuously pronounced with such treatment, suggesting that in this segment the tubular fluid composition must also play a decisive role in the functioning of the CNT cells.

Principal cells that are functionally associated with sodium reabsorption and potassium secretion, in addition to their responsiveness to ADH to increase water reabsorption, develop an increase in basolateral membrane area with high levels of plasma mineralocorticoids independent of the associated potassium intake.

Intercalated cells in the cortex reveal no significant alteration of basolateral membrane area, but react with changes in luminal area. In rabbits on a high-sodium, low-potassium diet, these cells displayed about the same pattern of axial changes as in control animals, but the luminal exposure of the cells in all measured portions of the cortex was less than in controls. With a low-sodium, high-potassium diet, the luminal exposure is higher than in controls. This is especially evident in the collecting duct within the medullary ray. A high mineralocorticoid plasma level with DOCA application, combined with a high sodium intake, is associated with structural changes in intercalated cells, but luminal exposure of the cells does not differ from that of controls.

These structural studies suggest that in addition to peritubular factors the tubular fluid composition can influence the transport capacity of the cells. Although there are no serious controversies concerning the possible functional stimuli for the DCT, CNT, and principal cells, the role of mineralocorticoid hormones and electrolytes on the assumed function of intercalated cells—such as hydrogen ion secretion and possibly potassium reabsorption—is still in question.

Next, the Workshop considered the role of adrenal hormones in regulating distal tubule structure and function. Several lines of evidence suggest that either mineralocorticoids, or glucocorticoids, or both classes of adrenal corticosteroids regulate sodium and potassium transport at the level of the initial and cortical collecting tubule. For example, some investigators have suggested that glucocorticoids, but not mineralocorticoids, produce a kaliuresis. It is apparent from these studies that the differential effects of mineralocorticoids and glucocorticoids on ion transport are controversial.

Several factors may be identified that have bearing on this controversy. *First,* in some studies either pharmacologic or supraphysiologic doses of hormone were used, and this may have resulted in nonspecific effects through binding to both types of renal corticosteroid receptors. *Second,* hormone treatment frequently leads to simultaneous changes in other factors, particularly urinary sodium concentration and flow rate, that are known to have a potent influence on sodium and potassium transport. *Third,* very few studies have examined the effects of adrenal corticosteroids at the level of the initial or cortical collecting tubule. In many experiments the function of these segments has been inferred from urinary excretion rates. This type of analysis may be misleading, since the rate of urinary sodium and potassium excretion reflects the sum of the contribution of several nephron segments that are likely to have very different responses to hormonal treatment.

Experiments were conducted to examine the differential effects of *low physiologic levels* of aldosterone and dexamethasone on ion transport and cellular ultrastructure of the initial collecting tubule. Ultrastructural studies were performed to determine whether regulation of sodium and potassium transport by adrenal corticosteroids involves specific changes in membrane area.

Rats were adrenalectomized and infused continuously for 10 days with low doses of aldosterone or dexamethasone. After 10 days of hormone treatment, standard electron microscopic and morphometric techniques were used to examine the cells of the initial collecting tubule; sodium and potassium transport was measured by micropuncture and microperfusion of single initial collecting tubules.

Adrenalectomy led to a sharp reduction in sodium reabsorption and potassium secretion. Basolateral membrane surface density of the principal cell fell from 3.05 $\mu m^2/\mu m^3$ in intact control animals to 2.11 $\mu m^2/\mu m^3$ in adrenalectomized animals. This change in cell structure was specific for the basolateral membrane of the principal cell; the intercalated cell structure was not affected. Dexamethasone replacement increased glomerular filtration rate, but had no direct effect on the transport of sodium or potassium when changes in tubular and urinary flow rate were held constant by experimental design. Dexamethasone had no effect on cell structure of either cell type. In contrast, aldosterone restored ion transport to control values and increased basolateral membrane surface density of principal cells to 3.25 $\mu m^2/\mu m^3$, a value similar to adrenal-intact controls.

These studies suggest that mineralocorticoids, but not glucocorticoids, regulate sodium and potassium transport by the initial collecting tubule. Aldosterone regulates ion transport in principal cells, in part, by determining the amount of basolateral membrane and, accordingly, the number of Na^+-K^+-ATPase pumps. These data also suggest that the glucocorticoid-induced kaliuresis at the level of the initial collecting tubule reported by others is an indirect, flow-induced phenomenon.

The final segment of the Workshop was devoted to a discussion of the use of immunocytochemistry and lectin-gold cytochemistry to map sites of carbonic anhydrase (CA-C) and calcium binding protein (CaBP) in the distal tubule and collecting duct. The distal nephron and collecting ducts of mammalian kidney are involved in specific functions that may be reflected in the specialization of their epithelial cell populations. Specific antibodies were used: carbonic anhydrase C (an enzyme involved in acidification processes) and the 28,000-molecular weight vitamin D-dependent calcium binding protein (CaBP, which may play a role in renal calcium handling). They were localized in rat kidney by using double immunostaining methods at the light (immunofluorescence, protein A peroxidase) and electron microscopic (protein A-gold) levels. Furthermore, a new cytochemical technique was used. It involves the direct application of lectin-gold complexes to thin and semithin tissue sections to examine the lectin-binding patterns of collecting tubule cells at both the light and electron microscopic level.

All intercalated cells were strongly positive for carbonic anhydrase C, and immunolabeling was distributed throughout the cytosol of these cells. It was not preferentially associated with the plasma membrane. In contrast, intercalated cells contained no detectable CaBP. Principal cells of parts of the distal convoluted tubule were positive for CaBP, but were most strongly reactive in the connecting segment. The antigen was present throughout the cytosol.

In this segment cells that were positive for CaBP were negative for CA-C and vice versa. In the cortical collecting duct, the number of CaBP-positive cells fell sharply, but many CA-C-positive cells were present, corresponding to the known distribution of intercalated cells in rat kidney. In this segment, principal cells also showed some reactivity toward the anti-CA-C antibody, but much less than the intercalated cells.

All intercalated cells, then, showed intense reactivity toward the CA-C antibody; but, in contrast, they demonstrated a distinct regional variation in their binding of *Helix pomatia* lectin. Cells from the cortex and outer stripe showed a heavy labeling of their apical plasma membrane and apical cytoplasmic vesicles, whereas in the inner stripe and inner medulla, intercalated cells were either unlabeled or very weakly labeled with this lectin. Principal cells, on the other hand, were positive for this lectin in all regions of the collecting duct.

The described heterogeneity in the tubular and cellular content of CA-C and CaBP probably reflects differential roles of these cell populations and nephron segments in urinary acidification and renal calcium handling, although the meaning of the nonhomogeneous lectin-binding pattern of the intercalated cells along the nephron is at present unknown.

A brief presentation by Bergeron concluded the Workshop. This investigator described two distinct patterns in the intracellular distribution of the endoplasmic reticulum in the rat CNT segment and the cortical collecting duct. In the intercalated cells, the amount of endoplasmic reticulum greatly exceeded that observed in either the principal cells or the CNT cells, and the pattern of distribution was more dispersed in the latter two cell types.

Control of Acid and Electrolyte Excretion

Acidification Mechanisms

Chairpersons: Thomas D. DuBose, Jr. and Michel Paillard
Discussants: Eberhard Frömter, Robert J. Alpern, David W. Good, and Dennis K. Stone

The role of the kidney in acid-base balance is to stabilize the plasma concentration of bicarbonate. This is accomplished by the reabsorption of all filtered bicarbonate and by the titration of urinary buffers and ammonia. The cellular mechanism of this process has been investigated extensively. Although there has been controversy regarding the distinction between proton secretion and bicarbonate reabsorption per se, the majority of studies in vivo and in vitro have firmly supported the view that bicarbonate reabsorption is mediated by hydrogen ion secretion.

Carbonic anhydrase (CA) accelerates the hydration (the reaction that governs the process of proton secretion) of carbon dioxide some 1000-fold. In the proximal tubule both cytoplasmic and membrane-bound fractions have been described by histochemical, biochemical, and membrane vesicle studies. Until recently, it has not been established whether or not the orientation of the luminal enzyme allows it to be active in the lumen of the tubule.

Recently, a high molecular weight dextran-bound carbonic anhydrase inhibitor (DBI) has been synthesized by Tinker, Coulson, and Weiner. In a recent series of studies in DuBose's laboratory, the effects of selective inhibition of luminal carbonic anhydrase were investigated. Comparison of the effects of the dextran-bound inhibitor (DBI) with those of the unbound inhibitor (STZ) on total carbon dioxide reabsorption and intraluminal pH were used as a pharmacologic means of comparing the specific role of the luminal enzyme to the cytoplasmic enzyme. In tubules perfused with artificial ultrafiltrate containing 1 mg/ml AED (vehicle, no CA activity), mean volume reabsorptive rate, J_v, was 2.5 ± 0.3 nl·mm^{-1}·min^{-1}, and the mean total carbon dioxide reabsorptive rate, J_{tCO2}, was 138 ± 10 pmoles·mm^{-1}·min^{-1}. Intraluminal pH measured in the proximal tubule loops immediately adjacent to the perfusion pipette were similar to those reported previously for superficial proximal tubules perfused with artificial ultrafiltrate solution (7.31 ± 0.03). The addition

---

This manuscript is a summary of a Workshop entitled *Acidification Mechanisms.*

of DBI to the perfusion solution resulted in a marked reduction of Jv (1.1 $\pm$ 0.2 nl·mm^{-1}·mm^{-1}) and J$_{tco2}$ (30 $\pm$ 5 pmoles·mm^{-1}·mm^{-1}) ($P < 0.001$). When DBI was added to the perfusate, intraluminal pH measured in superficial loops close to the perfusion pipette was significantly more acidic than in control tubules (6.80 $\pm$ 0.02). This degree of acidification occurred despite marked inhibition of bicarbonate transport.

When STZ, the unbound carbonic anhydrase inhibitor, was added to the perfusion solution (10^{-3} M), both bicarbonate and volume reabsorption were reduced significantly to values indistinguishable from the results obtained with DBI. However, the addition of STZ to the perfusate was not associated with significant acidification of tubule fluid (pH = 7.24 $\pm$ 0.04).

The studies described by DuBose demonstrate that proximal tubule fluid is in functional contact with luminal or "membrane-bound" carbonic anhydrase, which is responsible for mediating approximately 80% of the bicarbonate reabsorption and thus proton secretion normally achieved by this segment.

Frömter examined the mechanism of bicarbonate exit from rat proximal tubular cells by measuring cell membrane potentials (PD) and intracellular pH (pH$_c$) in vivo in response to fast peritubular perturbations of bicarbonate and OH$^-$/H$^+$ concentrations or of carbon dioxide pressure. From the dependence of the PD on peritubular bicarbonate concentration (30 mv, a 10-fold change in bicarbonate concentration) and from the resistance increase during inhibition of bicarbonate permeation, it was concluded that bicarbonate permeation was a conductive process. This was confirmed by pH$_c$ measurements, which showed a fast cell acidification in response to a sudden increase of bicarbonate (at constant P$_{CO2}$). The latter experiment is suggestive of a conductive (rheogenic) process. In further support of this conclusion, it was observed that the latter response (bicarbonate permeation) together with the PD change was abolished by the disulphonic stilbene SITS (10^{-3} moles/liter), whereas the former response (carbon dioxide permeation) was not.

From similar observations in amphibian kidney, Boron and Boulpaep concluded that two or more bicarbonate ions move together with one sodium ion. This model, however, does not seem to apply to the rat kidney, because neither was the PD response to a change in bicarbonate concentration affected significantly by sodium-free solutions nor did the change in sodium concentration produce similar PD changes as did the change in bicarbonate concentration; nor was the PD response to the change of sodium concentration abolished by SITS.

Frömter's data indicate that bicarbonate moves, either completely or to a greater extent, as OH$^-$ and CO$_2$. This is concluded from the observation that peritubular pH changes in well buffered bicarbonate-free solutions produced similar PD and/or pH$_c$ changes as peritubular bicarbonate concentration was altered in a stepwise fashion. This model explains why carbonic anhydrase is bound to the peritubular cell membrane (Wistrand and Kinne) and why carbonic anhydrase inhibitors inhibit bicarbonate permeation and increase the membrane resistance.

From the intracellular pH of 7.17 an intracellular bicarbonate concentration of 13.4 mmoles/liter was calculated, which indicates that bicarbonate exit is opposed by a small bicarbonate concentration gradient (or OH⁻ concentration gradient) and that the real driving force for bicarbonate exit is the cell membrane potential.

Modulation of proximal bicarbonate transport in response to alterations in bicarbonate delivery and systemic acid-base status was discussed by Alpern. He first pointed out that bicarbonate absorption in the rat proximal convoluted tubule can be described as active transcellular proton secretion in parallel with passive paracellular bicarbonate diffusion. The rate of passive bicarbonate diffusion is calculated from the bicarbonate permeability (3.5×10^{-5} cm/sec) and the transepithelial concentration gradient. The bicarbonate permeability is unaffected by changes in luminal flow rate and pH (luminal and peritubular), and is of similar magnitude in both the absorption and secretory direction.

Alpern pointed out that increases in luminal pH and bicarbonate concentration stimulate bicarbonate reabsorption, which can be attributed to an effect on active transcellular proton secretion. The rate of transcellular proton secretion is sensitive to luminal bicarbonate at low concentrations, but sensitivity decreases as luminal concentration increases. At luminal bicarbonate concentrations of 45 mEq/liter, proton secretion achieves a maximal rate and becomes independent of luminal concentration. This independence of luminal bicarbonate concentration (and pH) at high concentration has been useful in elucidating the regulation of acidification.

Increases in luminal flow rate enhance transcellular proton secretion. This stimulation is due to an effect on the luminal bulk-phase concentration profile; but, moreover, proton secretion is stimulated by flow per se. This latter stimulation occurs at low luminal bicarbonate concentrations, but does not occur at luminal concentrations associated with the maximal transport rate (45 mEq/liter). This kinetic behavior suggests an effect of flow rate on the bicarbonate concentration and pH of a luminal compartment that is not in the bulk-phase (that is, a luminal flow-dependent diffusion barrier).

Increases in peritubular bicarbonate concentration inhibit, and decreases in peritubular bicarbonate concentration stimulate active proton secretion. This effect occurs at all luminal bicarbonate concentrations, and thus, the maximal rate of proton secretion is altered.

The inhibition of volume absorption leads to the inhibition of net bicarbonate absorption. Prior inhibition of active proton secretion prevents this effect. Thus, this bicarbonate-water interaction is not due to solvent drag across the tight junction, but is due to an effect of volume flux on the rate of active proton secretion. The bicarbonate-water interaction increases in magnitude at high luminal bicarbonate concentrations, and thus affects the maximal rate. This kinetic behavior is similar to that of peritubular bicarbonate concentration changes and suggests that volume flux modifies the local pH on the peritubular side of the luminal membrane by a convective interaction in a cellular and/or peritubular diffusion barrier.

In summary, luminal and peritubular pH are important determinants of the rate of proximal tubular acidification. Their major effect is on active proton secretion, although they also affect the rate of paracellular bicarbonate diffusion. In addition to explaining the effect of acidosis and alkalosis on proximal acidification, changes in local pH mediate the effects of flow rate and volume flux on proton secretion.

The role of extracellular fluid volume (ECFV), parathyroid hormone (PTH), and serum calcium concentration (Ca^{++}) on renal bicarbonate transport was discussed by Paillard. He indicated that new work concerning the role of ECFV status, PTH, and calcium on the renal handling of bicarbonate has emerged. The role of PTH in the inhibition of renal reabsorption of bicarbonate was examined by him during isohydric volume expansion (VE). Two groups of rats were studied, intact and acutely TPTX, with the same degree of VE. In intact rats, plasma $[Ca^{++}]$ declined during VE, from 2.28 ± 0.06 to 2.11 ± 0.04 mEq/liter ($P < 0.01$), and PTH secretion increased as reflected by the increase in nephrogenous cyclic AMP from 29 ± 5 to 66 ± 10 pmoles/min $\cdot$ g kwt ($P < 0.02$). The inhibition of bicarbonate reabsorption in the proximal tubule during VE was reduced (11%) in TPTX rats compared to intact rats (30%), and the mean transepithelial concentration gradient for tCO_2 decreased by 21% in TPTX instead of 50% in intact rats. This suggests that the discrepancies observed among previous studies regarding the degree of inhibition of proximal bicarbonate reabsorption might be explained by differences in PTH activity during plasma repletion and/or VE. Paillard then examined whether PTH alters hydrogen ion secretion in the distal nephron by observing the urine-to-blood (U-B) P_{CO_2} difference in alkaline urine (pH > 7.8) in acutely TPTX rats before and after PTH infusion (2.3 U/hr/100 g of body wt). When U-B P_{CO_2} values were plotted against urinary bicarbonate concentration, two linear relationships of the same slope (0.22 vs. 0.20) but different intercepts on the y axis (13.3 vs. -1.6, $P <$ 0.01) were described. When the effect of PTH was examined at constant urinary phosphate concentration, no effect of PTH on U-B P_{CO_2} was observed. This observation rules out a direct effect of PTH on distal nephron hydrogen secretion. Paillard then tried to localize the previously observed reduction of urinary bicarbonate excretion induced by acute hypercalcemia. Hypercalcemia was induced by calcium chloride infusion in acutely TPTX rats. For a mild increase in plasma calcium (0.23 to 0.43 mM) the reduction in urinary bicarbonate excretion (166 ± 43 vs. 401 ± 90 nmol/min, $P < 0.05$) was due to an enhanced tubular reabsorption of bicarbonate, since whole kidney glomerular filtration rate (GFR) remained unchanged (1.02 ± 0.07 vs. 1.11 ml/min g of kidney wt). The increase in tubular reabsorption of bicarbonate was not localized to the superficial proximal tubule (end-proximal delivery 352 ± 32 vs. 328 ± 30 pmol/min g of kidney wt). The distal hydrogen secretion rate assessed by U-B P_{CO_2} in maximally alkaline urine was unchanged after sodium chloride infusion, as reflected by the same linear relationship between U-B P_{CO_2} and urinary bicarbonate concentration. In a second series of experiments, when the increase in plasma calcium was greater (by 0.79 mM), whole kidney GFR was reduced (0.96 ± 0.06 vs. $1.23 \pm$ 0.06 ml/min g of kidney wt, $P < 0.02$), without variation in superficial SNGFR (44.9 ± 1.7 vs. 46.0 ± 1.3 nl/min $\cdot$ g kwt). These findings suggest that hypercalcemia reduces urinary bicarbonate excretion by enhancing proximal bicarbonate reabsorption and by decreasing GFR in juxtamedullary nephrons.

Good emphasized that our present knowledge of the contribution of different nephron segments to renal ammonia excretion has come primarily from clearance and micropuncture experiments. These studies have shown that ammonia is secreted by the proximal tubule, the distal convoluted tubule, and the collecting ducts and is reabsorbed from the loops of Henle. Because of the limitations of micropuncture techniques, uncertainties remain about the direction and magnitude of ammonia transport in several nephron segments. Little direct information is available regarding mechanisms of ammonia transport across renal tubular epithelia. Good reviewed recent experiments from his laboratory in which ammonia production and mechanisms of ammonia transport were studied in isolated nephron segments in vitro.

To determine the relative importance of different nephron segments as sites of ammonia production, tubule segments were dissected from normal, acidotic, and alkalotic rats. The tubules were incubated in vitro with glutamine and absolute ammonia production rates were measured directly. The bulk of renal ammonia production was found to occur in the proximal tubule. Adaptive changes in production occurred only in specific segments of the proximal tubule:acidosis-increased production in S1 and S2, but not in S3; alkalosis decreased production only in S1. Acidosis had no detectable effect on segments of the thick ascending limb, the distal convoluted tubule, or the collecting duct.

To assess sites and mechanisms of ammonia transport in the loop of Henle, cortical and medullary thick ascending limbs of rats were perfused in vitro with 4 mM ammonia and 25 mM bicarbonate perfusion and bathing solutions. Both segments absorbed ammonia and bicarbonate. Because total ammonia concentration and pH were less in collected fluid than in the bath, ammonia was absorbed against a concentration gradient. The ammonia absorption most likely was due to passive absorption of NH_4^+, driven by the lumen-positive transepithelial voltage.

To examine mechanisms of ammonia secretion in cortical collecting ducts, tubules from DOC-treated rabbits were perfused by Good in vitro with 25 mM HCO_3 and 4 mM ammonia in perfusate and bath. The solutions were potassium-free. Under these conditions, the tubules secreted both ammonia and bicarbonate. Ammonia secretion was not inhibited by ouabain, thus excluding transport of NH_4^+ by Na^+-K^+-ATPase. Ammonia secretion was converted to ammonia absorption when carbonic anhydrase was added to the luminal perfusate. Good inferred that the development of an acid pH disequilibrium reduces lumen pH below that of the bath, resulting in secretion of ammonia by nonionic diffusion.

In summary, Good's experiments with isolated nephron segments in vitro have shown the following: (1) In the rat, alteration in ammonia production in response to systemic acid-base changes occurs only in specific segments of the proximal tubule; (2) the thick ascending limb contributes to loop ammonia absorption in rats by absorbing NH_4^+ directly; (3) ammonia transport in cortical collecting ducts of rabbits is influenced by a luminal acid disequilibrium pH and occurs predominantly by nonionic diffusion.

Mechanisms of collecting duct acidification were discussed by Stone. Studies from his laboratory have indicated that rabbit medullary collecting duct acidification occurs by means of an electrogenic, sodium-independent process that is modulated by aldosterone. Chloride serves a dual role in regulating acidification. Preliminary evidence by Stone indicates that intracellular base is extruded across the basolateral membrane of medullary collecting duct cells by means of a chloride-base exchange mechanism. Moreover, chloride is utilized preferentially as the co-ion counterbalancing electrogenic acidification; the bicarbonate-reabsorptive rate is matched by the chloride secretory rate in this segment.

Plasma membrane vesicles prepared from bovine renal medulla contain a nonmitochondrial proton-translocating ATPase, suggesting that the final effector of urinary acidification is a proton pump. Studies conducted with turtle bladder and rat collecting duct indicate that these proton pumps are maintained in a reservoir of secretory vesicles that reside in proximity to the luminal surface of the acidifying cells. With imposition of respiratory acidosis, these vesicles fuse with the luminal membrane to increase the number of pumps available for acidification. Moreover, it appears that these secretory vesicles are in communication with clathrin-coated vesicles that, in other systems, have been shown to be Golgi-derived. The demonstration that Golgi membranes and clathrin-coated vesicles contain proton pumps supports a model of acidification in which proton pumps are sequentially transferred from Golgi to clathrin-coated vesicles, to secretory vesicles, and finally to the luminal membrane of acidifying cells.

In further support of this model, Stone and his colleagues examined the characteristics of acidification in bovine brain clathrin-coated vesicles and bovine renal medulla vesicles of plasma membrane origin. Both vesicle populations contain proton pumps, as measured by ATP-generated acridine orange quenching, which are insensitive to oligomycin, efrapeptin, and mitochondrial ATPase inhibitor. These pumps, which at present are functionally indistinguishable, catalyze $^{32}P_i$-ATP exchange, have a strict ATP dependence, and are electogenic, as assessed by $[^{14}C]SCN$ uptake. In both systems, the electogenicity of the proton pump is dissipated by the parallel conductance of chloride through a specific chloride transporter. These findings serve, at a vesicle level, to characterize the mechanisms responsible for medullary collecting duct acidification.

Atrial Natriuretic Factor

Chairpersons: Adolfo J. de Bold and Harald Sonnenberg
Discussants: Uwe Ackermann, Edward H. Blaine, Josephine P. Briggs,
Barbara R. Cole, Ralph Keeler, Sidney Solomon, Frank Spinelli, Nick
C. Trippodo, and Thomas Maack

In 1980 it was first reported that injection of crude extracts of atrial heart muscle produced a powerful diuretic and natriuretic response in nondiuretic assay rats. This response was rapid in onset and decay. The increase in sodium excretion amounted to 30 times basal values and was accompanied by an equivalent increase in chloride excretion. Urine volume rose 10-fold. These changes took place without an observable difference in glomerular filtration rate (GFR) between the test animals and their controls, which were injected with either ventricular heart muscle extracts or phosphate-buffered saline. Animals injected with atrial extracts showed significantly lower blood pressure (BP) values and higher hematocrits by the end of the experimental period.

Testing of heart atrial extract for effect on kidney function was based on earlier observations, which indicated that the majority of muscle fibers (cardiocytes) in the mammalian atria appear to be morphologically differentiated as both contractile and secretory cells. As secretory cells, atrial cardiocytes contain numerous membrane-bound granules—the specific atrial granules—which are morphologically and histochemically similar to granules known to store polypeptide hormones. The number of granules in atrial cardiocytes varies in certain experimental situations in which water and electrolyte balance is manipulated.

The factor responsible for the natriuretic effect of atrial extract was named atrial natriuretic factor (ANF). ANF is stored mainly within the specific atrial granules as indicated by: (1) presence in atrial but not ventricular cardiocytes of mammals; (2) presence in both these cells in nonmammalian vertebrates which possess specific granules in atria and ventricles; (3) approximately direct correlation between ANF and granule number in the hearts of different species; (4) ANF and specific granules copurify in tissue fractionation procedures; and (5) antibodies against a synthetic 28 amino acid ANF selectively demonstrate the specific atrial granules by immunocytochemistry.

This manuscript is a summary of a Workshop entitled *Atrial Natriuretic Factor.*

The nature of ANF was shown to be proteinaceous and its elution from gel chromatography was shown to include several related peptides. Thus, natriuretic activity was recovered in several peaks with apparent molecular weights ranging from 15,000 to less than 5,000.

To date, much controversy surrounds the molecular weight distribution of the different native ANFs. Current amino acid sequence data show that these different peptides display: (1) precursor product interrelationships, and (2) several favored sites for proteolytic cleavage. Conversion of high molecular weight (HMW) form to low molecular weight (LMW) may be observed in extracts prepared in 0.1 M acetic acid. This conversion is mediated by a heat-labile factor likely present in membranes of atrial muscle cells. This conversion does not occur in 1.0 M acetic acid or after boiling extracts in 0.1 M acetic acid.

The number of LMW ANFs purified to homogeneity reported from different laboratories varies from 2 to 6. Extraction of atrial tissues under conditions which inactivate proteolytic activity from the onset consistently allows for the isolation of four forms of ANF. The most abundant of these is a 28 amino acid peptide containing a tyrosine at the carboxy terminus. All of these peptides have in common a 17-member amino acid sequence delimited by an internal disulfide bridge. Reduction of this disulfide bridge results in loss of natriuretic activity. The addition to the basic 17-member sequence of two Ser at the N-terminus and one Asp at the C-terminus results in a peptide which is natriuretic and relaxes intestinal smooth muscle. Further additions of Phe-Arg or Phe-Arg-Tyr result in peptides that cause internal muscle spasmolysis, relax vascular smooth muscle, and are natriuretic. A synthetic 26-residue peptide is an effective spasmolytic in the presence of catecholamines, serotonin, angiotensin II, and histamine. These effects are observable at peptide doses in the nanomolar range.

HMW ANF is not nearly as well defined as LMW forms. Work on the gene encoding for rat ANF suggests the existence of a precursor molecule of at least 150 amino acids; the LMW forms described above were located near the C-terminus of the precursor.

The mechanism of action of ANF in the kidney is not yet well defined. This situation may be partly due to the great diversity of approaches taken to isolate ANF and the expected differences in the extent of product degradation thus obtained, which, in turn, may result in different peptide sequences. Nevertheless, both tubular and vascular components are thought to be responsible for the natriuretic effect of crude preparations of ANF. The administration of low doses of partially purified native ANF allows for observable dissociation between vascular and transport actions. Low doses induce only natriuresis and diuresis, while with high doses a marked increase in GFR becomes evident. This is consistent with the idea that separate receptors for transport and vascular responses exist. The question of dosage may be relevant to the effect of synthetic ANF on GFR, which is reported to either increase or not affect this parameter.

Studies using hydronephrotic kidneys show a dose-dependent vasodilation in the preglomerular vascular bed but no effect in either the afferent or efferent arterioles. This effect may result in natriuresis.

Comparative studies on the effect of ANF and furosemide were carried out with special reference to chloride transport. Furosemide was shown to effect an increase in chloride excretion in tubular fluid and to augment chloride secretion in isolated renal cells, as well as in rat terminal colon. Such an effect was not shared by ANF. In addition, thiocyanate, which inhibits chloride secretion in some epithelia, did not prevent the renal effects of ANF. Furthermore, there may be differences in the renal response to synthetic peptides and atrial factor extracted from the heart.

In rats, negative pressure breathing, which is known to dilate the atria, induces a diuresis and natriuresis similar to that following injection of ANF. In addition, plasma samples taken at the beginning of the natriuresis showed natriuretic activity when injected into bioassay rats, suggesting that negative pressure breathing releases endogenous atrial natriuretic factor.

Studies on cardiac and peripheral effects of ANF were carried out in comparative studies utilizing chromatographically purified rat atrial and ventricular extracts. Both extracts produced falls in total peripheral resistance, but only atrial extract produced a significant fall in mean BP resulting from failure to increase cardiac output. Depression in heart rate and failure to increase cardiac performance were responsible for the latter effect. Studies of the reflexes involved suggest that ANF has peripheral actions that cause immediate fall in total peripheral resistance.

Regulation of Potassium Excretion

Chairpersons: Gerhard Giebisch and Lawrence Rabinowitz
Discussants: Fred S. Wright, Karol Bomsztyk, Stephen C. Hebert,
Bruce Stanton, John B. Stokes III, Bruce Koeppen,
and Roger G. O'Neil

Renal potassium excretion is modulated by a variety of factors including reabsorption along the proximal tubule and Henle's loop and secretion along the initial and cortical collecting tubule. This workshop reviews some of the recent advances that have provided new insights into the cellular transport processes that regulate tubular potassium transport at strategic sites along the nephron.

Potassium transport by the proximal tubule was surveyed by Wright and Bomsztyk. It was pointed out that filtered potassium is reabsorbed by the proximal tubule approximately in proportion to the reabsorption of sodium and water. The pathways and mechanisms involved in this quantitatively large transport process are not, however, clearly understood. For example, there is no agreement yet concerning the exact quantitative relations between potassium absorption and fluid absorption. The concentration of potassium in fluid reaching the end of the proximal convoluted tubule accessible to micropuncture has been reported to be higher than in plasma, to remain unchanged, or in some circumstances to be lower than in plasma.

Results of three previous studies indicated that potassium can be absorbed against a transepithelial concentration gradient. In the first, potassium ion concentration in tubule fluid was observed to decrease by approximately 10% between early and late proximal segments in rat kidneys. In the second study, the total potassium concentration in tubule fluid was observed to decline by 15% along the proximal tubule in dogs during an intravenous infusion of acetazolamide. Fluid, sodium, and calcium absorption was reduced, but not that of potassium; and potassium absorption continued from a lower concentration in tubule fluid to a higher concentration in plasma. A lumen-positive transepithelial voltage could have contributed to this potassium absorption but is unlikely to have been large enough to account for it entirely. In the third study, a dissociation between the effects on sodium and potassium transport was observed following contralateral nephrectomy. Fractional reab-

This manuscript is a summary of a Workshop entitled *Regulation of Potassium Excretion.*

sorption of fluid and sodium was reduced, but not that of potassium. Potassium concentrations declined along the proximal tubule, reaching values 10% below plasma. In this study, the glomerular filtration rate (GFR) was elevated following contralateral nephrectomy, and the absolute rate of fluid absorption did not change. It is possible that proximal potassium absorption may depend on the simultaneous rate of fluid absorption.

Wright and Bomsztyk examined this possibility by perfusing individual proximal tubules in vivo. By adding mannitol to a perfusion solution that otherwise resembled the fluid reaching the late proximal tubule, it was possible to reduce and then reverse the direction of net fluid transport. Stopping the net fluid absorption slowed but did not stop sodium absorption. In contrast, when the fluid absorption went to zero, the direction of potassium transport reversed from net absorption to net secretion. When the direction of fluid transport was reversed and fluid entered the tubule, the rate of potassium secretion increased. This dependence of potassium transport on fluid transport may indicate direct coupling through the same pathway: a solvent drag mechanism. Alternatively, it may be that fluid absorption raises potassium concentration immediately adjacent to the apical membrane of proximal cells and thus creates a concentration difference favoring potassium absorption. This mechanism would require the proximal tubule to be sufficiently permeable to potassium to allow rather modest passive driving forces to effect significant absorptive transport.

In further microperfusion experiments, the luminal potassium concentration and the transepithelial voltage were varied to study their effects on potassium absorption. The results showed that potassium transport was zero when the electrochemical driving force and the net fluid transport were both zero. With fluid absorption held at zero, the potassium transport changed in proportion to changes in the transepithelial electrochemical driving force; it did not change when the electrochemical driving force did not change. Calculations indicated a permeability coefficient for potassium of 3.0 μm/sec. This value is more than three times the value recently determined for the distal tubule of the rat. Together, the relatively high permeability, the lack of direct evidence for active transport in our experiments, and the symmetry of the correlation between the net potassium transport and the passive driving force are consistent with the concept that there is a mechanism for diffusing potassium through a single barrier: presumably the intercellular junctions. This paracellular movement of potassium appears to be importantly affected by the concurrent rate of net fluid transport.

The role of potassium in sodium chloride absorption by the mammalian thick ascending limb of Henle (TALH) was discussed by Hebert. He surveyed recent evidence that net transepithelial chloride absorption in the TALH involves a secondary active transport process in which luminal chloride entry into cells is mediated by an electroneutral [1 Na^+, 1 K^+, 2 Cl^-] cotransport mechanism. Studies assessing either tracer chloride uptake or the binding of the radiolabeled "loop" diuretic, tritiated bumetanide, by apical membrane vesicles prepared from medullary TALH segments have confirmed the dependence of chloride uptake and both sodium and potassium in this nephron segment.

The apical membranes of diluting segments including rabbit cortical TALH (cTALH), mouse medullary TALH (mTALH), and the *Amphiuma* diluting segment also contain a large barium-sensitive potassium conductance. Observations in the mouse mTALH indicate that the apical potassium conductance in this nephron segment has many of the characteristics (for example, both voltage and concentration dependence; competition effects between barium and potassium on conductance; and titration of potassium conductance with hydrogen ions) of barium/potassium and hydrogen ion interactions with potassium channels in other epithelia and in excitable tissues. Luminal solutions containing 5 mM barium at zero potassium increase the apical-to-basolateral membrane resistance ratio (R_a/R_{bl}) 6-fold and depolarize V_a, the apical membrane voltage. Furthermore, in this nephron segment, increasing the luminal potassium from 5 to 50 mM depolarizes V_a by 53 mV, or 87% of the expected ideal Nernstian value of 61.4 mV. These data indicate that the conductance of apical membranes in the mouse mTALH is attributable principally to potassium. Virtually identical results have been obtained by Greger and associates for the rabbit cTALH and by Oberleithner and associates for the amphibian diluting segment.

In addition to an *active* sodium chloride absorption, an *active potassium transport* has also been observed in in vitro microperfused mouse and rabbit mTALH segments and in the mouse cTALH. In the mouse mTALH, net potassium transport is in the secretory direction and amounts to approximately 10% of the magnitude of net chloride absorption of about 1000 $pEq \cdot sec^{-1} \cdot cm^{-2}$. In amphibian diluting segments, adaptation to a high-potassium diet stimulates net potassium secretion and is associated with the appearance of an amiloride-sensitive sodium/hydrogen ion exchanger in luminal membranes. Friedman and Andreoli have provided evidence both for a sodium/hydrogen and a chloride/bicarbonate double exchanger mechanism, which is responsible for 50% of sodium chloride absorption and for net potassium secretion in cTALH segments from mice fed a standard high-potassium diet. Whether there is a link between the magnitude of net potassium secretion and this amiloride-sensitive sodium chloride transport mechanism in the mouse cTALH is unknown.

Since dilution of the urine by the TALH occurs through the net absorption of equal quantities of sodium and chloride, a stoichiometry of 1 Na^+:2 Cl^- for the transcellular transport mechanism would require that one-half of net sodium absorption occur paracellularly. Two conditions must be met for such a model. First, the transepithelial voltage must result from a cellular electromotive force (EMF) rather than from dilution voltages caused by lateral interspace hypertonicity. Second, the magnitude of the paracellular conductance must be adequate to permit the required paracellular absorptive sodium flux.

An upper estimate of the resistance of the lateral intercellular space has been obtained using luminal barium to block the cellular conductance pathway and a reversed osmotic gradient (perfusate greater than peritubular osmolality) to open up the tight junctions. These studies indicated that the resistance of the lateral intercellular space is not sufficient to permit the development of interspace hypertonicity; in other words, the transepithelial voltage must arise from a cellular rather than a paracellular EMF.

Similar high concentrations of luminal barium and/or reductions in luminal pH sufficient to block the cellular conductance pathway have been used to determine the magnitude of the sodium-permselective shunt conductance in the mouse mTALH. The magnitudes of the lumen-positive transepithelial voltage and the calculated sodium conductance of the shunt pathway appear to be sufficient to drive a quantity of sodium though the paracellular route equal to about half of the rate of net chloride absorption.

Finally, estimates of the transepithelial currents during net chloride absorption in the mouse mTALH indicate that the rate of unidirectional potassium flux across the apical membrane from cell to lumen is 60% of the rate of net chloride absorption. Thus, about 90% of potassium secreted into the lumen must recycle across apical plasma membranes back into cells, presumably through the [1 Na^+, 1 K^+, 2 Cl^-] cotransporter. The combination of the electroneutral [1 Na^+, 1 K^+, 2 Cl^-] cotransporter and the apical membrane potassium conductance appears to provide a pathway for potassium to be recycled across apical membranes, resulting in a large transepithelial current that permits 50% of net sodium absorption paracellularly. The major advantage of this mode of sodium chloride absorption for the TALH appears to be that the combination of a lumen-positive transepithelial voltage and a high-shunt conductance reduces (with respect to exclusively transcellular, active sodium absorption) the metabolic energy expenditure for net sodium absorption.

Potassium Transport Across the Initial Collecting Tubule. It has long been recognized that the *initial collecting tubule*—the *"late" distal tubule* referred to in micropuncture experiments—is one of the main sites of tubular potassium secretion. Microperfusion studies have allowed the analysis of several factors that modulate potassium transport along this tubular segment. Potassium transport across this nephron segment was analyzed by Stanton. He surveyed the evidence based on a careful comparison of fine structural data with transport studies. The data indicate that potassium ions are secreted by principal cells in the latter half of the distal tubule, that is, in the initial collecting tubule. Physiologic, morphologic, and biochemical evidence suggests that the *initial* and *cortical* collecting tubules are functionally similar. Among the factors that affect potassium secretion along the initial collecting tubule, three are especially important: fluid flow rate, luminal sodium concentration, and acid-base balance. More recent studies have focused on the effects of adrenal corticosteroids, of plasma potassium levels, and of antidiuretic hormone (ADH) on potassium transport across this nephron segment.

Such experiments have shown that ADH stimulates potassium secretion at the level of the distal and initial collecting tubules. These observations help to explain why a water diuresis (low vasopressin levels) is not associated with a kaliuresis and why vasopressin-induced antidiuresis does not lead to potassium retention and hyperkalemia despite the sharp fall in distal tubular flow rate.

The effects of physiologic levels of mineralocorticoids and glucocorticoids on potassium transport were also examined by distal tubular microperfusion. Chronic (8 to 10 days) and acute (3 to 5 hr) infusion of aldosterone in rats stimulates potassium secretion by the distal tubule. The *chronic* effect of aldosterone on transport is mediated, in part, by an increase in Na-K-ATPase pump sites and by an increase in the basolateral membrane area of principal cells. Glucocorticoid (dexamethasone) treatment had no direct effect at the level of the distal tubule on potassium transport, basolateral membrane area, or ATPase activity. Thus, mineralocorticoids, but not glucocorticoids, regulate potassium secretion by a *direct* effect on the distal tubule. However, glucocorticoids may stimulate potassium excretion by elevating glomerular filtration rate and distal tubular flow rate.

Since alterations of plasma potassium levels are often associated with changes in adrenal corticosteroids, it has been difficult to examine the effects of plasma potassium changes themselves on potassium secretion. In adrenalectomized animals in which corticosteroid levels were held constant by implanted minipumps, hyperkalemia was shown to stimulate potassium secretion directly. Thus, both hyperkalemia and elevated aldosterone levels contribute to potassium secretion.

An additional site of regulation of potassium excretion is the cortical collecting tubule. Three presentations during the Workshop dealt with its permeability properties, its electrophysiology, and key aspects of transport-related enzyme (ATPase) adaptation.

Regulation of Potassium Permeability of the Cortical Collecting Tubule (*CCT*). Stokes pointed out that our current understanding of the mechanism of potassium secretion by the cortical collecting tubule cell includes a model whereby sodium is absorbed by two processes in series. The entry of sodium into the cell across the luminal membrane occurs via a sodium-selective pathway or "channel," and it is extruded across the basolateral membrane by Na-K-ATPase. The potassium that enters the cell via this exchange for sodium can then exit the cell across either the apical membrane or the basolateral membrane. The magnitude of potassium secretion is therefore regulated by at least two processes: the turnover rate of the sodium-potassium pump and the relative permeabilities of the apical and basolateral membrane for potassium.

Efforts by Stokes and his associates to characterize the nature of these pathways for potassium permeation across the apical and basolateral membranes have been conducted by using primarily two techniques. The first technique involves the elevation of the potassium concentration in either the lumen or the bath. This maneuver induces a diffusion voltage that reflects the transference number for potassium across the apical or basolateral membranes, respectively. The second is the use of tracer permeabilities or rate coefficients. The passive permeation of potassium as measured by tracer has a large cellular component that is, at least in part, a property of the conductive pathways of the apical and basolateral membranes. It appears that one or both of these permeabilities can be regulated by maneuvers that effect the magnitude of active transport.

Initially it was shown that the potassium diffusion voltage, estimated by raising potassium concentration in either the lumen or the bath, would not produce a stable or reproducible measurement. Because of the probability that this maneuver influenced the active transport voltage, active transport was eliminated with amiloride in the lumen, and stable diffusion voltages were obtained. Evaluating these potassium diffusion voltages, it was discovered that there were time-dependent and history-dependent effects. Exposure to elevated concentrations of potassium causes the diffusion voltage to increase gradually to a stable value over a period of 10 to 20 min. This effect was present from either the lumen or the bath surface. Furthermore, the time required to reach the steady state depended on the history of the tubule. A second exposure to potassium caused the tubule to reach the steady state much more rapidly than the first exposure. These results were among the first clues that the conductive pathways to potassium might be regulated by maneuvers that affect active transport.

In the presence of amiloride, the diffusion voltage from the bath was always larger than the diffusion voltage from the perfusate. This result indicated that the transference number for potassium was larger in the basolateral membrane than in the apical membrane and suggested that under these conditions basolateral membrane permeability might be larger than the apical membrane permeability. This finding was surprising in light of previous observations of Stokes and his colleagues. His previous results indicated that most of the potassium entering the cell via the pump exited across the apical membrane, suggesting that the apical membrane should be more permeable than the basolateral membrane. Analysis of the effects of amiloride on the lumen-to-bath tracer rate coefficient for potassium (K_K), a measure of passive transport, showed that amiloride treatment greatly increased K_K. This increase was out of proportion to the change in the transepithelial voltage, which might have accounted for some of the increase. One possible explanation for these observations was that amiloride secondarily increased the potassium permeability of the cell.

The passive permeability characteristics were examined more carefully by using tubules already treated with amiloride and examining the effect of inhibition of the sodium-potassium pump with either ouabain or a zero-potassium bath. Inhibition of the pump reduced the potassium-diffusion voltage, as measured from either the lumen or the bath. Likewise, pump inhibition reduced the potassium rate coefficient consistent with the notion that the apical- and/or the basolateral membrane-conductive permeability to potassium was inhibited following inhibition of the sodium-potassium pump. The time course for the changes in these permeabilities appeared to parallel the time course required for pump inhibition to alter the intracellular ion activities (approximately 20 min).

The evidence for a predominantly *cellular* pathway for passive potassium transfer in the amiloride-treated tubule is supported by the following evidence: (1) diffusion voltages from the lumen and bath are asymmetric, (2) there is a time- and history-dependent nature of the development of the potassium-diffusion voltage, (3) there is a larger increase in K_K following amiloride than would be expected for a paracellular pathway, (4) there was a differential change in the K_K following elevation of either lumen or bath potassium, (5) following symmetric depolarization (raising the potassium concentration equally in perfusate and bath), there is a reduction in K_K that is not accompanied by changes in the transepithelial voltage, and (6) with inhibition of the sodium-potassium pump, there are strikingly different effects on the passive sodium permeation and K_K.

In summary, several factors increase either the apical or the basolateral membrane potassium permeability. They include agents that inhibit the entry of sodium into the cell (such as amiloride), as well as aldosterone. A reduction in potassium permeability occurs following the inhibition of the sodium-potassium pump. Furthermore, other investigators have demonstrated that luminal acidification and barium likewise reduced potassium permeability.

Cellular Electrophysiology of Potassium Transport in the Collecting Duct. Significant advances have been made in the understanding of tubular potassium transport by measuring cell potentials of the cortical and medullary collecting tubules. Important differences between the electrical properties of different parts of the collecting duct and an analysis of the cellular electrophysiology of potassium transport in the collecting duct were presented by Koeppen. He pointed out that there are significant differences in several electrophysiologic parameters between the *cortical* and *medullary* collecting ducts. The transepithelial voltage is lumen-negative in the cortex, but positive in the outer medulla, particularly in the inner stripe. The cell potential is electrically more negative in the cortex than the medulla, and there is a significant increase of the transepithelial electrical resistance with the progression from cortical to medullary segments of the collecting tubule.

The cortical collecting duct of the rabbit is a major target for mineralocorticoid hormones. Their effect at this site is to increase both the net reabsorption of sodium and the net secretion of potassium. The transport rate of these cations is increased several times following chronic (7 to 14 day) treatment of rabbits with high doses (5 mg/day) of deoxycorticosterone acetate (DOCA). Both biochemical and morphologic changes occur during this time, including an increase in Na-K-ATPase activity and amplification of basolateral membrane area of the principal cells. Microelectrode studies indicate that important changes in membrane electrical properties also occur and likely contribute to increased cation transport. Specific changes that occur include: (1) an increase in the sodium- and potassium-conductive pathways of the luminal cell membrane, (2) a decrease in the conductance of the paracellular "shunt" pathway, (3) depolarization of the lumen membrane potential, and (4) hyperpolarization of the basolateral cell membrane. Taken together and within the context of the cellular mechanism of sodium and potassium transport, the effects of chronic high-dose DOCA treatment can be summarized as follows: Cellular uptake of potassium is increased both by the activity of Na-K-ATPase as well as by the altered electrochemical gradient across the basolateral cell membrane. Efflux of potassium across the luminal cell membrane is increased because of the increased conductance and a more favorable electrochemical gradient.

Regulation of Potassium Secretion and Na-K-ATPase Activity of Mammalian Collecting Tubule. Research in several laboratories has also shown that important changes in ATPase activity accompany alterations in potassium transport. These changes served as the topic of O'Neil's report. Recent studies of the rabbit-isolated cortical collecting tubule have revealed that potassium secretion is controlled by three separate steps: Potassium is actively taken up into the cell across the basolateral membrane via the sodium-potassium exchange pump (*step 1*), and then is either recycled across the basolateral membrane by diffusing down its electrochemical gradient through a potassium channel (*step 2*), or is secreted into the tubular lumen by diffusing down its electrochemical gradient through an apical membrane potassium channel (*step 3*). Potassium secretion can therefore be influenced by regulating any one of these three steps.

It has long been known that potassium secretion by the collecting duct is partially under the control of the mineralocorticoid aldosterone. Elevated plasma aldosterone levels are accompanied by an increased ability of the collecting ducts to secrete potassium (and reabsorb sodium), whereas depressed plasma aldosterone levels are accompanied by a reduced ability to secrete potassium. In animals with intact adrenal glands, chronic elevation of plasma mineralocorticoid levels for several days is accompanied by an elevation in the Na-K-ATPase activity of the cortical collecting tubule. The converse was observed with depressed plasma mineralocorticoid levels. This is consistent with the notion that the effect of mineralocorticoids is on the Na-K-ATPase activity of the collecting duct.

O'Neil and his colleagues recently extended the above studies to assess (1) the effects of mineralocorticoids on the Na-K-ATPase activity of the cortical collecting duct in greater detail and (2) the role that sodium entry into the cell may play on the mineralocorticoid-dependent regulation of the Na-K-ATPase. All studies were performed on rabbits with intact adrenal glands. First, the influence of endogenous plasma aldosterone levels on the Na-K-ATPase of the cortical collecting tubule was assessed. Initially, animals were maintained on a high-sodium diet to suppress endogenous aldosterone levels. Then, at a given time (day 0), they were switched to a low-sodium diet for 3 to 17 days (plus furosemide treatment at days 0 and 3) to elevate plasma aldosterone levels. With the high-sodium diet, the plasma aldosterone levels averaged 16 ng/dl. They increased nearly 4-fold after 3 to 4 days on the low-sodium diet and 16-fold after 15 to 17 days. The Na-K-ATPase activity of cortical collecting tubules isolated from these animals increased by over 2-fold after 3 to 4 days on the low-sodium regimen from the control values of 13 pmoles of ADP/mm/min for animals on the high-sodium regimen. Surprisingly, with continued treatment with the low-sodium regimen, the Na-K-ATPase activity declined, returning to control values after 2 or more weeks. It seemed likely that the decline in the ATPase activity was related to a reduced delivery of sodium to the cortical collecting tubule in the animal, which would reduce sodium entry into the cell. Indeed, when animals were maintained on a normal sodium diet to support a higher delivery of sodium to the collecting tubules, treatment with the mineralocorticoids, deoxycorticosterone acetate (DOCA, 2 mg/kg/day, i.m.), caused the Na-K-ATPase activity of the cortical collecting tubules to increase, after a 1-day latent period, to a 2-fold maximum value over control values after 3 to 4 days *without* evidence of a decline in activity with continued treatment.

These results indicate that the effects of mineralocorticoids on the Na-K-ATPase of the cortical collecting tubule may be related to sodium entry into the cell across the apical cell border.

The influence of the cellular entry of sodium on the mineralocorticoid-induced elevation of cortical collecting tubule Na-K-ATPase was assessed with the aid of amiloride, a sodium-channel blocker. Animals were simultaneously treated with both DOCA (2 mg/kg/day, i.m.) and amiloride (10 mg/kg/twice daily, i.m.) for 3 to 4 days. Amiloride completely abolished the effects of DOCA on Na-K-ATPase activity. Amiloride treatment alone had no influence on the control activity. These results demonstrate that the effect of mineralocorticoids on the Na-K-ATPase depends directly on sodium's entry into the cell, thereby indicating that the initial effect of mineralocorticoids may be on the sodium permeability of the apical cell border.

It was concluded that (1) by controlling the Na-K-ATPase activity, mineralocorticoids play an important role in the regulation of potassium secretion by the cortical collecting tubule, and (2) that regulation of the Na-K-ATPase levels is a secondary action of mineralocorticoids, the primary effect being the sodium permeability of the apical cell membrane.

Renal Metabolism, Prostaglandins, and Renin

Contemporary Issues in Renal Metabolism

Chairpersons: Richard L. Tannen and Brian A. Ross
Discussants: Anton C. Schoolwerth and Norman J. Siegel

This Workshop dealt with two major topics in renal metabolism: (1) The use of nuclear magnetic resonance (NMR) to investigate renal metabolic events and the insights gained from this approach, and (2) the effect of acute changes in pH on renal ammonia production.

The Impact of ^{31}P Nuclear Magnetic Resonance on Clinical Nephrology

Renal metabolism has been a study in its own right since Krebs defined the pathway of renal glutamine metabolism in 1935. Developments in microdissection, enzymatic analysis, and endocrinology have given us a more complete understanding of intermediary metabolism in the kidney, perhaps, than of any other organ of comparable complexity. From current work, we are approaching a synthesis of renal transport physiology with its underlying metabolic events. Nonetheless, the impact of all this information on clinical nephrology has been relatively slight, because the biochemical methods have been destructive. Direct examination of biochemistry in the kidney has not been possible and examination of blood and urine is no substitute. Now, with the advent of ^{31}P-NMR, we at last have a tool that will enable critical events in renal energy metabolism and in acid-base homeostasis to be followed continuously in "real-time."

The concept of ^{31}P-NMR for nephrology was introduced at the VIIIth Congress of the International Society of Nephrology in a previous Workshop on renal metabolism (Ross, 1981). The object of the first part of the present Workshop is to report the impact of ^{31}P-NMR on our understanding of

---

This manuscript is a summary of a Workshop entitled *Contemporary Issues in Renal Metabolism.*

some central problems of nephrology. Since we are clearly on the verge of an ability to monitor renal energy metabolism continuously in humans, we shall ask the question: What clinical problems can be addressed most profitably with this technique?

NMR. Within a powerful magnetic field the intrinsic magnetic properties of atomic nuclei become measurable. Three types of NMR experimentation are currently in use: (1) "pulse and collect" qualitative NMR, (2) quantitative NMR, and (3) saturation transfer NMR (STNMR).

"Pulse and collect" NMR involves irradiation of the sample with a radiofrequency pulse that excites specific nuclei; for example, ^{31}phosphorus. The signal is collected, subjected to Fourier transformation, and stored on a magnetic disc. The cycle is repeated many times, until the amplitude of the signal can be discriminated from the background noise. The result is a spectrum from which the qualitative determination of ATP, AMP, ADP, Pi, and quantitative measurement of intracellular pH can be made. Table 1 summarizes the wide range of experiments which have already been carried out using this form of ^{31}P-NMR. Siegel discussed one such study of this type, namely, one involving the diagnosis of acute renal failure and the direct monitoring of the effects of therapy.

Quantitative NMR has demanded some ingenuity, but it also involves "pulse and collect" experiments. An external reference standard is required. There are major differences between the NMR-determined values for ADP and Pi compared with classically accepted values.

Saturation transfer NMR is a third type of NMR experiment that is used extensively in the intact kidney. During a quantitative "pulse and collect" experiment, the rate of ATP synthesis can be determined directly if the γ-phosphorus of ATP is irradiated at *its* specific frequency (saturated). "Saturation" of the γ-phosphorus signal results in loss of this peak from the kidney spectrum. As is obvious intuitively, phosphorus from the saturated γ-ATP will transfer continuously to the Pi peak, that is, "saturation transfer." The proportion of the Pi signal which is saturated will be a measure of the continuous chemical exchange, and this in turn is obviously the rate of ATP synthesis.

These results and concepts are derived from studies of the rat kidney in vivo. However, there is little doubt that similar results will emerge in humans when wide-bore high-field magnet techniques have been extended. This certainty comes from preliminary studies with the intact human kidney.

Three selected applications or facets of NMR were discussed during this Workshop:

(1) *Acute renal failure (Dr. Norman Siegel):* (A) *^{31}P-NMR during ischemia.* The speed and versatility of the "pulse and collect" experiment is well demonstrated in its ability to monitor relative [ATP] concentrations and intracellular pH continuously, before, during, and after clamping of the renal pedicle. The percentage changes in [ATP] correlate closely with chemical assays of [ATP] determined in a parallel study. After 45 min of renal ischemia, animals treated with normal saline had a very slow and incomplete recovery of tissue [ATP] to 66 $\pm$ 2% of control values. The infusion of ATP-MgCl$_2$ or AMP-MgCl$_2$ resulted in a significant enhancement in the rate of recovery

Table 1. ^{31}P-NMR studies in nephrology

Investigation	Species	Model	Principal finding(s)	References[a]
Total ischemia	Rabbit	Auto-perfusion	Acidosis + ATP depletion	1
Renal preservation	Rat	Excised kidney	Infused buffer prevents pH-drop	2
Metabolic acidosis	Rat	Perfusion	Intracellular pH parallels extra-cellular, not urine pH	3
Respiratory acidosis	Rat	Perfusion	As metabolic acidosis, but [HCO$_3$] controls urine acidification, not ammoniagenesis	4
Intracellular pH gradients	Rabbit	Tubules	DMO and NMR give different pH: mitochondrial pH calculated 0.5 U above cytosol	5, 6
Ischemic acute renal failure	Rat	In vivo	3 models lose ATP; pH falls	7, 8
	Rat	In vivo	Mg-ATP infusion restores [ATP]	9
Nonischemic acute renal failure	Rat	In vivo	Glycerol depletes ATP, but other models show no NMR change despite severe ATN	7
Assigning NMR peaks	Rabbit	Isolated tubules	Glycerophosphoryl-choline identified in renal papilla	6
Assigning NMR peaks	Rat	Perfused	AMP identified as only 30% of 12 ppm peak; remainder unknown compound	4
Localization	Rat	In vivo	Noninvasive focusing identified kidney through muscle	3
Quantitation	Rat	Perfused	[Pi], [ADP] and phosphorylation potential redetermined	11
Quantitation	Rat	In vivo	Nucleotides similar to perfused; ATP exceeds enzymatic assay	12

Table 1. (*continued*)

Investigation	Species	Model	Principal finding(s)	References[a]
Saturation transfer (STNNR)	Rat	Perfusion	ATP:0 ratio directly determined = 2.5	11
Saturation transfer	Rat	In vivo	ATP:0 ratio between 1–2	12, 13
Saturation transfer	Rat	In vivo	Transfer observed α-ATP $\rightarrow$ Pi	8
Hemorrhagic hypotension (STNMR)	Rat	In vivo	Fall in metabolic rate by STNMR parallels O_2 consumption: [ATP] also falls indicating very early compromise of metabolism	12
Viability of donor kidney	Human	Excised kidney	pH and change in ATP correlated with outcome of transplant in clinical study	14
Acute ischemia	Human	Normothermic perfusion	Human ^{31}P-NMR spectrum identical to rat, rabbit and dog	15
Hypernephroma and Wilms Tumor	Human	Normothermic perfusion	Characteristic NMR peak at 4.2 ppm; tumors resist hypoxia; respond to drugs	15

[a] References: 1. SEHR PA, BORE PS, PAPATHEOPHANIS J, RADDA GK: *Br J Exp Pathol* 60:632–641, 1979   2. BORE PJ, SEHR PA, CHAN L, THULBORN KR, ROSS BD, RADDA GK: *Eur Surg Res* (suppl 1):20–21, 1980   3. ACKERMAN JJH, LOWRY M, RADDA GK, ROSS BD, WONG GG: *J Physiol* 319:65–79, 1981   4. FREEMAN DM, LOWRY M, RADDA GK, ROSS BD: *Biochem Soc Trans* 10:399, 1982   5. BALABAN RS: *Fed Proc* 41:42–47, 1982   6. ADLER S, SHORBRIDGE EA, RADDA GK: *Am J Physiol* (in press)   7. CHAN LC, LEDINGHAM JGG, DIXON JA, THULBOEN KR, WATERTON JC, RADDA GK, ROSS BD: in *Acute Renal Failure,* edited by ELIAHOU HE, London, Libbey, pp 35–41   8. KORETSKY AP, WANG S, MURPHY-BOESCH J, KLEIN MP, JAMES TL, WEINER MW: *Proc Natl Acad Sci USA* 80:7491–7495, 1983   9. SIEGAL NJ, AVISON MJ, REILLY HF, ALGER JR, SHULMAN RG: *Am J Physiol* 245:F530-F534, 1983   10. BALABAN RS, GADIAN DG, RADDA GK: *Kidney Int* 20:575–579, 1981   11. FREEMAN DM, BARTLETT SB, RADDA GK, ROSS BD: *Biochim Biophys Acta* 762:325–336, 1983   12. YAHAYA H, CHAN L, FREEMAN DM, HOLLOWAY P, ROSS BD: *Clin Sci* 66:358, 1984   13. ROSS BD, FREEMAN DM, CHAN LC: 6th International Workshop in Phosphate and Other Minerals, 1983   14. CHAN LK: PhD Dissertation. Oxford, England, University of Oxford, 1983   15. ROSS BD, MARSHALL VM, SMITH MB, BARTLETT SB, FREEMAN DM: *Lancet* i:641–646, 1984

of tissue [ATP] (83 ± 2%) and thus represented the metabolic and molecular basis of the salutary effect of these compounds. Moreover, the enhanced recovery of renal function and preservation of sublethally injured tubular cells that was previously demonstrated with this combination may be due to the provision of precursors that allow the resynthesis of tissue nucleotides following the ischemic insult. (*B*) *Other nuclei*. Preliminary studies in which 2-^{13}C-acetate was infused into animals in vivo enable ^{13}C spectra of kidney to be observed. This powerful application of NMR spectroscopy creates the possibility of observing many organic molecules of metabolic importance: glutamate and glutamine, C2 and C4, accumulated in kidney, together with C2 to C5 of glucose, and the original C2 of acetate. After infusion of ^{13}C-glucose (C-1), a small but significant peak for ^{13}C-labeled glucose (+ 98 ppm) can be seen in the kidney. After 20 min of ischemia, the third carbon of lactate becomes visible (+ 20 ppm) and then can be traced during the remaining 80 min of ischemic injury. This approach permits evaluation not only of changes in tissue pH, but also of the rate of lactate generation during an ischemic injury and subsequently during the recovery period.

(2) *Saturation transfer NMR in hemorrhagic hypotension*. The ATP:0 ratio has been determined directly for the first time and was approximately 2:0. As expected, blood pressure fell as the metabolic rate fell. Surprising, however, was the finding that ATP fell in parallel, a clear indication of renal metabolic impairment even in mild hypotension. This occurred before the appearance of acute tubular necrosis and may represent a prodromal phase.

(3) ^{31}*P-NMR of human kidney tumors*. Because of the expediency of isolated normothermic perfusion of carefully preserved human nephrectomy specimens, the "pulse and collect" NMR experiment has been applied to questions of human kidney preservation, acute renal ischemia (that is, ATN), hypoxia, and the metabolic response to chemotherapy in both hypernephroma and Wilms tumors. The human kidney spectrum is typical and the quantitative differences of both Pi and ADP using NMR are also present in humans. The changes in ^{31}P NMR appearance seen by Chan et al (1981) and Siegal et al (1983) in ischemic acute renal failure in the rat apply equally to this human kidney preparation. The prospects for in vivo monitoring of the response to cancer chemotherapy in humans are illustrated by studies of isolated normothermic human kidney perfusion.

Effect of Acute Changes in pH on Renal NH$_3$ Production

While it is well known that chronic metabolic acidosis and alkalosis result in adaptive changes which modify the capacity of the kidney to produce NH$_3$, the effect of acute changes in pH on NH$_3$ production has been appreciated more recently and important strides have been made in elucidating the underlying mechanisms. Acute refers to events within the first 2 hr of exposure to a modified pH in vivo, before the enzymatic adaptations which characterize the chronic response are initiated, and in vitro to the direct effects of an altered pH on ammonia metabolism.

As reviewed by Tannen, it seems clear, especially in the rat, that both acute metabolic and acute respiratory acidosis stimulate renal NH_3 production. Increased ammoniagenesis is demonstrable in the intact animal, with renal cortical tubules incubated in vitro and also with the isolated rat kidney perfused at physiologic concentrations of glutamine (0.5 mM). In both the intact animal and the perfused kidney, the response occurs rapidly (within 15 min) and is reversed with a similar time course. The increase in NH_3 production by the perfused kidney exposed to a low pH is inhibited by a factor excreted in the urine. Recent studies have shown that this urinary inhibitor is an arachidonic acid metabolite. The prostaglandin moiety which inhibits the ammoniagenic response to acute acidosis is not PGE_2 and appears to be $PGF_{2\alpha}$. The precise mechanism whereby acute acidosis alters renal ammonia metabolism was considered by Schoolwerth later in this Workshop.

The response to an acute increase in pH has not undergone as careful scrutiny as the response to acidosis, and Tannen focused on recent studies with the isolated perfused rat kidney during the remainder of his presentation. In the intact rat acute respiratory alkalosis inhibits ammoniagenesis, but the response to acute metabolic alkalosis is equivocal. NH_3 production by renal cortical tubules incubated in vitro is not altered by an alkaline pH.

Respiratory alkalosis (pH 7.75 or 7.58) has no effect on NH_3 production during the initial 45 min of perfusion at a high pH. However, during the subsequent 45 min of perfusion suppression of NH_3, production is clearly evident regardless of whether the pH had been returned to normal or the exposure to respiratory alkalosis sustained. When the studies in which the pH was returned to 7.4 were prolonged for an additional 45 min, NH_3 production returned to normal. Thus, in contrast to acute acidosis where NH_3 production increased rapidly (within 15 min), with acute alkalosis, 45 min is required for suppression of NH_3 production to be manifest and an equal length of exposure to a normal pH for the inhibition of ammoniagenesis to be reversed. This striking difference in time course suggests that acute acidosis and alkalosis modify ammoniagenesis by different metabolic mechanisms.

Exposure to metabolic alkalosis (pH 7.71) increased NH_3 production during the first 45 min of perfusion. However, if the pH was returned to normal, NH_3 production was suppressed in the same fashion as with an initial period of exposure to respiratory alkalosis. When exposure to metabolic alkalosis persisted, an inhibitory effect of the high pH on NH_3 production became apparent, but it took more than 90 min for the high pH to override the stimulatory effect of a high bicarbonate concentration. Thus, a high HCO_3 concentration results in transitory stimulation of ammoniagenesis, but a high pH resulting from either respiratory or metabolic alkalosis initiates the predominant, more slowly activated mechanism which suppresses NH_3 formation.

The precise metabolic events accounting for the high HCO_3 and high pH effects on renal ammonia production are unknown. However, as with acute acidosis, albeit by different mechanisms, acute alkalosis does alter NH_3 production. The unusual time course of the response to acute alkalosis, and especially to metabolic alkalosis, may account for the equivocal response in the intact animal and the inability to detect a change with renal tubules incubated in vitro.

Schoolwerth next reviewed the results of studies with isolated rat renal cortical mitochondria, which shed light on the mechanisms whereby acute acidosis stimulates renal ammonia production.

When renal cortical mitochondria are incubated with 1 mM glutamine as the sole substrate, a reduction in the pH of the medium from 7.4 to 6.8 results in inhibition of mitochondrial NH_3 production. However, when this identical maneuver is carried out with 0.5 mM alpha-ketoglutarate also present in the medium, the acidic pH stimulates ammonia formation by 66%. An analysis of the flux through the intramitochondrial ammonia-metabolizing pathways indicates that the stimulation of NH_3 formation is attributable entirely to increased flux through glutamate dehydrogenase. Flux through phosphate-dependent glutaminase is unchanged and there is no definite effect on the glutamate-oxaloacetate transamination pathway. In addition, the low pH also decreases the accumulation of glutamate in the incubation medium.

Thus, a low pH can stimulate mitochondrial ammoniagenesis, but this response is critically contingent on the presence of alpha-ketoglutarate in the incubation medium. The key ammonia-producing step stimulated by a low pH is glutamate deamination. To explain these observations further the following studies were carried out: an assessment of intramitochondrial pH, an evaluation of alpha-ketoglutarate flux, measurement of the mitochondrial matrix concentration of the key metabolites of the glutamate dehydrogenase flux, and an evaluation of mitochondrial glutamate transport.

Intramitochondrial pH is 0.6 U greater than the medium pH at pH 7.4. When the medium pH is reduced to 6.8 in the presence of alpha-ketoglutarate, matrix pH decreases by a smaller amount so that the gradient is increased to 0.9 pH U. By contrast, when glutamine is the only substrate, the decrease in matrix pH is more profound. Similarly, a more severe decrease in matrix pH occurs in the presence of alpha-ketoglutarate when arsenite, an inhibitor of alpha-ketoglutarate dehydrogenase, is added to the incubation medium, indicating that the metabolism of alpha-ketoglutarate maintains the matrix pH more alkaline.

Studies from several laboratories have shown that an acid pH alters the activity of alpha-ketoglutarate dehydrogenase by lowering the K_m. Incubation of mitochondria at pH 6.8 accelerates alpha-ketoglutarate flux as demonstrated by a more rapid disappearance of alpha-ketoglutarate from the medium and increased formation of $^{14}CO_2$ from 2-($1^{14}C$)-ketoglutarate.

Mitochondrial matrix concentrations of alpha-ketoglutarate and NH_3 are reduced at pH 6.8 and the concentration of glutamate is increased. These alterations all favor increased flux from glutamate to alpha-ketoglutarate. The decrease in alpha-ketoglutarate concentration results from the increase in alpha-ketoglutarate dehydrogenase activity induced by the decrease in matrix pH and the decrease in NH_3 concentration from the increased transmitochondrial pH gradient. Matrix glutamate concentration increases, because a low pH inhibits glutamate efflux from the mitochondrial matrix. The inhibition of glutamate efflux coupled with increased deamination by glutamic dehydrogenase can account for the decrease in renal tissue glutamate concentration found with acute acidosis.

The studies detailed above, which provide a rational framework for the stimulation of NH_3 formation by a low pH were all carried out in a bicarbonate-free medium. Additional studies investigating the effect of isohydric manipulations of bicarbonate on mitochondrial metabolism indicate that a high bicarbonate concentration inhibits flux through phosphate-dependent glutaminase by a mechanism that does not appear to represent a direct effect on the enzyme. Furthermore, a high bicarbonate concentration inhibits flux through succinate dehydrogenase. Hence, the decrease in bicarbonate concentration with acute metabolic acidosis might further enhance the ammoniagenic effect of a low pH by relieving inhibition at both the phosphate-dependent glutaminase and succinic dehydrogenase steps.

To summarize the cogent findings in this portion of the Workshop: Acute acidosis stimulates and acute alkalosis inhibits renal ammoniagenesis, but the involved metabolic mechanisms appear to differ. Acute acidosis stimulates ammonia production rapidly by accelerating glutamate deamination secondary to effects on alpha-ketoglutarate dehydrogenase, intramitochondrial pH, and glutamate efflux from the mitochondrial matrix. By contrast acute alkalosis inhibits ammoniagenesis by a slowly activated, currently uncharacterized process, which appears unrelated to the effects of pH on alpha-ketoglutarate metabolism.

Biochemistry of Renal Prostaglandins

Aubrey R. Morrison

The prostaglandins and eicosanoids produced by the kidney are oxygenated metabolites of the 20-carbon polyunsaturated fatty acids, which are important constituents of biological membranes. The major fatty acids which give rise to the oxygenated metabolites are dihomo gammalinolenic acid ($C_{20}:3$), arachidonic acid ($C_{20}:4$), and eicosapentaenoic acid ($C_{20}:5$), which give rise to the monoenic (series 1), the bisenoic (series 2), and trienoic (series 3) prostaglandins. In mammalian species the major fatty acid of biological importance under normal conditions is arachidonic acid. This fatty acid is a normal constituent of the mammalian phospholipids and is normally in the 2 position in an acyl linkage. Because prostaglandins are not stored [1], then the initial controlling step in the biosynthesis must be the release of arachidonic acid from membrane phospholipids. Several stimuli are coupled to the release of arachidonic acid through mechanisms which are not completely understood. Table 1 shows some stimuli which trigger the release of arachidonic acid. There are several features of the release which are worthy of some comment. Certain specific stimuli, for example, peptides, seem to be very tightly coupled to the specific release of arachidonic acid and not to the release of any other fatty acid. This was demonstrated by Schwartzman and Raz [2, 3] who showed bradykinin releases only arachidonate from membrane phospholipids. In contrast, however, nonspecific stimuli, for example, ischemia, released other fatty acids in addition to arachidonic acid [2, 4]. It is clear that the release of fatty acid is controlled in some way by calcium (Ca^{++}) since the removal of Ca^{++} from the external environment of cells decreases arachidonic acid release [5]. In addition the divalent ionophore A23187 stimulates arachidonate release and increases prostaglandin biosynthesis [6, 7]. Furthermore, there appears to be an endogenous inhibitor of the acylhydrolase, which is glucocorticoid-regulated [8]. This protein has been given the names macrocortin [9] or lipomodulin [10]. The cellular events involved in the release of arachidonic

This manuscript was presented as part of a Symposium on *Prostaglandins and the Kidney*.

acid from membrane phospholipids may involve either activation of an acylhydrolyse (phospholipase A_2), which then cleaves in a Ca^{++}-dependent step, that is, the release of arachidonic acid from the sn-2 position. Alternatively, as has been described in the platelet, the initial cleavage is through a phospholipase C which forms diacylglycerol and then subsequent release of arachidonic acid [9].

The arachidonic acid once released can be metabolized to biologically active prostaglandins and eicosanoids through a series of particulate and soluble enzymes. In the kidney there seems to be much regional specificity in the distribution of the enzymes. The enzymes can be described as the cyclooxygenase, the lipoxygenases, and the cytochrome P_{450} monooxygenases.

Cyclooxygenase

The enzyme activity is distributed in the kidney in medulla > papilla > cortex. In the medulla the enzyme appears to be localized to the collecting duct [12] and the medullary interstitial cells [13]. In the papilla it is in the thin loops of Henle, and in the cortex in the afferent glomerular arteriole [12] in glomerular epithelial [14, 15] and mesangial cells [14, 16]. This enzyme is membrane-bound and appears to be in greatest proportions in the microsomal fractions of the kidney. The enzymes acting on the substrate arachidonic acids insert a hydroperoxy function at C_{15}, remove a hydrogen from C_{13}, and insert oxygen at C_{11}; cyclization occurs to form the unstable intermediate PGG_2 which can then be converted to PGH_2 with a reduction of hydroperoxy function at C_{15} to a hydroxy function (Fig. 1). The intermediate PGH_2 is the unstable endoperoxide ($T_{1/2}$ in aqueous media 5 min), which is the substrate for the enzymatic conversion to the biologically active prostaglandins and thromboxanes. The cyclooxygenase is irreversibly inhibited by acetylsalicylic acid and reversibly by the nonsteroidal anti-inflammatory drugs (NSAID). From the endoperoxide several biologically active products are formed. In the kidney the most active is the prostaglandin E_2 (PGE_2) isomerase of the renal medulla, which utilizes glutathione (GSH) as a cofactor and converts the endoperoxide to PGE_2 (9-keto, 11,15 dihydroxy prosta 5,13, dienoic acid). In addition PGD_2 and prostaglandin $F_{2\alpha}$ ($PGF_{2\alpha}$) are also formed from the endoperoxide by renal medulla. The renal medulla also has the enzymes prostacyclin synthetase which converts the endoperoxide

Table 1. Stimuli which release arachidonic acid

A. Peptide	Angiotensin II	B. Others	Catecholamines
	Bradykinin		α-adrenergic
	Vasopressin		β-adrenergic
	Calcitonin		Adenosine triphosphate
			Ischemia
			Diuretics
			Mechanical

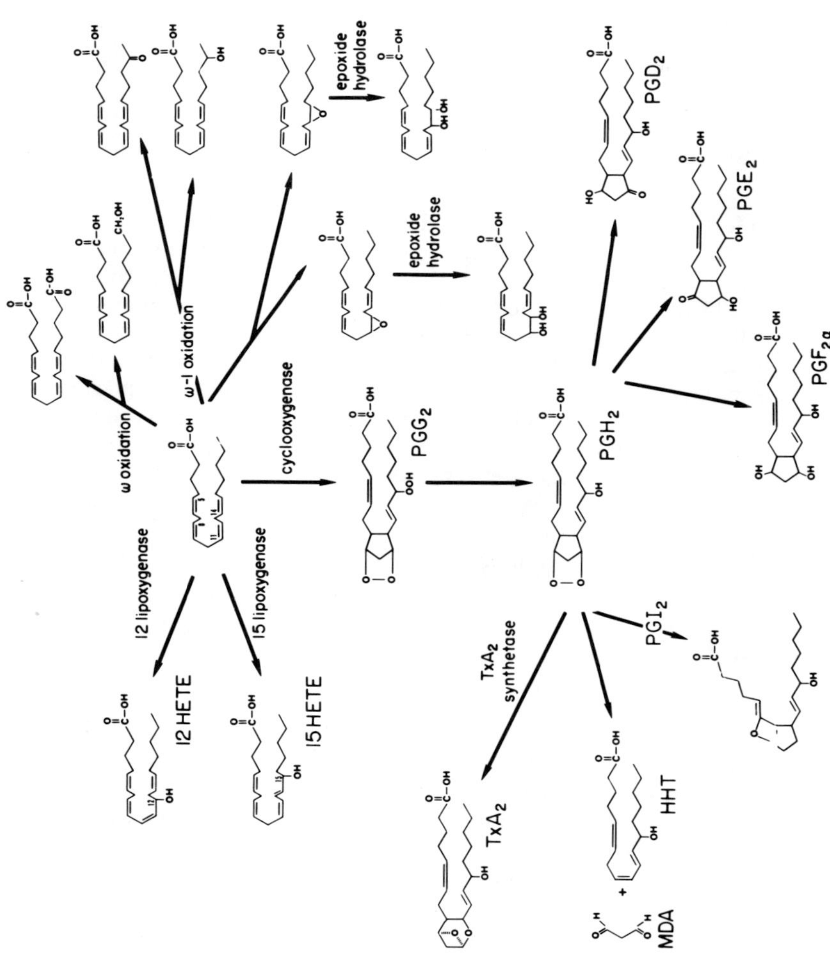

Fig. 1. Pathways of arachidonate metabolism by the kidney.

to prostacy clin (PGI_2) and thromboxane synthetase which converts PGH_2 to thromboxane A_2 (Fig. 1). Both PGI_2 and TxA_2 are unstable. PGI_2 easily forms the dehydration product 6-keto $PGF_{1\alpha}$ and TxA_2 breaks down with $T_{1/2}$ of 35 to 40 min in aqueous media to thromboxane B_2 (TxB_2). All of these enzymes have also been demonstrated to be present in the cortex of the kidney. PGH_2 to PGE_2 isomerase is particularly dominant in the cortical collecting duct while PGI_2, TxA_2, PGE_2, and $PGF_{2\alpha}$ are all produced by isolated glomeruli [17, 18].

Lipoxygenases

The unique feature of these enzymes is that on insertion of molecular oxygen into the fatty acid percursor the double bond is shifted to give a conjugated diene, which is a good ultra-violet (UV) chromophore and absorbs with a λ_{max} in the 235 nm range in methanol. The kidney has the enzymes which generate 15 hydroxy and 12 hydroxy eicosatetraenoic acids (15 and 12 HETE). The presence of these enzymes were first demonstrated in rabbit medulla [19], but subsequently investigators have documented the presence of the 12 lipoxygenase in murine species [19], and the 15 and 12 lipoxygenase enzymes in the human glomerulus [20]. The function of these compounds is somewhat unclear, since they are very weak chemoattractants [21]. These enzymes are soluble and appear to have a requirement for Ca^{++} similar to 5 lipoxygenase of neutrophils [22]. It is inhibited by nordihydroguiaretic acid (NDGA) and eicosatetraynoic acid (ETYA).

Cytochrome P_{450}

Two classes of enzymes have been described in the kidney cortex. The first class of enzymes are those that oxidize the fatty acid, for example, arachidonate, to form ω and ω-1 products. These products are 19, and 20 hydroxy eicosatetraenoic acid, 19-keto eicosatetraenoic acid, and eicosatetraen-1,20 dioic acid [23–25]. This enzyme has an obligatory requirement for NADPH and is inhibited by carbon monoxide [24], SKF525A, and metyrapone [23]. The other class of enzyme inserts oxygen across the double bonds to form epoxides. In the kidney the major epoxides formed are the 14,15 and 11,12 epoxides [24]. These are rapidly metabolized in vitro to form the vicinal diols 14,15,dihydroxy eicosatrienoic acid and 11,12 dihydroxy eicosatrienoic acid. Unlike the lipoxygenase, there is no requirement for Ca^{++} and no conjugated diene is formed; thus, the diols are poor UV chromophores. These enzymes can be inhibited by ETYA, metyrapone, SKF525A, and carbon monoxide. Figure 2 shows an HPLC tracing of a chromatogram of organic extract of arachidonate incubation with renal cortical microsomes in the presence of 1 mM NADPH. Compound I is 19-OH and 20-OH eicosatetraenoic acid; compound II, 19-keto eicosatetrienoic acid; compound III, eicosatetraen, 1,20 dioic acid; and compounds IV and V are 11,12 and 14,15 dihy-

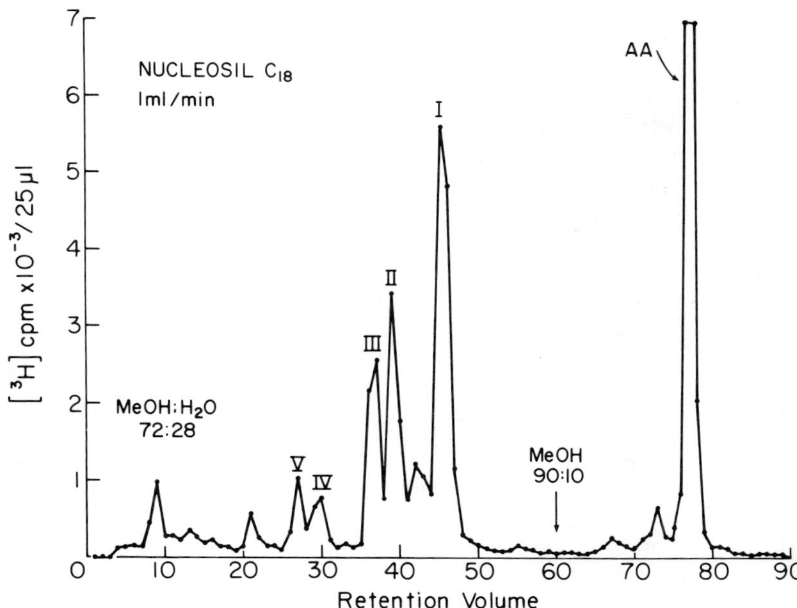

Fig. 2. HPLC tracing of incubation of ^{14}C arachidonate with renal cortical microsomes in presence of 1 mM NADPH.

droxy eicosatrienoic acids, respectively. Of some interest is that when we treat rabbits with hydrocarbon inducers of cytochromes, we can show differential induction of these two types of enzymes. Table 2 shows the percentage changes in in vitro activity using arachidonate as substrate. It can be seen that 3 methyl cholanthrene is a good inducer of diol formation and mild inducer of ω and ω-1 oxidation. On the other hand, benz[a]pyrene is a weak inducer of diol formation and does not appear to induce ω or ω-1 oxidation.

The formation of these metabolites of arachidonate in various regions of the kidney and their biological role in control of renal transport is of considerable interest and under active investigation.

Table 2. Percentage changes of in vitro activity using arachidonate as substrate

Treatment	Expt 1	Expt 2	Expt 3	Mean
		$\Delta\%$		$\Delta\% \pm$ SE
DIOL products				
3-MC	+405	+337	+244	329 ± 47
BP	+78	+204	+57	113 ± 46
ω and ω-1 products				
3-MC	+59	+61	+35	52 ± 8
BP	−10	−10	−33	−18 ± 8

Summary

Arachidonic acid $C_{20:4}$ is a substrate for a number of enzymes in the kidney cortex and medulla which convert the polyunsaturated fatty acid to unique metabolites through unstable intermediates. Cortex and medulla have a cyclo-oxygenase which metabolizes arachidonic acid to the unstable endoperoxide PGH_2 and then subsequently to PGE_2, $PGF_{2\alpha}$, PGI_2, TxA_2, and HHT. In the cortex, isolated glomeruli, glomerular epithelial, and mesangial cells also form prostanoids. In addition, the collecting duct (cortical) also appears to produce mainly PGE_2. In the medulla PGE_2 appears to be a major product with smaller amounts of $PGF_{2\alpha}$ and PGI_2. The cortex also metabolizes arachidonic acid through mixed-function oxidases which have an obligatory requirement for NADPH. Two types of metabolites are observed: (1) Metabolites derived from ω and ω-1 oxidatin, and (2) oxygenation reactions which involve the insertion of oxygen across the 11,12 and 14,15 double bonds to form intermediate epoxides. These latter compounds can be further converted to vicinal diols via an epoxide hydrolase. This pathway can be induced by some P_{450} inducers. There is now evidence for metabolism of $C_{20:4}$ via lipoxygenase (formation of conjugated dienes) in the soluble fraction of renal medulla with the formation of 15 and 12 HETE. In addition, the glomerulus also produces 12 and 15 HETE and there appears to be a species variation. Thus, arachidonic acid by the kidney produces a number of oxygenated compounds, the biology of which are currently under active investigation.

Acknowledgments. This study was supported by National Institutes of Health Public Health Award R0130542. Dr. Morrison is an Established Investigator of the American Heart Association.

References

1. PIPER P, VANE JR: Release of additional factor in anaphylaxis and its antagonism by antiinflammatory drugs. *Nature* 223:29–35, 1969
2. SCHWARTZMAN M, RAZ A: Prostaglandin generation in rabbit kidney. Hormone activated selective lipolysis coupled to prostaglandin biosynthesis. *Biochem Biophys Acta* 472:363–369, 1979
3. SCHWARTZMAN M, RAZ A: Biochemical action of vasoactive peptide hormones. Time synchronized activation of lipolysis and decreased fatty acid release by bradykinin in the perfused rabbit kidney. *Biochem J* 192:127–131, 1980
4. HSUEH W, ISAKSON PC, NEEDLEMAN P: Hormone selective lipase activation prostaglandins. *Prostaglandins* 13:1073–1091, 1977
5. ZENSER TV, DAVIS BB: Effects of calcium on prostaglandin synthesis by rat uiner medullary slices. *Am J Physiol* 235:F213–F218, 1978
6. ERMAN A, RAZ A: Effects of bivalent cations as prostaglandin biosynthesis and phospholipase A_2 activation in rabbit kidney medulla slices. *Biochem J* 182:821–828, 1978
7. KNAPP HR, OLEZ O, ROBERTS LJ, SWEETMAN BJ, OATES JA, REED P: Ionophores stimulate prostaglandin and thromboxane biosynthesis. *Proc Natl Acad Sci USA* 74:4251–4255, 1977

8. BLACKWELL GJ, FLOWER RJ, NIJKAMP FP, VANE JR: Phospholipase A_2 activity of guinea pig isolated perfused lungs: Stimulation and inhibition by anti-inflammatory steroids. *Br J Pharmacol* 62:79–89, 1978

9. BLACKWELL GJ, CARNUCCIO R, DIROSA M, FLOWER RJ, PARENTE L, PERSICO P: Macrocortin: A polypeptide causing the antiphopholipase effect of glucocorticoids. *Nature* 287:147–149, 1980

10. HIRATA F, SCHIFFMANN D, VENKOTASUBRAMANIAN K, SALOMON D, AXELROD J: A phopholipase A_2 inhibiting protein in rabbit neutrophils induced by glucocorticoids. *Proc Natl Acad Sci USA* 77:2533–2536, 1980

11. RITTENHOUSE-SIMMONS S: Production of diglyceride from phosphatidyl inositol in activated human platelets. *J Clin Invest* 63:580–587, 1979

12. SMITH WL, BELL TG: Immunohistochemical localization of the prostaglandin forming cyclooxygenase in renal cortexs. *Am J Physiol* 235:F451–F457, 1978

13. ZUSMAN RM, KEISER HR: Prostaglandin biosynthesis by rabbit renomedullary intenstitial cells in tissue culture. *J Biol Chem* 252:2069–2071, 1977

14. SRAER J, FORIDART J, CHANSEL D: Prostaglandin synthesis by mesangial and epithetial glomerular cultured cells. *FEBS Lett* 104:420–424, 1979

15. PETRULIS AS, AIKAWA M, DUNN MJ: Prostaglandin and thromboxane synthesis by rat glomerular epithetial cells. *Kidney Int* 20:469–474, 1984

16. SCHARSCHMIDT L, DUNN MJ: Prostaglandin synthesis by rat glomerulus mesangial cells in culture. The effects of sengiolensin II and organic vasopressin. *J Clin Invest,* in press

17. HASSID A, KONIECZKOWSKI M, DUNN MJ: Prostaglandin synthesis in isolated rat kidney glomeruli. *Proc Natl Acad Sci USA* 76:1155–1159, 1979

18. FOLKERT VW, SCHLONDORFF D: Prostaglandin synthesis in isolated glomeruli. *Prostaglandins* 17:79–86, 1979

19. WINOKUR T, MORRISON AR: Regional synthesis of monohydroxy eicosaroids by the kidney. *J Biol Chem* 256:10221–10223, 1981

20. JIM K, HASSID A, SUN F: Lipoxygenase activity in rat renal glomeruli. *J Biol Chem* 257:10249–10299, 1982

21. SRAER J, RIGAUD M, BENS M, RABINOVITCH H, ARDAILLOU R: Metabolism of arachidonic acid in the lipoxygenase pathway in human and murine glomeruli. *J Biol Chem* 258:4325–4330, 1983

22. GOETZL EJ, PICKETT WC: The human PNN leukocyte chemotactic activity of complex hydroxy eicosatetraenoic acids (HETES). *J Immunol* 125:1789–1791, 1980

23. JAKSCHIK BA, SAN FF, LIEH-LAUH LEE MM: Steinhoff calcium stimulation of a novel lipoxygenase. *Biochem Biophys Res Commun* 95:103–110, 1980

24. MORRISON AR, PASCOE N: Metabolism of arachidonate through NADPH-dependent oxygenase of renal cortexes. *Proc Natl Acad Sci USA* 78:7375–7378, 1981

25. OLIVER EH, LAWSON JA, BRASH AR, OATES JA: Arachidonic acid metabolism in rabbit renal cortex. *J Biol Chem* 256:9926–9931, 1981

26. CAPDEVILLA J, PARKHILL L, CHACOS N, OKITA R, MASTERS BS, ESTABROOK RW: The oxidative metabolism of arachidonic acid by purified cytochromes P_{-450}. *Biochem Biophys Res Commun* 101:1357–1363, 1981

From Molecular Biology to Antihypertensive Drugs: Current Research on Renin Inhibitors

Edgar Haber

The recent literature provides ample evidence for an intense interest in the structure of renin. A complete amino acid sequence of mouse submaxillary renin has been reported [1], as have the cDNA sequences of both mouse and human renins [2, 3]. Is this only the result of undirected curiosity, or does it have an end and a purpose in both the clinical investigation and the treatment of hypertension?

A central problem in renin research has been the lack of availability of adequate quantities of the enzyme. It is present in the kidney only in minute amounts and, thus, is very difficult to isolate from this source. Only quite recently has pure kidney renin been available in small quantities [4–7]. The realization that renin is produced in very large amounts in the salivary glands of certain strains of mice permitted the isolation of adequate quantities of renin for direct amino acid sequence analysis by conventional methods [8]. However, it later became apparent that submaxillary gland renin in this strain of mouse was the product of a different gene from that responsible for the synthesis of renal renin, and that there were differences in amino acid sequence [9, 10]. The abundant synthesis of renin in the submaxillary gland facilitated the isolation of renin's RNA and the consequent production of cDNA. The latter was sequenced [2], which generally confirmed the amino acid sequence of mouse submaxillary renin (there were a few errors) and provided a sequence of the pre- and prorenin segments of the molecule. At this point, we knew a great deal about the structure and biosynthesis of mouse submaxillary renin, but nothing about kidney renin. The function of submaxillary renin is still unknown, but everyone accepts a major role for renal renin in normal physiologic regulation of the cardiovascular system, as well as in the genesis of more than one form of hypertension [11]. It was the availability of the cDNA of mouse submaxillary renin that permitted the identification, isolation, and sequencing of the DNA of human renin.

This manuscript was presented as part of a Symposium on *Renin: Recent Advances.*

The two nucleotide sequences were sufficiently homologous, so that hybridization could be used as a tool for isolating human kidney cDNA and ultimately for sequencing it [3]. This was a very important short-cut to the difficult problem of isolating a very rare messenger from the kidney.

Thus, in a very few years, we proceeded from an understanding that renin was an enzyme of a given specificity to the availability of the detailed cDNA, and thereby to the inferred amino acid sequence of human renin. Of what value is this information?

Role of Renin-specific Antibodies

The pioneering work of Goldblatt in the 1930s allowed us to infer that renin played a central role in the genesis of renovascular hypertension; yet, the issue was not settled, and controversy concerning the mechanism for blood pressure elevation and maintenance continued for many years. It was not sufficient to show that renin or angiotensin II concentration increased in parallel with blood pressure, since this could be an association and not a cause. A variety of inhibitors of the renin-angiotensin system were examined in renovascular hypertension models, but the results could not be considered decisive because the inhibitors were not specific.

The interaction of angiotensin II with its receptor may be competitively inhibited by peptide analogs of the hormone. These have proven to be interesting diagnostic tools in renovascular hypertension; however, they are treacherous in clinical investigation, since they are partial agonists [12]. The conversion of the prohormone to the active peptide may be inhibited by converting enzyme inhibitors. Two compounds are now available as drugs: captopril and enalapril. Early clinical studies with converting enzyme inhibitors produced the unanticipated observation that patients with essential hypertension with normal or even depressed plasma renin levels showed a significant fall in blood pressure [13, 14]. It could not be determined whether these results suggested a hypertensive effect of renin acting in a compartment other than extracellular space or a manifestation of actions of these drugs apart from the renin-angiotensin system. A converting enzyme has at least one other role in addition to the conversion of angiotensin I to II. It metabolizes bradykinin, which is a potent vasodilator, to inactive peptide fragments. Could some of the effects of converting enzyme inhibitors be caused by the vasodilatory effects of bradykinin?

Another element of uncertainty in interpretation was added by the observation that the vasodilatory prostaglandin E_2 (PGE_2) increased in concentration in the plasma of patients having a hypotensive response to captopril that was associated with an increased urinary kinin excretion [15]. It was later shown that the inhibition of prostaglandin synthesis blunted the antihypertensive response to converting enzyme inhibition [16], as well as diminishing its hypotensive effect in sodium-depleted subjects [17].

Renin antibodies have been used as physiologic reagents for many years [18, 19]; yet, their specificity was in doubt, since we now know that the preparations then used as immunogens contained less than 1% of the enzyme. Dzau et al [5] purified canine renin some 600,000-fold in an eight-step process that yielded a product that was homogeneous by several criteria. Antibodies that were specific for purified canine renin raised in a goat were shown to be monospecific for renin, thereby providing a reagent that would interact with the enzyme alone. The antibodies and their Fab fragments proved to be a highly selective reagent for physiologic studies; there was no possibility of interaction with other systems. Renin-specific antibody [20] and Fab [21] inhibited the pressor action of the enzyme, but it did not modify the capacity of either angiotensin I or II to raise blood pressure. The hemodynamics of the unanesthetized, Na-replete dog were unchanged, while a significant hypotensive effect was noted in the Na-depleted dog. Parallel to the fall in blood pressure, a decrease in both plasma renin activity and angiotensin II concentrations was observed, indicating that the antibody was exerting its effect by inhibiting the enzymatic action of renin on its substrate. Thus, it could be concluded that renin played a role in normal cardiovascular homeostasis. During sodium restriction, it was essential for blood pressure maintenance.

The production of one-kidney, acute renovascular hypertension in the dog allowed questions about whether all of the blood pressure elevation observed was the consequence of increased renin secretion. Normal blood pressure was restored almost immediately after the intravenous (i.v.) administration of Fab, thus allowing a firm conclusion to be drawn concerning renin's role in this model of hypertension [21]. Thus, simply the purification of renin allowed for the production of a reagent more specific than any previously available.

These observations have now been applied by Corvol et al by using antihuman renin monoclonal antibodies as renin inhibitors in the marmoset, which is a primate that possesses renin with close structural similarity and immunologic cross-reactivity with human renin. Observations in this species were very similar to those described above in the dog—both in Na depletion and in renovascular hypertension [22].

Unanswered Questions: Renin in Human Essential Hypertension

Considerable progress has been made in understanding the relative roles of neural, endocrine, and renal control in the normal individual; however, the distortion of that control in essential hypertension has eluded the investigator. A major impediment is the lack of an animal model that is a convincing analog of the human disease. Clues must be sought in the observation and study of patients.

While renin was initially believed to be of relevance only in certain uncommon forms of secondary hypertension, such as renovascular hypertension, a flurry of interest was created by the demonstration that some patients with essential hypertension had abnormal plasma renin levels that were either elevated or depressed [23]. This observation did not lead to further insight until drugs became available that blocked the renin-angiotensin system by inhibiting the activity of angiotensin-converting enzyme. It was expected that the drugs would be effective in lowering blood pressure in those patients who had an elevated plasma renin, but investigators were soon surprised to find that some patients with normal or even depressed renin levels showed a significant fall in blood pressure [13, 14]. Unfortunately, as indicated above, converting enzyme inhibitors are relatively nonselective agents.

Thus far, the only convincingly specific inhibitor available is the antibody or its fragments. It is unlikely that widespread clinical investigation with the antibody will be possible when it derives from mouse immunoglobulin; the risk of immunization and its potential consequences are simply not warranted in the study of a chronic disease. Other, equally specific, and risk-free drugs must be sought.

Renin Inhibitors

Pepstatin and Its Congeners

Renin is an enzyme that—together with such enzymes as pepsin and cathepsin D—is considered to be an aspartyl protease because of the presence of two aspartic acid residues at the active site that are intimately involved in catalysis. In 1971, Umezawa et al discovered that the bacterial peptide they had been studying as an inhibitor of pepsin was also an effective blocker of a number of acid proteases [24]. Shortly thereafter, Gross et al [25, 26] demonstrated that in vivo inhibition of the renin-angiotensin system could be effected with pepstatin. This work was difficult to reproduce, probably because of the insolubility of the peptide [27, 28]; and, it did not lead to widespread adoption of pepstatin in physiologic experiments. Improvements in solubility—first by acetylation of pepstatin [29] and then by the substitution of hydrophilic amino acids at the carboxy terminus of the molecule [30]—yielded more convincing results. Although pepstatin derivatives may eventually prove to be adequate in vivo renin inhibitors, their use as investigative agents is limited conceptually by their lack of specificity for renin. Since all of the acid proteases studied are inhibited to varying degrees, how is a physiologic change to be interpreted as reflecting renin inhibition? May not some other acid proteases be involved in the regulation of the circulation? The desire to obtain an agent suitable for clinical investigation is certainly not satisfied by a general protease inhibitor, regardless of its efficacy.

Angiotensinogen Analogs

Skeggs et al [31] defined the minimal sequence from natural protein substrate that interacts strongly with renin. The octapeptide sequence extending from histidine-6 through tyrosine-13 (Table 1) [32] has kinetic parameters that are essentially the same as those of the full tetradecapeptide renin substrate [31]. Kokubu et al [33] synthesized a number of analogs of the tetradecapeptide that are found between residues 10 and 13 (Table 1) in the hope of

Table 1. Selected substrates and inhibitors of renin

Compound	Amino acid sequence	Reference
	1 2 3 4 5 6 7 8 9 10 11 12 13 14	
Equine substrate		
	Asp-Arg-Val-Tyr-Ile-His-Pro-Phe-His-Leu-Leu-Val-Tyr-Ser-	31
Human substrate		
	Asp-Arg-Val-Tyr-Ile-His-Pro-Phe-His-Leu-Val-Ile-His-	65
Minimal substrate		
	His-Pro-Phe-His-Leu-Leu-Val-Tyr	31
Early inhibitors	D	
	His-Pro-Phe-His-Leu-Leu-Val-Tyr	35
	D	
	Asp-Arg-Val-Tyr-Ile-His-Pro-Phe-His-Leu-Leu-Val-Tyr-Ser-	38
	Pro-His-Pro-Phe-His-Phe-Phe-Val-Tyr	34
In vivo inhibitors		
RIP:	Pro-His-Pro-Phe-His-Phe-Phe-Val-Tyr-Lys	44
	R	
	D-His-Pro-Phe-His-Leu-Leu-Val-Tyr	41
	Boc-His-Pro-Phe-His-Sta———Leu-Phe-NH$_2$	42
Potent inhibitors of human renin	R	
H-142:	Pro-His-Pro-Phe-His-Leu-Val- Ile-His-Lys	40
	Iva-His-Pro-Phe-His-Sta———Ile-Phe-NH$_2$	42
	Boc-Phe-His-Sta———Ala-Sta	43

	Amino acid sequence	Reference
	11 12 13 14 15 16 17 18 19	
Mouse submaxillary prosegment peptides		
	Boc-Leu-Lys-Lys-Met-Pro-OMe	51
	Boc-Glu-Arg-Ile-Pro- Leu-Lys-Lys-Met-Pro-OMe	51

D above an amino acid indicates the D stereoisomer.

R above a bond indicates a reduced peptide bond.

Sta indicates statine; Iva, isovaleryl; Boc, *tert*-butyloxycarbonyl; OMe, O-methyl.

creating an effective inhibitor. While inhibition could be shown, inhibitory constants were only in the millimolar range.

To produce more effective inhibitors, Burton et al [34, 35] synthesized analogs of a larger segment of renin substrate. Peptides were tested as renin inhibitors by using radioimmunoassay [36] to measure decreases in the generation of angiotensin I from either natural protein substrate or the tetradecapeptide. Addition of the octapeptide analogs to the standard assay mixture decreased the rate of formation of angiotensin I. Data from these tests fit the standard Michaelis-Menten equation [35], which indicates competitive inhibition.

The native octapeptide sequence is both a competitive inhibitor and a substrate for renin. Edman degradation of the reaction product shows that the enzyme quantitatively cleaves the leucyl-leucine bond in the octapeptide [35]. The first modifications made in the octapeptide sequence were aimed at producing peptides that would bind—but not be cleaved—by renin. Replacement of either leucyl residue (either 10 or 11 in the first sequence in Table 1) with the D-enantiomorph yields inhibitors that are not cleaved by renin. In addition, the (D-Leu^6)octapeptide binds renin one order of magnitude (3 μm) more tightly than does the parent octapeptide (39 μm).

K_I of the various inhibitors can be related to the lipophilicity of amino acid residues at the cleavage site. Replacement of the leucyl residues with phenylalanine yields an analog that binds about 40 times as well as Pro-octapeptide (K_I, 1 μm versus 39 μm) [37]. Chlorophenylalanine provides an even more hydrophobic residue at the cleavage site, and it yields a compound that is an even more potent inhibitor. Two chlorophenylalanines at the site yield an insoluble peptide.

Parikh and Cuatrecasas synthesized inhibitor peptides of greater length, but there was no apparent advantage with respect to enhanced inhibition (Table 1) [38].

Solubility of peptides is a requirement for a physiologically applicable inhibitor, since both a high concentration and tight binding to renin are required to compete with natural substrate. The effectiveness of an inhibitor is best judged by the ratio between solubility and K_I. Addition of a single prolyl residue to the (Phe^6)octapeptide doubled the solubility and decreased K_I so that this ratio increased from 6 to 100 [39]. A further improvement in the ratio was obtained by attaching a lysyl residue to the C-terminus of the (Pro)$_1$(Phe^{5}Phe^6) octapeptide (RIP) (Table 1). Solubility of this peptide was increased 8-fold with only a doubling of K_I, thus yielding a solubility/K_I ratio of 420:1. The pattern of solubility as a function of pH is also changed, which significantly enhances solubility at neutral pH as would be desirable in an inhibitor of physiologic usefulness.

Another approach to the construction of competitive inhibitors has been undertaken by Szelke et al [40]. Instead of substituting amino acids for those normally at the cleavage site of a substrate analog, the peptide bond (-CO-NH-) has been entirely replaced with a reduced bond (-CH$_2$-NH-). It is likely that the reduced peptide bond acts as a transition-state analog. One of these compounds (Table 1) has been shown to be an effective renin inhibitor in the dog [41]. Another is highly potent with respect to inhibiting human renin (Table 1).

If pepstatin derivatives could be rendered more specific by incorporating the recognition sequence of angiotensinogen, then useful inhibitors might be obtained. Pepstatin inhibits pepsin with a $K_I < 10^{-11}$ M. If a renin inhibitor could be constructed of similar potency, based on pepstatin's essential structures (such as the amino acid statine), one would have both a powerful and selective pharmacologic agent. Boger et al [42] and Evin et al [43] have inserted statine near the scissile bond of substrate analogs, thereby creating highly potent inhibitors of renin (Table 1). As in the instance of the reduced peptide bond, statine probably forms the tetrahedral configuration that mimics the transition state of an acid protease's substrate. This provides the high affinity of the inhibitor. It is the substrate sequence that determines selectivity for renin over other acid proteases. One of these compounds has been shown to be effective in blocking the hypertensive action of hog renin in the ganglion-blocked anesthetized rat [42].

Animal Studies

We have examined in vivo inhibition of renin by Pro-(Phe^{5}Phe^6)octa-peptidyllysine (RIP) (Table 1) in the monkey, *M. fascicularis* [44]. When infused into normotensive Na-replete monkeys, no significant change in blood pressure was observed. The pressor effect of purified human renin [45] was inhibited by an infusion of the peptide, but the effects of angiotensin I and angiotensin II were not. The peptide was then tested in normal Na-depleted animals. An i.v. bolus resulted in a prompt reduction in blood pressure; within 15 min, the pressure had returned to normal. An i.v. dose of the converting enzyme inhibitor teprotide resulted in an identical fall in pressure.

In Na-depleted renin-dependent hypertensive monkeys, the i.v. injection of RIP resulted in a prompt fall in blood pressure to normal levels. After hypertension was re-established, teprotide caused an identical fall in pressure (Fig. 1).

These experiments closely duplicate the observations previously described that used renin-specific antibody. The substrate inhibitor peptide acts specifically on renin, and it does not inhibit the pressor action of either angiotensin I or II. It appears to be well tolerated, without any hemodynamic consequences in the normotensive Na-replete animal. Of interest is the observation that at these doses of inhibitor, the effects are not significantly different from those of the converting enzyme inhibitor teprotide. At this point in the investigation, we had learned nothing that suggested that the inhibition of renin was different from the inhibition of converting enzyme. It was not until this compound was examined in humans that differences became apparent.

Human Studies

Normal, Na-depleted human volunteers, as well as a low-renin hypertensive patient, were studied [46]. Subjects were examined both in the supine position and after 1 min of upright tilting to 70°, following a 10-min infusion. Figure 2 shows the mean response of the normal subjects studied in the supine position. In the upright position, the hypotensive response was similar. The hypotensive response at higher doses of RIP was greater than that observed with the converting enzyme inhibitor captopril under the same conditions.

Captopril (up to 325 mg p.o. over 3 hr) reduced supine blood pressure (mm Hg) from 108 ± 2/68 ± 2 to 89 ± 6/48 ± 5 (P < 0.05); and, on upright tilting, blood pressure fell from 108 ± 2/76 ± 2 to 74 ± 5/41 ± 14 (P < 0.05). Captopril also had no effect on heart rate. In a low-renin hypertensive patient on a 10-mEq diet, RIP (1 mg/kg/min) reduced blood

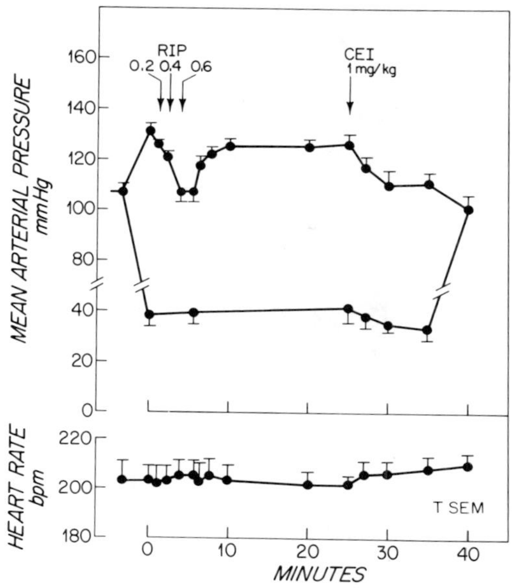

Fig. 1. After 1 hr of aortic cuff inflation, the mean arterial pressure (MAP) above the aortic cuff (*upper curve*) rose from 107 to 131 mm Hg in six studies of renin-dependent hypertension. Aortic pressure below the cuff was maintained at approximately 40 mm Hg (*lower curve*). Renin-inhibitory peptide (*RIP*) was given as a graded infusion of 0.2 mg/kg/min increments. At 0.6 mg/kg/min, MAP was restored to prehypertensive levels ($P < 0.004$). After a brief period, infusion was discontinued and MAP increased to 127 mm Hg. Converting-enzyme inhibitor (*CEI*), 1 mg/kg, reduced MAP to 111 mm Hg ($P < 0.002$). The MAP responses to renin-inhibitory peptide and to converting-enzyme inhibitor were similar (difference not statistically significant). The heart rate was consistent throughout. (Reprinted from [44] by permission of the National Academy of Sciences)

pressure on upright tilting from 135/113 mm Hg to an inaudible BP measurement; heart rate fell from 116 to 60 beats per min [47]. In contrast, the upright blood pressures following captopril administration are shown to exhibit a gradual fall, rather than the dramatic orthostatic changes observed with RIP.

Why had these effects not been observed in the monkey? We returned to the Maccac monkey and repeated our earlier experiments at higher infusion rates of the peptide. Striking hypotension was observed in both Na-depleted and Na-replete animals (Hartley, Zusman, and Haber, unpublished observations). There seems to be a differential dose response between humans and the Maccac, with humans being somewhat more sensitive to the effects of the peptide.

Why are the results with a renin inhibitor different from those observed with a converting enzyme inhibitor at the higher end of the dose-response range? Is RIP acting at a site of renin action other than plasma? Does renin

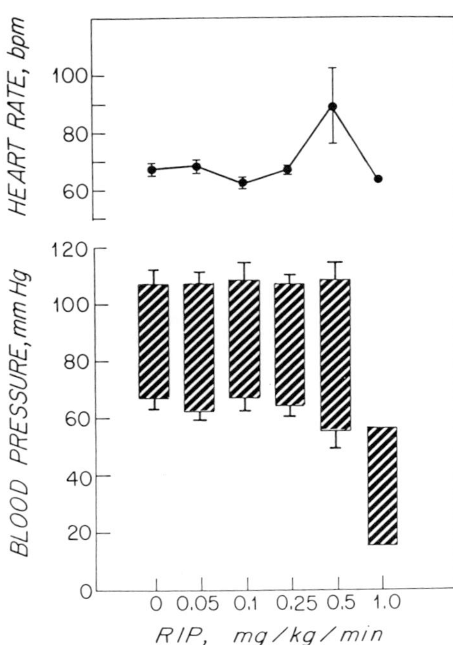

Fig. 2. The effect of RIP on heart rate and blood pressure in normal Na-depleted subjects in the supine position. (Reprinted with permission from [46])

have a role in the neural regulation of blood pressure, cardiac output, and peripheral resistance? Is the adrenergic facilitatory effect of angiotensin II selectively blocked by RIP entering a privileged site that is inaccessible to captopril? Or, has there simply been an element of nonspecificity uncovered at higher doses of RIP? Clearly, many more experiments need to be done before we understand the mechanism of action of RIP.

Recently, Webb et al [48] have examined one of the peptides described above in two normal Na-depleted human subjects. H-142 (Table 1) was ineffective in producing a blood pressure response at an infusion rate of up to 0.4 mg/kg/hr in one subject. When the dose was raised to 1.0 mg/kg/hr in the second subject, a fall in blood pressure from 104/56 mm Hg to 94/48 mm Hg was observed without a change in the pulse rate. There was an associated decrease in both angiotensin I and angiotensin II plasma concentrations. It is likely that these investigators observed only the results of inhibition of plasma renin activity and did not use sufficient doses of this compound to test whether a second effect—of the kind we observed—might be manifest.

Prorenin Peptides as Renin Inhibitors

Aspartyl proteases, such as pepsin and chymosin, are first synthesized as inactive zymogens and then are processed by the proteolytic release of an amino terminal peptide to yield the active enzyme [49–51]. There is significant homology between the prosegment of the renin precursor and that of pepsinogen [52]. The enzymatic activity of the pepsin is inhibited by fragments of the prosegment of pepsinogen [53, 54]. In light of these observations, Evin et al synthesized peptides from the prosegment of mouse submaxillary gland renin [52], as deduced from the nucleotide sequence of the cDNA [2]. Some of the peptides were inhibitors of moderate potency, thus demonstrating an IC_{50} of 2 to 3 μM with mouse renin (Table 1). It will be of great interest to see whether analogs of these compounds will yield more potent inhibitors and provide a new principle for effecting renin inhibition.

Thus, while there is some promise of attaining specificity that has eluded investigators with other simple compounds, at the present state of development within this field, more questions have been raised than answered.

The Three-dimensional Structure of Renin: A Route to More Specific Inhibitors

A detailed knowledge of the structure of the catalytic site of carboxypeptidase led to the synthesis of effective converting enzyme inhibitors. The practical result was the drug captopril. Analogously, if the structure of renin's active site were understood in detail, it would be possible to design inhibitors with greater precision than can be achieved simply by attempting mimicry of substrate. While adequate quantities of mouse submaxillary renin are available to provide material for an x-ray film crystallographic study, there are very substantial differences in specificity between human and mouse renin [55]. Optimal inhibitors for one enzyme may not be adequate for the other; 20 kg of human kidneys yields, at best, 1 μg of renin [5]. Even renin-secreting tumors—although their content of the enzyme is orders of magnitude greater than that contained in kidney—have not provided significant amounts of material. We can look forward in the near future to the use of the genomic or copy DNAs as a source of expression of renin either in mammalian cell cultures or in prokaryotes. Then, adequate amounts of material will certainly be available for x-ray film crystallography.

Meanwhile, rather reasonable three-dimensional structures can be built by using known crystallographic models of acid proteases [56, 57]. The modeling of potential inhibitors in these catalytic sites may provide powerful insights. Carlson, Karplus, and this author have most recently proposed a three-dimensional structure for human renin that is based on the available amino acid sequence, as well as on the structure of three acid proteases.

Three acid proteases have had atomic coordinates determined by x-ray film crystallographic procedures [58, 59]. As expected from the sequence homology [60], the three-dimensional structures of the acid proteases from *Rhizopus chinensis* (*RC*) and *Endothia parasitica* (*EP*) [58] are very similar. We have used these available coordinates to determine what parts of the three-dimensional structure are highly conserved and where significant differences occur. The results of this analysis were then applied in aligning the renin sequence and in building its structure. An important aspect of this approach was the application of energy minimization techniques to refine the proposed structure. This prevented forbidden orientations (such as an overlap of atoms or approach of two atoms within their van der Waals' radii) and, more importantly, arranged the structure in a conformation corresponding to its minimal energy level.

The renin model was built first by constructing the peptide backbone and then by adding the amino acid side chains. Coordinates of the *RC* backbone, which were obtained from the 1.8-Å electron density map, were used directly for all residues for which there was an overlap between renin and *RC* sequences. Additions and deletions were made at positions where they occurred in the sequence alignment. Each addition or deletion was visualized with the molecular graphics system, and an attempt was made to avoid obviously forbidden conformations. Bond distances and bond angles were set to those determined for a model peptide backbone; the backbone was rotated to avoid unfavorable dihedral angles or violations of van der Waals' radii.

When the peptide backbone was complete, the amino acid side chains were added. If the amino acids were identical for renin and *RC,* then the coordinates for the *RC* side chains were used directly. If the amino acids were different, then the renin residues were constructed by using the $\psi 1$ angle for the amino acids in the *RC* structure. If there was an additional degree of freedom in the renin amino acid, the c ψ angle was set as close as possible to that for the *RC* side chain. If the *RC* side chain was shorter than the corresponding residue in renin, the ψ angle was taken arbitrarily from model compounds. In certain cases, the side chain conformations that were chosen in this fashion caused steric conflicts. Side chains were then rotated about their C-α to C-β bond ($\psi 1$ angle) to minimize steric overlap.

There was very substantial structural homology among the acid proteases, particularly with respect to the core of the molecule. Atoms varied in position, with a mean distance of less than 1.0 Å at the core and in the region adjacent to the catalytic site, which was adjacent to the essential aspartic acids at positions 37 and 225 in the human sequence. At the surface of the molecule, particularly where there was little secondary structure (such as at the end of loops), there was considerably more variation. This is not at all surprising, since these regions are not essential in maintaining structure.

Since the renin structure is based on the *RC* structure, it is not surprising that there are similarities—many of which are common to all the acid proteases. The model has two lobes, with the active site cleft between them. There are two β-sheet structures in the amino terminal lobe, with the peptide backbone in one β-sheet running at right angles to the other. In the carboxy terminal lobe, the corresponding β-sheets make up the bulk of the structure, but they are less well defined. There are two aspartic acid residues juxtaposed in the active site (positions 37 and 225), and there is a flap at positions 75 to 85 of the amino terminal lobe that overlays the active site. This flap has been hypothesized as acting as a trap door that swings open to allow access to the active site and then closes when substrate is bound [61].

Of course, it is the active site that is of greatest interest in the design of renin-specific inhibitors. Models for pepstatin and for two hexapeptides (Pro-Phe-His-Leu-Leu-Val and Pro-Phe-His-Leu-Val-Ile) that reproduce the scissile region of natural substrate for renin were constructed in the active site of renin. It appeared that pepstatin could be accommodated easily at the active site of both mouse and human renin without steric conflicts.

Renin has a very different and more selective substrate requirement than that of the other acid proteases; and, there are significant differences in substrate requirements between mouse submaxillary renin and human renal renin as well. When we reported a model for the three-dimensional structure of mouse submaxillary renin [57], differences in active site structures between that enzyme and other acid proteases were noted. These differences were consistent with the species specificity both of a peptide inhibitor of renal renin (RIP) [55] and inhibitors containing modified peptide bonds at the cleavage site [40].

The model of human renin presented here differs little from that of the mouse submaxillary enzyme in the topology of the active site (Fig. 3). The two aspartic acid residues (37 and 225) at the active site have virtually the identical orientation as that in both the mouse renin model and the x-ray models of the acid proteases. The adjacent residues (Gly 39, Ser 40, Gly 227) stabilize the carboxyl groups of the aspartic acids by forming hydrogen (H) bonds with them, and they are fully conserved. However, there is one residue that is involved in this type of interaction; it is invariant in the structures of the other acid proteases, yet is changed in human renin. In all the other acid proteases, there is a threonine that forms a H bond to the essential aspartic acid in the carboxy terminal lobe (225 in human renin). This residue changes to a serine in the mouse renin and to an alanine in the human

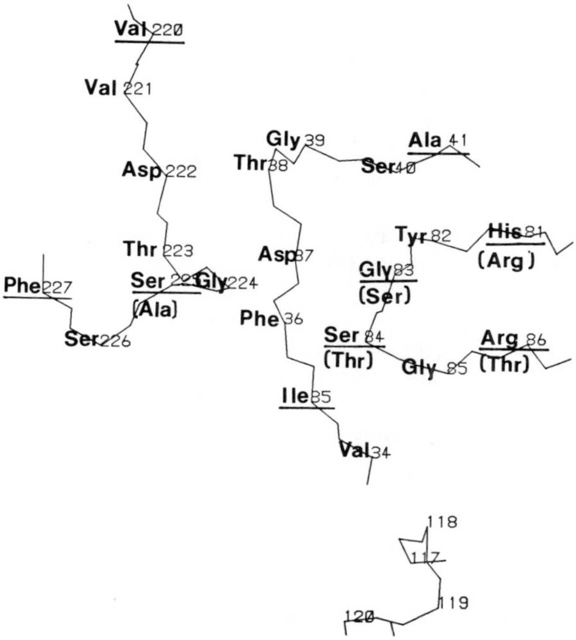

Fig. 3. Amino acids in the active site of the mouse renin model. Amino acids that differ in the human renin model are shown in parentheses beneath the corresponding mouse amino acid.

renin sequence. The change from a threonine to a serine would preserve the H bonding, but it would change the steric properties by eliminating an intervening methyl group. The change to an alanine of course would make H bonding impossible and, thus, change the electrostatic potential around the essential aspartic acids significantly.

The hydrophobic pocket hypothesized to form the S_1' subsite in the *RC* protease [58] is well conserved in the models of mouse and human renin. However, there are some small changes that may be significant. Valine (at position 223 in mouse renin) changes to leucine, which has a methylene group in its side chain that is not present in valine. The effect on the S_1' subsite would be to reduce its size in the human—as compared to the mouse—enzyme. However, because of other relative shifts in the backbones of the two structures, this change has little apparent effect on the size of the pocket, but it does alter its shape. The pocket is such that in the human renin structure, there is sufficient hydrophobic surface available to interact with the smaller valine side chain of the human substrate in the P_1' position, and there is still enough space to accommodate the larger side chains (such as leucine) that are present in the nonprimate renin substrates. This type of interaction would explain how human renin can act on a wide variety of renin substrates, while mouse renin cleaves human substrate only poorly [55, 62]. The residues that line the S_1 subsite, which are identified from the structure of pepstatin at the active site of *RC*, appear to be identical in both human and mouse renin. This is consistent with the data on the substrate specificity of renins, which demonstrates that the residues on the amino terminal side of the scissile bond of the substrates are identical, while the residues that differ are on the carboxy terminal side of the scissile bond [62].

Other significant differences between the human and mouse structures occur in the 75 to 85 flap. The residues on the protein side of this flap are identical in all of the acid proteases and in both renins (Fig. 3). A tyrosine, which has been preserved in both renin structures, was originally thought to be important as an H bond donor during catalysis [63]; however, it is now thought to form part of the hydrophobic pocket that binds the side chain in the P_1 position of the substrate. However, on the solvent-accessible surface of the 75 to 85 flap, there are a number of changes between the human and mouse renin structures. At position 81 in the human structure, there is an arginine that is replaced by a histidine in the mouse structure. At position 86 in the human sequence, there is a threonine where there is an arginine in the mouse structure. These amino acids have quite different properties, and they could inhibit activity by altering the interactions with an antibody that binds to these residues and sterically blocks the active site. This could easily explain the differences in the specificity of the antibodies that cause them to differentiate between the mouse renin and the human renin [64]. It is entirely possible that these changes account for the differences in substrate specificity as well, and that the alterations in the sequences of the substrate around the scissile bond are fortuitous.

The structure presented here is only a hypothetical model, although it is one that can be tested against experimental data. It may be possible to draw some inferences concerning renin's mechanism of action that can be tested directly by comparing the experimental behavior of model substrates. The final test, of course, will be a comparison of the model to a structure determined by x-ray film crystallography.

Thus, the impact of molecular biology on the study of renin is already apparent, as is the potential for future applications. This author has detailed the first—the role of renin purification in the genesis of antibodies (which became the first specific inhibitors of the enzyme), and also the importance of the amino acid sequence of renin (as first determined by the means of conventional protein chemistry and then by cDNA sequencing) in designing specific inhibitors that are potentially useful in the clinical investigation of essential hypertension. The amino acid sequence of human renin was a unique product of recombinant DNA research. It could not be obtained by the techniques of protein chemistry because of the minimal amounts of the enzyme obtainable. Nor was it likely that the RNA (from which the cDNA was transcribed) could be isolated without mouse submaxillary cDNA being used as a probe. The first models of the three-dimensional structure of renin are only extrapolations. It is the availability of human renin's DNA that will eventually allow for expression of adequate quantities of the enzyme for a formal crystallographic study. The accurate model that is attained will be of more specific help in the design of inhibitors.

Uncovering the details of renin biosynthesis is another issue that has not been discussed here. We already know the structure of prorenin from its cDNA. This information will lead to the chemical synthesis of peptides that may be used as immunogens to produce antibodies that differentiate between renin and prorenin. An important application of these selective probes will be to determine the relationship between prorenin, as defined biosynthetically, and the inactive renin of plasma—the nature of which has continued to elude investigators.

Summary

Does the availability of highly purified renin and the knowledge of the amino acid and cDNA sequences of this molecule and of its pre- and proenzymes, lead us to a further understanding of the role of renin in vascular homeostasis or in the genesis of human essential hypertension? Purified renin has led to monospecific—as well as to monoclonal—antibodies that have proven to be very selective physiologic probes in animal experiments. They do not, however, appear to be suitable for clinical investigation at present. Thus, greater selectivity than is presently available with converting enzyme inhibitors or angiotensin II antagonists is sought in a new class of compounds: peptide inhibitors of renin. Initially, these appeared to be very selective for renin, but the most recent clinical and nonhuman primate studies raise significant questions concerning their site of action. As a guide to the synthesis of new renin inhibitors, a model of human renin has been constructed that is based on the three-dimensional structures of other acid proteases and the amino acid sequence of human renin as deduced from its cDNA sequence. A detailed examination of the active site may lead to the design of new compounds that are highly specific inhibitors.

References

1. MISONO KS, CHANG JJ, INAGAMI T: Amino acid sequence of mouse submaxillary gland renin. *Proc Natl Acad Sci* 79:4858–4862, 1982
2. PANTHIER JJ, FOOTE S, CHAMBREAUD B, STROSBERG AD, CORVOL P, ROUGEON F: Complete amino acid sequence and maturation of the mouse submaxillary gland renin precursor. *Nature* 298:90, 1982
3. IMAI T, MIYAZAKI H, HIROSE S, HORI H, HAYASHI T, KAGEYAMA R, OHKUBO H, NAKANISHI S, MURAKAMI K: Cloning and sequence analysis of cDNA for human renin precursor. *Proc Natl Acad Sci USA* 80:7405–7409, 1983
4. MURAKAMI K, INAGAMI T: Isolation of pure and stable renin from hog kidney. *Biochem Biophys Res Comm* 62:757–763, 1975
5. DZAU VJ, SLATER EE, HABER E: Complete purification of dog renal renin. *Biochemistry* 18:5224–5229, 1979
6. YOKASAWA H, HOLLADAY LH, INAGAMI T, HAAS E, MURAKAMI K: Human renal renin: Complete purification and characterization. *J Biol Chem* 255:3498–3502, 1980
7. SLATER EE, STROUT VJ: Pure human renin: Identification and characterization of two major molecular weight forms. *J Biol Chem* 256:8164–8171, 1981
8. COHEN S, TAYLOR JM, MURAKAMI K, MICHELAKIS AM, INAGAMI T: Isolation and characterization of renin-like enzymes from mouse submaxillary gland. *Biochemistry* 11:4286–4293, 1972
9. PANTHIER JJ, ROUGEON F: Kidney and submaxillary gland renins are encoded by two non-allelic genes in Swiss mice. *Embo J* 2(Suppl 5):675–678, 1983
10. PICCINI N, KNOPF JL, GROSS KW: A DNA polymorphism, consistent with gene duplication, correlates with high renin levels in the mouse submaxillary gland. *Cell* 30(Suppl 1):205–213, 1982
11. HABER E: Specific inhibitors of renin. The fifth Volhard lecture. *Clin Sci* 59(Suppl 6):7s–19s, 1980
12. HOLLENBERG NK, WILLIAMS GH, BURGER B, ISHIKAWA I, ADAMS DF: Blockade and stimulation of renal, adrenal, and vascular angiotensin II receptors with 1-Sar, 8-ala angiotensin II in normal man. *J Clin Invest* 57:39–46, 1976
13. BRUNNER HR, GAVRAS H, WAEBER B, KERSHAW GR, TURINI GA, VUKOVICH RA, MCKINSTRY DN, GAVRAS I: Oral angiotensin-converting enzyme inhibitor in long-term treatment of hypertensive patients. *Ann Intern Med* 90:19–23, 1979
14. Captopril: benefits and risks in severe hypertension (*editorial*). *Lancet* 2:129–130, 1980
15. VINCI JM, HORWITZ D, ZUSMAN RM, PISANO JJ, CATT KJ, KEISER HR: The effect of converting enzyme inhibition with SQ 20881 on plasma and urinary kinins, prostaglandin E, and angiotensin II in hypertensive man. *Hypertension* 1:416–426, 1979
16. SWARTZ SL, WILLIAMS GH, HOLLENBERG NK, MOORE TJ, DLUHY RG: Converting enzyme inhibition in essential hypertension: The hypotensive response does not reflect only reduced angiotensin II formation. *Hypertension* 1:106–111, 1979
17. GOLDSTONE R, MARTIN K, ZIPSER R, HORTON R: Evidence for a dual action of converting enzyme inhibitor on blood pressure in normal man. *Prostaglandins* 22:587–598, 1981

18. DEODHAR SD, HAAS E, GOLDBLATT H: Production of antirenin to homologous renin and its effect on experimental renal hypertension. *J Exp Med* 119:425–432, 1964
19. WAKERLIN GE: Antibodies to renin as proof of the pathogenesis of sustained renal hypertension. *Circulation* 17:653–657, 1958
20. DZAU VJ, KOPELMAN RI, BARGER AC, HABER E: Renin-specific antibody for study of cardiovascular homeostasis. *Science* 207:1091–1093, 1980
21. DZAU VJ, KOPELMAN RI, BARGER AC, HABER E: A comparison of renin-specific IgG and Fab in studies of blood pressure regulation. *Am J Physiol* 246:H404–H409, 1984
22. CORVOL P, GALEN FX, DEVAUX C, GUYENE TP, MENARD J, BARIETY J, CAMILLERI JP, PHAT VN, NOCHY D: Human antirenin antibody: a new tool for studying the renin-angiotensin system. *Adv Nephrol* 12:3–17, 1983
23. BRUNNER HR, LARAGH JH, BAER L, NEWTON MA, GOODWIN FT, KRAKOFF LR, BARD RH, BUHLER FR: Essential hypertension: Renin and aldosterone, heart attack and stroke. *N Engl J Med* 286:441, 1972
24. AOYAGI T, KUNIMOTO S, MORISHIMA H, TAKEUCHI T, UMEZAWA H: Effect of pepstatin on acid proteases. *J Antibiot (Tokyo)* 24:687–694, 1971
25. GROSS F, LAZAR J, ORTH H: Inhibition of the renin-angiotensinogen reaction by pepstatin. *Science* 175:656, 1972
26. LAZAR J, OSTER P, GROSS F, HACKENTHAL E: Demonstration of *in vivo* action of pepstatin: Effects on plasma angiotensin II concentration. *Biochem Pharmacol* 23:2776–2778, 1974
27. KOKUBU T, HIWADA K, NAGASAKA Y, YAMAMURA Y: Effect of several protein-ase inhibitors on renin reaction. *Japan Circ J (English)* 38:955–958, 1974
28. MILLER RP, POPER CJ, WILSON CW, DEVITO E: Renin inhibition by pepstatin. *Biochem Pharmacol* 21:2941–2944, 1972
29. MYAZAKI M, OKUNISHI H, KOMORO T, YAMAMOTO K: Renin inhibitory effect of N-acetylpepstatin. *Japan J Pharmacol* 28:171, 1978
30. EID M, EVIN G, CASTRO B, MENARD J, CORVOL P: New renin inhibitors homologous with pepstatin. *Biochem J* 197:465–471, 1981
31. SKEGGS L, LENTZ K, KAHN J, HOCHSTRASSER H: Kinetics of the reaction of renin with nine synthetic peptide substrates. *J Exper Med* 128:13–34, 1968
32. HABER E: Peptide inhibitors of renin in cardiovascular studies. *Fed Proc* 43(Suppl 15):3155–3161, 1983
33. KOKUBU T, HIWADA K, ITO T, UEDA E, YAMAMURA Y, MIZOGUCHI T, SHIGEZANE K: Peptide inhibitors of renin angiotensinogen reaction system. *Biochem Pharmacol* 22:3217–3223, 1973
34. BURTON J, POULSEN K, HABER E: Competitive inhibitors of renin: Inhibitors effective at physiological pH. *Biochemistry* 14:3892–3898, 1975
35. POULSEN K, BURTON J, HABER E: Competitive inhibitors of renin. *Biochemistry* 12:3877–3882, 1973
36. POULSEN K, JORGENSEN K: An easy radioimmunological microassay of renin activity, concentration and substrate in human and animal plasma and tissues based on angiotensin I trapping by antibody. *J Clin Endocrinol Metab* 39:816–825, 1974
37. BURTON J, POULSEN K, HABER E: Solubility and lipophilicity relationships in the design of renin inhibitors, in *Polymeric Drugs,* edited by DONARUMA LG, VOGL O, New York, Academic Press, 1978, pp 219–237
38. PARIKH I, CUATRECASAS P: Substrate analog competitive inhibitors of human renin. *Biochem Biophys Res Commun* 54:1356–1361, 1973

39. HABER E, BURTON J: Inhibitors of renin and their utility in physiologic studies. *Fed Proc* 38:2768–2773, 1979

40. SZELKE M, LECKIE B, HALLETT A, JONES DM, SUEIRAS J, ATRASH B, LEVER AF: Potent new inhibitors of human renin. *Nature (London)* 299:555–557, 1982

41. SZELKE M, LECKIE BJ, TREE M, BROWN A, GRANT J, HALLETT A, HUGHES M, JONES DM, LEVER AF: H-77: A potent new renin inhibitor. *In vitro* and *in vivo* studies. *Hypertension* 4:59–69, 1982

42. BOGER J, LOHR NS, ULM EH, POE M, BLAINE EH, FANELLI GM, LIN TY, PAYNE LS, SCHORN TW, LAMONT BI, VASSIL TC, STABILITO II, VEBER DF, RICH DH, BOPARI AS: Novel renin inhibitors containing the amino acid statine. *Nature* 303(Suppl 5912):81–84, 1983

43. EVIN G, CASTRO B, DEVIN J, MENARD J, CORVOL P, GUEGAN R, DIAZ J, DEMARNE H, CAZAUBON C, GAGNOL JP: New potent inhibitors of human renin, in *Peptides: Structure and Function. Proceedings of the Eighth American Peptide Symposium,* edited by HRUBY VJ, RICH DH, Rockford Illinois, Pierce Chemical Co, 1984, pp 583–590

44. BURTON J, CODY RJ JR, HERD JA, HABER E: Specific inhibition of renin by an angiotensinogen analog: Studies in sodium depletion and renin-dependent hypertension. *Proc Natl Acad Sci USA* 77:5476–5479, 1980

45. SLATER EE, COHN RC, DZAU VJ, HABER E: Purification of human renal renin. *Clin Sci Mol Med* 55:117–120, 1978

46. ZUSMAN RM, BURTON J, CHRISTENSEN D, DODDS A, HABER E: Hemodynamic effects of a competitive renin inhibitory peptide in man: evidence for multiple mechanisms of action. *Trans Am Assoc Physicians* 96:365–374, 1983

47. HABER E, ZUSMAN R, BURTON J, DZAU VJ, BARGER AC: Is renin a factor in the etiology of essential hypertension? Proceedings of the Fifth Scientific Meeting of the Inter-American Society of Hypertension. Sao Paulo, Brazil. *Hypertension* V(Suppl):V8–V15, 1983

48. WEBB DJ, CUMMING AM, LECKIE BJ, LEVER AF, MORTON JJ, ROBERTSON JI, SZELKE M, DONOVAN B: Reduction of blood pressure in man with H-142, a potent new renin inhibitor (*letter*). *Lancet* 2(8365–8366):1486–1487, 1983

49. HARBOE M, FOLTMANN B: Bovine pepsin: The sequence of the first 65 amino acid residues (completing the sequence of the first 110 residues of bovine pepsinogen). *FEBS Letters* 60:133–135, 1975

50. SEPULVEDA P, MARCINISCZYN J, LIU D, TANG J: Primary structure of porcine pepsin III. *J Biol Chem* 250:5082–5088, 1975

51. FOLTMANN B, PEDERSEN VB, JACOBSEN H, KAUFFMAN D, WYBRANDT G: The complete amino acid sequence of prochymosin. *Proc Natl Acad Sci USA* 74:2321–2324, 1977

52. EVIN G, DEVIN J, CASTRO B, MENARD J, CORVOL P: Synthesis of peptides related to presegment of mouse submaxillary renin precursor: a new approach to renin inhibitors. *Proc Natl Acad Sci USA* 81:48–52, 1984

53. KUMAR H, KASSELL B: Improved pepsin inhibitor derived from activation peptide 1–16 of porcine pepsinogen. *Biochemistry* 16:3846–3849, 1977

54. DUNN BM, DEYRUP C, MOESCHLING WG, GILBERT WA, NOLAL RJ, TRACH ML: Inhibition of pepsin by zymogen activation fragments. Spectrum of peptides released from pepsinogen NH_2 terminus and solid phase synthesis of two inhibitory peptide sequences. *J Biol Chem* 253(Suppl 20):7269–7275, 1978

55. POULSEN K, HABER E, BURTON J: On the specificity of human renin: Studies with peptide inhibitors. *Biochim Biophys Acta* 452:533–537, 1976

56. BLUNDELL TL, SIBANDA L, PEARL LH: The three-dimensional structure, specificity and catalytic activity of renin. *Nature* 304:273–275, 1983

57. CARLSON WD, HABER E: A model for the three-dimensional structure of renin, in *Peptides: Structure and Function. Proceedings of the Eighth American Peptide Symposium,* edited by HRUBY VJ, RICH DH, Rockford Illinois, Pierce Chemical Co, 1984, pp 873–876
58. SUBRAMANIAN E, SWAN JDA, LIU M, DAVIES D, JENKINS JA, TICKLE IJ, BLUNDELL T: Homology among acid proteases: comparison of crystal structures at 3Å resolution of acid proteases from *Rhizopus chinensis* and *Endothia parasitica. Proc Natl Acad Sci USA* 74:556–559, 1977
59. HSU IN, DELBAERE LTJ, JAMES MNG: Penicillopepsin from *Penicillium janthinellum* crystal structure at 2.8Å and sequence homology with porcine pepsin. *Nature* 266:140, 1977
60. HOFMANN T: Structure and function of acid proteases, in *Advances in Chemistry Series: Food Related Enzymes* (vol 136), Washington, DC, Am Chem Soc, 1974, pp 146–185
61. JAMES MNG, SIELECKI A, SALITURO F, RICH DH, HOFMAN T: Conformational flexibility in the active sites of aspartyl proteinases revealed by a pepstatin fragment binding to penicillopepsin. *Proc Natl Acad Sci USA* 79:6137–6141, 1982
62. SMEBY RR, BUMPUS RM, PAGE JW, McCUBBIN JW: *Renal Hypertension,* Chicago, Chicago Yearbook Publishers, Inc, 1968, pp 27–29
63. JAMES MNG, HSU IN, DELBAERE LTJ: Mechanism of acid protease catalysis based on the crystal structure of penicillopepsin. *Nature* 267:808–813, 1977
64. DZAU VJ, DEVINE D, MUDGETT-HUNTER M, KOPELMAN RI, BARGER AC, HABER E: Antibodies as specific renin inhibitors: Studies with polyclonal and monoclonal antibodies and Fab fragments. *Clin Exper Hypertension* A5:1207–1220, 1983
65. TEWKSBURY DA, DART RA, TRAVIS J: The amino terminal amino acid sequence of human angiotensinogen. *Biochim Biophys Res Commun* 99:1311–1315, 1981

Inactive Renin

Jean E. Sealey

Human plasma contains a 58,000-dalton substance that appears to be enzymatically inactive, but which has characteristics very similar to those of the enzyme renin following limited proteolysis with trypsin [1–3]. This substance is called "inactive renin." It has also been called "prorenin" [4], but direct biochemical evidence is still lacking that inactive renin is, indeed, the biosynthetic precursor of active renin. However, most of the available information concerning inactive renin is consistent with this possibility, and its abundant presence in ectopic renin-secreting tumors [5] makes it highly likely that it is, indeed, prorenin.

Inactive renin was discovered in human amniotic fluid in 1971 [6] and in patients with Wilms tumors in 1974 [7]. However, several years passed before it was generally recognized that it is normally present in human plasma in amounts that average close to 10 times that of active renin. Prior to this time, the existence of inactive renin had not even been suspected; perhaps, because inactive renin is not normally converted to active renin in the blood. All of the active renin in the blood appears to be the result of renal secretion of the active form.

Shortly after inactive renin was discovered, two investigators demonstrated an activable form of renin in renal extracts of various animals [8, 9]. It was several years before it became clear that active renin can bind to a renal substance that is present in extracts of various animal kidneys; and, it can form a complex that has diminished activity [10, 11]. The binding protein is destroyed by acidification, resulting in an increase in activity. Whether this complex occurs in vivo is uncertain at present. It has not been shown to be present in the circulation. Whatever the case, the complex is not inactive renin, since it has intrinsic activity and can be biochemically distinguished from inactive renin. This renin complex will not be considered any further in this chapter.

This manuscript was presented as part of a Symposium on *Renin: Recent Advances.*

Inactive renin was discovered in blood, because two different techniques that were used to prepare samples for plasma renin activity measurement caused activation of some or all of the inactive renin [12–15]. A dialysis step to pH 3.3 was used in certain renin methods to destroy angiotensinases and to eliminate endogenous renin substrate [13, 14], so that incubation of renin could be performed in the presence of the same concentration of angiotensinogen (renin substrate), thus eliminating the effect of differences in renin substrate on the assay. The samples were subjected to a second step of dialysis to pH 7.4, at which the renin incubation was subsequently carried out in the presence of exogenous renin substrate. We now know that these two steps cause the complete and irreversible activation of inactive renin in plasma.

The other technique that activates inactive plasma renin, cryoactivation, causes only partial activation of inactive renin [12, 15]. When plasma samples are chilled, but not frozen, some of the inactive renin in plasma is activated irreversibly. Therefore, the commonly accepted practices of chilling blood or thawing frozen samples in the refrigerator results in activation of a variable portion of inactive renin, perhaps as much as 1/10th of the total. Also, storage of samples in freezers that do not maintain plasmas that are completely frozen (plasma is liquid at $-6°C$) also can result in cryoactivation; it was just this type of occurrence that led to our discovery of cryoactivation of inactive renin in the first place [12].

In this report, we will review our studies concerning the activation of inactive renin, the factors that influence its circulating levels, and some of the physicochemical characteristics of inactive and activated inactive renin.

Activation of Inactive Renin

Inactive renin can be activated in vitro by limited proteolysis with trypsin [16]. Unfortunately, this enzyme can destroy active renin at slightly higher concentrations than those needed to activate it; the presence of inhibitors and competing substrates markedly affect the potency of the enzyme and the degree to which activation and/or destruction occur [17, 18]. Therefore, the conditions for optimum activation of inactive renin by trypsin have to be modified, depending on the medium in which inactive renin is found [18]. We have never been able to maximally activate inactive renin with trypsin during a 37°C incubation, most likely because—at that temperature—destruction of renin occurs simultaneously with activation [17]. However, for pooled plasma, we found that the maximum degree of activation and the rate of activation were quite similar when using 1 mg/ml trypsin—whether we incubated at 25°C, 6°C, or −4°C. These results suggested that maximal activation had occurred at these temperatures and that no concurrent destruction was occurring (Fig. 1). Subsequently, however, we found that different plasmas contained variable concentrations of trypsin inhibitors; this could lead to occasional underestimation of inactive renin because of destruction (low inhibitor concentration) or incomplete activation (high inhibitor concentration). This problem was resolved by increasing the trypsin concentration

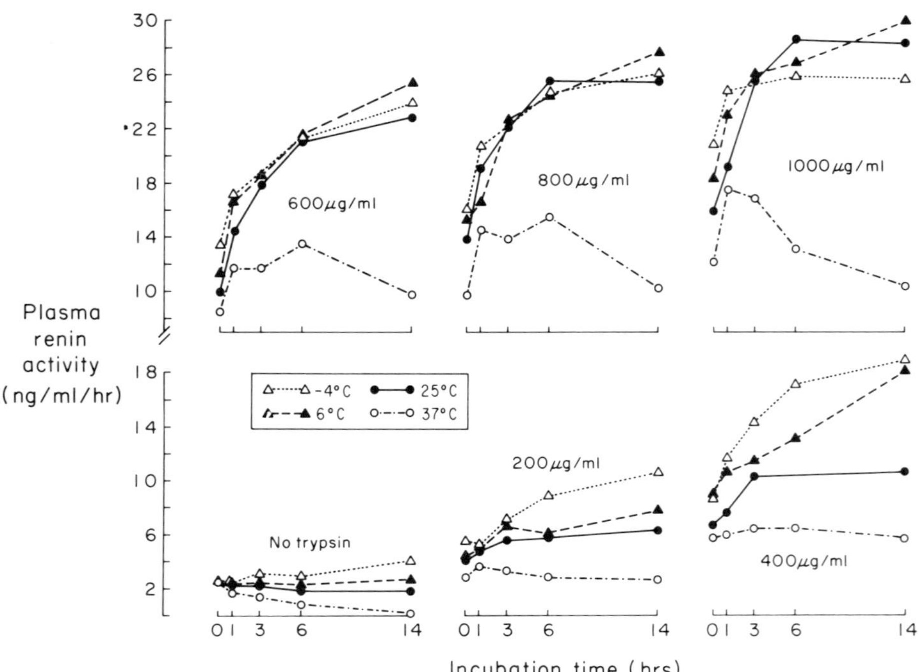

Fig. 1. To overcome trypsin inhibitors, very high concentrations of trypsin are required for activation of inactive renin in plasma. Illustrated here are the effects of different trypsin concentrations, incubation temperatures, and incubation times on the conversion of inactive-to-active renin in human plasma. For each point, 10 μl of trypsin (or 0.0025 N HCl) was added to 1 ml of plasma that had been preincubated for 1 hr at the appropriate temperature. The reaction was stopped at each time period via the addition of 100 μl maleic acid and 5 μl PMSF. For the zero incubation time, maleic acid and PMSF were added within 1 min after addition of trypsin. However, during this short time, disproportionately large amounts of inactive renin were activated, most likely because the plasma inhibitors required a finite time to bind to exogenous trypsin. (Reprinted with permission of the American Heart Assoc., Inc., from [17])

to 1.5 mg/ml and by adding 5 mM benzamidine, which is a competitive inhibitor of trypsin that seems to help protect the renin from concurrent destruction by the higher concentration of trypsin [19]. However, plasmas from third-trimester pregnant women contain double the normal concentration of trypsin inhibitors, and they require 2.5 mg/ml trypsin in the presence of 5 mM benzamidine for maximal activation [19].

Trypsin does not affect human renin substrate. Since inactive renin is quantitated by measuring the enzymatic activity of renin before and after activation and then by subtracting the active from the total renin, the lack of an effect of the activating enzyme on the renin substrate level can be an advantage.

In the purification of inactive renin from plasma and kidney [18], we encountered considerable difficulty in detecting inactive renin in chromatographic fractions, because the trypsin concentration required for optimal activation differed in each fraction; it also decreased markedly with each successive purification step, thus necessitating titration of the trypsin concentration. Upon further investigation, we found that a satisfactory estimate could be made of inactive renin levels in chromatographic fractions—resulting in activation that is approximately 80% of maximum, irrespective of the degree of purification—by incubating samples for 1 hr at 25°C with 100 μg/ml trypsin in buffer (between 7.5 and 8.0) containing 10 mM benzamidine and 0.5% BSA. The reaction was stopped by addition of 100 μg/ml SBTI and by further incubation for 15 min prior to pH adjustment and measurement of renin activity in the presence of exogenous homologous renin substrate [18].

Activation by trypsin, as has been described, provides the best approach thus far to reproducibly activating inactive renin in various media. Acid activation and cryoactivation have a disadvantage in that they require plasma cofactors; thus, they are only applicable to plasma samples. Nonetheless, the mechanisms involved in both cryoactivation and acid activation are worth examining, since they may provide clues about possible mechanisms of activation in vivo. As previously discussed, inactive renin can be activated in plasma by cryoactivation; that is, by incubation at −4°C [20]. Incubation for 4 days only activates about one-third of the inactive renin activated by trypsin [17]. We showed that cryoactivation does not occur in the presence of exogenous serine protein inhibitors [21] or at pH levels below 6 [20]; from this we deduced that it involves the participation of endogenous neutral serine proteases. However, it is, as yet, unclear which particular enzymes are involved in cryoactivation and whether or not cold changes the conformation of the inactive renin molecule to make it more accessible to proteolytic cleavage. The Hageman factor-kallikrein system appears to be involved in cryoactivation, since cryoactivation does not occur in plasmas lacking these enzymes [22]; however, plasmas that are deficient in certain other enzymes of the coagulation and fibrinolytic systems also fail to cryoactivate normally [19]. Cold is reported to affect circulating inhibitors of serine proteases [23], making them less effective. This situation most likely allows the endogenous activating enzymes to cleave inactive renin in the cold, while preventing such an effect at higher temperatures. Further studies are required to accurately define the mechanisms involved in cryoactivation.

More is known about the factors involved in acid activation [22, 24–26]. Acidification per se activates inactive renin, but acid activation is reversible; also, loss of activity occurs when the pH is restored towards neutrality [25, 26]. The reason is quite complicated as to why *irreversible* activation of inactive renin occurs when plasma is dialyzed to pH 3.3 and then back to pH 7.4, each for 24 hr. Besides activating inactive renin, dialysis to pH 3.3 destroys plasma inhibitors of the serine proteases of the coagulation and fibrinolytic systems. Then, during the second dialysis step to pH 7.4, a small amount of activated Hageman factor begins to convert prekallikrein to kallikrein; kallikrein then activates more Hageman factor. A positive feedback system develops, resulting in accumulation of large amounts of active plasma kallikrein. Kallikrein then cleaves the reversibly activated inactive renin and prevents the subsequent loss of activity [22, 24]. The cleavage of activated inactive renin by plasma kallikrein seems to occur as the pH rises during the dialysis step (before the activated renin begins to lose activity), so that dialysis to pH 3.3 followed by dialysis to pH 7.4 results in the same degree of activation of inactive renin as does incubation with trypsin.

As the phenomenon of the reversibility of activation of inactive renin was studied, it seemed possible that it could be due to the association-dissociation of active renin with an inhibitor. However, kinetic analysis of the reversal process indicated that only a single molecular species was involved [27], which suggests that this phenomenon is due to unfolding and refolding of the inactive renin molecule (Fig. 2). Kidney-, tumor-, and plasma-inactive renin all behave similarly in this regard [5, 27], thus reinforcing the similarity of the molecules from all three sources and making it unlikely that any of them are renin-inhibitor complexes.

The kidney enzyme kallikrein can activate inactive renin [28]. As with plasma kallikrein, this enzyme is more potent against the preacidified molecule than the native molecule. The tissue kallikreins are distinct enzymes from plasma kallikrein. They are neutral serine proteases that have quite restricted substrate specificity. As with renin, renal kallikrein is present in the kidney in high concentrations, and it is present in highest concentrations in the renal cortex. Therefore, its ability to activate inactive renin has provoked considerable interest and speculation that it might be the in vivo activator of inactive renin. Although there is, as yet, no direct evidence that it participates in the activation in vivo, the juxtaposition of these two enzyme systems in the kidney—that is, the renin-angiotensin system and the kallikrein-kinin system, with opposite vasoactive effects—led us to speculate about their possible inter-relationships [29]. If renal kallikrein is the in vivo converting enzyme for prorenin, its release might accompany renin release. In fact, such a possibility exists and is supported by our observation of a direct relationship between the daily excretion of urinary kallikrein and the proportion of active renin (active:total) in the circulation [17].

Activation of inactive renin does not appear to occur in the circulation. While enzymes of the coagulation [22, 24] and fibrinolytic [30, 31] systems were capable of activating inactive renin under certain circumstances and circulated with inactive renin in plasma, we were unable to activate inactive renin in vitro when the Hageman factor-prekallikrein system was activated by the addition of kaolin to plasma [32]. Plasmin also can activate inactive renin [30, 31]; however, the total absence of active renin in anephric plasma [33] argues against any of these enzymes playing a role in activating inactive renin in the circulation itself, unless the kidney participates in some way.

In summary, activation of inactive renin appears to involve the participation of neutral serine proteases. The predicted cleavage site for conversion of prorenin to renin is the C-terminal side of a pair of basic amino acid residues, which suggests that trypsin-like enzymes are likely to be involved [34]. However, additional tryptic cleavage sites occur within the prosequence of the human gene [35], which could explain how active renins might be

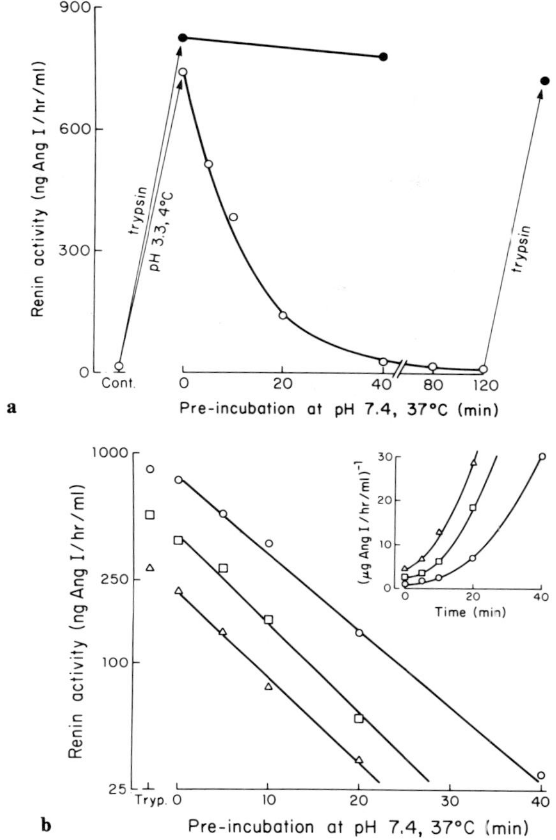

Fig. 2. Reversible acid activation of partially purified inactive renin from human kidney. **a** After dialysis to pH 3.3, samples were diluted on ice in pH 7.4 buffer containing 0.5% albumin, and then they were preincubated at 37°C for the various times indicated. Immediately thereafter, samples were adjusted to pH 5.7, angiotensinogen was added, and renin activity was determined during a 6 min incubation (○, *pH 3.3-dialyzed;* ●, *trypsin-treated*). After preincubation for 120 min, renin activity disappeared, but it was recovered after reacidification (not shown) or incubation with trypsin. **b** Semilogarithmic plot of the decline in activity during preincubation of 10 (△), 20 (□), or 40 (○) µl of pH 3.3-dialyzed inactive renin in a final reaction volume of 0.3 ml. The values for trypsin-activated enzyme (Tryp.) are plotted at −3 min to indicate that some inactivation occurred during the 6-min renin incubation; however, these points were not used in determining the best-fit regression lines. These data fit the first-order rate equation, $-dE/dt = kE$ (where E represents the remaining enzyme activity), which on integration yields the expression $\ln E = -kt + \ln E_o$. Values obtained for k were 0.095, 0.089, and 0.086 min⁻¹, respectively, with corresponding half-times of 7.3, 7.1, and 8.1 min. The inset demonstrates that the data do not fit the expression, $-dE/dt = kE^2$, which would be expected for a second-order reaction in which both reactants are equimolar—as in the case of a purified enzyme-inhibitor complex that has been dissociated. The integral, $E^{-1} = kt + E_o^{-1}$, indicates that the reciprocal of remaining activity should be a linear function of time, which it clearly is not (*Ang I, angiotensin I*). (Reprinted with permission from [27])

formed during incubation with trypsin-like enzymes in vitro that are larger than the native molecule (see below). Together, these findings again are compatible with the possibility that inactive renin is prorenin.

Factors That Influence Circulating Levels of Inactive Renin

Inactive renin measurements are affected by the methods used for measurement [1]. Thus, cryoactivation usually underestimates this level [17]. Perhaps more importantly, the measurement is markedly affected by differences in renin substrate concentration. Some methods get around this problem by adding a fixed amount of heterologous sheep substrate to samples before and after activation; thus, all incubations are carried out in the presence of the same effective substrate concentration [24, 25]. We do not do that; therefore, apparent changes in inactive renin might be due instead to changes in renin substrate. For this reason, we routinely measure renin substrate with inactive renin in plasma samples. Fortunately, renin substrate does not change markedly under most circumstances, and it is rare that a change in the inactive renin measurement can be ascribed to renin substrate changes. An exception may occur during both pregnancy [36, 37] and oral contraceptive therapy [38], when substrate concentration can increase by as much as 5-fold. Since the normal substrate concentration is close to K_m [38], such a change can cause a maximum 2-fold increase in the inactive renin measurement.

Most of the factors that affect active renin secretion seem to result in a similar directional change in inactive renin [1]; however, usually, the magnitude of the response of inactive renin is less than that of active renin. The result of this is that plasma levels of inactive renin generally bear a weak—although significant—direct relationship to the active renin level [5]. Patients who have low active renins usually have low inactive renin levels, and those patients with high active renin usually have high inactive plasma renin levels; however, the higher the active renin in the circulation (under steady-state conditions), the lower the proportion of inactive renin. This suggests, perhaps, that as the demand for active renin increases, a higher proportion of synthesized prorenin is converted to active renin, resulting in a lower proportion of inactive renin in the circulation.

The most consistent response of inactive renin is to changes in sodium balance [4, 20, 39–43]. Sodium depletion (either dietary or diuretic) raises inactive renin and sodium loading decreases it, but the effects on active renin are more pronounced. When we studied the effect of high, medium, and low dietary sodium intake in eight hypertensive patients, we found that inactive renin increased from 18.8 ± 9.7 ng/ml/hr to 26.4 ± 5.9 to 31.1 ± 6.4 ng/ml/hr with decreasing salt intake; however, the proportion of inactive renin in the circulation fell slightly from 94%, to 93% to 89%. The same patients on the same diets were studied again during administration of the diuretic indapamide for a minimum of 3 weeks. On each diet, inactive renin was higher during diuretic therapy. Thus, inactive renin increased from 29.9 ± 5.3 to 43.3 ± 7.7 to 53.6 ± 9.1 ng/ml/hr as sodium intake fell; the proportion of inactive renin in the circulation fell from 90% to 89% to 80%. Therefore, the lowest inactive renin occurred during placebo plus a high-salt diet (18.8 ng/ml/hr), and the highest occurred during indapamide plus a low-salt diet (53.6 ng/ml/hr). However, the proportion of inactive renin was highest during placebo plus a high-salt diet (94%) and was lowest during diuretic administration plus a low-salt diet (80%) (unpublished).

The lowest inactive renins that we have observed occurred in untreated patients with primary aldosteronism [1]. In 10 of a group of 11 such patients, inactive renin averaged only 4.7 ng/ml/hr; in five of these patients in whom inactive renin was measured pre- and postsurgery or during diuretic treatment, inactive renin increased from 3.7 to 11.2 ng/ml/hr. These results suggest that the volume expansion that accompanies primary aldosteronism causes suppression of inactive renin. Paradoxically, however, one patient had a normal inactive renin level of 21.1 ng/ml/hr, and it actually fell following removal of the tumor and cure of the hypertension to 8 ng/ml/hr (unpublished results). Therefore, sodium balance obviously is not the only factor determining circulating levels of inactive renin. There is some evidence that active [44] and inactive renins are synthesized in the adrenal glands [45]. It is possible that in this particular patient, the adrenal gland was the source of the unusually high inactive renin. We also have observed very high levels of circulating inactive renin (150 ng/ml/hr) in a patient with an adrenal carcinoma who had normal active renin values; again, this suggests that the adrenal gland occasionally may contribute to the plasma-inactive renin level.

It is quite clear that in humans, the kidney is not the only source of circulating inactive renin [12, 33, 46]. This is in contrast to active plasma renin, which appears to come entirely from the kidney. Inactive renin often is low in nephrectomized patients, but it is always detectable; in certain patients, it can be markedly elevated for unknown reasons. Renin has been identified in several extrarenal tissues [47] such as the submaxillary gland [48], brain [49], uterus [50], blood vessel walls [51], and adrenal glands [44]; but, so far, we do not know which tissues might secrete this putative precursor (prorenin) into the circulation. As already mentioned, the adrenal gland is one possible source [45]. Nephrectomized patients tend to have very low plasma levels of the adrenal steroid aldosterone; this is most likely due to the fact that they have undetectable levels of circulating renin [52]. However, we observed in one such patient that when plasma-inactive renin increased about 8-fold, plasma aldosterone also increased close to 8-fold, but there was no increase in plasma-active renin. This finding raises the possibility that adrenal renin may have played some role in the increase in aldosterone biosynthesis, and that the adrenal gland might also have been the source of the increased circulating inactive renin [52].

Measurement of inactive renin in renal vein samples has failed to give a clear answer to the question of whether inactive renin is normally secreted by the kidney or whether it is cleared or converted to active renin during passage through the renal circulation [28, 53–55]. Without question, inactive renin is present in extracts of human kidneys [56]. It is also released by human kidneys that have been perfused ex vivo [56]; occasionally, significant arteriovenous differences in inactive renin have been detected by renal venous sampling in vivo [28, 53]. On the other hand, many renal vein samples do not show a significant increment in inactive renin, compared to concurrently collected arterial samples; however, neither do many of them show a significant decrement in inactive renin. These inconsistent results could be due to many factors, including the inaccuracy of the measurement, the possibility that inactive renin is concurrently cleared (or taken up) and secreted by the kidney, or that it is secreted only intermittently. Perhaps more importantly, if the biologic half-life of inactive renin was an order of magnitude greater than that of active renin, one would not expect to be able to detect an increment in inactive renin concentration across the kidney (unless blood flow were markedly reduced). The normal increment of active renin averages only 25% of the arterial level [57]; if the clearance rate of inactive renin was 1/10th that of active renin, this increment would be expected to be only 2.5% of the peripheral level—well below the accuracy of the measurement. Fragmentary data following nephrectomy have suggested that the half-life may be close to 2 hr [53] (more than double that of active renin), but the accuracy of this type of estimation is questionable.

A striking (close to 10-fold) increase in inactive renin occurs during the early stages of pregnancy at a time when renin substrate has not increased very much (Fig. 3) [36, 37, 58]. Most of this rise is sustained throughout pregnancy, although there does appear to be a slight drop-off after the eighth week, despite the fact that renin substrate is rising. Thus far, it is unclear whether the increased levels of inactive renin that occur in the plasma during pregnancy are of renal or extrarenal origin. The chorion has been shown to synthesize inactive renin, and it could be a source [59, 60]. Also, inactive renin falls rapidly postpartum [61]. On the other hand, after the initial rise in inactive renin, the inactive and active renin levels tend to change in parallel throughout pregnancy; they respond together to changes in sodium balance and to development of hypertension [19, 36]. Therefore, these physiologic observations might be consistent with a renal source of inactive renin in pregnancy.

While most of the factors that acutely affect active renin release also induce changes in inactive renin, the time course of the inactive renin response usually is much slower; that is, over days rather than minutes [62]. When short-term changes in inactive renin have been reported, the magnitude of the observed changes often have been within the error of the method, which is very great when active renin is high in relation to inactive renin. Despite this problem, the report of Hsueh et al [63] presents convincing evidence for a marked and transient *fall* in inactive renin as active renin *increased* during short-term administration of the converting enzyme inhibitor captopril to sodium-depleted normal subjects. Over the long-term course, captopril increased both active and inactive renin. Therefore, it is possible that the transient fall in inactive renin may have been due to increased conversion of prorenin to renin as the stimulus for renin release occurred; however, it

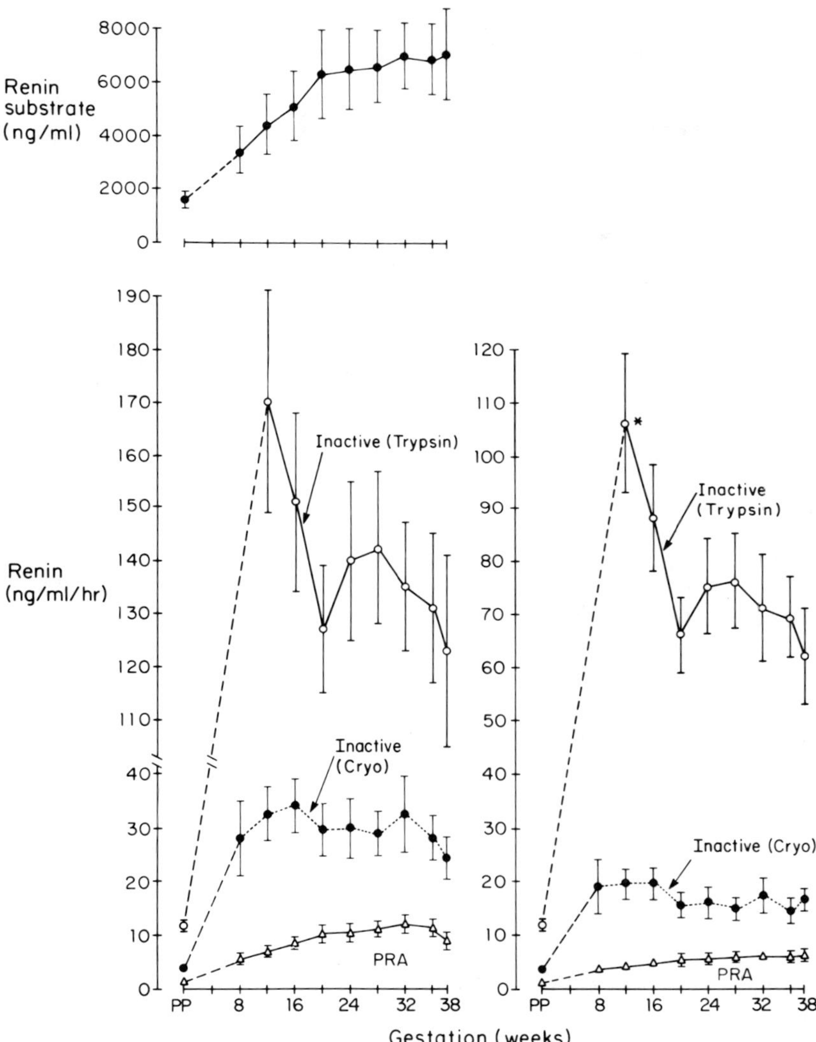

Fig. 3. Serial changes in active and inactive renin and in renin substrate throughout pregnancy. Inactive renin was measured by both trypsin and cryoactivation. In the *right-hand panel*, the values are normalized to the postpartum renin substrate concentration, assuming a Michaelis constant of 2700 ng/ml for endogenous renin substrate in undiluted plasma [38]. (Reprinted with permission from [37] by courtesy of Marcel Dekker, Inc.)

is possible that over the longer-term course, this was offset by increased biosynthesis and a restoration and then by an increase of the circulating inactive renin level.

The effect of beta blockade is unusual in that inactive renin remains essentially unchanged, while active renin falls [40, 64]. This has led to speculation that beta blockers do not reduce the rate of biosynthesis of renin, but they merely alter the degree of conversion of prorenin to renin. The lack of response of inactive renin resulted in some confusion in early studies of the effect of beta blockers on active renin, because (sometimes) an acid-dialysis step was used prior to measurement of active renin, leading to inadvertent measurement of total renin (which did not change) instead of active renin (which fell) [65].

Inactive renin measurements may be diagnostic in the detection of patients with ectopic renin-secreting tumors [5]. We found that two hypertensive patients with proven renin-secreting carcinomas of nonrenal origin (pancreas and ovary) had both high plasma-active renin (119 and 138 ng/ml/hr) and the highest inactive renin levels that we have ever observed (5200 and 14,300 ng/ml/hr; normal range is 3 to 50). The proportion of inactive renin (98 to 99%) far exceeded that found in other patients with high active-renin levels. A third hypertensive patient with a probable renin-secreting ovarian carcinoma exhibited a similar pattern. Both inactive renins isolated from plasma and tumors of these patients were biochemically similar to semipurified inactive renins from normal plasma or cadaver kidney (see below). Inactive renin from each source was activated irreversibly by trypsin and reversibly by dialysis to pH 3.3 at 4°C; the reversal process followed the kinetics of a first-order reaction in each instance. The trypsin-activated inactive renins all were identical to semipurified active renal renin in terms of their pH optimum (pH 5.5 to 6.0) and kinetics with homologous angiotensinogen (Michaelis constants, 0.8 to 1.3 μmoles), and also in terms of their inhibition by pepstatin or by serial dilutions of renin-specific antibody. These results suggest that a markedly elevated plasma-inactive renin level distinguishes patients with ectopic renin production from other high-renin hypertensive states [5]. Also, the coproduction of inactive and active renin by extrarenal neoplasms provides strong presumptive evidence that inactive renin is a biosynthetic precursor of active renin. The usually high proportion of inactive renin in plasma and tumor extracts from these patients is consistent with ineffective precursor processing by neoplastic tissue.

In summary, measurements of plasma-inactive renin in human subjects have demonstrated many similarities and a few differences, when compared to active renin. The major difference is its presence in nephrectomized subjects, which demonstrates clearly that renin is not synthesized only in the kidney in human subjects. However, the role of extrarenal renin is far from clear and is currently under investigation. The fact that active renin is not found in the circulation of nephrectomized subjects—even those with very high inactive renin levels—suggests that if "activation" is required for function, it most likely occurs at an extravascular site, perhaps inside the cell. It will be intriguing to find out what the extravascular function of renin might be.

Physicochemical Characteristics of Inactive Renin

Inactive renin differs from active renin in several respects, in addition to its apparent lack of catalytic activity [18, 19, 66]. Unlike active renin, inactive renin binds to Cibacron Blue-agarose and does not bind to pepstatin-amino-hexylagarose. Inactive renin has a weaker affinity for anion exchange resins than does the active form; it may be more hydrophobic, since unlike active renin, it could not be recovered from octyl-sepharose CL-4B (Pharmacia) [66]. Both active and inactive renin bind to concanavalin A-Sepharose and are eluted with α-methyl-mannoside, which suggests that they are both glyco-proteins.

Trypsin-activated inactive renin has catalytic properties that are indistin-guishable from those of active renin. Neither active nor activated renins hydrolyze hemoglobin. The pH optimum with homologous angiotensinogen for both is pH 5.5 to 6.0. The K_m for human angiotensinogen for both is 0.8 to 1.3 μmole/liter. They are inhibited noncompetitively by pepstatin at low (1 to 3 μmole/liter) concentrations of pepstatin with an apparent K_i of 2.6 to 3.2 μmole/liter, but at higher concentrations, a mixed pattern of inhibition is found. Both can be inhibited 100% by antirenin antibodies, and a 50% inhibition occurred for both at a dilution of 5×10^{-5} [66].

Trypsin-activated renin differs from active renin in that it has a greater apparent molecular weight via gel filtration on Sephadex G100 [18]. This holds true for plasma- and kidney-inactive renins, but it does not seem to affect the catalytic properties of the enzyme. Presumably, trypsin does not mimic exactly the activation process as it occurs in vivo.

Interestingly, there is one characteristic that distinguishes plasma-inactive renin from kidney-inactive renin and plasma-active renin from kidney-active renin. Both plasma renins have a greater apparent molecular weight via gel filtration on Sephadex G100 [18]. We found that plasma-inactive renin aver-aged 56,000 $\pm$ 1500, and plasma-active renin averaged 48,000 $\pm$ 2000, while kidney-inactive renin averaged 49,500 $\pm$ 1000 and kidney-active renin aver-aged 39,500 $\pm$ 500. Active and inactive renin from renal perfusate had elution characteristics similar to those of the renal substances, while active and inac-tive renin from ectopic renin-secreting tumors ran between plasma and renal forms. These findings do not necessarily suggest differences in primary struc-ture, since alterations in carbohydrate composition or molecular configuration perhaps could account for these differences.

With the recent availability of antirenin antibodies, it has been possible to demonstrate that activated "inactive renin," indeed, is renin and not a different enzyme with similar catalytic properties. It appears to be of larger molecular weight than the active counterpart. The fact that it is present in ectopic renin-secreting tumors suggests a tight genetic linkage with active renin [5]. The observation that all sources of human-inactive renin (kidney, tumor, and plasma) demonstrate reversible acid activation suggests that they are very similar substances; the demonstration that the reversal of activation follows first-order kinetics suggests that it is a unimolecular interaction and is not active renin bound to an inhibitor. Also, as mentioned above, activation of inactive renin by trypsin-like enzymes is consistent with the known molecular structure of prorenin. Therefore, most available evidence suggests that inactive renin, indeed, may be prorenin. Further studies are required to provide direct biochemical evidence on this point.

Summary and Conclusions

Inactive renin is a substance in human plasma with characteristics very similar to those that would be predicted for a biosynthetic precursor of active renin. The plasma level of inactive renin usually responds in the same way as active renin, but much slower, to stimuli that affect active renin secretion. One notable exception is that beta blockers consistently lower active renin, but they have little effect on inactive renin in plasma. Inactive renin is secreted from both renal and extrarenal sources, but renal-inactive renin has not been differentiated biochemically from extrarenal-inactive renin; therefore, we do not know the relative contribution of the kidney to the plasma level. The source of extrarenal-circulating inactive renin is also unknown, although it has been identified in several extrarenal tissues that include the brain and adrenal gland, and in the fetoplacental unit during pregnancy. Unlike inactive renin, active renin does not circulate in anephric subjects; therefore, the role of extrarenal-inactive renin is obscure. If activation is required for inactive renin to have an effect, then its actions may be confined to the extravascular space. Alternatively, reversible activation may occur at particular vascular sites that allow local activity, but result in no detectable increase in circulating active renin. Reversible activation of human-inactive renin has been shown to occur following acidification to pH 3.3; however, reversibility of activation has not yet been demonstrated under physiologic conditions. In summary, inactive renin is a fascinating substance that may be an important element of the renin-angiotensin system. The next few years should shed light on its function and whether or not it contributes to the cardiovascular and hormonal effects of the renin-angiotensin system.

References

1. SEALEY JE, ATLAS SA, LARAGH JH: Prorenin and other large molecular weight forms of renin. *Endocr Rev* 1:365–391, 1980
2. INAGAMI T, MURAKAMI K: Prorenin. *Biomed Res* 1:456–475, 1980
3. LECKIE BJ: Inactive renin: an attempt at a perspective. *Clin Sci* 60:119–130, 1980
4. SEALEY JE, LARAGH JH: Prorenin in human plasma? Methodological and physiological implications. *Circ Res* 36, 37(Suppl I):10–16, 1975
5. ATLAS SA, HESSON TE, SEALEY JE, DHARMGRONGARTAMA B, LARAGH JH: Characterization of inactive renin ("prorenin") from renin-secreting tumors of non-renal origin: Similarity to inactive renin from kidney and normal plasma. *J Clin Invest* 73:437–447, 1984
6. LUMBERS ER: Activation of renin in human amniotic fluid by low pH. *Enzymologia* 40:329–336, 1971
7. DAY RP, LUETSCHER JA: Big renin: a possible prohormone in kidney and plasma of a patient with Wilms tumor. *J Clin Endocrinol Metab* 38:923–926, 1974

8. BOYD GW: The nature of renal renin, in *Hypertension '72*, edited by GENEST J, KOIW JE, New York, Springer-Verlag, 1972, pp 161–169

9. LECKIE B: The activation of a possible zymogen of renin in rabbit kidney. *Clin Sci* 44:301–304, 1972

10. FUNAKAWA S, FUNAE Y, YAMAMOTO K: Conversion between renin and high-molecular-weight renin in the dog. *Biochem J* 176:977–981, 1978

11. SAGNELLA GA, CALDWELL PRB, PEART WS: Sub-cellular distribution of low- and high-molecular weight renin and its relation to a renin inhibitor in pig renal cortex. *Clin Sci* 59:337–345, 1980

12. SEALEY JE, MOON C, LARAGH JH, ATLAS SA: Plasma prorenin in normal, hypertensive and anephric patients and its effect on renin measurements. *Circ Res* 40(Suppl I):41–45, 1977

13. SKINNER SK: Improved assay methods for renin "concentration" and "activity" in human plasma. *Circ Res* 20:391–402, 1967

14. BROWN JJ, DAVIES DL, LEVER AF, ROBERTSON JIS, TREE M: The estimation of renin in human plasma. *Biochem J* 93:594–600, 1964

15. OSMOND DH, ROSS LJ, SCIAFF KD: Increased renin activity after cold storage of plasma. *Can J Physiol Pharmacol* 51:705–708, 1973

16. MORRIS BJ, LUMBERS ER: The activation of renin in human amniotic fluid by proteolytic enzymes. *Biochim et Biophys Acta* 289:385–391, 1972

17. SEALEY JE, ATLAS SA, LARAGH JH, OZA NB, RYAN JW: Activation of prorenin-like substance in human plasma by trypsin and by urinary kallikrein. *Hypertension* 1:179–189, 1979

18. ATLAS SA, SEALEY JE, DHARMGRONGARTAMA B, HESSON TE, LARAGH JH: Detection and isolation of inactive, large molecular weight renin in human kidney and plasma. *Hypertension* 3(Suppl I):30–40, 1981

19. SEALEY JE, ATLAS SA, LARAGH JH: Plasma prorenin: physiological and biochemical characteristics. *Clin Sci* 63:133s–145s, 1982

20. SEALEY JE, MOON C, LARAGH JH, ALDERMAN M: Plasma prorenin: cryoactivation and relationship to renin substrate in normal subjects. *Am J Med* 61:731–738, 1976

21. ATLAS SA, LARAGH JH, SEALEY JE: Activation of inactive plasma renin: evidence that both cryo- and acid-activation work by liberating a neutral serine protease from endogenous inhibitors. *Clin Sci Mol Med* 55:135s–138s, 1978

22. SEALEY JE, ATLAS SA, LARAGH JH, SILVERBERG M, KAPLAN AP: Initiation of plasma prorenin activation by Hageman factor-dependent conversion of plasma prekallikrein to kallikrein. *Proc Natl Acad Sci* 76:5914–5918, 1979

23. ARMSTRONG D, DASILVA WD: Kinin formation in human blood serum induced by cooling and by heat aggregated human gamma globulin preparations. *Adv Exper Med Biol* 8:31–37, 1970

24. DERKX FHM, BOUMA BN, SHALEKAMP MPA, SHALEKAMP MADH: An intrinsic factor XII-prekallikrein-dependent pathway activates the human plasma renin-angiotensin system. *Nature* 280:315–316, 1979

25. HSUEH WA, CARLSON EJ, ISRAEL-HAGMAN M: Mechanism of acid-activation of renin: role of kallikrein in renin activation. *Hypertension* 3(Suppl I): 22–29, 1981

26. LECKIE BJ, MCGHEE NK: Reversible activation-inactivation of renin in human plasma. *Nature* 288:702–704, 1980

27. ATLAS SA, HESSON TE, SEALEY JE, LARAGH JH: Reversible acid activation of inactive renin: evidence favoring a unimolecular reaction. *Clin Sci* 63:167–170, 1982

28. SEALEY JE, ATLAS SA, LARAGH JH, OZA NB, RYAN JW: Human urinary kalli-

316   Renal Metabolism, Prostaglandins, and Renin

krein converts inactive to active renin and is a possible physiological activator of renin. *Nature* 275:144–145, 1978

29. SEALEY JE, ATLAS SA, LARAGH JH: Linking the kallikrein and renin systems via activation of inactive renin: new data and a hypothesis. *Am J Med* 65:994–1000, 1978

30. SEALEY JE, ATLAS SA, LARAGH JH, SILVERBERG M, KAPLAN AP: Plasmin can activate plasma prorenin but is not required for the alkaline phase of acid activation. *Clin Sci* 57:97s–99s, 1979

31. OSMOND DH, LO EK, LOH AY, ZINGG EA, HEDLIN AH: Kallikrein and plasmin as activators of inactive renin (*letter*). *Lancet* 2:1375, 1978

32. BLUMBERG AL, SEALEY JE, ATLAS SA, LARAGH JH, DHARMGRONGARTAMA B, KAPLAN AP: Contact activation of human plasma prorenin in vitro. *J Lab Clin Med* 97:771–778, 1981

33. SEALEY JE, WHITE RP, LARAGH JH, RUBIN AL: Plasma prorenin and renin in anephric patients. *Circ Res* 41(Suppl II):17–20, 1977

34. PANTHIER JJ, FOOTE S, CHAMBRAUD B, STROSSBERG AD, CORVOL P, ROUGEON F: Complete amino acid sequence and maturation of the mouse submaxillary gland renin precursor. *Nature* 298:90–91, 1982

35. IMAI T, MIYAZAKI H, HIROSE S, HORI H, HAYASHI T, KEGEYAMA R, OHKUBO H, NAKANISHI S, MURAKAMI K: Cloning and sequence analysis of CDNA for human renin precursor. *Proc Natl Acad Sci* 80:7405–7409, 1983

36. HSUEH WA, LUETSCHER JA, CARLSON EJ, GRISLIS G, FRAZE E, MCHARGUE A: Changes in active and inactive renin throughout pregnancy. *J Clin Endocrinol Metab* 54:1010–1016, 1982

37. SEALEY JE, WILSON M, MORGANTI AA, ZERVOUDAKIS I, LARAGH JH: Changes in active and inactive renin throughout normal pregnancy. *Clin Exp Hyper* A4(11, 12):2372–2384, 1982

38. NEWTON MA, SEALEY JE, LEDINGHAM JGG, LARAGH JH: High blood pressure and oral contraceptives. *Am J Obstet Gynecol* 101:1037–1045, 1968

39. WEINBERGER M, AOI W, GRIM C: Dynamic responses of active and inactive renin in normal and hypertensive humans. *Circ Res* 41(Suppl II):21–25, 1977

40. ATLAS SA, SEALEY JE, LARAGH JH, MOON C: Plasma renin and "prorenin" in essential hypertension during sodium depletion, beta-blockade and reduced arterial pressure. *Lancet* II:785–789, 1977

41. HSUEH WA, LUETSCHER JA, CARLSON E, GRISLIS G, ELBAUM D, CHAVARRI M: A comparison of cold and acid activation of big renin and of inactive renin in normal plasma. *J Clin Endocrinol Metab* 47:792–799, 1978

42. MCKENZIE JK, REISIN E: Acid-activated renin responses to hydrochlorothiazide, propranolol and indomethacin. *Clin Sci Mol Med* 55:151s–153s, 1978

43. KAPPELGAARD AM, BIESE J, IBSEN H, NIELSEN MD, RABOL A: Different secretion patterns of active and inactive renin in man. *Clin Sci Mol Med* 55:143s–146s, 1978

44. RYAN JW: Renin-like enzyme in the adrenal gland. *Science* 158:1589–1590, 1967

45. MITSUHIDE N, SUSSMAN CR, NARUSE K, JACKSON RV, INAGAMI T: Renin exists in human adrenal tissue. *J Clin Endocrinol Metab* 57:482–487, 1983

46. WEINBERGER M, WADE MB, AOI W, USA T, DENTINO M, LUFT F, GRIM CE: An extrarenal source of "renin-like" activity in anephric man. *Circ Res* 40(Suppl I):1–4, 1977

47. GANTEN D, SCHELLING P, VECSEI P, GANTEN U: Iso-renin of extrarenal origin. "The tissue angiotensinase systems." *Am J Med* 60:760–765, 1976

48. WERLE E, VOGEL R, GOLDEL LF: Uber ein blutdrucksteigerndes Prinzip in Extrakten aus der Glandula submaxillaris der weissen Maus. *Arch Exp Pathol (Berlin)* 230:236–240, 1957

49. GANTEN D, MARQUEZ-JULIO A, GRANZER P, HAYDUK K, KARSUNKY KP, BOUCHER R, GENEST J: Renin in dog brain. *Am J Physiol* 221:1733–1737, 1971

50. GROSS F, SCHAECHTELIN G, ZIEGLER M, BERGER M: A renin-like substance in the placenta and uterus of the rabbit. *Lancet* 1:914–915, 1964

51. GOULD AB, SKEGGS LT, KAHN JR: The presence of renin activity in blood vessel walls. *J Exp Med* 119:389–399, 1964

52. SEALEY JE, WHITE RP, LARAGH JH, CASE DB, RUBIN AL: Studies of plasma aldosterone in anephric people: evidence for fundamental role of the renin system in maintaining aldosterone secretion. *J Clin Endocrinol Metab* 47:52–60, 1978

53. DERKX FHM, WENTING GJ, MAN IN'T VELD AJ, VERHOEVEN RP, SCHALE-KAMP MADH: Control of enzymatically inactive renin in man under various pathological conditions: implications for the interpretation of renin measurements in peripheral and renal venous plasma. *Clin Sci Mol Med* 54:529–538, 1978

54. BIRKENHAGER WH, DELEEUW PW, FALKE HE, VAN SOUST GAW: Renin secretion by the human kidney. *Clin Sci Mol Med* 55:147s–150s, 1978

55. GLORIOSO N, DESSI-FULGHERI P, MADEDDU P, URIGO F, TONOLO GC, OPPES M, PALERMO M, RAPPELI A: Active and inactive renin during acute reduction of renal perfusion pressure in essential hypertensives. *Clin Exp Hyper* A4(11, 12):2293–2302, 1982

56. ATLAS SA, LARAGH JH, SEALEY JE, HESSON TE: An inactive, prorenin-like substance in human plasma and kidney. *Clin Sci* 59:29s–33s, 1980

57. SEALEY JE, BÜHLER FR, LARAGH JH, VAUGHAN ED JR: The physiology of renin secretion in essential hypertension: estimation of renin secretion rate and renal plasma flow from peripheral and renal vein renin levels. *Am J Med* 55:391–401, 1973

58. SKINNER SL, CRAN EJ, GIBSON R, TAYLOR R, WALTERS WAW, CATT KJ: Angiotensins I and II, active and inactive renin, renin substrate. renin activity and angiotensinase in human liquor amnii and plasma. *Am J Obstet Gynecol* 121:626–630, 1975

59. SYMONDS EM, STANLEY MA, SKINNER SL: Production of renin by in vitro cultures of human chorion and uterine muscle. *Nature* 217:1152–1153, 1968

60. ACKER GM, GALEN FX, DEVAUX C, FOOTE S, PAPERNICK E, PESTY A, Menard J, Corvol P: Human chorionic cells in primary culture: a model for renin biosynthesis. *J Clin Endocrinol Metab* 54:902–910, 1982

61. BROUGHTON PIPKIN F, DATS JJN, SYMONDS EM: Sequential changes in the human renin-angiotensin system following delivery. *Br J Obstet Gynecol* 85:821–827, 1978

62. SEALEY JE, OVERLACK A, LARAGH JH, STUMPE KO, ATLAS SA: Effect of captopril and aprotonin on inactive renin. *J Clin Endocrinol Metab* 53:626–630, 1981

63. HSUEH W, GOLDSTONE R, CARLSON E, HORTON R: Reciprocal changes in active and inactive renin after converting enzyme inhibition in man. *Clin Sci* 63(Suppl 8):175s–177s, 1982

64. DERKX FHM, v GOOL JMG, WENTING GJ, VERHOEVEN RA, MAN IN'T VELD AJ, SCHALEKAMP MADH: Inactive renin in human plasma. *Lancet* 2:496–499, 1976

65. AMERY A, LIJNEN P, FAGARD R, REYBROUK T: Inactive renin in human plasma. *Lancet* 2:849–850, 1976

66. ATLAS SA, SEALEY JE, HESSON TE, KAPLAN AP, MENARD J, CORVOL P, LARAGH JH: Biochemical similarity of partially purified inactive renins from human plasma and kidney. *Hypertension* 4(Suppl II):86–95, 1982

The Renin Gene: Structure and Processing of Renin

Florent Soubrier, Joël Menard, and Pierre Corvol

A very long time elapsed between the discovery by two Danish investigators, Tigerstedt and Bergman, of the pressor effect of a kidney extract and the elucidation of the structure of both renin and its precursor. This was achieved in 1982 by amino acid sequencing and nucleotide analysis of the renin structural gene. Both the extremely low amount of renin in the kidney (less than 1/500,000 of total proteins) and its copurification with other proteases explain the difficulties encountered by previous investigators.

The knowledge of the primary structure of mouse and human renin and of its precursor by cDNA sequencing allows the construction of models of its processing. These models were evaluated by cellular biosynthetic experiments of renin in the mouse submaxillary gland (SMG) and in the human kidney. They show that renin is biosynthesized as an inactive preprorenin precursor and that it is likely processed into active renin within endocrine-type granules. The active site of renin is known and models are proposed for its organization in three dimensions. No doubt, this progress will help us considerably to understand the "molecular physiology" of renin; it will assist design of specific inhibitors of the renin-substrate reaction.

It is our purpose to review the progress made in the last 2 years in understanding the structure of the renin gene and the processing of the renin precursor, both in the mouse SMG and in the human kidney.

Renin Messenger RNA

Structure of Mouse Submaxillary Gland (SMG) Renin cDNA [1]

A "renin-like" enzyme, whose physiologic role is not known, is present in the submaxillary gland (SMG) of some mouse strains; it has biochemical,

---

This manuscript was presented as part of a Symposium on *Renin: Recent Advances.*

immunologic, and enzymatic preperties similar, but not identical, to that of the renal enzyme. It represents as much as 5% of the total protein content of the SMG, indicating a high level of renin mRNA in this gland.

RNA was extracted from the SMG of Swiss mice and was translated in vitro by using the mRNA-dependent rabbit reticulocyte lysate. The renin precursor was immunoprecipitated with a rabbit antiserum against mouse SMG renin that was purified according to Cohen et al [2]. A 45,000 (45 kd) molecular weight protein was detected on SDS-polyacrylamide gel electrophoresis, which is a molecular size 8-kd higher than the molecular weight of the mature protein. A cDNA library was constructed from SMG mRNA in the plasmid pBR322 and was used to transform host bacteria. Recombinant clones bearing the renin cDNA were identified by genetic screening. Indeed, renin mRNA in the SMG is present in great abundance in males of some strains of mice (Swiss, AKR), whereas it is in minute amounts in females and in some other strains (Balb/c). Renin clones hybridized with a ^{32}P-cDNA probe that was made with mRNA from renin-rich SMG and from kidney. They did not hybridize with a ^{32}P-cDNA probe made with mRNA from a renin-poor SMG. The renin cDNA clones also were able to hybridize with renin mRNA and to inhibit their in vitro translation. Two clones (pRn3-5 and pRn4-7) were identified.

Clones pRn3-5 and pRn4-7 shared an identical 900-nucleotide segment and represented an essentially complete transcript of renin mRNA. The amino acid sequence of the renin precursor was deduced from the nucleotide sequence of the two clones.

Comparison of the primary structure of renin with that of other aspartyl proteases revealed that mouse SMG renin contained the sequence Asp_{101}-Thr-Gly-Ser, which is homologous to the sequence containing the aspartyl residue 32 of penicillinopepsin. This residue is involved in the catalytic site. The sequence Asp_{286}-Thr-Gly is homologous to the sequence containing the second aspartyl residue (215) of the penicillinopepsin catalytic site. These sequences are found in all sequenced aspartyl proteases.

Residues Tyr 75 and Trp 39 of penicillinopepsin, which are thought to be implicated in the catalytic site, are conserved in preprorenin. They occur at positions 146 and 108, respectively, in the preprorenin molecule. The overall homology between prorenin and porcine pepsinogen is 37%. Together, these findings strongly support the contention that the amino acids involved in the catalytic mechanisms of renin are very similar to those of acid proteases.

The N-terminus sequence of the protein was also determined by Panthier et al [1]. They showed that mouse SMG renin consisted of two chains, A and B, linked by a disulfide bridge. At the same time, the complete amino acid sequence of active mouse SMG renin has been established by Misono, Chang, and Inagami [3], by using automatic Edman's degradation.

Model for Mouse SMG Renin Processing

A model for processing of the renin precursor has been proposed [1], based on the comparison of the nucleotide sequence of the SMG renin cDNA and the NH_2 terminus of the mature protein. This model involves at least two processing steps:

1. A signal peptide first is cleaved off by a signal peptidase from rough microsomes; these signal peptidases are able to cotranslationally hydrolyze the leader sequence from nascent polypeptide chains. The exact cleavage site is not known, since the NH_2 terminus of prorenin has not been determined yet.
2. Prorenin then is subjected to two sequential cleavages, leading to an active mature renin consisting of two chains linked by an interchain disulfide bond. Each of these proteolytic cleavages occur after a dibasic peptide: Lys_{62}-Arg_{63} and Arg_{352}-Arg_{353}. This mechanism of peptide maturation is similar to that described for most prohormone-hormone processing, in which the active hormone usually is released from an inactive precursor after a pair of basic amino acid residues [4].

In vitro experiments by Catanzaro, Mullins, and Morris [5] and Pratt, Ouelette, and Dzau [6] have further defined the biosynthetic pathway of renin. Pulse-labeling studies of minced SMG tissue and immunoprecipitation of labeled products have demonstrated the rapid intracellular synthesis of an immunoreactive ^{35}S-labeled precursor (molecular weight, 44 ± 2 kd). This renin is 3-kd lower than the preprorenin identified by cell-free translation of SMG mRNA. As early as 15 min, prorenin is converted to a 38 ± 2 kd molecular weight form of renin corresponding to a single chain. Finally, after several hours, the one-chain renin is converted into two-chain renin. Pratt et al [6] also found that enriched Golgi predominantly contained the one-chain renin and that mature granules contained mainly the two-chain form.

No N-glycosylation sites were found in the SMG renin primary structure. The observed microheterogeneity of mouse SMG renin, therefore, could be due to other post-translational events. Indeed, the dibasic pair Arg_{352}-Arg_{353}, deduced from the nucleotide sequence of the clone, is not present in the sequence determined by Misono et al [3] in the active enzyme. The presence of this dipeptide in some renin molecules could account for a charge difference.

Evidence for a Gene Duplication in Some Mice Strains

The variation in the organization of the renin gene that is associated with the synthesis of high or low levels of renin in the SMG of various mice strains has recently been elucidated.

It has been shown by Piccini, Knopf, and Gross [7] and by Panthier, Holm, and Rougeon [8] that the phenotypic groups of mice that have high levels of renin activity in the SMG regulated by androgen have two renin genes (AKR or Swiss). Inbred strains of mice that have a low renin activity possess a single renin gene. It also has been found [9] that in strains carrying two renin genes, renin mRNA in the kidney is transcribed mainly from one gene and the mRNA in the SMG is transcribed from the other.

Structure of Human Renal Renin cDNA

In normal human kidneys, renin represents approximately 1/100,000 to 1/500,000 of the total protein content. This very low amount has prevented the purification of human renin in quantities sufficient for the determination of its primary structure. The strategy used was to construct a cDNA library from kidney mRNA and to screen the recombinant clones with the mouse SMG renin cDNA probe.

Kidney mRNA was extracted from a surgically removed infarcted kidney, as its renin content is about 100-fold higher than in a normal kidney. Characterization of the renin mRNA was performed by the Northern Blot technique [10]; by hybridization with the mouse SMG renin cDNA as a probe, a unique mRNA of 1.6-kb length was detected similar to that of the mouse kidney and SMG renin. A cDNA library of approximately 10,000 clones was constructed. Colonies were screened by hybridization with the mouse ^{32}P-cDNA probe. One clone, which contained an 1100-base pair (bp) insert, was sequenced as previously reported [11]. Imai et al [12] have reported the sequence of an entire human renin mRNA transcript. The overall homology between human renal and mouse SMG renin is 76% in the coding region at the nucleotide level. At the amino acid level, the homology is 68%. Amino acid residues known to be involved in the catalytic mechanism are conserved when compared to SMG renin and to other aspartyl proteases. Two potential N-glycosylation sites are present in the sequence Asn-Gly-Thr (residue 138 to 140) and in the sequence Asn-Thr-Thr, which is located at residues 68 to 70. Renin was expected to have N-glycosylation sites, since human renal renin binds to Con A-sepharose.

The human renin clone was also used to investigate the extrarenal expression of renin [11]. Messenger RNA was extracted from fetal membranes. Via the Northern Blot technique, a unique mRNA that is the same size as renal renin mRNA hybridized with human renin cDNA probe. It has also been shown that there is only one renin gene in humans by using the Southern hybridization technique [11].

Model for Human Renal Renin Processing

The renin precursor and its processing have been studied with different methodologies: cell-free translation and the incorporation of ^{35}S-methionine into renin precursors in cell culture or tissue.

Imai et al [13] have used cell-free translation of kidney mRNA and immunoprecipitation of ^{35}S-labeled products by antirenin antibodies. A major band of Mr 43 kd was detected and was presumed to be the renin precursor. In the cell-free system, neither processing cleavage occurs nor does post-translational modification, such as glycosylation or phosphorylation. Biosynthesis of human renin in cellular translation systems have been studied by Galen et al [14] in renin secreting tissues and cells (Fig.1). Two models were used: the chorion, which is a rich source of inactive renin, and a renin-secreting tumor.

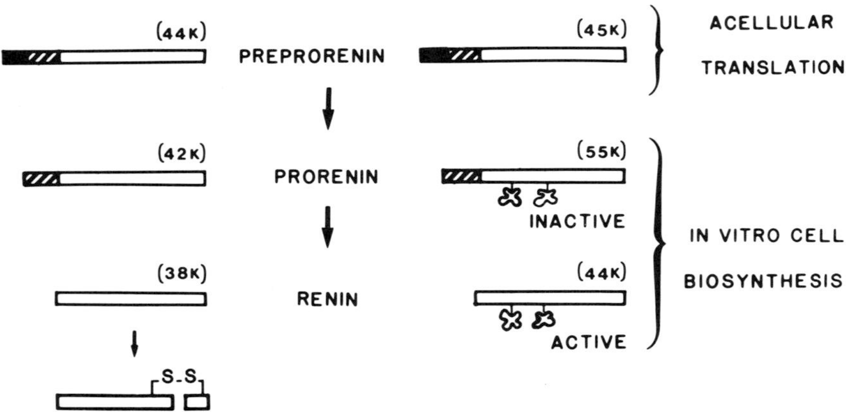

Fig. 1. Comparative schema for the structure and processing of mouse (*left panel*) submaxillary and human (*right panel*) renal renin precursors. ✸ : site of glycosylation; ■: prefragment; ▨: profragment. 38 kd, 42 kd, 45 kd, 55 kd, 38,000, 42,000, 45,000, 55,000 mol wt. (After Galen et al [14])

In chorionic-cultured cells, renin was secreted as an inactive precursor that could be activated by limited trypsinization into a 44-kd active renin.

Pulse-chase experiments were performed with tissue slices of a human juxtaglomerular tumor. Renin was synthesized as a high molecular weight form (55 kd), and then it was converted into a 44-kd protein. Juxtaglomerular tumoral cells also were cultured. Renin-producing cells in primary culture were pulsed with radiolabeled amino acids; immunoprecipitable radiolabeled renin was found in the culture media. Renin was rapidly released into the medium as an inactive 55-kd form, and no processing into a 44-kd active protein was detected. In the tumoral tissue, endocrine-type secretory granules were observed in the normal kidney, whereas in the chorionic and tumoral cultured cells, such granules could not be detected. The absence of granules was associated with the loss of capacity of packaging and processing 55-kd renin into the active 44-kd form.

The sites of processing of prorenin into renin still are speculative, because the N-terminus amino acid sequence of active human renin has not yet been reported. However, based on the structural homology between mouse SMG renin and human kidney renin cDNA and amino acid sequences, it can be speculated that human preprorenin is processed in a similar way to that of mouse renin:

1. Cleavage of a leader sequence with a putative length of 20 amino acids.
2. Prorenin processing into active renin. A dibasic pair, Lys_{62}-Arg_{63}, is located at almost the same position as the Lys_{65}-Arg_{66} of the mouse SMG renin. If this site is the main site of prorenin processing, a further step that converts a single-chain form into two chains is still unknown. Comparison with the mouse SMG renin sequence shows that the dibasic pair Arg_{352}-

Fig. 2. Proposed model of two pathways for the intracellular processing and release of renin. Pathway ① would be predominant in kidney and juxtaglomerular cell tumoral tissue. Pathway ② would be predominant in the renin-producing cells in culture. Inactive renin, 55,000 mol wt; active renin, 44,000 mol wt. (From Galen et al [14])

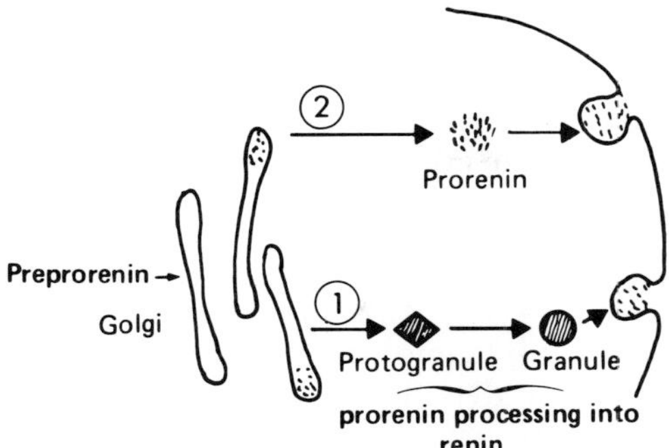

Arg_{353}, after which SMG renin is cleaved into chains A and B, might be replaced by the dibasic pair Lys_{354}-Lys_{355} in the case of human renin. Nevertheless, there is no evidence at present for such a processing of the human enzyme.

After removal of the signal peptide, prorenin could follow two pathways: (1) complete intracellular processing within the secretory granules and (2) direct release of the proform out of the cell, if there are no granules. These two pathways of externalization could correspond to the "regulated" and the "constitutive pathways" described by Gumbiner and Kelly [15]. In the regulated pathway, processing events would take place in the secretory granules, which store the material to be secreted. Proteins externalized by the constitutive pathway are not stored, but they reach the cell surface a few minutes after leaving the Golgi. This pathway would be predominant or even exclusive in poorly differentiated cells, such as renin secretory cells in primary culture and in trophoblastic cells (Fig. 2).

Structure of Mouse Kidney Renin

The structure of the mouse kidney renin has been recently reported by Holm et al [16]. It was deduced from the sequenced exons of the unique renin gene present in the Balb/c strain of mice. The mouse-genomic library was screened with the mouse SMG renin cDNA probe, and hybridizing clones were isolated. Exons were sequenced and the amino acid sequence of mouse kidney renin was predicted in view of the complete sequence of the SMG renin mRNA. The two dibasic residues Lys_{63}-Arg_{64} and Arg_{353}-Arg_{354} that are involved in the processing of SMG renin are found at identical positions in the renal renin. In contrast with the SMG enzyme, but as in the case of the human kidney renin, the mouse kidney renin is glycosylated; three potential glycosylation sites are located at amino acid positions 69, 139, and 319. Comparison of the amino acid sequence of mouse and human kidney renin showed that the proteins are 69.4% homologous. At the nucleotide level, the homology between the two enzymes is 77.5% in the coding region.

Structural Organization of the Renin Gene

The organization of the mouse renin gene was deduced from the approximate locations of the exons by Southern Blot analysis with the SMG cDNA probe [2]. The intron-exon junctions were located by comparing the sequences of the exons with the sequence of the SMG renin mRNA. The exact locations of the splice junctions have been assigned on the basis of the GT . . . AG rule [17]. The Balb/c renin gene coding for a 1.6-kb mRNA spans 9.6 kb, and it is split into nine exons by eight intervening sequences of various length.

Aspartyl proteases have a bilobal structure with the two topologically similar domains. The two lobes are connected by a short connecting peptide that is located at residues 244 to 248, which are encoded by the first half of exon six. The two active aspartates of the site are located on the second exon of each cluster of four exons (Fig. 3). These results show that each domain of renin is encoded by each of the two blocks of four exons. This 1-4-4 organization of the nine exons of the renin gene strongly supports and extends the duplication fusion hypothesis of Tang [18]. Holm et al [16] have suggested that the ancestral gene was divided into five exons by four intervening sequences. An unequal, meiotic cross-over between two direct repeats of DNA located, respectively, in the first intervening sequence and in the 3' region of the ancestral gene would have generated the aspartyl protease gene. The duplication model suggests that the ancestral gene encoded a polypeptide that corresponds to one lobe of pepsin. This polypeptide was active as a dimer with two identical subunits. After gene duplication and fusion, the two subunits were connected by the short peptide encoded by exon six. This gene fusion could have allowed divergent evolution between the two lobes and a better association between the two divergent subunits.

Conclusion

The mouse submaxillary gland (SMG) renin cDNA has been cloned, and its nucleotide sequence allowed the determination of the amino acid sequence

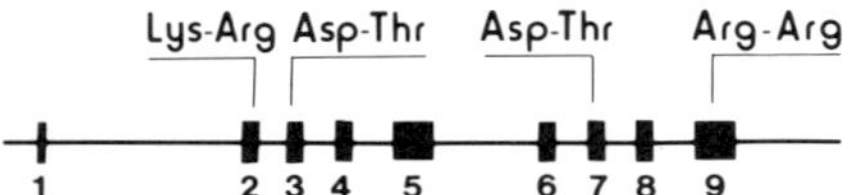

Fig. 3. Organization of the Balb/c mouse renin gene. This figure shows the location of the coding region in the renin gene. The exons are indicated by blocks numbered 1 to 9 in the 5' to 3' direction. Lys-Arg in exon 2 are homologous to the cleavage site between pro- and mature renin in the mouse SMG renin. Asp-Thr in exons 3 and 7 are the two aspartates of the active site and are homologous to pepsin. Arg-Arg in exon 9 are homologous to the site of cleavage between chain A and chain B in mouse SMG renin. (From Holm et al [16])

of its precursor, preprorenin. A model of processing of preprorenin into active renin has been proposed. The structure of human renin cDNA has been recently elucidated by using the mouse renin cDNA as a probe for identifying the human renin cDNA recombinant. Its processing has been examined both in a cell-free translation system and in cellular biosynthetic experiments, leading to a model of human renin processing. There is a strong homology between human and mouse renin and, to a lesser extent, between the proteins belonging to the aspartyl protease family. All of these proteins share the same catalytic site and have a bilobal structure. The structural organization of the renin gene in the mouse further supports the hypothesis that aspartyl proteases and renin result from a gene duplication of a single protein that corresponds to one lobe of the protein, having one aspartyl residue involved in the catalytic mechanism. Each lobe of this protein has an aspartyl residue involved in the catalytic mechanism.

References

1. PANTHIER JJ, FOOTE S, CHAMBRAUD B, STROSBERG AD, CORVOL P, ROUGEON F: Complete aminoacid sequence and maturation of the mouse submaxillary gland precursor. *Nature* 298:90–92, 1982
2. COHEN S, TAYLOR JM, MURAKAMI K, MICHELAKIS AM, INAGAMI T: Isolation and characterization of renin-like enzymes from mouse submaxillary gland. *Biochemistry* 19:2616–2622, 1980
3. MISONO KS, CHANG JJ, INAGAMI T: Amino acid sequence of mouse submaxillary renin. *Proc Natl Acad Sci USA* 79:4858–4862, 1982
4. CHRETIEN M, LI CH: Isolation, purification and characterization of alpha-lipotropic hormone from sheep pituitary glands. *Can J Biochem* 45:1163–1174, 1967
5. CATANZARO DF, MULLINS JJ, MORRIS BJ: The biosynthetic pathway of renin in mouse submandibular gland. *J Biol Chem* 258:7364–7368, 1983
6. PRATT RE, OUELETTE AJ, DZAU VJ: Biosynthesis of renin: multiplicity of active and intermediate forms. *Proc Natl Acad Sci USA* 80:6809–6813, 1983
7. PICCINI H, KNOPF JC, GROSS KW: A DNA polymorphism, consistent with gene duplication, correlates with high renin levels in the mouse submaxillary gland. *Cell* 30:205–213, 1982
8. PANTHIER JJ, HOLM I, ROUGEON F: The mouse Rn locus: S allele of the renin regulator gene results from a single structural gene duplication. *EMBO J* 1:1417–1421, 1982
9. PANTHIER JJ, ROUGEON F: Kidney and submaxillary gland renins are encoded by two non-allelic genes in Swiss mice. *EMBO J* 2:675–678, 1983
10. THOMAS P: Hybridization of denatured RNA and small DNA fragments transferred to nitrocellulose. *Proc Natl Acad Sci USA* 77:5201–5205, 1980
11. SOUBRIER F, PANTHIER JJ, CORVOL P, ROUGEON F: Molecular cloning and nucleotide sequence of a human renin cDNA fragment. *Nucl Acids Res* 11:7181–7190, 1983
12. IMAI T, MIYAZAKI H, HIROSE S, HORI H, HAYASHI T, KAGEYAMA R, OHKUBO H, NAKANISHI S, MURAKAMI K: Cloning and sequence analysis of cDNA for human renin precursor. *Proc Natl Acad Sci USA* 80:7405–7409, 1983
13. IMAI T, MIYAZAKI H, HIROSE S, MURAKAMI S: Cell-free translation of human renin mRNA. *Clin Exp Hypertension* A5:961–968, 1983
14. GALEN FX, DEVAUX C, HOUOT AM, MENARD J, CORVOL P, CORVOL MT,

Gubler NC, Mounier F, Camilleri JP: Renin biosynthesis by human juxtaglomerular cells. Evidences for a renin precursor. *J Clin Invest* 73:1144–1155, 1984
15. GUMBINER B, KELLY RB: Two distinct intracellular pathways transport secretory and membrane glycoproteins to the surface of pituitary tumor cells. *Cell* 28: 51–59, 1982
16. HOLM I, OLLO R, PANTHIER JJ, ROUGEON F: Evolution of aspartyl proteases by gene duplication: the mouse renin gene is organized in two homologous clusters of four exons. *EMBO J* 3:557–562, 1984
17. BREATHNACH R, BENOIST C, O'HARE K, GANNON F, CHAMBON P: Ovalbumin gene: evidence for a leader sequence in mRNA and DNA sequences at the exon-intron boundaries. *Proc Natl Acad Sci USA* 75:4853–4857, 1978.
18. TANG J, JAMES MNG, HSU IN, JENKINS JA, BLUNDELL TL: Structural evidence for gene duplication in the evolution of acid proteases. *Nature* 271:618–621, 1978

Intracellular Actions of Renin

Tadashi Inagami, James C. McKenzie, Kailash Pandey,
Mitsuaki Nakamaru, Daniel L. Clemens, Tomio Okamura,
Mitsuhide Naruse, and Kiyoko Naruse

Peptide hormones are produced from larger prohormone molecules by proteo-lytic degradation. Practically nothing is known about the enzymes that mediate peptide hormone formation. An exception is found in the production of the octapeptide angiotensin II (AII). All of the components have been identified and their structures have been determined. The decapeptide angiotensin I (AI) is first formed from the macromolecular prohormone angiotensinogen (molecular weight, 70,000) by the specific action of renin, which cleaves a unique leucyl peptide bond. Subsequently, AI is converted to AII by the angiotensin I-converting enzyme (ACE). Our complete knowledge of the components of this system makes it a unique model for the studies of peptide hormone formation. The renin-angiotensin system of renal origin functions within the vascular system; however, we are beginning to discover the endocrine mechanisms of AII formation in various tissues, in addition to the well-known extracellular function.

Methodologic Considerations

The measurement of specific renin activity in tissues other than the kidney is complicated by nonspecific renin-like activity of ubiquitous cathepsin D. Earlier reports of renin in extrarenal tissues, such as the brain [1] or adrenal gland [2], can be subject to severe criticisms, since the assay method employed did not take this problem into account [3, 4]. The renin-like activity of pure renal cathepsin D that was determined recently showed that at pH 5.5, cathepsin D is 1.6% as active as renin; at pH 7.0, cathepsin D is 0.1% as active as in producing AI from angiotensinogen renin [5]. Since concentrations of cathepsin D are several orders of magnitude greater than that of renin in

---

This manuscript was presented as part of a Symposium on *Renin: Recent Advances.*

various tissues, the majority of AI formed by tissue extracts will be due to cathepsin D.

To eliminate the contribution of cathepsin D, several measures must be used in combination. The use of affinity chromatography [6, 7], and specific renin antibody and assay at neutral pH are two of the key ingredients essential for the specific determination of renin [8, 9]. Contamination by blood-borne renin must also be carefully eliminated by nephrectomy and exhaustive perfusion of tissues before excision.

Intracellular Action of Renin in the Kidney

During the course of immunohistochemical studies of renin and angiotensin in 1980, Celio and Inagami found an AII-immunoreactive substance in renin-containing JG cells of rat kidneys [10]. Taugner and Hackenthal also reported similar findings [11].

The presence of AII in JG cells could be due either to intracellular production or to uptake by internalization of the AII-receptor complex. Angiotensin II has a strong action on JG cells in inhibiting renin release, and JG cells are considered to have a high concentration of AII receptors. To distinguish between these alternatives, other components of the renin-angiotensin system were investigated.

Immunoreactive AI was found in JG cells after treatment with the ACE inhibitor captopril for several days. In serial sections of rat kidney, renin and AII were always visible, although the latter became less visible after captopril treatment [12]. Since it was unlikely that JG cells have AI receptors, the appearance of AI indicated the presence of an AII synthesis pathway in JG cells. Earlier, Morris and Johnston reported the presence of angiotensinogen-containing particles in kidney homogenate [13].

Further confirmation of the coexistence of renin, AI, and AII was obtained by studies using cloned and cultured JG cells [14]. Rat JG cells that were cloned by Muirhead et al [14] were shown to contain characteristic myofibrils and dense granules. Although renin activity was decreased rapidly during repeated passages, the enzyme activity remained at detectable levels, even after 30 passages. Cells were lysed and extracted by a buffer containing a mixture of protease inhibitors, which were essential for preserving angiotensins and renin. These components were detected as shown in Table 1. Renin activity showed a neutral pH optimum, rather than the acidic pH optimum that is characteristic of cathepsin D [5]. Furthermore, the enzyme activity that was detectable in the neutral pH region was inhibited by specific antisera raised against rat renal renin [5]. The presence of a converting enzyme was determined by using the synthetic substrate hippuryl-histidyl-leucine; inhibition of the hydrolysis of the hippuryl-histidyl peptide bonds was determined by the ACE inhibitor captopril or by a chloride-free medium. The specific converting enzyme-catalyzed reaction is dependent on the chloride ion.

The combination of the immunohistochemical and cell biologic approaches suggests that AII is produced in JG cells. The use of cloned and cultured

Table 1. Renin-angiotensin system in cloned and cultured rat juxtaglomerular cells

Cell line	Renin (pg AI/hr per 10^6 cells)	ACE (pmole/min per 10^6 cells)	AI (pg/10^6 cells)	AII (pg/10^6 cells)
With serum	26	76	85	37
Without serum	87	76	193	63

From [3].

cells eliminate potential contamination by plasma AII. The fate and function of locally produced AII are not clear, but they may explain some observations to be discussed.

Intracellular Action of Renin in the Brain and Cultured Neuroblastoma Cells

Brain tissue has been known to contain AII receptors [15, 16], AII [17–19], AI [18], ACE [20, 21], and angiotensinogen [22]. Although a nonspecific renin-like action of cathepsin D [1, 3, 4] is present in the brain, the presence of a specific antibody-inhibitable renin was established by affinity-chromatographic separation of renin from the protease [6, 7, 23, 24]. Subsequently, regional distribution of renin has been determined for various nuclei or regions of the hog [8] and rat brain (K. Naruse, to be published). In the rat brain, regional distribution of renin in the spontaneously hypertensive rat (SHR) and the normotensive control strain (WKY) were compared. Surprisingly, renin in many regions of the SHR brain was found to be markedly lower compared with the normotensive strain. This observation is not in agreement with the currently held view that SHR (considered as a model of human essential hypertension) has an elevated cardiovascular sympathetic outflow that may be due to elevated levels of the brain renin-angiotensin system.

Because the brain consists of various regions that are contiguous to each other without clear-cut separation by membranes, it was not possible to identify the exact distributional relationship of the various components of the renin-angiotensin system in a given region of the brain. The presence of blood-borne renin and angiotensins in cerebral vessels also presents problems in identifying endogenous tissue components. The use of cloned and cultured cells in serum-free media provided a convenient model for neuronal cells that was free from the above technical problems.

Mouse cell lines that have been used have been derived from mouse C1300 neuroblastoma of peripheral (ganglionic) origin. Rat cell lines have been cloned from a rat neuroblastoma of central origin. After the culture reached confluency, the monolayer of cells was washed thoroughly with the medium free from the sera, and they were maintained for 24 hr in the serum-free medium until the determination of enzyme activities and angiotensins. Rat cells were harvested by treatment with 1 mM EDTA, and mouse cells were detached from culture flasks with 0.25% trypsin containing 1 mM EDTA. Cells were lysed by five cycles of freezing and thawing in the presence of 1 mM di-isopropylfluorophosphate, 1 mM captopril, 5 g/ml leupeptin, and 5 mM EDTA.

As shown in Table 2 [25, 26], all cell lines examined (except for B103 line from rat neuroblastoma) were found to contain renin, ACE enzyme, AI, and AII at variable levels. The renin-like activity was inhibited by specific antirenin antibodies in different degrees. The antibody-sensitive portion of the activity from each cell line showed a pH activity curve with an optimum near pH 7. The identity of immunoreactive angiotensins was confirmed via thin-layer chromatography. The identity of ACE, which was determined by the hydrolysis of hippuryl-histidyl-leucine by a fluorometric method, was confirmed by greater than 90% inhibition caused by 1 mM EDTA, captopril, or by the omission of sodium chloride (NaCl). Similar coexistence of renin and angiotensins in neuroblastoma-glioma hybrid has been reported by Fishman et al [27]. The presence of renin, AI, and AII in the same cell suggests the formation of AII, presumably by an intracellular mechanism involving renin and ACE that are present in the same cells. On the other hand, the inclusion of EDTA and captopril in the cell lysis medium decreased the amount of AII. It is possible that much of the converting enzyme is on the outside of the plasma membrane, and AII may be formed outside of the cell after the lysis of the cell.

Biosynthetic experiments using tritiated leucine in the culture medium indicated intracellular synthesis of angiotensinogen, since immunoprecipitable AI and AII labeled with tritium emerge within the cultured cells. However, angiotensinogen, which was isolated from rat plasma and added to culture medium, was also taken up slowly by neuroblastoma cells; it gave rise to some increase in angiotensin in the cell. These results indicate the possibility

Table 2. Renin-angiotensin system in cloned neuroblastoma cells

Cell line	Renin (pg AI/hr per 10^6 cells)	ACE (pmole/min per 10^6 cells)	AI (pg/10^6 cells)	AII[a] (pg/10^6 cells)
Mouse cells				
Neuro-2a	145	351	11.8	4.3
NB41A3	463	762	8.6	4.5
N4TG1	0.78		4.7	0
Rat cells				
B82	2.2	202	9.0	5.2
B50	1.2	0	5.3	0
B103	0	0	0	0
RT4E4	0.93	849	30	7.2

[a] Determined in the absence of EDTA and captopril [18, 19].

that the prohormone angiotensinogen may be produced endogenously by an intracellular synthesis and/or may be produced by other types of cells with neuronal cells taking it up by an internalization mechanism. Some glial cells seem to be able to produce angiotensinogen. Glioma cells were found to contain angiotensinogen at high concentrations, whereas no renin was found in these cell lines. It is intriguing to speculate that certain glial cells produce angiotensinogen, and that it is transferred to renin-containing neuronal cells for conversion to angiotensins.

Other Tissues

In addition to the brain and kidney, renin activity has been reported in many types of tissues [28]. These observations are largely based on measurements of renin-like activity at a slightly acidic pH near 5.5, and they are mostly due to the nonspecific action of the lysozomal protease cathepsin D. Shifting the assay pH to a neutral region (by using crude rat plasma taken from nephrectomized animals as the source of angiotensinogen and— most importantly—by distinguishing the nonspecific renin-like activity of proteases and renin by selective immunosuppression of angiotensin generation by antiserum to renin [7]), we have been able to identify renin in various tissues of mice as listed in Table 3 [29]. In addition to these tissues, blood vessel walls contain considerable amounts of renin [30], presumably on their luminal surface both by absorption [31] as well as by internal biosynthesis [32].

Pituitary Gland

Renin was detected in the pituitary gland in a relatively high concentration, as shown in Table 3. Its presence is limited to the anterior lobe in nephrectomized rats, and it is localized in luteinizing hormone (LH) containing gonadotrops. Coexistence of renin and LH were demonstrated by immunohistochemical staining of serial sections by using anti-rat renin antibodies and anti-LH antibodies. No other types of cells (such as those containing adrenocorticotropin, growth hormone, and thyroid-stimulating hormone) have been stained by antirenin antibodies [33]. The LH-containing ovoid cells were also found to contain AII via immunohistochemical methods [34, 35]. The reported observation of AII in prolactin-containing cells may have been due to misinterpretation of the characteristic processes of lactotrops, which often encircle LH-containing cells. These observations indicate that in the anterior pituitary, renin is either exclusively or mainly localized in the LH gonadotrops and AII is produced by an intracellular mechanism. This view is supported by the emergence of AI in LH gonadotrops upon captopril treatment.

Table 3. Immunosuppressible renin activity in various tissues and plasma of nephrectomized and sialoadenectomized mice

	Renin activity (ng AI/hr/mg protein)	Inhibition by antibody[a] (%)
Male		
Adrenal	571 ± 68.9[b]	98.2
Spleen	326 ± 45.1	98.4
Aorta	175 ± 27.6	98.8
Testis	138 ± 20.0	98.6
Liver	67.6 ± 6.3	99.6
Upper GI tract[c]	50.5 ± 16.2	98.8
Lung	48.2 ± 14.2	99.0
Skeletal muscle	41.5 ± 10.4	99.4
Lower GI tract[d]	27.9 ± 3.9	96.7
Heart	17.3 ± 4.1	97.2
Brain	7.6 ± 1.6	98.9
Anterior pituitary	2.2 ± 0.2	98.9
Posterior pituitary	Not detected	—
Plasma	0.7 ± 0.2	—
Kidney	188 ± 72.0 × 10^3	99.9
Submaxillary	1790 ± 185 × 10^3	99.9
Female		
Adrenal	496 ± 74.5[b]	98.1
Uterus	80.4 ± 11.5	98.4
Ovary	68.5 ± 8.7	97.9
Plasma	0.2 ± 0.1	—

Values are the means ± SEM of five animals.
[a] Inhibition of renin activity by homologous antirenin antibody.
[b] $P < 0.005$ versus other tissues and plasma.
[c] The esophagus, stomach, and duodenum were included.
[d] The small and large intestines were included.

Adrenal Medulla

Although a great majority of renin activity in the adrenal gland is found in the cortex, as discussed below, a small number of adrenal medullary cells are stained by antirenin antibodies.

Cloned pheochromocytoma cell line PC12 was used as a model for adrenal medullary cells. Again, coexistence of renin, ACE, AI, and AII has been demonstrated in the cells (Table 4). Although their levels are rather low, they again indicate the intracellular generation of AII [36].

Adrenal Cortical Cells

As shown in Table 3, renin concentration in the adrenal gland is among the highest of the various mouse tissues examined [29]. Rat adrenal also

Table 4. Renin-angiotensin system in cloned pheochromocytoma cell line PC12

Renin (pg AI/hr per 10^6 cells)	ACE (pmole/min per 10^6 cells)	AI (pg/10^6 cells)	AII (pg/10^6 cells)
4.4	400	7.2	5.2

contains renin at a very high concentration. More than 90% of the adrenal renin is present in the cortical capsule. Indeed, immunohistochemical examination localized renin in the zona glomerulosa. This is in agreement with earlier reports of renin-like activity in cortex and capsular layers [37, 38], even if not all the renin-like activity that was determined earlier may have been renin. Again, AII is found in the rat adrenal capsule, suggesting the synthesis of AII in the zona glomerulosa. Cells cloned from adrenocortical tumor (Y-1 cell line) have been grown and were shown to contain renin and AII.

Testis

Leydig cells of rat testis were found to stain intensely with anti-rat renin antibodies [39]. Leydig cells purified from normal rat testis also showed significant renin activity, which was completely abolished by antirenin antibodies [40]. These cells also contain AII, which can be identified by the combination of high-pressure liquid chromatography (HPLC) and radioimmunoassay.

Vascular Tissues

Vascular tissues present great difficulty in determining the presence of renin due to their extensive contact to blood and the possible adhesion of plasma renin to the vascular wall [41]; and, also due to a large amount of acid proteases when compared to renin. Although controversy still exists as to the nature of renin-like activity in the vascular wall [42], an observation of endogenous synthesis of renin in aortic smooth muscle cells has been reported by Re et al [24]. We have been able to determine immunosuppressible-specific renin and AII in cultured bovine aortic smooth muscle cells. Lilly et al have observed the coexistence of renin and AII in aortic endothelial cells [43]. Immunosuppressive renin was observed in the rat mesenteric artery [30].

What is Released from Cells Containing Renin and AII?

From the studies of renin and angiotensins in kidney JG cells, neuroblastoma cells (as the model of neuronal cells), pituitary cells, testis cells, adrenal cells, and vascular cells, it is now becoming clear that AII is present in many renin-containing cells. Many other tissues listed in Table 3 have not been studied yet. It is yet to be determined whether tissues such as the liver and spleen also contain AII. Although the mere coexistence does not necessarily imply intracellular biosynthesis of AII, identification of ACE and AI provides strong evidence for intracellular biosynthesis of AII. Moreover, as discussed above, direct evidence is obtained by radiolabeling AI and AII with tritium-labeled isoleucine with neuroblastoma cells.

Questions arise concerning the role of the tissue renin-angiotensin system. At present, it is reasonable to assume that renin and/or AII is secreted from these cells. Preliminary studies have been performed to determine whether it is renin or AII that is released from these cells.

Cultured JG cells release significant proportions of renin in the cells. However, studies with cells derived from extrarenal tissues (such as neuroblastoma cells, neuro 2a cells, adrenocortical Y-1 cells, and rat testicular Leydig cells) have revealed that little, if any, renin is released. Only negligible levels of renin activity have been found in the culture media.

Stronger evidence in support of the lack of renin release from these nonrenal tissues is provided by failure to observe an increase in renin release after the intracellular renin levels are rapidly increased (5- to 16-fold) by removing fetal calf serum from the culture medium. Further evidence for the lack of release of adrenal renin is provided by the failure to see a higher level of renin in the adrenal vein, compared with arterial blood.

Thus, renin in many of these extrarenal tissues does not seem to have the ability to leave the cells. This is in marked contrast to renin in JG cells of the kidney and placental chorionic cells. Since the amount of renin in these tissues is not as high as in the kidney, it may not appreciably affect the concentration of renin in plasma; it may also fail to elicit the physiologic response.

Factors determining renin secretion are not known. Both in renin-secreting JG cells and in nonsecreting cells (such as pituitary cells), renin is in a vesicular structure. Whether the ability to be secreted depends on the renin molecule or the storage vesicle is not known.

In contrast to renin, our preliminary studies are beginning to reveal that AII is released from cultured renin-containing cells. Culture media of neuroblastoma cell lines were shown to contain appreciable amounts of AII. Cultured Leydig cells also seem to release AII in culture media.

Functional Consideration

Plasma levels of renin and AII are largely maintained by storage of renin in the kidney and by a high capacity for the synthesis of angiotensinogen in the liver. Thus, it seems that angiotensin released from these tissues may exert its effect locally rather than contributing to circulating AII.

Angiotensin II in JG cells may affect intrarenal renin synthesis and may have a functional role in tubuloglomerular feedback [44–46]. It may also affect tubular function. In this context, it is interesting to note that a very high concentration of renin and angiotensins have been found in renal lymph [47].

Although the quantities of renin and AII in the various extrarenal tissues are small, their concentrations are sensitive to changes in cellular environment. For example, renin in neuroblastoma cells increases by more than 10-fold when fetal calf serum used for cell culture is removed from the medium. Renin in cultured JG cells increases by a factor of 3.0 upon removal of the serum from culture medium [14].

Renin in the adrenal cortex is also highly variable. Nephrectomy in rats causes a greater than 4-fold increase in 36 hr [9]. Renin in the adrenal glands of spontaneously hypertensive rats is seven times higher than that in normotensive controls [9]. Sodium loading markedly decreases adrenal renin, whereas sodium depletion, potassium loading, and aldosterone [48] increase it [37]. The hyperkalemia-induced increase in adrenal renin is considered to be the mechanism of adrenal renin elevation, which we have observed upon nephrectomy in rats [30].

As shown in Table 5, potassium loading caused a marked increase in both adrenal renin (10-fold) and adrenal aldosterone (3-fold), while not increasing plasma renin. When captopril was administered during the high potassium loading, adrenal aldosterone was normalized. This observation indicated that the increment of aldosterone above the normal level may be regulated by adrenal AII that is generated locally by the adrenal renin-angiotensin system [48].

Angiotensin II administered in the brain elicits various physiologic responses, which include dipsogenesis [49], direct pressor activity [50], and release of vasopressin [51, 52]. If these actions are mediated by receptors inside the blood-brain barrier, intracerebral AII seems to have important roles.

Angiotensin II has been reported to stimulate the release of adrenocorticotropin [51, 53], β-endorphine [53], prolactin [54], and LH [55] from the anterior pituitary gland. It is likely that part of AII may be supplied by LH-gonadotrops.

Angiotensin II stimulates steroidogenesis in the adrenal gland by stimulat-

Table 5.

Condition	Number	Adrenal renin (ng AI/ mg prot/hr)	Adrenal aldosterone (n/mg prot)	Plasma renin activity (ng AI/ml/hr)
Control	6	2.7 ± 0.2	24.2 ± 1.1	3.0 ± 0.4
Potassium-loaded	6	28.2 ± 1.5^b	69.8 ± 8.5^b	2.5 ± 0.3^a
Captopril	6	6.1 ± 1.0^b	21.0 ± 9.6	6.8 ± 0.5^b
Potassium + captopril	5	20.3 ± 2.9^b	29.6 ± 2.8^a	8.2 ± 1.9^b

Values are means $\pm$ SEM.
[a] $P < 0.05$.
[b] $P < 0.01$ versus control.

ing P-450 enzymes that catalyze the oxidative pathway for the formation of aldosterone by oxygenases [56, 57]. Locally generated AII in the adrenal gland and testis may play a role in the regulation of synthesis of aldosterone and testosterone.

Control of Renin Action in Cells

Plasma renin is regulated by a set of exquisite control mechanisms affecting renin secretion by JG cells. Intracellular renin cannot be regulated by a similar mechanism, but since renin and angiotensinogen are present in the same cell, a control mechanism is needed for homeostasis. Possible mechanisms may include compartmentalization of renin and/or angiotensinogen inhibition of renin synthesis. We have shown that renin in the anterior pituitary gland is in a particulate fraction [58]. We have also found that renin inhibitor exists in neuroblastoma [59], rat brain [60], and rat testicular Leydig cells. The inhibitor seems to bind to, and is dissociated from, renin in a reversible manner. The dissociation seems to be catalyzed by or accelerated by a sulfhydryl compound (such as dithiothreitol), whereas the binding is facilitated by an oxidant such as sodium tetrathionate. Although the complete picture of the regulation is not clearly delineated, relationship of the intracellular function of renin to the oxido-reduction state of cells is intriguing.

In summary, several specific types of cells contain intracellular renin and components of the angiotensin system that generate angiotensin II. Although intriguing roles for local angiotensin have been speculated, much work is required to clarify their functions in these tissues.

References

1. GANTEN D, MARQUEZ-JULIO A, GRANGER P, HAYDUCK K, KARSUNKY KP, BOUCHER R, GENEST J: Renin in dog brain. *Am J Physiol* 221:1733–1737, 1971
2. RYAN JW: Renin-like enzyme in the adrenal gland. *Science* 158:1589–1590, 1967
3. HACKENTHAL E, HACKENTHAL R, HILGENFELDT U: Purification and partial characterization of rat brain acid protease (isorenin). *Biochim Biophys Acta* 522:5576–5592, 1981
4. DAY RP, REID IA: Renin activity in dog brain: enzymological similarity to cathepsin D. *Endocrinology* 99:93–100, 1976
5. FIGUEREDO AFS, TAKII Y, TSUJI H, KATO K, INAGAMI, T: Rat kidney renin and cathepsin D: purification and comparison of properties. *Biochemistry* 22:5476–5481, 1983
6. INAGAMI, T, YOKOSAWA H, HIROSE S: Definitive evidence for renin in rat brain by affinity chromatographic separation from protease. *Clin Sci Mol Med* 55(Suppl): 121s–123s, 1978
7. HIROSE S, YOKOSAWA H, INAGAMI T: Immunochemical identification of renin in rat brain and distinction from acid proteases. *Nature* 274:392–393, 1978
8. HIROSE S, YOKOSAWA H, INAGAMI T, WORKMAN RJ: Renin and prorenin in

hog brain: ubiquitous distribution and high concentration in the pituitary and pineal. *Brain Res* 191:489–499, 1980

9. NARUSE H, INAGAMI T: Markedly elevated specific renin levels in the adrenal in genetically hypertensive rats. *Proc Natl Acad Sci USA* 79:3295–3299, 1982

10. CELIO MR, INAGAMI T: Angiotensin II immunoreactivity coexists with renin in the juxtaglomerular granular cells of the kidney. *Proc Natl Acad Sci USA* 78:3897–3900, 1981

11. TAUGNER R, HACKENTHAL E: Angiotensin II in epithelioid (renin containing) cells of rat kidney. *Histochemistry* 72:499–509, 1981

12. NARUSE K, INAGAMI T, CELIO MR, WORKMAN RJ, TAKII Y: Immunohistochemical evidence that angiotensin I and II are formed by intracellular mechanism in juxtaglomerular cells. *Hypertension* 4(Suppl II):70–74, 1982

13. MORRIS BJ, JOHNSTON CI: Renin substrate in granules from rat kidney cortex. *Biochem J* 154:625–637, 1976

14. RIGHTSEL WA, OKAMURA T, INAGAMI T, PITCOCK JA, BROOKS B, BROWN P, MUIRHEAD EE: Juxtaglomerular cells grown as monolayer culture contain renin angiotensin I and II/III. *Circ Res* 50:822–829, 1982

15. BENNETT JR, SNYDER SH: Angiotensin II binding to mammalian brain membranes. *J Biol Chem* 251:7423–7430, 1976

16. SIRET NE, MCLEAN AS, BRAY JJ, HUBBARD JI: Distribution of angiotensin II receptors in rat brain. *Brain Res* 122:299–312, 1977

17. CHANGARIS DG, SEVERS WB, KEIL LC: Localization of angiotensin in rat brain. *J Histochem Cytochem* 26:593–607, 1978

18. FISCHER-FERRARO C, NAHMOD VE, GOLDSTEIN DJ, FINKIELMAN S: Angiotensin and renin in rat and dog brain. *J Exp Med* 133:353–361, 1971

19. FUXE K, GANTEN D, HOKFELT T, BOLME P: Immunohistochemical evidence for the existence of angiotensin II containing nerve terminals in the brain and spinal cord in the rat. *Neurosci Lett* 2:229–234, 1976

20. YANG HYT, NEFF NH: Distribution and properties of angiotensin converting enzyme of rat brain. *J Neurochem* 19:2443–2450, 1972

21. POTH MH, HEATH RG, WARD M: Angiotensin converting enzyme in human brain. *J Neurochem* 25:83–85, 1975

22. PRINTZ MP, LEWICKI JA: Renin substrate in the CNS: potential significance to central regulatory mechanism, in *Central Action of Angiotensin and Related Hormones,* edited by BUCKLEY JP, FERRARIO CM, New York, Pergamon Press, 1977, pp 57–64

23. GANTEN D, SPECK G: The brain renin-angiotensin system: A model for the synthesis of peptides in the brain. *Biochem Pharmacol* 17:2379–2389, 1978

24. OSMAN MY, SMEBY RR, SEN S: Separation of dog brain renin-like activity from acid protease activity. *Hypertension* 1:52–60, 1979

25. OKAMURA T, CLEMENS DL, INAGAMI T: Renin, angiotensins and angiotensin-converting enzyme in neuroblastoma cells: evidence for intracellular formation of angiotensins. *Proc Natl Acad Sci USA* 78:6940–6943, 1981

26. INAGAMI T, OKAMURA T, HIROSE S, CLEMENS DL, CELIO MR, NARUSE K, TAKII Y, YOKOSAWA H: Identification characterization and evidence for intraneuronal function of renin in the brain and neuroblastoma cells, in *The Renin Angiotensin System in the Brain,* edited by GANTEN D, PRINTZ M, PHILLIPS MJ, Scholkens BA, Heidelberg, Springer-Verlag, 1982, pp 64–75

27. FISHMAN MC, ZIMMERMAN EA, SLATER EE: Renin and angiotensin: the complete system within the neuroblastoma x glioma cell. *Science* 214:921–923, 1981

28. GANTEN D, HUTCHINSON JS, SCHELLING P, GANTEN U, FISHER H: The isorenin

angiotensin systems in extrarenal tissue. *Clin Exp Pharmacol Physiol* 3:103–126, 1976

29. NARUSE M, NARUSE K, INAGAKI T, INAGAMI T: Immunoreactive renin in mouse adrenal gland. *Hypertension* 6:275–280, 1984

30. NARUSE M, INAGAMI T: Antibody-sensitive renin of adrenal and resistance vessels is markedly elevated in spontaneously hypertensive rats. *Clin Sci* 63:187s–189s, 1982

31. SWALES JD: Vascular renin in hypertension. *Hormone Res* 12:65–78, 1980

32. RE R, FALLON JT, DZAU VJ, QUAY SC, HABER E: Renin synthesis by canine aortic smooth muscle cells in culture. *Life Sci* 30:99–106, 1982

33. NARUSE K, TAKII Y, INAGAMI T: Immunohistochemical localization of renin in luteinizing hormones producing cells of rat pituitary. *Proc Natl Acad Sci USA* 78:7579–7583, 1981

34. STEELE MK, BROWNFIELD MS, GANONG WF: Immunocytochemical localization of angiotensin immunoreactivity in gonadotrops and lactotrops of the rat anterior pituitary gland. *Neuroendocrinology* 35:155–158, 1982

35. MCKENZIE JC, INAGAMI T: Immunocytochemical co-localization of renin and angiotensin II in cells of the anterior pituitary (*abstract*). *Fed Proc* 43:912, 1984

36. OKAMURA T, CLEMENS DL, INAGAMI T: Generation of angiotensin in cultured pheochromocytoma cells. *Neurosci Lett* 46:151–156, 1984

37. AGUILERA G, FUJITA K, SCHIRAR A, CATT K: Role of angiotensin II in the regulation of aldosterone secretion. *Proceedings of the VI International Congress of Endocrinology,* Melbourne, Australia, 1980, pp 389–392

38. DOI Y, ATARASHI K, FRANCO-SAENZ R, MURLOW P: Adrenal renin: a possible regulation of aldosterone secretion. *Clin Exp Hypertension* A5:1119–1126, 1983

39. PARMENTIER M, INAGAMI T, POCHET R, DESCLIN JC: Pituitary dependent renin-like immunoreactivity in the rat testis. *Endocrinology* 112:1318–1323, 1983

40. PANDEY K, MELNER M, PARMENTIER M, INAGAMI T: Demonstration of renin in purified rat Leydig cells: evidence for the existence of an endogenous inactive (latent) form of enzyme. *Endocrinology* (in press, 1984)

41. LOUDON M, BING RF, THURSTON H, SWALES JD: Arterial wall uptake of renal renin and blood pressure control. *Hypertension* 5:629–634, 1983

42. FORDIS CM, MEGORDEN JS, ROPCHAK TG, KEISER HR: Absence of renin-like activity in rat aorta and microvessels. *Hypertension* 5:635–641, 1983

43. LILLY LS, PATT RE, ALEXANDER RW, GIMBRONE MA, DZAU VJ: Cultured vascular endothelial cells contain the complete renin angiotensin system (*abstract*). *Clin Res* 31:332A, 1983

44. TURAU K: *Proceedings of the Second International Congress of Nephrology.* Prague, Amsterdam, Exerpta Medica, 1963, pp 33–38

45. GUYTON AC, LANGSTONE JB, NAVAR G: Theory for renal antoregulation by feedback at the juxtaglomerular apparatus. *Circ Res* 14/15(Suppl I):187–194, 1964

46. NAVAR LG, PLOTH DW, BELL PD: Distal tubular feedback control of renal hemodynamics and autoregulation. *Ann Rev Physiol* 42:557–571, 1980

47. PROUD D, NAKAMURA S, CARONE PL, HERRING M, KAWAMURA M, INAGAMI T, PISANO JJ: The kallikrein-kinin and renin-angiotensin systems in rat renal lymph. *Kidney Int* (in press, 1984)

48. NAKAMARU M, NARUSE M, NARUSE K, SHIZUME K, INAGAMI T: Regulation of adrenal renin: effect of sodium, potassium and captopril (*abstract*). *Fed Proc* 43:1077, 1984

49. EPSTEIN AN, FITZSIMONS JT, ROLLS BJ: Drinking induced by injection of angio-tensin into the brain of the rat. *J Physiol* 210:457–474, 1970

50. SMOOCKLER HH, SEVERS WB, KINNARD WJ, BUCKLEY JP: Centrally mediated cardiovascular effects of angiotensin II. *J Pharmacol Exptl Therap* 153:485–494, 1966
51. RAMSEY DJ, KEIL LC, SHARPE ML, SHINSAKO J: Angiotensin infusion increases vasopressin, ACTH and 11-hydroxycorticosteroid secretion. *Am J Physiol* R234:66–71, 1978
52. KEIL LC, SUMMY-LONG J, SEVERS WB: Release of vasopressin by angiotensin II. *Endocrinology* 96:1063–1065, 1975
53. KRAFT K, LANG RR, GAIDA W, UNGER T, GANTEN D: Angiotensin stimulates β-endorphine release from anterior pituitary gland cell culture of rats. *Neurosci Lett* 46:25–29, 1984
54. AGUILERA G, HYDE CI, CATT KJ: Angiotensin II receptors and prolactin release in pituitary lactotrophs. *Endocrinology* 111:1045–1050, 1982
55. STEELE MK, McCANN SM, NEGRO-VILLAR A: Modulation by dopamine and estradiol of the central effects of the angiotensin II on anterior pituitary hormone release. *Endocrinology* 111:722–729, 1982
56. AGUILERA G, MENARD RH, CATT KJ: Regulatory action of angiotensin II on receptors and steroidogenic enzymes in adrenal glomerulosa cells. *Endocrinology* 107:55–60, 1980
57. KRAMER RE, GALLANT S, BROWNIE AC: Actions of angiotensin II on aldosterone biosynthesis in the rat adrenal cortex. *J Biol Chem* 255:3442–3447, 1980
58. GRAMMER RT, NARUSE M, INAGAMI T: The subcellular distribution of renin in hog anterior pituitary. *Endocrinology* 113:344–347, 1983
59. INAGAKI T, OKAMURA T, INAGAMI T: Endogenous renin inhibitor in neuroblastoma cells. *Brain Res* 250:373–377, 1982
60. INAGAKI T, INAGAMI T: A new form of inactive renin in rat brain: a latent renin. *Hypertension* 6(Suppl I):I137–I142, 1984

The Endocrine System and the Kidney

Similarity of the Effects of Antidiuretic Hormone, Parathyroid Hormone, Calcitonin, and Glucagon on Rat Kidney

Christian de Rouffignac, Jean-Marc Elalouf, Nicole Roinel, Claire Bailly, and Claude Amiel

Recent developments in techniques for studying microdissected nephron segments have made it possible to know exactly where hormones act in the kidney [1]. Since 1976, our knowledge of the precise distribution of the target sites of peptide hormones along the nephron has been particularly enhanced by the elaboration and extensive exploitation of a biochemical approach, depending on the determination of the hormone-dependent activity of the adenylate cyclase system that is present in the target cell membranes [2]. This distribution was found to vary, to some extent, from one animal species to another, with different tubular segments containing adenylate cyclase that was responsive to several hormones [3]. The present report deals exclusively with the rat kidney—especially with the thick ascending limb (TALH) of the nephron, which raises important new problems in renal physiology. Rat TALH is a target site for many hormones, including antidiuretic hormone (ADH), parathyroid hormone (PTH), calcitonin (CT), and glucagon. From experiments designed to test the additive effects of these four hormones on the cyclase responsiveness of the TALH, Morel et al [4] concluded that PTH, CT, and glucagon may stimulate the same cyclase pool in the cortical portion of the TALH, and that ADH, CT, and glucagon should act similarly on its medullary portion. In other words, in both portions (which are homogeneous at the cell level), all of the hormones should induce adenylate cyclase activation in common target cells; since the cell type determines the nature of the response, these authors concluded that all of the active hormones in a given portion should induce the same physiologic responses.

From this conclusion, the need to develop a new approach to in vivo investigation of the renal effect of peptide hormones became evident [5]. To explore the effect of one of these hormones, it is not sufficient to suppress it in the circulating blood and then to administer it under appropriate conditions. It is also essential to eliminate the other hormones that could maintain

---

This manuscript was presented as a State-of-the-Art lecture.

the cyclase activity of the cells involved. Therefore, we studied the effects of the above four hormones on rats acutely deprived of these hormones. Rats with hereditary diabetes insipidus due to lack of vasopressin production (Brattleboro strain) were used. They were acutely thyroparathyroidectomized to suppress PTH and CT; and, they were given glucose or somatostatin to inhibit glucagon secretion. Those rats with suppressed levels of ADH, PTH, CT, and reduced levels of glucagon will be referred to as hormone-deprived animals. Clearance and micropuncture experiments were carried out on these rats during administration of either PTH or glucagon [6] (Bailly, Roinel, Amiel, submitted for publication), or of human calcitonin (HCT) [7] or dDAVP [5, 8] (an ADH analog) infused at rates eliciting plasma concentrations that were very close to the endogenous levels obtained during maximal stimulation of the secretory processes.

Methods

Experiments that were performed simultaneously in the two laboratories (Saclay and Faculté Xavier Bichat) were very similar in design. They were carried out on 200-g male homozygous DI Brattleboro rats bred at Saclay by Juvanon and Cayla. Rats were considered to be homozygous when their water intake was higher than 60 ml/100 g/24 hr, or when their urine osmolality was lower than 200 mOsm/kg H_2O and urine output was higher than 2 ml/hr. Anesthesia was achieved by intraperitoneal administration of Inactin, 8 to 10 mg/100 g body wt. Since the preparation of these rats has been described in detail elsewhere [5–8], we will only mention some essential points of the experimental procedure. The rats were prepared to reduce the plasma concentration of the three hormones that, in addition to ADH, act on the TALH. At the beginning of the surgical procedure, the parathyroid and thyroid glands were removed. During surgery, fluid losses were replaced by repeated intravenous (i.v.) injections of sodium chloride (NaCl) solutions. At the end of the preparation (time zero of the experiment), the rats were given a priming dose of tritiated inulin, which was immediately followed by the sustaining dose and the infusion of either glucose [5] or somatostatin [6–8] to reduce glucagon secretion. The administration rate of glucose was 1.08 mg/min, increasing the glycemia to values between 8 to 10 mmoles/liter. Somatostatin (Clin-Midy, France) was infused at a rate of 70 ng/min · 100 g body wt to reduce the plasma glucagon concentration to a level that no longer was detectable by a sensitive radioimmunoassay. The experiments were performed either on such hormone-deprived animals (controls) or on hormone-deprived animals to which one of the lacking hormones was administered. The administration rates of the peptides were as follows: dDAVP (Ferring, Sweden) was infused at 20 pg/min/100 g body wt, giving theoretic plasma dDAVP concentrations of 20 to 30 pg/ml—a concentration range comparable with the plasma vasopressin concentration of rats during maximal antidiuresis [9]. The glucagon administration rate (highly purified porcine glucagon, Novo Industri, Denmark) was 5 ng/min/100 g body wt, raising the plasma glucagon concentration from undetectable levels in hormone-deprived animals (detection limit of the radioimmunoassay—7×10^{-12} M) to 2.4×10^{-10} M after equilibration of the infusion; that is, to plasma concentrations only 2.5 times higher than the endogenous level in the rat after a 24-hr fasting [10]. Calcitonin (synthetic human calcitonin, Cibacalcin, C 47175 Ba) was infused at 1 mU/min/100 g body wt, increasing the plasma concentration from undetectable levels in hormone-deprived rats (detection limit of the radioimmunoassay, 0.15 ng/ml) to 11.8 ng/ml at equilibrium; that is, to levels similar to those observed in the rat during acute calcium (Ca) loading [11]. The rats were infused at 10 μl/min with a solution of 50 mmoles/liter Na_2HPO_4 and 10 mmoles/liter NaH_2PO_4, and with a further solution containing 25 mmoles/liter $CaCl_2$ to prevent reduction of plasma phosphate and calcium concentrations during sustained CT infusion. Parathyroid hormone (synthetic 1–34 fragments PTH, Beckman Instruments, USA) was administered at a rate of 5 mU/min/100 g body wt. In the absence of a sufficiently sensitive radioimmunoassay, there are indications that PTH was not given in excess. Plasma calcium concentrations—although significantly increased from 1.66 ± 0.04 mmoles/liter in hormone-deprived animals to 2.06 ± 0.14 mmoles/liter during PTH infusion—were still below the values of intact Brattleboro rats (2.21 ± 0.05 mmoles/liter); urinary excretion of phosphate was $15.9 \pm 2.5\%$ of the filtered load, as compared with $21.3 \pm 2.7\%$ in the intact Brattleboro rats (DiStefano, Elalouf, Garel, de Rouffignac, submitted for publication).

The only protocol difference between the experiments conducted at Faculté Xavier Bichat (glucagon and PTH) and those made at Saclay (dDAVP and HCT) concerns the state of hydration of the animals during the experiments. At Bichat, the rats were infused with a 0.45% NaCl solution at 0.100 ml/min/100 g body wt from time 0 to the end of the micropuncture experiment. At Saclay, diuretic animals were given a 0.4% NaCl solution at 62.5 μl/min during the first hour, and then again during micropuncture at a rate adjusted to compensate for water losses; that is, 50 μl/min/100 g body wt. Rats perfused with dDAVP did not receive such infusions. Therefore, the rats administered HCT and their controls received less water and NaCl than the PTH- and glucagon-treated rats and their respective controls.

To determine the hormonal influences on Henle's loop, the early accessible distal and late accessible proximal convolutions belonging to the same nephron were located via stereomicroscopic observation after injection of lissamine green solution in the proximal tubules with a 4 to 5 μm micropipette. The early distal convolution first was punctured; then, the late proximal convolution was punctured. Three to eight nephrons were punctured in each rat during four or five 30-min clearance periods.

The radioactivities of macro- and microsamples were determined by liquid scintillation counting (Intertechnique, France). The solute concentrations in plasma and urine samples were determined as follows: sodium and potassium by flame emission photometry (Netheler and Hinz, Hamburg, West Germany), calcium and magnesium by flame atomic absorption photometry (Perkin Elmer, USA, and Instrument Laboratory, USA), phosphate by photocolorimetry, and total solutes either by cryoscopy or with a vapor pressure osmometer (Wescor, Inc). Electrolytes in proximal and distal tubular fluid samples were determined with an electron probe analyzer (Camebax, Cameca, France) [12]. The results are expressed as means ± SEM.

Results

The Hormone-deprived Rat

Before considering hormonal effects, it is necessary to describe the main physiologic characteristics of our original experimental model. In these animals, the mean arterial blood pressure and the sodium, potassium, and total solute plasma concentrations were very similar to those measured in intact DI Brattleboro rats; whereas, as expected, the mean phosphate concentration was higher and the calcium concentration was lower than in the intact rats [5]. The glomerular filtration rate (GFR) and the excretion rate of water, sodium, potassium, and total solutes of the hormone-deprived rats were not significantly different from those of intact DI rats. Hormone-deprived rats excreted very large volumes of hypotonic urine. Phosphate excretion, on the other hand, was considerably lower (between 1 to 3% of the filtered load); and, magnesium and calcium excretions were, respectively, 1.5 and 10 times higher in hormone-deprived rats than in intact DI Brattleboro rats. The fluid composition at the late proximal site was similar to that measured in intact DI Brattleboro rats or in rats of other strains, except that the phosphate concentration was consistently low. At the early distal site, the magnesium and calcium concentrations were twice as high as those in thyro-parathyroidectomized rats of other strains. The amounts of water delivered to the late proximal tubule and early distal tubule represented 42 and 19% of the filtered amounts, respectively. In short, the kidney functions of hormone-deprived rats differ from those of intact rats, mainly by an extremely low phosphate urinary output and very high calcium and magnesium excretion rates. These differences were most probably due to PTH and CT suppression; however, the increases of magnesium and even more so of calcium excretion were much higher than those observed in rats of other strains after parathyroidectomy or thyroparathyroidectomy.

Effects of the Four Hormones on Plasma Composition and Kidney Function

None of the four hormones produced significant alterations of the sodium, potassium, and total solute plasma contents in hormone-deprived rats. Plasma magnesium concentration was increased by glucagon and PTH, and plasma calcium concentration was increased by PTH in all studies; whereas, the increase with glucagon achieved significance in one study (Bailly, Roinel, Amiel, submitted for publication), but not in the other [6]. The GFR was unchanged by dDAVP and PTH, but was increased by 40% by glucagon. In some instances, HCT also elicited a significant GFR rise, which was smaller than that induced by glucagon. The filtered load of electrolytes was unchanged by the administration of dDAVP and PTH, except in the case of magnesium, which was significantly—although slightly—increased by the peptides and calcium, which was increased by PTH. Human CT and glucagon tended to increase the filtered load of all electrolytes. As expected, dDAVP elicited antidiuresis and PTH phosphaturia. The sodium and potassium fractional excretion rates (as percentage of the filtered load) were unaltered by the administration of either hormone, as illustrated at the top of Figure 1. The higher sodium fractional excretion rate in the glucagon and PTH series, as

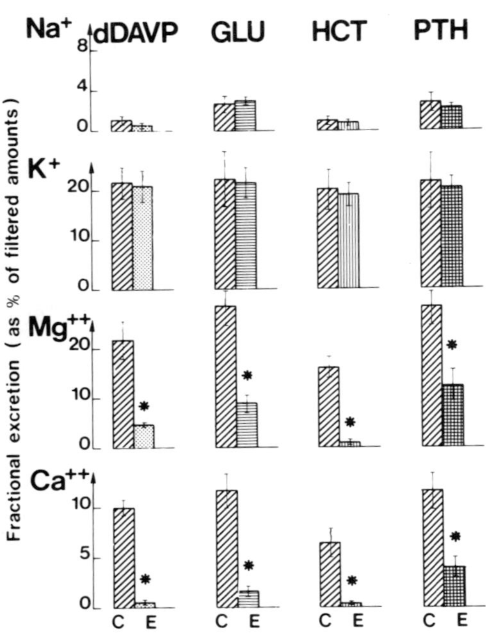

Fig. 1. Similarity of the effects of dDAVP, glucagon (*GLU*), human calcitonin (*HCT*), and parathyroid hormone (*PTH*) on the sodium (*Na*), potassium (*K*), calcium (*Ca*), and magnesium (*Mg*) fractional excretion rates. These effects were investigated in hormone-deprived rats; that is, in rats with suppressed (ADH, calcitonin, PTH) or reduced (glucagon) hormones. Each of the four experimental series comprised two groups of rats: hormone-deprived (controls, *C*) and hormone-deprived infused with one of the peptides (*E*). The administration rates per 100 g body wt were: dDAVP, 20 pg/min (1-desamino-8-D-arginine vasopressin, Ferring); glucagon, 5 ng/min (highly purified porcine glucagon, Novo Industri); calcitonin 1 mU/min (synthetic human calcitonin, Cibacalcin); and PTH, 5 mU/min (synthetic 1 to 34 fragment PTH, Beckman Instruments). These administration rates elicit concentrations in the rat plasma that are very close to the endogenous levels obtained during maximal stimulation of the hormonal secretory processes. All four peptides significantly (*) reduced magnesium and calcium excretion, but were without effect on sodium or potassium excretion. (Data from [6–8])

compared with the other series, was due to the fact that these rats were infused with a hypotonic sodium chloride solution at twice the rate of those in the dDAVP and HCT series (see the section on "Methods"). All four hormones, however, induced a marked fall in magnesium and calcium fractional excretion rates (Fig. 1, bottom). The absolute excretions of these ions were also considerably reduced, even with CT and glucagon, despite the filtered load increases.

Glomerular and Tubular Effects

In all studies, the apparent number of nephrons remained unchanged, indicating a lack of a significant redistribution of glomerular filtration. The single nephron glomerular filtration rate (SNGFR) and the electrolyte-filtered load were unchanged or only slightly modified by PTH and dDAVP, but were significantly increased by HCT and glucagon.

The four hormones did not significantly change the ratios of tubular fluid to plasma ultrafiltrate concentration (TF/UF) of any electrolyte at the late proximal site. However, the absolute amount of electrolyte delivered to the loop was increased by glucagon and HCT as a consequence of the SNGFR rise and of a significant decrease of the TF/UF in the case of HCT. In other words, three out of the four hormones left the electrolyte fractional reabsorption unchanged; HCT significantly diminished the fractional reabsorption of water, as well as that of sodium and chloride.

At the early distal site, on the other hand, the four hormones considerably modified the fluid composition. The TF/UF concentration ratios of potassium, magnesium, and calcium were systematically reduced by all hormones (Fig. 2). In addition, dDAVP and HCT also reduced the TF/UF for sodium and chloride, and glucagon that of chloride, whereas PTH was without effect on these parameters. The TF/UF phosphate was unchanged by dDAVP and HCT, but was augmented by glucagon and PTH. The fractions of filtered water remaining at the early distal site of HCT-treated rats were not significantly different from those of hormone-deprived rats. dDAVP reduced this fraction notably, whereas glucagon and PTH increased it.

Effects on the Loop of Henle

Our experimental protocol makes it possible to calculate, for each nephron, the amounts of water and electrolytes reabsorbed by Henle's loop, which is arbitrarily defined as the nephron segment located between the late-accessible proximal tubule and the early-accessible distal tubule. As reported above, the hormones considerably modified the fluid composition at the early distal site. If we consider the amounts reabsorbed by the loop as being percentages of the amounts delivered to it, it can also be seen that each of the four hormones enhanced the potassium, magnesium, and calcium reabsorptions (Fig. 3). Therefore, the hormone-dependent modification of early distal tubular fluid composition should be attributed to effects occurring in the loop. Reab-

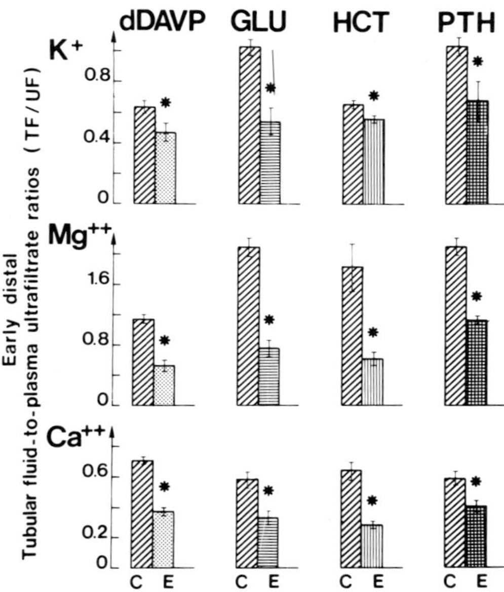

Fig. 2. Similarity of the effects of dDAVP, glucagon (*GLU*), human calcitonin (*HCT*), and parathyroid hormone (*PTH*) on the ratios of potassium (*K*), magnesium (*Mg*), and calcium (*Ca*) tubular fluid to plasma ultrafiltrate (*TF/UF*) in the first convolution of the distal tubule that is accessible to micropuncture. These effects were investigated in hormone-deprived rats; that is, in rats with suppressed (ADH, calcitonin, PTH) or reduced (glucagon) hormones. Each of the four experimental series comprised two groups of rats: hormone-deprived (controls, *C*) and hormone-deprived infused with one of the peptides (*E*). The administration rates per 100 g body wt were: dDAVP, 20 pg/min (1-desamino-8-D-arginine vasopressin, Ferring); glucagon, 5 ng/ min (highly purified porcine glucagon, Novo Industri); calcitonin, 1 mU/min (synthetic human calcitonin, Cibacalcin); and PTH, 5 mU/min (synthetic 1 to 34 fragment PTH, Beckman Instruments). All four peptides significantly (*) decreased the potassium, magnesium, and calcium TF/UF ratio. The amplitude of the effects on the calcium and magnesium TF/UF in relative terms (as compared with controls) were greater than those on the potassium TF/UF. (Data from [6–8])

sorption of sodium and chloride was also enhanced by dDAVP and HCT, whereas PTH and glucagon were without effect on the transport of these ions. Fractional reabsorption of the phosphate load that was delivered was unaltered by dDAVP, slightly but significantly decreased in the glucagon and CT series and was markedly decreased in the PTH series. Fractional reabsorption of water was only modified in the dDAVP series, the other hormones remaining without effect on this variable.

Therefore, it is clear that the administration of any of the lacking hormones to these hormone-deprived rats enhanced the reabsorptive capacity for potassium, magnesium, and calcium. Furthermore, irrespective of the amount delivered to the loop, the amount of potassium, calcium, and magnesium reabsorbed was definitely greater in hormone-treated rats than in hormone-

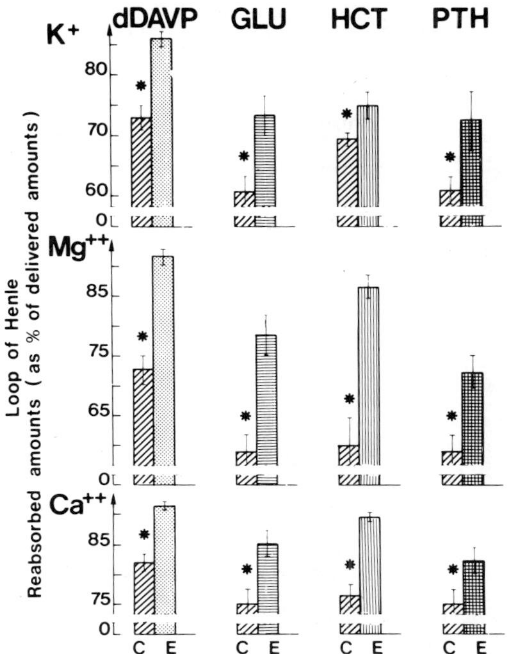

Fig. 3. Similarity of the effects of dDAVP, glucagon (*GLU*), human calcitonin (*HCT*), and parathyroid hormone (*PTH*) on the potassium (*K*), magnesium (*Mg*), and calcium (*Ca*) fractional reabsorption (as percentage of the delivered amounts) in the loop of Henle. These effects were investigated in hormone-deprived rats; that is, in rats with suppressed (ADH, calcitonin, PTH) or reduced (glucagon) hormones. Each of the four experimental series comprised two groups of rats: hormone-deprived (controls, *C*) and hormone-deprived infused with one of the peptides (*E*). The administration rates per 100 g body wt were: dDAVP, 20 pg/min (1-desamino-8-D-arginine vasopressin, Ferring); glucagon, 5 ng/min (highly purified porcine glucagon, Novo Industri); calcitonin, 1 mU/min (synthetic human calcitonin, Cibacalcin); and PTH, 5 mU/min (synthetic 1 to 34 fragment PTH, Beckman Instruments). The amounts that were reabsorbed in the loop were calculated by subtracting the deliveries at the early distal site from those measured at the late proximal site of the same nephron (3 to 8 nephrons per rat, 5 to 6 rats per group). All four peptides significantly (*) enhanced the potassium, magnesium, and calcium transport by the loop. (Data from [5–7])

deprived rats [5–7]. An example of this is given for the effects of the four hormones on magnesium reabsorption (Fig. 4).

Discussion

The effects of hormone administration on the proximal tubule and GFR have been described in some detail to differentiate hormonal effects on the

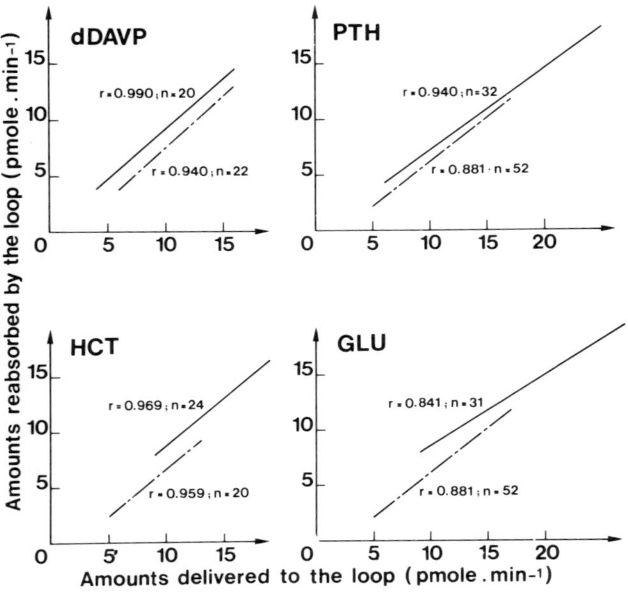

Fig. 4. Relationship between the amounts of magnesium delivered to the loop and the amounts reabsorbed by the loop. The studies were performed in hormone-deprived rats; that is, in rats with suppressed (ADH, calcitonin, PTH) or reduced (glucagon) hormones. Each of the four experimental series comprised two groups of rats: hormone-deprived (*dotted lines*) and hormone-deprived infused with one of the peptides (*solid lines*). The administration rates per 100 g body wt were: dDAVP, 20 pg/min (1-desamino-8-D-arginine vasopressin, Ferring); glucagon, 5 ng/min (highly purified porcine glucagon, Novo Industri); calcitonin, 1 mU/min (synthetic human calcitonin, Cibacalcin); and PTH, 5 mU/min (synthetic 1 to 34 fragment PTH, Beckman Instruments). The regression lines have the same slope, but a higher origin ordinate in the presence of peptides than in hormone-deprived rats (covariance analysis). (Data from [5–7])

loop itself from effects that are due to modification of the fluid delivered to the loop. In fact, the investigation of possible hormonal effects on the glomerulus or the proximal tubule is beyond the scope of this study. Nevertheless, we would like to draw attention to the fact that the adenyl cyclase of the rat proximal tubule (pars convoluta and pars recta) is only sensitive to PTH, which would explain the marked reduction of phosphate reabsorption in the loop that is associated with PTH infusion; the pars recta being the major site of inhibition of phosphate transport by PTH [13]. The absence of any physiologic change in net water and electrolyte transport along the proximal convoluted tubule after dDAVP administration is also relevant. The administration of CT and glucagon was associated in the proximal convoluted tubule with significant inhibition of water (and NaCl) and calcium transports, respectively; and, in the loop, with a reduction of phosphate transport (pars recta).

It is likely that these effects of HCT and glucagon were not fortuitous; some have already been reported in rats of other strains [14]. It would seem that these effects are the result of mechanisms that do not involve the intracellular production of cyclic AMP via the adenyl cyclase system since, in the proximal tubule, this system would not appear to be sensitive to CT or glucagon.

Comparative Effects of dDAVP, Glucagon, HCT, and PTH in the Loop of Henle

The fractional water delivery at the early distal site was reduced by dDAVP administration, whereas it was unaltered by the other hormones. A reduction, in fact, was only to be expected in the presence of dDAVP since, in these conditions, the fluid flowing down the descending limbs enters a steeper corticomedullary concentration gradient than in the other experimental conditions.

Regarding hormonal effects on electrolyte handling by the loop, the present data demonstrate that the administration of any hormone decreased the potassium, magnesium, and calcium concentration at the early distal site. Clearly, this was a consequence of enhanced reabsorption of these ions in the loop. In this structure, the thick ascending limb (TALH) is the main segment involved in magnesium reabsorption; and, it is the sole segment with a cyclase system sensitive to all four hormones. Therefore, the tubular localization of these physiologic processes is unequivocal, since the TALH is the only possible candidate. Are the effects the direct consequence of hormonal stimulation of the TALH? First, they were observed in the absence of a change in the plasma calcium concentration, except of course with PTH; thus, they could not be the result of such an alteration. Second, extracellular cyclic AMP could not be responsible for them—especially for those observed during CT, glucagon, and PTH administration—since cyclic AMP infused at a rate that raised the cyclic AMP plasma concentration to values as high as 1.3×10^{-6} M was strictly without any effect on potassium, calcium, and magnesium handling in the loop [6].

The hormone-dependent increase of the reabsorption rates in the loop were very different for the three ions, when expressed as percentages of the reabsorption rates measured in hormone-deprived rats. The effects were most marked for magnesium and were least for calcium ions. When expressed in absolute terms (Fig. 5), the calcium and magnesium reabsorption flux increases elicited in the loop by each of the hormones were strikingly similar. HCT, which elicited a 2 pmoles/min increase in the reabsorption fluxes of both calcium and magnesium, was the most potent hormone in this respect, whereas PTH was the least efficient. The similarity of their reactions strongly suggests the existence of a common mechanism governing the transport of these two ions; it suggests that the cortical portion of the TALH is the main target site responsible for such effects, since a cyclase sensitive to PTH in the rat only occurs in this cortical portion and not in the medullary portion. All four hormones also stimulated K^+ transport in the TALH. However, the amplitude of the effects did not parallel those observed for calcium and magne-

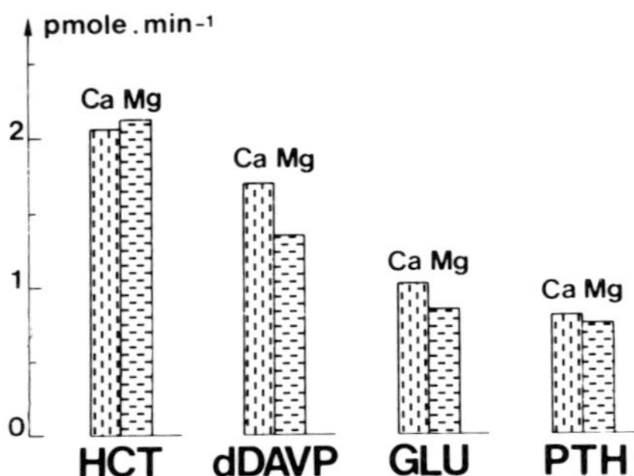

Fig. 5. Similarity of the hormone-dependent increases of calcium (*Ca*) and magnesium (*Mg*) reabsorption in the loop. Each column represents the difference between the amounts reabsorbed by the loop in the presence and absence of peptides. This difference was determined from the regression lines correlating the amounts reabsorbed by the loop to the load delivered to it. These correlations make it possible to calculate (for a same delivery) the amounts reabsorbed by the loop in the absence and presence of peptides. The deliveries used in these calculations are the means of values measured in rats receiving either calcitonin, dDAVP, glucagon, or PTH. The administration rates per 100 g body wt were: dDAVP, 20 pg/min (1-desamino-8-D-arginine vasopressin, Ferring); glucagon, 5 ng/min (highly purified porcine glucagon, Novo Industri); calcitonin, 1 mU/min (synthetic human calcitonin, Cibacalcin); and PTH, 5 mU/min (synthetic 1 to 34 fragment PTH, Beckman Instruments). (Data from [5–7])

sium ions. Parathyroid hormone produced the maximal stimulatory effect, whereas HCT induced the smallest response. Therefore, the situation was the reverse of that observed for calcium and magnesium ions.

Regarding sodium and chloride, dDAVP and HCT significantly increased the reabsorption of these ions in the loop, whereas glucagon and PTH did not. These responses are compatible with the distribution of cyclase responsiveness along the TALH, if we admit that sodium chloride reabsorption by the TALH predominates in the medullary portion of this segment. However, this is not true for glucagon, which is able to produce an even higher cyclase stimulation than vasopressin and CT in this portion; therefore, glucagon should have increased sodium chloride reabsorption in the loop. Differences in protocol (see the section on "Methods") were proposed as a possible source of this discrepancy, since in the glucagon and PTH experiments, a higher perfusion rate of a solution containing more sodium chloride was used; this led to a higher urinary output of sodium than during HCT and dDAVP administration. In fact, subsequent experiments showed that this slight difference in protocol could not account for the discrepancy. Administration of glucagon under conditions that were rigorously similar to those chosen for the dDAVP and HCT studies failed to produce a significant change of the TF/UF sodium at the beginning of the distal tubule. The values averaged 0.412 ± 0.013 ($N = 54$) for the hormone-deprived (control) rats and 0.377 ± 0.013 ($N = 53$) for the hormone-deprived + glucagon rats ($t = 1.882$, $0.05 < P < 0.10$) [6] (Bailly, Roinel, Amiel, submitted for publication).

It must be recalled at this point that the absolute amount of sodium chloride delivered to the loop was increased by almost 30% as a result of the increased GFR during glucagon administration. This increased sodium chloride delivery could itself have caused the TF/UF sodium rise at the end of the diluting segment, thus reducing the hormonal response. It is clear, therefore, that a glucagon effect on sodium transport cannot be either excluded or evidenced.

The cells of the medullary and cortical portions of the TALH, although possessing the same main morphologic organization, differ somewhat in that: (1) they contain cyclases of distinct responsiveness to hormones, and (2) they are very different in size—the cells of the cortical portion being narrower with a simpler ultrastructural organization than those of the medullary portion [15]. Since the specificity of the biologic response to intracellular cyclic AMP generation depends on the characteristics of the cell itself, it is likely that the response elicited by dDAVP, HCT, glucagon, and PTH in the cortical TALH, and that elicited by the first three hormones in the medullary TALH, are different. The present data interpreted in the light of cyclase distribution [3] suggest that in the rat, the response of the cortical part is mainly a stimulation of divalent ion transport; that of the medullary parts is rather a stimulation of monovalent ion transport. In vitro microperfusion studies should help to clarify the respective functions of these two nephron segments. Unfortunately, in the rat, few in vitro studies have been made. To our knowledge, it is only known that ADH increases the positive transepithelial potential difference (PD) of the medullary TAL in this species [16]; more recently, in the Brattleboro rat, this hormone enhances the PD and the net chloride reabsorption flux in this segment [17]. Two teams of authors examined, in the early 1970s, the possible effects of vasopressin on electrolyte transport by the loop in Brattleboro rats [18, 19]. They failed to find any effect. Very recently, re-examination of this question in the same strain of rat revealed that during ADH infusion, the early distal chloride concentration decreased by only 4 ± 1.7 mEq/liter and the fractional chloride reabsorption increased by 5.4 ± 2.5% [17]. In the presence of the other circulating peptide hormones that act on the TALH, the effects appear very limited in comparison with those described in the hormone-deprived rats; in these, ADH reduced the early distal chloride concentration by 17 mEq/liter. Very recently, Peterson et al [20] examined, in hormone-deprived rats, the electrolyte composition of the fluid trapped in the TALH lumen of single loops after stop-flow periods. Administration of dDAVP to these rats enhanced TALH sodium chloride reabsorption by about 25%, thus confirming the amplitude of the effect in the absence of the other hormones. Calcitonin administered to thyroparathyroidectomized rats enhanced calcium and magnesium reabsorption in the loop; but, at variance with the hormone-deprived rats, it did not affect the transport of potassium, sodium, and chloride [14].

The mouse and the rabbit are the two species most extensively studied with in vitro microperfusion techniques. They made it possible to establish the following facts. In the mouse, ADH [16, 21–23] and glucagon [24] enhance the transepithelial PD of the medullary TALH; ADH significantly increases sodium and chlorine reabsorption in the medullary TALH [16, 21–23], but not in the cortical TALH [22]. In the rabbit, ADH and CT exert no measurable effect on the TALH PD [16, 25]. Calcitonin stimulates calcium transport in the medullary portion of the TALH, but it is inactive in the cortical portion [25]. Parathyroid hormone stimulates calcium and magnesium transport in the cortical TALH [26–28], but not in the medullary TALH [27]. Although the results using the microperfusion technique are fragmentary, all of the hormonal effects on electrolyte transport thus far demonstrated agree with the general conclusions drawn from studies on hormone-deprived animals—that ADH and glucagon increase TALH PD in the mouse, while ADH and calcitonin do not change it in the rabbit suggests species differences in the transepithelial PD responsiveness to hormonal stimulation. This does not exclude the possibility that a stimulatory effect on electrolyte transport occurs in the rabbit, if the flux enhancements are concomitant with alteration of the ionic conductance.

The Effect of Hormone-mediated Responses of the Thick Ascending Limb on Kidney Excretory Functions

First, it is important to note that none of the hormones induced natriuresis (Fig. 1), indicating that undesirable pharmacologic effects were avoided as expected from the use of doses eliciting hormonal concentration variations in plasma within physiologic ranges. The fact that neither the sodium nor the potassium excretion rates were altered during hormone administration, in spite of concomitant stimulation of sodium and potassium reabsorption in the loop, was probably due to the intense reabsorptive and secretory processes taking place along the nephron terminal segments. The situation is different for magnesium and calcium ions. Each of the four hormones decreased urinary excretion of these ions. The extent to which they did so places them in the following order: HCT > dDAVP > glucagon > PTH. This also is the order of their effect in increasing the calcium and magnesium reabsorption in the loop (Fig. 5). There was, in fact, an inverse relationship between the amplitude of the loop response and the urinary excretion rate; the greater the stimulation, the lower the excretion rate. Thus, in hormone-deprived rats, the hormonal stimulations of loop function are most probably responsible for profound modifications of urine composition. Are these effects of physiologic significance? The first positive evidence is that they were observed at physiologic doses of the peptides. Second, very recently, Bailly et al [29] on the basis of cyclase data [30] reported that glucagon administered to rats diminished magnesium excretion. Bankir, Bouky, and Trinh [31] established that dDAVP administered to DI Brattleboro rats significantly reduced the daily calcium and magnesium urinary output. Since the hormone-dependent decrease of calcium and magnesium excretion elicited by CT and PTH in thyroparathyroidectomized rats is now clearly established, it is clear, therefore, that when administered individually to rats deprived of the hormone under consideration—but in the presence of the others—each of the four hormones produced a significant reduction of calcium and/or magnesium excretion, although quantitatively to a lesser extent than seen in hormone-deprived rats. It is interesting to note that the effects of glucagon and ADH on these parameters had never been suspected. Finally, it appears that the amplitude of electrolyte transport by the loop may be modulated by the circulating levels of the peptides. The transepithelial PD of the mouse medullary TALH varies in a dose-dependent manner with the ADH concentration applied to the basolateral medium [16, 22]; and, the magnesium and calcium excretions in hormone-deprived rats are closely related to the circulating levels of HCT (Di Stefano, Elalouf, Garel, de Rouffignac, submitted for publication). All of these observations are necessary prerequisites for affirming the physiologic significance of the observed effects.

Influence of Peptide Hormones on Other Tubular Segments

With the hormone-deprived model, several other functions can be studied in addition to hormonal effects on the TALH. Along the mammalian nephron, segments other than the TALH possess a cyclase system sensitive to more than one peptide hormone. These include the distal tubule and the cortical collecting duct. Our model has been successfully used for evaluating hormonal influences in these segments. On the cortical collecting duct, Morel et al [4] demonstrated that salmon CT and vasopressin produced nonadditive stimulation of cyclase responsiveness. The administration of salmon CT to hormone-deprived rats [32] reduced diuresis and increased the urinary osmolality (as also observed in Wistar rats [33]) as would be expected if CT was able to elicit the same final effect on the cortical collecting duct as vasopressin; that is, an increase in the permeability to water. The adenylate system of rat distal tubule is also sensitive to many hormones or agonists, including ADH, PTH, CT, glucagon, and isoproterenol. No additive experiments have, as yet, been made on this segment. In the distal tubule, micropuncture experiments in progress in our two laboratories indicate that in hormone-deprived rats, ADH elicited the expected increase in water permeability, whereas HCT, PTH, and glucagon had no detectable effect. Regarding sodium, chloride, magnesium, and potassium, the effects depended on the hormone administered. For example, ADH stimulated the reabsorption of sodium, chloride, and calcium and the secretion of potassium, but it was without effect on magnesium transport [8]. It is relevant to recall that in the intact DI Brattleboro rat (in the presence of PTH, CT, and glucagon), ADH had no effect on sodium and potassium transport [34]; whereas, in the TPTX Wistar rat (in the presence of glucagon only), ADH enhanced sodium but not calcium reabsorption [35]. Human calcitonin infused in hormone-deprived rats stimulated the reabsorption of sodium, chloride, calcium, and magnesium, and it reduced the secretion of potassium [36]. Neither ADH nor HCT affected phosphate movements. In these hormone-deprived rats, all four hormones stimulated calcium reabsorption [7–8, 36] (Bailly, Roinel, Amiel, submitted for publication). The distal tubule comprises five cell populations that show great differences in morphology, ultrastructural organization [15], and cyclase responsiveness [37]. In view of the common calcium transport response, it is likely that one of the cell populations is responsive to ADH, PTH, CT, and glucagon. It is likely that some of the other cell populations are not target sites for all four hormones, but only for a few of them, which would result in the occurrence of specific effects in this tubular segment that are related to target cell differentiation.

Finally, only those segments that are target sites for one single peptide hormone will give unambiguous responses when the functional characteristics of this hormone are investigated, since possible interference by other hormones activating the same cyclase pool will not confuse the issue. This is true for the proximal tubule, which contains a cyclase system responsive only to PTH, and for the medullary collecting duct, which is responsive almost exclusively to vasopressin. In this connection, it is significant that only the effects elicited by PTH on phosphaturia and by ADH on diuresis were immediately recognized and accepted, whereas those elicited by all of the other peptide hormones provoked numerous contradictory observations.

Conclusions

Antidiuretic hormone, PTH, calcitonin, and glucagon—four hormones that are believed a priori to play very different roles in body fluid homeostasis— may elicit similar responses in the TALH of Henle's loop; consequently, they could affect similarly the excretory function of the kidney. This similarity was revealed by a new procedure for investigating the renal effects of peptide hormones. When different hormones are thought to activate the same cyclase pool, the technique consists of studying the functional effects of a given hormone in the absence of the others that may interfere with it. The data presented here show that this approach clarifies the situation by giving unequivocal responses. This was not the case when classic methods were used; these frequently gave rise to contradictory conclusions.

The present study also indicates that these peptide hormones may alter the process of urine formation in several target segments of the kidney. It is very probable that all of the effects described here are of physiologic importance. Currently, however, speculation regarding the physiologic significance of such hormonal control of tubular function is premature in terms of body fluid homeostasis.

Summary

Micropuncture and clearance experiments were performed on rats that were deprived of the four hormones (ADH, PTH, calcitonin, and glucagon) that stimulate the same cyclase pool in the TALH. Therefore, with this material, the biologic effects of each hormone can be investigated in the absence of the others, which would maintain the cyclase activity of the TALH. DI Brattleboro rats (lacking vasopressin) were acutely thyroparathyroidecto-mized to suppress calcitonin and PTH, and then were infused with glucose or somatostatin to reduce glucagon secretion. Experiments were performed on these hormone-deprived rats in the absence (control) or presence of one of the four hormones acting on the TALH in concentrations within the physiologic range. All four hormones considerably reduced magnesium and calcium fractional excretion rates. At the same time, they significantly lowered magnesium, calcium, and potassium concentrations at the early distal site; and, they markedly increased the reabsorptive capacity of the loop for these ions. In view of this common response, it is concluded that all four hormones activating the cyclase system in rat TALH have the same physiologic effect on this segment. The hormone-deprived model can be used for studying hormonal influences on other target segments that possess a cyclase system sensitive to more than one hormone. Results concerning the distal tubule and the cortical collecting duct have been discussed.

References

1. MOREL F: Regulation of kidney functions by hormones: a new approach. *Rec Prog Horm Res* 39:271–304, 1983
2. IMBERT M, CHABARDES D, MONTEGUT M, CLIQUE A, MOREL F: Adenylate cyclase activity along the rabbit nephron as measured in single isolated segments. *Pflügers Arch* 354:213–222, 1975
3. MOREL F, IMBERT-TEBOUL M, CHABARDES D: Distribution of hormone-dependent adenylate cyclase in the nephron and its physiological significance. *Ann Rev Physiol* 43:569–581, 1981
4. MOREL F, CHABARDES D, IMBERT-TEBOUL M, LE BOUFFANT F, HUSCITHAREL A, MONTEGUT M: Multiple hormonal control of adenylate cyclase in distal segments of the rat kidney. *Kidney Int* 21:55–62, 1982
5. DE ROUFFIGNAC C, CORMAN B, ROINEL N: Stimulation by antidiuretic hormone of electrolyte tubular reabsorption in rat kidney. *Am J Physiol* 244:F156–F164, 1983
6. BAILLY C, ROINEL N, AMIEL C: PTH-like glucagon stimulation of Ca and Mg reabsorption in Henle's loop of the rat. *Am J Physiol* 246:F205–F212, 1984
7. ELALOUF JM, ROINEL N, DE ROUFFIGNAC C: ADH-like effects of calcitonin on electrolyte transport by Henle's loop of rat kidney. *Am J Physiol* 246:F213–F220, 1984
8. ELALOUF JM, ROINEL N, DE ROUFFIGNAC C: Effects of antidiuretic hormone on electrolyte reabsorption and secretion in distal tubules of rat kidney. *Pflügers Arch* (in press, 1984)
9. ROBERTSON GL, ATHAR S, SHELTON L: Osmotic control of vasopressin function, in *Disturbances in Body Fluid Osmolality,* edited by ANDREOLI TE, GRANTHAM JJ, RECTOR FC, Washington DC, American Physiological Society, 1977, pp 125–148
10. EMMANOUEL DS, JASPAN JB, RUBENSTEIN AH, HUEN AHJ, FINK E, KATZ AI: Glucagon metabolism in the rat. *J Clin Invest* 62:6–13, 1978
11. CRESSENT M, BOUIZAR Z, PIDOUX E, MOUKHTAR MS, MILHAUD G: Effet de l'ovariectomie sur le taux de calcitonine plasmatique chez le rat. *CR Acad Sci (Paris)* 289:501–504, 1979
12. MOREL F, ROINEL N: Application de la microsonde électronique à l'analyse élémentaire quantitative d'échantillons liquides d'un volume inférieur à 10^{-9} l. *J Chim Phys-Chim Biol* 66:1084–1091, 1969
13. DENNIS VW, BELLO-REUS E, ROBINSON RR: Response of phosphate transport to parathyroid hormone in segments of rabbit nephron. *Am J Physiol* 233:29–38, 1977

14. POUJEOL P, TOUVAY C, ROINEL N, DE ROUFFIGNAC C: Stimulation of renal magnesium reabsorption by calcitonin in the rat. *Am J Physiol* 239:F524–F532, 1980

15. KRIZ W, KAISSLING B, PSZOLLA M: Morphological characterization of the cells in Henle's loop and the distal tubule, in *New Aspects of Renal Function. Proceedings of the Workshop Conference* (vol 6), edited by VOGEL HG, ULLRICH KJ, Amsterdam, Excerpta Medica, 1978, pp 67–79

16. SASAKI S, IMAI M: Effects of vasopressin on water and NaCl transport across the in vitro perfused medullary thick ascending limb of Henle's loop of mouse, rat and rabbit kidneys. *Pflügers Arch* 383:215–221, 1980

17. WORK J, BOOKER B, SCHAFER JA, GULLA J, LUKE R: In vivo and in vitro effect of ADH on loop of Henle chloride reabsorption in the Brattleboro (DI) rat (*abstract*). *Kidney Int* 25:322, 1984

18. SCHNERMANN J, VALTIN H, THURAU K, NAGEL W, HORSTER M, FISCHBACH H, WAHL M, LIEBAU G: Micropuncture studies on the influence of antidiuretic hormone on tubular fluid reabsorption in rats with hereditary hypothalamic diabetes insipidus. *Pflügers Arch* 308:103–118, 1969

19. JOHNSTON P, LACY FB, JAMISON RL: Effect of antidiuretic hormone-induced antidiuresis on water reabsorption by the superficial loop of Henle in Brattleboro rats. *J Lab Clin Med* 90:1004–1011, 1977

20. PETERSON LN, DE ROUFFIGNAC C, LEVINE DZ: An in vivo assessment of the stimulatory effect of antidiuretic hormone (dDAVP) on NaCl reabsorption by the thick ascending limb (TAL) in the rat (*abstract*). *Kidney Int* 25:313, 1984

21. HALL DA, VARNEY DM: Effect of vasopressin on electrical potential difference and chloride transport in mouse medullary ascending limb of Henle's loop. *J Clin Invest* 53:393–402, 1980

22. HEBERT SC, CULPEPPER RM, ANDREOLI TE: NaCl transport in mouse medullary thick ascending limbs. I. Function nephron heterogeneity and ADH-stimulated NaCl cotransport. *Am J Physiol* 241:F412–431, 1981

23. HEBERT SC, CULPEPPER RM, ANDREOLI TE: NaCl transport in mouse medullary thick ascending limbs. II. ADH enhancement of transcellular NaCl cotransport; origin of transepithelial voltage. *Am J Physiol* 241:F432–F442, 1981

24. CULPEPPER RM, ANDREOLI TE: Site of PGE_2 inhibition of ADH-mediated NaCl transport in mouse medullary thick ascending limb (mTAL) (*abstract*). *Kidney Int* 23:253, 1983

25. SUKI WN, ROUSE D: Hormonal regulation of calcium transport in thick ascending limb renal tubules. *Am J Physiol* 241:F171–F174, 1981

26. BOURDEAU JE, BURG MB: Effect of PTH on calcium transport across the cortical thick ascending limb of Henle's loop. *Am J Physiol* 239:F121–F126, 1980

27. SUKI WN, ROUSE D, NG RCK, KOKKO JP: Calcium transport in the thick ascending limb of Henle. Heterogeneity of function in the medullary and cortical segments. *J Clin Invest* 66:1004–1009, 1980

28. SHAREGHI GR, AGUS ZS: Magnesium transport in the cortical thick ascending limb of Henle's loop of the rabbit. *J Clin Invest* 69:759–769, 1982

29. BAILLY C, AMIEL C: Effect of glucagon on magnesium renal reabsorption in the rat. *Pflügers Arch* 392:360–365, 1982

30. BAILLY C, IMBERT-TEBOUL M, CHABARDES D, HUS-CITHAREL A, MONTEGUT M, CLIQUE A, MOREL F: The distal nephron of rat kidney: a target site for glucagon. *Proc Natl Acad Sci USA* 77:3422–3424, 1980

31. BANKIR L, BOUBY N, TRINH MM: Effects of ADH on renal handling of electrolytes: evidence for a role in Ca and Mg excretion in the conscious rat (*abstract*). *Kidney Int* 25:294, 1984

32. DE ROUFFIGNAC C, ELALOUF JM: Effects of salmon calcitonin on the renal concentrating mechanism. *Am J Physiol* 245:F506–F511, 1983
33. CARNEY S, MORGAN T, RAY C, THOMPSON L: Effect of calcitonin on urine concentration in the rat. *Am J Physiol* 244:F432–435, 1983
34. FIELD MJ, STANTON BA, GIEBISCH GH: Influence of ADH on potassium handling by the distal nephron in Brattleboro rats (*abstract*). *Kidney Int* 23:254, 1983
35. COSTANZO LS, WINDHAGER EE: Effects of PTH, ADH and cyclic AMP on distal tubular Ca and Na reabsorption. *Am J Physiol* 239:F478–F485, 1980
36. ELALOUF JM, ROINEL N, DE ROUFFIGNAC C: Stimulation by human calcitonin of electrolyte transport in distal tubules of rat kidney. *Pflügers Arch* 399:111–118, 1983
37. MOREL F, CHABARDES D, IMBERT M: Functional segmentation of the rabbit distal tubule by microdetermination of hormone-dependent adenylate cyclase activity. *Kidney Int* 9:264–277, 1975

Brush Border and Basal-Lateral Membranes in the Action of Thyroid Hormone on the Proximal Tubule

Giovambattista Capasso and Rolf Kinne

In the last few years, the role of thyroid hormones in the regulation of kidney function has been studied by several investigators. Their reports have demonstrated that the lack of thyroid hormones induces dramatic changes in kidney function. Among these changes are: (1) a decrease in glomerular filtration rate (GFR) and renal plasma flow (RPF) and an increase in urine flow [1], (2) an inability to concentrate or dilute the urine [2], (3) impaired urinary acidification [3], and (4) decreased phosphate reabsorption [4].

In previous experiments [5], we have shown that in proximal tubules of thyroidectomized rats, there is a reduction of isotonic fluid reabsorption (J_v) and a reduction of histidine transport, which can be reversed by the administration of tri-iodothyronine (T_3) (5 μg/100 g body wt) for 7 days. However, proton secretion is only slightly affected by the hormonal status of the animal.

An understanding of the mechanism of action of thyroid hormones on the proximal tubule is hampered by several factors: (1) several studies employed thyroparathyroidectomized rats instead of thyroidectomized rats with intact parathyroid glands, (2) no distinction between acute and chronic effects of T_3 and of hypothyroidism is made, and (3) pharmacologic doses, instead of physiologic doses, of thyroid hormones are used that could elicit alterations superimposed on the physiologic effects of the hormone. In the following short review, therefore, we will try to always carefully define the status of the animal and the type of regimen used for hormone repletion.

In addition, we will focus on recent studies in which the site of action of thyroid hormones within the proximal tubule cell has been determined.

Action of Thyroid Hormones on the Luminal Membrane

Phosphate Transport

When chronically thyroparathyroidectomized rats are treated for 5 days with a dose of 200 μg of T_4/100 g body wt, brush border vesicles isolated from

This manuscript was presented as part of a Symposium on *Brush Border Transport Mechanisms*.

Table 1. Na uptake by brush border membranes isolated from kidney cortex of thyroidectomized rats (TX) or thyroidectomized rats treated for 3 days with 1 μg of T_3/100 g body wt (TX + 3 T_3)

Rats	Incubation time			
	15 sec	1 min	1 min 45 sec	2 min 30 sec
TX	65.7 ± 12.4	118.4 ± 21.2	144.7 ± 25.4	162.2 ± 35.2
TX + 3 T_3	70.9 ± 24.1	110.9 ± 34.9	144.2 ± 35.0	168.5 ± 40.2

Vesicles containing 100 mM mannitol and 20 mM Tris-HEPES, pH 7.4, were incubated in a medium additionally containing 0.4 M Na_2SO_4 and 10 μCi ^{22}Na. Data represent mean value $\pm$ SEM from six paired experiments and are expressed as percent of the uptake at equilibrium. (See [7] for further details)

the renal cortex show increased Na-dependent phosphate transport in both the presence and absence of a Na gradient [6]. The kinetic analysis revealed an increase in V_{max} (30%), but only a slight increase in affinity.

Sodium Transport

In brush border vesicles that are isolated from thyroidectomized rats supplemented for 3 days with 1 μg of T_3/100 g body wt, no change in Na permeability nor in the rate of Na-proton exchange could be detected (Tables 1 and 2) [7]. In accordance with these findings, perfusion of proximal tubules with amphotericin B, in a concentration that significantly increased Na efflux in isolated brush border membranes, did not change the rate of Na reabsorption [7].

Other Transport Systems

Short-term treatment of thyroidectomized rats with low doses of T_3 did not affect Na-gradient driven histidine uptake in isolated brush border membranes

Table 2. Amiloride-sensitive Na uptake by brush border membranes isolated from kidney cortex of thyroidectomized rats (TX) or thyroidectomized rats treated for 3 days with 1 μg of T_3/100 g body wt (TX + 3 T_3)

Rats	Incubation time		
	15 sec	1 min	1 min 45 sec
TX	0.080 ± 0.014	$0.120 + 0.016$	$0.134 + 0.018$
TX + 3 T_3	0.100 ± 0.033	0.141 ± 0.029	0.167 ± 0.028

Vesicles containing 100 mM mannitol and 20 mM Tris-HEPES, pH 7.4, were incubated in a medium additionally containing 10 μCi ^{22}Na, 0.4 mM Na_2SO_4, and 0.4 mM amiloride. The amiloride-sensitive NA uptake was calculated as the difference between the total Na uptake and the amiloride-insensitive Na uptake. Data are expressed as nmole/mg protein and represent mean values $\pm$ SEM from five paired experiments. (See [7] for further details)

[7], nor did the treatment of thyroparathyroidectomized rats for 5 days with 200 μg of T_4/100 g body wt change Na-gradient-dependent D-glucose or L-proline transport [6].

Action of Thyroid Hormones on the Contraluminal Membrane

A well-known action of thyroid hormones is the increase in Na-K-ATPase in renal cortical plasma membranes [9]. This response reaches its maximum after 48 hr, and it is evident when 25 μg of T_3/100 g body wt or more are injected once into hypothyroid animals [10]. The increase occurs in the proximal tubule, as is evident from studies on the Na-K-ATPase activity in tubules microdissected from thyroidectomized rats treated with 1 μg of T_3/100 g body wt for 7 days [8, 11]. It should be noted, however, that treatment with 1 μg of T_3/100 g body wt for a short period of time (1 to 4 days) does not elicit any increase in Na-K-ATPase activity in renal cortex homogenates, dissected tubules, or isolated plasma membranes (Fig. 1) [8, 12]. Recent micropuncture experiments demonstrated that valinomycin application can partly mimic the effect of thyroid hormones on Na transport (Table 3) [8]. This led to the suggestion that the K permeability of the basolateral plasma membrane might be altered by thyroid hormones.

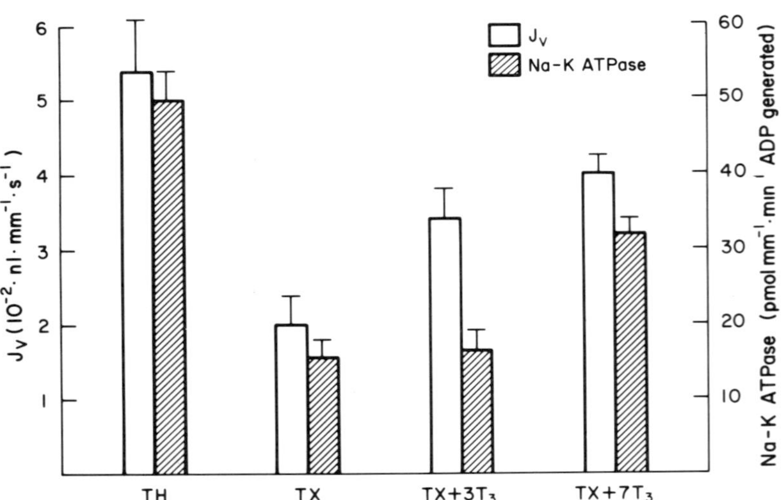

Fig. 1. Isotonic fluid reabsorption (J_v) and Na-K-ATPase activity in late proximal convoluted tubules of superficial nephrons (S_2 segments) of control rats (*TH*), thyroidectomized rats (*TX*), and TX rats treated for 3 days (*TX* + *3 T_3*) or for 7 days (*TX* + *7 T_3*) with 1 μg T_3/100 g body wt (See [8] for further details)

Table 3. Isotonic fluid reabsorption (J_v) in late proximal tubules of thyroidectomized rats (TX), TX rats treated for 3 days (TX + 3 T_3) with 1 μg of T_3/100 g body wt. The tubules were perfused from both the luminal and peritubular side with modified Ringer solution with and without valinomycin (1 μg/ml)

	Rats				
	TX	TX + 3 T_3	Δ	TX + valinomycin	Δ
J_v	1.81 ± 0.29	2.86 ± 0.31[a]	1.05	2.23 ± 0.37[a]	0.42
	n = 32	n = 31		n = 64	(40%)
	(11)	(8)		(11)	

Δ is the difference between the experimental J_v and that of TX. Data are expressed as $10^{-2} \cdot$ nl $\cdot$ mm$^{-1} \cdot$ sec^{-1} and represent mean values $\pm$ SEM. n indicates the number of tubules punctured. The number of rats is given in parentheses.
[a] $P < 0.005$ versus TX rats. (See [8, 12] for further details)

Action of Thyroid Hormones on Metabolic Reactions

One of the metabolic enzymes under the control of thyroid hormones is the α-glycerophosphate dehydrogenase. Its activity is increased significantly after 48 hr, when a single injection of 10 μg of T_3/100 g body wt is used [10].

Correlation Between Transport and Hormone Action

With regard to phosphate reabsorption, the results indicate that increased phosphate reabsorption by the kidney [6] and, thus, probably by the proximal tubule is accompanied by an increase in the activity of the luminal Na-phosphate cotransport system. Under the conditions employed in these studies, one also can assume that the activity of both the Na-K-ATPase and α-GPDH are increased. Thus, an additional stimulation of Na-gradient-dependent phosphate transport can be expected on the basis of an increased activity of the Na pump, which (as primary active transport system) provides the driving force for the secondary active Na cotransport systems. The latter might also be the cause for the increase in histidine transport without a change in the activity of the transport system, when studied in isolated brush border preparations. In contrast to the in vivo situation within in vitro studies, identical driving forces are used for the vesicles derived from hypothyroid- and hormone-treated animals.

The effect of thyroid hormones on Na reabsorption is readily explained for the situation in which an increase in Na-K-ATPase has been observed. In this instance, apparently only the activity of the contraluminal pump is increased—the luminal Na permeability not being affected by thyroid hormones and also not being rate-limiting for the transport [7]. When thyroidectomized animals are treated with low doses of hormone and only for a short period of time, the Na reabsorption is already markedly increased; however, no increase in Na-K-ATPase is detected in the same tubule when assayed in vitro (Fig. 1) [8, 12]. Under these circumstances, other factors have to be invoked in hormone action. Since no effects on the luminal entry step for Na are observed and metabolic stimulation probably is also small [10], the exit step has to be accelerated by other means for Na. One possibility for increasing the turnover number of the Na-K-ATPase in vivo is an increase in the K permeability of the basal-lateral plasma membrane, which would facilitate the exit of K from the cell [13]. Indirect evidence for such a mechanism can be deduced from the valinomycin experiments. However, it has to be noted that direct measurements of K permeability of the basal-lateral membranes of proximal tubules have not been performed at present. Furthermore, the interpretation presented above assumes that the Na permeability of the brush border membrane, as measured in vitro, can be correlated to the Na permeability in vivo, and that no changes in the paracellular pathways occur.

On the other hand, effects of thyroid hormones on membrane permeability have already been suggested in studies on thermogenesis [14]; also, they have been demonstrated in the rat diaphragm [15].

Conclusion

In summarizing the effect of thyroid hormones on the properties of luminal and contraluminal membranes of the proximal tubule in hypothyroid rats, only the Na-phosphate cotransport system has been demonstrated as being affected parallel to phosphate reabsorption by the kidney. Changes in the number of Na pump sites in the contraluminal membrane occur concomitantly with changes in Na reabsorption, if high doses of hormone or low doses for a longer period are used. The mechanism of increase of Na transport at low doses after short-term treatment remains to be elucidated. One possible explanation is an early change in the K permeability of the basal-lateral membrane.

References

1. HOLMES EW, DI SCALA VA: Studies on the exaggerated natriuretic response to a saline infusion in the hypothyroid rat. *J Clin Invest* 49:1224–1236, 1970
2. EMMANOUEL DS, LINDHEIMER MD, KATZ AI: Mechanism of impaired water excretion in the hypothyroid rat. *J Clin Invest* 54:926–934, 1974
3. MICHAEL UF, CHAVEZ R, COOKSON SL, VAAMONDE CA: Impaired urinary acidification in the hypothyroid rat. *Pfluegers Arch* 361:215–220, 1976
4. RITZ E, KREUSSER W, BOMMER J: Effects of hormones other than parathyroid hormones on renal handling of phosphate, in *Renal Handling of Phosphate*, edited by MASSRY SG, FLEISCH H, New York, Plenum Press, 1980, pp 137–194
5. DE SANTO NG, CAPASSO G, PADUANO C, CARELLA C, GIORDANO C: Tubular transport processes in proximal tubules of hypothyroid rats. Micropuncture studies

on isotonic fluid, amino acid and buffer reabsorption. *Pfluegers Arch* 384:117–122, 1980

6. ESPINOSA RE, KELLER MJ, YUSUFI ANK, DOUSA TP: Effect of thyroid administration on phosphate transport across renal cortical brush border membrane. *Am J Physiol* 246:F133–F139, 1984

7. CAPASSO G, KINNE-SAFFRAN E, DE SANTO NG, KINNE R: Regulation of volume reabsorption by thyroid hormones in the proximal tubule of rat: Minor role of luminal sodium permeability. *Pfluegers Arch* (submitted)

8. CAPASSO G, LIN JT, DE SANTO NG, KINNE R: Short term effect of low doses of tri-iodothyronine on proximal tubular membrane Na-K-ATPase and potassium permeability in thyroidectomized rats. *Pfluegers Arch* (submitted)

9. EDELMAN IS: Thyroid thermogenesis. *N Engl J Med* 290:1303–1308, 1974

10. SOMJEN D, ISMAIL-BEIGI F, EDELMAN IS: Nuclear binding of T_3 and effects on QO_2, Na-K-ATPase, and α-GPDH in liver and kidney. *Am J Physiol* 240:E146–E154, 1981

11. GARG LC, MACKIE S, TISHER CC: Site of action of thyroid hormones on Na^+-K^+-ATPase in rat nephron segments (*abstract*). *Kidney Int* 21:274, 1982

12. DE SANTO NG, CAPASSO G, KINNE R, MOEWES B, CARELLA A, ANASTASIO P, GIORDANO C: Tubular transport processes in proximal tubules of hypothyroid rats. Lack of relationship between thyroidal dependent rise of isotonic fluid reabsorption and Na^+-K^+-ATPase activity. *Pfluegers Arch* 394:294–301, 1982

13. SCHULTZ SC: Homocellular regulatory mechanism in sodium-transporting epithelia: Avoidance of extinction by "flush-through." *Am J Physiol* 241:F579–F590, 1981

14. EDELMAN IS: Receptors and effectors in hormone action on kidney. *Am J Physiol* 241:F333–F339, 1981

15. HABER RS, LOEB JN: Effect of 3,5,3'-triiodothyronine treatment on potassium efflux from isolated rat diaphragm: Role of increased permeability in the thermogenic response. *Endocrinology* 111:1217–1223, 1982

Binding of Aldosterone and Corticosterone Along the Nephron and Effects on Na-K-ATPase

Adrian I. Katz, Marcia A. Chekal, and Salim K. Mujais

Both mineralocorticoids and glucocorticoids influence numerous metabolic and transport functions of the kidney. That they exert a stimulatory effect on renal tubular Na-K-ATPase has been proposed as a possible mechanism of their action [1–4]; however, defining the role that each major class of corticosteroids plays in this process has met with considerable difficulty (reviewed in [5]). Two of the reasons for this difficulty have been as follows: (1) the frequent use in earlier studies of pharmacologic doses of hormone that could produce extrarenal alterations or nonspecific effects because of receptor cross-occupancy, and (2) the determination of enzyme activity in kidney homogenates that were heterogeneous and thus unlikely to reveal subtle effects in target segments of the nephron.

During the last few years, our laboratory has reexamined several aspects of the interaction of adrenal corticoids with the kidney. In these studies we have taken advantage of newer techniques, which have allowed us to analyze biochemical events in individual nephron segments with micromethods specifically adapted for this purpose [5–9]. First, we determined the binding profile of aldosterone and corticosterone along the nephron to determine their putative sites of action [7, 8]. After identifying the cortical collecting tubule (CCT) as the major target site for both hormones, we evaluated the role of physiologic replacement doses of either aldosterone or corticosterone in the maintenance and restoration of Na-K-ATPase in the CCT of adrenalectomized rats [5]. In studies still in progress, we are examining the effect of high physiologic doses of these two hormones on the enzyme from various nephron segments of intact animals [9]. A description of these studies, together with a brief survey of relevant recent literature, forms the basis of this article.

This manuscript was presented as part of a Symposium on *Aldosterone and the Kidney*.

Binding of Corticosteroid Hormones Along the Nephron

Because hormones must first bind to specific receptors before they can exert a physiologic effect, it is necessary to characterize and locate the corticosteroid binding sites in the nephron before the renal actions of these hormones can be understood.[1] In a series of landmark investigations, Funder, Feldman, an Edelman demonstrated a decade ago the existence of several distinct classes of steroid hormone receptors in the kidney. Using cell-free homogenates or tissue slices, they characterized the mineralocorticoid receptors ("type I") and glucocorticoid receptors (types II and III for dexamethasone and corticosterone, respectively) and thus helped to describe the initial sequence of events leading to the renal effects of corticosteroids [10–13]. However, despite the wealth of information generated by these studies, the precise localization of the receptors in the nephron has remained unknown until recently, when work reported concurrently by two groups of investigators has defined the binding profile of adrenal corticoids along the mammalian nephron.

We studied the binding of tritiated aldosterone [7] and corticosterone [8] in freshly dissected rabbit and rat tubules with a direct binding microassay. In this type of study, individual nephron segments are dissected freehand and incubated with the labeled hormone under conditions found to be optimal for binding (60 min, 25°C), with or without the addition of excess unlabeled homologous hormone or related steroids to determine binding specificity. The advantages of this technique are its conceptual simplicity, the possibility of quantitative measurement in well-defined nephron segments, and relative freedom from postbinding dissociation artifacts [16]. On the other hand, because the microassay examines only a few micrograms of tissue, it is not possible to determine with it the intracellular (for example, nuclear versus cytoplasmic) distribution of the receptors.

Results of these studies are summarized in Figure 1. Tritiated aldosterone binding to rabbit tubules showed a very distinct pattern. A high concentration of binding sites of high affinity and specificity for aldosterone was found only in anatomic subdivisions of the collecting tubule (branched, cortical, and outer medullary), whereas specific binding was negligible in all the more proximal segments of the nephron, including notably the distal convoluted tubule [7]. Although the nature of the corticosterone receptor is still uncertain [16], we have chosen this steroid because it is the main or only natural glucocorticoid in both the rat and rabbit. In contrast to aldosterone, and in keeping with the more protean actions of glucocorticoids in the kidney, specific tritiated corticosterone binding could be detected in proximal as well as distal nephron segments [8]. Nevertheless, by far the highest concentration

---

[1] Although the terms *receptor* and *binding site* are not identical, their meaning overlaps in this chapter. In a strict sense, the term *receptor* implies high affinity and specificity for the hormone, and that binding is followed by a specific biological event. At least in the case of aldosterone, the excellent correspondence between the nephron segments where its effects on tubular function are elicited [14, 15], and the location and steroid specificity of its binding sites [7], suggests that the latter are indeed true receptors.

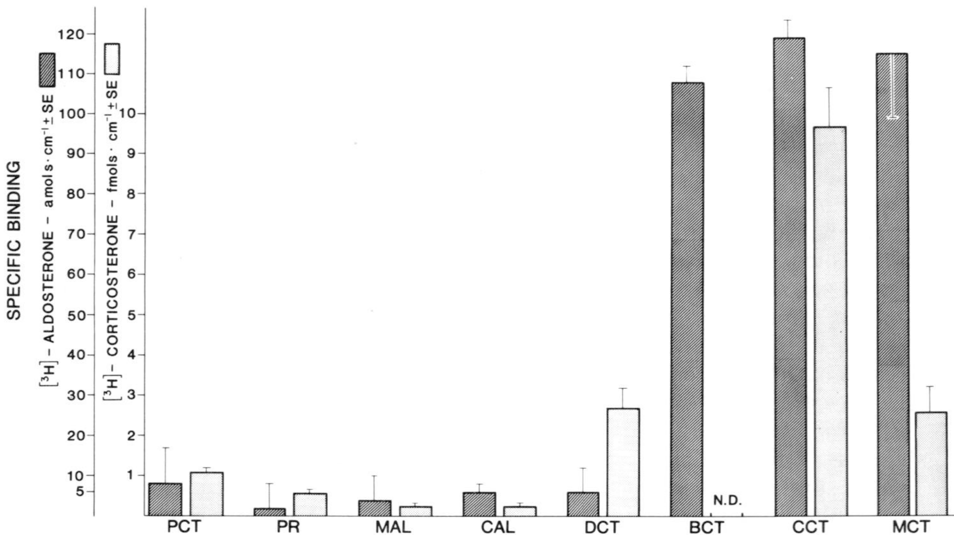

Fig. 1. Specific binding of aldosterone and corticosterone along the nephron. Significant binding of tritiated aldosterone was detected only in the branched (*BCT*), cortical (*CCT*), and medullary (*MCT*) portions of the collecting tubule. Tritiated corticosterone bound specifically to several additional nephron segments, but the concentration of binding sites was highest in the CCT. (*T bars* represent the SEM.) *DCT* is the distal convoluted tubule; *PCT,* proximal convoluted tubule; *MAL,* medullary thick ascending limb; *PR,* pars recta; *CAL,* cortical thick ascending limb.

of binding sites was also found in the CCT, suggesting that this nephron segment is a major target site for corticosterone as it is for aldosterone. The maximal binding capacity of the CCT for corticosterone was nearly two orders of magnitude higher than that for aldosterone (Fig. 1), which is in agreement with measurements by other investigators in kidney cytosol [10, 12] and with the relative abundance of the two hormones in the circulation.

A different approach to the localization of steroid binding sites in the nephron was chosen by Farman, Vandewalle, and Bonvalet, who studied the binding of aldosterone and dexamethasone to rabbit tubules with an autoradiographic technique [17–20]. In this procedure, kidney pyramids are incubated with the radioligand followed by microdissection and transfer of the tubule segments onto dry film; fixation and staining are done several months later, at the end of film exposure. Limitations of this method are the semiquantitative nature of the measurements of grain distribution, and the possibility of dissociation of radioactivity during tissue preparation [16]. Its advantage over the direct binding assay is its ability to estimate nuclear as opposed to cytosolic binding from visual inspection of grain distribution in the autoradiograph.

Initially, Farman et al found specific nuclear aldosterone binding to be highest and comparable in the CCT and distal convoluted tubules, but no distinction was attempted between the "bright" and "granular" portion of the latter; binding was low in the thick ascending limb and absent in proximal tubules [17, 18]. When more detailed studies analyzed the behavior of aldosterone binding in relation to ligand concentration and competition by various steroids, as well as examining separately the subdivisions of the distal convoluted tubule, the authors concluded that aldosterone binds to mineralocorticoid sites in the CCT, but to both mineralocorticoid and glucocorticoid receptor sites in other parts of the nephron [19]. Dexamethasone binding was demonstrated along the entire nephron, but in proximal tubules it occurred chiefly in the cytoplasm, as opposed to being mainly nuclear in all segments beyond the pars recta [20].

Work from the two laboratories just cited, despite widely divergent methodologic approaches, is in general agreement. It excludes the proximal nephron and identifies the collecting tubule (connecting segment, including "DCTg," and the cortical and medullary collecting tubule)[2] as the major site of aldosterone binding. Although not strictly comparable because of the existence of separate classes of receptor for each [11, 12], binding of the natural (corticosterone) and synthetic (dexamethasone) glucocorticoid could be demonstrated along the entire nephron, a pattern consistent with the broader spectrum of glucocorticoid effects on the kidney.

Regulation of Renal Na-K-ATPase by Adrenal Steroids

Under Basal Conditions

It has been established beyond doubt that renal Na-K-ATPase is under partial corticosteroid control, for its activity invariably declines to a substantial degree following adrenalectomy and is restored in part or in full by adrenal steroids (reviewed in [5, 16, 21]). However, the relative importance of the two major classes of corticosteroids in the regulation of renal Na-K-ATPase has long been debated, some studies attributing a predominant role to mineralocorticoids [1, 2, 22] and others to glucocorticoids [3, 23, 24]. There are numerous explanations for this controversy, including the explanations that kidney homogenates were used rather than the specific nephron segments that are the target sites of the hormone, and that synthetic steroids were used. The renal effects of the latter may not be identical to those of the native hormone. Another important limitation of earlier studies relates to the steroid dose used, which was often excessive and thus compromised the ability to distinguish between mineralocorticoid and glucocorticoid effects because of illicit cross-occupancy of each other's receptors, besides producing confounding extrarenal alterations. Even when a seemingly appropriate dose of hormone

---

[2] Doucet and Katz [7] reported high specific aldosterone binding in the medullary collecting tubule, whereas Farman et al [19] considered this segment to contain a mixture of mineralocorticoid and glucocorticoid sites. However, we examined the outer medullary collecting tubule, in contrast to the latter report in which the medullary collecting tubules were obtained from "the papillary portion or close to it."

was chosen, its administration by bolus injection probably produced transient pharmacologic levels in the circulation, and consequently at the receptor sites.

We attempted in a recent study [5] to circumvent these difficulties by evaluating the effect of aldosterone and corticosterone (the native mineralocorticoid and glucocorticoid in the rat) on Na-K-ATPase in the CCT, the major target site of both hormones in this species. In addition, each hormone was supplied in steady fashion by long-term s.c. delivery from pellets or osmotic minipumps in doses calculated to provide physiologic replacement; in these adrenalectomized animals, they restored aldosterone or corticosterone plasma levels to those seen in intact, unstressed animals (5 ng/dl and 7.4 μg/dl, respectively).

Adrenalectomy halved the Na-K-ATPase activity in CCT after 7 days, without further decline thereafter. When hormone replacement began at the time of surgery, aldosterone fully prevented this decline, whereas similar replacement with corticosterone was without effect (Fig. 2). Furthermore, when Na-K-ATPase was first allowed to reach its nadir and similar replacement of each hormone was started 1 week after adrenal ablation, aldosterone but not corticosterone restored enzyme activity to levels equal to or higher than those in adrenal-intact animals. These results strongly suggest that under basal conditions (that is, when physiologic hormone levels prevail) Na-K-ATPase activity in the CCT, a major target segment for both classes of hormone, is under mineralocorticoid rather than glucocorticoid control.

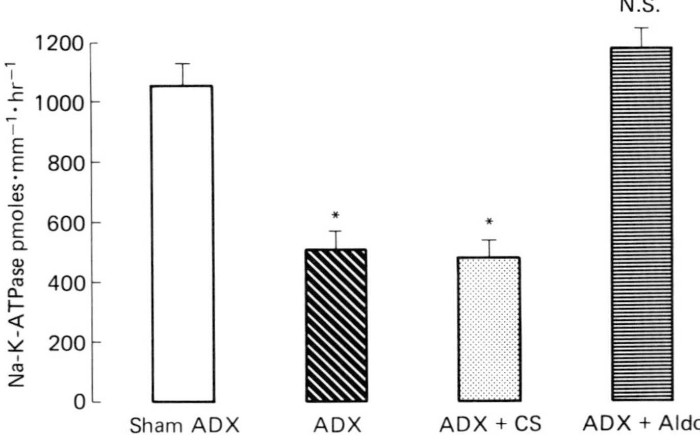

Fig. 2. Na-K-ATPase activity in the cortical collecting tubule of adrenal-intact (*Sham ADX; N* = 9), adrenalectomized but untreated (*ADX; N* = 9), and adrenalectomized rats treated with either corticosterone (*ADX + CS; N*= 8) or aldosterone (*ADX + Aldo; N* = 6), 7 days after adrenalectomy or a sham operation. Aldosterone, but not corticosterone, prevented the decline in enzyme activity. *, *P*<0.001. (Reproduced from [5] by permission of the American Society for Clinical Investigation)

Under Conditions That Mimic Stimulated Corticosteroid Production

Several investigators [25–27] demonstrated a stimulatory effect of chronic deoxycorticosterone administration on Na-K-ATPase in the rabbit collecting tubule, but the hormone was given in pharmacologic amounts (5 mg/day). We therefore sought to further clarify the interaction of native corticosteroids with rat nephron Na-K-ATPase in experiments in which the hormones were given in high physiologic doses. Specifically, we wished to determine whether sustained (7 days) "stimulated" levels of aldosterone, such as those achieved during potassium loading or sodium deprivation [28], and levels of corticosterone that might be expected from chronic ACTH stimulation modulate Na-K-ATPase activity in the cortical collecting tubule of adrenal-intact rats. To evaluate the specificity of this effect, we also measured Na-K-ATPase in two other nephron segments: the proximal convoluted tubule (PCT), because it has receptors for corticosterone but not for aldosterone, and the medullary thick ascending limb of Henle's loop (MAL) where receptors for either hormone are sparse or undetectable [7, 8]. We chose to give exogenous hormones rather than to manipulate their endogenous production, because maneuvers such as potassium loading or sodium deprivation likely influence Na-K-ATPase activity in their own right, and long-term ACTH excess stimulates the production of both corticosterone and aldosterone. Circulating levels of aldosterone simulating potassium loading and sodium deprivation were obtained by constant delivery from s.c. implanted osmotic minipumps of 5 and 50 $\mu g \cdot 100$ g$^{-1} \cdot$ day^{-1}, respectively, whereas those reflecting stimulated corticosterone production were produced with two s.c. pellets containing together 150 mg of the hormone. Because with even this dose of corticosterone no effect on Na-K-ATPase could be observed, we used larger pellets (total of 300 mg) in additional experiments designed to provide pharmacologic levels of the hormones. (It is recalled that 40 mg of corticosterone in pellets provide the equivalent of endogenous production of the hormone in adrenalectomized rats.)

Preliminary results of these studies are summarized in Fig. 3. Aldosterone administration caused a significant increment in Na-K-ATPase activity in the CCT, to approximately twice the control values, but did not alter the enzyme in proximal convoluted tubules and medullary thick ascending limb. This is consistent with the distribution of aldosterone receptors in the nephron. Moderately high doses of corticosterone, in contrast, did not stimulate Na-K-ATPase in CCT, but provision of pharmacologic amounts of the hormone did enhance the activity of the enzyme in this segment alone without affecting it in PCT and MAL. Because these regions of the nephron lack specific aldosterone receptors, which are present in abundance in the CCT, it is postulated that the effect of pharmacologic doses of corticosterone in the latter may be mediated by cross-occupancy of the mineralocorticoid receptor. These experiments demonstrate a segment-specific increase in Na-K-ATPase activity by circulating levels of aldosterone simulating those prevailing during potassium excess or sodium deprivation, and confirm the primacy of mineralocorticoid modulation of renal tubular Na-K-ATPase.

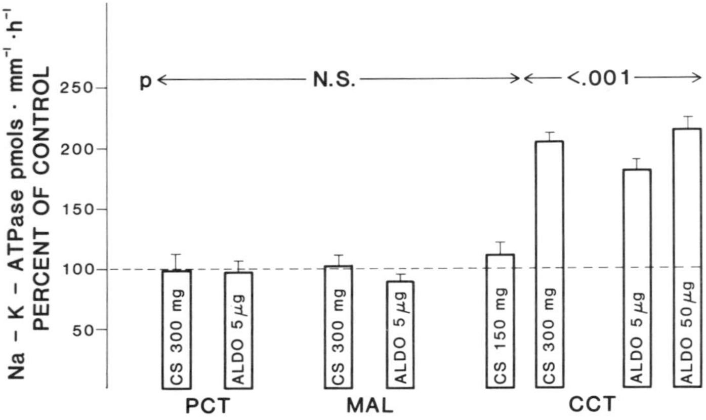

Fig. 3. Effect of long-term (7 days) administration of corticosterone and aldosterone on Na-K-ATPase in three nephron segments of the adrenal-intact rat. Aldosterone (*Aldo*) produced a significant increase in enzyme activity in the cortical collecting tubule (*CCT*), but only pharmacologic doses of corticosterone (*CS*) elicited this effect, possibly by cross-occupancy of aldosterone receptors; neither hormone influenced Na-K-ATPase in segments of the nephron where aldosterone receptors are absent.

Acknowledgments. Some of our studies were performed in collaboration with A. Doucet, J. P. Hayslett, W. J. Jones, and S. M.-K. Lee. This work was supported by National Institutes of Health Grant AM 13601 and by the Chicago Heart Association.

References

1. SCHMIDT U, SCHMID J, SCHMID H, DUBACH UC: Sodium- and potassium-activated ATPase: A possible target of aldosterone. *J Clin Invest* 55:655–660, 1975
2. PETTY KJ, KOKKO JP, MARVER D: Secondary effect of aldosterone on Na-K-ATPase activity in the rabbit cortical collecting tubule. *J Clin Invest* 68:1514–1521, 1981
3. RODRIGUEZ HJ, SINHA SK, STARLING J, KLAHR S: Regulation of renal Na$^+$-K$^+$-ATPase in the rat by adrenal steroids. *Am J Physiol* 241:F186–F195, 1981
4. RAYSON BM, EDELMAN IS: Glucocorticoid stimulation of Na-K-ATPase in superfused distal segments of kidney tubules in vitro. *Am J Physiol* 243:F463–F470, 1982
5. MUJAIS SK, CHEKAL MA, JONES WJ, HAYSLETT JP, KATZ AI: Regulation of renal Na-K-ATPase in the rat: Role of the natural mineralo- and glucocorticoid hormones. *J Clin Invest* 73:13–19, 1984
6. DOUCET A, KATZ AI: Short-term effect of aldosterone on Na-K-ATPase in single nephron segments. *Am J Physiol* 241:F273–F278, 1981
7. DOUCET A, KATZ AI: Mineralocorticoid receptors along the nephron: [³H]aldosterone binding in rabbit tubules. *Am J Physiol* 241:F605–F611, 1981
8. LEE SMK, CHEKAL MA, KATZ AI: Corticosterone binding sites along the rat nephron. *Am J Physiol* 244:F504–F509, 1983
9. MUJAIS SK, CHEKAL MA, JONES WJ, HAYSLETT JP, KATZ AI: Effect of adrenal

steroids on Na-K-ATPase in single segments of the rat nephron. *Clin Res* 31:781A, 1983

10. FUNDER JW, FELDMAN D, EDELMAN IS: The role of plasma binding and receptor specificity in the mineralocorticoid action of aldosterone. *Endocrinology* 92:994–1004, 1973

11. FUNDER JW, FELDMAN D, EDELMAN IS: Glucocorticoid receptors in rat kidney: The binding of tritiated dexamethasone. *Endocrinology* 92:1005–1013, 1973

12. FELDMAN D, FUNDER JW, EDELMAN IS: Evidence for a new class of corticosterone receptors in the rat kidney. *Endocrinology* 92:1429–1441, 1973

13. EDELMAN IS: Mechanism of action of steroid hormones. *J Steroid Biochem* 6:147–159, 1975

14. GROSS JB, KOKKO JP: Effects of aldosterone and potassium-sparing diuretics on electrical potential differences across the nephron. *J Clin Invest* 59:82–89, 1977

15. MARVER D, SCHWARTZ MJ: Identification of mineralocorticoid target sites in the isolated rabbit cortical nephron. *Proc Natl Acad Sci USA* 77:3672–3676, 1980

16. MARVER D: Evidence of corticosteroid action along the nephron. *Am J Physiol* 246:F111–F123, 1984

17. VANDEWALLE A, FARMAN N, BENCSATH P, BONVALET JP: Aldosterone binding along the rabbit nephron: An autoradiographic study on isolated tubules. *Am J Physiol* 240:F172–F179, 1981

18. FARMAN N, VANDEWALLE A, BONVALET JP: Aldosterone binding in isolated tubules: I. Biochemical determination in proximal and distal parts of the rabbit nephron. *Am J Physiol* 242:F63–F68, 1982

19. FARMAN N, VANDEWALLE A, BONVALET JP: Aldosterone binding in isolated tubules: II. An autoradiographic study of concentration dependency in the rabbit nephron. *Am J Physiol* 242:F69–F77, 1982

20. FARMAN N, VANDEWALLE A, BONVALET JP: Autoradiographic determination of dexamethasone binding sites along the rabbit nephron. *Am J Physiol* 244:F325–F334, 1983

21. KATZ AI: Renal Na-K-ATPase: Its role in tubular sodium and potassium transport. *Am J Physiol* 242:F207–F219, 1982

22. HORSTER M, SCHMID H, SCHMIDT U: Aldosterone in vitro restores nephron Na-K-ATPase of distal segments from adrenalectomized rabbits. *Pfluegers Arch* 384:203–206, 1980

23. CHIGNELL CF, TITUS E: Effect of adrenal steroids on a Na^+- and K^+-requiring adenosine triphosphatase from rat kidney. *J Biol Chem* 241:5083–5089, 1966

24. SINHA SK, RODRIGUEZ HJ, HOGAN WC, KLAHR S: Mechanisms of activation of renal $(Na^+ + K^+)$-ATPase in the rat. Effects of acute and chronic administration of dexamethasone. *Biochim Biophys Acta* 641:20–35, 1981

25. GARG LC, KNEPPER MA, BURG MB: Mineralocorticoid effects on Na-K-ATPase in individual nephron segments. *Am J Physiol* 240:F536–F544, 1981

26. LE HIR M, KAISSLING B, DUBACH UC: Distal tubular segments of the rabbit kidney after adaptation to altered Na- and K-intake: II. Changes in Na-K-ATPase activity. *Cell Tissue Res* 224:493–504, 1982

27. EL MERNISSI G, CHABARDÈS D, DOUCET A, HUS-CITHAREL A, IMBERT-TEBOUL M, LE BOUFFANT F, MONTÉGUT M, SIAUME S, MOREL F: Changes in tubular basolateral membrane markers after chronic DOCA treatment. *Am J Physiol* 245:F100–F109, 1983

28. MARTIN RS, JONES WJ, HAYSLETT JP: Animal model to study the effect of adrenal hormones on epithelial function. *Kidney Int* 24:386–391, 1983

Localization of Aldosterone Receptors Along the Nephron

Nicolette Farman and Jean-Pierre Bonvalet

This chapter is directed toward the localization of binding sites for aldosterone along the mammalian nephron. The main body of our data consists of autoradiographic detection of aldosterone receptors on intact tubular segments that were isolated by microdissection from kidney tissue incubated in vitro with tritiated aldosterone. Indeed, the finding of specific receptors for a hormone in a particular tubular epithelium is strong evidence for designating this epithelium as a site of action for the hormone, providing criteria for the presence of receptors are fulfilled: that is, high-affinity, low-capacity hormone and tissue specificity, and subsequent biologic response. Nevertheless, it should be emphasized that the binding of the hormone to its receptors is the very initial step of its cellular action. Following this step, multiple intracellular events (DNA transcription, RNA processing, and protein synthesis) lead to physiologic expression. This expression and its eventual modulation could vary among epithelial cells according to their metabolic and enzymatic equipment, and to the general organization of the epithelium, which largely differs along the nephron. Consequently, it should be kept in mind that different physiologic responses could be observed in two tubular segments that each present specific aldosterone binding.

Concerning aldosterone, it has been largely documented that it binds with a high affinity and specificity to a class of receptors considered to be its actual specific receptors, namely the type I or mineralocorticoid binding sites; and, also to at least another class of receptors with lower affinity and higher capacity. This second class of binding sites (type II sites) is generally considered to be representative of specific binding sites for glucocorticoids. Differentiation of binding of aldosterone to these two types of sites lies on indirect arguments drawn mainly from the observation of the dose-dependent increase in binding and steroid specificity.

We will report on experiments performed in the rabbit and the rat at concentrations ranging from 0.2 to 20 nM, including competition experiments.

This manuscript was presented as part of a Symposium on *Aldosterone and the Kidney*.

Methods

Experiments were done on rabbits that were fed a low-potassium, high-sodium diet and also on adrenalectomized rats. Isolated tubular segments [proximal convoluted tubule (PCT), pars recta (PR), thin descending limb (TDL), thin ascending limb (TAL), thick medullary (MAL) and cortical (CAL) ascending limbs of the loop of Henle, distal tubule in its initial (DCT$_b$) and late (DCT$_g$ or DCT$_l$) portion, cortical collecting tubule (CCT$_g$ or CCT$_l$), and medullary collecting tubule (MCT) in its papillary portion] were obtained via microdissection [1]. Microdissection was performed after previous in vitro incubation of kidney pyramids in the presence of collagenase and tritiated steroid ± an excess of unlabeled steroids to determine the specificity of the binding. In some cases, experiments were performed after in vivo injection of steroids.

Autoradiographs were done, using a dry x-ray film technique [1] that avoided diffusion of the marker. Quantification of labeling (silver grain density per 100 μm^2 over cytoplasmic or nuclear areas) was performed. Specific binding was calculated by subtracting nonspecific binding (tritiated steroid in presence of an excess unlabeled steroid) from total binding (tritiated steroid alone).

In one series, we determined specific nuclear binding of aldosterone by using microbiochemical methods on isolated tubules [2].

Results and Discussion

Figure 1 illustrates the labeling observed in a rabbit CCT and PCT, at 2 nM aldosterone. A clear, nuclear specific labeling, which was assessed by the displacement of label in presence of an excess-unlabeled aldosterone, is apparent in CCT; whereas, labeling is almost absent in PCT. This is in accordance with our microbiochemical results on specific nuclear binding in isolated CCT and PCT. This study [2] revealed the presence of specific receptors in CCT and not in PCT. The Kd was about 1 nM. The number of sites in the CCT has been estimated to be about 250×10^{-14} moles/mg DNA, or 10^5 per cell in this structure. These figures are much higher than those found in whole kidney tissue [3], which is an expected finding, since the kidney is presumably composed of a minority of target cells and a majority of nontarget cells for aldosterone.

Quantification of specific nuclear labeling by aldosterone at three concentrations (0.2 to 20 nM), is given in Figure 2 for the rabbit and the rat. In the rabbit [4], at the lowest concentration (0.2 nM), only DCT$_g$ and CCT$_g$ exhibited significant specific aldosterone nuclear binding. With increasing concentrations, specific nuclear labeling appeared in all nephron segments, except the proximal tubule. Saturation was reached at 2 nM in the DCT and CCT. In other segments (loop of Henle and the MCT), binding increased with concentration. Binding values equivalent to that of both the DCT and CCT were reached only in the CAL and MCT, but only at 20 nM. Some macula densae could be obtained that exhibited a clear nuclear labeling. The rat [5] resembles the rabbit, with some minor differences. At 0.2 nM, only CCT$_l$ and not DCT$_l$ was labeled. The specific nuclear labeling became equivalent

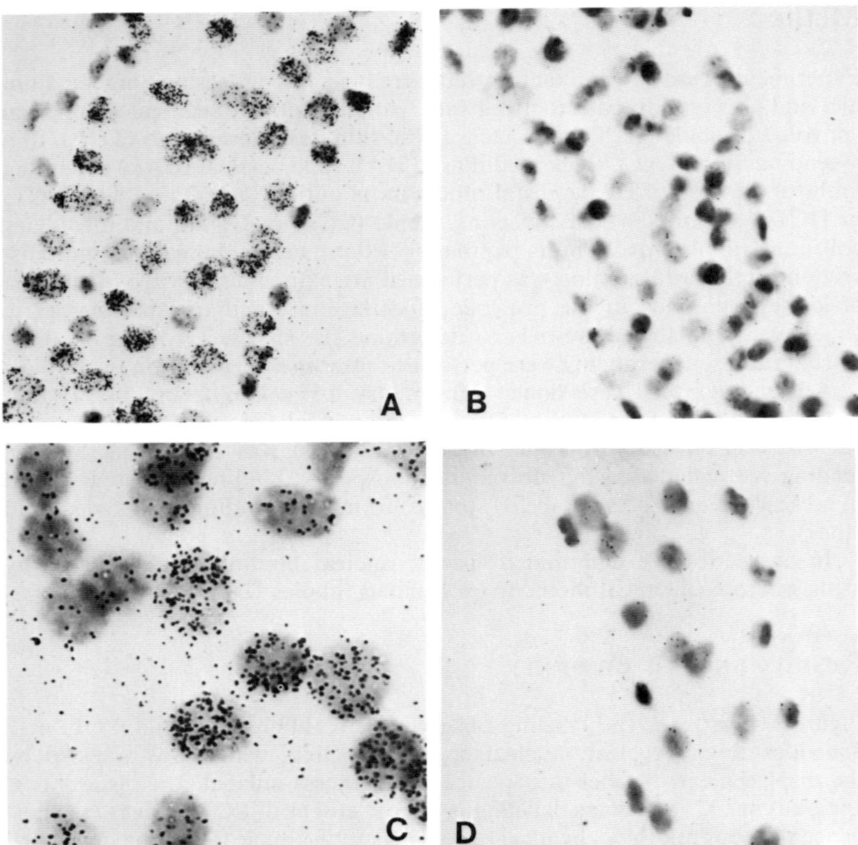

Fig. 1. Autoradiographs of CCT and PCT after incubation with 2 nM (^{3}H)-aldosterone. **A** CCT ($\times$490) incubated with (^{3}H)-aldosterone alone. A highly exclusive nuclear labeling is present, which is heterogeneous from one nucleus to another, as shown on an enlargement **(C)** ($\times$1300). **B** Displacement of the labeling by an excess of ($\times$200) unlabeled aldosterone in CCT. **D** in PCT, no labeling is present.

all along the loop and distal structures at 2 and 20 nM. As in the rabbit, no significant specific nuclear labeling was present at any concentration in the PCT and PR. Cytoplasmic-specific labeling was absent in all segments at any concentration in both species. However, some nonspecific labeling appeared at 20 nM, in the proximal tubule, particularly in the PR.

Competition studies revealed that in the CCT, aldosterone is unequivocally the best competitor in both species [4, 5]. Figure 3 illustrates steroid specificity of the binding along the rat nephron. In contrast with CCT$_l$, a mixed (dexamethasone and aldosterone) specificity was observed all along the loop of Henle and in the DCT$_b$, DCT$_l$, and MCT.

When all of these results are considered together, the CCT emerges as the most mineralocorticoid target segment, in the sense that specific binding appears at low concentrations; highest values of labeling are observed in

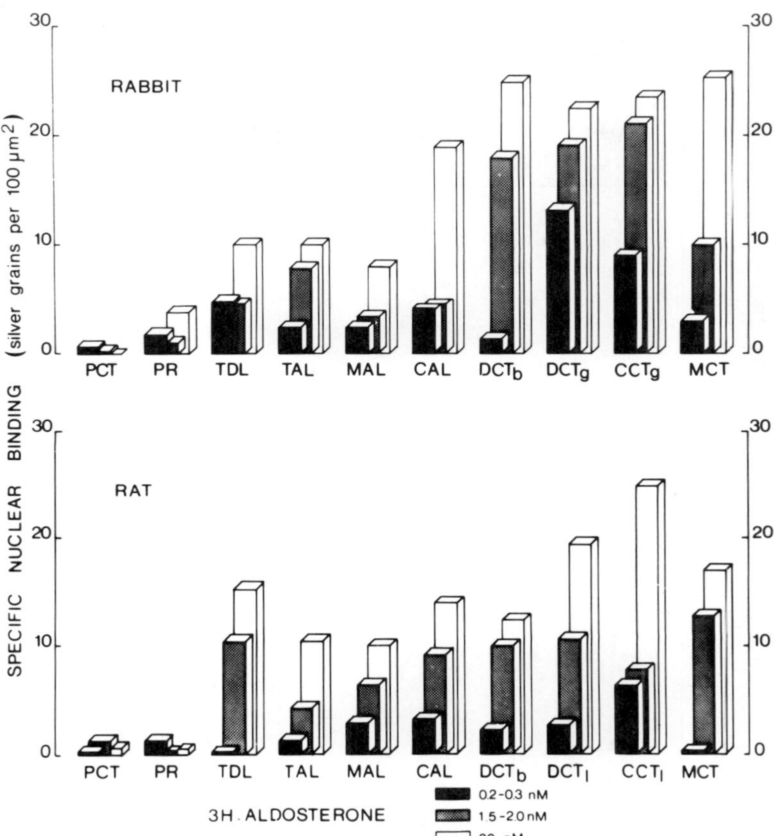

Fig. 2. Profiles of specific nuclear labeling along the nephron of the rat and the rabbit at three concentrations (0.2, 2, and 20 nM) of (^{3}H)-aldosterone.

this segment, with very selective mineralocorticoid specificity. This finding correlates with other studies on aldosterone binding [6, 7], enzyme induction [8–11], and aldosterone-modulated sodium and potassium transport [12–14]. In the DCT, some dissociation appears between these elements. At 2 nM, binding values are similar in the DCT_b, DCT_g, or DCT_l, and CCT_g, or CCT_l. Paired comparisons of specific nuclear labeling in the DCT and CCT from the same nephron revealed no difference [1]. However, at 0.2 nM, DCT_b (rabbit) or DCT_b and DCT_l (rat) did not exhibit significant specific nuclear labeling. In competition studies, dexamethasone displaced aldosterone binding in the DCT as well as aldosterone. All along the loop of Henle and the MCT, the appearance of specific nuclear labeling for higher concentrations than in the CCT—without saturation associated with a mixed steroid specificity—is in favor of an occupancy by aldosterone of type II sites in combination with a small number of type I sites. In fact, a clear prevalence of glucocorticoid binding sites is likely in these segments, as it can be seen on dexamethasone autoradiographs. For the DCT, the question is less clear due to the high

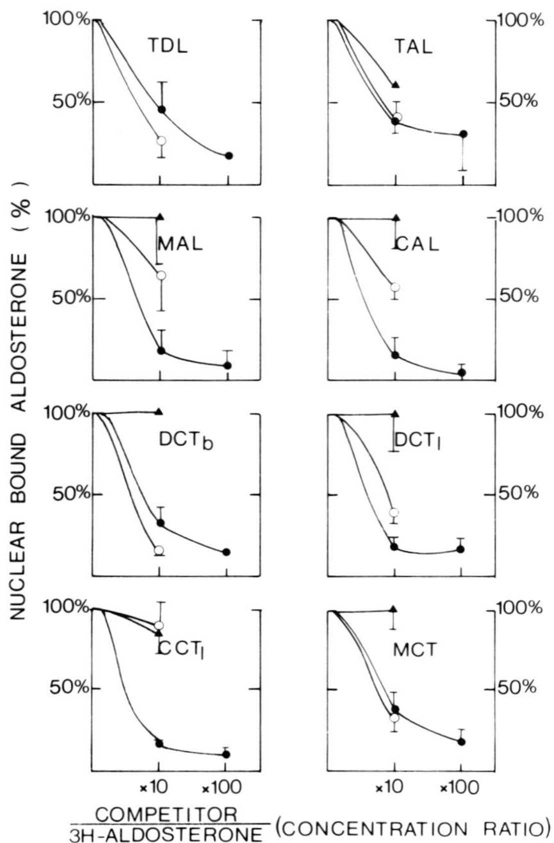

Fig. 3. Competition studies of nuclear (^{3}H)-aldosterone binding (20 nM) along the rat nephron, with 10- or 100-fold excess-unlabeled aldosterone (●), dexamethasone (○), and estradiol (▲). The best aldosterone specificity is in CCT. (Reprinted with permission from [5])

binding values, even at low concentration. This could suggest the presence of mineralocorticoid binding sites in the DCT, which are less abundant than in the CCT, but more than in the CAL and MCT. A low number of aldosterone binding sites, in comparison with glucocorticoid sites, could be at the origin of the failure to evidence aldosterone binding sites in another biochemical study [7] or aldosterone-modulated enzyme induction [8] or transport [12]. These aspects will be widely discussed by the other participants in this symposium.

We directly examined the distribution of binding sites for (^{3}H)-dexamethasone along the rabbit nephron [15]. Numerous specific nuclear binding sites are present along the nephron, except in the PCT and pars recta. The binding appeared at 3 nM, with no clear difference between segments; and no saturation was observed up to 53 nM. For comparable concentrations and specific activities, the intensity of specific nuclear labeling, which probably reflects the number of glucocorticoid binding sites, is much higher than for aldosterone. Therefore, if one compares the specific nuclear labeling for aldosterone and dexamethasone at concentrations of each hormone that correspond approximately to their respective Kd (2 nM for aldosterone and 20 nM for dexamethasone), the ratio of dexamethasone to aldosterone-specific labeling is about 4 in the DCT and CCT and 10 to 20 in the loop of Henle and the MCT. In the PCT and pars recta, the absence of specific nuclear labeling is contrasted with the existence of a diffuse specific cytoplasmic labeling. The significance of this cytoplasmic-specific labeling in the proximal tubule remains unclear. It could be related, for example, to differential nucleocytoplasmic kinetics in proximal and distal structures, to some metabolism of the hormone, or to nongenomic effects of steroids in the proximal tubule.

Some experiments were designed to check whether in vitro results actually correspond to the binding localization after in vivo injection of tritiated aldosterone or dexamethasone [15]. Fifteen min after injection, proximal tubules and cortical collecting ducts were processed for autoradiography without previous collagenase incubation. Nuclear labeling was present in the CCT and not in the PCT or pars recta. No cytoplasmic labeling appeared in the CCT, whereas it was present in the PCT and pars recta in dexamethasone-injected animals. These data are in very good accordance with in vitro findings.

The binding of aldosterone and dexamethasone to glomerular cells was examined in a particular series of autoradiographs [16]. No specific labeling by (^{3}H)-aldosterone was detectable in glomeruli or glomerular arterioles up to 24 nM. Some specific nuclear labeling by dexamethasone was present in glomerular cells, which increased from 4 to 110 nM. However, these values were about five times lower than those observed in the distal tubular structures. At 110 nM, glomerular arterioles also exhibited specific nuclear labeling. Our technique does not allow a distinction between the different glomerular cell types, thus precluding any detection of a preferential binding on one particular glomerular cell type.

Medullary structures are physiologically submitted to wide variations of osmolarity; and, conformational changes of receptor molecules have been described, depending on a low or high sodium environment. We examined whether incubation of kidney pyramids in isotonic (300 mOsm) or hypertonic (600 mOsm) solutions could result in changes in binding capacity of aldosterone in medullary structures (thin and thick medullary ascending limb and papillary collecting tubule). This was not the case. No difference in specific nuclear labeling by (^{3}H)-aldosterone (2 nM) was found for each of these structures after isotonic or hypertonic incubation (unpublished data).

The question of the appearance of specific binding sites for aldosterone during ontogenesis is of interest, since maturation of tubular structure and function is not achieved at birth in rats and rabbits, and homeostatic conditions are quite different before and after birth. In fetuses (1 to 3 days before birth), specific nuclear binding was present in amounts comparable to adult collecting tubules, and no binding was found in either fetus or adult proximal structures (unpublished data). The appearance of binding sites in the distal nephron, thus, is precocious, with a localization along the tubule that seems to be comparable to that of the adult.

Finally, we would like to comment about the heterogeneity of ^{3}H-aldosterone labeling from one collecting duct nucleus to another. This is particularly striking in Figure 1, where low-density labeled nuclei neighbor heavily labeled ones. It is unlikely that such heterogeneity depends on technical reasons (such as variable distances between nuclei and the film, leading to Gaussian distribution of labeling). Cell-to-cell heterogeneity also was observed for uridine incorporation in isolated tubular segments; statistical analysis of the distribution of labeling within the cell population of the CCT does not fit with a random distribution. In addition, this heterogeneity was also found on histologic slices (unpublished data). For aldosterone [4] as well as for uridine [17], heterogeneity of nucler labeling was not observed in the CAL (handled in conditions similar to the CCT, and known to be composed of only one cell type), in contrast to the CCT, which is composed of at least two main cell types. The question of a differential effect of steroids on these two cell types—light (principal) and dark cells that are clearly distinct, based on morphologic criteria—is open. Several lines of evidence indicate that a differential effect may be possible. Amplification of basolateral membranes after chronic deoxycorticosterone acetate (DOCA) treatment affects only principal cells [18]. Basal uridine incorporation reflecting RNA synthesis differs in the two cell types, and relative modulation of this incorporation is differently affected by DOCA treatment (unpublished data). Nevertheless, these experimental protocols do not distinguish between a mineralocorticoid and a glucocorticoid effect, or between a primary versus secondary effect. If these effects are really primary and mineralocorticoid-specific, it would be of great interest to determine whether they are due to different binding capacities or to modulation of intracellular steps that intervene beyond the binding of steroids to its receptors. This issue deserves further investigation.

Summary

The localization of aldosterone receptors along the nephron has been investigated on microdissected glomeruli and tubular segments of the rabbit and rat kidney. Biochemical methods and quantitative autoradiography on dry film have been used after in vitro incubation. Based on high specific nuclear binding values, dose response curves, and competition studies, the cortical collecting tubule (CCT) appears to be the most selective binding site for aldosterone. The distal convoluted tubule (DCT) also presents high binding, but with lower mineralocorticoid specificity. In the loop of Henle and the medullary collecting tubule (MCT), aldosterone binding is likely to be to a mixture of a few mineralocorticoid and abundant glucocorticoid sites, which have been demonstrated directly in all of these segments of the rabbit nephron by (^{3}H)-dexamethasone binding studies. No specific nuclear aldosterone or dexamethasone binding was detected in proximal tubules. Similar results were obtained after in vivo injections of steroids. No major difference in the localization of aldosterone binding sites along the tubule appears between the rat and the rabbit. In glomeruli or juxtaglomerular arterioles of the rabbit kidney, only dexamethasone binding was found. In the rabbit, aldosterone binding was already present in the CCT of fetal nephrons. Variation of osmolarity does not influence aldosterone binding in medullary structures. In the CCT, cell-to-cell heterogeneity of binding is clearly present; is discussed its function in light of the known cellular heterogeneity in this segment.

References

1. VANDEWALLE A, FARMAN N, BENCSATH P, BONVALET JP: Aldosterone binding along the rabbit nephron: an autoradiographic study on isolated tubules. *Am J Physiol* 240(9):F172–F179, 1981
2. FARMAN N, VANDEWALLE A, BONVALET JP: Aldosterone binding in isolated tubule: I/Biochemical determination in proximal and distal parts of the rabbit nephron. *Am J Physiol* 242(11):F63–F68, 1982
3. FARMAN N, VANDEWALLE A, BONVALET JP: Binding of aldosterone to cytoplasmic and nuclear receptors of the rabbit kidney. *Am J Physiol* 240(9):C20–C27, 1981
4. FARMAN N, VANDEWALLE A, BONVALET JP: Aldosterone binding in isolated tubules: II. An autoradiographic study of concentration dependency in the rabbit nephron. *Am J Physiol* 242(11):F69–F77, 1982
5. FARMAN N, BONVALET JP: Aldosterone binding in isolated tubules. III. Autoradiography along the rat nephron. *Am J Physiol* 245(14):F606–F614, 1983
6. SCHOLER DW, MISHINA T, EDELMAN IS: Distribution of aldosterone receptors in rat kidney cortical tubules enriched in proximal and distal segments. *Am J Physiol* 237(6):F360–F366, 1979
7. DOUCET A, KATZ AI: Mineralocorticoid receptors along the nephron: (^{3}H)-aldosterone binding in rabbit tubule. *Am J Physiol* 241(10):F605–F611, 1981
8. MARVER D, SCHWARTZ MJ: Identification of mineralocorticoid target sites in the isolated rabbit cortical nephron. *Proc Natl Acad Sci USA* 77:3672–3676, 1980
9. GARG LC, KNEPPER MA, BURG MB: Mineralocorticoid effects on Na-K-ATPase in individual nephron segments. *Am J Physiol* 240(9):F536–F544, 1981
10. PETTY KJ, KOKKO JP, MARVER D: Secondary effect of aldosterone on Na-K-ATPase activity in the rabbit cortical collecting tubule. *J Clin Invest* 68:1514–1521, 1981
11. EL MERNISSI G, DOUCET A: Short-term effect of aldosterone on renal sodium transport and tubular Na-K-ATPase in the rat. *Pflügers Arch* 399:139–146, 1983
12. GROSS JB, IMAI M, KOKKO JP: A functional comparison of the cortical collecting tubule and the distal convoluted tubule. *J Clin Invest* 55:1284–1294, 1975
13. SCHWARTZ GJ, BURG MB: Mineralocorticoid effects on cation transport by cortical collecting tubules in vitro. *Am J Physiol* 235(6):F576–F585, 1978
14. STOKES JB, INGRAM MJ, WILLIAMS AD, INGRAM D: Heterogeneity of the rabbit collecting tubule: localization of mineralocorticoid hormone action to the cortical portion. *Kidney Int* 20:340–347, 1981
15. FARMAN N, VANDEWALLE A, BONVALET JP: Autoradiographic determination of dexamethasone-binding sites along the rabbit nephron. *Am J Physiol* 244(Suppl 13):F325–F334, 1983
16. FARMAN N, VANDEWALLE A, BONVALET JP: Autoradiographic study of aldosterone and dexamethasone binding in isolated glomeruli of rabbit kidney. *Am J Physiol* 243(12):F235–F242, 1982
17. VANDEWALLE A, FARMAN N, CLUZEAUD F, BONVALET JP: Heterogeneity of uridine incorporation along the nephron. I. Autoradiographic study. *Am J Physiol* 246(15):F417–F426, 1984
18. WADE JB, O'NEIL RG, PRYOR JL, BOULPAEP EL: Modulation of cell membrane area in renal collecting tubules by corticosteroid hormones. *J Cell Biol* 81:439–445, 1979

Mechanism of Action of Aldosterone: Effects on Sodium, Potassium, and Hydrogen Transport

Juha P. Kokko

Selective hypoaldosteronism in patients is associated with hyperkalemia, hyperchloremic metabolic acidosis, and salt wastage, while opposite metabolic effects have been demonstrated in patients with elevated plasma concentrations of aldosterone. These clinical observations have led to the commonly accepted view that there is a direct link between sodium (Na), potassium (K), and hydrogen (H) transport; and also, that aldosterone affects the transport of these ions by a common or an interdependent mechanism. However, recent in vitro microperfusion studies proved that this view was no longer tenable. It is now accepted generally that significant structural functional heterogeneity exists along the collecting tubule and that aldosterone will have different physiologic effects on the specific segments of the collecting tubule. It is the purpose here to discuss the transport properties of the two major target segments of mineralocorticoids—the cortical and outer medullary collecting tubules—and to review current concepts regarding the effect of aldosterone on these transport properties.

Sodium Transport

It is now well appreciated that one of the major effects of aldosterone is to stimulate renal sodium reabsorption. Thus, renal salt wastage is one of the hallmarks of primary hypoaldosteronism.

It was first suggested by the studies of Gross, Imai, and Kokko [1] that the cortical collecting tubule (CCT) and not the distal convoluted tubule (DCT) is the primary target for the antinatriuretic effect of aldosterone. This was more extensively examined later by Schwartz and Burg [2], when they noted a positive correlation between plasma aldosterone concentrations and

This manuscript was presented as part of a Symposium on *Aldosterone and the Kidney*.

sodium flux in CCTs obtained from rabbits in which the endogenous aldosterone was changed by various physiologic perturbations. A consistent finding in studies using CCTs from chronically mineralocorticoid-stimulated rabbits has been the finding of an associated increase in lumen-negative potential. Thus, it appears that chronic deoxycorticosterone (DOCA) administration stimulates active electrogenic sodium reabsorption.

While agreement has been reached on the effect of chronic DOCA administration, the effect of acute aldosterone has been more controversial and difficult to demonstrate. Indeed, Schwartz and Burg [2] were unable to demonstrate any increase in sodium reabsorption due to acute administration of aldosterone; they concluded that their studies were not conducted under appropriate conditions. More recent preliminary studies by Wingo et al [3] have demonstrated increased reabsorption of sodium from 12.7 ± 3 to 23.5 ± 7 pEq/mm/min in CCTs from adrenalectomized rabbits after the addition of 10^{-6}M aldosterone to the bath. There was no change in transepithelial potential difference. Thus, these studies suggest that acute and chronic aldosterone administrations stimulate sodium reabsorption across CCTs via different mechanisms. Acute effects are nonelectrogenic, while chronic effects involve electrogenic mechanisms. Perhaps the chronic effects involve a decrease in chloride conductance as shown by O'Neil and Helman [4], while acute effects are not associated with such changes.

To understand how aldosterone might affect sodium transport across the CCT, it is pertinent to discuss the currently accepted model by which basal-active sodium transport occurs in this segment. In this model, it has been suggested that sodium moves from lumen to cell, down a favorable electrochemical gradient through conductive pathways. While many indirect studies have suggested the existence of these pathways, the intracellular microelectrode studies by Koeppen, Biagi, and Giebisch [5] directly demonstrated the presence of these pathways at the apical membrane of a rabbit CCT; and also, that the conductance of these pathways was inhibited by luminal amiloride. The concentration of intracellular Na in the cytoplasm of CCTs has not been measured directly when all transport determinants are known, but the electron microprobe studies by Beck et al [6] in superficial DCTs contaminated with an "occasional" CCT do suggest that the sodium concentration is roughly 10 to 15 mEq/liter. Thus, under normal expected physiologic conditions, there exists a favorable downhill electrochemical driving force for entry of sodium. The active extrusion of sodium across the basolateral membrane occurs via the well-characterized Na-K-ATPase.

The mechanism by which aldosterone stimulates Na transport has been examined via a number of physiologic and microenzymatic techniques. There are three basic ways that aldosterone could stimulate Na reabsorption: (1) a primary increase in Na-K-ATPase activity, (2) an increase in the synthesis of enzymes involved with transcellular transport, and (3) an increase in apical permeability to Na.

Several studies have demonstrated that treating animals either chronically or acutely increases Na-K-ATPase activity [7–13]. These results have been obtained by using physiologic concentrations of mineralocorticoid. The studies by Petty, Kokko, and Marver [9] further demonstrate that the rise in Na-

K-ATPase activity in response to mineralocorticoid can be blocked with spirolactone; and, it does not occur in response to dexamethasone. What these results are unable to address is whether the rise in Na-K-ATPase activity is a primary response to aldosterone or a secondary response to increased apical entry of sodium. The studies by Petty, Kokko, and Marver [9] address this issue, in which it is shown that pretreatment of rabbit with sodium channel-blocker amiloride blocks the otherwise increased Na-K-ATPase activity in response to aldosterone. Thus, the studies are consistent with the view that Na-K-ATPase activity rising in response to aldosterone is the secondary consequence of increased apical entry of sodium [9]. The mechanism by which sodium increases Na-K-ATPase activity is conjectural; it remains a fertile area for research in the future.

In the other medullary collecting tubule, the primary mechanism of sodium transport is diffusional [14]. This transport mechanism is passive; therefore, it is not expected to respond to either ouabain or to mineralocorticoids [14]. Thus, aldosterone does not have a major effect in Na transport across the outer medullary collecting tubule.

Potassium Transport

Hyperkalemia is a common finding in patients with hypoaldosteronism, while increased kaliuresis and hypokalemia is common in states of chronically elevated mineralocorticoid levels. However, whether mineralocorticoids have a direct effect on potassium secretion has been difficult to establish. From a clinical viewpoint, it has been repeatedly demonstrated that mineralocorticoids do not increase K secretion when intake and urinary excretion of sodium are minimal [15–17].

Potassium transport across the collecting duct occurs via both active and passive transport mechanisms. Grantham, Burg, and Orloff [18] initially demonstrated that potassium concentration in the lumen of isolated, perfused rabbit collecting ducts reached values higher than predicted by Nernst equilibrium potentials. They also were able to show that the potassium secretory rate was decreased with either peritubular ouabain, removal of sodium from the perfusate, or removal of potassium from the bath. Thus, these studies constitute strong evidence that there exists an active potassium secretory mechanism across the collecting duct and that this process depends on sodium (secondary active potassium secretion). Whether additional non-Na-dependent, active transport processes exist across the collecting duct has not been rigorously examined, although it is clear that fixed coupling of Na to K does not exist across the entire epithelium [4].

It also is clear that there is a strong dependence of potassium transport on the transepithelial potential difference across the rabbit CCT [19, 20]. Potassium secretion rates are increased as the lumen potential becomes more negative. Thus, these studies show that passive transport down a favorable electrochemical gradient is an important determinant of net potassium transport.

O'Neil and Helman [4] have shown that the rabbit (like humans) increases urinary potassium excretion and decreases serum potassium concentrations in response to chronic DOCA treatment. They further demonstrated a progressive increase in potassium secretion in CCTs dependent on the direction of DOCA administration to rabbits from whom the tubules were harvested. The increase in potassium secretion became maximal only after 11 to 18 days of DOCA treatment. Schwartz and Burg [2] have extended these findings, in which they compared the potassium secretory rates across CCTs obtained from various groups of rabbits when the endogenous aldosterone level was manipulated by dietary and pharmacologic means. The summary of their results demonstrates a nice correlation between endogenous aldosterone and potassium secretory rates. These results, therefore, provide convincing evidence that chronic mineralocorticoid treatment stimulates potassium secretion across the CCTs.

The mechanism by which chronic mineralocorticoid affects potassium secretion can be the result of a number of different factors: increase in lumen negativity, increase in Na-K ATPase, increase in driving forces for intracellular movement of potassium from the blood side, and increase in apical membrane conductance to potassium. It is now well established that the luminal PD becomes more negative with chronic mineralocorticoids [1, 2, 4, 21–24]. It also has been demonstrated that there is an increase in Na-K-ATPase activity in collecting ducts from animals receiving mineralocorticoids [7–13]. It is not known whether other factors contribute to the increased K secretion in response to mineralocorticoids. It is interesting to note from the studies by Koeppen, Biagi, and Giebisch [5] that the basolateral potential clearly becomes more negative (−105 mv) in collecting tubules from DOCA-treated rabbits, as compared to tubules from control animals [−84 mv]. Thus, there is an increased driving force for the influx of potassium from the blood side into the collecting tubule cells. They also noted a slight decrease in the apical-to-basolateral membrane resistance ratio, but (as pointed out by the authors) the significance of the resistance ratio is difficult to interpret. However, the studies by Koeppen et al [5] are consistent with the view that chronic DOCA may influence potassium secretion by mechanisms that are additional to the previously demonstrated effects of DOCA on the transepithelial PD and Na-K-ATPase.

No active transport processes for potassium secretion have been identified as existing in the medullary collecting duct obtained from regular rabbits or from rabbits that have received DOCA [14]. Thus, the medullary collecting duct has different transport characteristics for potassium, since it does not increase its secretion of potassium in response to chronic mineralocorticoid administration.

Hydrogen Transport

Hyperchloremic metabolic acidosis is a common metabolic abnormality with primary hypoaldosteronism. However, the direct role of mineralocorticoids in bicarbonate (HCO_3) reabsorption (or hydrogen secretion) across collecting duct segments has been difficult to establish prior to in vitro microperfusion studies. There are two general issues that have been the focus of recent research: (1) the site and mechanism of hydrogen transport, and (2) the effect of mineralocorticoids in these transport processes.

McKinney and Burg [25–27] were the first to demonstrate that the CCT of the rabbit could either secrete or reabsorb HCO_3, depending on the metabolic status of the rabbit from which the tubules were dissected. Thus, tubules obtained from rabbits who were made acidotic by receiving ammonium chloride reabsorbed HCO_3, while tubules from alkalotic rabbits secreted HCO_3. These findings were subsequently confirmed by Lombard, Kokko, and Jacobson [28].

The mechanism of HCO_3 reabsorption in the CCT is interesting in that McKinney and Burg [26] determined that it does not require sodium, is not inhibited by ouabain, but is inhibited by 10^{-4} M acetazolamide. Koeppen and Helman [29] also have shown that luminal acidification can occur in the absence of NaCl. However, in more recent studies, Laski and Kurtzman [30] have shown a decrease in the transepithelial potential difference and in HCO_3 reabsorption with replacement of 40 mM NaCl by LiCl in perfusate and bath. However, this decrease in bicarbonate reabsorption or acidification may reflect the secondary role of the transepithelial PD on acidification. Indeed, Koeppen and Helman [29] have found a nice correlation with increased luminal negativity induced by chronic DOCA and minimal pH of the collected fluid. Since the CCT is finitely permeable to H (1.3×10^{-3} cm/sec) [31], it is not surprising to see a positive relationship between lumen-negative PD and lumen-acidic pH. Why such a relationship has not been consistently demonstrated with ouabain [26] is not clear.

The characteristics of bicarbonate reabsorption differ in outer medullary tubules contrasted with the CCTs. When these two segments are studied under similar in vitro microperfusion techniques, the studies by Lombard, Kokko, and Jacobson [28] show that the outer medullary collecting tubule reabsorbs 4 to 7 times more HCO_3/mm of tubule length than does the CCT. Furthermore, these studies demonstrated that the medullary collecting tubule always reabsorbed bicarbonate irrespective of the acid-base status of the rabbit from which they were harvested [28]. Studies also have shown that the bicarbonate reabsorption is not dependent on luminal replacement of sodium with tetramethylammonium [32], is decreased with bath substitution of chloride with gluconate [33], and is associated with lumen-positive voltage [28, 30, 32, 33]. Furthermore, the studies have shown that the bicarbonate reabsorption is inhibited by 10^{-4} M acetazolamide [28].

Thus, the available data are consistent with the model of medullary collecting duct acidification in which the primary H secretory mechanism is located on the apical membrane, while the base exit at the basolateral membrane occurs in exchange for chloride. Due to the present uncertainty concerning the magnitude of apical chloride conductance, it is not known what fraction of chloride moves transcellularly when contrasted with paracellular routes. What is clear from the studies by Stone et al [33] is that chloride secretion occurred at the same rate as hydrogen secretion, indicating that the outer medullary collecting duct secretes HCl.

Further support for the model of medullary collecting tubule acidification are the recent studies by Stone et al [34] that used luminal fraction-enriched vesicles from bovine renal medulla. In these studies, they provided evidence for the existence of proton-translocating ATPase. Their studies suggest luminal membrane localization of the proton-translocating ATPase, since in their vesicle preparation, ouabain-sensitive ATPase was virtually eliminated [34]. Further studies nevertheless are necessary to rigorously prove the apical membrane localization of the proton-translocating ATPase.

The role of mineralocorticoid modulation of rabbit medullary-collecting duct acidification has been recently clarified. In the studies by Stone et al [32], they determined that chronic administration of DOCA to rabbits increased HCO_3 reabsorption significantly from medullary collecting tubule segments that were harvested from these rabbits. In addition to the chronic mineralocorticoid effect, they were able to show that acute addition of 5×10^{-8} M aldosterone to the bath of medullary collecting tubules caused a significant increase in HCO_3 reabsorption, and also that this increase was evident in the absence of luminal Na or in the presence of luminal amiloride [32]. Thus, mineralocorticoids increase medullary collecting duct acidification both acutely and chronically.

Summary

It is evident that aldosterone exerts major effects on Na, K, and H transport across cortical and outer medullary collecting tubules. Aldosterone stimulates primary active Na absorption across CCTs, while not influencing Na transport across outer medullary collecting tubules. The chronic effects of aldosterone on Na transport are electrogenic, while aldosterone stimulates Na reabsorption acutely by electroneutral mechanisms. Chronic mineralocorticoid exposure stimulates active and passive secretion of K across the CCT, but not the medullary collecting tubule. In CCT, chronic mineralocorticoid treatment causes the lumen pH to become more acidic, while in the outer medullary collecting duct, aldosterone stimulates a higher capacity system of Na-independent H secretion. Thus, aldosterone exerts different transport effects on specific segments of the collecting tubule system.

References

1. Gross JB, Imai M, Kokko JP: A functional comparison of the cortical collecting tubule and the distal convoluted tubule. *J Clin Invest* 55:1284–1294, 1975
2. Schwartz GJ, Burg MB: Mineralocorticoid effects on cation transport by cortical collecting tubules in vitro. *Am J Physiol* 235:F576–F585, 1978
3. Wingo CS, Kokko JP, Jacobson HR: Evidence for different acute and chronic

actions of mineralocorticoids on the rabbit cortical collecting tubule (*abstract*). *Clin Res* 29:481a, 1981

4. O'NEIL RG, HELMAN SI: Transport characteristics of renal collecting tubules: influences of DOCA and diet. *Am J Physiol* 233:F544–F558, 1977
5. KOEPPEN BM, BIAGI BA, GIEBISCH GH: Intracellular microelectrode characterization of the rabbit cortical collecting duct. *Am J Physiol* 244:F35–F47, 1983
6. BECK F, BAUER R, BAUER U, MASON J, DORGE A, RICK R, THURAU K: Electron microprobe analysis of intracellular elements in the rat kidney. *Kidney Int* 17:756–763, 1980
7. SCHMIDT V, SCHMID J, SCHMID H, DUBACH UC: Sodium and potassium activated ATPase. A possible target of aldosterone. *J Clin Invest* 55:655–660, 1975
8. KATZ AI, DOUCET A, MOREL F: Na-K-ATPase activity along the rabbit, rat, and mouse nephron. *Am J Physiol* 237:F114–F120, 1979
9. PETTY KJ, KOKKO JP, MARVER D: Secondary effect of aldosterone on Na-K ATPase activity in the rabbit cortical collecting tubule. *J Clin Invest* 68:1514–1521, 1981
10. GARG LC, KNEPPER MA, BURG MB: Mineralocorticoid effects on Na-K-ATPase in individual nephron segments. *Am J Physiol* 240:F536–F544, 1981
11. HORSTER M, SCHMID H, SCHMIDT U: Aldosterone in vitro restores nephron Na-K-ATPase of distal segments from adrenalectomized rabbits. *Pflügers Arch* 384:203–206, 1980
12. KNOX WH, SEN AD: Mechanism of action of aldosterone with particular reference to (Na + K)—ATPase. *Ann NY Acad Sci* 242:471–488, 1974
13. EL MERNISSI G, CHABARDES D, DOUCET A, HUS-CITHARD A, IMBERT-TEBOUL M, LE BOUFFANT F, MONTEGUT M, SIAUME S, MOREL F: Changes in tubular basolateral membrane markers after chronic DOCA treatment. *Am J Physiol* 245:F100–F109, 1983
14. STOKES JB: Na and K transport across the cortical and outer medullary collecting tubule of the rabbit: evidence for diffusion across the outer medullary portion. *Am J Physiol* 242:F514–F520, 1982
15. SELDIN DW, WELT LG, CORT JH: The role of Na salts and adrenal steroids in the production of hypokalemic alkalosis. *Yale J Biol Med* 29:229, 1956
16. RELMAN AS, SCHWARTZ WB: The effect of DOCA on electrolyte balance in normal man and its relation to sodium chloride intake. *Yale J Biol Med* 24:540, 1956
17. FINN A, WELT LG: Effect of aldosterone administration on electrolyte excretion and GFR in the rat. *Am J Physiol* 204:243–244, 1963
18. GRANTHAM JJ, BURG MB, ORLOFF J: The nature of transtubular Na and K transport in isolated rabbit renal collecting tubules. *J Clin Invest* 49:1815–1826, 1970
19. STOKES JB: Potassium secretion by cortical collecting tubule: relation to sodium absorption, luminal sodium concentration, and transepithelial voltage. *Am J Physiol* 241:F395–F402, 1981
20. WINGO CS, SELDIN DW, KOKKO JP: Dietary modulation of active potassium secretion in the cortical collecting tubule of adrenalectomized rabbits. *J Clin Invest* 70:579–586, 1982
21. GROSS JB, KOKKO JP: Effects of aldosterone and potassium-sparing diuretics on electrical potential differences across the distal nephron. *J Clin Invest* 59:82–89, 1977
22. STOKES JB, INGRAM MG, WILLIAMS AD, INGRAM D: Heterogeneity of the rabbit collecting tubule: localization of mineralocorticoid action in the cortical portion. *Kidney Int* 20:340–347, 1981

23. Holt WF, Lechene C: ADH-PGE$_2$ interactions in cortical collecting tubule. I. Depression of sodium transport. *Am J Physiol* 241:F452–F460, 1981
24. Wingo CS, Kokko JP, Jacobson HR: Effects of in vitro aldosterone on the rabbit cortical collecting tubule. *Kidney Int* (submitted, 1984)
25. McKinney TD, Burg MB: Bicarbonate transport by rabbit cortical collecting tubules. Effect of acid and alkali loads in vivo on transport in vitro. *J Clin Invest* 60:766–768, 1977
26. McKinney TD, Burg MB: Bicarbonate reabsorption by rabbit cortical collecting tubules in vitro. *Am J Physiol* 234:F141–145, 1978
27. McKinney TD, Burg MB: Bicarbonate secretion by rabbit cortical collecting tubules in vitro. *J Clin Invest* 61:1421–1427, 1978
28. Lombard WE, Kokko JP, Jacobson HR: Bicarbonate transport in cortical and outer medullary collecting tubules. *Am J Physiol* 244:F289–F296, 1983
29. Koeppen BM, Helman SI: Acidification of luminal fluid by the rabbit cortical collecting tubule perfused in vitro. *Am J Physiol* 242:F521–F531, 1982
30. Laski ME, Kurtzman NA: Characterization of acidification in the cortical and medullary collecting tubule of the rabbit. *J Clin Invest* 72:2050–2059, 1983
31. Hamm LL, Pucacco LR, Kokko JP, Jacobson HR: Hydrogen ion (H$^+$) permeability of isolated perfused tubules (*abstract*). *Am Soc Nephrology* 14:107A, 1981
32. Stone DK, Seldin DW, Kokko JP, Jacobson HR: Mineralocorticoid modulation of rabbit medullary collecting duct acidification: a sodium-independent effect. *J Clin Invest* 72:77–83, 1983
33. Stone DK, Seldin DW, Kokko JP, Jacobson HR: Anion dependence of rabbit medullary collecting duct acidification. *J Clin Invest* 71:1505–1508, 1983
34. Stone DK, Xie X-S, Wu L-T, Racker E: Proton translocating ATPases of clathrin-coated vesicles, renal medulla, and Erhrlich ascites tumor cells, in *Hydrogen Ion Transport in Epithelia,* edited by Forte J, Rector FC, New York, John Wiley & Sons (in press, 1984).

Mechanism of Action of Aldosterone: Role of Na-K-ATPase

Bernard C. Rossier, Käthi Geering, and Jean-Pierre Kraehenbuhl

It is our purpose to examine the mechanism of action of aldosterone and we will reassess the model proposed by Edelman, Bogoroch, and Porter more than 20 years ago [3]. We will also present our recent contribution in this field and discuss the effect of aldosterone on Na-K-ATPase synthesis and its cell surface expression.

Aldosterone-induced Proteins: A Model Revisited

Aldosterone increases sodium reabsorption across a variety of epithelia, including the distal part of the nephron or the colon. In the urinary bladder of the toad *Bufo marinus,* the physiologic response to aldosterone (80 nM) can be divided into three distinct phases: (1) a *latent* period (about 45 min), (2) an *early response* (up to 2.5 hr) during which sodium transport increases rapidly and total resistance falls concomitantly, and (3) a *late response* (up to 24 hr) during which sodium transport further increases without change in electrical resistance [1, 2, 28]. Like other steroid hormones, aldosterone exerts its action by interacting with cytoplasmic receptors, which subsequently bind to chromatin acceptor sites, thereby controlling the expression of various genes that encode specific proteins; namely, the aldosterone-induced (AIPs) or aldosterone-repressed proteins (ARPs). These AIPs and ARPs, in turn, are responsible for the observed changes of sodium transport across the target epithelial cells [3–6]. Like glucocorticoids [7], aldosterone appears to control the expression of a number of proteins localized in various cell organelles; that is, mitochondria plasma membrane, endoplasmic reticulum, Golgi, and cytosol [8–13], thus constituting a typical *pleiotropic* response [14]. Steroid

---

This manuscript was presented as part of a Symposium on *Aldosterone and the Kidney.*

and thyroid hormones can induce or repress the expression of a set of several specific proteins, thus constituting a hormonal *domain.* Induction and repression is restricted in our terminology to an increase or decrease in the rate of synthesis of individual proteins [7]. Pleiotropic responses at the translational level are best analyzed by two-dimensional gel analysis, which is a method developed by O'Farrell [15] and recently applied to the toad urinary bladder [16, 17]. The relationship between induced (or repressed) proteins and the physiologic response (increased sodium transport) is by no means easy to establish. One can expect, however, that various AIPs and ARPs act at different intracellular sites, mediating transepithelial sodium transport.

As illustrated in the model of Figure 1, one could divide AIPs (and ARPs) into two categories: those involved in a constitutive pathway for sodium transport and those involved in a regulatory pathway. The constitutive pathway is directly implicated in the translocation of sodium across the epithelial cell at three critical points; namely, the apical membrane (locus of the amiloride-sensitive *sodium channel*), the basolateral membrane (locus of the ouabain-sensitive *sodium pump*), and the tight junction that controls overall leakiness of the tissue. The regulatory pathway involves a set of molecular events (for example, phosphorylation-dephosphorylation, acylation, and transmethylation) that modulates the constitutive pathway.

Three sites of modulation can be envisaged. First, the insertion (and/or the expression) of the sodium channel at the apical membrane (site 2). Second, the insertion (and/or the expression) of the sodium pump at the basolateral membrane (site 4) could be modulated by regulatory AIPs or ARPs. Third, sodium transport also could be regulated by controlling either the energy supply (adenosine triphosphate) to the sodium pump or the adenosine triphosphate/adenosine diphosphate ratio, which (in turn) alters the apical sodium permeability. Mitochondrial enzymes involved in adenosine triphosphate production belong to this category of regulatory proteins. Finally, one should consider the possibility that the time course of induction (and repression) may vary for each protein under aldosterone control. Thus, the early or the late mineralocorticoid response could be sequentially controlled by different AIPs or ARPs.

A number of data from the literature and from our own laboratory are consistent with the proposed model. Recent experimental evidence indicates that aldosterone-regulated sodium transport is mediated by complex mechanisms involving the apical [18–20] or the basolateral membrane permeability [21–25] as well as the supply of energy [26, 27]. Finally, the whole process appears to be finely tuned in a time-dependent manner, as evidenced by the selective inhibition of the late mineralocorticoid response by agents such as tri-iodothyronine (T_3) [2] or sodium butyrate [28].

The Sodium Pump as a Target for Aldosterone

We decided to focus our attention on Na-K-ATPase and its possible control by aldosterone for two main reasons. First, Na-K-ATPase, which is the molec-

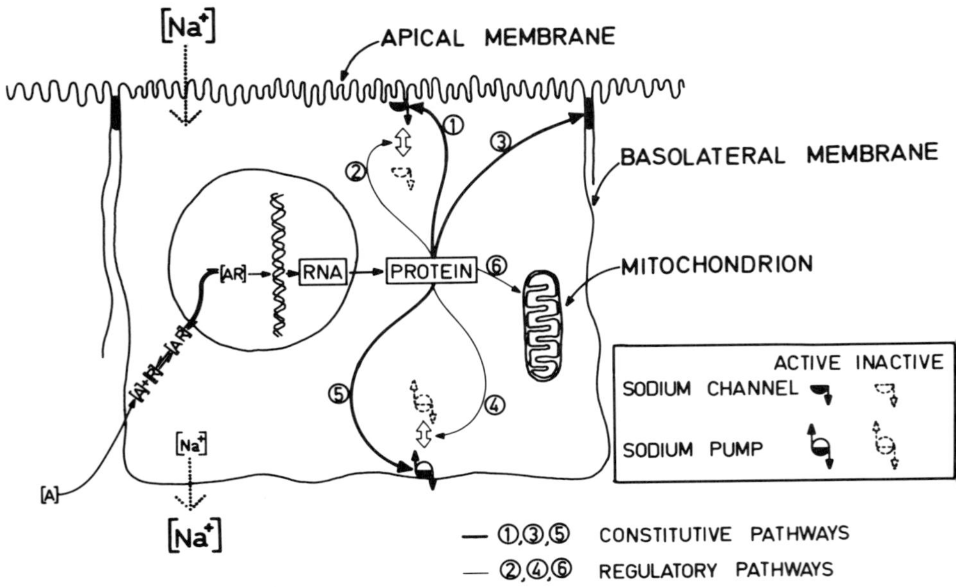

Fig. 1. Model of the mechanisms of action of aldosterone. An epithelial cell is
schematically represented. Aldosterone (*A*) crosses the plasma membrane and binds
to its cytosolic receptor (*R*). The complex (*AR*) is translocated into the nucleus,
where it binds to chromatin and induces and/or represses the transcription of genes
that encode proteins, thus mediating an increased transepithelial sodium transport
(sites *1* to *6*). The net transport of sodium across an epithelial cell is determined
by three factors: the apical membrane, the basolateral membrane, and the tight junction
permeability to sodium. Altogether, these three factors are the major determinants
of the *constitutive* pathway for sodium transport. Aldosterone-induced proteins (AIPs)
or aldosterone-repressed proteins (ARPs) would be directly part of this pathway,
with 1 as a sodium channel (or one of its components), 3 as a tight junction (or
one of its components), and 5 as a sodium pump (or one of its components).
Aldosterone-induced proteins could be regulatory proteins (phosphorylases?
methylases? acyclases? phospholipases?) that control the constitutive pathway, with
2 via activation of an inactive sodium channel pool, 4 via activation of an inactive
sodium pump pool, and 6 via increasing the supply of energy to the sodium pump
(increased ATP synthesis) or via changing the ATP/ADP ratio, which in turn alters
the apical permeability to sodium. Finally, a set of AIP or ARP (early AIP or early
ARP) could determine the early response (2, 4, or 6), while other AIPs or ARPs
(late AIP or late ARP) will determine the late response (1, 5, or 3).

ular counterpart of the Na pump, is the major (if not unique) determinant
of the active sodium transport across epithelial cells. Therefore, it is a potentially important site for regulation. Second, Na-K-ATPase is an oligomeric
plasma membrane enzyme—the subunits of which [the α (catalytic and β
(glycoprotein) subunits] have been purified to homogeneity, thus allowing
the preparation of polyclonal or monoclonal antibodies [29, 30]. Such probes

then serve to study the biogenesis and the cell surface expression of each
enzyme subunit and their assembly into an active enzyme complex. Clearly,
aldosterone could control Na-K-ATPase at different sites (see Fig. 1):
(1) transcriptionally by increasing the de novo synthesis of sodium pumps
(site 5), (2) post-translationally by inducing (and/or repressing) regulatory proteins that control the expression of the sodium pump at the cell
surface (site 4), and (3) by a combination of the two effects in a coordinate
manner to adapt the sodium transport capacity of the cell in a well-timed
fashion.

Na-K-ATPase: A Late Aldosterone-induced Protein

We have measured the effect of aldosterone on the relative rate of synthesis
of each subunit of Na-K-ATPase by using monospecific polyclonal antibodies
directed against either the α subunit (Mr 96 kd) or the β subunit (Mr 60
kd) in the urinary bladder of the toad [29, 30].

At supramaximal concentration of aldosterone, the synthesis of both subunits increased 2- to 3-fold after 18 hr of incubation [31]. That Na-K-ATPase
was indeed an AIP was tested according to the following criteria: (1) de
novo RNA synthesis dependency, (2) mineralocorticoid receptor dependency,
and (3) sodium transport dependency. Actinomycin D, which is a transcrip-
tional inhibitor, added 30 min before aldosterone selectively inhibited the
aldosterone-induced Na-K-ATPase synthesis [29]. The dose-response curve
showed that the effect of aldosterone on Na-K-ATPase synthesis occurred
at low hormone concentrations (0.4 to 7 nmol) corresponding to the saturation
of type I binding sites (kd $\sim$ 0.5 to 3.7 mM) [32]. In addition, the synthesis
induction was antagonized by spironolactone (at a 500:1 molar ratio), which
completely blocks the aldosterone-dependent sodium transport [31]. Finally,
amiloride did not block the induction of Na-K-ATPase synthesis by aldosterone. Thus, the increase in Na-K-ATPase synthesis can be considered as a
primary steroid effect that is independent of any transepithelial sodium transport [31].

Based on these pharmacologic evidences, we propose that Na-K-ATPase
is part of the constitutive pathway (site 5, Fig. 1), which does not imply
that induction of Na-K-ATPase synthesis is a prerequisite for the increased
sodium transport. A time course of induction showed that increased synthesis
was a late event that was not significant earlier than 6 hr after aldosterone
addition [31]. Therefore, the induction cannot be responsible for the early
changes in sodium transport and transepithelial electrical resistance; still, it
could play a role in maintaining high sodium transport, which is characteristic
of the late response. The selective effect of sodium butyrate, which blocks
both the induction of Na-K-ATPase synthesis and the late effect on sodium
transport, is consistent with this concept [28]. Thus, we propose that Na-
K-ATPase is a late AIP.

Recently, we have extended our observations to the TBM (Rossier et al, unpublished results) and A6 cell lines [33].[1] However, it is not yet known whether aldosterone displays similar effects in other classes of vertebrates, especially in mammals such as the rat or the rabbit—the most widely used experimental models for studying the effects of aldosterone. In these species, however, a number of studies have recently shown that aldosterone can rapidly restore (after 60 min) the enzymatic activity of Na-K-ATPase, which had fallen to very low levels after adrenalectomy [23, 24]. Such a rapid reversal by aldosterone in the adrenalectomized rat is not likely to be linked to a de novo synthesis of the sodium pump, since the transit time (20 to 60 min) required to insert a new protein into the plasma membrane is relatively long. In addition, the turnover of Na-K-ATPase in the kidney appears to be slow ($t\frac{1}{2} \cong 3.5$ days in the rat) [34]; and, it is not really compatible with such fast induction kinetics. In our opinion, these data suggest the existence of a precursor (inactive) pool of Na-K-ATPase (Fig. 1, site 4), which could be located intracellularly (vesicles) or within the basolateral membrane. An early AIP (a regulatory protein) that is yet to be identified would rapidly control the activity of the sodium pump at the cell surface.

Expression of Na-K-ATPase at the Cell Surface

In view of the considerations mentioned above, the expression of the sodium pump at the surface of epithelial cells involved in sodium transport becomes a biologic problem that merits investigation. The activity of the pump, measured by ion fluxes, should be correlated to the number of pump sites estimated by ouabain binding and/or by immunologic probes. Although there is a lack of information on this question, one study reports that the mineralocorticoid status modulates the pump activity at the basolateral membrane of the isolated, perfused cortical collecting tubule (CCT) [35]. It also has been shown recently that aldosterone induces a 40% increase in ouabain binding sites on A6 cells after 18 hr of stimulation [22]. During the last 2 years, we have investigated the expression of the two Na-K-ATPase subunits at the surface of TBM cells, which is a cell line that exhibits (in culture) transepithelial Na transport similar to that observed in the intact tissue [36]. In a first approach, the subunits were recovered by immunoprecipitation from cells radioiodinated by the glucose-oxidase-lactoperoxidase procedure at 4°C [37]—a temperature that prevents internalization of cell surface constituents. The major advantage of the culture system is that it allows selective labeling of the apical membrane as the result of the establishment of a tight monolayer. The protein pattern, revealed by two-dimensional gel analysis, was clearly different between cells that were labeled selectively at their apical surface

---

[1] TBM [36] and A6 [22] are continuous amphibian cell lines. A6 is derived from an unknown site in the kidney of *Xenopus laevis* and TBM is from the urinary bladder of *Bufo marinus*. When grown collagen coats the millipore filters, both cell lines display high electrical resistance ($\geq 5000\ \Omega \cdot cm^2$) and amiloride-sensitive sodium transport, which is increased 2- to 3-fold on stimulation by aldosterone.

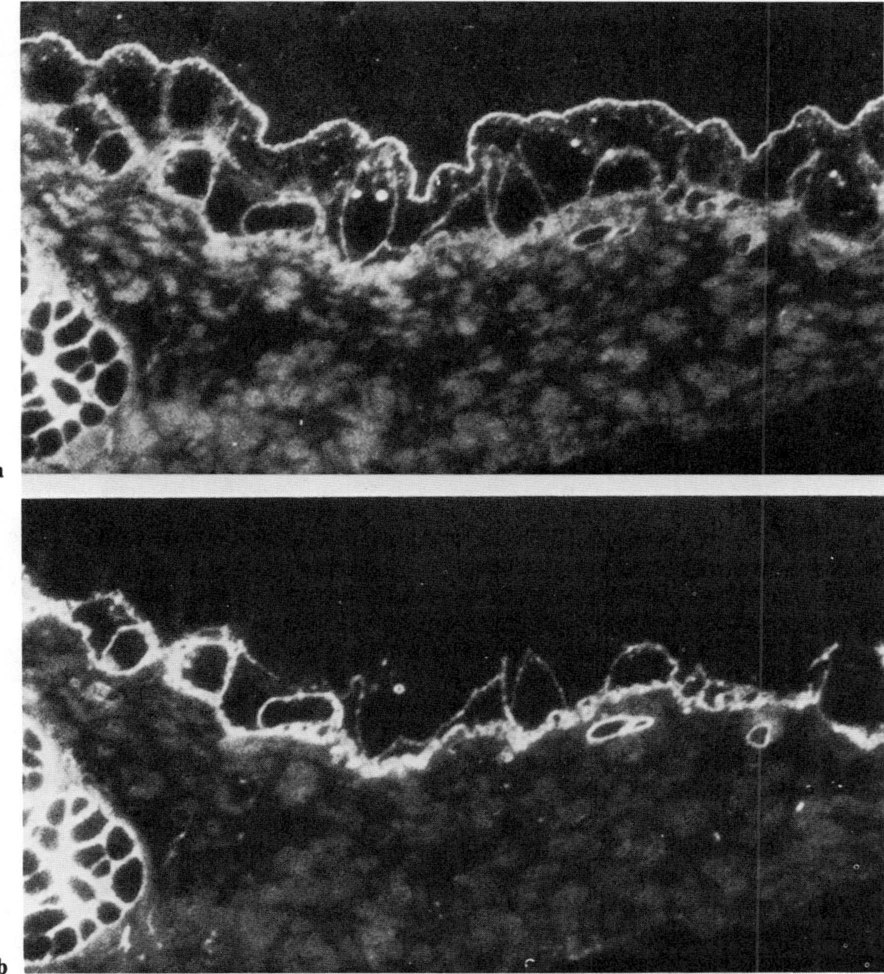

Fig. 2. Immunocytochemical localization of the Na-K-ATPase subunits on 0.5-μm thick frozen sections of toad bladder stimulated in vitro for 20 hr with aldosterone. The sections were first incubated with a biotinylated monoclonal antibody directed against the β subunit, revealed with streptavidine coupled to lissamine; then, with a biotinylated polyclonal antibody directed against cytoplasmic and ectoplasmic epitopes of the α subunit, revealed with streptavidin coupled to FITC.
a Immunofluorescence localization of the α subunit epitopes. Both the apical and basolateral membrane of the epithelial cells are labeled. Several apical vacuoles and vesicles also are labeled. Smooth muscle cells reacted intensively with the antibody.
b Immunofluorescence localization of the β subunit. The labeling is coincidental with the α subunit basolateral membrane labeling and with that of the smooth muscle. The apical membrane of the epithelial cells remains unlabeled.

and cells that were radioiodinated on their entire surface. The β subunit (Mr 60 kd) was recovered only from cells that were radioiodinated on their entire cell surface, but not from cells that were apically labeled; this indicates that this subunit is restricted to the basolateral cell surface. The α subunit was recovered from the basolateral membrane as a 96-kd polypeptide. A significant portion of the specific immunoprecipitated radioactivity was not resolved on the SDS-PAGE gel system, indicating the presence of aggregate and/or high Mr entities. This high Mr material, but not the 96-kd subunit, was also immunoprecipitated with the anti-α subunit antibodies from the apically labeled cells. Aldosterone stimulation (24 hr) increased the surface expression of the β subunit ($\cong$ 3-fold), as well as that of the basolateral 96-kd α subunit and the apical high Mr species. These results indicate that the α subunit, like the β subunit, is restricted to the basolateral membrane, thus reflecting the functional polarity of the sodium pump; whereas, aldosterone-inducible epitopes recognized by antibodies directed against cytoplasmic determinants of the α subunit are also associated with the apical membrane of TBM cells. In our second approach, we have localized α and β subunit antigenic determinants on the surface of 0.5 μm-thick frozen sections of TBM monolayers by using lissamine- or fluorescein-labeled antibodies. Morphologically, the β subunit was again restricted to the basolateral cell surface of the bladder epithelial cells (Fig. 2b), in contrast to α-subunit determinants that were also associated with the apical membrane (Fig. 2a). In the unstimulated state, both the α and β subunits were barely detectable on the basolateral membrane. Upon aldosterone stimulation, there was a significant increase in the surface expression of both subunits. The apical α-subunit epitopes also were modulated by aldosterone, with a drastic increase during the early response and no significant change at a later time.

We have recently postulated, as a working model [29, 38], that the sodium channel at the apical membrane and the α subunit of the sodium pump at the basolateral membrane share structural homology that is recognized by antibodies directed against the α subunit of the Na-K-ATPase. This model, which we termed the sodium pump-channel hypothesis, predicts that the genetic information needed to form a Na-K pump also serves to build an Na or K channel. Several possibilities can be envisaged. The sodium channel and the α subunit of the sodium pump are encoded by genes that belong to the same gene family—the structure of which are closely related. Alternatively, the apical sodium channel and the basolateral α subunit are encoded by a single gene that is processed differentially at the post-transcriptional level (different splicing) or at the post-translational level (different covalent modifications of the gene product).

References

1. SPOONER PM, EDELMAN IS: Further studies on the effect of aldosterone on electrical resistance of toad bladder. *Biochim Biophys Acta* 406:304–314, 1975
2. GEERING K, GAEGGELER HP, ROSSIER BC: Effects of thyromimetic drugs on aldosterone-dependent sodium transport in the toad bladder. *J Membr Biol* 77:15–23. 1984

3. EDELMAN IS, BOGOROCH R, PORTER GA: On the mechanism of action of aldosterone on sodium transport: the role of protein synthesis. *Proc Natl Sci USA* 50:1169–1177, 1963
4. PORTER GA, BOGOROCH R, EDELMAN IS: On the mechanism of action of aldosterone on sodium transport: the role of RNA synthesis. *Proc Natl Acad Sci USA* 52:1326–1333, 1964
5. LUDENS JH, FANESTIL DD: The mechanism of aldosterone function. *Pharmacol Ther B* 2:371–412, 1976
6. MARVER D: Aldosterone action in target epithelia. *Vitam Horm* 38:55–117, 1980
7. IVARIE RD, BAXTER JD, MORRIS JA: Interaction of thyroid and glucocorticoid hormones in rat pituitary tumor cells. *J Biol Chem* 256:4520–4528, 1981
8. BENJAMIN WB, SINGER I: Aldosterone-induced protein in toad urinary bladder. *Science* 186:269–272, 1974
9. SCOTT WN, SAPIRSTEIN VS: Identification of aldosterone-induced proteins in the toad's urinary bladder. *Proc Natl Acad Sci USA* 72:4056–4060, 1975
10. SCOTT WN, REICH IM, BROWN JA JR, YANG CPH: Comparison of toad bladder aldosterone-induced proteins and proteins synthesized in vitro using aldosterone-induced messenger RNA as template. *J Membr Biol* 40(special issue):213–220, 1978
11. SCOTT WN, REICH IM, GOODMAN DBP: Inhibition of fatty acid synthesis prevents the incorporation of aldosterone-induced protein into membranes. *J Biol Chem* 254:4957–4959, 1979
12. LAW PY, EDELMAN IS: Effect of aldosterone on incorporation of amino acids into renal medullary proteins. *J Membr Biol* 41:15–40, 1978
13. LAW PY, EDELMAN IS: Induction of citrate synthase by aldosterone in the rat kidney. *J Membr Biol* 41:41–64, 1978
14. IVARIE RD, MORRIS JA, EBERHARDT NL: Hormonal domains of response: Actions of glucocorticoid and thyroid hormones in regulating pleiotropic responses in cultured cells, in *Recent Progress in Hormone Research* (vol 36), edited by GREEP RO, New York, Academic Press, 1980, pp 195–239
15. O'FARRELL PH: High resolution two-dimensional electrophoresis of proteins. *J Biol Chem* 250:4007–4021, 1975
16. GEHEB M, HUBER G, HERCKER E, COX M: Aldosterone-induced proteins in toad urinary bladders. *J Biol Chem* 256:11716–11723, 1981
17. TRUSCELLO A, GEERING K, GAEGGELER HP, ROSSIER BC: Action of aldosterone (A) and thyroid hormone (T3) in regulating pleiotropic responses in the toad urinary bladder. *Experientia* 39:675, 1983
18. SARIBAN-SOHRABY S, BURG MB, TURNER RJ: Apical sodium uptake in toad kidney epithelial cell line A6. *Am J Physiol* 245:C167–C171, 1983
19. GARTY H, EDELMAN IS: Amiloride-sensitive trypsinization of apical sodium channels. Analysis of hormonal regulation of sodium transport in toad bladder. *J Gen Physiol* 81:785–803, 1983
20. PALMER LG, EDELMAN IS: Control of apical sodium permeability in the toad urinary bladder by aldosterone. *Ann NY Acad Sci* 372:1–14, 1981
21. BEAUWENS R, CRABBE J: Evidence for concerted effects of aldosterone on a target sodium-transporting epithelium. *J Clin Invest* 72:928–934, 1983
22. HANDLER JS, PRESTON AS, PERKINS FM, MATSUMURA M, JOHNSON JP, WATLINGTON CO: The effect of adrenal steroid hormones on epithelia formed in culture by A6 cells. *Ann NY Acad Sci* 372:442–454, 1981
23. DOUCET A, KATZ AI: Short-term effect of aldosterone on Na$^+$-K$^+$-ATPase in single nephron segments. *Am J Physiol* 241:F273–F278, 1981
24. PETTY KJ, KOKKO JP, MARVER D: Secondary effect of aldosterone on Na-K

ATPase activity in the rabbit cortical collecting tubule. *J Clin Invest* 68:1514–1521, 1981

25. GARG LC, KNEPPER MA, BURG MB: Mineralocorticoid effects on Na⁺-K⁺-ATPase in individual nephron segments. *Am J Physiol* 240:F536–F544, 1981

26. GARTY H, EDELMAN IS, LINDEMANN B: Metabolic regulation of apical sodium permeability in toad urinary bladder in the presence and absence of aldosterone. *J Membr Biol* 74:15–24, 1983

27. CORTAS N, ABRAS E, ARNAOUT M, MOORADIAN A, MUAKASAH S: Energetics of sodium transport in the urinary bladder of the toad. Effect of aldosterone and sodium cyanide. *J Clin Invest* 73:46–52, 1984

28. TRUSCELLO A, GEERING K, GÄGGELER HP, ROSSIER BC: Effects of butyrate on histone deacetylation and aldosterone-dependent Na⁺ transport in the toad bladder. *J Biol Chem* 258:3388–3395, 1983

29. ROSSIER BC: Biosynthesis of Na⁺,K⁺-ATPase in amphibian epithelial cells. *Curr Top Membr Transp* 20:125–145, 1984

30. GIRARDET M, GEERING K, FRANTES JM, GESER D, ROSSIER BC, KRAEHENBÜHL JP, BRON C: Immunochemical evidence for a transmembrane orientation of both the (Na⁺,K⁺)-ATPase subunits. *Biochemistry* 20:6684–6691, 1981

31. GEERING K, GIRARDET M, BRON C, KRAEHENBÜHL JP, ROSSIER BC: Hormonal regulation of (Na⁺,K⁺)-ATPase biosynthesis in the toad bladder. Effect of aldosterone and 3,5,3′-triiodo-L-thyronine. *J Biol Chem* 257:10338–10343, 1982

32. GEERING K, CLAIRE M, GAEGGELER HP, GIRARDET M, ROSSIER B: Stimulation of Na⁺ transport and Na⁺,K⁺-ATPase synthesis by aldosterone: correlation with occupancy of hormone binders. *Experientia* 39:663, 1983

33. PACCOLAT MP, GEERING K, GAEGGELER HP, ROSSIER BC: A toad kidney epithelial cell line (A6): a suitable experimental model for studying the late mineralocorticoid response with regard to sodium transport and (Na⁺,K⁺)ATPase biosynthesis. *Kidney Int* (in press, 1984)

34. LO CS, EDELMAN IS: Effect of triiodothyronine on the synthesis and degradation of renal cortical (Na⁺⁺K⁺)-adenosine triphosphatase. *J Biol Chem* 251:7834–7840, 1976

35. NATKE E JR, STONER LC: Na⁺ transport properties of the peritubular membrane of cortical collecting tubule. *Am J Physiol* 242:F664–F671, 1982

36. HANDLER JS, STEELE RE, SAHIB MK, WADE JB, PRESTON AS, LAWSON NL, JOHNSON JP: Toad urinary bladder epithelial cells in culture: maintenance of epithelial structure, sodium transport, and response to hormones. *Proc Natl Acad Sci USA* 76:4151–4155, 1979

37. GIRARDET M, TRUSCELLO A, GEERING K, ROSSIER BC: Effects of aldosterone on surface-exposed (Na⁺,K⁺)-ATPase and plasma membrane proteins (PMP). *Experientia* 39:664, 1983

38. KRAEHENBUHL JP, BONNARD C, GEERING K, GIRARDET M, ROSSIER BC: The sodium channel on the apical membrane of epithelial cells. Role of antigenic determinants of the catalytic subunit of (Na⁺,K⁺)-ATPase (*abstract*). *J Cell Biol* 97:310a, 1983

Renal Actions by Which Vasopressin May Aid the Concentration of Urine

Heinz Valtin

Any discussion of the various means by which vasopressin might aid the concentration of urine must be based on an understanding of the renal countercurrent mechanisms. I would like to begin, therefore, with a very brief review of these mechanisms.

Countercurrent Mechanisms

Figure 1 portrays some of the important anatomic features, especially of the renal medulla, which have been described so well by Jamison and Kriz [1]. The mammalian kidney is divided into the major zones of: cortex, outer medulla (which itself is subdivided into an outer and an inner stripe), inner medulla, and the inner medulla's tip, called the papilla. There are at least two types of nephron: the outer (or superficial) cortical nephron, whose short loop of Henle turns in the inner stripe of the outer medulla; and the juxtamedullary nephron, whose long loop of Henle turns in the inner medulla.[1] The so-called "single effect" of a countercurrent multiplier, which is the reabsorption of sodium chloride to the exclusion of water in the ascending limbs of Henle [2], gets multiplied in the loops of Henle. As a result, there is a buildup of the corticopapillary interstitial osmotic gradient, rendering the interstitium in the outer and inner medulla hypertonic to plasma. Reabsorption of urea from collecting ducts in the inner medulla adds to the interstitial hyperosmolality. Then, in the presence of vasopressin, the late distal

---

This manuscript was presented as part of a Symposium on *Vasopressins: Diverse Actions.*

[1] Most experts recognize the so-called midcortical nephrons in addition to the two mentioned; I have lumped these with the outer cortical nephrons. Strictly speaking, outer cortical and midcortical nephrons do not necessarily give rise to short loops of Henle; and juxtamedullary nephrons, to long loops. By and large, however, that organization is correct (see pp. 35–39 of [1]).

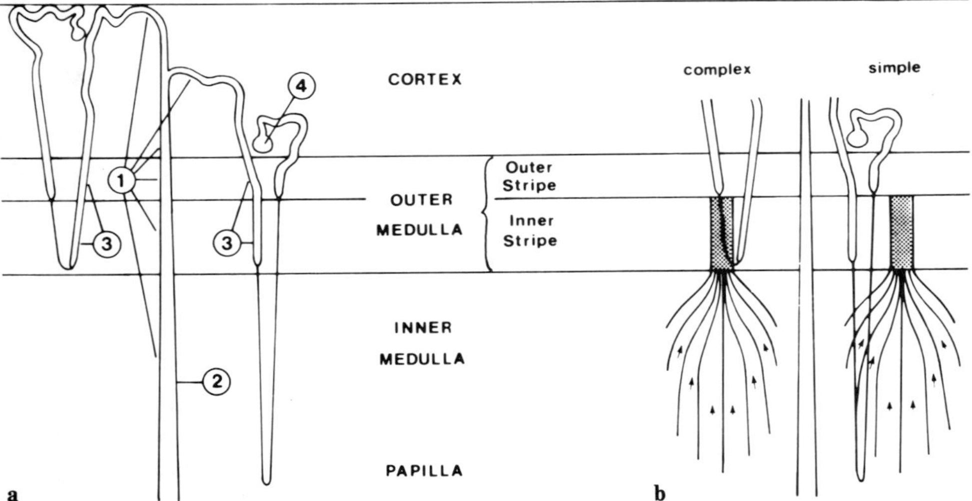

Fig. 1. Diagramatic representation of some of the important anatomic features of mammalian kidneys. Part **a** shows the sites for four major actions of vasopressin on the nephron (itemized in text). Part **b** shows the ascending vasa recta (*upward arrows*). They join with the descending vasa recta (not shown) to form the vascular bundles in the inner stripe of outer medulla (*stippled rectangles*). Simple bundles contain only vasa recta, whereas complex vascular bundles contain, in addition, descending limbs of short loops of Henle, but not of long loops. Long descending limbs run alongside thick ascending limbs of Henle. (Slightly modified from [35] and partly adapted from [22])

tubules and all portions of the collecting ducts are rendered highly permeable to water, causing water to flow out of these structures until osmotic equilibration between tubular fluid and the surrounding hypertonic interstitium has been attained.

Countercurrent multiplication may occur by two means: through active reabsorption of sodium chloride from thick ascending limbs of Henle; and, possibly, through passive reabsorption of sodium chloride from long, thin ascending limbs. The latter process, referred to as the *passive model* (references cited in [1]), is restricted to the inner medulla and may operate as follows: Urea, which has been concentrated within collecting ducts in the cortex and outer medulla through vasopressin-mediated withdrawal of water, is reabsorbed from inner medullary collecting ducts. The resulting urea in the interstitium, for which the long, thin descending limbs of Henle have a high reflection coefficient, causes water to be reabsorbed from these limbs, thereby concentrating sodium chloride within them. As a result, the sodium chloride concentration of tubule fluid in long, thin ascending limbs of Henle exceeds the concentration of sodium chloride in the adjacent interstitium, so that the single effect for the countercurrent multiplier can now be created through the passive reabsorption of sodium chloride—still to the exclusion of water reabsorption, since the thin ascending limbs, like the thick limbs, are virtually impermeable to water.

Renal Actions of Vasopressin

For many years, it was believed that the major, possibly the sole, action of vasopressin on the kidney was to increase the water permeability of the late distal tubules and collecting ducts. In 1961, Jaenike [3] suggested, on the basis of indirect evidence, that vasopressin increases the urea permeability of collecting ducts, a suggestion for which more direct evidence was adduced some years later by Morgan and Berliner [4]. Shortly thereafter, Atherton, Green, and Thomas described a stepwise time course for the action of vasopressin on the kidney, and they presciently suggested not only that the hormone might influence the nephron through actions in addition to altering water and urea permeabilities, but also that the recruitment of these additional effects might depend on the dose of vasopressin [5] (also discussed at length in chapter 7 of [1]). All of these suggestions were greatly strengthened by the studies of Morel, Imbert, and Chabardès [6, 7], who showed that vasopressin can activate adenylate cyclase in the medullary portion of thick ascending limbs of Henle, in thin ascending limbs, in glomeruli, as well as in late distal tubules and collecting ducts.

We now recognize at least four influences of vasopressin on the nephron, designated by the corresponding numbers in Figure 1: (1) to increase the water permeability along the late distal tubules and the entire length of collecting ducts; (2) to increase the urea permeability of inner medullary collecting ducts; (3) to stimulate sodium chloride reabsorption from medullary thick ascending limbs of Henle; and (4) to raise the glomerular filtration rate in juxtamedullary nephrons. I shall describe each of these actions in turn and make an attempt to show how they might mesh with the complex but beautifully integrated system by which mammalian urine is rendered hypertonic to plasma.

Increased Water Permeability

The effect of vasopressin to increase the water permeability of sensitive epithelia was inferred for many years (references cited in [1] and [7]) before it was demonstrated directly in anuran membranes [9, 10] as well as in distal tubules [11] and collecting ducts [12]. It is this all-important action of vasopressin that is responsible for rendering tubular fluid isosmotic at the beginning of cortical collecting ducts (in most species) and hypertonic at the end of papillary collecting ducts—all through passive transport of water. Without this action, urine cannot be concentrated. In contrast, the other three renal effects to be described are probably adjuncts that make the urine more concentrated than it otherwise would be, but are not essential to forming urine with an osmolality greater than that of plasma.

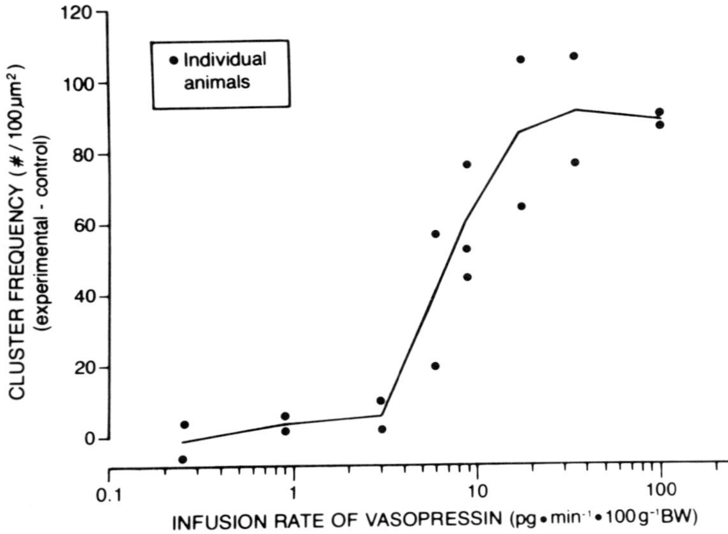

Fig. 2. Frequency of aggregation of intramembranous particles within luminal membranes of collecting duct cells in response to vasopressin in Brattleboro homozygotes [33]. The steep portion of this dose-response curve coincides with rates of vasopressin infusions that led to physiologic plasma concentrations of the hormone. (Reprinted with permission from [16])

Although there have been many exciting developments in elucidating the mechanisms by which vasopressin increases water permeability, I shall restrict my comments to just one phenomenon that is involved: the aggregation of intramembranous particles within the luminal (apical) membrane of collecting duct cells. These aggregates, which are induced by neurohypophyseal hormones [13, 14] and which involve specifically that action of vasopressin that increases water permeability [15], may reflect the insertion of specialized water-permeable patches into the apical plasma membranes of target epithelia. It is likely, therefore, that the aggregation phenomenon affords a means for directly visualizing water permeability. Using this assumption, my colleagues and I [16] have been able to construct a reasonable dose-response curve for the intensity of aggregation in response to vasopressin (Fig. 2). Given this relationship, the aggregation phenomenon is probably a direct end-point that we can measure to gauge the water permeability that existed in inaccessible portions of the distal nephron in situ; we have now begun to use the phenomenon for this purpose [17, 18].

Increased Urea Permeability

Deposition of urea in the medullary interstitium is essential for full concentration of urine. This process is greatly aided by a differential effect of vasopressin on the water versus the urea permeability of the collecting ducts [2]: vasopressin increases the water, but not the urea, permeability of the cortical and outer medullary collecting ducts (top five lines emanating from point 1 in Fig. 1) (for a list of permeability characteristics and references, see Tables A-1 and A-2 of [1], pp. 290–291). As a consequence, the urea concentration within the cortical and outer medullary collecting ducts rises, so that when the fluid reaches the inner medullary collecting ducts—which are rendered permeable by vasopressin not only to water but also to urea (point 2 in Fig. 1)—urea can diffuse down its concentration gradient into the interstitium of the inner medulla.

Medullary Recycling of Urea

The responses to vasopressin just described, abetted by a countercurrent exchange for urea in the vasa recta [2], cause urea to exist within the inner medullary interstitium in a gradient of ever-increasing concentration [5]. There is therefore a constant tendency for urea to be dissipated from that area, in part by diffusion through the interstitium toward the cortex, but mainly by entering the ascending vasa recta (Fig. 1b). For the urine to be concentrated maximally, this dissipated urea must be returned to the inner medullary interstitium. It turns out that this task is best accomplished if urea re-enters (that is, is recycled into) short loops of Henle, but not long loops [19, 20]. Once urea has entered short loops (probably mainly the thin descending short limbs in the inner stripe of outer medulla; Fig. 1a), it encounters urea-impermeable segments of the nephron, namely, thick ascending limbs of Henle, distal tubules, and cortical and outer medullary collecting ducts (see Table A-1 of [1], p. 290). Therefore, urea cannot again be reabsorbed from the tubular system until it reaches the inner medullary collecting ducts, which are rendered more permeable to urea by vasopressin (point 2 in Fig. 1a). In contrast, were urea to be recycled into long loops of Henle, the passive mode of countercurrent multiplication in the inner medulla would be defeated, since it is urea in the interstitium that is thought to remove water from the descending long limbs and thereby concentrate sodium chloride within those limbs (Fig. 1a).

There are some fascinating anatomic relationships that are highly consistent with the view of urea recycling, preferentially via short loops of Henle. These have been described principally by Kriz [21, 22] and by deRouffignac [23] and their associates. These workers have described two types of vascular bundles in the inner stripe of the outer medulla (shaded areas in Fig. 1b): (a) simple bundles, which contain only descending and ascending vasa recta; and (b) complex bundles, in which descending limbs of short loops of Henle (but not of long loops) are intermingled with the vasa recta. Complex bundles are thus ideally suited for a direct transfer of the urea that has been dissipated from the inner medulla via ascending vasa recta (denoted by the arrows in Fig. 1b) into descending thin limbs of short loops—and hence for eventual return to the inner medulla, as just described. In fact, a rough correlation has been drawn between the size and prevalence of complex bundles in several mammalian species and the degree of urea recycling (and hence of the ability to concentrate urine) in those species [23] (summarized in [20]).

Increased Sodium Chloride Reabsorption

Following the demonstration by Morel et al [6] that vasopressin stimulates adenylate cyclase in thick ascending limbs of Henle, two groups showed that the hormone enhances the reabsorption of sodium chloride from this part of the nephron [24, 25]. Shortly thereafter, Hebert, Culpepper, and Andreoli [26] found that this effect of vasopressin is limited to the medullary (as opposed to the cortical) portions of thick ascending limbs (point 3 in Fig. 1a)—again, in consonance with the site for activation of adenylate cyclase in thick limbs [6]. de Rouffignac, Elalouf, and DiStefano have reported a higher threshold for this effect of vasopressin than for its influence on water permeability, a finding they have interpreted as possibly reflecting the primacy of the latter effect [27].

The action of vasopressin on the thick ascending limbs of Henle, which amounts to an augmentation of the "single effect" of the countercurrent multiplier, might abet the concentration of urine in at least three interrelated ways: (1) Being confined to the medulla, where blood flow is greatly reduced over that of the cortex, it will enhance countercurrent multiplication, whereas were the stimulatory effect of vasopressin to occur in the cortical portion of thick ascending limbs (Fig. 1a), the very high rate of cortical blood flow would probably dissipate any interstitial osmotic gradient that might be built up. (2) The enhancement of countercurrent multiplication in the outer medulla might aid the passive mode of countercurrent multiplication in the inner medulla, in the following manner: By increasing the interstitial osmolality of the outer medulla (Fig. 1a), the enhancement might increase reabsorption of water from outer medullary collecting ducts, which would raise the concentration of urea in collecting duct fluid and hence increase the deposition of urea in the inner medulla; other things being equal, that deposition should lead to increased withdrawal of water from long, descending thin limbs of Henle in the inner medulla, which is the first step that enables countercurrent multiplication through passive transport of sodium chloride [2]. (3) The vasopressin-mediated stimulation of sodium chloride reabsorption from medullary thick ascending limbs might further enhance passive countercurrent multiplication through direct transfer of sodium chloride into long, thin descending limbs of Henle. Again, the special anatomic relations shown in Fig. 1b— where thick ascending limbs of Henle in the inner stripe of outer medulla are apposed to long, thin descending limbs [22, 28]—would favor such direct transfer. It has even been suggested that the localization of Na-K-ATPase in the outer medullary portion of long, thin descending limbs of Henle might reflect active secretion of sodium chloride into those limbs and thus promote the direct transfer [28]. Once sodium chloride has entered the long, thin descending limbs, there is likely to be an augmentation of the single effect through passive sodium chloride reabsorption from thin ascending limbs.

Increased Juxtamedullary Filtration Rate

Several workers [29–31], though not all [32], have found that vasopressin increases the glomerular filtration rate selectively in juxtamedullary nephrons. The evidence for this effect, which was adduced in Brattleboro rats, is summarized in Figure 3. Heterozygotes of the Brattleboro strain, which have vasopressin [33] and served as controls for this study, manifest the normal situation in which the single nephron glomerular filtration rate (SNGFR) is higher in juxtamedullary than in superficial cortical nephrons. In Brattleboro homozygotes, which lack vasopressin [33], this nephron heterogeneity is absent. And when homozygotes are treated with vasopressin, or with its analog, 1-deamino-8-D-arginine vasopressin (dDAVP), the heterogeneity is restored. Note that vasopressin induces the difference in SNGFR by selectively increasing that of juxtamedullary nephrons, not by influencing the filtration rate of superficial nephrons. Thus, this effect of vasopressin, like the one on thick ascending limbs of Henle, would be expected to increase delivery of sodium chloride selectively to long, thin descending limbs (Fig. 1a) and thereby aid countercurrent multiplication by the mechanisms described under *3* in the preceding section.

The mechanism by which vasopressin increases SNGFR is not yet known. We have done experiments that seem to rule out a direct action on blood vessels [31]; mice with nephrogenic diabetes insipidus [34] lack heterogeneity for SNGFR, whereas normal mice demonstrate such heterogeneity [35]. Inas-

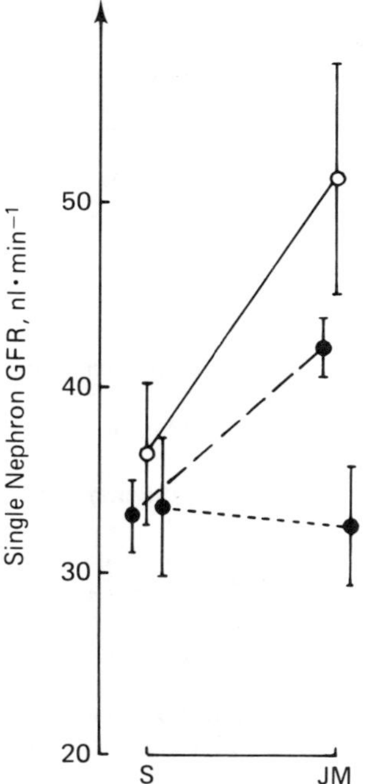

Fig. 3. Lack of nephron heterogeneity for single nephron glomerular filtration rate in homozygotes of the Brattleboro strain of rats (●- - - - -●, Brattleboro homos), which lack vasopressin. Such heterogeneity is present in heterozygotes of the same strain
(○———○, Brattleboro heteros), which do have vasopressin; and heterogeneity is restored when Brattleboro homozygotes are treated with the synthetic analog of vasopressin, 1-deamino-8-D-arginine vasopressin (●– – –● dDAVP-treated homos). *S* denotes superficial cortical nephrons; *JM*, juxtamedullary nephrons. (Adapted from [31])

much as the diseased mice have ample vasopressin in their plasma [36], and since they have intact vascular receptors for vasopressin as reflected in a rise of systemic arterial pressure when they are given high doses of vasopressin (Valtin and Veale, unpublished observations), they should show heterogeneity if it were due to a direct vascular effect. The fact that they lack heterogeneity may thus be a function of their deficient corticopapillary interstitial osmotic gradient [30], or of a high tubuloglomerular feedback signal [37], or of other, as yet unidentified, factors [35].

Concluding Comments

There are at least four discrete influences of vasopressin on the kidney which, acting together, aid the concentration of urine. Virtually all of these actions utilize differences between nephrons and thus give us a hint about the biological importance of nephron heterogeneity [38, 39]. It is in large measure because of the selective nature of vasopressin action—on water permeability only of late distal tubules and collecting ducts; on urea permeability only of inner medullary collecting ducts; on sodium chloride reabsorption only of medullary thick ascending limbs of Henle; and on filtration rate only of juxtamedullary nephrons—that vasopressin can exert its integrated, salutary influence on the concentrating mechanism. The fact that medullary recycling of urea probably occurs predominantly via short loops of Henle not only reinforces this view but also points up the importance of the short loops to the total concentrating process. No longer can we say, as we once did, that in respect to urinary concentration, the outer cortical nephrons are parasitic on the juxtamedullary nephrons. Rather, all nephrons contribute importantly, but in different ways, to this beautifully integrated system.

Acknowledgments. Work in my laboratory has been supported mainly by USPHS Research Grant AM 08469.

References

1. JAMISON RL, KRIZ W: *Urinary Concentrating Mechanism: Structure and Function.* Oxford, Oxford University Press, 1982
2. VALTIN H: Chap 8 of *Renal Function. Mechanisms Preserving Fluid and Solute Balance in Health* (2nd ed). Boston, Little, Brown, 1983
3. JAENIKE JR: The influence of vasopressin on the permeability of the mammalian collecting duct to urea. *J Clin Invest* 40:144–151, 1961
4. MORGAN T, BERLINER RW: Permeability of the loop of Henle, vasa recta, and collecting duct to water, urea and sodium. *Am J Physiol* 215:108–115, 1968
5. ATHERTON JC, GREEN R, THOMAS S: Influence of lysine-vasopressin dosage on the time course of changes in renal tissue and urinary composition in the conscious rat. *J Physiol* 213:291–309, 1971
6. MOREL F, IMBERT-TEBOUL M, CHABARDÈS D: Distribution of hormone-dependent adenylate cyclase in the nephron and its physiological significance. *Ann Rev Physiol* 43:569–581, 1981

7. IMBERT M, CHABARDÈS D, MOREL F: Hormone-sensitive adenylate cyclase in isolated rabbit glomeruli. *Mol Cell Endocrinol* 1:295–304, 1974
8. SMITH HW: *The Kidney: Structure and Function in Health and Disease.* New York, Oxford University Press, 1951, pp 256–263
9. SAWYER WH: Effect of posterior pituitary extract on permeability of frog skin to water. *Am J Physiol* 164:44–48, 1951
10. KOEFOED-JOHNSEN V, USSING HH: The contributions of diffusion and flow to the passage of D_2O through living membranes: Effect of neurohypophyseal hormone on isolated anuran skin. *Acta Physiol Scand* 28:60–76, 1953
11. ULLRICH KJ, RUMRICH G, FUCHS G: Wasserpermeabilität und transtubulärer Wasserfluss corticaler Nephronabschnitte bei verschiedenen Diuresezuständen. *Pfluegers Arch* 280:99–119, 1964
12. GRANTHAM JJ, BURG MG: Effect of vasopressin and cyclic AMP on permeability of isolated collecting tubules. *Am J Physiol* 211:255–259, 1966
13. CHEVALIER J, BOURGUET J, HUGON JS: Membrane associated particles: Distribution in frog urinary bladder epithelium at rest and after oxytocin treatment. *Cell Tiss Res* 152:129–140, 1974
14. KACHADORIAN WA, WADE JB, DiSCALA VA: Vasopressin: Induced structural change in toad bladder luminal membrane. *Science* 190:67–69, 1975
15. HAYS RM, LEVINE SD: Pathophysiology of water metabolism, in *The Kidney* (2nd ed), edited by BRENNER BM, RECTOR FC JR, Philadelphia, Saunders, 1981, pp 795–796
16. HARMANCI MC, STERN P, KACHADORIAN WA, VALTIN H, DiSCALA VA: Vasopressin and collecting duct intramembranous particle clusters: A dose-response relationship. *Am J Physiol* 239: F560–F564, 1980
17. BROWN D, VALTIN H, MORRIS J, ORCI L: Lack of intramembrane particle aggregates in collecting ducts of mice with nephrogenic diabetes insipidus. *Abst Proc IX Int Cong Nephrol.* Los Angeles, 1984, p. 407a
18. EDWARDS BR, HARMANCI MC: Intramembranous particle clusters in collecting duct cells of rats: Influence of water balance. *Renal Physiol* 6:275–280, 1983
19. STEWART J: Urea handling by the renal countercurrent system: Insights from computer simulation. *Pfluegers Arch* 356:133–151, 1975
20. VALTIN H: Structural and functional heterogeneity of mammalian nephrons. *Am J Physiol* 233:F491–F501, 1977
21. LEVER AF, KRIZ W: Countercurrent exchange between the vasa recta and the loop of Henle. *Lancet* 1:1057–1060, 1966
22. KRIZ W, BARRETT JM, PETER S: The renal vasculature: Anatomical-functional aspects. *Int Rev Physiol* 11:1–21, 1976
23. DE ROUFFIGNAC C, IMBERT M: Role of sodium and urea in the renal concentrating mechanism. *Proc II Eur Colloq Renal Physiol, Balatonfüred, Hungary,* 1977
24. SASAKI S, IMAI M: Effects of vasopressin on water and NaCl transport across the in vitro perfused medullary thick ascending limb of Henle's loop of mouse, rat and rabbit kidneys. *Pfluegers Arch* 383:215–221, 1980
25. HALL DA, VARNEY DM: Effect of vasopressin on electrical potential difference and chloride transport in mouse medullary thick ascending limb of Henle's loop. *J Clin Invest* 66:792–802, 1980
26. HEBERT SC, CULPEPPER RM, ANDREOLI TE: NaCl transport in mouse medullary thick ascending limbs: I. Functional nephron heterogeneity and ADH-stimulated NaCl cotransport. *Am J Physiol* 241:F412–F431, 1981
27. DE ROUFFIGNAC C, ELALOUF JM, DiSTEFANO A: Renal effects of ADH on water permeability and electrolyte transport: Evidence for different thresholds of stimulation, in *Proc XXIX Cong Int Un Physiol Sci,* 1983, vol 15, pp 343, abstract #419.02

28. ERNST SA, SCHREIBER JH: Ultrastructural localization of Na$^+$, K$^+$-ATPase in rat and rabbit kidney medulla. *J Cell Biol* 91:803–813, 1981
29. HORSTER M, SCHNERMANN J, THURAU K: Die Funktion der juxtamedullären Nephrone in Wasserdiurese und ADH-induzierter Antidiurese, in *Proc VI Symp Ges Nephrologie,* edited by WATSCHINGER B, Vienna, Wiener Mediz Akad, 1968, pp 609–614
30. DAVIS JM, SCHNERMANN J: The effect of antidiuretic hormone on the distribution of nephron filtration rates in rats with hereditary diabetes insipidus. *Pfluegers Arch* 330:323–334, 1971
31. TRINH-TRANG-TAN MM, SOKOL HW, BANKIR L, VALTIN H: Homozygous Brattleboro rats lack normal nephron heterogeneity as a consequence of their urine concentrating defect. *Ann NY Acad Sci* 394:524–534, 1982
32. JAMISON RL, BUERKERT J, LACY F: A micropuncture study of Henle's thin loop in Brattleboro rats. *Am J Physiol* 224:180–185, 1973
33. VALTIN H: The discovery of the Brattleboro rat, recommended nomenclature, and the question of proper controls. *Ann NY Acad Sci* 394:1–9, 1982
34. KETTYLE WM, VALTIN H: Chemical and dimensional characterization of the renal countercurrent system in mice. *Kidney Int* 1:135–144, 1972
35. VALTIN H: How nephron heterogeneity abets the concentration of mammalian urine, in *One Medicine,* edited by RYDER OA, BYRD ML, New York, Springer-Verlag, 1984, pp 309–320
36. STERN P, FAHEY JV, LAROCHELLE FT JR: Excretion of prostaglandins E$_2$ and F$_{2\alpha}$ is urine flow dependent in the mouse (*abstract*). *Kidney Int* 21:266, 1982
37. BANKIR L, TRINH MM, BOUBY N, DOUTÉ M: Functional consequences of ADH-induced thick ascending limb (TAL) hypertrophy in Brattleboro rats with diabetes insipidus (DI). *Abst XV Ann Mtg Am Soc Nephrol,* 1982, p 156A
38. WALKER LA, VALTIN H: Biological importance of nephron heterogeneity. *Ann Rev Physiol* 44:203–219, 1982
39. KNEPPER M, BURG M: Organization of nephron function. *Am J Physiol* 244:F579–F589, 1983

Cellular Modes of Action of Vasopressin

Rui C. de Sousa

The neurohypophyseal hormone, vasopressin, exerts a variety of biologic effects in several cell systems [1, 2]. Two of these effects were well recognized from the beginning, as evidenced by the names currently used to designate this hormone: (1) vasopressin (VP), denoting its effect on vascular smooth muscle fibers, and (2) antidiuretic hormone (ADH), denoting its effect on the concentration and output of urine.

For many years, the antidiuretic effect monopolized the attention of most investigators who were interested in VP. Several reasons contributed to this situation: (1) the VP-induced pressor effect appeared to be a pharmacologic action with little or no physiologic significance, (2) the antidiuretic effect was clearly involved in the pathophysiology of many clinical situations characterized either by polyuria (for example, diabetes insipidus) or by inappropriate secretion of ADH, (3) VP was taken up by the shock wave of research generated by the discovery of the countercurrent mechanism in the 1950s, and (4) the use of VP-sensitive epithelia from amphibians, as in vitro models, gave great impetus to the study of the cellular events underlying the hydrosmotic effect and consequently the antidiuretic effect.

Vasopressin and Its Target Cells

In the last few years, the biologic actions of VP, other than those related to water transport, have been intensively investigated. We will briefly review some of the effects associated with four main target cells for VP: epithelial cells, hepatocytes, smooth muscle fibers, and nerve cells.

There are three classic VP-sensitive epithelia: the collecting duct of the mammalian kidney, and the skin and the urinary bladder of amphibians.

This manuscript was presented as part of a Symposium on *Vasopressin: Diverse Actions.*

Vasopressin causes several permeability changes in these epithelial structures; namely, an increase in permeability to water, sodium, urea, and lipophilic molecules [1]. In amphibian membranes, all of these permeability changes can be elicited in a single epithelium, whereas the collecting duct shows a segmental specialization in the expression of such actions (for details, see the preceding chapter by Valtin in this volume). Concerning the VP-induced enhancement of water permeability, available data indicate that this phenomenon is cell-specific [3]. In fact, the granular cell of either toad bladder or toad skin and its counterpart in the collecting duct epithelium—the principal or clear cell—are the cell types most clearly, if not exclusively, involved in the hydrosmotic action of VP.

Vasopressin has a glycogenolytic effect on hepatocytes, and it causes contraction of vascular smooth muscle fibers. In both instances, the hormone apparently binds to a type of receptor—the V_1 or liver isoreceptor—that differs from the one found in epithelia—the V_2 or kidney isoreceptor—as shown by studies with extensive series of VP structural analogs ([2] and the following chapter by Sawyer and Manning in this volume). It also should be noted that current work suggests that the VP pressor effect does participate in the physiologic regulation of blood pressure; it may even be involved in certain types of hypertension (see the article by Johnston, Hivatari, and Abrahams in this section).

Work on the effects of VP on the central nervous system also developed into a very important line of research ([1, 2] and the chapter by Sawyer and Manning). It is possible that VP, like many other neuropeptides, acts either as a true neurotransmitter or as a neuromodulator; the latter is a regulatory function similar to the paracrine secretion in non-neural tissues. In any case, the reported effects of VP and oxytocin on memory, learning, and behavior are most challenging and have opened a new field in neurobiology.

Vasopressin and Its Messengers

Vasopressin is a typical example of a polypeptide hormone whose action on a target cell starts with the occupancy of specific receptors embedded in the plasma membrane. From that point on, two basic mechanisms have been disclosed in the cascade of events that couples the hormonal stimulus with the biologic response: (1) cyclic AMP-dependent, and (2) cyclic AMP-independent.

The cyclic AMP-dependent mechanism underlies the well-known permeability changes induced in VP-sensitive epithelia. The corresponding membrane receptor—the V_2—is a membrane component that is functionally coupled to an adenylate cyclase that generates the intracellular messenger, cyclic AMP, in a dose-dependent manner [2]. Interestingly, toad bladder was among the first biologic systems in which the criteria or postulates of Sutherland for the messenger role of cyclic AMP were established firmly [4].

The cyclic AMP-independent mechanism underlies the glycogenolytic and pressor effects of VP on liver and smooth muscle cells, respectively. In this case, the membrane receptor is not functionally coupled to an adenylate cyclase (V_1). As is well known, the study of the glycogenolytic effect of beta-adrenergic agents on liver led to the first demonstration of the messenger role of cyclic AMP. With time, however, it became apparent that the effect of other glycogenolytic agents, (namely, alpha$_1$-adrenergic agents, angiotensin, and VP) was mediated by Ca^{++} instead of cyclic AMP. The exact nature of this cyclic AMP-independent mechanism has been debated, particularly with regard to the factors promoting the rise in intracellular Ca^{++}: increased Ca^{++} influx and/or release of Ca^{++} from intracellular stores [2]. In a recent paper, Thomas, Alexander, and Williamson [5] reported that in the range of 0.2 to 1.0 nM, VP significantly increased cytosolic free Ca^{++} from 160 to 400 nM as measured with the fluorescent Ca^{++} indicator Quin 2. Such Ca^{++} changes correlated with hormone-induced changes in lipid metabolism, which resulted in the breakdown of phosphatidylinositol compounds and the production of inositol triphosphate. This latter product appears to be a major link between the hormone stimulus and the rise in intracellular Ca^{++} by mobilizing intracellular Ca^{++} stores; the nature of this is still controversial.

The Stimulus-Hydrosmotic Response

It generally is accepted that the enhancement of water permeability (hydrosmotic response) in VP-sensitive epithelia is triggered by the occupancy of V_2 receptors and is mediated by cyclic AMP [1, 3, 4]. This messenger role of cyclic AMP has been recently corroborated by the use of the diterpene, forskolin, which is a direct activator of adenylate cyclase [6]. Figure 1 shows a hydrosmotic response elicited by forskolin in toad bladder.

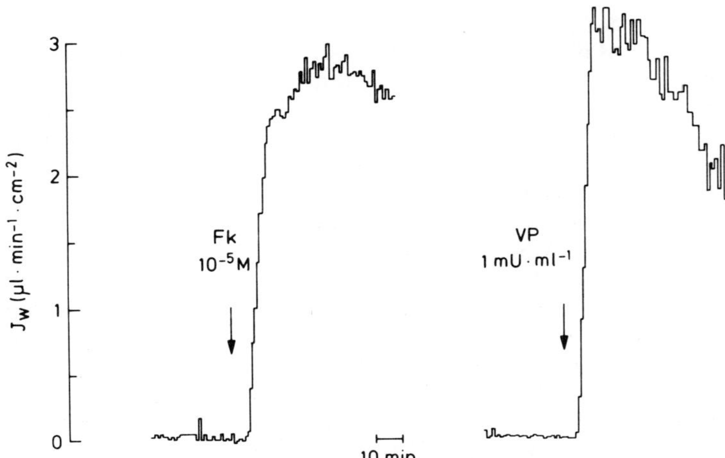

Fig. 1. Water flow (J_w) across two paired quarter-bladders of a toad *Bufo marinus*. Jw was averaged over 1-min periods by means of an automatic technique (see [17]). Note the similar pattern of hydrosmotic response elicited by forskolin (*Fk*), which is a diterpene that directly activates adenylate cyclase, and by vasopressin (*VP*).

In a polar epithelial cell, the hormonal stimulus triggers a vectorial flow of biologic information that goes from the basolateral to the apical portion of the plasma membrane, where it promotes the transition from a low to a relatively high state of water permeability of the rate-limiting barrier. Several biophysical models have been proposed over the years to account for this striking change in permeability [1]. In essence, the propositions changed from a model of enlargement of pre-existing aqueous pores in the apical membrane to a model postulating the increase in the number of narrow aqueous pores so narrow ($< 2\text{Å}$) that water molecules cannot overtake each other inside this pathway (single-file diffusion) [1]. This last model could account for features of transepithelial water flow, such as the high transport selectivity, the high activation energy, and the discrepancy between diffusional (P_d) and osmotic water permeability (P_f) coefficients. Such a discrepancy has been interpreted as being evidence of positive isotope interaction; the actual value of P_f/P_d has been interpreted as being equal to the number of water molecules inside the pore [1].

The pore theory, which was advanced as an attempt to explain the permeability changes underlying the hydrosmotic response, implied a restructuring of the apical membrane of the pertinent epithelial cell. Consequently, a great deal of interest was generated by the observation showing that the VP-induced increase in water permeability was indeed associated with a well-defined ultrastructural modification—the appearance of intramembrane particle aggregates in the apical epithelial membrane, which were detectable with the freeze-fracture technique [7, 8].

The Intramembrane Particle Aggregates

Work from several laboratories strongly suggests that the appearance of IMP aggregates is a hallmark of the hydrosmotic response elicited in VP-sensitive epithelia. To date, this ultrastructural feature has been observed in the amphibian bladder [7, 8], amphibian skin [9, 10], and kidney collecting duct [11–13], whenever the epithelia were stimulated by a hydrosmotic agent. This includes not only VP, but also cyclic AMP [14, 15], isoproterenol (in toad skin) [9, 10], and even serosal hypertonicity [14].

The appearance of IMP aggregates showed the same type of cellular specificity that was previously noted for the hydrosmotic response: the granular cell [7–10] and the clear or principal cell [11–13]. There is a strong correlation between the surface occupied by IMP aggregates and the transepithelial water flow values in both the bladder [15] and the skin [10] of amphibians. The restructuring of the apical membrane is reversible, and it follows a time course compatible with the development of the physiologic response [16]. Blockers of the hydrosmotic action induce a parallel decrease in water flow and in the appearance of IMP aggregates [10, 17–19].

A second ultrastructural feature of paramount importance was independently reported by two laboratories: the presence of IMP aggregates in intracytoplasmic vacuolar structures [20, 21]. Subsequently, it was shown that these intracytoplasmic structures "fuse" with the apical membrane, and a correlation was found between the number of "fusion events" and the development of the hydrosmotic response [22]. Moreover, the physiologic response was accompanied by a significant decrease in the number of intracytoplasmic structures containing IMP aggregates [23] and by a concomitant increase in membrane capacitance [24, 25]. Collectively, these observations suggest that VP induces the insertion, by an exocytosis-like process, of membrane patches that are water permeable [1, 17]. Withdrawal of the hydrosmotic stimulus results in a decrease in water permeability towards baseline values, which is a phenomenon paralleled by the gradual disappearance of IMP aggregates from the apical membrane [16]. During this phase, there is a marked increase in the apical uptake of horseradish peroxidase into vesicular structures that resemble those decorated with IMP aggregates [26]. Consequently, the reversal of the hydrosmotic response seems to be accompanied by an endocytosis-like process that leads to the retrieval of membrane patches containing IMP aggregates from the apical membrane.

Two Emerging Concepts

The insertion of transport units from intracytoplasmic reservoirs, which was first observed in connection with the VP-induced hydrosmotic response, apparently is a rather general mechanism for the modulation of cell permeability. In fact, there are some indications that the VP-induced stimulus-natriferic response possibly follows a similar pattern [1, 27, 28]. However, a most convincing series of observations came from other cell systems that include: (1) the transport of glucose by the adipose cell [29, 30], (2) the reabsorption of potassium (K) by the medullary collecting duct [31], (3) the secretion of H^+ by turtle bladder [32, 33], and (4) the reabsorption of sodium by rabbit urinary bladder [34, 35]. It also is possible that a similar mechanism applies to the H^+-K^+-ATPase involved in hydrogen chloride (HCl) secretion by the gastric mucosa [36].

Two concepts emerge from current work on the modulation of membrane permeability: (1) the gating versus the insertion mechanism of control, and (2) the similarity between the stimulus-secretion coupling and the stimulus-permeability response.

According to time course and residency of membrane components involved in the control of membrane permeability, two basic mechanisms can be identified:

1. In excitable cells, a very rapid modulation of membrane permeability, with a time course on the order of milliseconds, is achieved by a gating mechanism that controls the on-off stages of transport units residing in the plasma membrane.
2. In nonexcitable cells, the relatively slow time course (seconds to minutes) of permeability changes that is induced by hormones or neurotransmitters is compatible with the insertion of transport units that are recruited from intracytoplasmic vesicular stores. From the viewpoint of cellular energetics, this mechanism—like the secretion of products stored in granular form— allows for an efficient and quantal regulation of cell functions.

The second emerging concept pertains to the striking similarity between the stimulus-secretion response and the stimulus-permeability response in nonexcitable cells. The same fundamental building blocks (membrane receptors, intracellular messengers, and cytoskeleton) appear to assure the basic steps of the cellular stimulus-effect coupling process, whether the biologic response is the secretion of a packaged product released by exocytosis or a change in permeability induced by the addition to the plasma membrane of preformed intracytoplasmic transport units (exocytosis-like process). The parietal cell of the gastric mucosa probably is the first example in which these two processes occur simultaneously: release of intrinsic factor and addition of H^+/K^+ pumps to the apical membrane from the same vesicular structures [37].

Ca^{++}, Depolarizing Agents and Water Transport

The synarchic regulation exerted by cyclic AMP and Ca^{++} on a great variety of cell processes [38] raised the question of whether Ca^{++} also might be involved in the hydrosmotic and natriferic responses to VP. This topic has been recently reviewed [1, 39]. Mention should also be made here to the possible involvement of calmodulin in the hydrosmotic response, as reported by several laboratories [19, 40, 41].

Membrane depolarization is a classic trigger of secretion processes. Since the mechanisms underlying the secretion and permeability responses of the cell are so similar, we looked at the effects of depolarizing agents on the hydrosmotic action of VP. In toad bladder, high potassium [42] as well as ouabain and veratridine (unpublished observations), significantly enhanced the hydrosmotic response to submaximal concentrations of VP. Interestingly, high potassium [43] and ouabain and veratridine elicited by themselves a hydrosmotic response in toad skin. An example is shown in Figure 2, in which rubidium mimics the effect of potassium. Most importantly, the potassium-induced hydrosmotic effect was accompanied by the appearance of IMP aggregates similar to those observed with either VP or a beta-adrenergic agonist [9, 10].

Conclusion

In VP-sensitive epithelia, the increase in water permeability induced by the hormonal stimulus apparently depends on an exocytosis-like process that allows for the quantal insertion of permeable membrane patches in the apical membrane. It is likely, although not proven, that such patches contain water channels behaving as osmotic shunts across the lipid bilayer of the rate-limiting barrier to water flow. Isolation of these putative water channels will certainly be one of the most exciting lines of research in the future.

Acknowledgment. Work in the author's laboratory has been supported mainly by the Swiss National Science Foundation, grant no. 3.342.0.82.

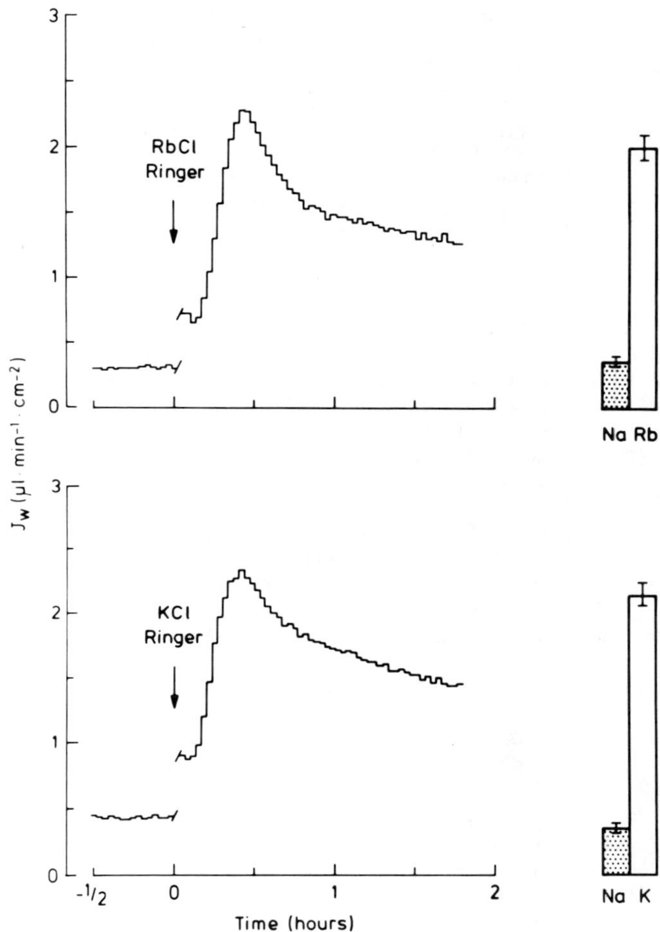

Fig. 2. Hydrosmotic effect induced in toad skin (*Bufo marinus*) by replacement of K (or Rb) for Na in the bathing Ringer solutions (Δ Osm = 200 mOsm). Typical automatic recordings of J_w are shown on the left. A statistical summary of six paired experiments is shown on the right. The *stippled columns* represent average basal J_w in control Na-Ringer; the *white columns* represent average peak J_w during K (or Rb) exposure.

References

1. DE SOUSA RC, GROSSO A: The mode of action of vasopressin: membrane microstructure and biological transport. *J Physiol* (*Paris*) 77:643–669, 1981
2. JARD S: Vasopressin isoreceptors in mammals: relation to cyclic AMP-dependent and cyclic AMP-independent transduction mechanisms. *Curr Topics Membr Transp* 18:255–285, 1983

3. DIBONA DR, CIVAN MM, LEAF A: The cellular specificity of the effect of vasopressin on toad urinary bladder. *J Membr Biol* 1:79–91, 1969

4. STREWLER GJ, ORLOFF J: Role of cyclic nucleotides in the transport of water and electrolytes. *Adv Cycl Nucl Res* 8:311–361, 1977

5. THOMAS AP, ALEXANDER J, WILLIAMSON JR: Relationship between inositol polyphosphate production and the increase of cytosolic free Ca^{2+} induced by vasopressin in isolated hepatocytes. *J Biol Chem* 259:5574–5584, 1984

6. GROSSO A, DE SOUSA RC: Forskolin increases the water permeability of the skin and the bladder of toads Bufo marinus (*abstract*). *Experientia* 39:633, 1983

7. CHEVALIER J, BOURGUET J, HUGON JS: Membrane associated particles: distribution in frog urinary bladder epithelium at rest and after oxytocin treatment. *Cell Tissue Res* 152:129–140, 1974

8. KACHADORIAN WA, WADE JB, DISCALA VA: Vasopressin: induced structural change in toad bladder luminal membrane. *Science* 190:67–69, 1975

9. BROWN D, GROSSO A, DE SOUSA RC: Isoproterenol-induced intramembrane particle aggregation and water flux in toad epidermis. *Biochim Biophys Acta* 596:158–164, 1980

10. BROWN D, GROSSO A, DE SOUSA RC: Correlation between water flow and intramembrane particle aggregates in toad epidermis. *Am J Physiol* 245:C334–C342, 1983

11. HARMANCI MC, KACHADORIAN WA, VALTIN H, DISCALA VA: Antidiuretic hormone-induced intramembranous alterations in mammalian collecting ducts. *Am J Physiol* 235:F440–F443, 1978

12. HARMANCI MC, STERN P, KACHADORIAN WA, VALTIN H, DISCALA VA: Vasopressin and collecting duct intramembranous particle clusters: a dose-response relationship. *Am J Physiol* 239:F560–F564, 1980

13. BROWN D, ORCI L: Vasopressin stimulates formation of coated pits in rat kidney collecting ducts. *Nature* 302:253–255, 1983

14. BOURGUET J, CHEVALIER J, HUGON JS: Alterations in membrane-associated particle distribution during antidiuretic challenge in frog urinary bladder epithelium. *Biophys J* 16:627–639, 1976

15. KACHADORIAN WA, WADE JB, UITERWYK CC, DISCALA VA: Membrane structural and functional responses to vasopressin in toad bladder. *J Membr Biol* 30:381–401, 1977

16. KACHADORIAN WA, CASEY C, DISCALA VA: Time course of ADH-induced intramembranous particle aggregation in toad urinary bladder. *Am J Physiol* 234:F461–F465, 1978

17. DE SOUSA RC, GROSSO A: Osmotic water flow across the abdominal skin of the toad *Bufo marinus:* effect of vasopressin and isoprenaline. *J Physiol* 329:281–296, 1982

18. KACHADORIAN WA, ELLIS SJ, MULLER J: Possible role for microtubules and microfilaments in ADH action on toad urinary bladder. *Am J Physiol* 236:F14–F20, 1979

19. LEVINE SD, KACHADORIAN WA, LEVIN DN, SCHLONDORFF D: Effects of trifluoperazine on function and structure of toad urinary bladder. *J Clin Invest* 67:662–672, 1981

20. HUMBERT F, MONTESANO R, GROSSO A, DE SOUSA RC, ORCI L: Particle aggregates in plasma and intracellular membranes of toad bladder (granular cell). *Experientia* 33:1364–1367, 1977

21. WADE JB: Membrane structural specialization of toad urinary bladder revealed by freeze-fracture technique. III. Location, structure and vasopressin dependence of intramembrane particle arrays. *J Membr Biol* (special issue) 40:281–296, 1978

22. Muller J, Kachadorian WA, di Scala VA: Evidence that ADH-stimulated intramembrane particle aggregates are transferred from cytoplasmic to luminal membranes in toad bladder epithelial cells. *J Cell Biol* 85:83–95, 1980
23. Wade JB: Hormonal modulation of epithelial structure. *Curr Topics Membr Transp* 13:123–147, 1980
24. Stetson DL, Lewis SA, Alles W, Wade JB: Evaluation by capacitance measurements of antidiuretic hormone induced membrane area changes in toad bladder. *Biochim Biophys Acta* 689:267–274, 1982
25. Palmer LG, Speez N: Modulation of antidiuretic hormone-dependent capacitance and water flow in toad urinary bladder. *Am J Physiol* 246:F501–F508, 1984
26. Wade JB, Stetson DL, Lewis SA: ADH action: Evidence for a membrane shuttle mechanism. *Ann NY Acad Sciences* 372:106–117, 1981
27. Li JHY, Palmer LG, Edelman IS, Lindemann B: The role of sodium-channel density in the natriferic response of the toad urinary bladder to an antidiuretic hormone. *J Membr Biol* 64:77–89, 1982
28. Garty H, Edelman IS: Amiloride-sensitive trypsinization of apical sodium channels. *J Gen Physiol* 81:785–803, 1983
29. Karnieli E, Zarnowski MJ, Hissin PJ, Simpson IA, Salans LB, Cushman SW: Insulin-stimulated translocation of glucose transport systems in the isolated rat adipose cell. *J Biol Chem* 256:4772–4777, 1981
30. Kono T, Robinson FW, Blevins TL, Ezaki O: Evidence that translocation of the glucose transport activity is the major mechanism of insulin action on glucose transport in fat cells. *J Biol Chem* 257:10942–10947, 1982
31. Stetson DL, Wade JB, Giebisch G: Morphologic alterations in the rat medullary collecting duct following potassium depletion. *Kidney Int* 17:45–56, 1980
32. Gluck S, Cannon C, Al-Awqati Q: Exocytosis regulates urinary acidification in turtle bladder by rapid insertion of H^+ pumps into the luminal membrane. *Proc Natl Acad Sci USA* 79:4327–4331, 1982
33. Stetson DL, Steinmetz PR: Role of membrane fusion in CO_2 stimulation of proton secretion by turtle bladder. *Am J Physiol* 245:C113–C120, 1983
34. Lewis SA, de Moura JLC: Incorporation of cytoplasmic vesicles into apical membrane of mammalian urinary bladder epithelium. *Nature* 297:685–688, 1982
35. Loo DDF, Lewis SA, Ifshin MS, Diamond JM: Turnover, membrane insertion, and degradation of sodium channels in rabbit urinary bladder. *Science* 221:1288–1290, 1983
36. Diamond JM, Machen TE: Impedance analysis in epithelia and the problem of gastric acid secretion. *J Membr Biol* 72:17–41, 1983
37. Levine JS, Nakane PK, Allen RH: Human intrinsic factor secretion: immunocytochemical demonstration of membrane-associated vesicular transport in parietal cells. *J Cell Biol* 90:644–655, 1981
38. Rasmussen H: *Calcium and cAMP as Synarchic Messengers.* New York, John Wiley & Sons, 1981, p 124
39. Taylor A, Palmer LG: Hormonal regulation of sodium chloride and water transport in epithelia, in *Biological Regulation and Development,* vol 3A, chap 7, edited by Goldberger RF, Yamamoto K, New York, Plenum Press, 1982, p 253
40. Grosso A, Cox JA, Malnoë A, de Sousa RC: Evidence for a role of calmodulin in the hydrosmotic action of vasopressin in toad bladder. *J Physiol (Paris)* 78:270–278, 1982
41. de Sousa RC, Grosso A, Malnoë A, Cox JA: Vasopressin and its intracellular messengers, in *Neuroendocrinology of Vasopressin, Corticoliberin and Opiomelano-*

cortins, edited by BAERTSCH AJ, DREIFUSS JJ, London, Academic Press, 1982, p 199
42. GROSSO A, DE SOUSA RC: High [K^+] alters the stimulus-hydrosmotic response coupling in toad bladder. *Pflügers Arch* 400:349–355, 1984
43. GROSSO A, BROWN D, DE SOUSA RC: Cellular and membrane events involved in the K-induced increase in water permeability of toad skin. *Pflügers Arch* 395:145–151, 1982

Specificity of Agonistic and Antagonistic Analogues of Vasopressin

Wilbur H. Sawyer and Maurice Manning

What we had long considered to be solely an antidiuretic hormone has recently been recognized to contribute significantly to cardiovascular regulation as well. Also, we are only now beginning to appreciate that vasopressin may serve a variety of functions within the central nervous system as a neuromodulator or neurotransmitter. The development of structural analogues of vasopressin with specific agonistic or antagonistic activities can provide valuable pharmacologic methods for exploring the diversity of vasopressin's actions and the receptors that mediate them. We plan to consider here the types of vasopressin receptors that have been well characterized and to mention a few examples suggesting the existence of additional classes of receptors. We shall also recount our progress in the development of specific vasopressin receptor blockers and point out why we feel that specificity is an important goal.

Vasopressin Receptor Types

Structural analogues of arginine-vasopressin (AVP) differ markedly in their relative antidiuretic and vasopressor potencies [1]. A well-known example is dDAVP (1-deamino [8-D-arginine] vasopressin), which has more antidiuretic activity than AVP and only about 1/1000 as much vasopressor activity (Table 1). This diversity of action shows that antidiuretic and vasopressor receptors are activated by different structural features of the AVP molecule. In vitro binding studies using agonistic analogues of AVP also clearly demonstrate that these receptors differ in their specificities. In general, the affinities of various agonists for each receptor type in vitro correspond well with their respective activities in vivo [2, 3].

This manuscript was presented as part of a Symposium on *Vasopressin: Diverse Actions.*

Table 1. Relative agonistic potencies of some vasopressin analogues on rat V_1 and V_2 receptors

| | V_1 Receptors | | |
Analogue[a]	Vasopressor[b] (in vivo)	Glycogenolytic[c] (in vitro)	V_2 Receptors[b] (antidiuretic; in vivo)
AVP	100	100	100
dDAVP	0.1	0.06	370
dVDAVP	Antagonist	Antagonist	380
[Phe²]OVT	34	—	0.2
OT	1.1	0.3	1.2

[a] Abbreviations are AVP, arginine-vasopressin; dDAVP, 1-deamino [8-D-arginine] vasopressin; dVDAVP, 1-deamino [4-valine, 8-D-arginine] vasopressin; [Phe²]OVT, [2-phenylalanine, 8-ornithine] vasotocin; and OT, oxytocin. Relative activities are expressed as the percentage of the activity of AVP.

[b] Data on rat assays are from Sawyer, Grzonka, and Manning [1].

[c] Assayed on isolated rat hepatocytes; data from Keppens and de Wulf [30].

Antidiuretic and vasopressor receptors also differ in the manner in which they affect cellular responses to AVP. The antidiuretic response involves activation of membrane-bound adenylate cyclase and the generation of cyclic AMP as a second messenger [2]. The contractile response of vascular smooth muscle and the glycogenolytic response of hepatocytes do not involve cyclase activation [3]. This has led to the designation of vasopressor and hepatocyte receptors as *V_1-receptors* and antidiuretic receptors as *V_2-receptors* [4]. This is analogous to the designation of histamine receptors as H_1 and H_2. H_1 receptors do not appear to mediate the activation of adenylate cyclase, but H_2 receptors do.

Thus, the classical peripheral vasopressor and antidiuretic responses to AVP are mediated by V_1 and V_2 receptors that have been clearly differentiated in structure-activity studies with AVP analogues and on the basis of their mode of action. There are suggestions, however, that there may be other AVP receptor types that do not fall neatly into V_1 or V_2 categories. Such still-unclassified receptors may be involved in some of the diverse actions of AVP on the release of adrenocorticotropic hormone (ACTH), behavior, temperature regulation, and cardiovascular reflexes.

ACTH Release by AVP

AVP alone can cause ACTH release from the adenohypophysis, and it also potentiates release of ACTH by corticotropin releasing factor (CRF) [5]. Limited studies with agonistic AVP analogues in rats pretreated to prevent release of endogenous CRF indicate that the ACTH-releasing potencies of analogues parallel their vasopressor potencies. Release of ACTH by AVP could also be blunted with specific V_1 antagonists. V_1 receptors may thus be involved in the stimulation of ACTH release by systemically administered AVP [6]. Studies on isolated rat adenohypophyseal cells, however, indicate that the ACTH-releasing activities of AVP analogues are not correlated with either their vasopressor or antidiuretic activities or with their V_1 and V_2 agonistic activities determined by in vitro assays [7]. It is not clear whether ACTH release by AVP involves the generation of cyclic AMP [7, 8]. It seems possible, therefore, that AVP may influence ACTH release indirectly by acting on V_1 receptors and directly by acting on one or more types of receptors on adenohypophyseal cells that differ from the known V_1 and V_2 types [7].

Behavioral Effects of AVP

Although vasopressinergic fibers project from the ventral hypothalamus into many other areas of the central nervous system [9], their functions remain largely unknown. Exogenous AVP can exert a variety of behavioral effects. Limited studies with agonistic analogues suggest that different receptor types may be involved depending on the particular behavioral model studied [10].

One rat model that has been explored in some detail is the conditioned avoidance response. If vasopressin is administered soon after a rat has been conditioned to avoid a noxious stimulus, it delays the rate at which the conditioned avoidance behavior disappears. AVP thus appears to improve the consolidation and retention of memory. This effect of AVP can be blocked with V_1 antagonists [11]. In fact, a V_1 antagonist given alone has been shown to hasten extinction of the conditioned response. This "amnestic" effect could be due to blockade of endogenous vasopressin acting on V_1 receptors within the central nervous system. Studies using agonistic analogues, however, do not support the hypothesis that typical V_1 receptors are involved (Table 2). The desglycinamide vasopressins that have almost no vasopressor activity can also delay extinction of the avoidance response [12]. Recently, a desglycinamide metabolite of AVP, pyroglutamyl-asparagyl-cystinyl-prolyl-arginine, has been found much more potent than AVP itself in delaying extinction of an avoidance response [13]. This analogue has undetectable vasopressor

Table 2. Relative activities of several vasopressin analogues on some rat assays

Analogue[a]	Vasopressor (V_1) activity[b] (U/mg)	Antipyretic[c]	Consolidation of memory[c]	Antidiuretic (V_2) activity[b] (U/mg)
AVP	370	+++	++	320
OT	4	+	—	4
desGly(NH$_2$)^{9}AVP	0	0	+	6
[pGlu^4-Cys(Cys)^6]AVP(4–8)	0	0	++++	?[d]

[a] Abbreviations are AVP, arginine-vasopressin; OT, oxytocin; desGly(NH$_2$)^{9}AVP, desglycinamide-arginine-vasopressin; and [pGlu^4-Cys(Cys)^6]AVP(4–8), pyroglutamyl-asparagyl-cystinyl-prolyl-arginine.

[b] Data are from Sawyer et al [1] and Manning et al [31].

[c] Data adapted from Kovács and de Wied [12] and Burbach et al [13]. Peptides were injected into the lateral cerebral ventricles. "Consolidation of memory" was estimated from the retention of a conditioned passive-avoidance response for 24 and 48 hr.

[d] Not reported for this analogue, but [pGlu^4-Cys(Cys)^6]AVP(4–9) has an antidiuretic activity of 0.001 U/mg (unpublished). The desglycinamide AVP(4–8) analogue would be expected to be even less active on antidiuretic assays [31].

activity. Its action can, however, be blocked by a "specific" V_1 antagonist [14]. The antagonist studies suggest that the effects of AVP on memory in these rat models may be mediated by receptors resembling the V_1 type. The effectiveness of analogues lacking V_1 agonism, however, clearly shows that their receptors are not the same as the classical peripheral V_1 receptors. Another conclusion is that we have overrated the "specificity" of our V_1 antagonists by defining it only from measurements of blood pressure, urine flow, and uterine activity.

Antipyretic Action of AVP

AVP administered into the cerebral ventricles can decrease or prevent the febrile response of rats to bacterial endotoxin [12]. This central action of AVP appears to involve a different receptor type than does its action on memory. Desglycinamide analogues that are active in behavioral tests of memory consolidation lack detectable antipyretic activity. Only a few analogues have been tested, but their antipyretic activities seem to parallel their vasopressor activities (Table 2). The receptors involved may be the V_1 type, but more detailed studies are needed to confirm this. In any event, this is another clear indication that vasopressin receptors within the brain may differ among themselves in their pharmacologic characteristics.

AVP and Baroreceptor Reflexes

Although AVP is the most potent vasoconstrictor agent known, it has much less effect on systemic blood pressure in intact animals than one might expect from its direct vascular effects. AVP appears to produce an exaggerated reflex decrease in cardiac output that effectively buffers the influence of increased peripheral vascular resistance [15]. Injected or endogenous AVP appears to enhance the gain of the baroreceptor reflex, probably by acting somewhere on the lower brainstem [16]. Although the effect of AVP on peripheral resistance is clearly mediated by V_1 receptors, its effects on baroreceptor reflex sensitivity may involve a different receptor type. Brattleboro homozygous rats lacking AVP have depressed baroreceptor sensitivity [17]. This can be restored to normal by treatment with AVP or dDAVP, which is almost devoid of V_1 agonistic activity. A V_1 antagonist fails to block the effects of either endogenous or exogenous AVP on baroreceptor sensitivity. Thus, the effect of AVP on baroreflex activity does not appear to involve V_1 receptors. Further studies are needed to determine whether V_2 receptors or some other type may mediate this interesting action of AVP.

Development of Specific Antagonists

Antagonists of the diverse actions of AVP can be useful pharmacologic tools, particularly for studies on the actions of endogenous AVP. They can be used acutely in intact animals to block a particular response. This avoids many problems inherent in experiments involving neurohypophyseal ablation or the use of Brattleboro rats.

V_1 Antagonists

Vasopressor responses appear to be blocked relatively easily. The earliest antagonistic analogue reported by du Vigneaud's group over 20 years ago, [2-O-methyltyrosine]oxytocin, was a weak antagonist of the vasopressor response in rats [18]. Subsequently, this group reported that a vasopressin analogue containing a dialkyl substitution on the β carbon of the residue in the 1-position—[1-(β-mercapto-β, β-diethylpropionic acid)]lysine-vasopressin—was a much more potent vasopressor antagonist [19]. When we combined both types of modification into the same molecules, we found that their effects on antagonistic potency appeared additive. The most potent V_1 antagonist yet reported is an analogue of AVP with a cyclopentamethylene substitution on the β carbon of the residue in position 1 and a 2-O-methyltyrosine; namely, $d(CH_2)_5[Tyr(Me)^2]AVP$ ([1-β-mercapto-β,β-cyclopentamethyl-enepropionic acid, 2-O-methyltyrosine]arginine-vasopressin) [20]. This analogue, in terms of our standard assays, is also highly specific for V_1 receptors (Table 3). It is a weak antidiuretic agonist. It does not block antidiuretic responses to AVP, and it is about 100 times as effective in blocking vasopressor

Table 3. Specificities of some representative antagonists of vasopressin

	Antagonistic "effective doses,"[b] (nmoles/kg)		
Analogue[a]	Antivasopressor (V_1)	Antiantidiuretic (V_2)	Antioxytocic (in vivo)
$d(Ch_2)_5[Tyr(Me)^2]AVP^c$	0.16	Agonist	17
$d(CH_2)_5[Tyr(Et)^2]VAVP$	0.49	1.9	13
$d(CH_2)_5[D\text{-}Phe^2]VAVP$	0.58	0.67	8.9
$d(CH_2)_5[D\text{-}Ile^2,Ile^4]AVP$	26	0.67	9.4

[a] Abbreviations are defined as follows: $d(CH_2)_5[Tyr(Me)^2]AVP$ is [1-(β-mercapto-β,β-cyclopentamethylenepropionic acid), 2-O-methyltyrosine]-arginine-vasopressin; $d(CH_2)_5[Tyr(Et)^2]VAVP$ is [1-(β-mercapto-β,β-cyclopentamethylenepropionic acid), 2-O-ethyltyrosine, 4-valine]arginine-vasopressin; $d(CH_2)_5[D\text{-}Phe^2]VAVP$ is [1-(β-mercapto-β,β-cyclopentamethylenepropionic acid), 2-D-phenylalanine,4-valine]arginine-vasopressin; and $d(CH_2)_5[D\text{-}Ile^2,Ile^4]AVP$ is [1-(β-mercapto-β,β-cyclopentamethylenepropionic acid, 2-D-isoleucine,4-isoleucine]arginine-vasopressin.

[b] The "effective dose" of an antagonist is one that effectively reduces the response to 2 $\times$ units of agonist to equal the response to 1 $\times$ units in the absence of antagonist. For these antagonists, 1 nmole equals 1.1 to 1.2 μg. Data are from [20, 24–27].

[c] The structure of $d(CH_2)_5[Tyr(Me)^2]AVP$ is represented by the following diagram:

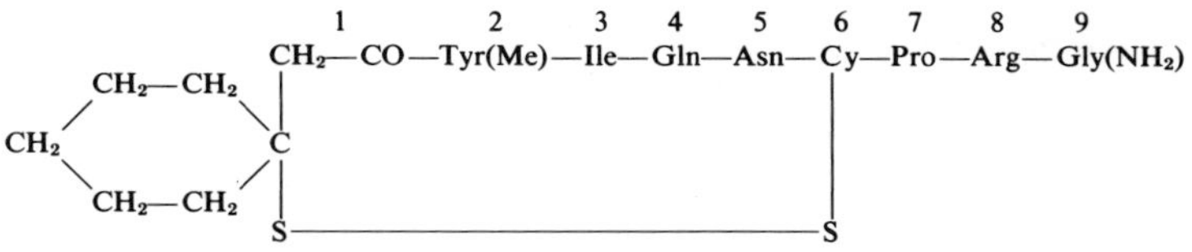

$$\begin{array}{cccccccccc}
 & & 1 & 2 & 3 & 4 & 5 & 6 & 7 & 8 & 9 \\
 & & CH_2\text{—}CO\text{—}Tyr(Me)\text{—}Ile\text{—}Gln\text{—}Asn\text{—}Cy\text{—}Pro\text{—}Arg\text{—}Gly(NH_2)
\end{array}$$

<pre>
      CH₂—CH₂ |
     /   \ |
CH₂   C
     \   / |
      CH₂—CH₂ |
                 S————————————————————————S
</pre>

responses to AVP as it is in blocking uterine responses to oxytocin. The combination of potency and specificity as a V_1 antagonist has made $d(CH_2)_5[Tyr(Me)^2]AVP$ a powerful tool for probing the contributions AVP makes to cardiovascular regulation. Studies using this peptide, and related V_1 antagonists, have established that AVP is an important factor in maintaining systemic blood pressure in conditions involving modest volume depletion, such as nonhypotensive hemorrhage, dehydration, and adrenocortical insufficiency [21–23].

V_2 Antagonists

The design of effective blockers of antidiuretic responses to AVP has been a long-sought goal. We were finally successful when we combined cyclopentamethylene substitution on the β carbon of the residue at position 1 with O-alkylation of the 2-tyrosine in analogues of 1-deamino[4-valine]arginine-vasopressin [24]. The best among the earliest V_2 antagonists reported was $d(CH_2)_5[Tyr(Et)^2,Val^4]AVP$, or [1-($\beta$-mercapto-$\beta$,$\beta$-cyclopentamethylene-propionic acid), 2-O-ethyltyrosine, 4-valine]arginine-vasopressin (Table 3). This was not a pure antagonist, for it caused a brief antidiuresis that was followed by a period in which it effectively blocked antidiuretic responses to exogenous AVP. It also blocked endogenous AVP. When given to normally hydrated rats, it caused a dramatic diabetes insipidus-like diuresis. This analogue was far from being a specific V_2 antagonist. It was, in fact, about four times more potent as a V_1 blocker.

In subsequent efforts to improve on both potency and specificity of V_2 antagonists, we have tried a large number of substitutions in the basic framework of $d(CH_2)_5[Tyr(Et)^2, Val^4]AVP$ [25]. We have found that substitution of 2-D-(O-alkyl)tyrosines improved potency and that some other D-amino acids in the 2-position were consistent with potent antagonistic activity. For example, $d(CH_2)_5[D\text{-Phe}^2, Val^4]AVP$ is more potent and is also devoid of detectable agonistic activity [26]. It is still far from specific, however, and retains V_1 antagonistic activity approximately equal to its V_2 antagonistic activity. When a 2-D-isoleucine is substituted, there is a dramatic jump in specificity (Table 3). $d(CH_2)_5[D\text{-Ile},Val^4]AVP$ is about 12 times more active as a V_2 than as a V_1 antagonist [26]. Substitution of other amino acids in the 4-position with hydrophobic side chains for the 4-valine led to even greater V_2-specificity [27]. $d(CH_2)_5[D\text{-Ile}^2, Ile^4]AVP$ is about 40 times as potent a V_2 as a V_1 antagonist is and is also without agonistic activity (Table 3). Although we have not yet managed to achieve absolute V_2 specificity, we have attained a level of selectivity that should allow one to use this antagonist in doses that block antidiuretic responses without significantly depressing vascular responses to AVP.

Effective V_2 antagonists should be powerful pharmacologic tools for assessing the contribution of AVP to water retention in a variety of pathophysiologic states. The only published report of such an application is one by Ishikawa and Schrier [28], who used $d(CH_2)_5[Tyr(Et)^2, Val^4]AVP$ to demonstrate the contribution of AVP to impaired water excretion by rats with adrenocorticosteroid deficiencies. As V_2 antagonists become more freely available, they should find widespread use in studies of this type.

Effective V_2 antagonists should provide the first specific means for treating the syndrome of inappropriate ADH secretion (SIADH). Although such analogues have not yet reached clinical trial, László, Csáti, and Baláspiri [29] found one that was effective in preventing hyponatremia and cerebral edema in rats treated with vasopressin tannate and given repeated water loads over a 5-day period.

The Importance of Specificity

We have emphasized the desirability of producing more specific V_1 and V_2 antagonists. These would obviously be useful experimentally for selectively blocking one or another of the diverse actions of AVP. They would also be useful in efforts to classify receptor types. Selectivity could also become important when antagonists are used clinically. For example, if a V_2 antagonist were used to treat water retention, it could be potentially troublesome if it also blocked central nervous system receptors associated with memory and possibly other cerebral functions. It thus seems important that we try to learn more about the characteristics of AVP receptors other than the well-known peripheral V_1 and V_2 receptors. This would let us attempt to design antagonists that can be targeted more sharply against the specific AVP receptors that we wish to block without the danger of undesirable side effects from blocking some of the other varied and largely unknown actions of AVP.

Acknowledgments. Unpublished findings of the authors reported here result from studies supported in part by research grants from the National Institute of Arthritis, Diabetes, Digestive and Kidney Diseases (AM-01940) and the National Institute of General Medical Sciences (GM-25280).

References

1. SAWYER WH, GRZONKA Z, MANNING M: Neurohypophysial peptides: Design of tissue-specific agonists and antagonists. *Mol Cell Endocrinol* 22:117–134, 1981
2. BUTLEN D, GUILLON, G, RAJERISON RM, JARD S, SAWYER WH, MANNING H: Structural requirements for activation of vasopressin-sensitive adenylate cyclase, hormone binding, and antidiuretic actions: Effects of highly potent analogues and competitive inhibitors. *Mol Pharmacol* 14:1006–1017, 1978
3. PENIT J, FAURE M, JARD S: Vasopressin and angiotensin II receptors in rat aortic smooth muscle cells in culture. *Am J Physiol* 244:E72-E82, 1983
4. MICHELL RH, KIRK CJ, BILLAH MM: Hormonal stimulation of phosphatidyl inositol breakdown with particular reference to the hepatic effects of vasopressin. *Biochem Soc Trans* 7:861–865, 1979
5. GILLIES GE, LINTON EA, LOWRY PJ: Corticotropin releasing activity of the new CRF is potentiated several times by vasopressin. *Nature (Lond)* 299:355–357, 1982

6. AIZAWA T, YASUDA N, GREER MA, SAWYER WH: In vivo adrenocorticotropin-releasing activity of neurohypophysial hormones and their analogs. *Endocrinology* 110:98–104, 1982

7. KNEPEL W, HOMOLKA L, VLASKOVSKA M, NUTTO D: In vitro adrenocorticotropin/β-endorphin-releasing activity of vasopressin analogs is related neither to pressor nor to antidiuretic activity. *Endocrinology*, in press

8. GIGUERE V, LABRIE F: Vasopressin potentiates cyclic AMP accumulation and ACTH release induced by corticotropin-releasing factor (CRF) in rat anterior pituitary cells in culture. *Endocrinology* 111:1752–1754, 1982

9. SOFRONIEW M: Projections from vasopressin, oxytocin, and neurophysin neurons to neural targets in the rat and human. *J Histochem Cytochem* 28:475–478, 1980

10. WALTER R, VAN REE JM, DE WIED D: Modification of conditioned behavior of rats by neurohypophysial hormones and analogues. *Proc Natl Acad Sci USA* 75:2493–2496, 1978

11. KOOB GF, LE MOAL M, GAFFORI O, MANNING M, SAWYER WH, RIVIER J, BLOOM FE: Arginine vasopressin and a vasopressin antagonist peptide: Opposite effects on extinction of active avoidance in rats. *Reg Peptides* 2:153–163, 1981

12. KOVÁCS GL, DE WIED D: Hormonally active arginine-vasopressin suppresses endotoxin-induced fever in rats: Lack of effect of oxytocin and a behaviorally active vasopressin fragment. *Neuroendocrinology* 37:258–261, 1983

13. BURBACH JPH, KOVÁCS GL, DE WIED D, VAN NISPEN JW, GREVEN HM: A major metabolite of arginine vasopressin in the brain is a highly potent neuropeptide. *Science* 221:1310–1312, 1983

14. DE WIED D, GAFFORI O, VAN REE JM, DE JONG W: Pharmacological evidence for brain receptors mediating the behavioral effects of vasopressin neuropeptides. *Nature (Lond)*, in press

15. MONTANI J-P, LIARD J-F, SCHOUN J, MÖHRING J: Hemodynamic effects of exogenous and endogenous vasopressin at low plasma concentrations in conscious dogs. *Circ Res* 47:346–355, 1980

16. LIARD JF, DÉRIAZ O, TSCHOPP M, SCHOUN J: Cardiovascular effects of vasopressin infused into the vertebral circulation of conscious dogs. *Clin Sci* 61:345–347, 1981

17. IMAI Y, NOLAN PL, JOHNSTON CI: Restoration of suppressed baroreflex sensitivity in rats with hereditary diabetes insipidus (Brattleboro rats) by arginine-vasopressin and DDAVP. *Circ Res* 53:140–149, 1983

18. LAW HD, DU VIGNEAUD V: Synthesis of 2-*p*-methoxyphenylalanine oxytocin (*O*-methyl-oxytocin) and some observations on its pharmacological behavior. *J Am Chem Soc* 82:4579–4581, 1960

19. DYCKES DF, NESTOR JJ JR, FERGER MF, DU VIGNEAUD V: [1-β-Mercapto-β,β-diethylpropionic acid]-8-lysine-vasopressin, a potent inhibitor of 8-lysine-vasopressin and of oxytocin. *J Med Chem* 17:250–252, 1974

20. KRUSZYNSKI M, LAMMEK B, MANNING M, SETO J, HALDAR J, SAWYER WH: [1-(β-Mercapto-β,β-cyclopentamethylenepropionic acid), 2-*O*(methyl)tyrosine]-arginine-vasopressin and [1-(β-mercapto-β,β-cyclopentamethylenepropionic acid)]-arginine-vasopressin, two highly potent antagonists of the vasopressor response to arginine vasopressin. *J Med Chem* 23:364–368, 1980

21. SCHWARTZ J, REID IA: Effect of vasopressin blockade on blood pressure regulation during hemorrhage in conscious dogs. *Endocrinology* 109:1778–1780, 1981

22. ANDREWS CE JR, BRENNER BM: Relative contributions of arginine vasopressin and angiotensin II to maintenance of systemic arterial pressure in the anesthetized water-deprived rat. *Circ Res* 48:254–258, 1981

23. SCHWARTZ J, KEIL LC, MASELLI J, REID IA: Role of vasopressin in blood

pressure regulation during adrenal insufficiency. *Endocrinology* 112:234–238, 1983
24. SAWYER WH, PANG PKT, SETO J, McENROE M, LAMMEK B, MANNING M: Vasopressin analogs that antagonize antidiuretic responses by rats to the antidiuretic hormone. *Science* 212:49–51, 1981
25. MANNING M, LAMMEK B, KOLODZIEJCZYK A, SETO J, SAWYER WH: Synthetic antagonists of in vivo antidiuretic and vasopressor responses to arginine vasopressin. *J Med Chem* 24:701–706, 1981
26. MANNING M, OLMA A, KLIS WA, SETO J, SAWYER WH: Potent antagonists of the antidiuretic response to arginine-vasopressin based on modifications of [1-(β-mercapto-β,β-cyclopentamethylenepropionic acid), 2-D-phenylalanine, 4-valine]-arginine-vasopressin (d(CH$_2$)$_5$ D-Phe^2-VAVP) at position four. *J Med Chem* 26:1607–1613, 1983
27. MANNING M, NAWROCKA E, MISICKA A, OLMA A, KLIS WA, SETO J, SAWYER WH: Potent and selective antagonists of the antidiuretic response to arginine-vasopressin based on modifications of [1-(β-mercapto-β,β-cyclopentamethylene-propionic acid), 2-D-isoleucine, 4-valine] arginine-vasopressin at position 4. *J Med Chem,* in press
28. ISHIKAWA S-E, SCHRIER RW: Effect of arginine vasopressin antagonist on renal water excretion in glucocorticoid and mineralocorticoid deficient rats. *Kidney Int* 22:587–593, 1982
29. LÁSZLÓ FA, CSÁTI S, BALÁSPIRI L: Prevention of hyponatremia and cerebral oedema by the vasopressin antagonist d/CH$_2$/$_5$ Tyr/Et/VAVP in rats treated with pitressin tannate. *Acta Endocrinol,* in press
30. KEPPENS S, DE WULF H: The nature of the hepatic receptors involved in vasopressin-induced glycogenolysis. *Biochim Biophys Acta* 588:63–69, 1979
31. MANNING M, OLMA K, KLIS W, KOLODZIEJCZYK A, NAWROCKA E, MISICKA-KESIK A, SETO J, SAWYER WH: Carboxy terminus of vasopressin required for activity but not binding. *Nature (Lond),* in press

Cardiovascular Effects of Vasopressin

Colin I. Johnston, Masao Hiwatari, and Josephine M. Abrahams

Vasopressin has diverse actions on the cardiovascular system (see Table 1). For many years, most of these actions were regarded as pharmacologic effects of little physiologic importance. This was because the dose of vasopressin required to produce a rise in blood pressure was a hundred times greater than that needed for maximal antidiuresis. However, many recent studies have demonstrated the importance of its cardiovascular effects in the physiologic control of the circulation and in blood pressure homeostasis [1–4]. The two major biological actions of vasopressin, that of vasoconstriction and antidiuresis to maintain volume, are similar to those of the renin-angiotensin-aldosterone system, another powerful vasoactive hormonal system important in blood pressure control.

Direct Vasoconstrictor Activity

Vasopressin is the most potent known vasoactive vasoconstrictor both in vitro and in vivo [5]. It constricts a variety of smooth muscle, including

Table 1. Circulatory effects of vasopressin

1. Vasoconstriction
2. Antidiuresis—volume
3. Modulation of baroreflex
4. Cardiac effects
   a. Chronotropic
   b. Inotropic
5. Interaction with sympathetic nervous system
   a. Peripheral
   b. Central
6. Interaction with renin-angiotensin system

This manuscript was presented as part of a Symposium on *Vasopressin: Diverse Actions.*

vascular smooth muscle, by activation of specific vasopressin plasma membrane receptors known as V_1 receptors (Fig. 1). Activation of the membrane receptor leads to contraction of smooth muscle owing to increases in cytoplasmic calcium. This vasoconstrictor action of vasopressin can be attenuated by calcium antagonists. When exogenous vasopressin is infused i.v. into intact humans and animals, it leads to increases in total peripheral resistance (TPR). The degree of vasoconstriction varies for different vascular beds: the skin, muscle, and splanchnic circulations contribute most to the increase; the coronary and renal beds are less sensitive; and the cerebral circulation is not affected [4, 6, 7]. The vasoconstriction and increase in TPR can be shown to occur with only small increases in plasma vasopressin levels, similar to concentrations seen during dehydration [8].

The resultant rise in blood pressure is, however, greatly attenuated in the intact animal, and plasma vasopressin concentrations of 100 pg or more (10 to 20 times normal) are needed to achieve a significant 10-mm Hg rise in arterial blood pressure (Fig. 2). The compensatory mechanisms buffering the increase in blood pressure following vasopressin infusion include specific activation of the baroreflex, which causes bradycardia and a fall in cardiac output, a direct negative chronotropic effect [9]. Compensatory mechanisms also include suppression of renin release from the kidney, and a resulting fall in plasma renin and angiotensin II levels (see Fig. 2) [10]. In animals in whom the autonomic nervous system has been either ablated [11] or blocked [12], there is increased sensitivity to vasopressin; there is a marked shift to the right in the pressor dose response curve and a rise in arterial blood pressure at low infusion rates. In this case, rises in blood pressure can be achieved within the physiologic concentration range for plasma vasopressin.

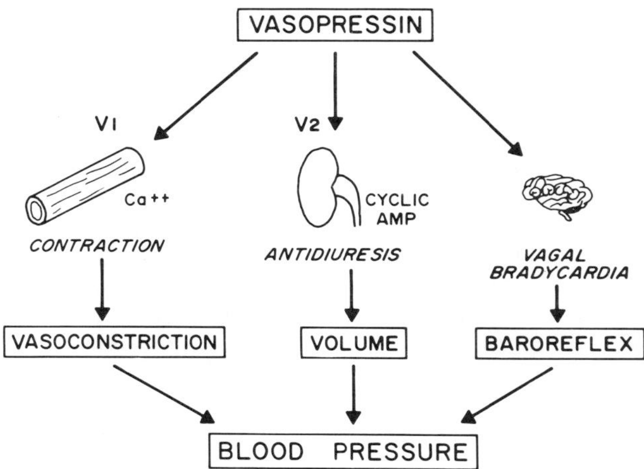

Fig. 1. Physiologic actions of vasopressin that influence the cardiovascular system and blood pressure.

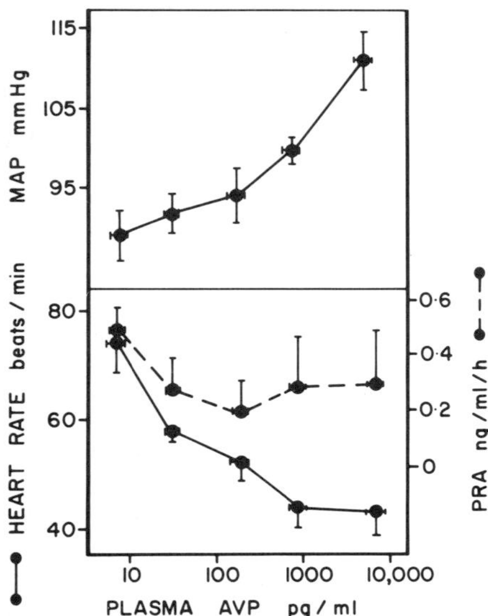

Fig. 2. Plasma vasopressin (*AVP*) concentration after infusion of synthetic arginine vasopressin into conscious dogs and the relation to mean arterial pressure (*MAP*), heart rate, and plasma renin activity (*PRA*).

Physiologic Importance of Vasopressin Vasoconstriction

Vasopressin is released from the posterior pituitary by both osmotic and nonosmotic stimuli. The low-pressure and high-pressure baroreceptors and volume receptors are activated when the volume state of the organism is threatened. The vasopressin released by these stimuli helps to maintain blood pressure by direct vasoconstriction.

During dehydration over a number of days, there is a progressive increase in plasma vasopressin even when maximal antidiuresis is achieved after the first 12 hr [13]. The importance of vasopressin in maintaining blood pressure during dehydration has now been demonstrated in several ways: (a) by showing a drop in blood pressure with specific vascular receptor antagonist to vasopressin [14, 15], (b) by showing the failure of the Brattleboro diabetes insipidus rat to maintain blood pressure during dehydration [16], and (c) by showing that the hemodynamic changes produced by dehydration can be mimicked in the rats by the infusion of exogenous vasopressin.

Similarly, vasopressin is important in the circulatory response to hemorrhage [17–19], orthostasis [20], and adrenal insufficiency [21].

Antidiuretic Volume Effects

Blood pressure is proportional to both the total peripheral resistance and the cardiac output. The cardiac output is dependent on adequate venous return and, hence, on blood volume. Vasopressin, through its antidiuretic activity, is essential for maintaining both a correct plasma osmolality and sodium concentration as well as a correct extracellular fluid volume. Hence, its antidiuretic action of influencing the extracellular and blood volume is an important component in blood pressure hemostasis.

A similar analogy can be drawn with the renin-angiotensin system, where angiotensin, through both its vasoconstrictor action and its stimulation of aldosterone and sodium retention, is an important hormone in the control of blood pressure.

In dehydration, the long-term maintenance of blood pressure is therefore dependent on both the antidiuretic as well as the vasoconstrictor properties of vasopressin. We have recently demonstrated this using dDAVP, a peptide analogue with antidiuretic properties but minimal vascular effects. In one-kidney one-clip experimental renal hypertension in rats [22], achieving the absolute hypertensive blood pressure was dependent on the antidiuretic properties of vasopressin rather than on its pressor properties [23]. Recent studies in deoxycorticosterone (DOCA)-salt hypertension support the same conclusion [24, 25]. Vasopressin appears to be necessary in this experimental model of hypertension, not for its vascular action as was proposed previously [25, 26], but for its antidiuretic action.

Cardiac Effects

Vasopressin has been shown to have only a weak direct negative chronotropic effect and a small inotropic effect in vitro [9]. But in vivo, it causes a marked bradycardia even before there is any rise in blood pressure and activation of baroreceptors. The bradycardia persists even after total autonomic blockade [10] and therefore consists of baroreceptor-dependent and -independent components. The direct negative chronotropic effect demonstrable in vitro at only high vasopressin concentrations may be of little physiologic importance unless some form of sensitization occurs.

Modulation of the Baroreflex Function

Vasopressin causes a greater decrease in heart rate for a given increase in blood pressure than do either angiotensin or adrenergic agonists (phenylephrine, methoxanine). This suggests that it may have some direct actions on the baroreflex. The importance of vasopressin in modulating the baroreflex has recently been established using the Brattleboro vasopressin-deficient rat. This animal has a depressed baroreflex; that is, for any rise in blood pressure, there is little reflex slowing of the heart rate. Imai, Nolan, and Johnston [27] further showed that the baroreflex in this animal could be corrected by either the i.v. or intracerebroventricular infusion of vasopressin or dDAVP. Whether the effect is on the carotid body, the afferent limb, the central connections, or the efferent limb of the baroreflex still needs establishing.

However, recent anatomic studies have established that there are noradrenergic pathways from the medullary cardiovascular centers (including the nucleii of the tractus solatarius) to the hypothalamus and, conversely, that there are vasopressinergic neurones from the paraventricular nucleus passing down to cardiovascular centers in the midbrain and spinal cord [28, 29]. These important pathways provide neuronal circuits by which vasopressin can influence central cardiovascular control.

Cowley, Quillen, and Skelton [3], using a more direct approach with an isolated carotid sinus of the dog, have also established the importance of vasopressin on the baroreflex.

Interaction with the Sympathetic Nervous System and the Renin-Angiotensin System

Vasopressin has some important interactions with the other two major systems involved in blood pressure regulation. As has been known for a long time, it potentiates the vascular action of either sympathetic nerve stimulation or noradrenaline [30]. Conversely, the sympathetic nervous system affects its vascular action [19], which has already been mentioned. The mechanism (or mechanisms) by which vasopressin potentiates the sympathetic nervous system is not known and requires further study. In a series of studies conducted over a long period of time, McNeill has elegantly shown how the three systems interact to maintain peripheral resistance, particularly after hemorrhage or volume depletion [4].

Vasopressin also suppresses renin release from the kidneys both in humans and animals. This appears to be both a direct action as well as an indirect action via the renal baroreceptors. The direct action has been demonstrated on the isolated perfused rat kidney. Angiotensin has also been reported to cause vasopressin release from the posterior pituitary. Share [31] has recently concluded that this is most likely a central effect of angiotensin. Interestingly, angiotensin receptors have been found in the supraoptic and paraventricular nuclei of the hypothalamus, which suggests some interrelationship between the two peptides.

Thus, the sympathetic nervous system, the renin-angiotensin system, and vasopressin seem to act in an integrated and coordinated manner to maintain the blood pressure and regulate blood flows to organs within normal limits.

References

1. MOHRING J: Neurohypophyseal vasopressor principle: Vasopressor hormone as well as antidiuretic hormone? *Klin Wochenschr* 56(Suppl. 1):71–79, 1978
2. JOHNSTON CI, NEWMAN M, WOODS RL: Role of vasopressin in cardiovascular homeostasis and hypertension. *Clin Sci* 61:129s–139s, 1981
3. COWLEY AW JR, QUILLEN EW, SKELTON MM: Role of vasopressin in cardiovascular regulation. *Fed Proc* 42:3170–3176, 1983

4. McNeil JR: Role of vasopressin in the control of arterial pressure. *Can J Physiol Pharmacol* 61:1226–1235, 1983
5. Altura BM, Altura BT: Vascular smooth muscle and neurohypophyseal hormones. *Fed Proc* 36:1867–1871, 1977
6. Liard JF, Deriaz O, Schelling P, Thinbonnier M: Cardiac output distribution during vasopressin infusion or dehydration in conscious dogs. *Am J Physiol* 243:H663–H669, 1982
7. Hoffman WE: Regional vascular effects of antidiuretic hormone in normal and sympathetic blocked rats. *Endocrinology* 107:334–341, 1980
8. Montani J, Liard JF, Schoun J, Mohring J: Hemodynamic effects of exogenous and endogenous vasopressin at low plasma concentrations in conscious dogs. *Circ Res* 47:346–355, 1981
9. Nakashima A, Angus JP, Johnston CI: Chronotropic effects of angiotensin I, angiotensin II, bradykinin and vasopressin in guinea pig atria. *Eur J Pharmacol* 81:479–485, 1982
10. Pullan PT, Johnston CI, Anderson WP, Korner PI: The role of vasopressin in blood pressure control and in experimental hypertension. *Clin Sci Mol Med* 55:251s–254s, 1978
11. Cowley AW Jr, Monroe E, Guyton AD: Interaction of vasopressin and the baroreceptor reflex system in the regulation of arterial blood pressure in the dog. *Circ Res* 34:505–514, 1974
12. Pullan PT, Johnston CI, Anderson WP, Korner PI: Plasma vasopressin in blood pressure homeostasis and in experimental renal hypertension. *Am J Physiol* 239:H81–H87, 1980
13. Johnston CI, Woods RL, Nolan PL, Imai Y: Vasopressin in blood pressure regulation, in *Proc 7th Asia & Oceania Congress of Endocrinology*, edited by Shizume E, Imura H, Shimizu N. Excerpta Medica Int Congress Series 598, 1982, pp. 349–354
14. Aisenbrey G, Manning M, Schrier R: Specific inhibitor of the vascular effect of exogenous and endogenous arginine vasopressin (AVP). *Kidney Int* 19:229, 1981
15. Andrews CE Jr, Brenner BM: Relative contributions of arginine vasopressin and angiotensin II to maintenance of systemic arterial pressure in the anaesthetised water-deprived rat. *Circ Res* 48:254–258, 1981
16. Woods RL, Johnston CI: Contribution of vasopressin to the maintenance of blood pressure and during dehydration. *Am J Physiol* 254:F615–F621, 1983
17. Cowley AW Jr, Switzer SJ, Guinn MM: Evidence and quantification of the vasopressin arterial pressure control system in the dog. *Circ Res* 46:58–66, 1980
18. Laycock J, Penn W, Shirley DG, Walter SJ: The role of vasopressin blood pressure regulation immediately following acute hemorrhage in the rat. *J Physiol* 292:267–275, 1979
19. Johnston CI, Imai Y, Woods RL: Regulation of blood pressure by vasopressin, in *Topics in Pathophysiology of Hypertension*, edited by Villereal H, Sambhi MP. Boston, Martinus Nighoff Publishers, 1984, pp 485–499
20. Davies R, Forsling ML, Slater JDH: The interrelationship between the release of renin and vasopressin as defined by orthostasis and propranolol. *J Clin Invest* 60:1438–1441, 1977
21. Schwartz J, Keil LC, Maselli J, Reid IA: Role of vasopressin in blood pressure regulation during adrenal insufficiency. *Endocrinology* 112:234–238, 1983
22. Woods RL, Johnston CI: The role of vasopressin in hypertension: Studies using the Brattleboro rat. *Am J Physiol* 242(6):F727–F732, 1982

23. Woods RL, Johnston CI: Importance of antidiuretic properties of vasopressin experimental renal hypertension. *Clin Exp Pharmacol Physiol* 8:519–523, 1981
24. Bereck KH, Murray RD, Cross F, Brody MJ: Vasopressin and vascular reactivity in the development of DOCA hypertension in rats with hereditary diabetes insipidus. *Hypertension* 4:3–12, 1982
25. Share L, Crofton JT: Contribution of vasopressin to hypertension. *Hypertension* 4(Suppl. 3):85–92, 1982
26. Mohring J, Mohring B, Petri M, Haack D: Vasopressor role of ADH in the pathogenesis of malignant DOC hypertension. *Am J Physiol* 232:260–269, 1977
27. Imai Y, Nolan PL, Johnston CI: Restoration of suppressed baroreflex sensitivity in rats with hereditary diabetes insipidus (Brattleboro rats) by arginine vasopressin & DDAVP. *Circ Res* 53:140–149, 1983
28. Sawochenko PE, Swanson LW: Central noradrenergic pathways for the integration of hypothalamic neuroendocrine and autonomic responses. *Science* 214:685–687, 1981
29. Sofroniew MV: Projections from vasopressin oxytocin and neurophysic neurons to neural targets in the rat and human. *J Histochem Cytochem* 28:475–478, 1980
30. Bartelstone HJ, Nasmyth PA: Vasopressin potentiation of catecholamine actions in dog, rat, cat and rat aortic strip. *Am J Physiol* 308:754–762, 1965
31. Share L: Interrelations between vasopressin and the renin angiotensin system. *Fed Proc* 38:2267–2271, 1979

Alterations of Extracellular Fluid Volume

Edema

Newer Concepts of Starling Equilibrium at the Capillary Level in the Production of Edema

Knut Aukland

The commonly used term *regulation of extracellular fluid volume* suggests that there is some kind of monitor of this volume that can provide adequate signals for the regulation of fluid intake and output. Only about one-fourth of the extracellular volume (ECV) is contained in the blood vessels (that is, the plasma volume), and the remainder is spread throughout the interstitium, which has greatly varying properties among organs and tissues. It is therefore difficult to imagine the kind of physiologic monitor that could be used to observe the extracellular volume, and just where it should be placed. Since changes in the ECV do not regularly imply variations in ionic composition or osmolality, a concentration receptor seems inappropriate. As for plasma volume, however, receptors that react to pressure, or rather to stretch, have been located in the atria and in the large intrathoracic veins, which are certainly strategic positions for the control of filling pressure for the heart. One might imagine similar stretch receptors in the interstitia, and suggestions to that effect have been made [1]. Yet, because the challenge to interstitial fluid balance is often local or regional (the feet in orthostasis, the lungs in pulmonary hypertension, and so on), there would have to be a large set of widespread interstitial-fluid-volume (IFV) receptors, each responding to local changes and causing appropriate local responses, for instance, through local or segmental nervous reflexes acting through circulatory control. At present, there is no evidence for such a complicated system.

The normal constancy of ECV, and accordingly of intracellular fluid volume (IFV), must therefore be provided by other mechanisms. It is the aim of this presentation to show that an important contribution is provided by local automatic adjustments of the transcapillary Starling forces and by lymph flow.

This manuscript was presented as part of a Symposium on *Pathogenesis of Edema in Cirrhosis and Nephrotic Syndrome.*

Determinants of Transcapillary Fluid Flow

As formulated by Starling [2], the requirement for having no net fluid transfer between plasma and interstitium is that there be a balance between hydrostatic and colloidal osmotic forces on the two sides of the capillary wall:

$$P_c - P_i = COP_p - COP_i \qquad (1)$$

where P_c and P_i are hydrostatic pressures in capillaries and interstitial fluid, respectively, and COP_p and COP_i are the colloidal osmotic pressures in plasma and free interstitial fluid, respectively. It is implicit in this formulation that it is possible to define these parameters in such a way that they are representative for a given tissue or region. In the case of P_c, there is necessarily a pressure drop along the capillaries, but this drop in pressure may vary greatly from site to site, even among neighboring capillaries [3]. Furthermore, the venules may well participate in transcapillary water transport because of their large surface area and hydraulic conductivity. In brief, P_c should be considered as an average, weighted by segmental surface area and hydraulic conductivity of the microvessels [4].

P_i and COP_i are even more suspect parameters. With the advance in knowledge during the last 10 to 20 years, there is an increased awareness of the complexity of the interstitium. Because it contains glycosaminoglycans (GAGs), the interstitium probably has gel properties, and the immobilized GAGs may exert an appreciable osmotic pressure. In addition, GAGs and collagen probably exclude plasma proteins from a sizeable portion of the interstitial fluid volume. In spite of these complexities, which have been thoroughly treated in several recent papers [1, 5–11], it seems still permissible to define P_i and COP_i as the pressures in the potential free-fluid phase, which in turn is in thermodynamic equilibrium with the gel phase. Although simple calculations suggest that plasma proteins are close to diffusion equilibrium within the interstitium [12, 13], appreciable gradients may occur in transitional states and under high net filtration or absorption. Furthermore, it is possible that net capillary filtrate may have preferential routes to the lymphatics, leading to COP gradients and a lymph protein concentration different from that of average interstitium [10, 11, 14]. Nevertheless, the available evidence suggests roughly parallel changes in lymph and interstitial COP.

In the case of P_i, micropipette measurements at random locations in skin and skeletal muscle suggest that any hydrostatic pressure gradients within the interstitium do not exceed a few tenths of 1 mm Hg [15]. Therefore, for the purpose of discussing IFV regulation, it seems permissible to assume that the interstitium is homogeneous with respect to COP_i and P_i.

The filtration equilibrium described by Eq. 1 could be maintained only if the capillary wall were completely impermeable to plasma proteins. Because it is not, a continuous net transfer of proteins from plasma requires their removal by lymph, and accordingly results in net filtration. Net filtration (J_F) is determined as

$$J_F = CFC\ [P_c - P_i - (COP_c - COP_i)\sigma] \qquad (2)$$

where CFC, the capillary filtration coefficient, is the product of the capillary hydraulic conductivity and the capillary surface area in a given volume of tissue, and σ is the osmotic reflection coefficient for plasma proteins, usually assumed to be 1.00. Various estimates suggest that σ may be lower, 0.8 to 0.9, but an absolute value is not required for a discussion of principles. If J_F differs from lymph flow, J_L (the IFV) will change as follows:

$$\Delta\, IFV = CFC \int_{t_1}^{t_2} [P_c - P_i - (COP_p - COP_i)\sigma]dt - \int_{t_1}^{t_2} J_L dt \qquad (3)$$

Edema-preventing Mechanisms

The contribution of lymph flow in maintaining constant IFV (that is, an IFV of zero in Eq. 3) may be better illustrated by rearranging Eq. 3 as follows:

$$\Delta\, IFV = CFC \int_{t_1}^{t_2} [P_c - P_i - (COP_p - COP_i)\sigma - J_L/CFC]dt \qquad (4)$$

The term J_L /CFC has the dimension of pressure and tells directly how large a net filtration pressure is when it is compensated by lymph flow. Various estimates suggest that J_L /CFC rarely exceeds 3 to 5 mm Hg in the absence of gross edema [11, 16, 17]. This means that a rise in P_i or fall in COP_i of more than 3 to 5 mm Hg should increase IFV and lead to edema, unless other parameters are changed. Clinical experience, however, tells us that this prediction is faulty: It is well known that patients with the nephrotic syndrome may have a 10-mm Hg reduction of COP_p without a development of edema and that lung edema may be absent at an estimated rise in capillary pressure of 15 mm Hg. The explanation is clearly that one or more of the remaining Starling forces have changed to compensate for the rise in P_i or the fall in COP_p. This is by no means a new idea. Starling observed a fall in lymph protein concentration during venous stasis, and he presumed a similar fall occurred in tissue fluid protein. In 1896, he wrote, "With increased capillary pressure there must be transudation, until equilibrium is established at a somewhat higher point, where there is more dilute fluid in the tissue-spaces, and therefore higher absorbing force to balance the increased capillary pressure" [2]. But this is not the only automatic counterpressure, and in the following 50 to 60 years, more emphasis was placed on a rise in P_i. Guyton introduced the terms *edema-preventing mechanisms* and *safety factors* and initiated systematic studies of these mechanisms [6, 18–20]. Even though local vasomotor responses were usually not included in these concepts, they may be of great importance and are therefore added in the schematic summary in Figure 1.

As shown in this scheme (Fig. 1), a rise in local arterial or venous pressure, or both, may cause vessel distension that will encroach upon IFV and thereby cause a rise of P_i in rigid tissues. Furthermore, the rise in transmural vascular pressure may elicit precapillary constriction and thereby limit the rise in P_i

and also reduce CFC by closure of precapillary sphincters. These mechanisms are rapid and do not depend on a primary rise in net filtration and IFV, but they will not be activated by hypoproteinemia. On the other hand, an increase in net filtration pressure (ΔP) and net filtration (J_F) caused by increased capillary pressure (P_c) as well as by reduced plasma colloidal osmotic pressure (COP_p) will increase P_i and reduce COP_i, thus constituting negative feedback loops that tend to reduce net filtration pressure and edema formation. To the same effect, a rise in lymph flow (J_L) will balance a net filtration pressure, corresponding to J_L /CFC. Finally, a high net filtration relative to plasma flow (high filtration fraction) will increase COP_p, as in the glomerular capillaries, and thereby impede further filtration. Many of these mechanisms reverse during net absorption and thereby act to resist fluid removal from the interstitium.

Although the existence of the mechanisms outlined in Figure 1 may be generally accepted, there is no agreement about their relative importance. The main reason for disagreement is probably methodologic differences, especially in the measurement of interstitial hydrostatic and colloidal osmotic pressures. In addition, there are large differences among various organs and tissues, and probably also among species.

Several reviews of the extensive literature are available [4, 6, 9, 11, 14, 17, 20], and the following text should be considered as a personal distillation, probably biased toward the studies performed by my collaborators in the

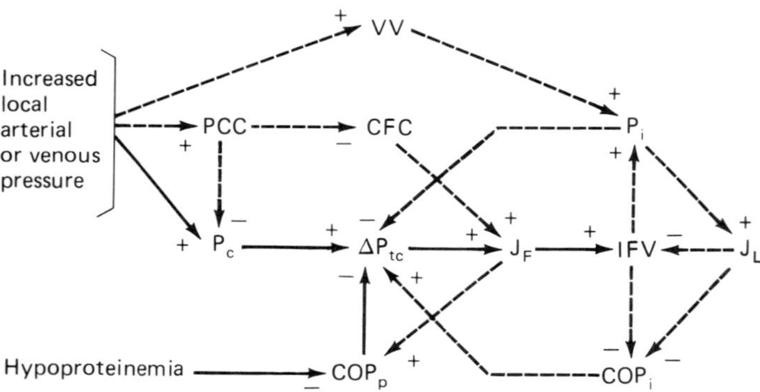

Fig. 1. Local automatic mechanisms opposing changes in interstitial fluid volume (*IFV*) at increased local arterial or venous pressure and during hypoproteinemia. An increase in the parameter at origin of an error will increase (+) or reduce (−) the parameter at the arrow head. *Solid arrows* denote primary edema-provoking sequences; *broken arrows,* edema-preventing effects. VV is local vascular volume; PCC, precapillary vasoconstriction; CFC, capillary filtration coefficient; P_c, average "capillary" pressure; P_{tc}, net transcapillary filtration pressure; COP_p and COP_i, colloid osmotic pressure of capillary plasma and interstitial fluid; J_F, net capillary filtration rate; P_i, interstitial fluid pressure; J_L, lymph flow rate. (Modified from Aukland and Nicolaysen [11])

Department of Physiology at the University of Bergen. The main emphasis is placed on skin and skeletal muscle because these tissues together contribute about two-thirds of the total IFV. Also, when available, observations in humans are used for illustrations, even when they may be less clear-cut than the experimental animal studies.

"Washdown" of Interstitial Protein Concentration

Starling's basis for postulating a washdown of protein as an important edema-preventing mechanism was his assumption that the interstitial fluid protein concentration was equal to that of lymph, which he had found was about one-half that of plasma. Accordingly, there was plenty of protein to dilute or remove by increased lymph flow, and thereby a potential for marked reduction in COP_i. When Krogh, Landis, and Turner [21], Landis and Pappenheimer [22] and Guyton, Granger, and Taylor [20] arrived at much lower estimates for the normal interstitial protein concentration, there was little to gain by washdown, and the mechanism was considered relatively unimportant. During the last 10 to 20 years, however, Starling's estimate of interstitial protein concentration has been corroborated for skin and muscle by a variety of techniques: by protein content of lymph and excised tissues, protein dilution, and kinetic studies, as well as by sampling of interstitial fluid by micropipettes, implanted wicks or perforated capsules, and by suction blister technique. Only a few direct comparisons have been made between these techniques, but most estimates give an interstitial protein concentration in skin and skeletal muscle of 40 to 70% of that in plasma and are somewhat higher for albumin than for the larger globulins (for review, see [11]).

Measurements in humans are scarce. Using nylon wicks implanted subcutaneously [23], Noddeland [24] obtained an average COP_i of 16 mm Hg at the chest and about 11 mm Hg at the ankle in healthy humans (compare with Fig. 2), in fair agreement with measurements on excised skin [25] and in peripheral lymph [26]. Thus, the potential for washout exists and does occur during hypoproteinemia and venous stasis both in experimental models and human disease (for review, see [11, 17]). As is evident from Figure 2, patients with the nephrotic syndrome showed a numerical reduction of subcutaneous COP_i that was practically identical to a fall in COP_p of 8 to 10 mm Hg [27]. Edema was detected only when COP_i flattened out, indicating that protein washdown alone might explain most of the edema resistance in subcutaneous tissue in humans.

The reduction of interstitial protein concentration ("protein washdown") is effected both by dilution and by washout of protein, that is, by a net removal of protein through an increased lymph flow. The repletion of intravascular protein mass resulting from interstitial washout may be of considerable importance after acute protein loss. As an additional mechanism, not included in Figure 1, hypoproteinemia may reduce capillary protein permeability, which will help to retain protein in the plasma [28]. Protein dil-

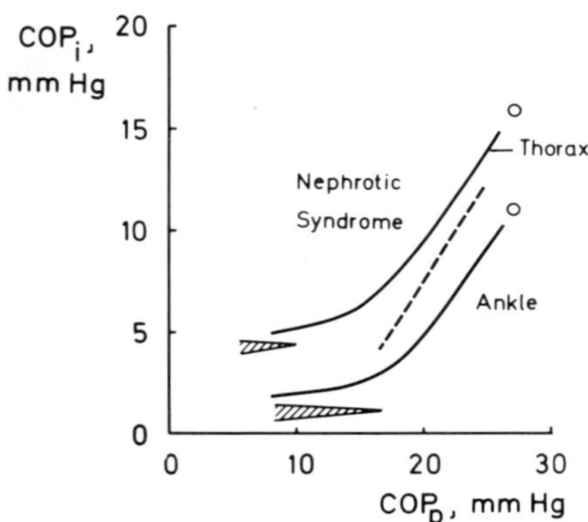

Fig. 2. Washdown of interstitial proteins in human subcutaneous interstitium in nephrotic syndrome. COP_i and COP_p are the colloidal osmotic pressures of interstitial fluid and plasma, respectively. *Open circles* denote healthy controls. *Hatched wedges* denote the appearance of clinical edema (pitting on pressure). *Broken line* denotes numerically equal change in COP_i and COP_p. (Data are derived from [27])

ution effected by an increased IFV may also be potentiated by a relative reduction of the protein-excluded volume created by GAGs and collagen [9, 29, 30].

Washdown of protein at an increased local venous pressure has been demonstrated in skin, muscle, lung, and intestine in experimental animals [11, 17]. It is also well known that edema fluid of decompensated heart failure is practically devoid of protein. However, protein washdown in skin has also been demonstrated prior to edema development, and even before a clinical diagnosis of heart failure can be made [31].

Increased Interstitial Fluid Pressure (P$_i$)

An increased net filtration and a beginning increase of IFV will cause a rise in P_i, depending on the distendability or compliance of the interstitium, defined as $\Delta IFV/\Delta P_i$. Again, diverging results have been obtained by various methods and in different tissues. The most direct and complete measurements of compliance have recently been presented by Reed and Wiig [32–34], who measured the P_i in vivo by glass micropipettes (outer diameter, 2 to 3 μm) and the IFV as extravascular ^{51}Cr-EDTA space on excised skin and muscle. Their volume–pressure curves obtained over a wide range of tissue hydration in rats and cats are shown in Figure 3. The compliance (the inverse slope of the curves) increases greatly at increasing hydration, which is in agreement with the classical study on dog hindlimb by Guyton [19]. The physiologic range, arbitrarily indicated in Figure 3 as $\pm10\%$ variation of IFV, is too narrow for an exact determination of compliance in the control state. The best estimate appears to be the compliance measured during dehydration, even if this is likely to underestimate the true compliance under control condition. Calculated as volume change in milliliters per 100 g of tissue per millimeter of mercury, the compliances were 5.4 and 1.4 in rat skin and skeletal muscle, respectively [32, 33]. The corresponding values in cats were somewhat lower, 3.2 and 1.0 ml $\times$ mm Hg^{-1} $\times$ 100 g^{-1} [34] (Wiig and Reed, personal communication). Although these values are greater than those obtained by Guyton in the dog hindlimb [19], they still indicate that adjustments of P_i may be about as important as adjustments of COP_i in dehydration and in the normal range of hydration in rats and cats.

Figure 3 and the numbers just quoted show that 100 g of skin will give off or accumulate a three to four times greater fluid volume than will 100 g of muscle at a given change in P_i. This does not mean that the interstitium as such is more compliant in skin than in muscle but follows from the three to four times greater IFV in skin than in muscle. Thus, if expressed as interstitial volume change relative to control IFV, the compliances in both tissues are about 14% per 1 mm Hg in the rat and 5 to 10% in the cat. Because of the much greater mass of muscle in the whole body, the two tissues will contribute about equally to total IFV and to accommodation or removal of fluid at a given change in P_i.

As is evident from Figure 3, the maximum hydrostatic counterpressure elicited by overhydration in rats and cats was only 1 to 2 mm Hg. Similar micropipette measurements in skin and muscle in dogs gave values of 2 to 3 mm Hg (Wiig, personal communication), and wick-in-needle measurements in human skin indicated a similar modest rise in subcutaneous P_i even in clinical edema [27]. Accordingly, the hydrostatic counterpressure is small

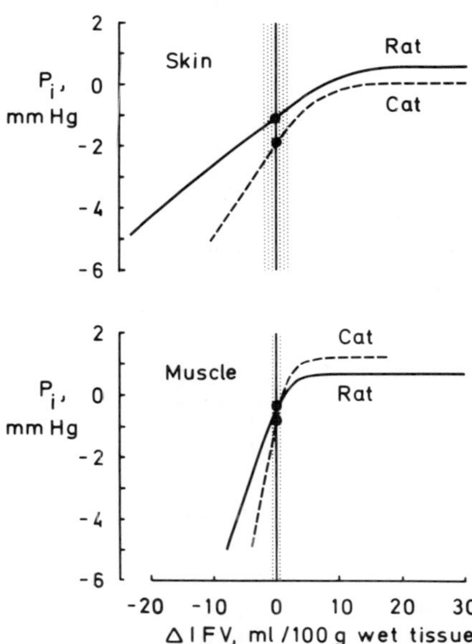

Fig. 3. Skin and skeletal muscle interstitial volume–pressure curves in cats and rats. Interstitial pressure (P_i) was measured through micropipettes; interstitial fluid volume (*IFV*) was measured as extravascular ^{51}Cr-EDTA space. *Solid circles* denote P_i during control conditions. *Solid vertical line and dotted column* denote the control IFV $\pm$ 10%. (Data are from Reed and Wiig [32–34] [personal communication])

compared with the edema-preventing effect of protein washdown that may contribute 7 to 8 mm Hg in rats and 10 to 12 mm Hg in humans. These estimates differ markedly from the classical study of Guyton [19], where the pressure in perforated capsules chronically implanted in dog subcutaneous tissue rose from a subatmospheric pressure of 7 mm Hg to about zero at relative modest overhydration. However, recent measurements by Wiig (personal communication) have shown control capsule pressures in anesthetized and unanesthetized dogs of about -1 to -2 mm Hg, in good agreement with micropipette and wick-in-needle measurements. Furthermore, a very low dehydration compliance as estimated by perforated capsules appears to result from a colloidal osmotic pressure over the capsule lining, as previously proposed by others [1, 35].

Little is known of long-term changes in interstitial compliance. It is widely believed that long-lasting edema leads to stretching of the formed tissue elements and thereby increases the compliances, but it is hard to find direct evidence for this. Lucas and Floyer [36] advanced the interesting hypothesis that interstitial compliance could be regulated by some renal factor. The supporting estimates of compliance were rather indirect, however, and later attempts to confirm their findings have given somewhat inconclusive results.

The conclusion that hydrostatic counterpressure has a quantitatively minor edema-preventing capacity in skin and muscle cannot be directly extrapolated to other tissues. Thus, a lower compliance and a greater hydrostatic counterpressure has been observed in the dog hindpaw [37] and in muscle compartments [38]; and in encapsulated organs a very slight increase of IFV is required to cause a large increase in P_i. In fact, dilatation of the blood vessels suffices to cause a marked increase of P_i in the brain [39] and in the rat tail [40]. Because this effect does not depend on an initial net filtration and increase of IFV, it is almost instantaneous and may in fact completely prevent a rise in IFV.

Vascular Adjustments in Orthostasis

Whereas hypoproteinemia and heart failure are the main clinical challenges to the edema-preventing mechanisms, the great physiologic challenge is orthostasis. In the sitting and standing position, the weight of the heart-to-foot blood column is completely transmitted to the foot veins, and will in the first place increase all the vascular pressures in the feet, including P_c, by 60 to 90 mm Hg. Net filtration seems inevitable and is not much opposed by the mechanisms discussed above; Olzewski and Engeseth [26] found a fall in lymph COP of 5 to 10 mm Hg in patients subjected to 12 hr of passive sitting, and tilting experiments have shown very little increase of P_i (unpublished data). Obviously, more rapid and powerful mechanisms are needed to keep the feet dry. Circulatory responses may provide at least a partial answer.

It has been well documented that a transition from the horizontal to a sitting or a standing position causes an increase in vascular resistance and a reduction of blood flow in the human legs. The vasoconstriction occurs in precapillary vessels and thereby tends to reduce local capillary pressure [41, 42]. In fact, Lewick and Michel [42] found by micropuncture of nailfold capillaries in the toes that the rise in capillary pressure in the upright position was only two-thirds of that expected had there been no change in vascular resistance; that is, the pressure rose by 60 mm Hg instead of 87 mm Hg. Whereas Mellander, Øberg, and Odelram [41] proposed that the vasoconstriction was elicited by a myogenic response to an increased arterial and arteriolar transmural pressure, Henriksen [43] provided strong evidence for local venoarterial reflex.

Mellander et al [41] also reported a marked reduction in the capillary filtration coefficient in the legs in orthostasis, down to 20% of horizontal control, presumably reflecting a closure of capillary sphincters and a reduction of effective capillary surface area. This would serve as an excellent mechanism to reduce net filtration and thereby enable the lymphatics to cope with a larger net filtration pressure (an increased J_L/CFC in Eq. 4). But in more recent experiments, Sejrsen, Hendriksen, and Paaske [44] found only a very slight reduction of CFC.

Increase of Capillary COP_p

It is generally taken for granted that COP of capillary blood equals that of arterial blood, that is, that the net filtration rate is negligible compared with the plasma flow. As demonstrated by Youmans et al in 1934 [45], this may not hold true for the capillaries in the feet in the upright position. We have recently repeated the experiments of Youmans et al and found that during a reduction of blood flow and a closure of the cutaneous arteriovenous anastomosis by general cooling, the COP of foot venous blood in the sitting position might exceed that of arm venous blood by up to 16 mm Hg [46] (similar to that of efferent glomerular plasma). Since the venous blood samples represent a flow average of all drained foot capillaries, it is possible that a large proportion of capillaries with sluggish flow could have a much greater increase of COP. Obviously, this effect approaches that of closing off a large number of capillaries (reduced CFC) and may contribute greatly to impede edema formation. Unfortunately, the opening of an arteriovenous anastomosis in warm environments prevents the demonstration of this phenomenon, and we therefore do not know how important it is in more normal conditions. In fact, it is possible that the increased foot blood flow and the reduction of capillary COP toward the arterial level may in part explain the greater tendency for orthostatic edema to occur in warm feet.

Why the Dependent Localization of Edema in Heart Failure and Hypoproteinemia?

That everybody seems to know the answer to this question may be a good reason for a closer analysis. In spite of all edema-preventing mechanisms, we are probably left with a high net filtration pressure in the feet for up to two-thirds of a 24-hr period. The so-called muscle pump acts efficiently to reduce leg venous pressure during walking and running, but the weight of the heart-to-foot blood column is fully transmitted to the feet during standing or sitting. Thus, ankle vein pressure is not reduced by moving the feet around in the sitting position [47]. If we roughly assume that the edema-preventing mechanisms discussed above could compensate for half of the theoretical rise in net filtration pressure (70 mm Hg), we would still be left with 35 mm Hg. It is therefore not surprising that even physically active normal persons accumulate fluid in the legs and feet during the day [48]. Obviously, they remove the same amount of fluid during the night by capillary absorption or by lymph flow. In comparison, a severely hypoproteinemic patient with his plasma COP reduced by 15 mm Hg would have an additional rise of net filtration pressure of 7 mm Hg after washout of interstitial proteins (compare with Fig. 2). In the upright position, the net filtration pressure in the feet would be increased from 35 to 42 mm Hg; that is to say, it would be 20% higher than that in the control subject but lower than that of a healthy, extra-tall person. It is therefore likely that a dependent edema in this patient is not caused so much by excessive filtration during the day as it is by insufficient net absorption pressure in the horizontal position during night. At heart level, the edema-preventing mechanisms are not overwhelmed by a hydrostatic pressure rise during the day, and there is accordingly no demand for a great absorption during night.

Regulation of Plasma Volume Versus Interstitial Fluid Volume: Conflicting Interests?

For the maintenance of cardiac output, arterial pressure, and renal function, it is obviously more important to regulate the plasma volume than the IFV. It may therefore be pertinent to consider how the local adjustments of the Starling forces just described will interact with the regulation of plasma volume, especially since any restriction on transcapillary fluid movement a priori would seem to exaggerate both physiologic and pathologic variations in it.

As emphasized above, the IFV-conserving mechanisms are not under central control in the sense that they can be used as effector mechanisms to create primary changes in IFV. Their main goal is to prevent or reduce the changes in IFV that result from changes in COP and local vascular pressure and thereby help to maintain a healthy *milieu interieur* for the cells by preventing the interstitium from drying up or flooding. However, this restraint on net capillary filtration and reabsorption also implies less buffering of changes in plasma volume by the interstitial space. Thus, in dehydration, the net absorption pressure caused by an increased COP_p or by reflex or humorally controlled precapillary vasoconstriction will be counteracted. Similarly, during an acute increase in plasma volume caused by a large salt and water load or by a primary salt and water retention, the rise in P_c and the fall in COP_p will be opposed by parallel changes in interstitial colloidal osmotic and hydrostatic pressures. Thus a rapid normalization of plasma volume is prevented.

The wisdom of this construction becomes clearer when one considers what would happen without the edema-preventing mechanisms. Primary retention of salt and water in plasma would be rapidly dissipated by overflowing into the interstitium. Plasma volume would remain unchanged, and the kidney would receive no signal to increase its water and salt excretion. In other words, the edema-preventing mechanisms will ensure changes in plasma volume that may serve as an error signal for activating better ways to dispose of a volume surplus than to store it away in the interstitia. To be sure, some overflow does occur, because the interstitial edema-preventing mechanisms are activated only in proportion to a change in IFV. Thus, the interstitium acts as a buffer for the plasma volume, but with increasing restraint at increasing the IFV. As a general result, changes in the plasma volume result in about proportional changes in IFV.

Also, in pathologic situations the local adjustments of the Starling forces may help the long-term regulation of plasma volume and total extracellular fluid volume. In hypoproteinemia the local adjustments of COP_i and P_i will oppose the threatening fall in plasma volume and thereby improve the conditions for maintaining adequate salt and water excretion. In congestive heart failure, the edema-preventing mechanisms will help to maintain a high blood volume and ventricular filling pressure by preventing too easy an overflow to the interstitium. Some increase of IFV is necessary for this function. But when the capacity of the edema-preventing mechanisms is exhausted, a further increase of IFV and overt edema formation does not provide any additional assistance to the heart.

In conclusion, local adjustments of the transcapillary Starling forces act to preserve a normal IFV, but they indirectly also contribute to a proper regulation of plasma volume through salt and water excretion.

References

1. ZWEIFACH BW, SILBERBERG A: The interstitial-lymphatic flow system, in *Cardiovascular Physiology III,* chapter 6, edited by GUYTON AC, YOUNG DB, Baltimore, University Park Press, 1979, vol 18, pp 215–260
2. STARLING EH: On the absorption of fluids from the connective tissue spaces. *J Physiol (Lond)* 19:312–326, 1896
3. ZWEIFACH BW: Quantitative studies of microcirculatory structure and function: II. Direct measurement of capillary pressure in splanchnic mesenteric vessels. *Circ Res* 34:858–866, 1974
4. WIEDERHIELM CA: Dynamics of capillary fluid exchange: A nonlinear computer simulation. *Microvasc Res* 18:48–82, 1979
5. GARLICK DG, RENKIN EM: Transport of large molecules from plasma to interstitial fluid and lymph in dogs. *Am J Physiol* 219:1595–1605, 1970
6. GUYTON AC, TAYLOR AE, GRANGER HJ: *Circulatory Physiology II: Dynamics and Control of the Body Fluids.* Philadelphia, W. B. Saunders Company, 1975

7. COMPER WD, LAURENT TC: Physiological function of connective tissue polysaccharides. *Physiol Rev* 58:255–315, 1978
8. WATSON PD, GRODINS FS: An analysis of the effects of the interstitial matrix on plasma-lymph transport. *Microvasc Res* 16:19–41, 1978
9. GRANGER HJ: Physiochemical properties of the extracellular matrix, in *Tissue Fluid Pressure and Composition,* edited by HARGENS AR, Baltimore, London, Williams & Wilkins, 1981, pp 43–61
10. BELL DR, WATSON PD, RENKIN EM: Exclusion of plasma proteins in the interstitium of tissues from the dog hindpaw. *Am J Physiol* 239 (Heart Circ Physiol 8): H532–H538, 1980
11. AUKLAND K, NICOLAYSEN G: Interstitial fluid volume: Local regulatory mechanisms. *Physiol Rev* 61:556–643, 1981
12. WIEDERHIELM CA: Dynamics of transcapillary fluid exchange. *J Gen Physiol* 52:29–63, 1968
13. AUKLAND K: Autoregulation of interstitial fluid volume: Edema-preventing mechanisms. *Scand J Clin Lab Invest* 31:247–254, 1973
14. RENKIN EM: Lymph as a measure of the composition of interstitial fluid, in *Pulmonary Edema,* edited by FISHMAN AP, RENKIN EM, Bethesda, Maryland, American Physiological Society, 1979, pp 145–159
15. WIIG H, REED RK, AUKLAND K: Micropuncture measurement of interstitial fluid pressure in rat subcutis and skeletal muscle: Comparison to wick-in-needle technique. *Microvasc Res* 21:308–319, 1981
16. NICOLL PA, TAYLOR AE: Lymph formation and flow. *Ann Rev Physiol* 39:73–95, 1977
17. TAYLOR AE: Capillary fluid filtration: Starling forces and lymph flow. *Circ Res* 49:557–575, 1981
18. GUYTON AC: A concept of negative interstitial pressure based on pressures in implanted perforated capsules. *Circ Res* 12:399–414, 1963
19. GUYTON AC: Interstitial fluid pressure: II. Pressure-volume curves of interstitial space. *Circ Res* 16:452–460, 1965
20. GUYTON AC, GRANGER HJ, TAYLOR AE: Interstitial fluid pressure. *Physiol Rev* 51:527–563, 1971
21. KROGH A, LANDIS EM, TURNER AH: The movement of fluid through the human capillary wall in relation to venous pressure and to the colloid osmotic pressure of the blood. *J Clin Invest* 11:63–95, 1932
22. LANDIS EM, PAPPENHEIMER JR: Exchange of substances through the capillary walls, in *Handbook of Physiology,* Section 2: Circulation, edited by HAMILTON WF, DOW P, Washington DC, American Physiological Society, 1963, pp 961–1034
23. AUKLAND K, FADNES HO: Protein concentration of interstitial fluid collected from rat skin by a wick method. *Acta Physiol Scand* 88:350–358, 1973
24. NODDELAND H: Influence of body posture on transcapillary pressures in human subcutaneous tissue. *Scand J Clin Lab Invest* 42:131–138, 1982
25. BERT JL, MATHIESON JM, PEARCE RH: The exclusion of human serum albumin by human dermal collagenous fibres and within human dermis. *Biochem J* 201:395–403, 1982
26. OLSZEWSKI WL, ENGESET A: Immune proteins, enzymes and electrolytes in human peripheral lymph. *Lymphology* 11:156–164, 1978
27. NODDELAND H, RIISNES SM, FADNES HO: Interstitial fluid colloid osmotic and hydrostatic pressures in subcutaneous tissue of patients with nephrotic syndrome. *Scand J Clin Lab Invest* 42:139–146, 1982

28. KRAMER GC, HARMS BA, BODAI BI, DEMLING RH, RENKIN EM: Mechanisms for redistribution of plasma protein following acute protein depletion. *Am J Physiol* 243 (Heart Circ Physiol 12): H803–H809, 1982

29. PARKER JC, FALGOUT HJ, PARKER RE, GRANGER DN, TAYLOR AE: The effect of fluid volume loading on exclusion of interstitial albumin and lymph flow in the dog lung. *Circ Res* 45:440–450, 1979

30. BELL DR, MULLINS RJ: Effects of increased venous pressure on albumin- and IgG-excluded volumes in muscle. *Am J Physiol* 242 (Heart Circ Physiol 11): H1044–H1049, 1982

31. NODDELAND H, OMVIK P, LUND-JOHANSEN P, OFSTAD J, AUKLAND K: Interstitial colloid osmotic and hydrostatic pressures in human subcutaneous tissue during early stages of heart failure. *Clin Physiol,* in press

32. REED RK, WIIG H: Compliance of the interstitial space in rats: I. Studies of hindlimb skeletal muscle. *Acta Physiol Scand* 113:297–305, 1981

33. WIIG H, REED RK: Compliance of the interstitial space in rats: II. Studies on skin. *Acta Physiol Scand* 113:307–315, 1981

34. WIIG H, REED RK: Interstitial compliance in cat skin and skeletal muscle (*abstract*). *Acta Physiol Scand* 120:38A, 1984

35. STROMBERG DD, WIEDERHIELM CA: Effects of oncotic gradients and enzymes on negative pressures in implanted capsules. *Am J Physiol* 219:928–932, 1970

36. LUCAS J, FLOYER MA: Changes in body fluid distribution and interstitial tissue compliance during the development and reversal of experimental renal hypertension in the rat. *Clin Sci Mol Med* 47:1–11, 1974

37. CHEN HI, GRANGER HJ, TAYLOR AE: Interaction of capillary, interstitial, and lymphatic forces in the canine hindpaw. *Circ Res* 39:245–254, 1976

38. HARGENS AR, MUBARAK SJ, OWEN CA, GARETTO LP, AKESON WH: Interstitial fluid pressure in muscle and compartment syndromes in man. *Microvasc Res* 14:1–10, 1977

39. WIIG H, REED RK: Rat brain interstitial fluid pressure measured with micropipettes. *Am J Physiol* 244 (Heart Circ Physiol 13): H239–H246, 1983

40. AUKLAND K, WIIG H: Hemodynamics and interstitial fluid pressure in the rat tail. *Am J Physiol,* in press

41. MELLANDER S, ØBERG B, Odelram H: Vascular adjustments to increased transmural pressure in cat and man with special reference to shifts in capillary fluid transfer. *Acta Physiol Scand* 61:34–48, 1964

42. LEVICK JR, MICHEL CC: The effects of position and skin temperature on the capillary pressures in the fingers and toes. *J Physiol* 274:97–109, 1978

43. HENRIKSEN O: Local sympathetic reflex mechanisms in regulation of blood flow in human subcutaneous adipose tissue. *Acta Physiol Scand* 450(Suppl):1–48, 1977

44. SEJRSEN P, HENRIKSEN O, PAASKE WP: Effect of orthostatic blood pressure changes upon capillary filtration-absorption rate in the human calf. *Acta Physiol Scand* 111:287–291, 1981

45. YOUMANS JB, WELLS HS, DONLEY D, MILLER DG, FRANK H: The effect of posture (standing) on the serum protein concentration and colloid osmotic pressure of blood from the foot in relation to the formation of edema. *J Clin Invest* 13:447–459, 1934

46. NODDELAND H, AUKLAND K, NICOLAYSEN G: Plasma colloid osmotic pressure in venous blood from the human foot in orthostasis. *Acta Physiol Scand* 113:447–454, 1981

47. NODDELAND H, INGEMANSEN R, REED RK, AUKLAND K: A telemetric tech-

nique for studies of venous pressure in the human leg during different positions and activities. *Clin Physiol* 3:573–576, 1983
48. HANDS L, COLLIN J: Legs that swell and ache: Volume changes during the day in healthy young adults. *Br Med J* 288:447–448, 1984

Pathogenesis of Edema in Cirrhosis

Murray Epstein

One of the most vexing problems afflicting patients is the occurrence of edema. By definition, edema is an excessive accumulation of fluid within the interstitial space (that is, within the nonvascular portion of the extracellular fluid volume). Although the pathogenesis of generalized edema has attracted much scientific inquiry, perhaps the most attention has been focused on the pathogenesis of ascites and peripheral edema in the patient with advanced liver disease [1], which will be the subject of this paper.

The pathogenetic events leading to the deranged sodium homeostasis of cirrhosis can be considered most simply as afferent events and efferent events. A discussion of afferent events usually includes a consideration of the detector element that is responsible for the recognition of the degree of volume alterations, as well as a consideration of the extracellular fluid's translocation or sequestration into serous spaces or interstitial fluid compartments, which characterize advanced liver disease.

Afferent Events

Two concepts are frequently cited to explain the pathogenesis of abnormal sodium retention in liver disease: (a) the role of a diminished "effective" volume and (b) the "overflow" theory of ascites formation.

Role of Diminished "Effective" Volume

Traditionally, ascites formation in cirrhotic patients is considered to begin when a critical imbalance of Starling forces in the hepatic sinusoids and

This manuscript was presented as part of a Symposium on *Pathogenesis of Edema in Cirrhosis and Nephrotic Syndrome.*

splanchnic capillaries results in an increase in the rate of lymph formation that exceeds the capacity of the thoracic duct [2, 3]. Consequently, lymph accumulates in the peritoneal space as ascites, with a subsequent contraction of circulating plasma volume. Thus, as ascites develops, there is a progressive redistribution of plasma volume.

Although an imbalance of Starling forces in the hepatosplanchnic microcirculation is an important factor contributing to the relative decrease in effective blood volume, it is not the sole mechanism. An additional determinant is total peripheral resistance, which is diminished significantly in most edematous cirrhotic patients (Fig. 1). This is no doubt related partially to the increase in the vascular capacity of the splanchnic and pulmonary circulation. When widely developed, these vascular changes may assume the proportion of arteriovenous shunts and contribute to the reduced systemic vascular resistance that is characteristic of patients with cirrhosis [4, 5] and animals with toxic cirrhosis [6] or with bile duct ligation [7]. It has also been proposed that

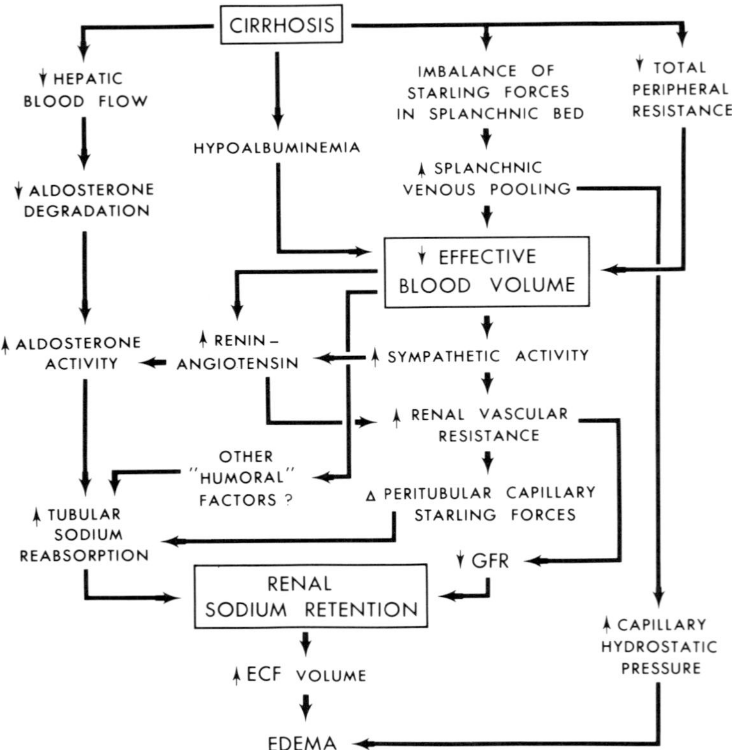

Fig. 1. Schematic drawing of the factors operative in the traditional or "underfilling" theory of sodium retention in cirrhosis. As can be seen, an imbalance of Starling forces in the hepatosplanchnic microcirculation is not the sole mechanism. Acting in concert, these factors promote a reduction in effective plasma volume.

some undefined endogenous vasodilator (either produced by or not inactivated by the diseased liver) plays a role. The decrease in effective volume is compounded further by an impaired pressor response to vasoactive agents including exogenous angiotensin II and noradrenaline [8]. Thus, despite an increase in total plasma volume, the relative "fullness" of the arteriovenous tree is decreased. In summary, several hemodynamic events act in concert to reduce effective blood volume in cirrhotic patients, thereby activating the mechanisms promoting sodium retention. Regardless of the cause, the resultant diminution of effective volume appears to constitute an afferent signal to the renal tubule to augment salt and water reabsorption.

This theory provides a possible explanation for why fluid retention may fail to modify the stimulus for continuing sodium and water retention. Despite a progressive increase in total extracellular fluid volume, fluid is sequestered into one or more of the other fluid compartments without normalizing effective blood volume. Only a correction of the disturbance in the forces governing fluid distribution will permit a reexpansion of effective blood volume to normal.

Although total plasma volume may be increased in this setting, the physiologic circumstance may mimic a reduction in plasma volume (a reduced *effective* plasma volume). As a consequence of the diminished effective volume, renal tabular salt and water reabsorption is enhanced. Thus, the traditional formulation suggests that the renal retention of sodium is a *secondary* rather than primary event.

In this context, it is important to underscore that the term *effective plasma volume* refers to that part of the total circulating volume that is effective in stimulating volume receptors. The concept is elusive because the actual volume receptors are defined incompletely. A diminished effective volume may reflect subtle alterations in systemic hemodynamic factors such as decreased filling of the arterial tree, a diminished central blood volume [9], or both. Because the stimulus is unknown and the afferent receptors are incompletely elucidated, alterations in effective volume must be defined in a functional manner, such as the kinetic response to volume manipulation (see below).

"Overflow" Theory

Over the past decade, Lieberman et al [10, 11] have proposed an alternative hypothesis to the diminished effective volume theory: the "overflow" theory for ascites formation. In contrast to the traditional formulation, the overflow theory postulates that the primary event is the inappropriate retention of excessive sodium by the kidneys. In the setting of abnormal Starling forces in the portal venous bed and hepatic sinusoids (both portal venous hypertension and a reduction in plasma colloid osmotic pressure), the expanded plasma volume is sequestered preferentially in the peritoneal space, with ascites formation. Thus, renal sodium retention and plasma volume expansion *precede rather than follow* the formation of ascites.

The promulgation of the overflow theory of ascites formation has engendered much controversy. The demonstration that plasma volume is increased in cirrhosis with ascites and that a spontaneous diuresis and natriuresis have been found to occur independent of measurable changes in the volume of the nonsplanchnic vascular compartment have been cited as evidence in support of the overflow hypothesis. Additional support derives from a series of elegant investigations carried out by Levy et al [12, 13] on dogs with portal cirrhosis produced by the feeding of dimethylnitrosamine. He demonstrated in sequential studies that renal sodium retention is the initial event that precedes ascites formation. Also, elimination of ascites in these cirrhotic dogs with the LeVeen shunt did not prevent sodium retention during liberal sodium intake [13]. Taken together, therefore, these studies support the view that the initiating event in the renal sodium retention of cirrhosis is not related to "underfilling." A cautionary note has been sounded, however, pointing out that an important, albeit undetectable, increase in vascular capacity (that is, peripheral vasodilatation) could have initiated the early sodium retention [14].

Of interest, in a recent study of cirrhotic patients, Decaux et al [15] observed a significant increase in the clearance of urea and uric acid, which they attributed to an increase in effective vascular volume. Although their interpretation may be correct, it is also possible that the changes in these clearances represented, at least in part, primary defects of renal tubular function.

Although collectively these observations support the overflow theory of ascites formation, a number of clinical observations in *humans* are inconsistent with such a formulation. Thus, rapid volume expansion with exogenous solutions including saline, mannitol, and albumin frequently results in a transient improvement in renal sodium and water handling [16–18]. Similarly, infusion of metaraminol to counteract the peripheral vasodilatation induces a natriuresis [19]. Finally, normalization of Starling forces by surgical decompression of the portal bed in certain patients with cirrhosis may be associated with mobilization of ascites, improvement in renal function, and natriuresis [20]. Of note, all these maneuvers may overcome the circulatory disturbance without improving the function of the cirrhotic liver.

Nevertheless, the fact that several of the utilized maneuvers nonspecifically increase the volume of all fluid compartments, along with the presumed concomitant alterations in plasma composition, has precluded definitive statements regarding the etiologic role of a diminished effective plasma volume. Thus, the results of many earlier studies must be considered inconclusive because of the confounding effects of the experimental designs.

Studies from our laboratory over the past 15 years have circumvented many of these problems by applying a unique investigative tool, the water immersion model, to the assessment of renal function and volume hormonal relationships [21–23]. Before proceeding to enumerate these findings, I shall briefly underscore the differences between water immersion and the more traditional attempts to achieve extracellular volume expansion.

In contrast to saline administration, water immersion is associated with a decrease in body weight rather than the increase that attends saline infusion. In addition, the "volume stimulus" of immersion is promptly reversible after cessation of immersion, which is in contrast to the relatively sustained hypervolemia that follows saline administration [24] and thus constitutes an important attribute in minimizing any risk to the patient. Also in contrast to saline administration, the "volume stimulus" of immersion occurs in the absence of changes in plasma composition [21, 23].

The delineation of the immersion model and the demonstration that it represents a potent "central volume stimulus" without the necessity of infusing exogenous volume expanders commended its use for assessing the role of alterations of *effective* plasma volume in the derangements of renal sodium homeostasis in cirrhosis. Studies in 32 patients with decompensated cirrhosis demonstrated a striking "normalization" of renal sodium handling. As shown in Figure 2, immersion resulted in marked natriuresis and kaliuresis in the majority of these patients. During the final hour of immersion, the urinary

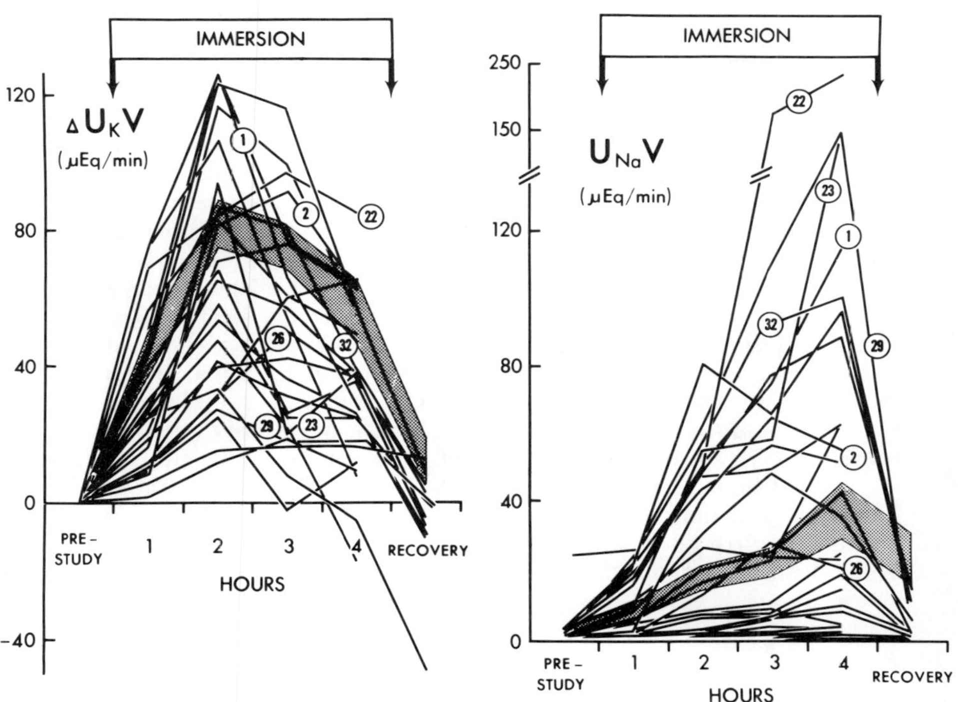

Fig. 2. Effects of water immersion following 1 hr of quiet sitting (*prestudy*) on rate of sodium excretion ($U_{Na}V$) and potassium excretion ($U_K V$) in a large group of patients with alcoholic liver disease. The *circled numbers* represent individual patients. Data for $U_K V$ are expressed in terms of absolute changes from prestudy hour ($\Delta U_K V$). The *shaded area* represents the mean ± SEM for 14 normal controls undergoing an identical immersion study while ingesting an identical diet containing daily 10 mEq of sodium and 100 mEq of potassium. Over half of the cirrhotic patients manifested an appropriate or "exaggerated" natriuretic response. In general, the increase in $U_{Na}V$ was associated with a concomitant increase in $\Delta U_K V$.

excretion of sodium ($U_{Na}V$) was 20-fold greater than it was during the prestudy hour. Thus, the marked antinatriuresis of cirrhosis was promptly reversed by a manipulation that merely altered the distribution of plasma volume without increasing (and often decreasing) total plasma volume. Indeed, in many instances the natriuresis of such patients exceeded markedly that manifested by normal subjects. Taken together, these studies lend strong support to the concept that a diminished effective intravascular volume is a major determinant of the enhanced tubular reabsorption of sodium in cirrhosis.

Further evidence that the immersion-induced natriuretic response is indeed supportive of a role for diminished effective volume and not merely an appropriate response comparable to that of normal subjects can be adduced from the concomitant changes in creatinine clearance (C_{Cr}) during immersion [25]. In marked contrast to the findings in normal persons [26], immersion was associated with significant increments in C_{Cr} in a majority of cirrhotic patients [25]. Two-thirds of them manifested increments in C_{Cr} (3-fold to 5-fold) that exceeded markedly the increments observed in sodium-depleted normal subjects. These observations suggest that immersion tends to "normalize" the diminished effective volume of cirrhotic humans with a resultant normalization of renal vascular tone.

Although I believe that the presently available evidence favors a prominent role for diminished effective volume in mediating the avid sodium retention of many cirrhotic patients, it should be emphasized that these two formulations (that is, diminished effective volume vs. overflow) may not be mutually exclusive. As noted above, cirrhosis is not a *static* disease, but rather a constantly evolving clinical disorder. Yet, virtually all the available clinical studies of deranged sodium homeostasis were carried out at a single stage of the disease, a time when decompensation was well established, with little information available during the incipient stage of sodium retention. In contrast, the studies with the canine cirrhosis model deal with the relatively early stage of sodium retention. Any formulation that suggests that the same antinatriuretic forces are operative throughout the evolution of sodium retention in cirrhotic humans is probably a marked oversimplification. Rather, one should adopt a more global view of the pathogenesis of abnormal sodium retention in cirrhosis in which differing forces participate in varying degrees as the derangement in sodium homeostasis evolves.

Efferent Factors

Initial attempts to explain the abnormalities of renal sodium handling focused on the decrement in glomerular filtration rate (GFR) that occurs frequently in patients with advanced liver disease. A number of observations indicate, however, that a decrease in GFR cannot constitute the major determinant of the abnormalities in renal sodium handling. Not only does sodium retention often occur despite preserved GFR, but avid sodium reabsorption has been observed even in the face of supranormal GFR [27, 28].

Although the weight of evidence demonstrates that the renal sodium retention accompanying cirrhosis is attributable primarily to enhanced tubular reabsorption rather than to alterations in the filtered load of sodium, the precise nephron sites operative remain the subject of continuing controversy [27–29].

The mediators of the enhanced tubular reabsorption of sodium in cirrhosis and their relative participation in the avid sodium retention have not been elucidated completely. Several hormonal, neural, and hemodynamic mechanisms have been suggested. Those mechanisms for which there is some evidence and their interrelationships are summarized schematically in Figure 3.

Since my recent editorial provided an in-depth review of the possible effectors mediating the enhanced sodium reabsorption [30], I will not consider all of them in this chapter. Rather, the focus here will be on the current reappraisal of our thinking regarding these efferent events. Specifically, I will emphasize that the attribution of deranged sodium handling to abnormalities of aldosterone metabolism is a gross oversimplification. It is now apparent that sodium retention is due to the combined and interacting abnormalities of several regulatory systems. Evidence supporting the postulate that aberrations in renal prostaglandin metabolism play a key role will be stressed.

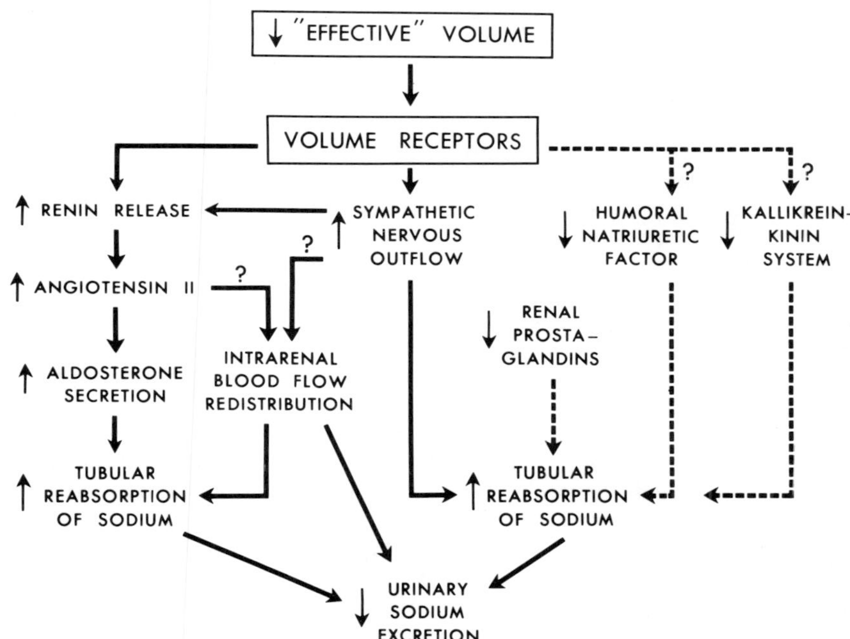

Fig. 3. Schematic drawing of possible mechanisms whereby a diminished *effective* volume results in sodium retention. The *solid arrows* indicate pathways for which evidence is available. The *dashed lines* represent proposed pathways, the existence of which remain to be established. (Reproduced from [36] with permission of the American Gastroenterological Association, Inc.)

Role of Hyperaldosteronism

With the isolation and characterization of aldosterone in the early 1950s, the task of explaining the abnormal sodium retention of cirrhosis was ostensibly rendered simple. Initially, several investigators documented increased levels of aldosterone in the urine of cirrhotic patients, as well as increased adrenal secretion of aldosterone [31, 32]. With the development of radioimmunoassay techniques, aldosterone was demonstrated to be markedly elevated in peripheral plasma [25, 33]. Many observers seized on these observations and proposed that aldosterone is a major determinant of sodium retention. For example, Wilkinson et al [34] demonstrated a hyperbolic relationship between both plasma aldosterone and aldosterone excretory rate on the one hand, and sodium excretion on the other. Furthermore, these workers extended the interpretation of their data to suggest an increased renal tubular sensitivity to the effects of aldosterone. Unfortunately, the demonstration of an inverse relationship between aldosterone and sodium excretion does not suggest necessarily that the hyperaldosteronism is responsible for the sodium retention. Rather, it is probable that a common pathogenetic mechanism was responsible for both phenomena.

In contrast to the above findings, many lines of evidence have challenged the etiologic role of elevated plasma aldosterone levels in mediating the sodium retention of cirrhosis. First, the widely held view that plasma aldosterone levels are elevated in advanced liver disease is probably an oversimplification. We have recently reexamined this question and have been unable to confirm the putative high frequency with which they are increased [35]. We observed that the basal plasma concentrations of 21 of 28 cirrhotic patients were within the normal range for seated normal subjects. Of the remaining 7 patients, 3 manifested suppressed levels, and 4 had distinctly elevated levels. Finally, the changes in levels varied independently of the degree of ascites [35].

Even in patients whose plasma aldosterone concentrations are elevated, many recent studies have suggested that these elevations and the sodium retention of cirrhosis may be pari passu events and not necessarily related etiologically. As detailed in a recent review [36], several investigators have demonstrated a dissociation between sodium excretion and plasma aldosterone in cirrhotic patients. Thus, renal sodium excretion has been demonstrated to vary independently of plasma aldosterone concentrations in patients undergoing a spontaneous diuresis [33], following aminoglutethimide administration [33], and following chronic oral sodium loading [37].

A kinetic assessment of the relationship of plasma aldosterone to renal sodium handling during acute volume expansion was clearly important, but methodologic considerations precluded investigations of the renal and hormonal response to acute volume expansion in cirrhotic humans. Such an approach using rapid volume expansion with saline, mannitol, or albumin has been hindered by the difficulties attending attempts to achieve extracellular fluid volume expansion (ECVE). First, such investigations are associated with the hazard of additional volume expansion. Second, interpretation of the results of rapid volume expansion is confounded by the nonspecific expansion of all fluid compartments. Third, attempts at ECVE with exogenous volume expanders are accompanied by concomitant alterations in plasma composition that might result in alterations of a number of effector systems, including the renin-angiotensin-aldosterone axis.

An immersion study demonstrated a dissociation between the suppression of circulating aldosterone and the absence of a natriuresis in one-half of the patients with decompensated cirrhosis [25]. These observations are consistent with the interpretation that aldosterone is not the primary determinant of the impaired sodium excretion of many cirrhotic patients.

Additional studies utilizing the immersion model [38] complemented this conclusion. It was demonstrated that spironolactone administration without immersion resulted in only a modest increase in sodium excretion. If the encountered sodium retention was attributable to the elevated aldosterone levels themselves, one would have anticipated a more marked natriuresis with spironolactone administration alone. In contrast, there was a dramatic increase in sodium excretion when immersion was carried out during chronic spironolactone administration, thereby indicating that the major contribution to the natriuresis was an enhanced distal delivery of filtrate. This explanation was supported by the documentation of a concomitant kaliuresis and an increase in free-water clearance [38].

Finally, a number of important observations were made when immersion followed acute deoxycorticosterone (DOCA) administration (10 mg i.m.) in cirrhotic patients with ascites and edema [1]. Immersion induced a clear-cut increase in sodium excretion despite the acute administration of pharmacologic doses of mineralocorticoid, supporting the concept that enhanced sodium reabsorption and elevated circulating mineralocorticoid levels are independent events.

Taken together, the evidence presently available therefore favors the postulate that the hyperaldosteronism of cirrhosis is a permissive factor only, and that the predominant component of the abnormal renal sodium handling is a diminished distal delivery of filtrate. Only when distal filtrate delivery is enhanced by an experimental or pharmacologic maneuver does aldosterone exert a major role in the renal sodium handling in cirrhosis.

The demonstration that hyperaldosteronism cannot account completely for sodium retention in cirrhosis has prompted a search for other hormonal mediators that participate in this derangement. Within the past 3 years, increasing evidence has accumulated suggesting that renal prostaglandins are important contenders in this regard. Recently, several investigators have demonstrated that the administration of inhibitors of prostaglandin synthetase (both indomethacin and ibuprofen) resulted in significant decrements in GFR and renal plasma flow (ERPF) in patients with alcoholic liver disease [39, 40]. Of interest, the decrement in renal hemodynamics varied directly with the degree of sodium retention; the patients with the most avid sodium retention manifested the largest decrements in GFR [40].

We believe that the above findings are not isolated observations. As noted in a recent formulation [41], one may conceive of renal prostaglandins as constituting critical modulators of renal function during conditions or disease states involving volume contraction. The demonstration that synthetase inhibition affected renal function only in decompensated (presence of ascites or edema or both) cirrhotic patients but not compensated cirrhotic patients, and that the effects of synthetase inhibition vary as a function of the degree of renal sodium avidity is consistent with this formulation.

Just as the studies just cited have examined the effect of inhibiting endogenous production of renal prostaglandins, it would be of great interest to assess the effect of augmenting endogenous prostaglandins on renal functional alterations. Our recent demonstration that head-out water immersion constitutes a unique means of augmenting urinary PGE excretion, and presumably renal PGE synthesis [41], prompted an examination of the relationship of immersion-induced changes in PGE and renal function. Immersion of cirrhotic patents was associated with prompt and marked increments in PGE excretion [41]. The observation that the same patients manifested a marked natriuresis and diuresis is consistent with the interpretation that an augmentation of renal PGE synthesis participates in the observed natriuresis.

Summary

It is apparent that renal sodium retention in patients with advanced liver disease constitutes a fascinating abnormality with numerous and diverse causes and an elusive pathophysiology. The dissociation between hyperaldosteronism and the attendant changes in renal sodium handling points to the participation of several hormonal and neural effectors acting in concert. Additional insight into this fascinating problem must await further biochemical characterization of the mediators and a delineation of their pathophysiologic role.

Finally, it must be emphasized that the questions raised by attempts to elucidate the mechanisms mediating sodium retention of liver disease are not restricted to this disorder. Rather, the lessons learned from such a reappraisal may provide us with a provocative framework with which to reassess the pathophysiology of deranged sodium homeostasis in other disease states characterized by altered volume regulation.

References

1. EPSTEIN M: Renal sodium handling in cirrhosis, in *The Kidney in Liver Disease* (2nd ed), edited by EPSTEIN M, New York, Elsevier Biomedical, 1983, pp 35–53
2. CONN HO: The rational management of ascites, in *Progress in Liver Disease*, edited by POPPER H, SCHAFFNER F, New York, Grune & Stratton, 1972, vol 4, pp 269–288
3. WITTE MH, WITTE CL, DUMONT AE: Progress in liver disease: Physiological factors involved in the causation of cirrhotic ascites. *Gastroenterology* 61:742–750, 1971
4. COHN JN: Renal hemodynamic alterations in liver disease, in *The Kidney in Systemic Disease* (2nd ed), edited by SUKI WN, EKNOYAN G, New York, John Wiley & Sons, 1981, pp 509–519
5. BREDFELDT JE, GROSZMANN RJ: Hemodynamic aspects of portal hypertension,

in *The Kidney in Liver Disease* (2nd ed), edited by EPSTEIN M, New York, Elsevier, 1983, pp 281–292

6. LEVY M: Sodium retention in dogs with cirrhosis and ascites: Efferent mechanisms. *Am J Physiol* 233:F586–F592, 1977

7. SHASHA SM, BETTER OS, CHAIMOVITZ C, DOMAN J, KISHON Y: Hemodynamic studies in dogs with chronic bile duct ligation. *Clin Sci* 50:533–537, 1976

8. AMES RP, BORKOWSKI AJ, SICINSKI AM, LARAGH JH: Prolonged infusions of angiotensin II and norepinephrine and blood pressure, electrolyte balance, and aldosterone and cortisol secretion in normal man and in cirrhosis with ascites. *J Clin Invest* 44:1171–1186, 1965

9. GAUER OH: Mechanoreceptors in the intrathoracic circulation and plasma volume control, in *The Kidney in Liver Disease* (1st ed), edited by EPSTEIN M, New York, Elsevier, 1978, pp 3–17

10. LIEBERMAN FL, DENISON EK, REYNOLDS TB: The relationship of plasma volume, portal hypertension, ascites and renal sodium retention in cirrhosis: The overflow theory of ascites formation. *Ann NY Acad Sci* 170:202–212, 1970

11. LIEBERMAN FL, ITO S, REYNOLDS TB: Effective plasma volume in cirrhosis with ascites: Evidence that a decreased value does not account for renal sodium retention, a spontaneous reduction in glomerular filtration rate (GFR) and a fall in GFR during drug-induced diuresis. *J Clin Invest* 48:975–981, 1969

12. LEVY M: Observations on renal function and ascites formation in dogs with experimental portal cirrhosis, in *The Kidney in Liver Disease* (1st ed), edited by EPSTEIN M, New York, Elsevier, 1978, pp 131–142

13. LEVY M, WEXLER MJ, MCCAFFREY C: Sodium retention in dogs with experimental cirrhosis following removal of ascites by continuous peritoneovenous shunting. *J Lab Clin Med* 94:933–946, 1979

14. BETTER OS, SCHRIER RW: Disturbed volume homeostasis in patients with cirrhosis of the liver. *Kidney Int* 23:303–311, 1983

15. DECAUX G, DUMONT I, NAEIJE N, MOLS P, MELOT C, MOCKEL J: High uric acid and urea clearance in cirrhosis secondary to increased "effective vascular volume." *Am J Med* 73:328–334, 1982

16. SCHEDL HP, BARTTER FC: An explanation for and experimental correction of the abnormal water diuresis in cirrhosis. *J Clin Invest* 39:248–261, 1960

17. VLAHCEVIC ZR, ADAM NF, JICK H, MOORE EW, CHALMERS TC: Renal effects of acute expansion of plasma volume in cirrhosis. *N Engl J Med* 272:387–391, 1965

18. TRISTANI FE, COHN JN: Systemic and renal hemodynamics in oliguric hepatic failure: Effect of volume expansion. *J Clin Invest* 46:1894–1906, 1967

19. GORNEL DL, LANCESTREMERE RG, PAPPER S, LOWENSTEIN LM: Acute changes in renal excretion of water and solute in patients with Laennec's cirrhosis induced by administration of the pressor amine, metraraminol. *J Clin Invest* 41:594–603, 1962

20. SCHROEDER ET, ANDERSON GH, SMULYAN H: Effect of peritoneovenous shunt on renin in the hepatorenal syndrome. *Kidney Int* 15:54–61, 1979

21. EPSTEIN M: Renal effects of head-out water immersion in man: Implications for an understanding of volume homeostasis. *Physiol Rev* 58:529–581, 1978

22. EPSTEIN M, PINS DS, ARRINGTON R, DENUNZIO AG, ENGSTROM R: Comparison of water immersion and saline infusion as a means of inducing volume expansion in man. *J Appl Physiol* 39:66–70, 1975

23. EPSTEIN M, RE R, PRESTON S, HABER E: Comparison of the suppressive effects of water immersion and saline administration on renin-aldosterone in normal man. *J Clin Endocrinol Metab* 49:358–363, 1979

24. LEVINSON R, EPSTEIN M, SACKNER MA, BEGIN R: Comparison of the effects of water immersion and saline infusion on central hemodynamics in man. *Clin Sci Mol Med* 52:343–350, 1977

25. EPSTEIN M, LEVINSON R, SANCHO J, HABER E, RE R: Characterization of the renin-aldosterone system in decompensated cirrhosis. *Circ Res* 41:818–829, 1977

26. EPSTEIN M, LEVINSON R, LOUTZENHISER R: Effects of water immersion on renal hemodynamics in normal man. *J Appl Physiol* 41:230–233, 1976

27. KLINGLER EL JR, VAAMONDE CA, VAAMONDE LS, LANCESTREMERE RG, MOROSI HJ, FRISCH E, PAPPER S: Renal function changes in cirrhosis of the liver. *Arch Intern Med* 125:1010–1015, 1970

28. CHAIMOVITZ C, SZYLMAN P, ALROY G, BETTER OS: Mechanism of increased renal tubular sodium reabsorption in cirrhosis. *Am J Med* 52:198–202, 1972

29. EPSTEIN M, RAMACHANDRAN M, DENUNZIO AG: Interrelationship of renal sodium and phosphate handling in cirrhosis. *Mineral Electrolyte Metab* 7:305–315, 1982

30. EPSTEIN M: Pathogenesis of renal sodium handling in cirrhosis. *Am J Nephrol* 3:297–309, 1983

31. COPPAGE WS JR, ISLAND DP, COONER AE, LIDDLE GW: The metabolism of aldosterone in normal subjects and in patients with hepatic cirrhosis. *J Clin Invest* 41:1672–1680, 1962

32. VECSEI P, DUSTERDIECK G, JAHNECKE J, LOMMER D, WOLFF HPD: Secretion and turnover of aldosterone in various pathological states. *Clin Sci* 36:241–256, 1969

33. ROSOFF L JR, ZIA P, REYNOLDS T, HORTON R: Studies of renin and aldosterone in cirrhotic patients with ascites. *Gastroenterology* 69:698–705, 1975

34. WILKINSON SP, JOWETT TP, SLATER JDH, ARROYO V, MOODIE H, WILLIAMS R: Renal sodium retention in cirrhosis: relation to aldosterone and nephron site. *Clin Sci* 56:169–177, 1979

35. EPSTEIN M: Aldosterone in liver disease, in *The Kidney in Liver Disease* (2nd ed), edited by EPSTEIN M, New York, Elsevier North Holland, 1983, pp 377–394

36. EPSTEIN M: Deranged sodium homeostasis in cirrhosis. *Gastroenterology* 76:622–635, 1979

37. CHONKO AM, BAY WH, STEIN JH, FERRIS TF: The role of renin and aldosterone in the salt retention of edema. *Am J Med* 63:881–889, 1977

38. EPSTEIN M, PINS DS, SCHNEIDER N, LEVINSON R: Determinants of deranged sodium and water homeostasis in decompensated cirrhosis. *J Lab Clin* 87:822–839, 1976

39. BOYER TD, ZIA P, REYNOLDS TB: Effect of indomethacin and prostaglandin A_1 on renal function and plasma renin activity in alcoholic liver disease. *Gastroenterology* 77:215–222, 1979

40. ZIPSER RD, HOEFS JC, SPECKART PF, ZIA PK, HORTON R: Prostaglandins: Modulators of renal function and pressor resistance in chronic liver disease. *J Clin Endocrinol Metab* 48:895–900, 1979

41. EPSTEIN M, LIFSCHITZ M, RAMACHANDRAN M, RAPPAPORT K: Characterization of renal PGE responsiveness in decompensated cirrhosis: Implications for renal sodium handling. *Clin Sci* 63:555–563, 1982

Renal Handling of Sodium in Hepatic Diseases Other than Cirrhosis

J. Rapaport and Cidio Chaimovitz

Although alcoholic cirrhosis is the hepatic disease most notably associated with renal salt and water retention, abnormal renal salt handling also occurs in other liver diseases. It has been studied both in rat and in various animal models. This presentation will focus on its occurrence in the following conditions: (a) chronic biliary obstruction, (b) hepatic venous outflow obstruction, (c) isolated portal hypertension, and (d) primary biliary cirrhosis.

Chronic Biliary Obstruction

Abnormalities of renal sodium reabsorption in chronic biliary obstruction have been studied in the experimental model of chronic bile duct ligation (CBDL) in various animals, but notably in the rat and dog [1]. CBDL results in jaundice, usually more pronounced in the rat than in the dog, but in the former animals, the bilirubin reverts to normal levels after several weeks due to recanalization [1]. Histologic changes in the liver vary. They are milder in the rat and more severe and reminiscent of human Laennec's cirrhosis in the dog. Salt retention is usually more common and more marked in CBDL dogs. There are some striking differences obtained in studies in the two animals, and we will discuss them separately and then compare them.

Chronic Bile Duct Ligation in Rats

Bank and Aynedjian performed a micropuncture study on six ascitic rats 10 to 14 days after bile duct ligation [2]. Glomerular filtration rate (GFR) and renal blood flow (RBF) did not vary significantly from control animals.

This manuscript was presented as part of a Symposium on *Pathogenesis of Edema in Cirrhosis and Nephrotic Syndrome.*

The micropuncture study showed an increased sodium reabsorption in the proximal tubule of these animals. This was explained by an afferent arteriolar vasoconstriction in cortical nephrons leading to increased single nephron filtration fraction and elevated peritubular capillary oncotic pressure. A marked reduction in surface nephron blood flow occurred in the absence of any decrease in overall RBF.

Yarger studied the intrarenal mechanism of renal salt retention in CBDL rats by means of micropuncture and regional analysis of renal blood flow by labeled microspheres [3]. Rats were studied in the early stages of salt retention, before the appearance of significant ascites. Plasma volume was reduced, and hematocrit slightly increased. GFR and renal plasma flow (RPF) were both markedly reduced to a similar extent, 59% and 57% respectively, so that filtration fraction was unchanged. Absolute sodium secretion was unchanged. The micropuncture study showed that SNGFR of cortical nephrons was reduced to 70% of control values. Fractional reabsorption was increased at all accessible sites. Blood flow was reduced by 49% in superficial nephrons, by 59% in intermediate nephrons, and by 73% in juxtamedullary nephrons. The author thus concluded that sodium retention in the early stages after CBDL was due to (a) a decrease in filtered sodium load and (b) an increased fractional reabsorption by superficial nephrons.

Subsequently, Allison et al studied 50 Sprague-Dawley rats after CBDL [4]. All rats became jaundiced, and micropuncture studies were performed an average of 26 days after CBDL. Only 10 of the 50 rats developed ascites. Twenty-one (42%) of the rats became hypotensive and died during the surgery prior to the micropunctive study, including 9 of the 10 animals with ascites. Micropuncture studies were performed in 10 animals, none of whom had ascites. In the surviving rats, there was no significant change in blood pressure, whole-kidney GFR, or single nephron GFR (SNGFR) from control animals. However, RPF was increased so that the whole kidney filtration fraction was low. Proximal tubular reabsorption in the jaundiced group was not different from control rats. However the urine-to-plasma (U/P) inulin ratio was reduced, which, in the face of unchanged proximal tubular reabsorption, indicates diminished distal reabsorption. Thus, the micropuncture study did not indicate increased reabsorption at any nephron site. It should be noted, however, as already mentioned, that none of the rats studied by micropuncture had ascites. Electron microscopy of the kidneys of the CBDL animals showed marked changes in glomeruli 20 to 30 days after ligation, consisting of swelling in endothelial cells, with increased density of cytoplasm in both epithelial and endothelial cells. The significance of these morphologic changes is unclear.

In a more recent study, Better et al studied urinary dilution in CBDL rats, comparing Sprague-Dawley rats with congenital diabetes insipidus rats (Brattleboro) following CBDL [5]. None of the rats developed ascites after ligation. In contrast to the previously quoted studies, RBF in both groups of rats was markedly reduced compared with controls, with a significant increase in renal vascular resistance, but GFR was unchanged. Micropuncture studies were not performed, but clearance studies indicated that distal delivery of sodium and diluting segment function were unchanged after CBDL. These results thus suggest normal tubular sodium reabsorption after CBDL.

Chronic Bile Duct Ligation in Dogs

The model of CBDL in dogs provides a more consistent model of renal salt retention, and has been studied by numerous workers.

Mullane and Gliedman studied the renal response to saline loading following double ligation and division of the common bile duct [6]. The dogs were studied 2 to 5 weeks after ligation, and most were not ascitic at this time. No information was given about bilirubin levels. No significant change was found in RPF or GFR, and there was a blunted natriuretic response to saline infusion.

Better and Massry performed a more sophisticated study of chronic bile duct ligated dogs, which were studied 2 to 7 weeks following double ligation. Two of the nine dogs studied developed ascites within 2 months of ligation. Serum bilirubin rose to maximum levels of 2.5 to 9.1 mg/dl within 2 weeks, and gradually fell to 0.8 to 4.5 mg/dl. GFR and RPF did not change after ligation. The natriuretic response to hypotonic saline infusion was markedly blunted by CBDL. Calculated distal delivery was significantly less after CBDL, and fractional sodium reabsorption at the diluting segment for any given rate of distal delivery was enhanced by CBDL. Furthermore, free water formation at any given rate of distal delivery was increased after CBDL. These clearance studies thus indicate enhanced proximal and distal sodium reabsorption following CBDL.

The influence of systemic hemodynamics on renal sodium retention in CBDL dogs was studied by Shasha et al [8]. Following ligation, there was an insignificant fall in mean arterial pressure, a significant rise in mean cardiac index, and a significant fall in mean total peripheral resistance. Central venous pressure was not elevated. RBF remained similar to control levels, despite the fall in total peripheral resistance, suggesting that renal vasodilatation did not occur. These results thus indicate that heart failure is not a factor in the salt retention of CBDL dogs.

The possible contribution of a redistribution of cortical blood flow following CBDL was studied by Shalev and Chaimovitz, using radiolabeled microspheres to measure regional renal blood flow after CBDL [9]. No redistribution of blood flow between outer and inner cortex was found to occur after CBDL in dogs.

Chaimovitz et al studied the role of the sympathetic system by evaluating the effect of renal denervation and alpha-adrenergic blockade on renal handling of sodium in CBDL dogs [10]. Both renal denervation and infusion of dibenzyline into the renal artery produced a slight but significant increment in urinary sodium excretion, but these changes were not different from those observed after renal denervation in normal animals. Furthermore, these procedures did not improve the impaired natriuretic response to saline volume expansion in CBDL dogs. It was concluded that renal sympathetic innervation and augmented alpha-adrenergic activity does not appear to play an important role in the salt retention of CBDL dogs.

Since renal vasodilatation is known to play a significant role in the natriuresis that follows extracellular volume expansion (ECVE), the blunted response to ECVE in CBDL dogs could be theoretically due to a failure of renal vasodilatation in these animals, or to an inability of the renal arteries to respond to vasodilators in the circulation. This question was addressed by Melman and Massry [11], who found that during ECVE, significant increases in RPF and urinary sodium excretion occurred in control animals, but not in CBDL dogs, in whom RPF did not change and natriuresis was blunted. Intrarenal administration of acetylcholine produced a normal increase in RPF in CBDL dogs, but the natriuretic response to ECVE remained blunted. Thus, the failure of CBDL dogs to vasodilate in response to ECVE does not appear to be a major factor in the antinatriuresis of these animals.

The effect of beta-adrenergic blockade was then studied by Winaver, Chaimovitz, and Better, who administered propranolol to dogs following CBDL and found that this partially reversed the antinatriuresis after CBDL [12]. The mechanism of the effect of propranolol, however, was not clear. The natriuretic effect of propranolol in CBDL dogs was associated with a fall in plasma renin activity. However, it is unlikely that the antinatriuresis itself was related to the renin-angiotensin system since no consistent change in plasma renin activity occurred with sodium retention after BDL. Thus, propranolol probably did not reverse the antinatriuresis via an effect on the renin system, and the authors postulated a systemic effect, with an improvement of renal hemodynamics consequent on beta-blockade, attributable to a hypothesized "normalization of disturbed autonomic activity" in CBDL dogs.

The joint findings of raised cardiac output, absence of heart failure, normal renal hemodynamics, and lack of effect of renal denervation indicate that the renal salt retention of CBDL is probably not secondary to changes in renal hemodynamics. This suggests that some humoral factor may be involved. This contention was studied by Chaimovitz, Alon, and Better, who investigated the role of mineralocorticoids [13]. They found that the antinatriuresis following CBDL was associated with a 3-fold rise in plasma aldosterone concentration. Ascites was present in all salt-retaining CBDL dogs. Bilateral adrenalectomy resulted in the disappearance of ascites and an improvement in the natriuretic response to extracellular volume expansion. Sodium balance studies in adrenalectomized CBDL dogs during chronic DOCA treatment showed that these dogs failed to escape from the mineralocorticoid-induced sodium retention. GFR and RPF did not change during these studies. The authors concluded that sodium retention in the CBDL dogs was due to an excess of circulating aldosterone, together with an extrarenal factor that prevents escape from the salt-retaining effect of mineralocorticoids in the CBDL dogs, thereby perpetuating the antinatriuresis in these animals.

CBDL results in histologic changes in the liver of dogs similar to those of Laennec's cirrhosis (Chaimovitz C, unpublished observation). Thus, the systemic and renal effects of CBDL in dogs could be due to cirrhotic changes, or they could be due to the hyperbilirubinemia itself. To determine the effects of isolated cholemia, Alon et al performed choledochocaval anastomosis in dogs [14]. These animals became deeply jaundiced, but the hepatocellular function remained substantially unchanged. After choledochocaval anastomosis, the mean arterial pressure and the total peripheral resistance decreased significantly, whereas cardiac index and plasma volume did not change. GRF and RPF were unchanged. The natriuretic response to ECVE was impaired.

Tubular dysfunction was manifested by impaired maximal urinary concentration and dilution. Thus, cholemia itself appears to cause systemic vasodilatation, hypotension, and renal tubular dysfunction, and may well be a factor in the antinatriuresis of CBDL dogs.

In summary, it is apparent that a large number of observations have been obtained following CBDL in different animals, in many cases conflicting. Better has summarized and discussed these differences [1]. In general, rats develop a predominantly hyperbilirubinemic picture initially, with mild histologic changes of prolification of bile canaliculi and early fibrosis [5]. Salt retention is highly variable, but appears to be much less common than it is in CBDL dogs [1]. The rat model thus appears to be more typical of pure biliary obstruction without salt retention. However, systemic hemodynamics and renal function vary enormously from study to study. RBF has been found to be normal [2], decreased [3, 5], or increased [4]. Superficial nephron blood flow when measured has been found to be decreased [2, 3], with relative sparing of SNGFR, suggesting efferent vasoconstriction. Systemic hemodynamics are also variable. Mean arterial pressure has been found to be normal [5], or reduced [4]. Better suggested that these wide variations are due to the effects of anesthesia and that conscious animals should be studied [1]. The wide variations in salt retention may also be related to differing salt intake after CBDL [4]. The variability of these results suggests that this model is not sufficiently consistent for the purpose of studying the relation between salt retention and liver disease. In the CBDL dog, on the other hand, the histology is more similar to human cirrhosis, with marked fibrosis (Chaimovitz C, unpublished observation). Hyperbilirubinemia is relatively mild, and salt retention frequent and marked, again similar to Laennec's cirrhosis in humans [7]. Studies of systemic hemodynamics show mild hypotension with peripheral vasodilatation and increased cardiac output, and normal GFR and RPF [8]. This appears to be a reliably reproducible model of renal salt retention associated with hepatic disease similar to cirrhosis, and results suggest that the avid salt retention appears in large part to be due to secondary hyperaldosteronism with loss of mineralocorticoid escape, with hyperbilirubinemia itself possibly also playing a role.

Hepatic Venous Outflow Obstruction

Obstruction to hepatic venous outflow is an extremely potent stimulus to renal salt and water retention. Hepatic venous congestion appears to be necessary, because obstruction of the abdominal inferior vena cava does not cause ascites [15]. Generally in these conditions, substantial systemic hemodynamic changes occur, which by themselves could affect renal salt handling.

To obviate these changes in systemic hemodynamics, Levy, in an elegant study, injected histamine base directly into the portal vein of dogs to cause a selective hepatic venous outflow obstruction [16]. The dosage used did not cause any changes in mean arterial blood pressure, cardiac output, or pulse rate. However, there was a significant decrease in RBF and sodium excretion. GFR was unchanged. Filtration fraction increased from 0.33 to 0.47. Despite this, proximal sodium reabsorption, as indexed by the tubular fluid-to-plasma (TF/P) inulin, did not change. Denervation of one kidney, continuous angiotensin infusion, adrenalectomy, and alpha-adrenergic blockade did not diminish the blunted natriuresis seen after acute hepatic venous obstruction. The author thus concluded that the efferent limb for the decreased sodium excretion in this condition did not involve mineralocorticoids, catecholamines, angiotensin, the renal nerves, or altered hemodynamics. It was postulated that hepatic congestion caused the liver to release humoral factors, which acted on both the renal vasculature and renal tubules and caused renal vasoconstriction and sodium retention.

Acute hepatic venous obstruction in humans, or the Budd-Chiari syndrome, results in very severe and rapid salt retention. A patient suffering from this condition was studied by Schramek et al, utilizing clearance techniques [17]. Both inulin and PAH clearances were reduced. Free water formation was normal, but the diluting site function, as indicated by the fraction of distally delivered sodium absorbed at this site, was supranormal. The authors concluded that the enhanced sodium reabsorption in this condition occurs mainly in the distal nephron.

Portal Hypertension

Since cirrhosis is so commonly associated with portal hypertension, the question arises as to the effect of portal hypertension itself on renal function and sodium excretion. Since portal hypertension often occurs together with marked abnormalities in systemic hemodynamics, which directly alter renal perfusion pressure, Anderson et al studied the effects of increasing the portal vein pressure on renal hemodynamics while maintaining a constant renal perfusion pressure [18]. This maneuver was associated with marked decreases in GFR and RPF and increases in renal vascular resistance. Since GFR and RPF fell concomitantly, the afferent arteriolar vasoconstriction was presumably the cause of the increased renovascular resistance. Because the renal perfusion pressure was maintained constant throughout, the increased portal vein pressure could not alter renal hemodynamics directly. The finding that renal denervation abolished the effects of increased portal vein pressure in GFR and RPF suggests that an adrenergically mediated splanchnic-renal reflex may be involved. The effect on salt excretion was not studied directly. However, renin secretion was increased in innervated kidneys. Furthermore, a linear correlation between changes in urine flow rate and free water clearance (C_{H2O}) were observed in hypophysectomized dogs during portal vein construction. These results suggest that elevated portal vein pressure diminishes water excretion by decreasing the rate of tubular fluid delivery to the distal nephron. Since this effect was found in both innervated and denervated kidneys, it suggests enhanced proximal reabsorption independent of an effect on GFR.

Primary Biliary Cirrhosis

Despite extensive hepatic damage and the existence of portal hypertension, it is well known that patients with this condition are much less subject to salt retention than are those suffering from alcoholic cirrhosis. Chaimovitz et al compared the renal response to ECVE in a group of patients with primary biliary cirrhosis to that in patients with Laennec's cirrhosis and to that in normal subjects [19]. They found an augmented natriuretic response to ECVE in these patients compared both to patients with Laennec's cirrhosis and to normal subjects. Segmental analysis of sodium handling by clearance methods under conditions of maximal ADH suppression suggested a reduced proximal sodium reabsorption in this condition, which may explain the late and uncommon appearance of ascites and edema.

References

1. BETTER OS: Bile duct ligation: An experimental model of renal dysfunction secondary to liver disease, in *The Kidney in Liver Disease* (2nd ed). New York, Elsevier, 1983, pp 295–311
2. BANK N, AYNEDJIAN H: A micropuncture study of renal salt and water retention in chronic bile duct obstruction. *J Clin Invest* 55:994–1002, 1975
3. YARGER WE: Intrarenal mechanisms of salt retention after bile duct ligation in rats. *J Clin Invest* 57:408–418, 1976
4. ALLISON MEM, MOSS NG, FRASER MM, DOBBIE JW, RYAN CJ, KENNEDY AC, BLUMGART LH: Renal function in chronic obstructive jaundice: A micropuncture study in rats. *Clin Sci Mol Med* 54:649–659, 1978
5. BETTER OS, AISENBREY GA, BERL T, ANDERSON RJ, HANDELMAN, WA, LINAS SL, GUGGENHEIM SJ, SCHRIER RW: Role of antidiuretic hormone in impaired urinary dilution associated with chronic bile-duct ligation. *Clin Sci* 58:493–500, 1980
6. MULLANE JF, GLIEDMAN ML: Renal response to saline load in experimental liver disease. *J Surg Res* 10:519–523, 1970
7. BETTER OS, MASSRY SG: Effect of chronic bile duct ligation on renal handling of salt and water. *J Clin Invest* 51:402–411, 1972
8. SHASHA SM, BETTER OS, CHAIMOVITZ C, DOMAN J, KISHON Y: Haemodynamic studies in dogs with chronic bile-duct ligation. *Clin Sci Mol Med* 50:533–537, 1976
9. SHALEV S, CHAIMOVITZ C: Renal hemodynamic studies in dogs with bile duct ligation. *Proc 34th ACEMB* 1984, p 350
10. CHAIMOVITZ C, MASSRY SG, FRIEDLER RM, COBURN JW: Effect of renal denervation and α-adrenergic blockade on sodium excretion in dogs with chronic ligation of the common bile duct. *Proc Soc Exp Biol Med* 146:764–800, 1974
11. MELMAN A, MASSRY SG: Role of renal vasodilatation in the blunted natriuresis of saline infusion in dogs with chronic bile duct obstruction. *J Lab Clin Med* 89:1053–1065, 1977
12. WINAVER J, CHAIMOVITZ C, BETTER OS: Natriuretic effect on propranolol on dogs with chronic bile-duct ligation. *Clin Sci Mol Med* 54:603–607, 1978
13. CHAIMOVITZ C, ALON U, BETTER OS: Pathogenesis of salt retention in dogs with chronic bile-duct ligation. *Clin Sci* 62:65–70, 1982

14. Alon U, Berant M, Mordechovitz D, Hashmonai M, Better OS: Effect of isolated cholaemia on systemic haemodynamics and kidney function in conscious dogs. *Clin Sci* 63:59–64, 1982

15. Lieberman FL, Ito S, Reynolds TB: Effective plasma volume in cirrhosis with ascites: Evidence that a decreased value does not account for renal sodium retention, a spontaneous reduction in GFR and a fall in GFR during drug-induced diuresis. *J Clin Invest* 48:975–981, 1969

16. Levy M: Renal function in dogs with acute selective hepatic venous outflow block. *Am J Physiol* 227:1074–1083, 1974

17. Schramek A, Better OS, Brook JG, Allroy GG, Gellei B: New observations on the clinical spectrum of the Budd-Chiari syndrome. *Ann Surg* 180:368–372, 1974

18. Anderson RJ, Cronin RE, McDonald KM, Schrier RM: Mechanisms of portal hypertension-induced alterations in renal hemodynamics, renal water excretion and renin secretion. *J Clin Invest* 58:964–970, 1976

19. Chaimovitz C, Rochman J, Eidelman S, Better OS: Exaggerated natriuretic response to volume expansion in patients with primary biliary cirrhosis. *Am J Med Sci* 274:173–178, 1977

Primary Renal Sodium Retention in the Nephrotic Syndrome

David B. Bernard

Edema, the clinical manifestation of an expanded interstitial fluid volume, is present in almost all patients with nephrotic syndrome (NS) at some time during the course of the disease. Indeed, swelling of the lower limbs or weight gain are the complaints that most often lead patients to seek medical advice. The basic processes that result in expansion of the interstitial space may be grouped into two interrelated categories: alterations occurring at the local tissue level, and alterations in the renal excretion of salt and water. The first of these, which involves an imbalance in Starling's forces across the capillary wall, is discussed elsewhere in this Section. In any edematous state, progressive expansion of the extracellular fluid compartment ultimately requires concomitant retention of salt and water by the kidneys. The current concepts of the pathophysiology of this avid renal salt retention in nephrotic edema is the subject of this review.

The traditional view of the pathway involved in the renal retention of sodium and water in the NS is shown in Fig. 1. The key alteration thought to initiate the process is a lowering of the plasma albumin concentration [1]. Hypoalbuminemia results in a reduction in the effective colloid oncotic pressure of the blood and favors movement of water from intravascular to interstitial spaces; hypovolemia is produced and becomes the afferent stimulus in the reflex arc whose ultimate effect is to promote enhanced salt and water retention by the kidneys. It is presumed that the contracted intravascular volume and its effects on arterial blood pressure and cardiac output would activate certain volume receptors and baroreceptors, and that through a variety of intrarenal and extrarenal neurohumoral and hemodynamic mechanisms, these receptors signal the kidney to retain salt and water [1]. In this way, sodium retention would be viewed as the expected and physiologically appropriate response by the kidney to the reduced circulation, serving to protect the organism from progressive plasma volume contraction. The sodium and

This manuscript was presented as part of a Symposium on *Pathogenesis of Edema in Cirrhosis and Nephrotic Syndrome.*

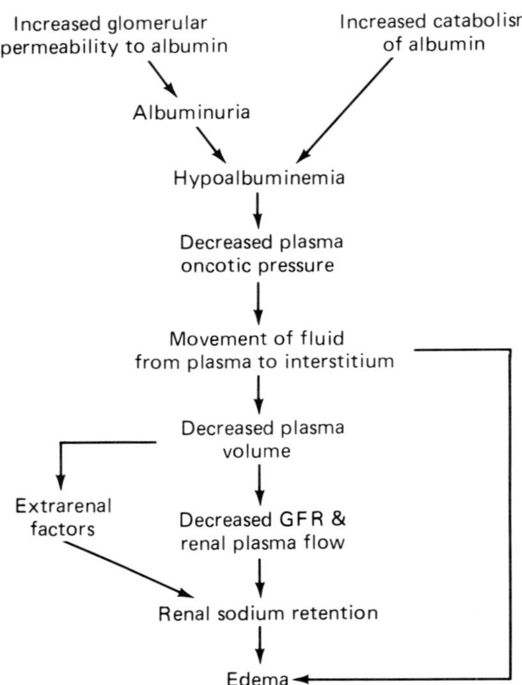

Fig. 1. Classic theory of the pathophysiologic mechanisms of edema formation in nephrotic syndrome. Hypoalbuminemia is viewed as the key alteration which initiates the process.

water retained initially dilutes plasma proteins and lowers intravascular oncotic pressure further, which accelerates the translocation of fluid from the intravascular to the interstitial compartment and results in only partial restoration of blood volume. This sequence of events continues until a new steady state is achieved in which sodium and water balance are reestablished, this time at the expense of a marked increase in interstitial volume.

Unequivocal confirmation of the validity of this hypothesis requires demonstration of the following events: (a) that blood and plasma volumes are reduced during the accumulation of edema; (b) that maneuvers that increase plasma volume into a clearly normal range in edematous nephrotic patients should invoke a natriuretic response; (c) that the functional importance of hypovolemia can be demonstrated by a circulatory and/or neurohumoral response to its presence. Over recent years, several important studies were unable to document these critical findings, and the classical theory, albeit logical and convenient, is now being brought into question. Several recent publications argue strongly in favor of an alternative hypothesis to explain edema in NS, namely, that retention of sodium by the kidney is a primary phenomenon occurring in response to intrarenal rather than systemic mechanisms [2–7]. Evidence in support of this hypothesis will be reviewed.

Blood Volume

The failure to demonstrate consistent reductions in blood and plasma volumes in nephrotic patients forms the basis for concluding that a primary reduction in renal sodium excretion may be a better explanation for the development of edema in many of these patients. In a recent review of this topic, the authors found reference to over 250 patients with NS in whom blood volumes had been measured; regardless of the method used, it was reduced in only 30%, being normal or increased in the rest [6]. Several more recent studies not only confirmed this general observation but reported an even higher percentage of normal or elevated blood volume measurements [4, 5, 8–10]. One possible criticism of these findings is that changes in albumin kinetics in NS, such as the rate of transcapillary escape of albumin or its distribution, may lessen the accuracy of blood volume measurements. However, in a preliminary report, one group of workers found that such changes introduced an error of no more than 1 to 2% in these measurements even when studied by standard techniques [9]. Of additional interest is the results from studies in NS which measured blood and plasma volumes during the phase of edema and again later in the same patients after they had undergone remission. In several of these, intravascular volume did not change, or was lower, once edema had resolved [6, 10–13]. Additionally, even in those studies in which plasma volume was found to be low during the phase of active sodium retention, it frequently remained low at the time of onset of a steroid-induced diuresis [7, 14].

In most blood volume studies in NS, measurements were made with the patient sitting or lying. The possibility that hypovolemia was missed in these cases is suggested by the observation that nephrotic patients have an exaggerated drop in plasma volume when standing [15]. Although normal values were obtained for blood or plasma volumes during recumbency in patients with NS, when plasma volume was measured after 20 min in an upright posture, it had fallen by 16%, significantly greater than the 7% decline noted in normal individuals [15]. Does this mean that hypovolemia is in fact present in nephrotic patients when they are standing and is then critical in stimulating renal salt and water retention? This possibility has not been studied extensively, although a recent preliminary report, while confirming an exaggerated fall in plasma volume with upright posture (16.8% in NS vs. 11.7% in control), nevertheless considered it of no "functional" significance because other parameters of hypovolemia such as changes in plasma renin activity (PRA), catecholamines, blood pressure, or heart rate were no different from normal [16]. An alternative recent suggestion is that there are actually two groups of nephrotic patients, separable according to their blood volume levels: those with low levels, generally represented by patients with minimal change disease and having normal renal function; and those with normal or elevated blood volumes, who are more likely to have reduced renal function and structural renal disease [7]. Other studies, however, have not been able to classify their patients in this way [4, 6, 9]. In summary, the majority of patients with NS have blood and plasma volumes that are normal or high rather than low, a finding in clear conflict with traditional concepts of edema formation.

On the other hand, in most studies of blood and plasma volumes in NS, a small percentage of the patients had low measurements together with a tendency for an increase toward normal values when a remission was entered, features in keeping with the classical theory of edema formation. Two possible interpretations could be made of this observation: (a) that in a certain number of cases, the classical theory is correct and hypovolemia is the afferent stimulus to renal sodium retention; or (b) that primary renal salt retention is in fact present in these cases and hypovolemia is a *secondary* phenomenon consequent on a more critical decline in plasma albumin concentration. That is to say, severe hypoalbuminemia, from enhanced losses and catabolism of albumin, leads to a fall in blood volume in spite of intrarenal mechanisms promoting sodium retention. Examining the renal response to volume expansion in these patients may allow these possibilities to be differentiated. An increase in urinary sodium excretion following intravascular volume expansion would favor the former; a lack of natriuresis, the latter.

Renal Response to Volume Expansion

The likelihood that hypovolemia is not the stimulus to renal sodium retention in all cases of NS was initially suggested by the variable natriuresis noted in response to hyperoncotic plasma infusion. Studies with plasma infusions were first performed over 30 years ago, soon after human plasma albumin became available for clinical use [17, 27], and showed that despite adequate volume expansion, diuresis and natriuresis occurred in only half of the treated cases, with a urinary sodium excretion response that varied from minimal to vigorous. In a more recent study, three patients with nephrotic edema were given 40 g of salt-poor albumin each day for 3 consecutive days [5]. The plasma volume was measured and shown to have increased into a normal or an above-normal range in all patients; yet the urine sodium excretion, although tending to increase somewhat, remained below daily intake, and all of them gained weight. The authors concluded that while a reduction in blood volume may have been a partial stimulus to sodium retention in their patients, an overriding mechanism, presumably intrarenal and independent of blood volume, had been promoting renal sodium avidity. Further confirmation of this notion is available from a study that examined the renal response to hyperoncotic plasma infusions given to patients with diuretic-resistant nephrotic edema [18]. In it, a successful natriuretic response was seen only if the patient was given potent diuretics with the infusion. In one patient for example, vigorous albumin infusions resulted simply in weight gain without any renal response, until doses of furosemide, smaller than those previously shown to be ineffective, were added. A brisk diuresis then occurred, clearly suggesting that some primary renal sodium retentive stimulus, blocked by the diuretic, had overcome the potential natriuretic effect of the volume expansion successfully.

Several recent studies in nephrotic patients examined the renal effects of immersion in a water bath for several hours (neck-out water immersion [8, 19, 20]), a well-established method of inducing central volume expansion [21]. In all patients, an increase in urinary sodium excretion was noted, although the individual response seemed to vary widely. For example, in one study, the overall mean increase in sodium excretion was 5-fold, but the peak response varied from 55 to 488 μEq/min despite the demonstration of normal or high blood volumes before the immersion in 7 of 8 subjects [8]. Another interesting observation in these studies was the fact that free water clearance (C_{H_2O}) increased markedly in the first 2 hr, whereas sodium excretion increased less. At least one interpretation of these findings is that both distal delivery and distal sodium chloride reabsorption had been enhanced during the early period of immersion despite significant volume expansion [19]. Only toward the end of the immersion period, when volume expansion had presumably been present for several hours (although not measured) did the urinary sodium excretion peak, again suggesting that some stimulus apart from hypovolemia had been responsible for the antinatriuresis present earlier [8, 19, 20].

Finally, if it cannot be shown consistently that absolute blood volume is reduced in NS, how consistently can evidence be documented for a humoral response to hypovolemia—namely, stimulation of the renin-angiotensin-aldosterone axis, and/or circulatory effects of hypovolemia?

Renin-Angiotensin-Aldosterone

Several studies measured plasma renin activity (PRA) and aldosterone concentrations or aldosterone excretion rates in patients with NS and reported variable results. This may be partly because of the many factors present in nephrotic subjects apart from blood volume that can affect this system, such as dietary sodium intake, the clinical stage of edema, and the presence of diuretics, making it difficult to compare different series [4, 6, 22, 23]. A review of available studies shows that PRA and plasma aldosterone concentrations or urinary excretion rates of aldosterone are high in about 50% of the patients [4, 6, 22, 23]. Since a smaller fraction of patients with NS has been found to have low blood volumes (about 30%), the possibility has been raised that PRA is stimulated in some patients by nonvolume-related factors. In support of this, several studies have been unable to demonstrate any close correlation between changes in PRA or aldosterone and blood volume [4, 6, 8], and in another study, salt loading produced an increase in blood volume and weight gain without a measurable decline in PRA [7]. An early suggestion that alterations in plasma renin substrate may complicate the interpretation of PRA [22] has not been confirmed [23].

In summary, it appears that PRA is increased in many but not all patients with NS and that although the stimulus for this is not well defined, it does not consistently indicate the presence of hypovolemia. It is also not clear whether either renin or aldosterone has anything to do with the sodium retention of NS: (1) Many patients have normal levels of these hormones during the phase of edema formation. (2) In several studies it has been shown that renin levels rise rather than fall with the onset of a remission [6, 23]. (3) Pharmacologic interruption of the renin-angiotensin system has had no effect on sodium excretion [5, 24]. (4) Patients with NS given a high-salt diet may retain sodium and gain weight despite suppression of their renin and aldosterone levels [25]. These data suggest that although aldosterone may contribute to the sodium retention in NS, it is not an essential factor.

There is further evidence in support of the notion that blood volume is functionally increased rather than reduced during the edematous phase of NS. It is the changes that occur in blood pressure when edema is gone. In a recent study of adults with minimal change disease, fully half the patients had a blood pressure of over 150/90 during relapse, although the mean blood pressure was lower following remission in 12 of 13 episodes [6]. This finding has been reported previously but was dismissed as being due to an overcompensation for hypovolemia, even though blood volumes had not been measured [26].

Taken together, the above data suggest that the commonly held view of hypovolemia being responsible for the onset and maintenance of renal sodium retention and edema in patients with NS cannot be supported in many cases. A clear, consistent relation between blood volume, plasma renin activity, and urinary sodium excretion is often lacking, and a more tenable explanation for the findings would frequently invoke primary renal retention of sodium as the initiating factor in edema. At first, blood volume would become expanded, and this would elevate blood pressure and suppress PRA and aldosterone levels. Edema now develops by "overflow," the expanded plasma volume leaking into the interstitium under the influence of altered Starling forces at a local tissue level. Later, as plasma albumin concentration falls further, expansion of the interstitial space increases and, depending on the balance between rate of movement of fluid out of the vascular tree and the degree of renal fluid retention, absolute hypovolemia may develop in some patients.

Even though this scenario clearly has considerable experimental support, pathophysiologic mechanisms in some cases of nephrotic edema may still be fitted more conveniently into the traditional view. Indeed, it seems most reasonable to suggest that no single mechanism can be invoked to explain all cases of renal sodium retention all of the time. Perhaps different mechanisms are operative in different patients. Or perhaps several mechanisms may be operative in any one patient at different times, depending on such factors as the specific underlying pathologic process, the stage of evolution of the sodium retentive disease, dietary salt intake, the posture of the patient, presence and severity of associated heart or liver disease, occult or evident, and a host of additional, as yet undefined factors.

What direct evidence is available in support of primary renal salt retention in NS?

Evidence for Primary Renal Salt Retention

Two recent studies of experimental NS used puromycin aminonucleoside (PAN) to induce the NS, a model of minimal change disease. They have produced clear evidence of renal sodium retention from local intrarenal cause(s) [2, 3]. These elegant studies have yielded critically important data that have greatly clarified our understanding of how nephrotic patients accumulating edema may develop the apparently confusing picture of normal blood volume or hypervolemia. In each case, only one kidney of each animal was perfused with PAN so that unilateral proteinuria was produced and hypoalbuminemia did not develop. Sodium excretion was normal or high from the nonperfused or saline-perfused control kidneys, but was reduced significantly from the PAN-perfused, proteinuric kidneys at a time when systemic plasma protein concentration, and presumably blood volume, was normal. Also, systemic factors that may stimulate secondary renal sodium retention should have been absent, clearly suggesting that sodium retention was a primary phenomenon caused by local intrarenal influences. In one of these studies [3], a compensatory increase in sodium excretion occurred in the contralateral, nonproteinuric (non-PAN perfused) kidneys, which maintained the animals in normal sodium balance. In the other [2], sodium excretion in the nonproteinuric kidneys of the experimental rats was not increased above control, and the rats were thus presumably in positive sodium balance. These studies have thus offered the first strong evidence for the presence of some local intrarenal factor or factors promoting avid sodium retention by proteinuric kidneys. It also offers a satisfactory explanation for the observation that the first change noted frequently in an edematous nephrotic prior to the onset of a diuresis is a reduction in urinary protein excretion and not an elevation in plasma albumin concentration or blood volume [14].

Renal sodium retention, whether a primary or secondary phenomenon, could arise because of changes in glomerular filtration, tubular function, or both. The next paragraphs analyze these aspects of renal function in NS.

Glomerular Filtration

Although a reduction in glomerular filtration rate (GFR) is not considered an important feature of idiopathic NS, at least when it is due to minimal change disease, most of the published series do, in fact, document a transient decrease in most patients [4, 6, 8, 13, 26]. Additionally, in many of these patients, GFR returned to normal with the onset of a remission [6, 13, 26]. Two questions arise from this observation: (1) What is the cause of the reduced GFR, and, specifically, does it reflect hypovolemia? (2) What role does the reduced GFR play in renal sodium retention?

As evidence against an important role for hypovolemia, several studies in patients with NS demonstrated that volume expansion large enough to raise blood volume to well above normal—by either hyperoncotic albumin infusion or water immersion—did not often increase GFR [8, 17, 21, 27]. Also, renal plasma flow was found to be within normal limits during the phase of edema and to fall with recovery [6], arguing against renal hypoperfusion as a cause of reduced GFR.

Several other studies offer suggestions as to the possible causes of the reduced GFR in nephrotic subjects. Hypoalbuminemia, at least when induced acutely, reduced the glomerular basement membrane ultrafiltration coefficient and could be a cause of reduced filtration in NS [28]. However, this seems unlikely to be an important mechanism on its own because, in several cases, GFR increased to normal with the onset of diuresis, whereas plasma albumin concentration was still markedly reduced [6, 14]. In a recent study of experimental NS in rats, the infusion of saralasin, a specific angiotensin II (AII) antagonist, led to a significant increase in whole kidney and single nephron glomerular filtration rate (SNGFR), suggesting that AII had contributed to the reduced filtration [2]. On the other hand, GFR was not returned to normal by saralasin, emphasizing that some other factor was also involved. Finally, two groups studied the clearance of macromolecules by the nephrotic glomerulus in minimal change disease and found a reduction in the clearance of molecules smaller than 44 Å [29, 30]. In concert with this, inulin clearances were reduced by 24% in untreated NS, and these returned to normal with steroid-induced elimination of proteinuria [29]. That lowered filtration rates in NS are not found more often may be due to the fact that GFR is usually estimated in these cases by the endogenous creatinine clearance. A recent report suggested that creatinine is an unreliable filtration marker in NS and may substantially overestimate true GFR [31]. In confirmation of this point, one group found their patients to have normal creatinine clearances on average, yet inulin clearance was reduced in many cases [8]. Whether this discrepancy between inulin and creatinine clearances in NS is important, and which is a more correct measure of true GFR, has not yet been established.

Assuming GFR is reduced in most patients with NS, albeit to a small degree, how important is this in the sodium retentive process? Studies are available both to suggest a role for reduced filtration in sodium retention and to deny such a role, and the matter cannot now be definitively resolved. For example, some studies demonstrated a progressive decline in GFR during the phase of active salt retention [13, 14], with a prompt increase to normal at the onset of diuresis, implying a key role for reduced filtration of sodium in the edematous process [6, 13]. On the other hand, several other studies drew opposite conclusions. Some examples are as follows: Elevation of GFR with saralasin in experimental NS failed to enhance sodium excretion [2]. In the water immersion studies, the increased sodium excretion occurred without any significant change in GFR, at least in the latter part of the immersion period [8, 19, 20], and similar observations were made after plasma infusion [17, 27]. Many patients have an elevated GFR during relapse, with a fall toward normality in remission [13]. In some studies, the expansion of plasma volume to levels normal or above normal with plasma infusions failed to increase sodium excretion [5] or did so only in the presence of powerful diuretics [18], favoring a more important role for primary tubular sodium retention rather than reduced glomerular filtration. On balance, although mild primary reductions in GFR may play some role in the fluid retention in NS, it seems far more likely that the excess accumulation of sodium and water is due predominantly to enhanced tubular reabsorption.

If primary renal sodium retention is present in many cases of NS, what are the intrarenal mechanisms responsible? Can we obtain some clues of what these might be by identifying the nephron segments where sodium avidity is occurring?

Potential Mechanisms of Intrarenal Sodium Retention

In the absence of available data, one can only speculate at this stage about the potential primary intrarenal mechanisms that may be promoting enhanced sodium reabsorption from proteinuric kidneys. That local angiotensin production is probably not involved is suggested by the study that failed to demonstrate increased sodium excretion in response to saralasin in unilateral proteinuria [2], or to converting enzyme inhibition in human NS [5, 24]. Although increased resistance to intratubular flow, thought to be attributable to the intraluminal albumin, was blamed for increased proximal fractional fluid reabsorption in one study [32], this observation could not be confirmed in normal animals [33]. Nevertheless, because a reduction in proteinuria is frequently the first sign that a nephrotic patient is about to enter a diuretic phase, it does seem as if the presence of albumin within the tubular lumen may itself in some direct way increase tubular sodium reabsorption. For example, reabsorption of albumin by tubular epithelial cells may damage key transport processes and prevent tubular rejection of the sodium needed to maintain normal homeostasis. The potential role of other factors remains to be defined, factors such as the failure to generate a locally produced natriuretic substance, as suggested by one study [34], or alterations in certain hormonal or enzyme systems known to influence renal sodium excretion, such as the prostaglandins [35] or kallikrein-kinin system [36].

Tubular Site of Sodium Retention

Proximal tubular function has been studied directly in a number of animal models of NS. In all cases, the *absolute* reabsorption of fluid in this segment of the nephron was found to be decreased whereas the *fractional* reabsorption was generally normal. In a recent micropuncture study of nephrotoxic nephritis, the proximal fractional reabsorption was reported to be increased [32], but because the GFR was markedly reduced, in agreement with other studies, the absolute proximal sodium reabsorption was significantly lower than the control. We found both fractional and absolute proximal sodium reabsorption to be reduced in a model of experimental NS studied during volume expansion [37]. The model used was that of autologous immune complex nephropathy, or Heymann nephritis, in which the glomerular lesion is indistinguishable from that of idiopathic membranous nephropathy in humans. The features of NS were well developed, and renal function was normal after saline expansion. In an indirect clearance study of human NS using the technique of distal tubular blockade, proximal tubular fractional reabsorption was also found to be lower than normal [38]. The sum of these experiments clearly suggests that the site of enhanced sodium reabsorption in NS is beyond the proximal tubule.

Two studies performed segmental analysis of sodium transport at segments beyond the late proximal tubule [2, 37]. In studies of rat membranous nephropathy, we showed that tubular handling of sodium in the loop of Henle and distal convoluted tubule was the same in experimental and control animals [37]. As shown in Fig. 2, filtered sodium was slightly, although not significantly, lower in the nephrotic rats (7.23 ± 0.23 vs. 8.12 ± 0.65 nEq/min) but this was offset by the reduction in proximal reabsorption in these animals, so that delivery of sodium to the loop of Henle was the same in both groups. Delivery of sodium to the early distal tubule on the surface of the kidney and reabsorption along the superficial distal tubule were also similar in both groups. By the time tubular fluid had reached the end of the superficial late distal tubule, both fractional and absolute amounts of sodium remaining were virtually identical in experimental and control animals—yet sodium excretion in the final urine was markedly different. Thus, in nephrotic rats, about 47% of the sodium passing beyond the superficial late distal tubule (or 0.17 ± 0.04 nEq/min) was reabsorbed, whereas in the control rats, only 8% (or 0.03 ± 0.04 nEq/min) was removed ($P < 0.05$). The final urinary sodium excretion was 4.7 ± 1.1 μEq/min (or 2.2 ± 0.5% of the filtered sodium) in nephrotic animals and 9.2 ± 1.2 μEq/min (or 4.0 ± 0.6% of the filtered load) in control animals ($P < 0.02$). We concluded that the site of enhanced sodium reabsorption in this model of experimental NS was either the nephron segments beyond the superficial late distal tubule (such as the collecting tubule) or it was in some undefined segment of deeper nephrons. Identical results were recently obtained in the model of PAN-induced unilat-

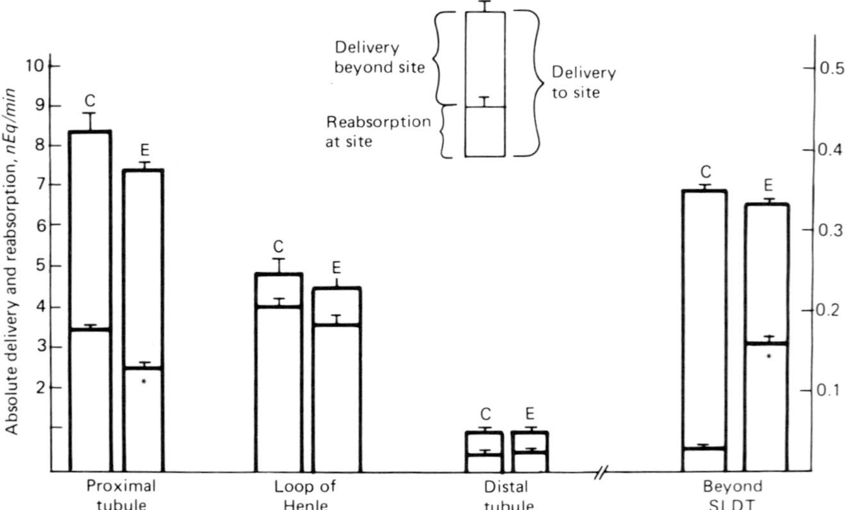

Fig. 2. Absolute sodium delivery to, reabsorption by, and delivery beyond various nephron segments in control animals (*C*) and animals with nephrotic syndrome (*E*). SLDT denotes the superficial late distal tubule. The *right-hand scale* applies only to the last pair of bars. *Asterisk* indicates $P < 0.05$ for C versus E. (Reproduced from [37] with permission)

eral proteinuria [2]. Although SNGFR in the PAN-perfused, proteinuric kidneys was reduced significantly, absolute proximal tubular and loop of Henle reabsorption was decreased as well, such that the amount of sodium reaching the early distal tubule was the same in proteinuric and nonproteinuric kidneys. Reabsorption of sodium along the superficial distal tubule and delivery of sodium beyond this site were also the same in experimental and control kidneys. However, sodium excretion in the final urine was markedly lower from the proteinuric side, again suggesting that the site of enhanced sodium reabsorption was either the segments of nephron beyond the micropunctured superficial late distal tubule or that altered function in deep nephrons was responsible.

Information currently available about the factors that control sodium reabsorption in the more terminal parts of the nephron does not offer immediate suggestions as to the likely defects in NS [39]. Changes in tubular fluid sodium chloride concentration, flow rate, local hormone or nerve action, or alterations in intrarenal hemodynamics may all be important. Additional studies are clearly needed to clarify this point further.

In 1950, Luetscher and colleagues [17] observed the variable natriuretic response to albumin infusion in patients with NS and wrote, "These observations suggest that the inability of the kidneys to excrete normal quantities of sodium and water in nephrosis may be a cause, not a consequence of the edema," an opinion we are only now beginning to share.

References

1. BERNARD DB, ALEXANDER EA: Edema formation in the nephrotic syndrome: Pathophysiologic mechanisms. *Cardiovasc Med* 4:605–625, 1979
2. ICHIKAWA I, RENNKE HG, HOYER JR, BADR KF, SCHOR N, TROY JL, LECHENE CP, BRENNER BM: Role for intrarenal mechanisms in the impaired salt excretion of experimental nephrotic syndrome. *J Clin Invest* 71:91–103, 1983
3. CHANDRA M, HOYER JR, LEWY JE: Renal function in rats with unilateral proteinuria produced by renal perfusion with aminonucleoside. *Pediatr Res* 15:340–344, 1981
4. BROWN EA, MARKANDU ND, ROULSTON JE, JONES BE, SQUIRES M, MACGREGOR GA: Is the renin-angiotensin-aldosterone system involved in the sodium retention in the nephrotic syndrome? *Nephron* 32:102–107, 1982
5. BROWN EA, MARKANDU ND, SAGNELLA GA, SQUIRES M, JONES BE, MACGREGOR GA: Evidence that some mechanism other than the renin system causes sodium retention in nephrotic syndrome. *Lancet* 2:1237–1240, 1982
6. DORHOUT MEES EJ, ROOS JC, BOER P, YOE OH, SIMATUPANG TA: Observations on edema formation in the nephrotic syndrome in adults with minimal lesions. *Am J Med* 67:378–384, 1979
7. MELTZER JI, KEIM HJ, LARAGH JH, SEALEY JE, JAN K-M, CHIEN S: Nephrotic syndrome: Vasoconstriction and hypervolemic types indicated by renin-sodium profiling. *Ann Intern Med* 91:688–696, 1979
8. KRISHNA GG, DANOVITCH GM: Effects of water immersion on renal function in the nephrotic syndrome. *Kidney Int* 21:395–401, 1982
9. GEERS AB, KOOMANS HA, BOER P, DORHOUT MEES EJ: A survey of plasma volume (PV) measurements in patients with nephrotic syndrome (NS): The labeled albumin method. *Kidney Int* 23:781, 1983

10. DORHOUT MEES EJ, GEERS AB, KOOMANS HA, ROOS JC: Changes in plasma volume and renin activity during correction of edema in the nephrotic syndrome (NS). *Kidney Int* 25:163, 1984
11. EISENBERG S: Blood volume in persons with the nephrotic syndrome. *Am J Med Sci* 255:320–326, 1968
12. KELSCH RC, LIGHT GS, OLIVER WJ: The effect of albumin infusion upon plasma norepinephrine concentration in nephrotic children. *J Lab Clin Med* 79:516–525, 1972
13. OLIVER WJ: Physiologic responses associated with steroid-induced diuresis in the nephrotic syndrome. *J Lab Clin Med* 62:449–464, 1963
14. OLIVER WJ, OWINGS CL: Sodium excretion in the nephrotic syndrome: Relation to serum albumin concentration, glomerular filtration rate, and aldosterone excretion rate. *Am J Dis Child* 113:352–362, 1967
15. EISENBERG S: Postural changes in plasma volume in hypoalbuminemia. *Arch Intern Med* 112:544–549, 1963
16. GEERS AB, DORHOUT MEES EJ, KOOMANS HA, BOER P: Postural changes in the nephrotic syndrome (NS). *Kidney Int* 25:165, 1984
17. LUETSCHER JA, HALL AD, KREMER VL: Treatment of nephrosis with concentrated human serum albumin: II. Effects on renal function and on excretion of water and some electrolytes. *J Clin Invest* 29:896–905, 1950
18. DAVISON AM, LAMBIE AT, VERTH AH, CASH JD: Salt-poor human albumin in management of nephrotic syndrome. *Br Med J* 1:481–484, 1974
19. BERLYNE GM, SUTTON J, BROWN C, FEINROTH MV, FEINROTH M, ADLER AJ, FRIEDMAN EA: Renal salt and water handling in water immersion in the nephrotic syndrome. *Clin Sci* 61:605–610, 1981
20. BERLYNE GM, BROWN C, ADLER A, FEINROTH MV, FEINROTH M, HIRSCH S, FRIEDMAN EA: Water immersion in nephrotic syndrome. *Arch Intern Med* 141:1275–1278, 1981
21. EPSTEIN M: Renal effects of head-out water immersion in man: Implications for an understanding of volume homeostasis. *Physiol Rev* 58:529–581, 1978
22. MEDINA A, DAVIES DL, BROWN JJ, FRASER R, LEVER AF, MALLICK NP, MORTON JJ, ROBERTSON JIS, TREE M: A study of the renin-angiotensin system in the nephrotic syndrome. *Nephron* 12:233–240, 1974
23. BOER P, ROOS JC, GEYSKES GG, DORHOUT MEES EJ: Observations on plasma renin substrate in the nephrotic syndrome. *Nephron* 26:121–125, 1980
24. DÜSING R, VETTER H, KRAMER HJ: The renin-angiotensin-aldosterone system in patients with nephrotic syndrome: Effects of 1-SAR-8-ALA-Angiotensin II. *Nephron* 25:187–192, 1980
25. CHONKO AM, BAY WH, STEIN JH, FERRIS TF: The role of renin and aldosterone in the salt retention of edema. *Am J Med* 63:881–889, 1977
26. CAMERON JS, TURNER DR, OGG CS, SHARPSTONE P, BROWN CB: The nephrotic syndrome in adults with minimal change glomerular lesions. *Q J Med* 171:461–488, 1974
27. ORLOFF J, WELT LG, STOWE L: The effects of concentrated salt-poor albumin on the metabolism and excretion of water and electrolytes in nephrosis and toxemia of pregnancy. *J Clin Invest* 29:770–780, 1950
28. BAYLIS C, ICHIKAWA, I, WILLIS WT, WILSON CB, BRENNER BM: Dynamics of glomerular ultration: IX. Effects of plasma protein concentration. *Am J Physiol* 232:F58–F71, 1977
29. ROBSON AM, GIANGIACOMO J, KIENSTRA RA, NAQVI ST, INGELFINGER JR:

Normal glomerular permeability and its modification by minimal change nephrotic syndrome. *J Clin Invest* 54:1190–1199, 1974
30. CARRIE BJ, SALYER WR, MYERS BD: Minimal change nephropathy: An electrochemical disorder of the glomerular membrane. *Am J Med* 70:262–268, 1981
31. CARRIE BJ, GOLBETZ HV, MICHAELS AS, MYERS BD: Creatinine: An inadequate filtration marker in glomerular diseases. *Am J Med* 69:177–182, 1980
32. KURODA S, AYNEDJIAN HS, BANK N: A micropuncture study of renal sodium retention in nephrotic syndrome in rats: Evidence for increased resistance to tubular fluid flow. *Kidney Int* 16:561–571, 1979
33. CARMINES PK, TANNER GA: Effect of albumin microinfusion on proximal tubular pressure. *Renal Physiol* 5:85–87, 1982
34. FAVRE H, GOURJON M: Absence of production of natriuretic factor following acute saline expansion in nephrotic rats. *Clin Sci* 63:317–319, 1982
35. GARIN EH, SAUSVILLE PJ, RICHARD GA: 6 Keto prostaglandin F_{1a} plasma levels in aminonucleoside nephrosis in the rat. *Prostaglandins* 23:391–395, 1982
36. BROUHARD BH, CUNNINGHAM RJ, PETRUSICK TW, BERGER M, TRAVIS LB: Urinary kallikrein excretion in idiopathic nephrotic syndrome. *J Urol* 121:672–674, 1979
37. BERNARD DB, ALEXANDER EA, COUSER WG, LEVINSKY NG: Renal sodium retention during volume expansion in experimental nephrotic syndrome. *Kidney Int* 14:478–485, 1978
38. GRAUSZ H, LIEBERMAN R, EARLEY LE: Effect of plasma albumin on sodium reabsorption in patients with nephrotic syndrome. *Kidney Int* 1:47–54, 1972
39. BURG MB: Renal handling of sodium, chloride, water, amino acids, and glucose, Chapter 7 in *The Kidney* (2nd ed), edited by BRENNER BM, RECTOR FC, Philadelphia, Saunders, 1981, vol 1, pp 353–365

Causes and Mechanisms
of Renal Injury

Immunologic Mechanisms in Renal Disease

Alfred F. Michael

Evidence that immunologic mechanisms play a role in human renal disease is derived from a number of observations. First, the characterization of certain experimental models, which are similar immunologically and morphologically to human glomerulonephritis, has provided a firm basis for this contention. Second, the recognition of deposits of immunoglobulin (Ig) and complement components within renal extracellular matrices and basement membranes is compelling evidence for the participation of humoral immunity in these diseases. Third, the presence of certain serologic abnormalities—antinuclear antibodies in lupus erythematosus, antibasement membrane antibodies in antiglomerular basement membrane (anti-GBM) nephritis, and immune complexes and complement component changes in a variety of diseases—provides additional support for this view. The reason for the association of complement-deficient states with certain types of glomerulonephritis has not been determined. Finally, cell-mediated immunity has been shown to have a dominant role in tubulointerstitial nephritis associated with homograft rejection, but its participation in the other forms of human glomerulonephritis is much less clear. However, cell-mediated injury has been implicated in certain experimentally induced forms of renal disease—acute serum sickness, anti-GBM nephritis, and tubulointerstitial disease.

In this chapter, emphasis will be placed primarily on the pathogenesis of glomerular disease; the mechanisms for immune injury to tubular structures are similar in many respects, but will not be discussed. No attempt will be made to exhaustively review the contributions of all investigators, since this is beyond the scope of this discussion.

Structural Characteristics of the Glomerular Capillary

The glomerular capillary is a unique structure consisting of endothelial and epithelial cells, with an interposed glomerular basement membrane (GBM).

This manuscript was presented as part of a Symposium on *Prostaglandins and the Kidney*.

In the peripheral region of the capillary, filtration of various molecules occurs, which is partly controlled by the hemodynamic factors that determine glomerular filtration as well as characteristics of the molecule—specifically, its size and charge. In the more centrolobular part of the glomerulus, the mesangium is bounded by the reflections of the GBM and the overlying endothelial cell that separates it from the capillary lumen [1–3]. The mesangium consists of mesangial cells and extracellular matrix material. Studies in rats by Schreiner et al [4] have demonstrated the presence of another cell within this region—a bone marrow-derived, Ia-positive phagocytic cell that is present in very small numbers. The mesangial cells and matrix are in close contiguity to elements of the juxtaglomerular apparatus, particularly the lacis cells.

The peripheral capillary and mesangium are common regions for immunologic injury—especially injuries related to the deposition of immune complexes, but also the interaction of antibody with structural or planted in situ antigens. Inflammatory cells and monocytes also may be recognized adjacent to or within these regions.

Antigenic and Macromolecular Components of Renal Basement Membranes

The human glomerular capillary wall contains arrays of distinct antigens that are identified by immunohistochemical techniques (Table 1) [5–7]. These antigens are distributed with a characteristic topography (Fig. 1). For example, certain antigens (types IV and V collagen, fibronectin) are present along the internal aspect of the GBM in contiguity with similar sites in the mesangium, whereas other antigens (antigenic sites reactive with human anti-GBM antibody) are located within the GBM exclusively. Antigenic heterogeneity of basement membranes is further suggested by studies using monoclonal

Table 1. Components of human glomerular basement membrane[a]

Collagen
  Types IV and V
Glycoproteins
  Fibronectin
  Laminin
  Entactin
  Antigen(s) reactive with autoantibodies
Proteoglycan
  Heparan sulfate
Anionic plasma proteins
Undefined antigens recognized by monoclonal antibodies

[a] Mesangial matrix contains types IV and V collagen, fibronectin, laminin, and proteoglycan (heparan sulfate and chondroitin sulfate).

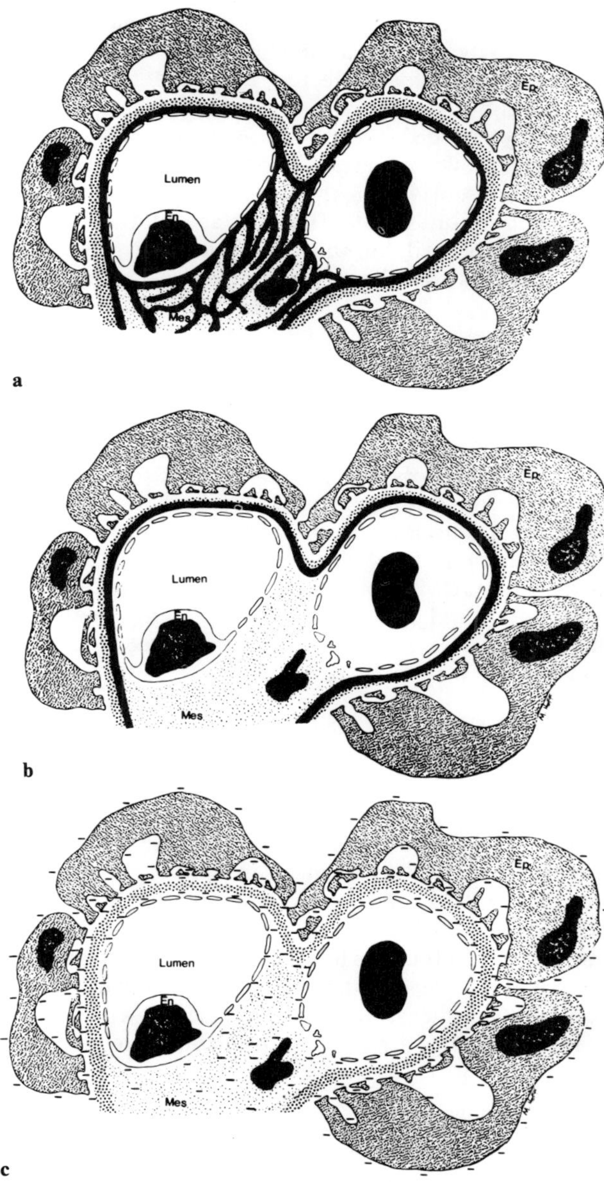

Fig. 1. The distribution of certain human basement membrane antigen(s) is illustrated in black. **a.** Type IV collagen and fibronectin; laminin has a similar distribution, but in addition is present along the lamina rara externa. **b.** Antigen(s) reactive with autoantibodies in anti-GBM nephritis or Goodpasture's syndrome. **c.** Negatively charged sites in the lamina rara interna and externa (heparan sulfate proteoglycan), the mesangial matrix (heparan and chondroitin sulfate), and along the visceral epithelial cell (sialic acid containing polyanion).

antibodies developed in mice against human or rat basement membranes. The reactivity of these antibodies reveal a number of different immunohisto-chemical phenotypes reflecting noncharacterized antigenic components.

Studies by Kanwar and Farquhar [8] have demonstrated the presence of negatively charged sites in the lamina rara externa and interna, and these have been shown to be related to heparan sulfate proteoglycan (Fig. 1). Similar sites are present within the mesangial matrix, which contains both heparan and chondroitin sulfate. The surface of the visceral epithelial cell is also negatively charged, but this is related to the presence of a sialic acid glycopro-tein, which is the glomerular polyanion—more recently called podocalyxin [9, 10].

Thus, there appears to be a remarkable heterogeneity and complexity of basement membrane components. In addition, studies from our laboratory have demonstrated that various human anti-GEM antibodies react differently with fetal GBM, suggesting the presence of more than one antigenic determi-nant.

The presence of plasma proteins in basement membrane has been demon-strated by immunohistochemical techniques and by direct immunoassay. Re-cently, it has been demonstrated that proteins with relatively low isoelectric points (albumin, IgG_4) are present in normal GBM and in increased amounts in diabetic GBM, whereas the more cationic species are not (for example, IgG_1, IgG_2, and IgG_3) [11]. These findings suggest that the GBM contains intrinsic positive charges that are abrogated by the binding of anionic plasma proteins in vivo.

Immunologic Mechanisms of Renal Disease

As discussed above, evidence of the participation of immune mechanisms in the pathogenesis of human renal disease is derived from a variety of experi-mental, immunohistochemical, morphologic, and serologic studies (Table 2) (reviewed in [12–22]). In certain human diseases (for example, anti-GBM nephritis and lupus nephritis), there appears to be sufficient evidence to impli-cate a specific process. However, the picture is far from clear in other diseases, such as dense deposit disease and other forms of glomerulonephritis. It has been erroneously assumed that all diseases with granular nonlinear deposition of immunoglobulin reflect the localization of circulating immune complexes.

Table 2. Immunologic mechanisms of renal disease

Deposition of circulating immune complexes
Interaction of antibody with an in situ antigen
Intrinsic or structural antigen
Exogenous-planted antigen
Cell-mediated immunity
Tubulointerstitial nephritis induced experimentally or
in homograft rejection
Participation in models of immune complex disease
and in situ antigen antibody interaction

The picture is further confused by a heavy reliance on comparisons with experimental models and our incomplete understanding and ignorance regarding the pathogenesis of human glomerulonephritis.

Deposition of Circulating Immune Complexes

The classic model for this form of glomerular or vascular injury is acute serum sickness in the rabbit, extensively studied over 2 decades ago by Dixon, Feldman, and Vasquez [21] and Germuth [22]. Following the administration of a foreign protein antigen (for example, bovine serum albumin or BSA), there is an initial period of equilibration followed by a linear logarithmic decline in plasma concentration for a period of approximately 9 to 12 days; then, by a rapid clearance from the plasma that is coincident with the appearance of antibody. During this period, antibody appears initially in an environment of excess antigen, leading to the formation of soluble antigen-antibody complexes. These complexes are biologically active and have the ability to fix complement. For reasons that are not completely clear, complexes localize within the mesangial and subendothelial regions of the glomerular capillary as well as in vessels in other parts of the body; they produce both vasculitis and glomerulitis (Fig. 2). The vasculitis is characterized by infiltration of polymorphonuclear leukocytes, whereas the glomerular lesion is associated primarily with mononuclear cell infiltration, as demonstrated by Hunsicker et al [23]. If this infiltration is abrogated by antimacrophage serum, there is a striking decrease in the amount of proteinuria that indicates the importance of these cells in the pathogenesis of glomerular capillary injury.

Glomerular Localization of Complexes

The mechanisms leading to or promoting the glomerular localization of these complexes or any macromolecule are incompletely understood (Table 3).

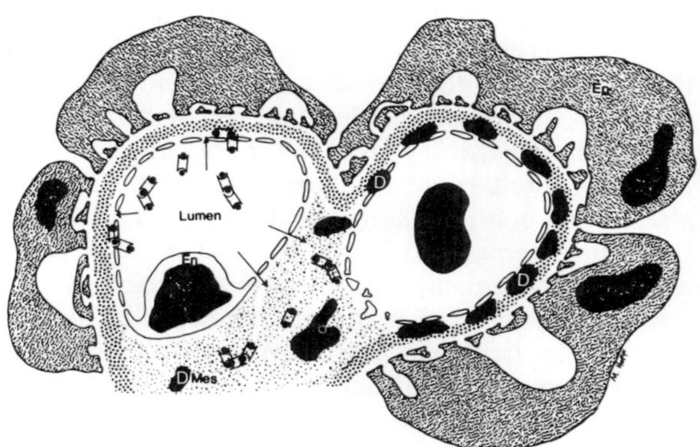

Fig. 2. The localization of immune complexes in the subendothelial and mesangial zones, with formation of immune deposits (*D*) containing immunoglobulin and complement components.

Table 3. Determinants of glomerular localization of macromolecules or immune complexes

Properties of the complex
  Size
  Antibody avidity
  Charge
  Plasma concentration—controlled in part by the
    mononuclear phagocytic system

Characteristics of the glomerulus
  Mesangial sequestration
  Electrostatic charge

Hemodynamic determinants

Biologically active mediators
  Angiotensin II, prostaglandins

The properties of the complex itself (size, antibody avidity, charge, and plasma concentration) are important determinants of this process [18, 24–31]. Thus, small complexes containing antibody of relatively low avidity or affinity tend to localize in the peripheral capillary, whereas larger-sized complexes made with antibody of high affinity become sequestered within the mesangium. There obviously are many variables in this process that make it difficult to construct precise laws governing the localization of immune complexes. Some conclusions have been predicated on analysis of the size and constituency of complexes in the plasma; however, these studies give incomplete information regarding the nature of the complexes that have become deposited within the kidney.

The plasma concentration appears to be an important variable, especially with respect to the uptake of macromolecules by the mesangium. Following the administration of immune complexes or macromolecules, there is engulfment by components of the mononuclear phagocytic system and ultimate clearance from the circulation. With respect to immune complexes, this uptake is largely dependent on Fc receptors, as well as on complement receptors (CR). Some complexes are also removed from the circulation by receptors that are specific for the antigen, as demonstrated by Finbloom et al [32]. However, other macromolecules (such as ferritin, colloidal carbon, and aggregated albumin) are phagocytosed by mechanisms that do not involve Fc receptors. Studies by Haakenstad, Striker, and Mannik [33] have demonstrated that complexes made with reduced and alkylated antibody are poorly taken up by mononuclear cells, which leads to an increased plasma level and (as a consequence) to an increased localization within glomeruli. Therefore, any consideration of immune complex disease must take into account the overall reticuloendothelial system as an important variable in this process.

The demonstration that the glomerular capillary wall contains negatively charged molecules has led to important studies regarding the influence of charge on immune complex localization. Thus, Gallo et al [34, 35] demonstrated that passive administration of cationic immune complexes resulted in diffuse localization within the subendothelial and subepithelial regions—

loci that are rich in the glycosaminoglycan, heparan sulfate. Similarly, Border et al [36] demonstrated that active immunization with cationic bovine serum albumin leads to the development of a membranous disease with peripheral capillary localization of immune complexes. Using this model in normal and C6-deficient rabbits, Groggel et al [37] demonstrated a requirement for terminal complement components in the development of capillary injury that appeared to be independent of mononuclear cells and neutrophils.

In addition, cationized human IgG binds to negatively charged sites of the rat glomerular capillary after in vivo perfusion-administered—and in this locus, it can bind passively—or actively induced antibody, resulting in glomerulonephritis [38, 39].

As indicated above, the mesangial zone is a common site for the deposition of immune complexes. There is abundant evidence, based largely on morphologic studies using various tracers, that this region is normally perfused by plasma (evidence reviewed in [3]). However, the inaccessibility of the mesangium has not permitted appropriate physiologic studies to define the rate or extent of plasmic flow. The uptake of macromolecules is conditioned by the various factors indicated above that are related to localization of immune complexes. In addition, certain experimental manipulations are known to affect mesangial kinetics. For example, induction of proteinuria by aminonucleoside or anti-GBM antibody results in increased localization of macromolecules within the mesangial zone. The mechanism of this phenomenon is unknown, but it may reflect increased mesangial perfusion in nephrotic states.

Macromolecules enter the mesangial zone at the endothelial-mesangial interface. However, the exit of complexes from the mesangium or degradation is much less clear. Phagocytosis by mesangial cells and infiltrating monocytes has been clearly demonstrated in a number of experimental situations. In addition, the presence of a small number of Ia-positive phagocytic cells also has been demonstrated in this region [4]. Another route of egress is via the glomerular stalk to the hilum of the glomerulus, although the route thereafter is more obscure—possibly into the interstitium or the lymphatic system. It is also possible that complexes or macromolecules may enter the mesangial zone in one region and return to the circulation by way of another.

The role of various hemodynamic factors in the localization of immune complexes in human renal disease is unknown. However, certain clinical observations suggest an influence. For example, it has been shown in both human and experimental situations that renal artery stenosis protects the kidney in immune complex disease. Administration of angiotensin II has been shown to result in an increase in mesangial sequestration of macromolecules [40, 41].

Immune Complex Disease as a Cause of Chronic Glomerulonephritis

The repetitive administration of an antigen over a period of weeks to a rabbit ultimately leads to a spectrum of morphologic changes similar to those observed in various forms of chronic glomerulonephritis in humans. The early observations of Dixon et al and Germuth et al described above have led to many of our concepts regarding the pathogenesis of glomerulonephritis. The antibody response of the animal plays a role in the ultimate clinical and morphologic picture in that nonantibody producers or aggressive antibody producers had no or minimal disease, whereas rabbits producing small amounts of antibody and being maintained by repetitive antigen administration in antigen excess had more severe disease.

Although most of the models of experimental renal disease involve the administration of a foreign antigen, the immune complex disease occurring in female NZB/NZW mice (and in more recently described mouse strains) reflect the interaction of host antigens (for example, native DNA and so on) with antibody. The spectrum of immune complex lupus nephritis in these mice is typical of that observed in human lupus erythematosus. This fascinating disease has been studied extensively by a number of investigators, as reviewed by Steinberg et al at the National Institutes of Health, Bethesda, Maryland, USA [42].

Another model that has resulted in considerable controversy is one initially described by Heymann 25 years ago. The administration of a crude tubular antigen, termed Fx1A, to a rat leads to the evolution of membranous nephropathy over a period of weeks to months [43]. Although there was initial evidence supporting the role of circulating immune complexes in this process, more recent studies suggest that this disease is a consequence of in situ antigen-antibody interaction [44].

Interaction of Antibody with an In Situ Antigen

Intrinsic or Structural Antigens

The recognition that a circulating antibody can interact directly with the kidney was first recognized at the turn of this century (Table 4). Although

Table 4. Interaction of antibody with an in situ antigen

Intrinsic or structural antigen
  Basement membrane or matrix component
    Type IV collagen, laminin
      Antigen(s) involved in experimental anti-GBM nephritis or Steblay's nephritis
      Antigen(s) involved in human anti-GBM nephritis or Goodpasture syndrome
    Subepithelial antigen(s)—passive Heymann nephritis and possibly other forms of
      membranous nephropathy

Exogenous-planted antigen
  Aggregated IgG in mesangium
  Concanavalin A on endothelium
  Cationized antigen on negatively charged (heparan sulfate proteoglycan) sites
    in basement membrane
  Heterologous antibody on the basement membrane or in epimembranous deposits

---

intensively studied during the last 2 decades, the model is incompletely understood. Two phases in this disease are recognized. In the *heterologous* phase, anti-GBM antibody made in one animal is administered to an animal of a different species, and it promptly binds to the GBM. After a period of time, the *autologous* phase appears, in which the recipient animal develops antibody to the fixed heterologous IgG—compounding the initial injury.

A number of mechanisms lead to glomerular capillary injury resulting in proteinuria. Activation of complement has been recognized as playing a role in some models, although there is considerable variation depending on the animal used and the type of antibody employed. The complement-dependent injury is a consequence of polymorphonuclear leukocyte infiltration that is related to the generation of chemotactic substances such as C5a, since this injury is partly inhibited by complement depletion using cobra venom factor or by neutrophil depletion using nitrogen mustard. Recently, Groggel et al [45] have demonstrated a requirement of the terminal complement sequence for the mediation of proteinuria and decreased renal function in the heterologous phase of anti-GBM nephritis in the rabbit. This injury was independent of C3 deposition and leukocyte infiltration, and it was not observed in C6-deficient rabbits. Therefore, complement plays a role in at least two ways: (1) the generation of chemotactic substances leading to leukocyte infiltration, and (2) activation of the terminal complement sequence. The mechanism of injury induced by the latter process is unknown. Thus, complement-independent mechanisms are related to monocyte infiltration as described above, as well as to other mechanisms that have not been defined [46].

Monocytes have been recognized in diseased glomeruli by morphologic techniques in glomerular cultures during the autologous phase of anti-GBM nephritis [47]. In an accelerated model of anti-GBM nephritis in the rat, Schreiner et al [48] demonstrated that the proteinuria appearing during the initial 24 hr correlated with polymorphonuclear leukocyte infiltration, whereas the proteinuria that developed between 48 to 96 hr was associated with infiltration mononuclear cells; during both time periods, rat IgG was present on the GBM in this accelerated model.

In a passive model of the autologous phase of anti-GBM nephritis (produced by injection of a subnephritic dose of horse antirabbit GBM antibody into rabbits, followed 15 hr later by rabbit antihorse Ig), depletion of monocytes by antimacrophage serum strikingly diminished monocyte infiltration, proteinuria, and histologic injury [49]. It is likely that macrophage accumulation is dependent on immune adherence to the Fc portion of the IgG molecule [50]. There is also evidence for infiltration of cells resembling lymphocytes during the heterologous phase of anti-GBM nephritis [51].

The precise structural antigens against which anti-GBM antibodies are directed have not been defined. As described above, the GBM contains a number of defined antigens, including type IV collagen and laminin; and, it is probable that most anti-GBM antisera contain antibodies to these and to other known antigens, as well as to undefined components.

Administration of antilaminin antibody to rats fails to induce acute proteinuria despite fixation of the antibody to GBM and the development of glomerular alteration [52]. Low-grade proteinuria did develop after 2 weeks and was unassociated with deposition of autologous rat IgG. Studies in mice following the administration of antibody to laminin or type IV collagen revealed basement membrane changes and relatively low-grade proteinuria [53].

Steblay's Nephritis

A variant of this disease was described by Steblay [54] in 1962. He observed that sheep immunized with heterologous GBM in adjuvant developed a progressive, severe form of glomerulonephritis as a consequence of fixation of autologous IgG to the sheep's own basement membrane. This autoimmune disease probably reflects the breaking of tolerance induced by immunization with basement membrane antigens—some of which are similar and others dissimilar to antigens of the sheep—resulting in production of autoantibodies and severe anti-GBM nephritis. A Steblay antibody similar to that seen in human anti-GBM nephritis has recently been observed [55].

Human Anti-GBM Nephritis and Goodpasture Syndrome

The presence of circulating or bound antibody to GBM is the hallmark of human anti-GBM nephritis or, if associated with pulmonary hemorrhage, Goodpasture syndrome. The cause of this loss of tolerance to the antigen(s) is unknown. The disease especially occurs in young adults, presents a clinical picture of rapidly progressive glomerulonephritis, and often is severe, leading to renal failure. Recent studies by Wieslander et al [56] have demonstrated that the putative antigen is collagenase-resistant, has a molecular weight of 26,000 and may be located in the noncollagen region of type IV collagen. However, studies from our laboratory have demonstrated that various human anti-GBM antibodies react differently—some identify basement membrane antigens in the fetal kidney and others do not react at all (Fig. 3).

In certain patients receiving renal homografts for familial nephritis, anti-GBM nephritis has been observed in the transplanted kidney. The formation of antibodies in these patients after transplantation and the inability to detect the nephritogenic antigen in the patients' own kidney suggests that there may be a genetic deletion in this structural component.

Experimentally Induced Membranous Nephropathy

It has been recognized for some time that the infusion into rats of heterologous antibody to a proximal tubular brush border antigen (Fx1A) leads to the relatively rapid development of epimembranous deposits (passive Heymann's nephritis). Largely through the efforts of Couser et al [44, 57] as well as Van Damme et al [58], this disease has been shown to develop as a consequence of in situ interaction of heterologous antibody, with an antigen located in the glomerular capillary wall (Fig. 4a). Although no inflammatory cells partic-

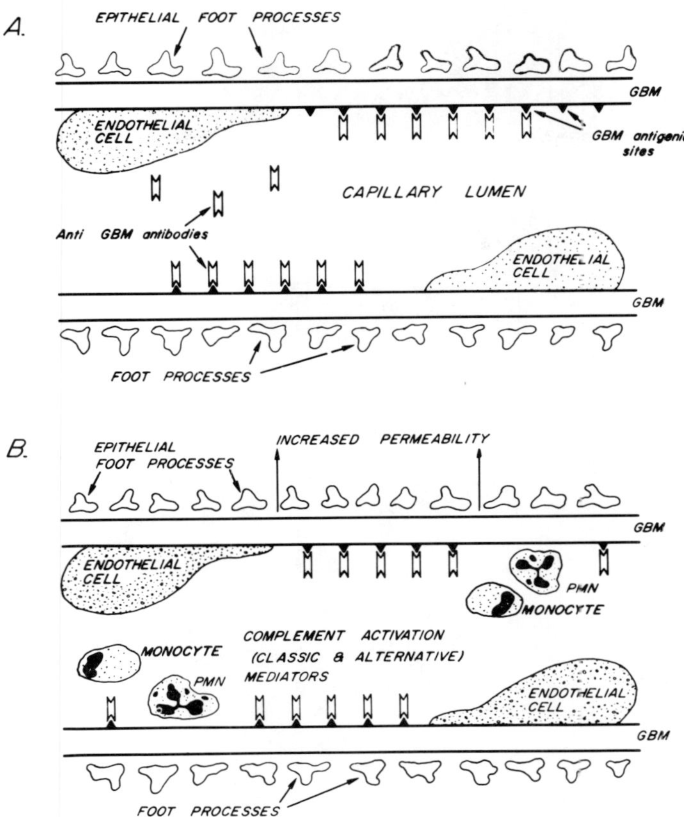

Fig. 3. In situ reactivity of antibody with antigen(s) located along the GBM in experimentally induced anti-GBM nephritis.

ipate in the injury leading to increased glomerular permeability to protein, a complement-dependent mechanism plays a role, since the proteinuria at 4 to 5 days is inhibited following complement depletion with cobra venom factor [59]. When sheep γ-2 antirat Fx1A IgG is administered to a rat, it becomes "planted" in the subepithelial region, where it is able to combine with passively administered or actively induced rat antisheep IgG; this results in proteinuria [60]. This latter injury also is cell-independent and complement-dependent. There is considerable evidence that the membranous nephropathy in active Heymann's nephritis (or autologous immune complex nephritis) represents a similar in situ mechanism, rather than reflecting the deposition of circulating immune complexes [44].

The nature of the glomerular antigen and the relationship to the tubular brushborder has been obscure. However, Kerjaschki and Farquhar [61] have isolated a large glycoprotein with a molecular weight of 330,000 (gp 330), and they have recently localized this antigen to coated pits on epithelial

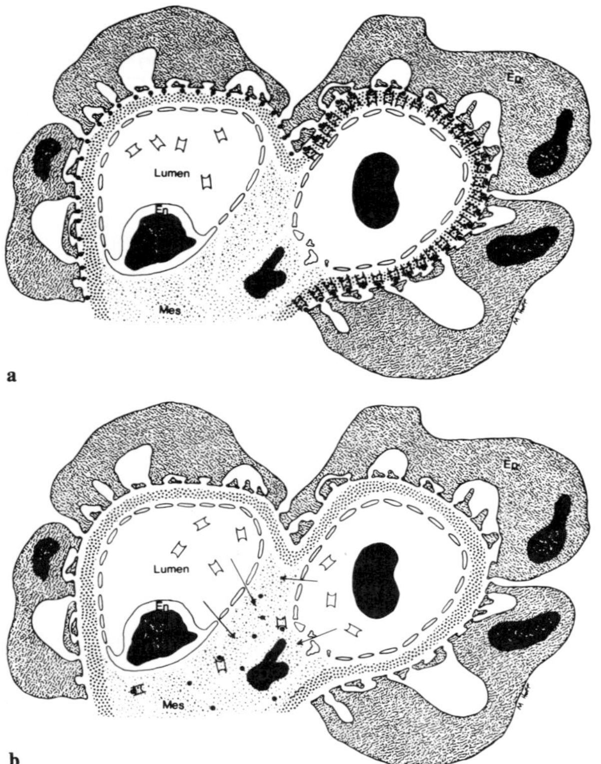

Fig. 4. Two illustrations of in situ antigen antibody interaction. In **a,** an antigen is located in the lamina rara externa adjacent to the foot processes. Antibody from the circulation fixes to the antigen, inducing membranous nephropathy. This mechanism is most likely responsible for the development of Heymann's nephritis. In **b,** an antigen either is a resident structural component of the mesangial matrix (indicated by *solid, dark spheres*) or has been "planted" in this region. In situ fixation occurs following administration or development of antibody.

cells. Maaker and Singh [62] have isolated a larger antigen (gp 600), and they suggest that gp 330 is a subunit of this molecule.

Exogenous-planted Antigens

Experimental studies have demonstrated that it is possible to plant an antigen in the glomerulus. Then, the subsequent interaction with an actively produced or passively administered antibody can be evaluated. Conceptually, this may be a potentially relevant mechanism in human disease, although there is no incontrovertible proof, at present, that it is operative in humans.

The demonstration of this process in experimental animals generally requires a contrived protocol. This is essential, since it is necessary to exclude the antigen from the circulation after planting it in the glomerulus to avoid formation of circulating immune complexes after passive administration or active formation of antibody.

In a model of acute mesangiitis, aggregated human IgG is administered to an animal (for example, rabbit or rat); following localization within the mesangium, the kidney is transplanted to another animal, and then rabbit antiserum to IgG is passively administered and binds to the antigen in the mesangium [63] (Fig. 4b). This results in acute mesangial injury with infiltration of polymorphonuclear leukocytes. When concanavalin A (Con A) is infused, it binds to endothelial surfaces; the subsequent administration of anti-Con A antiserum leads to in situ antigen-antibody interaction [64].

In the same vein, studies by Oite et al have demonstrated that renal perfusion of a cationized protein (ferritin or IgG) leads to binding to negatively charged sites in the capillary wall [38, 39]. The systemic passive administration of antibody or its active formation by the animal leads to glomerulonephritis as a consequence of in situ binding of antibody to the planted cationized antigen.

Cell-mediated Immunity (CMI)

As described above, humoral mechanisms (antibody mediated) have been shown to play a crucial role in the pathogenesis of various forms of glomerulonephritis. In earlier studies, there was little information regarding the relative importance of CMI in the development and progression of renal injury. It is accepted that T-cell regulatory mechanisms are necessary for immune responsiveness to certain antigens and to the ultimate development of antibody. What is at issue is whether cell-mediated mechanisms participate in the development of nephritis. Within the last 10 to 15 years, a number of observations have supported a role for cellular immunity in the development of renal disease [14, 65].

1. Monocytes have been demonstrated within diseased glomeruli of both experimental animals and patients by a number of investigators using standard light and electron microscopic techniques [3, 13, 49, 66].

2. The incisive experiments of Schreiner et al [48] and Hunsicker et al [23] have shown glomerular infiltration of monocytes, respectively, in an accelerated form of anti-GBM nephritis in rats and in acute serum sickness in rabbits. The infiltration was responsible for the development of proteinuria. This macrophage-dependent injury was abrogated by pretreatment with anti-macrophage serum [49].

3. Compelling evidence for CMI was derived from studies by Bhan et al [67, 68], who administered sensitized lymphocytes to rats with fixed heterologous anti-GBM antibody or immune complexes localized to the mesangium. This maneuver led to morphologic changes in both glomeruli and monocyte infiltration.

4. Cyclosporin A, which is thought to act on proliferating T cells, has

been shown by Neild et al [69] to inhibit glomerular injury in acute serum sickness in rabbits. Furthermore, in acute poststreptococcal glomerulonephritis, we have recently demonstrated the presence of small numbers of T cells as well as monocytes within glomeruli. The surface phenotype of these cells appear to distinguish tissue obtained early (OKT4 > OKT8) from late-obtained tissue (OKT8 > OKT4) in the course of the disease.

5. A number of studies have been carried out that evaluated the responsiveness of lymphoid cells in patients to GBM antigens by using assays measuring leukocyte migration inhibition and lymphocyte blastogenesis [65]. The antigens have included collagenase-digested GBM and tubular basement membrane (TBM), fetal kidney homogenates, trypsinized GBM, and glycosidase-treated membranes. These studies have demonstrated variable results in nephritic patients; in some instances, positive results in non-nephritic diseases have been demonstrated. The studies of Fillet et al [70] demonstrated responsiveness only to glycosidase-treated GBM in patients with proliferative glomerulonephritis. All of these studies may be criticized because of the impurity and recognized heterogeneity of the antigenic materials. In addition, there is no proof that the identified responses play a role in the development or progression of glomerulonephritis. Nevertheless, these observations are important, since they likely reflect systemic cellular autoimmune responses that develop as a consequence of glomerular injury.

6. The production of tubulointerstitial disease in mice, rats, and guinea pigs after immunization with xenogeneic TBM is characterized by the presence of anti-TBM antibodies and an interstitial mononuclear infiltrate. A review of the various model systems is beyond the scope of this chapter, but the reader is referred to other sources [14, 70–72]. Susceptibility to induction of the disease is linked to the major histocompatibility complex. The relative importance of antibodies versus CMI has been unclear, although both processes appear to be operative in the rat and guinea pig. In the mouse, Neilson et al have shown that the nephritis is not dependent on the generation of anti-TBM antibodies, but that susceptibility is largely a consequence of T-cell function linked to the major histocompatibility complex.

7. There is evidence and conjecture that CMI may be involved in the pathogenesis of idiopathic nephrotic syndrome. This syndrome, which occurs predominantly in young children, has not been associated with any of the hallmarks of a humoral (that is, antibody-mediated) immune process. However, a number of curious observations suggest participation of some cellular mechanism:

a. Recurrence or exacerbations are frequently associated with infections.
b. Prompt response to steroid therapy occurs in over 95% of the patients.
c. Alkylating agents, such as nitrogen mustard and cytoxan, also lead to remission of the syndrome. In addition, a short course of cytoxan has been shown to effect a prolonged remission in patients with frequent relapses.
d. The disorder may be associated with Hodgkin's disease. In addition, a similar syndrome also has been observed in acquired immune deficiency syndrome (AIDS) [73] and following the treatment of mycosis fungoides

with interferon [74]. We also have observed it after autologous bone marrow transplantation for leukemia.

e. Patients who are steroid-resistant and who develop progressive sclerosis with renal failure necessitating transplantation may develop recurrences of the disease in 20 to 30% of the instances.

A number of immunologic studies have been carried out on the lymphoid cells from these patients; however, no clear-cut consistent findings have been described that bear directly on altered glomerular permeability [75]. Some of the described immune abnormalities appear to be a consequence of the hyperlipidemia or are present in other forms of the nephrotic syndrome. Beale et al [76] have recently demonstrated increased immunoglobulin synthesis by mononuclear cells from patients with this syndrome, which suggests that these cells may be "turned on." In addition, a slight increase in glomerular lymphoid-monocytic cells has been observed in some patients with this syndrome, especially if mesangial proliferation is present [77].

Nonantibody-dependent Complement Activation

There is some suggestive evidence that nonantibody-dependent complement activation may play a role in some renal disease. Prior studies have suggested this possibility, primarily in diseases in which there is a dominant presence of complement components with minimal amounts of immunoglobulin (for example, dense deposit disease and some instances of acute glomerulonephritis). Recent studies have demonstrated the presence of the membrane attack complex of complement in the kidney in progressive renal disease of varied etiology—usually in extracellular matrices [78]. The mechanism and significance of these observations awaits further study and clarification.

Acknowledgments. This research was supported by grants AI10704, AM26149, and AM25518 from the National Institutes of Health and the Minnesota Vikings' Children's Fund.

References

1. FARQUHAR MG, PALADE GE: Functional evidence for the existence of a third cell type in renal glomerulus. *J Cell Biol* 13:55–87, 1962
2. LATTA H, MAUNSBACH AB, MADDEN SC: The centrolobular region of the renal glomerulus studied by electron microscopy. *J Ultrastruct Res* 4:455–472, 1960
3. MICHAEL AF, KEANE W, RAIJ L, VERNIER RL, MAUER SM: The glomerular mesangium (*editorial review*). *Kidney Int* 17:141–154, 1980
4. SCHREINER GF, KIELY JM, COTRAN R, UNANUE ER: Characterization of resident glomerular cell in the rat expressing Ia determinants and manifesting genetically restricted interactions with lymphocytes. *J Clin Invest* 68:920–931, 1981
5. MICHAEL AF, YANG J-Y, FALK RJ, BENNINGTON MJ, SCHEINMAN JI, VERNIER RL, FISH AJ: Monoclonal antibodies reactive with human kidney: Heterogeneity and ontogenic changes. *Kidney Int* 24:74–86, 1983
6. MICHAEL AF, FALK RJ, PLATT JL, MELVIN T, YANG J-Y: Antigens of the

human glomerulus, in *Advances in Nephrology,* Chicago, Year Book Medical Publishers, vol 13, 1983, pp 203–218

7. HOUSER M, SCHEINMAN JI, BASGEN J, STEFFES MW, MICHAEL AF: Preservation of mesangium and immunohistochemically-defined antigens in glomerular basement membrane isolated by detergent extraction. *J Clin Invest* 68:1169–1175, 1982

8. KANWAR YS, FARQUHAR MG: Presence of heparan sulfate in the basement membrane. *Proc Natl Acad Sci USA* 76:1303–1307, 1979

9. NEVINS TE, MICHAEL AF: Isolation of rat glomerular polyanion. *Kidney Int* 19:553–563, 1981

10. KERJASCHI D, SHARKEY DJ, FARQUHAR MG: Identification and characterization of Podocalyxin—The major sialoprotein of the renal glomerular epithelial cell. *J Cell Biol* 98:1591–1596, 1984

11. MELVIN T, KIM Y, MICHAEL AF: Selective binding of IgG_4 and other negatively-charged plasma proteins in normal and diabetic human kidneys. *Am J Pathol,* in press

12. WILSON CB, DIXON FJ: The renal response to immunologic injury, in *The Kidney,* edited by BRENNER BM, RECTOR FC, Philadelphia, W.B. Saunders & Co, 1981, p 1237

13. CAMERON JS: Glomerulonephritis: Current problems and understanding. *J Lab Clin Med* 99:755–787, 1982

14. MCCLUSKEY RT, BHAN AK: Cell-mediated mechanisms in renal diseases. *Kidney Int* 11:S6–S12, 1982

15. COUSER WG, SALANT D: In situ complex formation and glomerular injury. *Kidney Int* 17:1, 1980

16. DIXON FJ: The pathogenesis of glomerulonephritis. *Am J Med* 44:493–498, 1968

17. GLASSOCK RJ, COHEN AH, BENNETT CM, MARTINEZ-MALDONADO M: Primary glomerular diseases, in *The Kidney* (ed 2), edited by BRENNER BM, RECTOR FC, Philadelphia, W.B. Saunders & Co, 1981, pp 1351–1489

18. COCHRANE CG, KOFFLER D: Immune complex disease in experimental animals and man. *Adv Immunol* 16:185–264, 1973

19. WILSON CB: Nephritogenic antibody mechanisms involving antigens within the glomerulus. *Immunol Rev* 55:257–297, 1981

20. HAMMER DK, DIXON FJ: Experimental glomerulonephritis. II. Immunologic events in the pathogenesis of nephrotoxic serum nephritis in the rat. *J Exp Med* 117:1019–1034, 1963

21. DIXON FJ, FELDMAN JD, VASQUEZ JJ: Experimental glomerulonephritis. The pathogenesis of a laboratory model resembling the spectrum of human glomerulonephritis. *J Exp Med* 113:899–919, 1961

22. GERMUTH FG: A comparative histologic and immunologic study in rabbits of induced hypersensitivity of the serum sickness type (*abstract*). *J Exp Med* 97:275, 1953

23. HUNSICKER L, SHEARER T, PLATTNER SB, WEISENBERER D: The role of monocytes in serum sickness nephritis. *J Exp Med* 150:413–425, 1979

24. GERMUTH FG, RODRIGUEZ E: *Immunopathology of the Renal Glomerulus.* Boston, Little Brown & Co, 1973, pp 15–43

25. GERMUTH FG, SENTERFIT LB, DREESMAN GR: Immune complex disease: V. The nature of the circulating complexes associated with glomerular alterations in the chronic BSA-rabbit system. *Johns Hopkins Med J* 130:344–357, 1972

26. GERMUTH FG, RODRIGUEZ E, SIDDIQUI SY, LORELLE CA, MCGEE S, MILANO LL, WISE OL: Immune complex disease: VII. Experimental mesangiopathic glo-

merulonephritis produced by chronic immunization with thyroglobulin. *Lab Invest* 38:404–408, 1978

27. KOYAMA A, NIWA Y, SHIGEMATSU H, TANINGUCHI M, TADA T: Studies on passive serum sickness: II. Factors determining the localization of antigen-antibody complexes in the murine renal glomerulus. *Lab Invest* 38:253–262, 1978

28. KURIYAMA T: Chronic glomerulonephritis induced by prolonged immunization in rabbits. *Lab Invest* 28:224–235, 1973

29. FRIEND P, DONADIO J, KIM Y, MICHAEL AF: Pathogenesis of membranous nephropathy in systemic lupus erythematosus: Possible role of nonprecipitating DNA antibody. *Br Med J* 1:25–27, 1977

30. OOI YM, OOI BS, POLLAK VE: Relationship of levels of circulating immune complexes to histologic patterns of nephritis: A comparative study of membranous glomerulonephropathy and diffuse proliferative glomerulonephritis. *J Lab Clin Med* 90:891–898, 1977

31. ISKANDER SS, JENNETTE JC: Influence of antibody avidity on glomerular immune complex localization. *Am J Pathol* 112:115–159, 1983

32. FINBLOOM DS, MAGILAVY DB, HARFORD JB, RIFAI A, PLATZ PH: Influence of antigen on immune complex behavior in mice. *J Clin Invest* 68:214–224, 1981

33. HAAKENSTAD AO, STRIKER GE, MANNIK M: The glomerular deposition of soluble immune complexes prepared with reduced and alklyated antibodies and with intact antibodies in mice. *Lab Invest* 35:293–301, 1976

34. GALLO GR, CAULIN-GLASER T, LAMM ME: Charge of circulating immune complexes as a factor in glomerular basement membrane localization in mice. *J Clin Invest* 67:1305–1313, 1981

35. GALLO GR, CALIN-GLASER T, EMANCEPATOR SN, LAMM ME: Nephritogenicity and differential distribution of glomerular immune complexes related to immunogen charge. *Lab Invest* 48:353–362, 1983

36. BORDER WA, WARD HJ, KAMIE ES, COHEN AH: Induction of membranous nephropathy in rabbits by administration of an exogenous cationic antigen. *J Clin Invest* 69:451–461, 1982

37. GROGGEL GC, ADLER S, RENNKE HG, COUSER WG, SALANT DJ: Role of terminal complement pathway in experimental membranous nephropathy in rabbits. *J Clin Invest* 72:1948–1957, 1983

38. OITE T, BATSFORD SR, MIHATSCH MJ, TAKAMIYA MH, VOGT A: Quantitative studies of in situ immune complex glomerulonephritis in the rat induced by planted cationized antigen. *J Exp Med* 155:460–474, 1982

39. OITE T, SHIMIZU F, KIHARA I, BATSFORD SR, VOGT A: An active model of immune complex glomerulonephritis in the rat employing cationized antigen. *Am J Pathol* 112:185, 1983

40. KEANE W, RAIJ L: Angiotensin II modifies mesangial afferent and efferent limb (*abstract*). *Kidney Int* 23:184, 1983

41. STEIN HD, FEDDERGREN W, KASHGARIAN M, STERZEL RB: Role of angiotensin II—induced renal functional changes in mesangial deposition of exogenous ferritin in mesangial deposition of exogenous ferritin in rats. *Lab Invest* 49:270–280, 1983

42. STEINBERG A, RAVECHE EA, LASKIN CA, SMITH HR, SANTORO T, MILLER ML, PLATZ PH: Systemic lupus erythematosus: Insights from animal models. *Ann Int Med* 100:714, 1984

43. EDGINGTON TS, GLASSOCK RJ, DIXON FJ: Autologous immune complex nephritis induced with renal tubular antigens. I. Identification and isolation of the pathogenetic antigen. *J Exp Med* 12:555–572, 1968

44. MADAIO MP, SALANT DJ, COHEN AJ, ADLER S, COUSER WG: Comparative study of in situ immune deposit formation in active and passive Heymann's nephritis. *Kidney Int* 23:498–505, 1983
45. GROGGEL GC, SALANT DJ, DARBY C, RENNKE HA, COUSER WG: Role of terminal complement pathway in the heterologous phase of anti-glomerular basement membrane nephritis in the rabbit (*abstract*). *Kidney Int* 25:212, 1984
46. PILIA PA, BOACKLE RJ, SWAIN RP, AINSWORTH SR: Complement-independent nephrotoxic serum nephritis in Munich Wistar rats. *Lab Invest* 48:585–597, 1983
47. HOLDSWORTH SR, THOMPSON SN, GLASGOW JR, DOWLING JR, ATKINS RC: Tissue culture of isolated glomeruli in experimental crescentric glomerulonephritis. *J Exp Med* 147:98–109, 1978
48. SCHREINER GF, COTRAN R, PARDO V, UNANUE ER: A mononuclear component in experimental immunologic glomerulonephritis. *J Exp Med* 147:39–384, 1978
49. HOLDSWORTH SR, NEALE TJ, WILSON CB: Abrogation of macrophage-dependent injury in experimental glomerulonephritis in the rabbit. *J Clin Invest* 68:686–697, 1981
50. HOLDSWORTH SR: Fc dependence of macrophage accumulation and subsequent injury in experimental glomerulonephritis. *J Immunol* 130:735–739, 1983
51. KREISBERG JI, WAYNE DB, KARNOVSKY MJ: Rapid and focal loss of negative charge associated with mononuclear cell infiltration early in nephrotoxic serum nephritis. *Kidney Int* 16:290–300, 1979
52. ABRAHAMSON DR, CAULFIELD JP: Proteinuria and structural alteration in rat glomerular basement membranes induced by intravenously injected antilaminin immunoglobulin G. *J Exp Med* 156:128, 1982
53. YAAR M, FOIDART JM, BROWN KS, RENNARD SL, MARTIN GR, LIOTTA L: The Goodpasture-like syndrome in mice induced by intravenous injections of anti-type IV collagen and anti-laminin antibody. *Am J Pathol* 107:79–91, 1982
54. STEBLAY RW: Glomerulonephritis induced in sheep by injections of heterologous glomerular basement membrane and Freund's adjuvant. *J Exp Med* 116:253–272, 1962
55. JERAJ K, MICHAEL AF, FISH AJ: Immunologic similarities between Goodpasture's and Stabley's antibodies. *Clin Immunol Immunopathol* 23:408–413, 1982
56. WEISLANDER J, BYGREN P, HEINEGARD D: Isolation of the specific glomerular basement membrane antigen involved in Goodpasture's syndrome. *Proc Natl Acad Sci USA* 81:1544–1548, 1984
57. COUSER WG, STEINMULLER DR, STILMANT M, SALANT DJ, LOWENSTEIN LM: Experimental glomerulonephritis in the isolated perfused rat kidney. *J Clin Invest* 62:1275–1287, 1978
58. VAN DAMME BJC, FLEUREN CJ, BAKKER W, VERNIER RL, HOEDEMAEKER PJ: Experimental glomerulonephritis in the rat induced by antibodies directed against tubular antigens. V. Fixed glomerular antigens in the pathogenesis of heterologous immune complex glomerulonephritis. *Lab Invest* 38:502–510, 1978
59. SALANT DJ, BELOK S, MADAIO MP, COUSER WG: A new role for complement in experimental membranous nephropathy in rats. *J Clin Invest* 66:1339–1350, 1980
60. ADLER S, SALANT DJ, DITTMAN JE, RENNKE HG, MADAIO MP, COUSER WG: Mediation of proteinuria in membranous nephropathy due to planted glomerular antigen. *Kidney Int* 23:807–815, 1983
61. KERJASCHKE D, FARQUHAR M: The pathogenetic antigen of Heymann nephritis is a membrane glycoprotein of the renal proximal tubular brush border. *Proc Natl Acad Sci USA* 79:5557–5561, 1982

62. MAAKER SP, SINGH AK: Characterization of the antigen (gp 600) of Heymann nephritis. *Lab Invest* 50:287–293, 1984
63. MAUER SM, SUTHERLAND DER, HOWARD R, FISH AJ, NAJARIAN JS, MICHAEL AF: The glomerular mesangium. III. Acute immune mesangial injury: A new model of glomerulonephritis. *J Exp Med* 137:533–570, 1973
64. GOLBUS S, WILSON CB: Experimental glomerulonephritis induced by in situ formation of immune complexes in glomerular capillary wall (*abstract*). *Kidney Int* 16:148, 1979
65. FILLIT HM, ZABRISKIE JB: Cellular immunity in glomerulonephritis. *Am J Pathol* 109:227–243, 1982
66. ATKINS RC, HOLDSWORTH SR, HANCOCK WW, THOMSON NM, GLASGOW EF: Cellular immune mechanisms in human glomerulonephritis. The role of mononuclear leukocytes. *Springer Sem Immunopathol* 5:269–296, 1982
67. BHAN AK, COLLINS AB, SCHNEEBERGER EE, MCCLUSKEY RT: Evidence for a pathogenic role of a cell mediated immune mechanism in experimental glomerulonephritis. *J Exp Med* 148:246–260, 1978
68. BHAN AK, COLLINS AB, SCHNEEBERGER EE, MCCLUSKEY RT: A cell mediated reaction against glomerular bound immune complexes. *J Exp Med* 150:1410–1420, 1979
69. NEILD GH, IVORY K, HIRAMATSU M, GWYN WILLIAMS D: Cyclosporin A inhibits acute serum sickness in rabbits. *Clin Exp Immunol* 52:586–594, 1983
70. FILLIT HM, READ SE, SHERMAN RL, ZABRISKIE JB, VANDE RIJN I: Cellular reactivity to altered glomerular basement membrane in glomerulonephritis. *N Engl J Med* 298:235–242, 1975
71. NEILSON EG, ZAKHEIM B: T cell regulation, antiidiotypic immunity and the nephritogenic immune response. *Kidney Int* 24:289–302, 1983
72. MAMPASO FM, WILSON CB: Characterization of inflammatory cells in autoimmune tubulointerstitial nephritis in rats. *Kidney Int* 23:448–457, 1983
73. RAO TKS, FILIPPONE EJ, NICASTRI AD, LANDESMAN SH, FRANK E, CHER CK, FRIEDMAN EA: Associated focal and segmental glomerulosclerosis in the acquired immunodeficiency syndrome. *N Engl J Med* 310:669–673, 1984
74. AVERBUCH SD, AUSTIN HA, SHERWIN SA, AUTONOVYCH T, BUNN PA, LONGO DL: Acute interstitial nephritis with nephrotic syndrome following recombinant leukocyte A interferon therapy for mycosis fungoides. *N Engl J Med* 310:32–34, 1984
75. MELVIN T, SIBLEY R, MICHAEL AF: Nephrotic syndrome, in *Contemporary Issues in Nephrology*, New York, Churchill Livingstone, Inc, 1984, pp 191–230
76. BEALE MG, NASH GS, BERTOVICH MJ, MACDERMOTT RP: Immunoglobulin synthesis by peripheral blood mononuclear cells in minimal change nephrotic syndrome. *Kidney Int* 23:380–386, 1983
77. NAGATA K, PLATT JL, MICHAEL AF: Interstitial and glomerular immune cell populations in idiopathic nephrotic syndrome. *Kidney Int* 25:88–93, 1984
78. FALK RJ, DALMASSO AP, KIM Y, TSAI CH, SCHEINMAN JI, GEWURZ H, MICHAEL AF: A neoantigen of the polymerized ninth component of complement: Characterization of a monoclonal activity and immunohistochemical localization in renal disease. *J Clin Invest* 72:560–573, 1983

Cellular and Humoral Mediators of Renal Injury

Chairpersons: D. Keith Peters and Curtis B. Wilson
Discussants: David J. Salant, Roland C. Blantz, Robert C. Atkins,
Kym M. Bannister, Andrew J. Rees, George F. Schreiner,
R. Bernd Sterzl, Michael J. Dunn, Raymond Ardaillou,
and Roger C. Wiggins

Humoral and cellular mediators of inflammation cause both acute and progressive glomerular and tubular injury and overlap the various mechanisms of (usually immunologic) induction. Understanding the mediation pathways offers the opportunity of therapeutic manipulation without the necessity for completely identifying the immunopathogenetic mechanisms.

Salant reported a new role for complement (C) in glomerular injury. Based on classical studies of the Arthus reaction and heterologous anti-GBM nephritis, complement-mediated glomerular injury has been traditionally regarded as being cell-dependent. Observations in the passive Heymann nephritis model of rat membranous nephropathy demonstrated the role of complement in the pathogenesis of glomerular injury. Proteinuria was unaffected by depleting rats of inflammatory cells, whereas complement depletion with cobra venom factor (CVF) abrogated its development. The need for terminal C components in such complement-mediated injury was examined in membranous nephropathy induced in rabbits by immunization with cationized bovine serum albumin (BSA). C6-deficient rabbits showed no proteinuria, whereas 75% of control C6-sufficient animals developed heavy proteinuria. These observations, together with the recent findings of the membrane attack complex (MAC) and poly C9, suggest that the MAC may have a pathogenic role in glomerular disease.

Blantz studied the role of C in inducing alterations in glomerular hemodynamics. Complement depletion with CVF was found to eliminate renal vasoconstriction and to ameliorate the reductions in glomerular ultrafiltration coefficient (LpA) that follow the acute administration of large doses of anti-glomerular basement membrane (GBM) antibody. The decrease in LpA correlated with the elimination of polymorphonuclear leukocytes from the glomerular capillaries. Recent studies indicated that leukocyte depletion in the presence of a normal complement system also prevents the anti-GBM-induced

This manuscript is the summary of a Workshop entitled *Cellular and Humoral Mediators of Renal Injury.*

reductions in LpA. These observations were extended by examining the acute effects of an intrarenal arterial infusion of the anaphylotoxin C5a (1.25 μg/min $\times$ 12 min) on glomerular hemodynamics. Nephron filtration rate (SNGFR) was unchanged, but nephron plasma flow decreased from 225 $\pm$ 18 to 182 $\pm$ 11 nl/min. SNGFR was maintained by increases in glomerular capillary hydrostatic pressure ($\overline{P}_{GC}$) from 51 to 56 mm Hg and the hydrostatic pressure gradient ($\Delta\overline{P}$). C5a was shown to exert an effect on glomerular hemodynamics in the absence of immune injury. These experiments reproduce two of the major findings characteristic of an infusion of anti-GBM antibody: decreased nephron plasma flow and increased $\overline{P}_{GC}$ and $\Delta\overline{P}$.

Atkins reported the characterization of glomerular and tubulointerstitial infiltrating cells using monoclonal antibodies in human glomerulonephritis. Macrophages and neutrophils dominate in postinfectious, lupus, and crescentic nephritis. No T cells were identified. An association was noted between macrophages and fibrin deposition, which was further correlated with the presence of macrophage-related tissue factor or procoagulant activity. In contrast to the glomerular lesions, T cells were the predominant infiltrating cells in the interstitium of all of the glomerulonephritides studied. These studies raise the possibility that glomerular fibrin deposition may be directly mediated by macrophage activity under some circumstances.

Bannister and Wilson described a new model of tubulointerstitial nephritis (TIN) which allows the dissection of the cells responsible for a cell-mediated form of renal injury. TIN in humans was characterized by an extensive mononuclear cell infiltration, which included T cells that were usually without antibody fixation. Models of experimental TIN mediated by anti-TBM antibody are established in rats, mice, and guinea pigs, and are also characterized by mononuclear cell infiltrates. In the rats, such infiltrates contain T cell subsets, and although direct transfers of lymphoid cells have produced mild or no lesions, there is in vitro evidence of sensitized cells in some of the models. The Lewis (Lew) rat lacks the TBM antigen reacting with anti-TBM antibody in this model. Immunization with the homologous TBM antigen thus gives rise to sensitization and production of a circulating antibody that cannot react with the target antigen. In this model, a distinctive nodular TIN resulted, in which no fixation of anti-TBM were identified. Adoptive transfer of lymphoid cells to normal Lew rats reproduced lesions that were characterized by predominantly T-helper cells, a few T-suppressor cells, and a majority of Ia-positive cells. A transfer of serum caused the disease in the TBM antigen-positive BN strain, but not in Lew rats. Thus, this model of TIN allows dissection of T cell subsets responsible for a form of cell-mediated renal injury.

Rees reported that low doses of lipopolysaccharide (LPS) augmented proteinuria and diminished renal function in the heterologous phase of anti-GBM antibody-induced glomerulonephritis in rabbits. Higher doses of the LPS preparation induced a cortical necrosis when administered with the anti-GBM antibody. The augmentation by LPS may have bearing on infection factors previously found to worsen anti-GBM antibody-induced injury in humans.

To evaluate the potential effects of humoral and cellular immune mediators on the biology of mesangial cells, Schreiner investigated the modulation of angiotensin II (AII) receptors of mesangial cells isolated from animals with acute nephrotoxic nephritis. Loss of up to 50% of AII receptors was found, peaking at 16 hr and returning to normal by 48 hr. This was not prevented by complement depletion with CVF, which itself was found to induce a similar effect. In vitro, the reaction was clearly dependent on complement activation. The return to normal at 48 hr of AII receptors in nephrotoxic nephritis was not observed in experiments where monocyte infiltration was prevented, for example, by total body irradiation. The mechanisms relating monocyte infiltration to expression of mesangial AII receptors is not known.

Sterzl reported that macrophages located in glomeruli may contribute to enhanced proliferation of glomerular cells. He studied the effects of conditioned media from LPS-activated rat peritoneal macrophages on growth kinetics of cultured mesangial cells obtained from collagenase-treated isolated rat glomeruli. Conditioned media markedly increased mesangial cell growth measured by tritiated thymidine uptake. The mitogenic factor in conditioned media copurified with interleukin-I activity was similar by the several characteristics that were studied. These findings identify a mechanism by which macrophages in combination with platelet factors may cause mesangial cells to proliferate.

Dunn reported studies of glomerular arachidonic acid metabolism in nephrotoxic serum nephritis in the rat. Isolated rat glomeruli were shown to have the capacity to convert arachidonic acids to biologically active products of both the cyclooxygenase and lipoxygenase pathways. These two pathways were studied before and after the induction of nephrotoxic serum nephritis. Within 2 to 3 hr, thromboxane A2 was increased. The use of two distinct inhibitors, OKY1581 and UK38485, prevented thromboxane A2 production and simultaneously abrogated the effect of nephrotoxic serum on GFR and renal plasma flow. On day 14, increased synthesis of thromboxane was not accompanied by hemodynamic changes. This was shown to be due to an accompanying and striking increase in PGE_2 production: inhibition of PGE_2 by indomethacin at this stage led to a greater than 50% fall in GFR and renal plasma flow. It was concluded that glomerular cyclooxygenase and lipoxygenase pathways therefore exert important inflammatory hemodynamic and pathophysiologic actions in immune glomerular injury. Compensatory increases in glomerular PGE_2 maintained the GFR and the renal plasma flow, and the use of nonsteroidal antiinflammatory drugs may therefore reduce renal function under these circumstances.

To study the accumulation of macrophages in Bowman space, Ardaillou examined the binding of labeled macrophages to isolated glomeruli. Inhibition studies suggested that macrophage adherence was dependent on glomerular lipoxygenase activity, but not glomerular cyclooxygenase activity. Glomeruli interacted with macrophages in converting arachidonic acid to prostaglandins since the generation of 6-keto $PGF_{1\alpha}$, TXB_2, and PGD_2 by glomeruli and macrophages incubated in combination was greater than the sum of their production by either glomeruli or macrophages alone. Pretreatment of macrophages with aspirin abolished the production of prostaglandins. Reduction of prostaglandins and of 12-HETE by macrophages was stimulated by a lipid extract of glomeruli containing the oxygenated metabolites of arachidonic acid. Stimulation of macrophages by glomeruli was blunted by pretreatment of glomeruli with nordihydroguaiaretic acid. These data suggest that macrophage attachment to glomeruli and macrophage stimulation in the presence of glomeruli depend on glomerular lipoxygenase activity.

Wiggins addressed the role of oxygen preradicals in acute glomerular injury against the background of their studies in which antioxidant enzymes were shown to inhibit tissue injury. In the heterologous phase of nephrotoxic nephritis in rats (a complement- and polymorph-dependent injury), proteinuria was reduced by the administration of catalase, which inhibits H_2O_2-dependent injury, but not by treatment with superoxide dismutase or dimethylsulphoxide. By morphologic criteria, catalase reduced endothelial cell injury but it had no effect on neutrofil accumulation. The effects of oxidants on enzyme interactions, and particularly on inhibitors of proteases such as elastase, were postulated as being one mechanism by which tissue injury could be brought about.

Mechanisms of Immune Complex Formation and Deposition in Glomeruli

William G. Couser, Stephen Adler, Patricia J. Baker,
Richard J. Johnson, and Diana A. Perkinson

Immunologic mechanisms have been suspected to cause glomerulonephritis since the observations of Schick and Van Pirquet in the early 1900s [1, 2]. The nature of these mechanisms was substantially clarified with the advent of immunofluorescence (IF) microscopy as a diagnostic tool in human renal disease in the 1950s. This technique quickly revealed that the histologic changes characteristic of many forms of glomerulonephritis were associated with widespread deposits of immunoglobulin and complement in glomerular capillaries, usually in a discontinuous or a granular pattern [3, 4]. The pioneering studies of Germuth and Dixon in the late 1950s and early 1960s provided experimental evidence that these deposits represented antigen-antibody containing immune complexes (ICs). Their studies, done in acute and chronic serum sickness models in rabbits induced by bovine serum albumin (BSA), demonstrated that immunization with a foreign serum protein (after a latent period) led to the appearance of circulating, soluble ICs of the protein antigen and antibody to it, that glomerular IC deposits appeared coincident with the presence of circulating ICs, that deposits in glomeruli contained the same antigen and antibody present in the circulating ICs, and that the histologic and immunopathologic features of the glomerular lesions produced closely resembled those seen in several human glomerular diseases [5–7]. Since neither antigen nor antibody could be demonstrated by IF techniques to localize alone in glomeruli, it was concluded that the deposits originated exclusively from the passive trapping of preformed ICs from the circulation. The site and quantity of IC deposits in glomeruli were noted to vary with the ratio of antigen to antibody in the circulation and therefore were presumed to reflect primarily differences in the size of the circulating ICs formed with consequent differences in their site of glomerular localization [5–7].

Since that time, a large amount of work has been done to define

---

This manuscript was presented as part of a Symposium by the same title.

the determinants that affect circulating IC trapping in glomeruli. In another presentation in this section, Mannik will review recent studies related to factors that regulate the glomerular localization of circulating ICs.

After about two decades during which the pathogenesis of IC glomerulonephritis was believed to be reasonably well understood, a resurgence of research activity in this area began in the late 1970s and 1980s and continues today. The primary stimulus for this renewed interest came from observations made in the so-called Heymann nephritis models of membranous nephropathy in rats, a lesion characterized by diffuse subepithelial deposits of IgG and C3 in a granular pattern indistinguishable from membranous nephropathy in humans. This model was long considered a prototype of glomerular disease, produced by the passive trapping of small lattice preformed ICs containing a circulating tubular brushborder antigen and antibody to it [8, 9]. However, in 1978, studies by Hoedemaeker and his colleagues in the Netherlands and others from our laboratory in Boston demonstrated that this same pattern of glomerular immune deposits could be produced by free antibody reacting directly with a fixed glomerular antigen—an antigen apparently produced locally by glomerular epithelial cells [10, 11]. This is situ mechanism of glomerular IC formation was not a new concept; it had been previously demonstrated to occur within the glomerular mesangium [12] and to be operative in the well-studied autologous phase of nephrotoxic anti-GBM nephritis [13]. However, the recognition that a prototypic IC lesion similar to that in the chronic BSA serum sickness models could be produced by ICs forming locally rather than being trapped from the circulation prompted an extensive reexamination of how glomerular IC deposits form in all other circumstances. These recent studies have revealed several new mechanisms by which IC deposits may form in glomeruli. It is now apparent that in situ IC formation occurs not only with insoluble-fixed glomerular antigens as in the Heymann and anti-GBM models but also with a variety of soluble endogenous and exogenous nonrenal antigens that first become localized in free form, or "planted," in the glomerulus to initiate IC formation. Antibody may also localize independently and then bind antigen in situ. It is further clear that different mechanisms of deposit formation predominate at different sites in the glomerulus, and that the mediators of tissue injury activated and the resulting histologic and functional glomerular lesions produced depend in large part on the site and mechanism of deposit formation as well as on the nature of the specific reactants involved.

What follows is a simplified overview of the currently established mechanisms by which renal antigens, nonrenal antigens, and preformed ICs contribute to glomerular immune deposit formation at subepithelial, subendothelial, and mesangial sites and what is currently known of the mediation of glomerular injury as a result of IC deposit formation at each of these sites. Mechanisms related to conventional GBM antigens and anti-GBM antibody disease are not discussed.

Mechanisms of Glomerular Immune Deposit Formation

Subepithelial Deposits

Fixed Glomerular Antigens

The classical subepithelial fixed glomerular antigen is the Heymann antigen, which was first demonstrated by perfusing the IgG fraction of antibody to a crude proximal tubular brushborder fraction (Fx1A) into rat kidneys to produce the typical subepithelial deposits that occur over a longer period of time when rats are actively immunized with Fx1A [10, 11]. Subsequent work has identified the responsible antigen as a glycoprotein product of glomerular epithelial cells, where it has been reported in endoplasmic reticulum, Golgi elements, and in coated pits along the epithelial cell surface [14, 15]. Thus, immune deposit formation occurs when free antibody reacts with antigen along the basal surface of the epithelial cell, a process similar to that by which tubular basement membrane deposits develop in the ascending limb of Henle's loop with antibody to Tamm-Horsfall protein [16]. Deposit formation by this mechanism is reduced when glomerular permeability is increased by administration of aminonucleoside of puromycin or anti-GBM antibody, which reduce glomerular net negative charge [17–19], but not by adriamycin, which causes proteinuria primarily by altering the size-selective portions of the filter [20]. The reasons for these differential effects on the fixed epithelial antigen mechanism are unclear.

The marked change in glomerular permeability resulting from this process is dependent on complement fixation but not on effector cells, and is probably a terminal complement mechanism involving the membrane attack complex [21, 22]. Transplant studies in rats suggest that an antigen similar to the Heymann antigen may exhibit allospecificity independent of major histocompatibility system differences [23]. Another apparently different but obviously related antigen has been localized in a discontinuous distribution along the epithelial cell foot processes of rabbits by Neale and Wilson and is apparently involved in the development of a spontaneous nephropathy associated with proteinuria in that species [24]. A related but apparently distinct antigen has been reported to cause development of subepithelial deposits in mice injected with antibody to a pronase-digested fraction of mouse Fx1A [25].

Although no antibody reactive with intrinsic glomerular antigens has yet been identified in diseases associated with subepithelial deposits in humans, the rapid increase in understanding of glomerular structural components resulting from biochemical analyses and monoclonal antibody technology makes it highly likely that similarly distributed antigenic epitopes will be identified. The probability of such antigens gives increasing credibility to the hypothesis that subepithelial immune deposits in diseases such as idiopathic membranous nephropathy may form by antibody binding to a fixed glomerular antigen as they do in the Heymann models [26]. For example, some of the etiologic factors to be discussed by Hoedemaeker elsewhere in this volume lead to auto-antibody production with an associated membranous glomerular lesion.

Subepithelial Immune Deposit Formation Caused by Planted Nonrenal Antigens

It is now well established that the glomerular subepithelial deposits character-istic of membranous nephropathy can also be induced by the reaction of free antibody with a variety of nonrenal antigens that localize in free form in a subepithelial distribution. The major mechanism for antigen localization at this site appears to be an electrostatic interaction between charged proteins and oppositely charged sites in the glomerulus. The reasons for charge interac-tions to predominate at a subepithelial site probably reflect the density of negative charges along the subepithelial surface of the capillary wall conferred by the sialoprotein surface of the epithelial cell foot processes and slit dia-phragms and the negatively charged heparan sulfate containing glycosamino-glycans in the lamina rara externa of the capillary wall. Possible increases in capillary permeability that may precede immune deposit formation [27], and the forces of filtration that transport smaller molecules across the capillary wall where they may be restricted and concentrated in areas beneath the slit pore diaphragms undoubtedly also influence the site and pattern of deposits formed [28]. Both endogenous and exogenous nonrenal antigens have been implicated in this process. Moreover, deposit formation at this site may also be initiated by prior localization of antibodies rather than antigens, which will be discussed later. Subepithelial deposits induced by planted nonrenal antigens also cause proteinuria by a complement-dependent, cell-independent mechanism probably involving terminal complement components [22, 29].

Subepithelial Deposits Induced by Cationic Nonglomerular Antigens

Following recognition that subepithelial deposits in the Heymann models formed on an in situ basis, and a review of the literature noting that subepithe-lial deposits had not been demonstrated in numerous studies of the glomerular localization of infused preformed ICs, it was predicted that the subepithelial deposits caused by exogenous antigens probably also form locally, perhaps by antigen localization on a charge basis [30]. This hypothesis has now been verified by a number of different laboratories. Fleuren, Grond, and Hoede-maeker first demonstrated in situ subepithelial immune deposit formation with an exogenous antigen using an alternate perfusion system to show that subepithelial deposits of native BSA and anti-BSA could form locally [31]. Border et al subsequently used a model of chronic serum sickness induced with cationized BSA to show that antigens of appropriate positive charge could localize directly in the glomerulus and that deposit formation in the subepithelial space induced by cationic BSA was dependent on antigen charge rather than on antibody response, antigen-antibody ratio, or circulating IC size as had been concluded from the earlier serum sickness studies [32]. The current status of charge-charge interactions between the glomerulus and pathogenic antigens and antibodies is reviewed more extensively by Border elsewhere in this section. Numerous other investigators have also produced subepithelial deposits in situ using a variety of antigens with mol wts usually in excess of 100,000 daltons and chemically modified to achieve isoelectric points of over 8.5 [33]. These have included BSA, IgG, horse spleen ferritin, and others (reviewed in [34]). Native cationic molecules such as lysozyme and avidin have also been shown to exhibit this capacity [31, 35]. For these antigens to persist at a subepithelial site and form electron-dense deposits, they must be complexed with specific antibody [34, 36]. Moreover, they must be composed of multivalent antigens capable of rearrangement to form immune precipitates so that a lattice structure large enough to be visible by conventional transmission electron microscopy is achieved [36, 37].

For lower molecular weight antigens such as lysozyme or BSA, it is probable that subepithelial localization occurs directly. However, with larger antigen molecules, or large lattice ICs that cannot penetrate the capillary wall, Vogt et al have provided evidence that ICs may first be formed or trapped at a subendothelial site and then dissociated into smaller ICs or free antigen and antibody to reform in situ in a subepithelial distribution [33].

The role of such highly cationized antigens in the pathogenesis of subepithelial immune deposit disease in humans remains speculative. The finding of deposits confined entirely to the subepithelial space as seen in idiopathic membranous nephropathy is more consistent with the presence of an auto-antibody to a fixed glomerular antigen, perhaps induced by mechanisms analogous to those discussed by Hoedemaeker. When deposits are present at mesangial and subendothelial sites as well as in the subepithelial space, as in poststreptococcal glomerulonephritis, type I MPGN, and lupus nephritis, a nonrenal antigen mechanism seems more probable. Recently, Vogt et al have used the antibodies to several cationic extracellular protein antigens produced by streptococci and found such antigens localized in immune deposits in early poststreptococcal glomerulonephritis in 8 of 18 patients studied [38]. Endostreptosin is a streptococcal cytoplasmic antigen with a mol wt of about 43,000 daltons which is also cationic and has also been identified in early biopsy examinations of patients with poststreptococcal glomerulonephritis, although usually in a subendothelial and mesangial distribution rather than in the subepithelial space [39]. Others have implicated an IgG molecule made cationic by loss of a sialic acid residue as a potential antigen in poststreptococcal glomerulonephritis [40]. More studies will be required to determine if such cationic proteins are playing a pathogenic role in human glomerulonephritis or are localized nonspecifically because of their charge affinity for anionic sites in the glomerular capillary wall.

Subepithelial Deposits Induced by Initial Localization of Anionic Nonglomerular Antigens

There is now considerable evidence that in situ subepithelial IC formation can also occur with anionic antigens and that charge mechanisms are sometimes operative in this process. Since some of these mechanisms involve initial glomerular localization of cationic macromolecules, increases in glomerular permeability that are due to a reduction in the charge barrier preceding immune deposit formation may also contribute to IC formation at a subepithelial site [27].

Two endogenous anionic antigens have been shown to localize directly in glomeruli. Abrass and Cohen have demonstrated that a purified renal tubular brushborder antigen that is anionic and has a mol wt of about 240,000 daltons may bind directly in the subepithelial space; they have suggested that this mechanism, as well as the fixed antigen mechanism just described, may contribute to subepithelial deposit formation in the Heymann models [41]. Since this antigen is clearly related to a fixed antigenic component of the capillary wall, an internal imaging mechanism independent of charge may contribute to its glomerular localization [42]. DNA has also been demonstrated in subepithelial immune deposits in patients with membranous lupus nephropathy [43] and has been shown to localize in the glomerulus in free form [44], although it, too, is anionic. Other endogenous antigens such as C3 convertase proteins reactive with C3 nephritic factor [45] or neoantigens of the membrane attack complex of complement in glomerular deposits [46] may also serve as a nidus for in situ IC formation. As already mentioned, Fleuren et al have demonstrated in situ subepithelial IC formation with native BSA with a pI of only 4.6 [31].

The mechanism by which localization of anionic nonglomerular antigens is achieved in the subepithelial space, or at other capillary wall sites, is a subject of active investigation. One way this can occur is by immune binding of anionic antigen to specific cationic antibodies that themselves may localize on a charge basis as already discussed for cationic antigens. This mechanism appears to account for the finding of Fleuren, Grond, and Hoedemaeker with native BSA [31]. Alternatively, anionic antigens may bind electrostatically to nonimmune cationic proteins that bind to glomerular anionic sites prior to immune deposit formation. Compelling evidence that such a mechanism can be operative has been provided by Chan, Boyd, and Fritzler who produced typical subepithelial BSA IC deposits in mice by first administering cationized nonantibody IgG followed by anionic BSA and then anti-BSA antibody [47]. Injection of the polycation polyethyleneimine (PEI) has been shown by Barnes, Radnik, and Venkatachalam to increase glomerular formation of ICs induced by injection of anionic ferritin followed by antibody to it [48]. PEI also markedly increases deposition of native BSA-containing preformed ICs along the glomerular capillary wall and results in some formation of subepithelial IC deposits [48]. Whether these immune deposits represent subepithelial localization of the preformed ICs themselves or in situ formation of dissociated components of the injected ICs has not been established [49]. Evidence that some mechanism involving exposure of the glomerulus to cationic molecules or other processes leading to loss of anionic sites before immune deposit formation begins has been provided in the NZB/W model of murine SLE, in which loss of glomerular anionic sites and increased glomerular permeability appear to precede the development of glomerular IC deposits [27]. A variety of biologic proteins involved in immune reactions are cationic and may have such effects including neutrophil cationic proteins [50], cationic products of complement activation [51], platelet-activating factor [52], and platelet factor 4 [53]. Additional evidence for the potential of this mechanism has been provided by Batsford et al who altered net negative charge by infusion of cationized ferritin and produced nephrotic syndrome 5 to 7 days later in the apparent absence of persistent ferritin or subsequent IC formation in glomeruli [54]. In contrast to the fixed antigen mechanism of in situ subepithelial IC formation in which deposit formation is decreased by aminonucleoside of puromycin or anti-GBM antibody [17–19], increased glomerular permeability induced by anti-GBM antibody facilitates glomerular IC formation in BSA-serum sickness [55] and in NZB/W mice [56], although it is unclear if this represents in situ IC formation or simply increased mesangial uptake of preformed ICs as occurs when glomerular permeability is increased with aminonucleoside of puromycin [57].

Subepithelial Immune Deposits Induced by Initial Localization of Antibody

As just mentioned, chemically cationized IgG can localize in a subepithelial distribution in the glomerulus [58] and presumably, if it represented antibody, could then bind antigen and initiate in situ IC formation. Some evidence that this may happen with native IgG as well has been provided by Fleuren et al who have found that subepithelial deposits induced by alternate perfusion with native BSA (pI 4.6) and anti-BSA antibody develop only if the anti-BSA antibody contains IgG fractions with relatively cationic isoelectric points, suggesting that it is the antibody rather than the antigen that is localizing first (Fleuren, personal communication). Thus, in states of antibody excess or alternating antibody and antigen excess, it may be antibody rather than antigen localization that initiates in situ subepithelial immune deposit formation. However, glomerulonephritis mediated by prior localization of naturally occurring cationic IgG has not yet been described.

Subepithelial Deposits Induced by Preformed Immune Complex Trapping

A principal stimulus for the work that led to recognition of the in situ mechanism of subepithelial immune deposit formation was the consistent failure by a number of investigators to produce subepithelial deposits by infusion of a variety of different types of preformed ICs (reviewed in [30]). However, this mechanism has been investigated with renewed interest since 1980. Germuth et al produced subepithelial deposits by infusing preformed ovalbumin-antiovalbumin ICs made of low-avidity antibody [59]. However, the fact that these complexes were in 80-fold antigen excess and made of low-avidity antibody would favor their dissociation in the circulation and thereby make in situ deposit formation an equally plausible mechanism for the development of the deposits observed [60]. Gallo, Caulin-Glaser, and Lamm infused preformed ICs of cationized BGG and cationic anti-BGG IgG and also reported subepithelial localization of antigen and antibody [58]. However, the ICs used were in antigen excess, cationized antigen showed similar localization by itself, and the possibility of in vivo dissociation of the infused ICs with subsequent in situ formation of the glomerular deposits was not excluded. In a subsequent study, the same investigators reported similar experiments infusing covalently linked ICs that could not dissociate and again produced subepithelial deposits of complexes containing cationic BGG [61]. However, studies were reported at only 1 hr, and the ability of such ICs to produce persistent subepithelial deposits was not established. Similar deposits occurred with microgram injections of free antigen which could have been present in the milligram quantities of ICs infused, and the molecular weight of the ICs studied was larger than molecules that would normally be expected to penetrate to the subepithelial space. However, as discussed above, events that alter glomerular permeability are known to alter glomerular localization and distribution of macromolecules and can lead to patterns of deposition of preformed ICs not seen in normal glomeruli [17, 49]. At the present time, the question of whether circulating preformed ICs of the size and charge known to be present physiologically can localize intact in the subepithelial space remains unresolved. The characteristics of ICs that deposit in glomeruli is reviewed in more detail by Mannik elsewhere in this volume.

Subendothelial Immune Deposit Formation

Fixed Glomerular Antigens

There is currently little evidence for the formation of the traditional granular type of subendothelial IC deposits on the basis of antibody reacting with an endogenous antigen at this site. The anti-GBM antibody in Goodpasture syndrome has been reported to bind to an antigen in the lamina rara interna of the GBM by some [62]. By current terminology this phenomenon could be considered an example of in situ IC formation. However, anti-GBM antibody does not produce granular or electron-dense deposits. Antibodies to endothelial cell surface and Ia antigens have been reported in lupus and may localize on the inner surface of the glomerular capillary wall by such a mechanism [63, 64]. At that site, they might form granular deposits by an antigen-redistribution phenomenon as shown by Barba et al in other organ systems [65]. However, this sequence has not yet been clearly demonstrated to occur in glomerular disease.

Planted Nonrenal Antigens

The best example of this phenomenon comes from the studies of Goldus and Wilson, who used the plant lectin concanavalin A (con A) as an antigen. Con A binds directly to glucose and mannose constituents of capillary wall glycoproteins. When anti-con A antibody is injected, a linear-granular pattern of IC deposits along the inner surface of the capillary wall is produced accompanied by an acute proliferative glomerulonephritis [66]. Electron microscopy studies of this model suggested a predominantly subendothelial localization of deposits [66]. Viruses and other materials are known to contain such lectin-like components and may therefore have the potential for producing deposits by this mechanism in humans [22]. Charge also appears to contribute to in situ formation of subendothelial ICs by facilitating initial antigen localization at that site. Thus, subendothelial IC deposits have been produced in situ with cationized ferritin [33] and with avidin, a lower molecular weight, naturally occurring cationic protein [35]. As mentioned above, some of these subendothelial IC deposits may dissociate to cross the capillary wall and contribute to local formation of ICs in the subepithelial space as well [33]. Additional subendothelial IC formation may occur if IgG deposited at that site reacts with antibodies to IgG in the form of either rheumatoid factors [67] or anti-idiotypic antibodies [68].

Since granular subendothelial IC deposits are rarely seen in the absence of mesangial deposits, it is unlikely that subendothelial planting of antigens with subsequent in situ IC formation is a common pathogenetic event in the absence of a similar process in the mesangium.

Subendothelial Deposits Caused by Preformed Immune Complex Trapping

In contrast to the situation with subepithelial deposits, numerous studies have demonstrated that preformed ICs can localize along the subendothelial surface of the glomerular capillary wall (reviewed in [30]). Subendothelial deposits are generally not seen in the absence of substantial mesangial IC deposition as well. The localization of deposits in a subendothelial distribution usually reflects an increased glomerular delivery of ICs compared to situations where only mesangial deposits are seen, and may be contributed to by impaired mesangial clearing function [69] and by capillary wall charge alterations [49]. The factors that regulate mesangial and subendothelial trapping of circulating ICs are therefore discussed in more detail later under mesangial immune deposit formation. Because of their proximity to the circulation, antigen-antibody complexes in the subendothelial area are in dynamic equilibrium with the same reactants in free or complex form in the circulation [70, 71]. Accretion of additional antigen or antibody may therefore occur by immune interaction with free binding sites within the IC lattice structure, and preformed ICs may also be immunologically bound to tissue deposits [72]. Therefore, both in situ deposit formation and circulating IC trapping mechanisms likely contribute to deposit formation at this site. In addition, the relative accessibility of subendothelial deposits, and complement-derived chemotaxins generated by them, to circulating inflammatory cells is probably the principal reason why deposits in a subendothelial distribution are generally associated with a relatively severe inflammatory glomerulonephritis in diseases such as class IV SLE and type I membranoproliferative glomerulonephritis.

The models most relevant to subendothelial IC disease in which mediation mechanisms have been studied are the autologous phase models of nephrotoxic or anti-GBM nephritis in which IC deposits are actually formed in situ within the glomerular capillary wall itself. These studies implicate complement, neutrophils, and macrophages in the pathogenesis of proteinuria induced by IC deposit formation at that site [73–75]. It should be noted that it is the site of glomerular IC formation, and hence, too, the way by which the deposits form, which appears to determine the mediation mechanisms involved and thereby the type of histologic and clinical glomerular disease produced. This is well illustrated by the studies of Couser and Salant showing that when a specific antigen-antibody system produces IC deposits in the subepithelial space, a result is proteinuria that is complement-mediated but cell-independent [76]. However, exactly the same quantity of the same antigen and antibody interacting within the glomerular capillary wall closer to the circulation produce a proteinuria that is neutrophil- as well as complement-dependent [75].

Mesangial Immune Complex Deposits

Fixed Mesangial Antigens

The mesangium exhibits a variety of antigenic determinants that are quite accessible to circulating antibodies, including actin, myosin, glycosaminoglycans, fibronectin, laminin, type V collagen, procollagen type IV, and other less well-defined antigenic structures [77–79]. However, to date, no substantial clinical or experimental evidence has been reported for mesangial injury or glomerulonephritis caused by antibody reacting directly with such intrinsic mesangial structures [79].

Planted Mesangial Antigens

Because the mesangium has the capacity to take up and accumulate a wide variety of macromolecules of various sizes and characteristics, it serves as a likely site for exogenous antigen localization, followed by in situ IC formation. The classic studies of Mauer et al were the first to demonstrate that this can occur and to document the nephritogenic potential of this mechanism [12]. Aggregated human IgG with the properties of circulating ICs was injected into rabbits; it localized without causing injury in the glomerular mesangium. Rabbit kidneys containing mesangial IgG deposits were then transplanted into normal recipients who were passively administered antibody to human IgG. The recipients developed an acute focal proliferative glomerulonephritis much like that associated with mesangial deposits in diseases such as IgA nephropathy or lupus nephritis in humans [12]. Similar degrees of histologic and functional glomerular injury have not been produced by preformed IC infusion [12, 30]. Although other models of in situ IC formation in the mesangium have not been well studied, the mesangium clearly has the capacity to trap a variety of circulating potentially antigenic macromolecules with less restricted characteristics than those which may become localized in subepithelial or subendothelial areas. These have included material such as thorotrast, various aggregated serum proteins and ICs, colloidal carbon, myeloperoxidase, catalase, dextran, iron-dextran, and others (reviewed in [77, 80]). Charge has also been shown to play a role in mesangial trapping of potential antigens. Cationic antigens apparently localize better and persist longer at this site [81, 82]. The fact that severe glomerular injury has not been produced by infusions of preformed ICs but does occur acutely when similar quantities of ICs form in situ in the mesangium suggests that in situ mechanisms may be operative in producing the acute inflammatory glomerular lesions associated with mesangial IC deposits in diseases such as systemic lupus, IgA nephropathy, and Henoch-Schönlein purpura. Evidence that a nonrenal antigen mechanism is involved in the formation of IgA-containing mesangial IC deposits in IgA nephropathy and Henoch-Schönlein purpura has been reported in humans [83].

No studies of the mediation of mesangial IC disease have been reported, although the prominence of neutrophils and macrophages derived from the circulation in this lesion suggests that conventional complement and cell-dependent mechanisms of humoral tissue injury are probably operative [12]. The recently recognized potential of mesangial cells alone to produce a variety of potential inflammatory mediators including prostaglandins [84], reactive oxygen species [85], acidic and neutral proteases [86], and interleukin-like proinflammatory cytokines [87] suggest that products of local immune reactions in the mesangium such as complement-activation proteins may stimulate such local destructive mechanisms to be initiated. Moreover, the presence of some Ia antigen-bearing cells within the mesangium also suggests that some antigenic macromolecules trapped at that site may be presented in a genetically restricted fashion to sensitized T lymphocytes, which may then participate in the mediation of mesangial immune complex disease [88].

Mesangial Immune Complex Deposits Caused by Trapping of Circulating Immune Complexes

In all studies of preformed IC localization in the kidney, the major site of deposition has been within the glomerular mesangium, and this immunopathologic pattern of glomerular deposits can clearly be reproduced by circulating IC trapping. Because of the preferential localization of large macromolecules in the mesangium, most studies of factors that regulate the glomerular localization of ICs presumably have studied primarily mesangial uptake and egress of complexes. Briefly, mesangial uptake of macromolecules including ICs is determined by a combination of variables. These variables include systemic factors that determine glomerular delivery of ICs and local characteristics, both of the complexes themselves and of the glomerulus, that alter the extent to which complexes delivered to the kidney may deposit [60, 89]. The blood level of ICs is determined by the amount of antigen and antibody available for IC formation and their relative avidity, as well as by the efficiency with which such molecules are removed by the systemic mononuclear phagocyte system (MPS), a factor dependent on both IC characteristics and MPS clearing function [60, 89]. For any given blood level of ICs, glomerular deposition is generally related to glomerular delivery and the capacity to enter the mesangium, variables that are altered by renal blood flow, the glomerular hydrostatic pressure gradient, and local intraglomerular IC concentration as reflected by the filtration fraction [90, 91]. Intrinsic glomerular properties also influence this process, including permeability and charge characteristics of the glomerular capillary wall, charge sites within the mesangium, mesangial cell endocytic activity, and mesangial clearing function [77, 80]. Under some circumstances, increased glomerular permeability is associated with a marked increase in mesangial uptake of IC-like material [17, 77, 92], whereas other diseases such as experimental membranous nephropathy, with comparable increases in capillary wall permeability, exhibit an apparent reduced capacity of the mesangium to accumulate macromolecules [93]. Finally, although ICs with a wide range of sizes and composition localize within the mesangium, characteristics of the IC itself can also alter mesangial uptake owing to differences in their relative ability to deposit within the mesangium or to be handled by it, as well as to differences in systemic clearance rate and, hence, glomerular delivery. These properties include the size and composition of the IC, its relative electrical charge, relative biodegradability and chemotactic and phlogogenic potential, including complement fixing capacity [60, 89, 94]. Obviously, studies to assess any of these variables individually are difficult because they are so extensively interrelated.

Understanding the pathophysiology of mesangial IC deposition still leaves unresolved the ways in which preformed ICs might induce glomerular damage. Mesangial uptake of ICs appear to be a normal aspect of mesangial clearing function, with IC trafficking occurring largely through the mesangial matrix rather than mesangial cells [77, 80]. ICs are cleared by several mechanisms, including phagocytosis by infiltrating mononuclear cells [95] and perhaps to a small extent by mesangial cells themselves, by movement down the mesangial stalk to the juxtaglomerular zone, or perhaps by regurgitation from the mesangium back into the glomerular capillary [80]. Although phagocytizing cells themselves may cause tissue damage, significant inflammatory tissue injury has not been shown to result from the trapping of preformed ICs, which apparently behave as relatively inert macromolecules with respect to their ability to cause damage when formed in the circulation and then trapped in the glomerulus [30]. The possibility that exposure of mesangial cells to ICs may trigger local release of pathogenic mediators by the cells themselves as discussed above is a possibility that requires additional investigation. It must further be appreciated that deposits within the mesangium, like subendothelial deposits, are in dynamic equilibrium with antigen and antibody in the circulation, so that local immune interaction can take place as already described with subendothelial deposits. This process of on-going in situ IC formation and accretion within the mesangium appears to lead to greater persistence of the deposits as it does in the subepithelial space and to be a more nephritogenic process than the passive trapping of antigen and antibody in soluble IC form [12].

Relation Between In Situ Immune Complex Formation Involving Nonrenal Antigens and Circulating Immune Complex Trapping

When antigen and antibody combine locally in a tissue such as the glomerulus to produce in situ IC formation, the same reactants must obviously also be present in the circulation, and hence circulating ICs would be anticipated. The quantitative relationship between antigen and antibody in free and complex form represents a dynamic equilibrium (antigen + antibody $\rightleftharpoons$ ICs). The absolute amounts of each reactant are dependent on several factors, including the relative amounts and concentrations of each and the affinity of antigen and antibody for each other. Circumstances that facilitate IC formation or removal tend to shift this equilibrium to the right and consequently to diminish the amount of free antigen or antibody present. These include high-avidity antibody, multivalent antigens capable of extensive lattice formation and precipitation and enhanced MPS clearing function. Conversely, factors that reduce antigen-antibody union or impair IC removal tend to shift the equilibrium to the left, thereby increasing the amount of free antigen and antibody available. These include low-avidity antibodies and reduced MPS clearing function as noted in several IC diseases [96, 97]. These circumstances therefore favor in situ IC formation with nonrenal antigens [30]. For tissue injury to occur from in situ deposit formation, free antigen or antibody must also have the capacity to leave the circulation and localize in tissues. With respect to the glomerulus, the principal factor that facilitates this is the relation between antigen or antibody charge and the charge of the glomerular capillary wall or of proteins localized on it as described above. Other factors that lead to nonimmune interaction with endogenous or trapped glomerular constituents may also contribute to this process. Thus, when the antigen-antibody system involved has the appropriate characteristics for glomerular localization of antigen or antibody to occur, in situ deposit formation is facilitated by factors that increase the amount of uncomplexed reactants available to localize, and these include high levels of circulating ICs. However, glomerular trapping of circulating ICs is also increased by higher blood levels and renal delivery [69]. Therefore, measurements of circulating IC levels, and correlations between these levels and disease activity, cannot distinguish between these two mechanisms of glomerular deposit formation since they are directly related. However, the absence of circulating complexes in an IC glomerulonephritis may be more suggestive of deposit formation involving insoluble fixed renal antigens.

References

1. SCHICK B: Die nachkrenkheiten des scharlachs. *Jahrb Kinderheit* 65:132–173, 1907
2. VON PIRQUET CE: *Allergy Arch of Intern Med* 7:259–288, 383–436, 1911
3. MELLORS RC, SIEGEL M, PRESSMAN D: Analytical pathology: I. Histochemical

demonstration of antibody localization in tissues, with special reference to the antigenic components of kidney and lung. *Lab Invest* 4:69–89, 1955

4. MELLORS RC, ORTEGA LG: Analytical pathology: III. New observations on the pathogenesis of glomerulonephritis, lipoid nephrosis, polyarteritis nodosa and the secondary amyloidosis in man. *Am J Pathol* 32:455–499, 1956

5. GERMUTH GF JR, PACE MG, TIPPETT JC: Comparative histologic and immunologic studies in rabbits of induced hypersensitivity of the serum sickness type: II. The effect of sensitization to homologous and cross-reactive antigens on the rate of antigen elimination and the development of allergic lesions. *J Exp Med* 101:135–150, 1955

6. GERMUTH FG JR, FLANAGAN C, MONTENEGRO MR: The relationships between the chemical nature of the antigen, antigen dosage, rate of antibody synthesis and the occurrence of arteritis and glomerulonephritis in experimental hypersensitivity. *Johns Hopkins Med J* 101:149–169, 1957

7. DIXON FJ, FELDMAN JD, VAZQUEZ JJ: Experimental glomerulonephritis: The pathogenesis of a laboratory model resembling the spectrum of human glomerulonephritis. *J Exp Med* 113:899–920, 1961

8. EDGINGTON TS, GLASSOCK RJ, DIXON FJ: Autologous immune complex nephritis induced with renal tubular antigen: I. Identification and isolation of the pathogenetic antigen. *J Exp Med* 127:555–572, 1968

9. EDGINGTON TS, GLASSOCK RJ, DIXON FJ: Autologous immune complex pathogenesis of experimental allergic glomerulonephritis. *Science* 155:1432–1434, 1967

10. VAN DAMME BJC, FLEUREN GJ, BAKKER WW, VERNIER RL, HOEDEMAEKER PJ: Experimental glomerulonephritis in the rat induced by antibodies directed against tubular antigens: IV. Fixed glomular antigens in the pathogenesis of heterologous immune complex glomerulonephritis. *Lab Invest* 38:502–510, 1978

11. COUSER WG, STEINMULLER DR, STILMANT MM, SALANT DJ, LOWENSTEIN LM: Experimental glomerulonephritis in the isolated perfused rat kidney. *J Clin Invest* 62:1275–1287, 1978

12. MAUER SM, SUTHERLAND DER, HOWARD RJ, FISH AJ, NAJARIAN JS, MICHAEL AF: The glomerular mesangium: III. Acute immune mesangial injury: A new model of glomerulonephritis. *J Exp Med* 137:553–570, 1973

13. VAN ES LA, BLOK APR, SCHOENFELD L, GLASSOCK RJ: Chronic nephritis induced by antibodies reacting with glomerular-bound immune complexes. *Kidney Int* 11:106–115, 1977

14. KERJASCHKI D, FARQUHAR MG: The pathogenic antigen of Heymann nephritis is a membrane glycoprotein of the renal proximal tubule brush border. *Cell Biol* 79:5557–5561, 1982

15. KERJASCHKI D, FARQUHAR MG: Immunocytochemical localization of the Heymann nephritis antigen (GP330) in glomular epithelial cells of normal Lewis rats. *J Exp Med* 157:667–685, 1983

16. HOYER JR: Tubulointerstitial immune complex nephritis in rats immunized with Tamm-Horsfall protein. *Kidney Int* 17:284–292, 1980

17. COUSER WG, HOYER JR, JERMANOVICH NB, BELOK S, STILMANT MM: Effect of aminonucleoside nephrosis on immune complex localization in autologous immune complex nephropathy in rats. *J Clin Invest* 61:561–572, 1978

18. COUSER WG, SALANT DJ, STILMANT MM, ARBEIT LA, DARBY C, SLIOGERIS VS: The effects of aminonucleoside of puromycin and nephrotoxic serum on subepithelial immune-deposit formation in passive Heymann nephritis. *J Lab Clin Med* 94:917–932, 1979

19. SALANT DJ, BELOK S, DARBY C, STILMANT MM, COUSER WG: Determinants of glomerular localization of subepithelial immune deposits: Effects of altered antigen:antibody ratio, steroids, vasoactive amine antagonists and aminonucleo-

side of puromycin on passive Heymann nephritis in rats. *Lab Invest* 41:89–99, 1979

20. WEENING JJ, GROND J, HOEDEMAEKER PJ: Effect of increased glomerular permeability on the localization of immune aggregates and protamine-heparin aggregates in the rat. *Lab Invest* 49:619–615, 1983

21. SALANT DJ, BELOK S, MADAIO MP, COUSER WG: A new role for complement in experimental membranous nephropathy in rats. *J Clin Invest* 66:1339–1350, 1980

22. ADLER S, SALANT DJ, DITTMER JE, RENNKE HG, MADIO MP, COUSER WG: Mediation of proteinuria in membranous nephropathy due to a planted glomerular antigen. *Kidney Int* 23:807–815, 1983

23. THOENES GH, PIELSTICKER K, SCHUBERT G: Transplantation-induced immune complex kidney disease in rats with unilateral manifestation in the allografted kidney. *Lab Invest* 41:321–333, 1979

24. NEALE TJ, WILSON CB: Non-GBM glomerular antigen and spontaneous nephritis in rabbits. *Kidney Int* 14:715, 1978

25. ASSMANN KJM, TANGELDER MM, LANGE WBJ, TADEMA TM, KOENE RAB: Membranous glomerulonephritis in the mouse. *Kidney Int* 24:303–312, 1983

26. NEALE TJ, WILSON CB: Glomerular antigens and glomerulonephritis. *Springer Semin Immunopathol* 5:221–249, 1982

27. CAVALLO T, GOLDMAN M, GRAVES K, LAMBERT P-H: Altered glomerular permeability in the early phase of immune complex nephritis. *Kidney Int* 24:632–637, 1983

28. EVANS DJ: Pathogenesis of membranous glomerulonephritis. *Lancet* 2:1143–1144, 1974

29. GROGGEL GC, SALANT DJ, DARBY C, RENNKE HG, COUSER WG: Role of the terminal complement pathway in the heterologous phase of anti-glomerular basement membrane nephritis in the rabbit. In press

30. COUSER WG, SALANT DJ: In situ immune complex formation and glomerular injury (*editorial review*). *Kidney Int* 17:1–13, 1980

31. FLEUREN G, GROND J, HOEDEMAEKER PJ: In situ formation of subepithelial glomerular immune complexes in passive serum sickness. *Kidney Int* 17:631–637, 1980

32. BORDER WA, WARD HJ, KAMIL ES, COHEN AH: Induction of membranous nephropathy in rabbits by administration of an exogeneous cationic antigen: Demonstration of a pathogenic role for electrical charge. *J Clin Invest* 69:451–461, 1982

33. VOGT A, ROHRBACH R, SHIMIZU F, TAKAMIYA H, BATSFORD S: Interaction of cationized antigen with rat glomerular basement membrane: In situ immune complex formation. *Kidney Int* 22:27–35, 1982

34. VOGT A: New aspects of the pathogenesis of immune complex glomerulonephritis: Formation of subepithelial deposits. *Clin Nephrol* 21:15–20, 1984

35. KASEDA N, YAMAMOTO Y, TANAKA K: Demonstration of native cation macromolecule induced in situ immune complex glomerulonephritis in rat. In press

36. MANNIK M, AGODOA LYC, DAVID KA: Rearrangement of immune complexes in glomeruli leads to persistence and development of electron-dense deposits. *J Exp Med* 157:1516–1527, 1983

37. AGODOA LYC, GAUTHIER DJ, MANNIK M: Precipitating antigen-antibody systems are required for the formation of subepithelial electron-dense immune deposits in rat glomeruli. *J Exp Med* 158:1259–1271, 1983

38. VOGT A, BATSFORD S, RODRIGUEZ-ITURBE B, GARCIA R: Cationic antigens in poststreptococcal glomerulonephritis. *Clin Nephrol* 20:271–279, 1983

39. LANGE K, SELIGSON G, CRONIN W: Evidence for the in situ origin of poststrepto-

coccal glomerulonephritis: Glomerular localization of endostreptosin and the clinical significance of the subsequent antibody response. *Clin Nephrol* 19:3–10, 1983
40. MCINTOSH RM, GARCIA R, RABIDEAU D, RODRIGUEZ-ITURBE B: Evidence for an autologous immune complex pathogenic mechanism in acute poststreptococcal glomerulonephritis. *Kidney Int* 14:501–510, 1978
41. ABRASS CK, COHEN AH: Direct binding of renal tubular antigen to the subepithelial space of the glomerulus. In press
42. BONA CA, FINLEY S, WATERS S, KUNKEL HG: Anti-immunoglobulin antibodies: III. Properties of sequential anti-idiotypic antibodies to heterologous anti-globulins; detection of reactivity of anti-idiotype antibodies with epitopes of Fc fragments (homobodies) and with epitopes and idiotopes (epibodies). *J Exp Med* 156:986–999, 1982
43. KOFFLER D, SCHUR PH, KUNKEL HG: Immunologic studies concerning the nephritis of systemic lupus erythematosus. *J Exp Med* 126:607–623, 1967
44. IZUI S, LAMBERT PH, MIESCHER PA: In vitro demonstration of a particular affinity of glomerular basement membrane and collagen for DNA: A possible basis for local formation of DNA-anti-DNA complexes in systemic lupus erythematosus. *J Exp Med* 144:428–443, 1976
45. SCHREIBER RD, MULLER-EBERHARD HJ: Complement in renal disease, in *Contemporary Issues in Nephrology,* edited by WILSON CB, BRENNER BM, STEIN JH, New York, Churchill Livingstone, vol 3, pp 67–105
46. BIESECKER G, KATZ S, KOFFLER D: Renal localization of the membrane attack complex in systemic lupus erythematosus nephritis. *J Exp Med* 154:1779–1794, 1981
47. CHAN EKL, BOYD ND, FRITZLER M: In vivo anionic immune complex deposition in the murine glomerulus (*abstract*). *Clin Res* 31:448, 1983
48. BARNES JL, RADNIK RA, VENKATACHALAM MA: Enhancement of glomerular immune complex deposition by a circulating polycation, polyethyleneimine (*abstract*). *Kidney Int* 21:196, 1982
49. BARNES JL, VENKATACHALAM MA: Enhancement of glomerular immune complex deposition by a circulating polycation. *J Exp Med,* in press
50. CAMUSSI G, TETTA C, SEGOLONI G, KODA R, VERCELLONE A: Localization of neutrophil cationic proteins and loss of anionic charges in glomeruli of patients with systemic lupus erythematosus. *Clin Immunol Immunopathol* 24:299–314, 1982
51. HUNSICKER LG, SHEARER TP, SHAFFER SJ: Acute reversible proteinuria induced by infusion of the polycation hexadimethrine. *Kidney Int* 20:7–17, 1981
52. CAMUSSI G, TETTA C, KODA R, SEGOLONI GP, VERCELLONE A: Platelet-activating factor-induced loss of glomerular anionic charges. *Kidney Int* 25:73–81, 1984
53. BARNES JL, LEVINE SP, VENKATACHALAM MA: Binding of platelet factor 4 (PF4) to glomerular polyanion. *Kidney Int,* in press
54. BATSFORD SR, SASAKI M, TAKAMIYA H, VOGT A: Cationic macromolecule-induced nephrotic syndrome in rabbits: Lack of immune complex involvement. *Lab Invest* 49:260–269, 1983
55. TREVILLIAN P, CAMERON JS: The interaction of anti-glomerular basement membrane antibody deposition with immune elimination of bovine serum albumin in the rabbit. *Clin Exp Immunol* 35:338–349, 1979
56. RUDOFSKY UH: Murine lupus nephritis is accelerated by anti-glomerular basement membrane autoantibodies. *Clin Exp Immunol* 44:18–23, 1981
57. MAUER SM, FISH AJ, BLAU EB, MICHAEL AF: The glomerular mesangium: I. Kinetic studies of macromolecular uptake in normal and nephrotic rats. *J Clin Invest* 51:1092–1099, 1972
58. GALLO GR, CAULIN-GLASER T, LAMM ME: Charge of circulating immune com-

plexes as a factor in glomerular basement membrane localization in mice. *J Clin Invest* 67:1305–1313, 1981

59. GERMUTH FG JR, RODRIGUEZ E, LORELLE CA, TRUMP ER, MILANO LL, WISE O: Passive immune complex glomerulonephritis in mice: Models for various lesions found in human disease: II. Low avidity complexes and diffuse proliferative glomerulonephritis with subepithelial deposits. *Lab Invest* 41:366–371, 1979.

60. MANNIK M: Pathophysiology of circulating immune complexes. *Arthritis Rheum* 25:783–787, 1982

61. CAULIN-GLASER T, GALLO GR, LAMM ME: Nondissociating cationic immune complexes can deposit in glomerular basement membrane. *J Exp Med* 158:1561–1572, 1983

62. FISH AJ, CARMODY KM, MICHAEL AF: Spatial orientation and distribution of antigens within glomerular basement membrane. *J Lab Clin Med* 94:447–454, 1979

63. CINES DB, LYSS AP, REEBER MB, DEHORATIUS RJ: Presence of complement-fixing anti-endothelial cell antibodies in systemic lupus erythematosus. *J Clin Invest* 73:611–625, 1984

64. OKUDAIRA K, SEARLES RP, CEUPPENS JL, GOODWIN JS, WILLIAMS RC JR: Anti-Ia reactivity in sera from patients with systemic lupus erythematosus. *J Clin Invest* 69:17–24, 1982

65. BARBA LM, CALDWELL PRB, DOWNIE GH, CAMUSSI G, BRENTJENS JR, ANDRES GA: Lung injury mediated by antibodies to endothelium: I. In the rabbit repeated interaction of heterologous anti-angiotensin-converting enzyme antibodies with alveolar endothelium results in resistance to immune injury through antigenic modulation. *J Exp Med* 158:2141–2158, 1983

66. GOLBUS SM, WILSON CB: Experimental glomerulonephritis induced by in situ formation of immune complexes in the glomerular capillary wall. *Kidney Int* 16:148–157, 1979

67. FORD PM, KOSATKA I: In situ immune complex formation in the mouse glomerulus: Reactivity with human IGM rheumatoid factor and the effect on subsequent immune complex deposition. *Clin Exp Immunol* 51:285–291, 1983

68. ZANETTI M, WILSON CB: Participation of auto-anti-idiotypes in immune complex glomerulonephritis in rabbits. *J Immunol* 131:2781–2783, 1983

69. HAAKENSTAD AO, STRIKER GE, MANNIK M: The glomerular deposition of soluble immune complexes prepared with reduced and alkylated antibodies and with intact antibodies in mice. *Lab Invest* 35:293–301, 1976

70. WILSON CB, DIXON FJ: Quantitation of acute and chronic serum sickness in the rabbit. *J Exp Med* 134:7S–18S, 1971

71. HAAKENSTAD AO, STRIKER GE, MANNIK M: Removal of glomerular immune complex deposits by excess antigen in chronic mouse model of immune complex disease. *Lab Invest* 48:323–331, 1983

72. FORD PM, KOSATKA I: A mechanism of enhancement of immune complex deposition following in situ immune complex formation in the mouse glomerulus. *Immunology* 43:433–438, 1981

73. NAISH PF, THOMSON NM, SIMPSON IJ, PETERS DK: The role of polymorphonuclear leucocytes in the autologous phase of nephrotoxic nephritis. *Clin Exp Immunol* 22:102–108, 1975

74. HOLDSWORTH SR, NEALE TJ, WILSON CB: Abrogation of macrophage-dependent injury in experimental glomerulonephritis in the rabbit. Use of an antimacrophage serum. *J Clin Invest* 68:686–698, 1981

75. SALANT DJ, ADLER S, DARBY C, GROGGEL GC, RENNKE HG, DITTMER JE: Is the mediation of immunologic glomerular injury influenced by the distribution of antigen (*abstract*)? *Kidney Int* 25:218, 1984

76. COUSER WG, SALANT DJ: Immunopathogenesis of glomerular capillary wall injury in nephrotic states. *Contemp Issues Nephrol* 9:47–83, 1982
77. MICHAEL AF, KEANE WF, RAIJ L, VERNIER RL, MAUER SM: The glomerular mesangium (*editorial review*). *Kidney Int* 17:141–154, 1980
78. BATSFORD SR, ROHRBACH R, TAKAMIYA H, KLUTHE R, VOGT A: Autoantibodies specific for the glomerular mesangium and Bowman's capsule in man. *Clin Nephrol* 12:163–167, 1979
79. SEELIG HP, SEELIG R, ROTH E, ROTH E: Antibodies reacting with the glomerular mesangium. Isolation and immunopathology. *Virchows Arch A Path Anat Histol* 366:313–330, 1975
80. STERZEL RB, LOVETT DH, STEIN HD, KASHGARIAN M: The mesangium and glomerulonephritis. *Klin Wochenschr* 60:1077–1094, 1982
81. COHEN S, VERNIER RL, MICHAEL AF: The effect of charge on the renal distribution of ferritin. *Am J Pathol* 110:170–181, 1983
82. BORDER WA, KAMIL ES, WARD HJ, COHEN AH: Antigenic charge as a determinant of immune complex localization in the rat glomerulus. *Lab Invest* 40:442–449, 1981
83. TOMINO Y, ENDOH M, NOMOTO Y, SAKAI H: Specificity of eluted antibody from renal tissues of patients with IgA nephropathy. *Am J Kidney Dis* 1:276–280, 1982
84. SCHARSCHMIDT LA, DUNN MJ: Prostaglandin synthesis by rat glomerular mesangial cells in culture: Effects of angiotensin II and arginine vasopressin. *J Clin Invest* 71:1756–1764, 1983
85. BAUD L, HAGEGE J, SRAER J, RONDEAU E, PEREZ J, ARDAILLOU R: Reactive oxygen production by cultured rat glomerular cells during phagocytosis is associated with stimulation of lipoxygenase activity. *J Exp Med* 158:1836–1852, 1983
86. LOVETT DH, RYAN JL, KASHAGARIAN M, STERZEL RB: Lysosomal enzymes and glomerular cells of the rat. *Am J Pathol* 107:161–166, 1982
87. LOVETT DH, RYAN JL, STERZEL RB: A thymocyte-activating factor derived from glomerular mesangial cells. *J Immunol* 130:1796–1801, 1983
88. SCHREINER GF, KILEY J-M, COTRAN RS, UNANUE ER: Characterization of resident glomerular cells in the rat expressing Ia determinants and manifesting genetically restricted interactions with lymphocytes. *J Clin Invest* 68:920–931, 1981
89. MANNIK M: Physicochemical and functional relationships of immune complexes. *J Invest Dermatol* 74:333–338, 1980
90. HEBERT LA, ALLHISER CL, KOETHE SM: Some hemodynamic determinants of immune complex trapping by the kidney. *Kidney Int* 14:452–465, 1978
91. WARD DM, BLANTZ RC: Uptake of macromolecules by the glomerular mesangium is increased by angiotensin II (*abstract*). *Clin Res* 29:479, 1981
92. HOYER JR, MAUER SM, MICHAEL AF: Unilateral renal disease in the rat: I. Clinical, morphologic and glomerular mesangial functional features of the experimental model produced by renal perfusion with the aminonucleoside of puromycin. *J Lab Clin Med* 85:756–764, 1975
93. SCHNEEBERGER EE, COLLINS AB, STAVRAKIS G, McCLUSKEY RT: Diminished mesangial accumulation of intravenously injected soluble immune complexes in rats with autologous immune complex nephritis. *Lab Invest* 42:440–449, 1980
94. HEBERT LA, WAXMAN FJ, BIRMINGHAM DJ, KORNACOFF JB, VAN AMAN MA, SMEAD WL, KRAUT EH: Complement depletion accelerates the clearance of immune complexes from the circulation of primates (*abstract*). *Kidney Int* 23:183, 1983
95. STRIKER GE, MANNIK M, TUNG MY: Role of marrow-derived monocytes and

      mesangial cells in removal of immune complexes from renal glomeruli. *J Exp Med* 149:127–136, 1979

96. LAWLEY TJ: Immune complexes and reticuloendothelial system function and human disease. *J Invest Dermatol* 74:339–343, 1980

97. LAWRENCE S, PUSSELL BA, CHARLESWORTH JA: Mesangial IGA nephropathy: Detection of defective reticulophagocytic function in vivo. *Clin Nephrol* 16:280–283, 1983

Characteristics of Circulating Immune Complexes That Deposit in Renal Glomeruli

Mart Mannik and V. Joyce Gauthier

Experimental models of acute and chronic serum sickness have clearly established the relation between the presence of antigen–antibody complexes in renal glomeruli and the development of glomerulonephritis. In acute models of serum sickness, a large dose of antigen is required for induction of the disease. Concurrent with the development of antibody response to the antigen and the resulting immune clearance of the antigen, deposits of immune complexes arise in renal glomeruli. The induced alterations in glomeruli are transient since further formation of immune deposits ceases after all the available antigen has combined with antibodies. Acute serum sickness, however, can be converted to a chronic model by frequent, repeated antigen administration.

The chronic serum sickness models with reproducible renal disease have been achieved in many laboratories in rabbits, rats, and mice (for review, see [1]). With repeated injections of antigen the continued availability of endogenous antibodies leads to continued formation of immune complexes either in circulation or in tissues. In these chronic models, comparable to glomerulonephritis in humans, the antigen–antibody deposits in glomeruli are located in the mesangial, subendothelial, or subepithelial areas. The mesangial immune deposits are associated with increased cellularity of the mesangium, in part due to infiltration of monocytes, but renal function is minimally altered. When subendothelial deposits of immune complexes are present, then deposits also exist in the mesangial area, suggesting a relation between the two. The inflammatory process and alterations of renal function are extensive when substantial subendothelial deposits have formed. Subepithelial immune deposits are not associated with infiltrating inflammatory cells, but complement components are present, proteinuria develops, and renal function declines with chronic lesions. The mechanisms by which immune complexes deposit in these three different locations and the composition of deposited complexes could not be determined in active serum sickness.

This manuscript was presented as part of a Symposium on *Mechanisms of Immune Complex Formation and Deposition in Glomeruli.*

For these reasons, investigators turned to experiments with preformed immune complexes with known composition and lattice to examine the variables that may alter their localization in glomeruli. This approach has limitations in that the duration of experiments is usually short to avoid new variables introduced by the endogenous immune response and therefore extensive lesions might not be expected. The purpose of this review is to briefly consider the information gained by administration of preformed immune complexes.

Removal of Circulating Immune Complexes by the Mononuclear Phagocyte System

A substantial proportion of preformed immune complexes injected into experimental animals is removed from circulation by protective mechanisms. Soluble immune complexes are largely removed by the Kupffer cells in the liver. With the IgG class of antibodies in immune complexes, the removal is mediated by Fc receptors, provided the lattice of immune complexes has attained a sufficient size (that is, that it contains more than two IgG molecules) (for review, see [2]). When the lattice is even larger and efficient complement activation occurs by the complexes, then complement receptors on Kupffer cells may contribute to the removal of circulating, soluble immune complexes.

An interesting event has been suggested as a requirement for interiorization of immune complexes attached to the Fc receptors on macrophages. The process of attachment of immune complexes with sufficient lattice leads to increased local concentration of immune complexes on the cell surface. Thereafter, the complexes form even larger immune aggregates and then become phagocytized. When the formation of larger immune aggregates is prevented by stabilizing the lattice with covalent bonds between the antigen and antibody molecules, interiorization does not occur [3]. As will be explained later, similar events of rearrangement of immune complexes also occur in renal glomeruli.

In mice, Kupffer cells possess specific receptors for IgA molecules (Rifai and Mannik, submitted for publication). When immune complexes with IgA class of antibodies reach a size containing 8 or more IgA molecules, achieved either by 8 monomeric IgA molecules or 4 dimeric IgA molecules, then these immune complexes are quickly removed from circulation by Kupffer cells [4].

The nature of antigens in immune complexes can hasten the removal of immune complexes from circulation independently of lattice. For example, if exposed galactose groups are present on the antigen molecules, even small-latticed immune complexes are quickly removed from circulation by hepatocytes owing to the interaction with receptors that recognize the galactose groups [5]. Similarly, immune complexes containing single-stranded DNA are very rapidly removed from circulation owing to the rapid removal of DNA itself [6].

Particulate immune complexes (for example, red blood cells coated with IgG molecules) are preferentially removed from the circulation by the spleen and not the liver, depending on the average number of antibody molecules per cell (for review, see [7]). Very large immune complexes, large enough to be cosedimented with red blood cells that possess no complement receptors, bind to the CR1 (C3b) receptor on primate red blood cells and are then delivered to Kupffer cells for removal. Evidence for this mechanism was provided by injecting the complexes directly into the aorta of baboons [8]. In other species of animals, immune complexes of this enormous size become entrapped in pulmonary capillaries when administered into the venous circulation.

As will be emphasized next, the large-latticed immune complexes that are efficiently removed from circulation also are the immune complexes that have the potential for deposition in glomeruli. Only a small percentage of immune complexes deposit in renal glomeruli, either injected as preformed complexes or estimated to form in serum sickness [9, 10].

The foregoing comments serve to emphasize the dynamic state of immune complexes in circulation. The load of circulating immune complexes capable of deposition in glomeruli varies on one hand with the events that lead to their formation and on the other hand with the protective mechanisms that remove them from circulation. In human diseases, we are far from being able to measure and predict these variables.

Deposition of Circulating Immune Complexes in Mesangial and Subendothelial Areas

Experiments in which preformed immune complexes are injected into experimental animals, using protein antigens and IgG antibodies to these antigens, lead to predominantly mesangial deposition of the complexes (for review, see [11]). Most of this work has been done in mice since substantial doses of immune complexes (complexes containing 2 to 5 mg of antibodies) are needed to achieve significant deposition in glomeruli. The lattice of the injected complexes, the ability of the involved complexes to form immune precipitates, and the charge of antibodies or antigens influence the deposition and persistence of the immune complexes in mesangial and subendothelial areas. The structural features of glomeruli undoubtedly contribute to some of these findings. The glomerular endothelium has open fenestrations with a diameter of 43.6 ± 9.8 nm in rats [12]. Fixed negative charges exist in the lamina rara interna (subendothelial area) and lamina rara externa (subepithelial area) of the glomerular basement membrane [13]; the latter have rather regular spacing with a distance of 42 ± 12 nm in humans as determined with polyethyleneimine as a cationic probe [14]. In addition, glomeruli are important filtering structures where fluid is removed and macromolecules are retained.

The Role of Lattice of Immune Complexes in Glomerular Deposition

The lattice of immune complexes is defined as the number of antigen and the number of antibody molecules in a given complex. The lattice can be expressed with formulations like Ag_1Ab_1, Ag_2Ab_2, Ag_3Ab_4, and so on.

Several lines of experiments have indicated that small-latticed immune complexes—defined as Ag_1Ab_1, Ag_2Ab_2, or some other combinations with one or two antibodies per complex—do not deposit in renal glomeruli. Large-latticed complexes—defined as containing more than two antibody molecules (that is, greater than Ag_2Ab_2)—have the potential for deposition in glomeruli. *First,* when mixtures of large- and small-latticed immune complexes were administered to mice, glomerular deposition progressed only as long as large-latticed complexes persisted in the circulation [15]. These glomerular deposits declined whereas small-latticed complexes persisted in circulation. When antibodies in the immune complexes were altered to prolong the circulation of large-latticed complexes, then deposition in glomeruli was enhanced. *Second,* when only small-latticed antigen–antibody complexes (Ag_1Ab_1 and mostly Ag_2Ab_2) of the same system were injected into mice, no deposition occurred in glomeruli, even though large amounts of complexes persisted in circulation [16]. *Third,* when in vivo the immune complexes were converted into large antigen excess, the already deposited complexes promptly disappeared from glomeruli [17]. In these experiments, preformed immune complexes were injected into mice and were allowed to form extensive deposits in glomeruli. Twelve hr after the injection of the initial complexes, a large excess of free antigen (for example, a 40-fold antigen excess) was administered, and the persistence of immune deposits in glomeruli was examined. Already by 6 hr after excess antigen injection, most of the deposits had disappeared from glomeruli, and by 12 hr the glomeruli contained no deposits by immuno-fluorescence or electron microscopy. In control mice, however, the extensive deposits persisted. These experiments indicated that the already deposited immune complexes were released from the mesangial and subendothelial areas, when converted in vivo to small-latticed immune complexes.

In the experiments described above and studies reviewed by Couser and Salant [11], the deposits identified by immunofluorescence microscopy were located mostly in the mesangial matrix by electron microscopy. Sequential studies performed after the injection of complexes suggested that a progression occurred from early subendothelial and mesangial deposits to the presence of only mesangial deposits [15]. Of note was that the subendothelial deposits were always adjacent to the mesangium and not in the periphery of the capillary loop. Subepithelial electron-dense deposits were not found during these experiments or by other investigators in similar experiments (reviewed in [11]).

These observations indicate that immune complexes with a lattice of more than two antibody molecules have the potential of deposition from circulation transiently into the subendothelial and more prominently into the mesangial area. The mesangial deposits in these experiments with unaltered antibodies reached a maximum in about 12 hr and then declined and were largely gone by 96 hr [15]. Some hypercellularity of the mesangial area was observed and was due to an influx of monocytes from circulation [18]. The relatively transient presence of preformed immune complexes in the mesangium, the short persistence of protein aggregates in the mesangium (reviewed in [19]), as well as the relatively benign course of predominantly mesangial deposits of immune complexes in chronic serum sickness suggest that effective mechanisms exist for disposal of these deposits. Phagocytosis of mesangial immune deposits by monocytes is one mechanism for their disposal [18]. Endocytosis of protein molecules by resident mesangial cells is well established [20]. Other mechanisms for removal of mesangial immune deposits may exist as well. An abnormality of the mechanisms responsible for disposal of mesangial immune deposits might contribute to the development of extensive subendothelial deposits.

Precipitating Antigen–Antibody Systems Cause Persistence of Immune Complexes in Glomeruli

The electron-dense deposits of immune complexes, as seen on electron microscopy, achieve substantial size in mesangial, subendothelial, and subepithelial areas. The maximum dimension of Fab arms on IgG molecules on high-resolution electron microscopy is about 19 nm [21], whereas the diameters of immune deposits in glomeruli reach several hundred nanometers. The preformed, large-latticed immune complexes injected into mice do not reach such dimensions. This suggested that after the initial deposition in glomeruli, immune complexes rearrange or condense into larger complexes. Proof for this event was obtained in experiments that compared the glomerular deposition of immune complexes with comparable lattice, but in one preparation the lattice was fixed permanently by covalent bonds established between the antigen and the antibody [22]. The covalently cross-linked, soluble, large-latticed immune complexes remained stable in the absence of excess antigen and did not precipitate upon concentration. When the covalently cross-linked and non-cross-linked complexes were injected into mice in identical dosages, both preparations showed comparable deposition in glomeruli by immunofluorescence microscopy at 1 hr after injection. Thereafter, the deposition of the covalently cross-linked complexes declined, and the non-cross-linked complexes increased. Furthermore, the deposits of non-cross-linked complexes became visible as electron-dense deposits in the subendothelial and mesangial areas. On the other hand, the glomerular deposits of cross-linked complexes that were transiently present by immunofluorescence microscopy could not be seen with electron microscopy.

The requirement of precipitating antigen–antibody systems for the persistence of immune deposits and for the formation of electron-dense deposits was also illustrated by another series of experiments [23]. By varying hapten density on a carrier protein molecule, the experimenters were able to create precipitating and nonprecipitating antigen–antibody systems. For this process, they used antibodies to the hapten. The antigens were then cationized to plant them in the glomerular basement membrane, and antibodies specific to the hapten were administered. The antibodies were initially demonstrable in glomeruli by immunofluorescence microscopy for both the precipitating and nonprecipitating systems. After 4 hr, the presence of antibodies and antigen declined in the nonprecipitating systems. On the other hand, with the precipitating antigen–antibody system, the immune deposits persisted by immunofluorescence microscopy and became visible by electron microscopy in the subepithelial area. The transient deposits of antigen and antibody with nonprecipitating systems were not visible as electron-dense deposits.

These experiments indicate that after the initial attachment of immune complexes in the mesangium or on the glomerular basement membrane the complexes undergo further rearrangement or condensation into larger deposits. One factor that would contribute to rearrangement of immune complexes is an increased local concentration. The density of the fixed negative charges may play a crucial role in the initial, local concentration of immune complexes that allows their condensation into larger deposits. The concept of local rearrangement of deposits is supported also by earlier observations of Kubes [24]. When animals were immunized with two antigens identifiable by electron microscopy (ferritin and fibrinogen), single electron-dense deposits contained either fibrinogen or ferritin, not both. If the immune complexes had randomly polymerized into immune deposits in glomeruli, both antigens would have been expected in some deposits.

The Role of Charge on Circulating Immune Complexes on Deposition in Glomeruli

Several investigators have examined the role of charge–charge interactions in the deposition or formation of immune complexes in glomeruli as reviewed by Border in this symposium. The remarks in this section will be limited to observations made with preformed immune complexes.

Gallo, Caulin-Glaser, and Lamm [25] were first to examine the role of charge of immune complexes on deposition in glomeruli, using rabbit antibodies to bovine gamma globulin in mice. They used various combinations of isoelectrically focused antigen, chemically cationized antigen, and isoelectrically focused antibodies. Most of the prepared immune complexes caused mesangial deposits, and capillary loop deposition of immune complexes was found when a chemically cationized antigen was used in immune complexes. This study concentrated on mice examined 1 hr after the administration of immune complexes. The electron-dense deposits decorated the fixed anionic sites both in the lamina rara interna and the lamina rara externa. Electron-dense deposits were not predominantly at the slit pore membrane in the subepithelial areas as seen in other models with planted cationic antigens [26]. The presence of electron-dense deposits principally at the anionic sites in the first cited study most likely is due to the short period of time after injection of immune complexes and the lack of sufficient rearrangement to form immune deposits.

The role of charge on immune complexes was examined in a model system with chemically cationized rabbit antibodies to human serum albumin [27]. Immune complexes prepared and injected at 5-fold antigen excess with the cationized antibodies, containing large-latticed and small-latticed immune complexes, were present at the anionic sites in the lamina rara interna at 1 min and 1 hr after injection with formation of larger subendothelial deposits at the 1-hr time point. At 12 hr and later time points after injection of these complexes, the anionic sites in the lamina rara interna were no longer decorated with electron-dense material, and large subendothelial deposits were present along with mesangial deposits. Only few and small subepithelial deposits were noted. With the injection of the cationized antibodies alone in the same dosage as present in immune complexes, electron-dense deposits decorated the anionic sites at 1 min and 1 hr after injection and were not visualized at later time points. When small-latticed immune complexes, prepared at 50-fold antigen excess with the same cationized antibodies, were injected into mice, immunofluorescence microscopy demonstrated that these immune complexes persisted in glomeruli comparable to cationized antibodies alone.

These experiments with cationized antibodies are consistent with the concept described in the preceding section, suggesting that after the initial interaction with glomerular structures the immune complexes must undergo rearrangement to persist and to become visible as electron-dense deposits in the subendothelial and mesangial areas. The large-latticed immune complexes with cationized antibodies, made at 5-fold antigen excess, would become attached to the anionic sites in the lamina rara interna and result in increased local concentration. As a result of this, the complexes become condensed and after 1 hr become visible as extensive subendothelial and mesangial deposits. Of note is that the immune complexes with cationized antibodies constitute the first model of preformed immune complexes with persistence of extensive subendothelial deposits. In contrast, when complexes made at 50-fold antigen excess were injected, these also were transiently attached to the glomerular basement membrane. Owing to the very large amount of antigen present in circulation, these complexes were not able to rearrange or condense into larger deposits. The mechanisms that remove cationic macromolecules from the anionic sites in the glomerular basement membrane are not known at this time.

Large-latticed, preformed immune complexes with chemically cationized antibodies caused extensive immune deposits in the subendothelial and mesangial areas, as described above. Therefore, it became of interest to see if immune complexes with chemically anionized antibodies but with comparable lattice would deposit in glomeruli. When such preparations were injected into mice, the pattern of deposition with immune complexes made with chemically anionized antibodies was comparable to the deposits seen with complexes prepared with unaltered antibodies of comparable lattice [28]. By electron microscopy, the deposits were in the mesangial matrix. These studies indicate that the deposition of immune complexes in the mesangium does not depend on charge–charge interactions. The mechanisms involved in mesangial deposition of immune complexes or other large protein aggregates remain unknown [19].

Deposition of Preformed IgA Immune Complexes in Glomeruli

The study of experimental models with IgA immune complexes has considerable relevance to human IgA nephropathy and helps to clarify the mechanisms of glomerular deposition of these immune complexes. The use of discrete sizes of dextran molecules, ranging in mol wt from 10,000 to 500,000 daltons, with cationic, neutral, and anionic isoelectric points as antigens for serum sickness resulted in production of IgA antibodies and IgA deposition in glomeruli [29]. Furthermore, the deposits were primarily in the mesangium, and no subepithelial deposits were found, even though the study used cationized dextrans with average mol wts of 10,000, 70,000, and 500,000 daltons. The reasons for these differences as compared to protein antigens remain to be determined.

Dextrans of the same sizes and isoelectric points were used to prepare preformed immune complexes with IgA antibodies specific to 1,6-linked dextrans, produced by a mouse myeloma cell line [30]. Soluble immune complexes were prepared at 40-fold antigen excess with nine different dextran antigens, three sizes at each isoelectric point, and injected into mice. The deposition in glomeruli was examined only 18 hr after injection of the IgA immune complexes. Varying degrees of mesangial deposition were found with all preparations. Subendothelial deposits were present only with the 10,000-dalton cationized dextran. In this study the possible effects of clearance from circulation of the immune complexes prepared with the dextrans were not examined in relation to the degree of glomerular deposition.

Both of the described models, using dextran antigens and IgA class of antibodies, hold considerable promise for further elucidation of the mechanisms involved in the deposition of IgA immune complexes in glomeruli.

Role of Rheumatoid Factors and Anti-Idiotypic Antibodies in Glomerular Deposition of Circulating Immune Complexes

Rheumatoid factor activity has been demonstrated in glomeruli of patients with systemic lupus erythematosus and in other patients with chronic glomerulonephritis, by using fluoresceinated, aggregated IgG on tissue sections. In several experimental models of immune complex deposition, the injection of human IgM rheumatoid factors resulted in glomerular deposition of human IgM (reviewed in [31]). Furthermore, once the IgM rheumatoid factors were present in glomeruli of mice, additional circulating immune complexes were able to localize in glomeruli, presumably because of free combining sites on the IgM rheumatoid factors already bound to the glomeruli. IgM rheumatoid factors are antibodies specific to the Fc portion of the IgG molecule. Owing to their valence of 5, they bind firmly to polymeric IgG. The latter can be achieved either by nonspecific aggregation or by formation of immune complexes. In the circulation of patients, IgM rheumatoid factors are complexed with normal, monomeric IgG, but by weak interactions. When immune complexes with IgG are present in glomeruli and accessible to the IgM rheumatoid factor, the latter will dissociate from normal IgG and bind to the polymeric IgG in glomerular deposits. This occurs in experimental models as described above and may well occur in human diseases.

Another area of considerable interest is the role of auto-anti-idiotypic antibodies in glomerular deposition of circulating immune complexes. The presence of these antibodies has been demonstrated in two experimental models [32, 33]. The auto-anti-idiotypic antibodies could have opposing effects on glomerular deposition of antigen–antibody systems. On one hand, as previously suggested [33], the auto-anti-idiotypic antibodies could combine with the antigen–antibody complexes in circulation or in glomeruli and increase thereby the size and the pathogenicity of the complexes. On the other hand, one study has shown that specific antibodies and anti-idiotypic antibodies can form stable dimers owing to monogamous bivalent interaction [34]. Such complexes might not deposit in renal glomeruli. Furthermore, the formation of thermodynamically stable complexes between the specific antibodies and auto-anti-idiotypic antibodies might disrupt the already formed, large antigen–antibody deposits in glomeruli.

Do Circulating Immune Complexes Form Subepithelial Immune Deposits?

In chronic serum sickness models, subepithelial immune deposits develop in some animals, particularly when associated with the presence of relatively small, circulating immune complexes [35]. It was assumed that the relatively small immune complexes passed through the glomerular basement membrane and formed immune deposits in the subepithelial area. The finding that in a number of experiments with passive administration of immune complexes no subepithelial deposits evolved indicated that other mechanisms may be responsible for the formation of these deposits [11]. Local immune complex formation with development of subepithelial deposits has been documented with antibodies to endogenous antigens [36, 37], by alternating the administration of antigen and antibody [38] and by planting of cationic antigens [26]. In view of the available data and concepts, it is possible that with chronic antigen administration, particularly when relatively low-affinity antibodies are produced, an alternating presence of free antibodies and free antigens is reproduced, leading to local immune deposit formation in the subepithelial area. Alternatively, small immune complexes may pass through the lamina densa and condense to large deposits in the lamina rara externa. In considering these possibilities, one would suppose that the lamina densa most likely will limit the size of complexes that can pass to the lamina rara externa. For example, cationized horse spleen ferritin was able to pass through the lamina densa, but cationized human IgM was not able to reach this area [39]. These findings suggest that the limiting molecular size is between 400,000 and 900,000 daltons. For comparison, the size of immune complexes with albumin and IgG class of antibodies is 212,000 daltons for Ag_1Ab_1 and 424,000 daltons for Ag_2Ab_2. In addition, a precipitating antigen–antibody system is needed for the development of electron-dense deposits in the subepithelial area [23].

As already pointed out, the administration of preformed immune complexes with albumin and IgG antibodies and containing large-latticed complexes (greater than Ag_2Ab_2) caused mesangial and transient subendothelial deposits, but no subepithelial deposits. The size of the complexes greater than Ag_2Ab_2 may prevent their passage through the lamina densa. The injection of only small-latticed immune complexes with the same system caused no glomerular deposition, including the absence of subepithelial deposits. If these small-latticed (Ag_1Ab_1 and Ag_2Ab_2) complexes passed through the lamina densa, their condensation into larger lattices and electron-dense deposits could have been prevented by the presence of a large amount of free antigen. Thus, these experiments do not exclude the possibility of small complexes reaching the lamina rara externa.

One set of well-conducted experiments concluded that small-latticed immune complexes, prepared with low-avidity antibodies, were able to form subepithelial immune deposits [40, 41]. In these studies, high-avidity and low-avidity antibodies to ovalbumin (mol wt, 40,000) were prepared in rabbits. Soluble immune complexes were formed at 80-fold antigen excess and repeatedly administered to mice. The complexes prepared with high-avidity antibodies resulted in mesangial deposits, whereas complexes prepared with low-avidity antibodies resulted in subepithelial deposits. This difference was initially attributed to the differences in avidity, and it was suggested that the small complexes passed through the lamina densa. Alternative explanations, however, exist for these findings. Owing to the small size, ovalbumin is quickly removed from circulation, thus diminishing the degree of antigen excess. With the high-avidity antibodies, larger lattices would form by loss of the excess antigen, causing mesangial deposition. With the low-avidity antibodies, free antibody would be present in circulation, thus creating the possibility of local immune complex formation by the alternating presence of antigen and antibody [38]. Subsequent studies with these immune complexes indeed suggested that local immune complex formation may have occurred [42].

In detailed studies with cationized horse spleen ferritin and antibodies to this protein, an interesting possibility was raised [39]. In sequential studies, immune deposits were first seen in the subendothelial area when the cationized ferritin was injected and followed by specific antibodies. With passage of time, subepithelial deposits increased as subendothelial deposits diminished. These observations suggested that with passage of time, the subendothelial deposits dissociated and the antibodies alone or in the form of small immune complexes passed through the lamina densa to form large deposits in the subepithelial area where the cationized ferritin had bound to the fixed anionic sites.

Caulin-Glaser, Gallo, and Lamm examined the possibility that covalently cross-linked immune complexes might pass through the lamina densa of the mouse glomerular capillary wall [43]. Bovine IgG and rabbit IgG antibodies were used. The antigen to be used or the prepared complexes were cationized to assure localization in the glomeruli. The immune complexes were made at 70-fold antigen excess. The covalent cross-linking was accomplished with toluene-2,4-diisocyanate, which establishes covalent bonds between adjacent molecules but not necessarily in the antibody-combining site. The cross-linked complexes were gel filtered, and only a heterogeneous pool of relatively large complexes was used for injection into mice. By sedimentation velocity ultracentrifugation, the average sedimentation coefficient was 28S. One hour after the injection of 1 mg of these complexes, mice were sacrificed. By electron microscopy, the injected material decorated the anionic sites in the lamina rara interna and the lamina rara externa. Furthermore, with immunoelectron microscopy, rabbit IgG was present in lamina rara interna, lamina densa, and lamina rara externa in mice given immune complexes made with cationized antigen, unaltered antibodies, and cross-linked after the formation of complexes. These data indicate that immune complexes can pass through the glomerular basement membrane to reach the subepithelial area. Some uncertainty, however, remains in that the injected complexes were heterogeneous in size. As already discussed, one would expect that large complexes could not pass through the lamina densa and only small complexes might reach the subepithelial area.

In view of the available data, the possibilities for formation of subepithelial immune deposits include the following: (a) antigen or antibody may reach the subepithelial area alone and then combine with the other reactant to form immune deposits; (b) circulating immune complexes may bind to the lamina rara interna and then dissociate and migrate through the lamina densa individually to reform in the subepithelial area; and (c) small-latticed immune complexes may pass through the lamina densa and form large immune deposits in the subepithelial area. Future work should clarify if some or all of these mechanisms are operative in the genesis of subepithelial deposits of immune complexes.

References

1. WILSON CB, DIXON FJ: The renal response to immunological injury, in *The Kidney*, edited by BRENNER BM, RECTOR FC JR, Philadelphia, WB Saunders, 1981, pp 1237–1350
2. MANNIK M: Pathophysiology of circulating immune complexes. *Arthritis Rheum* 25:783–787, 1982
3. DOWER SK, DELISI C, TITUS JA, SEGAL DM: Mechanism of binding of multivalent immune complexes to Fc receptors: 1. Equilibrium binding. *Biochemistry* 20:6326–6334, 1981
4. RIFAI A, MANNIK M: Clearance kinetics and fate of mouse IgA immune complexes prepared with monomeric or dimeric IgA. *J Immunol* 130:1826–1832, 1983
5. FINBLOOM DS, MAGILAVY DB, HARTFORD JB, RIFAI A, PLOTZ PH: The influence of antigen on immune complex behavior in mice. *J Clin Invest* 68:214–224, 1981
6. EMLEN W, MANNIK M: Clearance of circulating DNA-antiDNA immune complexes in mice. *J Exp Med* 155:1210–1215, 1982
7. FRANK MM: Immunoglobulin G Fc receptor-mediated clearance in autoimmune diseases. *Ann Intern Med* 98:206–218, 1983
8. CORNACOFF JB, HEBERT LA, SMEAD WL, VANAMAN ME, BIRMINGHAM DJ, WAXMAN FJ: Primate erythrocyte-immune complex-clearing mechanism. *J Clin Invest* 71:236–247, 1983

9. MANNIK M, AREND WP: Fate of preformed immune complexes in rabbits and rhesus monkeys. *J Exp Med* 134:19s–31s, 1971

10. WILSON CB, DIXON FJ: Quantitation of acute and chronic serum sickness in the rabbit. *J Exp Med* 134:7s–18s, 1971

11. COUSER WG, SALANT DJ: In situ immune complex formation and glomerular injury. *Kidney Int* 17:1–13, 1980

12. BULGER RE, EKNOYAN G, PURCELL DJ, DOBYAN DC: Endothelial characteristics of glomerular capillaries in normal, mercuric chloride-induced, and gentamicin-induced acute renal failure in the rat. *J Clin Invest* 72:128–141, 1983

13. KANAWAR YS, FARQUHAR MG: Anionic sites in the glomerular basement membrane: In vivo and in vitro localization of the lamina rarae by cationic probes. *J Cell Biol* 81:137–153, 1979

14. VERNIER RL, KLEIN DJ, SISSON SP, MAHAN JD, OEGEMA TR, BROWN DM: Heparan sulfate-rich anionic sites in the human glomerular basement membrane: Decreased concentration in congenital nephrotic syndrome. *N Engl J Med* 309:1001–1009, 1983

15. HAAKENSTAD AO, STRIKER GE, MANNIK M: The glomerular deposition of soluble immune complexes prepared with reduced and alkylated antibodies and with intact antibodies in mice. *Lab Invest* 35:293–301, 1976

16. HAAKENSTAD AO, STRIKER GE, MANNIK M: The disappearance kinetics and glomerular deposition of small-latticed soluble immune complexes. *Immunology* 47:407–414, 1982

17. MANNIK M, STRIKER GE: Removal of glomerular deposits of immune complexes in mice by administration of excess antigen. *Lab Invest* 42:483–489, 1980

18. STRIKER GE, MANNIK M, TUNG MY: Role of marrow-derived monocytes and mesangial cells in removal of immune complexes from renal glomeruli. *J Exp Med* 149:127–136, 1979

19. MICHAEL AF, KEANE WF, RAIJ L, VERNIER RL, MAUER SM: The glomerular mesangium. *Kidney Int* 17:141–154, 1980

20. FARQUHAR MG, PALADE GE: Functional evidence for the existence of a third cell type in the renal glomerulus: Phagocytosis of filtration residues by a "distinctive third" cell. *J Cell Biol* 13:55–87, 1962

21. SEEGAN GW, SMITH CA, SCHUMAKER VN: Changes in quarternary structure of IgG upon reduction of the interheavy-chain disulfide bond. *Proc Natl Acad Sci USA* 76:907–911, 1979

22. MANNIK M, AGODOA LYC, DAVID KA: Rearrangement of immune complexes in glomeruli leads to persistence and development of electron dense deposits. *J Exp Med* 157:1516–1528, 1983

23. AGODOA LYC, GAUTHIER VJ, MANNIK M: Precipitating antigen-antibody systems are required for the formation of subepithelial electron dense immune deposits in rat glomeruli. *J Exp Med* 158:1259–1271, 1983

24. KUBES L: Experimental immune complex glomerulonephritis in the mouse with two types of immune complexes. *Virchows Arch [Cell Pathol]* 24:343–354, 1977

25. GALLO GR, CAULIN-GLASER T, LAMM ME: Charge of circulating immune complexes as a factor in glomerular basement membrane localization in mice. *J Clin Invest* 67:1305–1313, 1981

26. OITE T, BATSFORD SR, MIHATSCH MJ, TAKAMIYA H, VOGT A: Quantitative studies of in situ immune complex glomerulonephritis in the rat induced by planted, cationized antigen. *J Exp Med* 155:460–474, 1982

27. GAUTHIER VJ, MANNIK M, STRIKER GE: Effect of cationized antibodies in preformed immune complexes on deposition and persistence in renal glomeruli. *J Exp Med* 156:766–777, 1982

28. GAUTHIER VJ, STRIKER GE, MANNIK M: Glomerular localization of immune complexes prepared with anionic antibodies or with cationic antigen. *Lab Invest,* in press

29. ISAACS KL, MILLER F: Role of antigen size and charge in immune complex glomerulonephritis: I. Active induction of disease with dextran and its derivatives. *Lab Invest* 47:198–205, 1982

30. ISAACS KL, MILLER F: Antigen size and charge in immune complex glomerulonephritis: II. Passive induction of immune deposits with dextran-anti-dextran immune complexes. *Am J Pathol* 111:298–306, 1983

31. FORD PM: Interaction of rheumatoid factor with immune complexes in experimental glomerulonephritis: Possible role of antiglobulins in chronicity. *J Rheumatol* 10(Suppl 11):81–84, 1983

32. GOLDMAN M, ROSE LM, HOCHMANN A, LAMBERT PH: Deposition of idiotype-anti-idiotype immune complexes in renal glomeruli after polyclonal B cell activation. *J Exp Med* 155:1385–1399, 1982

33. ZANETTI M, WILSON CB: Participation of auto-anti-idiotypes in immune complex glomerulonephritis in rabbits. *J Immunol* 131:2781–2783, 1983

34. ROUX KJ, METZGER DW: Immunoelectron microscopic localization of idiotypes and allotypes on immunoglobulin molecules. *J Immunol* 129:2548–2553, 1982

35. GERMUTH FG JR, RODRIGUEZ E: *Immunopathology of the Renal Glomerulus.* Boston, Little, Brown and Co, 1973

36. VAN DAMME BJC, FLEUREN GJ, BAKKER WW, VERNIER RL, HOEDEMAEKER PJ: Experimental glomerulonephritis in the rat induced by antibodies directed against tubular antigens: V. Fixed glomerular antigens in the pathogenesis of heterologous immune complex glomerulonephritis. *Lab Invest* 38:502–510, 1978

37. COUSER WG, STEINMULLER DR, STILMENT MM, SALANT DJ, LOWENSTEIN LH: Experimental glomerulonephritis in the isolated perfused rat kidney. *J Clin Invest* 62:1275–1287, 1978

38. FLEUREN G, GROUD J, HOEDEMAEKER PJ: In situ formation of subepithelial glomerular immune complexes in passive serum sickness. *Kidney Int* 17:631–637, 1980

39. VOGT A, ROHRBACH R, SHIMIZU F, TAKAMIYA H, BATSFORD S: Interaction of cationized antigen with rat glomerular basement membrane: In situ immune complex formation. *Kidney Int* 22:27–35, 1982

40. GERMUTH FG JR, RODRIGUEZ E, LORELLE CA, TRUMP EI, MILANO L, WISE O'L: Passive immune complex glomerulonephritis in mice: Models for various lesions found in human disease: I. High avidity complexes and mesangiopathic glomerulonephritis. *Lab Invest* 41:360–365, 1979

41. GERMUTH FG JR, RODRIGUEZ E, LORELLE CA, TRUMP EI, MILANO LL, WISE O'L: Passive immune complex glomerulonephritis in mice: Models for various lesions found in human disease: II. Low avidity complexes and diffuse proliferative glomerulonephritis with subepithelial deposits. *Lab Invest* 41:366–371, 1979

42. GERMUTH FG JR, RODRIGUEZ E, WISE O'L: Passive immune complex glomerulonephritis in mice: III. Clearance kinetics and properties of circulating complexes. *Lab Invest* 46:515–519, 1982

43. CAULIN-GLASER T, GALLO GR, LAMM ME: Nondissociating cationic immune complexes can deposit in glomerular basement membrane. *J Exp Med* 158:1561–1572, 1983

Etiologic Factors in Immunologically Mediated Glomerulonephritis

Philip J. Hoedemaeker, Gert J. Fleuren,
and Jan J. Weening

The rationale of the study of experimental glomerulonephritis is to learn and to understand the etiologic factors and pathogenetic mechanisms that may also operate in human kidney disease.

It is now generally accepted that binding of antibodies to antigens presenting along or within the glomerular capillary wall can result in either an anti-GBM glomerulonephritis or an immune complex glomerulopathy; the latter especially in forms that are associated with the development of epimembranous immune aggregates [1].

The antigens involved in these models belong to either the antigenic structure of the glomerular basement membrane (GBM) as in the heterologous phase of nephrotoxic serum nephritis (NSN) [2] or the glomerular capillary cells as in Heymann nephritis [3, 4]; or, they are not related to intrinsic capillary wall antigens, but have been planted there from the circulation. Subsequently, antibodies may bind to these antigens, as in autologous phase NSN, passive serum sickness glomerulopathy [5, 6], or con-A glomerulonephritis [7]. When antigens belong to the intrinsic antigenic structure of the glomerulus, the glomerulonephritis resulting from the binding of antibodies to these antigens has to be regarded as an *autoimmune* glomerulonephritis. Induction of this type of glomerulonephritis requires termination of tolerance to these autoantigens. In experimental studies, this usually is achieved by (hyper)immunization of the animals with the antigens involved. This procedure may result either in fulminant glomerulonephritis with a rapid deterioration of renal function and death of the animals [8] or in no disease at all [9], depending on the species used.

In Heymann nephritis, the animals initially develop membranous glomerulopathy in which an autoantigen is involved that is present on cell membranes of several organs that are associated with absorption and excretion [10],

This manuscript was presented as part of a Symposium on *Mechanisms of Immune Complex Formation and Deposition in Glomeruli.*

and also along the visceral glomerular epithelial cell surface [11]. In the majority of cases, this membranous glomerulopathy is self-limited, and the autoallergic reaction against the glomerulotubular antigen wanes [12]. Apart from autoantibody activity, changes in cellular immunity have also been described in Heymann nephritis [13]; however, it is uncertain whether these changes bear any pathogenetic significance or merely represent an epiphenomenon.

In addition to (hyper)immunization resulting in cross-reacting antibodies or in termination of tolerance, a genetically determined defect in immunoregulation seems to be important in the pathogenesis of autoimmune disease. This is consistent with the fact that certain rat strains are susceptible to induction of autoimmune diseases, including membranous glomerulopathy, while others are not [14]. In several mice strains suffering from SLE-like disease, immune dysregulation has been demonstrated, which results in uncontrolled expression of autoreactive B lymphocytes [15].

In this chapter, two approaches leading to a disturbance of immunoregulation and immunologically mediated glomerulonephritis will be discussed:

1. Chronic administration of small quantities of $HgCl_2$ to certain susceptible strains of rats results in autoallergic phenomena, including glomerulonephritis, through polyclonal stimulation of B lymphocytes [16].
2. Administration of parental lymphocytes to F1 hybrids results in polyclonal stimulation of B lymphocytes leading to autoallergic phenomena, including glomerulonephritis as a part of an allogeneic disease [17, 18]. It is further demonstrated that both procedures can result in either anti-GBM nephritis or membranous glomerulopathy.

Methods

Mercuric chloride glomerulopathy was induced in Brown Norway (BN), PVG/c, Lewis (Lew), and Lewis/Brown Norway (Lew/BN) F1 hybrid rats.

The rats were given 0.1 to 0.2 mg $HgCl_2$/100 g body wt via alternate-day subcutaneous injections for at least 8 weeks. Allogeneic disease or graft versus host reaction (GvHR) was induced in Lew/BN, AO/BN, and AO/Lew F1 hybrids with one injection containing 3.5×10^8 thoracic duct lymphocytes (TDL) from either Lew or AO rats, with or without pretreatment of the animals with complete Freund adjuvant. Groups of rats were sacrificed at 2-week intervals. The maximal observation period was 16 weeks. Proteinuria was measured every other day in urine collected during 24 hr by using the biuret method. At the time of sacrifice, kidney specimens were processed for light microscopy, immunofluorescence, and electron microscopy. Kidney specimens were used for elution studies by using the two-step method of Bartolotti [19]. Serum samples were tested for the presence of autoantibodies by using indirect immunofluorescence on normal rat tissues.

Results

Mercuric Chloride (HgCl₂) Glomerulopathy

Administration of HgCl$_2$ to BN rats resulted in heavy proteinuria in all animals after 12 to 14 days. Marked lymphadenopathy and splenomegaly was found. Light microscopy of kidney specimens showed no abnormalities. Immunofluorescence revealed a linear distribution of IgG and C3 along the glomerular capillary walls (Fig. 1). Electron microscopy revealed a widespread fusion of epithelial cell foot processes.

Notwithstanding continuation of mercury administration, proteinuria subsided after 23 days (Fig. 2)—at which time the immunofluorescent pattern in the glomeruli had changed from *linear* to *granular* and electron microscopy revealed electron-dense aggregates exclusively localized at the epithelial side of the GBM.

In the PVG/c rats, administration of HgCl$_2$ did not result in significant proteinuria. After 8 weeks, a membranous glomerulopathy had developed that was associated with a granular pattern of IgG deposits along the glomerular capillary walls. In electron microscopy, the aggregates were found subepithelially [20].

In these animals, the renal lesions were associated with circulating antinu-

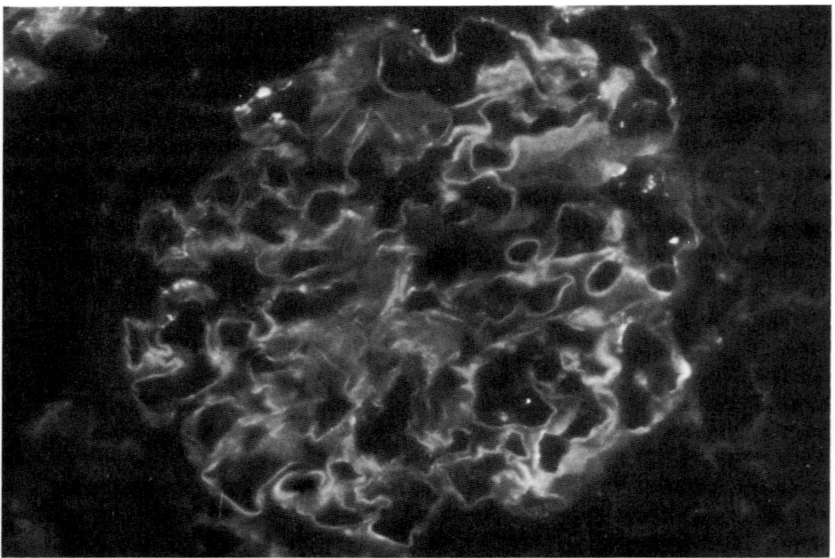

Fig. 1. Immunofluorescence micrograph showing linear staining of rat IgG along the glomerular and tubular basement membranes of a Brown Norway rat with HgCl$_2$ nephrosis at day 15 (×400).

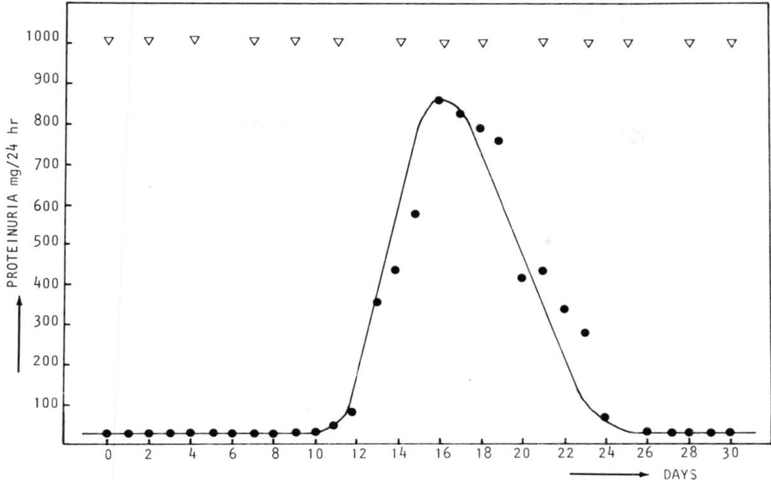

Fig. 2. 24-hr urine protein excretion in a Brown Norway rat during alternate-day HgCl₂ administration (∇). ∇, 0.2 mg HgCl₂ per 100 g body wt.

clear antibodies (ANA). Elution studies showed that the mercury-induced ANA were present in the glomerular-bound immune aggregates. The ANA activity was found to be directed against nonhistone nucleoprotein [21].

Administration of HgCl₂ to Lew rats did not result in renal lesions or proteinuria. Lew/BN F1 hybrids reacted the same as the BN rats to the administration of HgCl₂.

Allogeneic Disease

Administration of 1 to 2×10^8 parental TDL from Lew or AO rats to Lew/BN and AO/BN F1 hybrids respectively resulted in a chronic GvHR. A variety of autoantibodies were found that were directed against nuclear proteins, renal tubular epithelial (RTE) antigens, tubular basement membranes, and collecting duct cells.

A faint binding of autologous IgG along the GBM could be observed. No proliferative changes were found in the glomeruli, and proteinuria did not occur.

In the animals pretreated with complete Freund's adjuvant, the induction of GvHR, using 2.0 to 3.5×10^8 TDL, resulted in a heavy linear deposition of IgG along the GBM and occasionally in the mesangial area. In these animals, a transient proteinuria was noted that started on day 16, reaching levels as high as 600 mg/24 hr, and disappeared after day 23. IgG eluted from the kidneys of these animals bound to normal GBM in a linear pattern.

AO/LEW F1 hybrids injected with parental TDL from AO did not show renal binding of autoantibodies, and no proteinuria was observed in these animals.

Discussion

Chronic administration of $HgCl_2$ and induction of a GvHR led to strikingly similar autoallergic phenomena in rats.

In both cases, polyclonal stimulation of B lymphocytes resulted in autoantibody formation, anti-GBM nephritis, lymphadenopathy, and splenomegaly [22, 23]. Both procedures resulted in transient proteinuria, starting on day 16 and disappearing on day 23 (Fig. 2). Moreover, evidence was presented that incompatibility with BN rats seemed to be necessary for the development of anti-GBM nephritis as part of the allogeneic disease. Using both procedures, Lew rats seemed to be refractory for the development of these lesions.

Renal lesions following chronic administration of $HgCl_2$ have been studied extensively. In 1971, Bariéty et al [24] described a membranous glomerulopathy in outbred Wistar rats during chronic administration of $HgCl_2$. Druet et al [25] and Weening [26] extended these observations in several other rat strains and found that the susceptibility for the induction of glomerulonephritis by mercury is genetically restricted [26–29]. As reviewed recently [25, 26], rat strains can be divided into three groups as far as their susceptibility for the induction of mercury nephritis is concerned:

1. BN rats bearing the RT1n haplotype develop antibodies directed against glomerular and tubular basement membranes, which results in anti-GBM nephritis with massive proteinuria [30].
2. Several strains of rats bearing various RT1 haplotypes, such as the Wistar and the PVG/c rat, develop an immune complex glomerulopathy associated with ANA—usually without or with low proteinuria [29, 31].
3. Rat strains bearing the RT1l or RT1u haplotypes were found to be resistant to the development of glomerulonephritis upon mercury administration [28].

Susceptibility for the renal lesions seems to be determined primarily by the interaction of mercury with immunocompetent cells, since susceptibility can be induced in resistant Lew rats via transfer of immunocompetent cells from moderately susceptible Lew/BN rats [31]. The GBM antigen involved in the mercury-induced anti-GBM antibody response is present in both susceptible and resistant rats [27].

A normal BN rat kidney transplanted into a proteinuric rat during the first phase of the disease has been shown to bind IgG in a linear pattern along the GBM; however, when transplanted into a host after disappearance of proteinuria, the graft will develop subepithelial immune aggregates [32] that resemble Heymann nephritis. This sequence of anti-GBM nephritis followed by immune complex glomerulopathy has also been reported in New Zealand White rabbits that were exposed to mercury [33].

Anti-GBM antibodies have also been reported in BN rats that were treated with D-penicillamine [34]; whereas most rat strains are resistant to the induction of autologous anti-GBM nephritis, the BN rat seems to be an exception [35].

Mercury-induced anti-GBM nephritis in the BN rat is associated with lymphadenopathy, splenomegaly, high serum IgE levels, and low-titered antinuclear antibodies directed against single-stranded DNA [36, 37]. The production of autoantibodies against basement membrane and nuclear antigens in this model can be explained by a direct effect of the metal on lymphocytes and macrophages, as demonstrated in drug-induced autoimmune reactions in humans [38, 39].

In this way, $HgCl_2$ may interfere with immune regulation. This type of mechanism is supported by recent studies in PVG/c and BN rats [22, 37]. In vitro spontaneous- and mitogen-induced T-cell proliferation and suppressor cell function were found to be significantly reduced in mercury-treated rats [22]. In addition, neonatal thymectomy, which lowered suppressor cell population, enhanced mercury-induced disease [22] in a manner similar to that found after neonatal thymectomy in mice with spontaneous autoimmune disease [40].

A polyclonal activation of B cells and a striking increase in serum IgE levels were reported in mercury-diseased BN rats [37]. Recently, increased suppressor cell function was demonstrated in convalescent BN rats that were in the postproteinuric phase of mercury nephrosis [41]. Administration of lymphocytes from convalescent animals prevented mercury-induced disease in BN rats, which suggests a crucial role for suppressor cells in the "spontaneous" recovery of the animals [41].

Allogeneic disease results in various autoallergic phenomena, such as antibodies directed against single-stranded DNA, erythrocytes, and a hyperplasia of lymphoid tissues. Gleichmann et al [17] demonstrated that in selected parent-F1 hybrid combinations in mice, the GvHR was associated with an epimembranous glomerulonephritis, provided that donor and recipient differed at histocompatibility loci controlled by the MHC-complex [23]. In these cases, eluted antibodies from the glomeruli are directed against nuclear proteins and murine leukemia virus [42]. Some of these antibodies may be of pathogenetic significance in the resulting glomerulonephritis [43].

A GvHR is either associated with hypoplasia of the lymphoreticular tissues—and with hypogammaglobulinemia and aplastic anemia (acute GvHR)—or with stimulating phenomena, including polyclonal stimulation and autoantibody formation (chronic GvHR); this depends on the selection of parent F1 hybrid combination and the amount of TDL used for the induction of the disease. In chronic GvHR, the production of autoantibodies is thought to result from a stimulation of autoreactive B cells by allogeneic helper cells [23].

As with mercury-induced glomerulonephritis, the GvHR resulted in a transient proteinuria, although a change in glomerular fluorescence pattern to a granular distribution in the postproteinuric phase was not observed. To try to induce a more chronic renal lesion, we searched for a parent-F1 combination as well as an amount of parent lymphocytes that would result in a more continuous polyclonal stimulation and in a chronic glomerulopathy.

rats resulted, after 8 months, in a clear membranous glomerulopathy (Fig. 3) that was associated with a constant proteinuria with a maximum of 180 mg/24 hr.

The antigens involved in the GvHR-induced anti-GBM nephritis and membranous glomerulopathy have not yet been identified, but they presumably are autoantigens. This finding indicates that a chronic polyclonal stimulation of B cells may result in a membranous glomerulopathy that is associated with proteinuria. This situation may be induced by changes on lymphocyte membranes, particularly of MHC-coded class I and class II antigens that are induced either by drugs [17, 44] or by viral infections, which results in immune dysregulation and (probably) in a situation comparable to a chronic GvHR.

Conclusions

Mercuric chloride administration as well as GvHR have been shown to induce autoimmune phenomena and glomerulonephritis in several strains of rats. The response seems to be genetically restricted. The renal lesions are accompanied by T- and B-cell abnormalities, including a reduction in suppressor

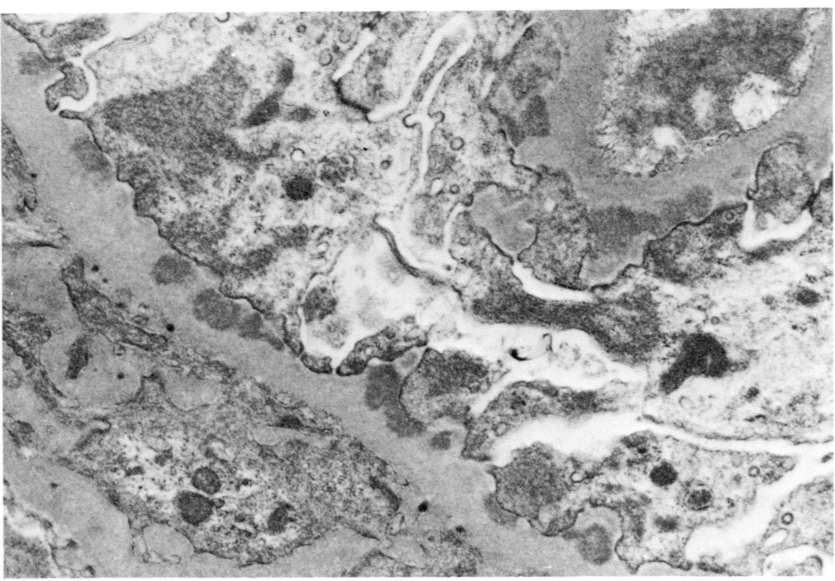

Fig. 3. Electron micrograph of a glomerulus of a rat with chronic allogeneic disease showing immune aggregates along the epithelial side of the GBM (uranyl nitrate, lead citrate, ×40,500).

cell function, polyclonal stimulation, lymphadenopathy, and splenomegaly. Possibly, mercury binds to lymphocytes and induces abnormal lymphocyte interactions that lead to autoimmune reactions. In GvHR, an allogeneic stimulation of helper lymphocytes might result in autoantibody production [42].

In humans, these mechanisms, induced either by drugs [44] or by virus infections [45], may play an important role in the etiology and pathogenesis of glomerulonephritis.

References

1. CAMERON JS: Pathogenesis and treatment of membranous nephropathy. *Kidney Int* 15:88–103, 1979
2. ALLISON MEM, WILSON CB, GOTTSCHALK CW: Pathophysiology of experimental glomerulonephritis in rats. *J Clin Invest* 53:1402–1423, 1974
3. DAMME BJC VAN, FLEUREN GJ, BAKKER WW, VERNIER RL, HOEDEMAEKER PHJ: Experimental glomerulonephritis in the rat induced by antibodies directed against tubular antigens. V. Fixed glomerular antigens in the pathogenesis of heterologous immune complex glomerulonephritis. *Lab Invest* 38:502–510, 1978
4. COUSER WG, STEINMULLER DR, STILMANT MM, SALANT DJ, LOWENSTEIN LM: Experimental glomerulonephritis in the isolated perfused rat kidney. *J Clin Invest* 62:1275–1287, 1978
5. FLEUREN GJ, GROND J, HOEDEMAEKER PHJ: In situ formation of subepithelial glomerular immune complexes in passive serum sickness. *Kidney Int* 17:631–637, 1980
6. BORDER WA, WARD H, KAMIL E, COHEN AH: Induction of membranous nephropathy in rabbits by administration of an exogenous cationic antigen. Demonstration of a pathogenic role for electrical charge. *J Clin Invest* 69:451–461, 1982
7. GOLBUS SM, WILSON CB: Experimental glomerulonephritis induced by in situ formation of immune complexes in glomerular capillary wall. *Kidney Int* 16:148–157, 1979
8. STEBLAY RW, RUDOFSKY UH: Experimental autoimmune antiglomerular basement membrane antibody-induced glomerulonephritis. I. The effects of injecting sheep with human, homologous or autologous lung basement membranes and complete Freund's adjuvant. *Clin Immunol Immunopath* 27:65–80, 1983
9. FLEUREN GJ, HOEDEMAEKER PHJ: Experimental anti-basement membrane renal disease: A linear glomerular and tubular immunofluorescence pattern caused by antibodies directed against endothelial antigens (*abstract*). *Proc 8th Int Congr Nephrol* Athens, 1981
10. MIETTINEN A, LINDER E: Membrane antigens shared by renal proximal tubules and other epithelia associated with absorption and excretion. *Clin Exp Immunol* 23:568–577, 1976
11. KERJASCHKI D, FARQUHAR GM: The pathogenetic antigen of Heymann nephritis in a membrane glycoprotein of the renal proximal tubule brush border. *Proc Natl Acad Sci USA* 79:5557–5561, 1982
12. FLEUREN GJ, GROND J, HOEDEMAEKER PHJ: The pathogenetic role of free-circulating antibody in autologous immune complex glomerulonephritis. *Clin Exp Immunol* 41:205–217, 1980
13. LITWIN A, ADAMS LE, LEVY R, CLINE S, HESS EV: Cellular immunity in experimental glomerulonephritis of rats. I. Delayed hypersensitivity and lymphocyte stimulation studies with renal tubular antigens. *Immunology* 20:755–766, 1971

14. STENGLEIN B, THOENES GH, GUNTHER E: Genetically controlled autologous immune complex glomerulonephritis in rats. *J Immunol* 115:895–897, 1975
15. NEILSON EG, ZAKHEIM B: T cell regulation, anti-idiotypic immunity, and the nephritogenic immune response. *Kidney Int* 24:289–303, 1983
16. DRUET P, BERNARD A, HIRSCH F, WEENING JJ, GENGOUX P, MAHIEU P, BIRKELAND S: Immunologically mediated glomerulonephritis induced by heavy metals. *Arch Toxicol* 50:187–194, 1982
17. GLEICHMANN H, GLEICHMANN E, ANDRE-SCHWARTZ J, SCHWARTZ RS: Chronic allogenic disease. III. Genetic requirements for the induction of glomerulonephritis. *J Exp Med* 135:516–532, 1972
18. FLEUREN GJ, HOEDEMAEKER PhJ, DE VRIES L, NIEUWENHUIS P: Graft-versus-host reaction in rats: Development of anti-kidney antibodies and glomerulonephritis. *Nieren- und Hochdruck Krankheiten* 12:361, 1983
19. BARTOLOTTI SR: Quantitative elution studies in experimental immune complex and nephrotoxic nephritis. *Clin Exp Immunol* 29:334–341, 1977
20. WEENING JJ, FLEUREN GJ, HOEDEMAEKER PhJ: Demonstration of antinuclear antibodies in mercuric chloride-induced glomerulopathy in the rat. *Lab Invest* 39:405–411, 1978
21. WEENING JJ, GROND J, VAN DER TOP D, HOEDEMAEKER PhJ: Identification of the nuclear antigen involved in mercury-induced glomerulopathy in the rat. *Invest Cell Pathol* 3:129–134, 1980
22. WEENING JJ, HOEDEMAEKER PhJ, BAKKER WW: Immunoregulation and anti-nuclear antibodies in mercury-induced glomerulopathy in the rat. *Clin Exp Immunol* 45:64–71, 1981
23. ROLINK AG, GLEICHMANN H, GLEICHMANN E: Diseases caused by reactions of T lymphocytes to incompatible structures of the major histocompatibility complex. VII. Immune-complex glomerulonephritis. *J Immunol* 130:209–215, 1983
24. BARIÉTY J, DRUET P, LALIBERTÉ F, SAPIN C: Glomerulonephritis with y and B1C-globulin deposits induced in rats by mercuric chloride. *Am J Pathol* 65:293–302, 1971
25. DRUET P, HIRSCH F, SAPIN C, DRUET E, BELLON B: Immune dysregulation and auto-immunity induced by toxic agents. *Transpl Proc* 14:482–484, 1982
26. WEENING JJ: Autoimmune reactions and glomerulonephritis caused by heavy metals and other toxins. *Proc 3d Int Congr Toxicol* Amsterdam, Elsevier Medical Press, 1983
27. DRUET E, SAPIN C, GUNTHER E, FEINGOLD N, DRUET P: Mercuric chloride-induced anti-glomerular basement membrane antibodies in the rat. Genetic control. *Eur J Immunol* 7:348–351, 1977
28. DRUET E, SAPIN E, FOURNIE G, MANDET C, GUNTHER E, DRUET P: Genetic control of susceptibility to mercury-induced immune nephritis in various strains of rat. *Clin Immunol Immunopathol* 25:203–212, 1982
29. DRUET P, AYED K, BARIÉTY J, BERNANDIN JF, DRUET E, GIRARD JF, HINGLAIS N, SAPIN C: Glomerulonephrite immunes experimentales indrutes par le bichlorure de mercure chez le rat. *Actualites Nephrologiques de l'Hopital Necker,* Paris, Flammarion, 1978, pp 245–264
30. SAPIN C, DRUET E, DRUET P: Induction of anti-glomerular basement membrane antibodies in the Brown-Norway rat by mercuric chloride. *Clin Exp Imm* 28:173–179, 1977
31. SAPIN C, DRUET P, MANDET C: Induction of susceptibility to $HgCL_2$ immune glomerulonephritis in the Lewis rat by immunocompetent cells from susceptible F1 hybrids. *Eur J Immunol* 10:371–374, 1980
32. BELLON B, CAPRON M, DRUET E, VERROUST P, VIAL MC, SAPIN C, GIRARD JF, FOIDART JM, MAHIEN P, DRUET P: Mercuric chloride induced autoimmune

disease in Brown-Norway rats: sequential search for anti-basement membrane antibodies and circulating immune complexes. *Eur J Clin Invest* 12:127–133, 1982

33. ROMAN-FRANCO AA, TURIELLO M, ALBINI B, OSSI E, MILGROM F, ANDRES GA: Anti-basement membrane antibodies and antigen-antibody complexes in rabbits injected with mercuric chloride. *Clin Immunol Immunopathol* 9:464–481, 1978

34. DONKER AJM, BRENTJENS JR, PAWLOWSKI JB, VENUTO RC, ANDRES GA: Development of autoantibodies and diffuse intravascular coagulation in D-penicillamine-treated Brown Norway rats. *Clin Immunol Immunopathol* 30:142–155, 1984

35. STUFFERS-HEIMAN M, GUNTHER E, ES LA VAN: Induction of autoimmunity to antigens of the glomerular basement membrane in inbred Brown-Norway rats. *Immunology* 36:759–767, 1979

36. PROUVOST-DANON A, ABADIE A, SAPIN C, BAZIN H, DRUET P: Induction of IgE synthesis and potentiation of antialbumin IgE antibody response by HgCl$_2$ in the rat. *J Immunol* 126:699–702, 1981

37. HIRSCH F, COUDERC J, SAPIN C, FOURNIE G, DRUET PH: Polyclonal effect of HgCL$_2$ in the rat. Its possible role in an experimental auto-immune disease. *Eur J Immunol* 12:620–625, 1982

38. KIRTLAND HH, MOHLER DH, HORWITZ DA: Methyldopa inhibition of suppressor-lymphocyte function. A proposed cause of auto-immune hemolytic anemia. *N Engl J Med* 302:825–832, 1980

39. BLUESTEIN HG, ZVAIFLER NJ, WEISMAN MH, SHAPIRO RF: Lymphocyte alteration by procainamide: Relation to drug-induced lupus erythematosus syndrome. *Lancet* II:816–819, 1979

40. ROUBINIAN JR, PAPOIAN R, TALAL N: Effects of neonatal thymectomy and splenectomy on survival and regulation of autoantibody formation in NZB/NZW F1 mice. *J Immunol* 118:1524–1529, 1977

41. LOCKWOOD CM, MASON DW, BOWMAN C: Suppressor cell function in mercuric chloride-induced autoimmune nephritis in the Brown Norway rat (*abstract*). *Kidney Int* 24:406, 1983

42. RAPPARD-VANDERVEEN FM, ROLINK AG, GLEICHMANN E: Diseases caused by reactions of T lymphocytes towards incompatible structures of the major histocompatibility complex. VI. Autoantibodies characteristic of systemic lupus erythematosus induced by abnormal T-B-cell cooperation across I-E. *J Exp Med* 155:1555–1560, 1982

43. FLEUREN GJ, WARNAAR SO, HOEDEMAEKER PHJ: Glomerulonephritis induced by heterologous antibodies against gp-70. (*abstract*). *IXth Int Cong Nephrol* Los Angeles, 1984

44. GLEICHMANN H: Studies on the mechanism of drug sensitization: T-cell-dependent popliteal lymphnode reaction to diphenylhydantoin. *Clin Immunol Immunopathol* 18:203–211, 1981

45. ZINKERNAGEL RM: H-2 restriction of cell-mediated virus-specific immunity and immunopathology: Self-recognition, altered self, and auto-aggression, in *Auto-Immunity*, edited by TALAL N, New York, Academic Press, 1977, p 363

Role of Antigen and Antibody Charge in Immune Complex Disease

Wayne A. Border

In the early 1970s, investigators in cell biology, pathology, and physiology simultaneously discovered and elucidated the electrical charge barrier of the glomerular capillary wall and mesangium [1, 2]. It was shown that anionic sites are distributed throughout the glomerular basement membrane (GBM), mesangial matrix, and also along the surfaces of the glomerular endothelial and epithelial cells. It became apparent that in addition to molecular size, electrical charge influenced the filtration of carbohydrate [3] and protein [4] molecules. For molecules of similar molecular size, a positive charge enhanced the filtration, whereas a negative charge decreased it. In 1975, Rennke, Cotran, and Venkatachalam showed that the ability of ferritin molecules to penetrate the glomerular capillary wall of the mouse directly correlated with molecular charge [5]. Native molecules with an isoelectric point (pI) of 4.6 barely entered the lamina rara interna, whereas with increasing pI there was deeper penetration into the GBM. Above a pI of 8, ferritin molecules regularly were found in the lamina rara externa and next to epithelial cell walls. The discovery that electrical charge influenced the ability of a molecule to penetrate the glomerular capillary wall had profound importance for renal immunopathology.

Historically, it was thought that the molecular size of soluble immune complexes (ICs), as determined by the size of the antigen and antibody and the antigen-antibody ratio, was the most important factor that determined nephritogenicity. Other factors included antibody avidity, immunoglobulin class, ability to fix complement, reticuloendothelial function, and IC load. The relevance of these factors had been questioned by investigators studying the mechanism of IC formation in passive Heymann nephritis. In this model, subsequent work would show that the IC formed in situ rather than being deposited from the circulation [6]. The discovery of the glomerular charge barrier added another dimension to the study of glomerular IC formation.

This manuscript was presented as part of a Symposium on *Mechanisms of Immune Complex Formation and Deposition in Glomeruli.*

The following discussion will review the evidence that electrical interaction between antigen or antibody and the anionic sites of the GBM or mesangial matrix can be a powerful force for initiating IC localization by either in situ formation or deposition from the circulation.

Nephritogenicity of Cationic Proteins. Investigators have cationized several molecules—including ferritin, bovine serum albumin (BSA), human serum albumin (HSA), ovalbumin, bovine gamma globulin, rabbit IgG, human IgG, and human IgM—to study their interaction with the glomerular capillary wall. Cationization is usually carried out by a standard chemical method that replaces hydroxyl groups with amines [7]. The chemical reaction can be controlled to select the degree of cationization. Chemical cationization does not change the molecular size or immunogenicity of the molecule [8]. Studies of molecules chemically cationized and native cationic molecules of the same pI have shown no differences. In the early studies, the cationic molecules, including the immunoglobulins, were used as antigens.

Cationic Antigens. When cationic molecules are administered systemically or directly into the renal artery of rats, rabbits, or mice, they bind to the anionic network of the GBM and mesangial matrix. This binding causes the anionic sites to coalesce or precipitate, making them visible by electron microscopy, a process commonly called *decoration.* In the absence of antibody, the decoration persists for 1 to 6 hr and disappears by 24 hr, and even large molecules do not produce electron-dense deposits. Antibody is required to anchor the cationic antigen and allow formation of an electron-dense deposit.

Batsford, Takamiya, and Vogt [9] produced glomerulonephritis in the rat by perfusing cationized ferritin (pI > 9.5) directly into the renal artery followed by systemic administration of anti-ferritin antibody. One hour later, both ferritin and IgG were detected by immunofluorescence to be uniformly deposited along the glomerular capillary wall. By 16 to 24 hr, the immunofluorescence pattern had become mesangial, but electron microscopy showed subepithelial deposits. Similar results were obtained by Ward, Cohen, and Border [10], who infused cationized BSA followed by sheep anti-BSA antibody directly into the renal artery of rabbits and then reestablished the circulation. Initially, the antigen and antibody were detected in a linear pattern along the glomerular capillary wall, but within hours the pattern became more granular. By 24 hr, small subepithelial electron-dense deposits were noted. Most experiments of this type have shown a similar sequence of early linear staining with the development of more granular staining as time passes. This phenomenon is attributed to immune reactants being driven deeper into the glomerular capillary wall, possibly by forces of filtration, and becoming localized against the epithelial cell wall.

The nephritogenic potential of a cationic antigen has been quantified by Oite et al [11]. These investigators perfused cationized human IgG (pI > 9.5) directly into the renal artery, and 1 hr later injected anti-human IgG systemically. At the onset of proteinuria, approximately 4 μg of human IgG and 30 μg of anti-human IgG antibody were present in the perfused kidney.

The 4 μg of cationic antigen can be compared to the 12 to 40 μg of kidney-fixing antibody per kidney required in heterologous nephrotoxic serum sickness and the 10 μg of antigen demonstrated in acute serum sickness. Thus, the requirements for proteinuria produced by cationic antigens seem to be in the same range as they are in other models of experimental glomerulonephritis.

One difficulty in using passive models, in which immunologic materials are injected directly into the kidney, is the possibility of nephrotoxicity. Earlier studies have shown that the polycation protamine sulfate, when directly perfused into the renal artery of rats, can produce abnormalities of the foot processes and proteinuria. This appears to be a dose-dependent phenomenon because systemic administration of smaller doses of protamine showed only decoration of the anionic network without morphologic changes or induction of proteinuria [12]. Similar results have been shown with other polycations, such as hexadimethrine and polyethyleneimine. To avoid the technical problems of direct renal artery administration of cationic substances, researchers have turned to active models, in which the cationic antigen is administered systemically and the host is allowed to form endogenous antibody against it.

The most thoroughly studied active model used cationic BSA in a modified model of chronic serum sickness induced in the rabbit [13]. Rabbits were immunized with native BSA (pI 4.5) or cationic BSA (pI > 9.5). One week later, daily 25-mg injections of the respective antigens were begun and continued for 6 weeks. Serial renal biopsy examinations were performed, along with measurements of renal function and immunologic studies to quantify the antibody response and the size of detectable circulating ICs. A separate group of animals received 1-mg daily antigen injections so that it could be determined whether larger complexes, formed in antibody excess, deposited in the mesangium. The effect of antigen charge on the development and morphology of the glomerular lesion was profound. With anionic BSA, mesangial deposits appeared after 2 weeks of injections and increased to 6 weeks. Ultrastructural examination showed numerous deposits within the mesangium and only rare deposits along the GBM. In contrast, animals receiving cationic BSA immediately developed granular capillary wall deposits that were maximal by 4 weeks. These deposits were located in a uniform manner in the subepithelial space. The cationic BSA induced an ultrastructural and histologic pattern of pure membranous nephropathy. The lesion appeared independently of antigen dose, for animals receiving 25 mg (antigen excess) or 1 mg (antibody excess) daily all developed the same lesion. Although circulating ICs were detected in the animals, the size did not correlate with the site of glomerular formation. In experiments to determine the mechanism by which the membranous deposits form, kidneys of nonimmunized rabbits were perfused with five alternating cycles of saline, antigen, and antibody, or saline and antigen alone were used in immunized rabbits [12]. Results showed that BSA and rabbit IgG localized along the GBM only after exposure to cationic BSA and antibody. Initially the deposits were linear, but after reestablishment of the circulation they became progressively more granular [10]. Ultrastructural examination showed effacement of foot processes and isolated subepithelial and occasional subendothelial deposits. Control experiments using native

BSA were negative. It was concluded that the membranous deposits formed in situ and were initiated by binding of the cationic BSA to the GBM. Separate studies showed that in contrast to the initial idea that membranous deposits form slowly, these deposits developed rapidly [14]. Ten minutes after the administration of the antigen to immunized animals, IgG was present in a trace granular pattern along the glomerular capillary wall. Within 24 hr, it was present in 2+ quantities and showed maximal staining 48 to 72 hr later. Electron-dense deposits were visible within 48 hr of the initial antigen administration.

Cationic Molecules and the Mesangium

Because the mesangial matrix also possesses anionic sites, it was interesting that mesangial deposits were not observed in the rabbit after an administration of cationic BSA [13]. This observation was pursued by using an identical protocol with cationic BSA in rats [15]. After 2 weeks of administration, immunofluorescence showed heavy, capillary, and mesangial deposits of BSA, IgA, and C3. At the same time, rats receiving native BSA showed only sparse mesangial deposits. By 6 weeks, rats receiving cationic BSA showed uniform small subepithelial dense deposits with associated foot process effacement and numerous subendothelial and mesangial deposits. No subepithelial deposits were present in rats receiving anionic BSA. Massive albuminuria occurred in rats injected with cationic BSA, whereas after 6 weeks of native BSA only trace albuminuria and no azotemia were seen. Unlike the results in the rabbit, the rat showed individual variation and localization of capillary wall deposits and marked formation of mesangial deposits. This work seems to demonstrate an interspecies difference in the glomerular IC formation between the rat and the rabbit.

It is known that the mesangial matrix possesses anionic sites rich in heparan sulfate similar to the GBM. It is likely that the electrical charge of circulating macromolecules might also be a factor in mesangial IC deposition. In rats, the injection of native ferritin (pI 4.5) was compared to slightly cationic ferritin (pI 7.0) and highly cationic ferritin (pI 8.5) [16]. After injection it was shown that native ferritin was cleared more rapidly and blood levels were significantly lower than they were for either of the cationic ferritins. The more rapid clearance of the native ferritin correlated with increased uptake by Kupffer cells in the liver and macrophages in the spleen. The higher blood levels of cationic ferritin seemed directly related to the poor uptake of this material by the liver and spleen. After 6 hr, deposition of both species of ferritin was similar in the kidney, but by 36 hr the native ferritin was significantly diminished, whereas the presence of cationic ferritin, particularly in the mesangium, persisted through 72 hr. The distribution of the two ferritins in the mesangium was different in that the cationic ferritin was diffuse throughout the mesangial matrix, whereas the anionic ferritin was more segmental in pattern. The persistence of cationic ferritin in the mesangium was attributed to the higher blood levels. Whether electrostatic binding played a role could not be determined. When native or cationic ferritin was injected into mice, the results were similar in terms of more rapid clearance of native ferritin with persistently higher blood levels of cationic ferritin [17]. Interestingly, in addition to a decreased uptake of cationic ferritin by the liver, spleen, and circulating leukocytes, there was also a decreased deposition in the kidney.

To study the effect of electrical charge on mesangial deposition independently of blood levels, Kamil and I injected cationic- and anionic-aggregated BSA directly into the renal artery of rats and then reestablished the circulation and quantified the disappearance from the kidney [18]. A dramatic increase in glomerular binding of cationic over negatively charged anionic BSA aggregates of comparable size was demonstrated. Thirty minutes after perfusion, glomeruli from rats receiving cationic BSA showed a 70-fold increase in binding of aggregates when compared to the rats receiving the anionic aggregates. On immunofluorescence microscopy, the anionic aggregates localized within the mesangium and were visually cleared from glomeruli by 4 hr. In contrast, cationic aggregates localized initially in the capillary wall and as the deposits cleared, definite mesangial staining could be detected that persisted for 4 days. The clearance of the cationic aggregates from glomeruli showed two compartments demonstrating rapid clearance from the capillary wall and delayed clearance from the mesangium. This delayed mesangial clearance could not be attributed to uptake from the blood since serum levels remained low and no uptake in the contralateral kidney was demonstrated. These findings indicate that cationic macromolecules can interact with the mesangium and that electrical charge plays an important factor in the enhanced uptake.

Cationic Antibody

Bovine gamma globulin [19] and human IgG and IgM [20] have been cationized and used as antigens to produce glomerular IC formation. Theoretically, the antibody properties of these immunoglobulins could have been exploited by allowing them to combine with their respective antigens, after binding to the GBM. The idea that a cationic antibody can start the process of IC formation is intriguing because naturally occurring immunoglobulins have a range of pIs from 5 to 9. The first demonstration of the nephritogenic potential of a cationic antibody was shown by Fleuren, Grond, and Hoedemaeker who perfused rat kidneys with alternating cycles of anionic BSA and anti-BSA antibody [21]. The perfusions resulted in the formation of subepithelial deposits, and the mechanism was interpreted initially to be simply one of diffusion of the antigen and antibody into the subepithelial space. In retrospect, however, it became clear that the anti-BSA antibody used in the experiment had a pI of 8.0 to 8.5. The authors now think that the mechanism of in situ formation in the perfused rat kidneys was the local binding of native BSA to cationic anti-BSA antibody that had bound to the anionic sites (personal communication). Subsequent work has confirmed that perfusion with cycles of an anionic antibody and anionic antigen do not result in subepithelial IC formation [10].

Ebling and Hahn have studied the pI of anti-DNA antibodies in three different strains of mice with systemic lupus [22]. The pI of the anti-DNA antibodies ranged from 5.5 to 9.0 with the highest frequency being between 8.0 and 8.5. Glomerular eluates from the mice showed that the anti-DNA antibody deposited in the kidney was more cationic than that found in the serum with a pI of 8.0 to 9.0. This suggests that cationic anti-DNA antibody may play a pathogenic role in the development of nephritis. The role of cationic antibody has also been demonstrated in passive Heymann nephritis and heterologous anti-GBM nephritis. Madaio et al have separated sheep anti-Fxla antibody [23] and anti-GBM antibody [24] into relative cationic and anionic fractions. The cationic and anionic antibodies were labeled with iodine 131 and 125, respectively, and administered to rats. At similar blood levels, the binding of cationic anti-Fxla antibody was two to three times greater than that of its anionic counterpart. It was even greater for cationic anti-GBM antibody, which was four times greater than that of the anionic antibody. The logical conclusion from these data is that antibody charge may determine the severity of disease, with cationic antibody producing more severe disease despite equal levels in the blood.

Given that one component of an antigen–antibody system is cationic, it would seem to make little difference whether it is the antigen or the antibody. The important thing is that the cationic component can bind to the anionic sites and then combine with its partner to initiate local IC formation. The experiments already cited show that both a cationic antigen or a cationic antibody can produce glomerulonephritis. The mechanism by which this would occur appears to be in situ formation. Initially, the cationic component binds throughout the GBM, and unless its corresponding partner is present, antigen or antibody alone cannot produce deposits. When both are present, deposits are seen earliest in both the lamina rara interna and externa, but with time there is movement resulting in the formation of subepithelial deposits. The exact mechanism of the formation of these deposits is speculative. Whether both antigen and antibody reach the subepithelial space and combine or whether they pass intact through the GBM is unknown. In any event, the power of a cationic protein to initiate in situ IC formation is clear, and it appears not to matter greatly whether it functions as an antigen or antibody.

Cationic Immune Complexes

Given the historical importance of circulating IC, one must consider the role of cationic IC. Although this is an attractive concept, there are technical difficulties in studying the effects of cationic IC. This is due to the fact that IC easily dissociate, and if the components are cationic, then direct binding to the glomerular wall can occur. Early work by Gallo, Caulin-Glaser, and Lamm [19] was criticized because there was free cationic antigen simultaneously present capable of initiating in situ IC formation. The same investigators repeated the work using covalently cross-linked cationized IC [25]. When these IC were injected into mice, they produced both subendothelial and subepithelial deposits; special studies showed that the material was distributed throughout the GBM. Although the exact characteristics of the complexes were not specified, it appears that their molecular weight was greater than 1 million and that they were highly cationic. Consistent with other observations was the fact that covalently linked anionic IC produced only mesangial or no deposits.

In studying the pathologic role of cationic IC, one must be aware of certain limitations. It is the net charge of the IC that is important, and the net charge will depend on the charge of the antigen and antibody and the manner in which they combine rather than the simple arithemetic sum of their charge. If the antigen and antibody are of similar pI, then electrostatic repulsion can facilitate the dissociation of the IC in the circulation as though it were formed with low-avidity antibody. Recent work with low-avidity antibody IC systems has shown that the major mechanism of glomerular IC formation is probably through dissociation and subsequent in situ IC formation [26].

IC prepared with cationized antibody and HSA at 5 and 50 times antigen excess have been injected into mice and their glomerular localization observed [27]. Large IC produced diffuse glomerular capillary wall staining with numerous subendothelial deposits. Subepithelial deposits were rare. By 14 days after injection, only mesangial deposits were present. IC prepared at 50 times antigen excess behaved similarly to cationic antibody alone in that both were cleared within 12 hr from the glomerulus and did not produce deposits. Other workers have used ferritin to prepare anionic IC (pI 5.0 to 6.5) and cationic IC (pI 6.5 to 7.5) [17]. Both species of complexes activated complement equally, and after their injection into mice, no differences in liver, spleen, or renal uptake were noted. These findings were interpreted as indicating that electrical charge of circulating IC did not play as important a role in their clearance from the blood as their ability to interact with FC and C3 receptors. In further investigating the BSA anti-BSA system, Wang and I prepared IC using cationic or anionic BSA [28]. The net charge of the resulting IC appeared to be unaffected by the charge of the antigen, with the pI being 4.6 to 4.8 with either antigen. After injection of cationic BSA IC, diffuse glomerular capillary staining was observed, but this cleared rapidly, leaving mesangial deposits. Anionic BSA containing IC resulted in only granular mesangial deposits. After cross-linking of the cationic BSA IC, the capillary wall staining was abolished and only mesangial deposits were detected. Finally, when aggregated cationic BSA was injected, it produced both glomerular capillary wall and mesangial deposits.

It would seem that electrical charge is a less important factor for determining the deposition of circulating IC. When complexes are prepared with a cationic constituent, the most likely event is that free cationic material will initiate in situ IC formation. Only when immune complexes are highly cationic and of high molecular weight have they been shown to produce direct GBM deposition with the formation of subendothelial and subepithelial deposits.

Neutralization of the Glomerular Charge Barrier

Recent experiments have shown that polycations acting either as an antigen or an antibody can neutralize the glomerular charge barrier resulting in increased permeability to macromolecules [29]. The mechanism of this effect is a distortion of the GBM structure, resulting in changes in charge and size permselectivity. The neutralization of the charge barrier makes it easier for IC to penetrate and deposit in the GBM. Cavallo et al have shown in a model of murine lupus nephritis that the changes in GBM permeability antedate the development of IC deposits [30]. The mechanism of this effect is unknown. It thus appears that an intact charge and size barrier is important in protecting the glomerular capillary wall from IC deposition.

Electrical Charge and the Glomerulus

The evidence is clear that electrostatic interaction between cationic immune reactants and the glomerular anionic network is a powerful force for initiating

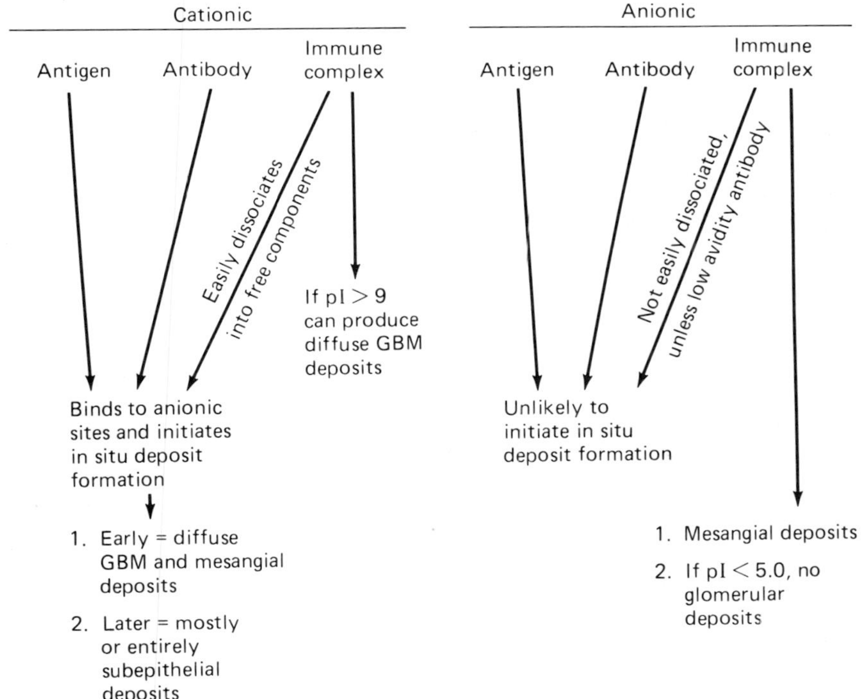

Fig. 1. Electrical charge and glomerular localization of immune reactants.

IC localization. The effect of electrical charge can be integrated with additional knowledge of factors affecting IC deposition to provide a comprehensive understanding of this subject (Fig. 1). Anionic antigen or antibody acting alone does not produce IC formation. Anionic IC either do not deposit in the glomerulus or are confined to the mesangium. If either the antigen or antibody is cationic, it can initiate in situ IC formation either in the GBM or in the mesangial matrix. In the GBM, the initial binding will be throughout the lamina densa, and subendothelial deposits will be present. With time, the deposits move toward the subepithelial space, and within 24 hr in most experimental models subepithelial deposits are dominant. Depending on the species, cationic reactants can also induce mesangial deposits that are distributed throughout the mesangial matrix in a pattern mimicking the anionic network. Cationic IC seem prone to dissociation and initiation of in situ IC formation as separate antigen or antibody. If cationic complexes have a sufficiently high pI and do not dissociate, they can bind directly to the GBM and produce both subendothelial and subepithelial deposits. It seems likely that electrical charge has its major nephritogenic effect through binding of antigen or antibody and in situ IC formation rather than deposition of intact IC.

References

1. VENKATACHALAM MA, RENNKE HG: The structural and molecular basis of glomerular filtration. *Circ Res* 43:337–347, 1978
2. BRENNER BM, HOSTETTER TH, HUMES HD: Molecular basis of proteinuria of glomerular origin. *N Engl J Med* 298:826–833, 1978
3. BENNETT CM, GLASSOCK RJ, CHANG RLS, DEEN WM, ROBERTSON CR, BRENNER BM: Permselectivity of the glomerular capillary wall. *J Clin Invest* 57:1287–1294, 1976
4. RENNKE HG, PATEL Y, VENKATACHALAM MA: Glomerular filtration of proteins: Clearance of anionic, neutral, and cationic horseradish peroxidase in the rat. *Kidney Int* 13:324–328, 1978
5. RENNKE HG, COTRAN RS, VENKATACHALAM MA: Role of molecular charge in glomerular permeability. *J Cell Biol* 67:638–646, 1975
6. COUSER WG, SALANT DJ: In situ complex formation and glomerular injury (*Editorial review*). *Kidney Int* 17:1–13, 1980
7. DANON D, GOLDSTEIN L, MARIKOVSKY Y, SKUTELSKY E: Use of cationized ferritin as a label of negative charges on cell surfaces. *J Ultrastruct Res* 38:500–510, 1972
8. BORDER WA, KAMIL ES, WARD HJ, COHEN AJ: Antigenic charge as a determinant of immune complex localization in the rat glomerulus. *Lab Invest* 40:442–449, 1981
9. BATSFORD SR, TAKAMIYA H, VOGT A: A model of in situ immune complex glomerulonephritis in the rat employing cationized ferritin. *Clin Nephrol* 14:211–216, 1980
10. WARD HJ, COHEN AH, BORDER WA: In situ formation of subepithelial immune complexes in the rabbit glomerulus: Requirement of a cationic antigen. *Nephron* 36:257–264, 1984
11. OITE T, BATSFORD SR, MIHATSCH MJ, TAKAMIYA H, VOGT A: Quantitative studies of in situ immune complex glomerulonephritis in the rat induced by planted, cationized antigen. *J Exp Med* 155:460–474, 1982

 559

12. ADLER SG, WANG H, WARD HJ, COHEN AH, BORDER WA: Electrical charge: Its role in the pathogenesis and prevention of experimental membranous nephropathy in the rabbit. *J Clin Invest* 71:487–499, 1983
13. BORDER WA, WARD HJ, KAMIL ES, COHEN AH: Induction of membranous nephropathy in rabbits by administration of an exogenous cationic antigen. *J Clin Invest* 69:451–461, 1982
14. WANG H, ADLER S, COHEN A, BORDER W: Rapid development of membranous deposits in serum sickness induced by a cationic antigen. *Kidney Int* 21:207, 1982
15. KAMIL ES, BORDER WA: Effect of electrical charge on serum sickness nephritis in the rat (*abstract*). *Clin Res* 20:451, 1982
16. COHEN S, VERNIER RL, MICHAEL AF: The effect of charge on the renal distribution of ferritin. *Am J Pathol* 110:170–181, 1983
17. GENIN C, COSIO F, MICHAEL AF: Macromolecular charge and reticuloendothelial function: Comparison between the kinetics of administered native and cationized ferritins and the corresponding immune complexes in the mouse. *Immunology* 54:225–238, 1984
18. KAMIL E, BORDER W: The effect of electrical charge on glomerular clearance of macromolecules. *Kidney Int* 21:200, 1982
19. GALLO GR, CAULIN-GLASER T, LAMM ME: Charge of circulating immune complexes as a factor in glomerular basement membrane localization in mice. *J Clin Invest* 67:1308–1313, 1981
20. VOGT A, ROHRBACH R, SHIMIZU F, TAKAMIYA H, BATSFORD S: Interaction of cationized antigen with rat glomerular basement membrane: In situ immune complex formation. *Kidney Int* 22:27–35, 1982
21. FLEUREN G, GROND J, HOEDEMAEKER PJ: In situ formation of subepithelial glomerular immune complexes in passive serum sickness. *Kidney Int* 17:631–637, 1980
22. EBLING F, HAHN BH: Restricted subpopulations of DNA antibodies in kidneys of mice with systemic lupus. *Arthritis Rheum* 23:392–402, 1980
23. MADAIO MP, SALANT DJ, COUSER WG, DARBY C, COPPARELL N: Influence of antibody charge and concentration on subepithelial immune deposit formation. *Kidney Int* 19:186, 1981
24. MADAIO MP, SALANT DJ, ADLER S, DARBY C, COUSER WG: Effects of antibody charge and concentration on glomerular deposition of anti-GBM antibody. *Kidney Int* 21:201, 1982
25. CAULIN-GLASER T, GALLO GR, LAMM ME: Nondissociating cationic immune complexes can deposit in glomerular basement membrane. *J Exp Med* 158:1561–1572, 1983
26. GERMUTH FG, RODRIGUEZ E, WISE O: Passive immune complex glomerulonephritis in mice: III. Clearance kinetics and properties of circulating complexes. *Lab Invest* 46:515–519, 1982
27. GAUTHIER VJ, MANNIK M, STRIKER GE: Effect of cationized antibodies in preformed immune complexes on deposition and persistence in renal glomeruli. *J Exp Med* 156:766–777, 1982
28. WANG H, BORDER WA: Influence of antigen charge on isoelectric point and biologic properties of preformed immune complexes. *Kidney Int* 26:191, 1982
29. BARNES JL, RADNIK RA, GILCHRIST EP, VENKATACHALAM MA: Size and charge selective permeability defects induced in glomerular basement membrane by a polycation. *Kidney Int* 25:11–19, 1984
30. CAVALLO T, GOLDMAN M, GRAVES K, LAMBERT PH: Altered glomerular permeability in the early phase of immune complex nephritis. *Kidney Int* 24:632–637, 1983

Pathogenic Antigen of Heymann Nephritis (gp330): Identification, Isolation, and Localization

Dontscho Kerjaschki and Marilyn Gist Farquhar

Heymann nephritis (HN) is an experimental model of human membranous glomerulonephritis that was originally induced by immunization of rats against homologous kidney cortex preparations [1]. The hallmark of both the human and experimental disease is the accumulation of endogenous IgG in a granular pattern in the lamina rara externa of the glomerular basement membrane (GBM) [2, 3]. Morphologic changes are followed by the onset of proteinuria. Heymann nephritis and membranous nephropathy have been considered typical autoimmune complex diseases [4]. Whereas apparent various antigens may be involved in the human disease [5–7], the pathogenic antigen(s) of Heymann nephritis (HN) was found to be restricted to the brushborder region of proximal tubule cells [8–10]—as shown by the fact that IgG from the serum of rats with HN or IgG eluted from isolated glomeruli of diseased kidneys bound to this region via immunofluorescence.

Identification of the HN Antigen

The similar morphology of HN and membranous glomerulonephritis suggested that similar mechanisms of development of immune deposits could be involved in both diseases. Identification and localization of the responsible antigen(s) are necessary for the understanding of these processes. Several previous attempts have been made to identify and to characterize the putative antigen. For example, a subfraction called RTEα5 was prepared from a crude cortical extract known as Fx1A (which has been widely used for the induction of HN); it was found to contain a 28s lipoprotein complex with pathogenic activity [11]. Other investigators have used pronase-digested subfractions of

This manuscript was presented as part of a Symposium on *Recent Advances in the Structure, Biochemistry and Function of the Glomerulus.*

Fx1A [12] or isolated microvilli of kidney brushborder and glycoprotein fractions derived from them [13] to induce HN. Collectively, these data indicated that the pathogenic antigen(s) of HN is located in the membranes of proximal tubule microvilli, and it probably is glycoprotein in nature [14].

We have isolated microvillar fractions from rat kidney cortex and have labeled the proteins facing the exterior via lactoperoxidase-glucose oxidase-mediated radioiodination [15]. Subsequently, the proteins were solubilized with detergents and were subjected to immunoprecipitation [16]. As sources of antibodies for this procedure, we have used: (1) serum of Fx1A-immunized rats with HN, (2) heterologous rabbit IgG directed against rat Fx1A, and (3) endogenous rat IgG eluted from diseased glomeruli of HN-nephritic rats. The two former preparations of IgGs precipitated several glycoproteins that were visualized as bands by SDS-PAGE (Fig. 1). By contrast, eluted IgG selectively recognized a large glycoprotein with an apparent molecular weight (Mr) of about 330,000, as determined by comparison with its electrophoretic mobility to that of a polymerized β-galactosidase standard. Because of its apparent Mr, this molecule was called gp330 [17].

Isolation of gp330

To prove that gp330 is the pathogenic antigen of HN, it was necessary to purify this protein and to induce HN with it. For this purpose, isolated microvillar membranes were solubilized in detergent, the soluble components were fractionated by gel filtration, and gp330 was isolated either by preparative

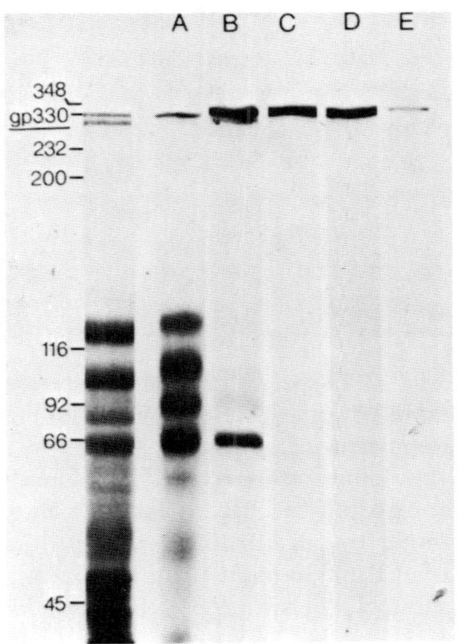

Fig. 1. Autoradiograms of ^{125}I-labeled microvillus proteins extracted with RIPA-buffer (*lane A*) and immune precipitates (*lanes B–E*) obtained from them with: rabbit IgG raised against a crude fraction from rat kidney cortex (Fx1A) (*lane B*), immunoglobulins eluted from isolated rat glomeruli with active HN induced by Fx1A (*lane C*), serum from a rat immunized against isolated gp330 (*lane D*), immunoglobulins eluted from glomeruli of a rat immunized against isolated gp330 (*lane E*). The lane on the far left is a Coomassie blue-stained SDS-PAGE pattern obtained from rat kidney brushborders; protein bands are given in kd.

SDS-PAGE or by affinity chromatography on either lentil lectin [17] or mono-clonal anti-gp330 IgG [18] affinity columns. The purity of these preparations was determined by SDS-PAGE.

Induction of HN by gp330

When rats were immunized against preparations of gp330 that had been prepared by any of these three methods, granular immune deposits were observed in the lamina rara externa (Fig. 2) [17]; after 2 months, mild protein-uria occurred (unpublished data).

To exclude the possibility that deposition of another unrelated IgG in the glomeruli had been triggered by immunization with purified gp330, glo-meruli of the immunized rats that developed HN were isolated; also, the

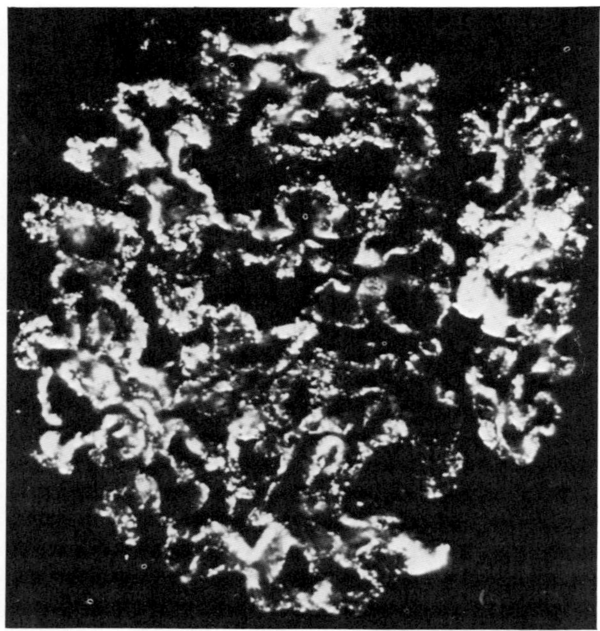

Fig. 2. Direct immunofluorescence of a glomerulus from a rat immunized against isolated gp330 stained with rhodaminated antirat IgG. Endogenous rat IgG is deposited in a granular pattern in the glomerular basement membrane, thus fulfilling the definition of active HN. The deposited IgG has been shown to be monospecific for gp330 (see Fig. 1, lane E). Similar results were obtained with gp330 purified either by gel filtration and lentil-lectin affinity chromatography, by direct isolation of the gp330-band from SDS-gels, or by affinity purification using immobilized monoclonal anti-gp330 IgG (×900).

nature of the accumulated pathogenic IgG was determined via immunoprecipitation. It was again specific for gp330 [17].

In addition to active immunization, HN could be passively transferred into healthy animals via intravenous (i.v.) injection of IgG prepared from rats that had developed HN after immunization with gp330. Overt passive HN also developed after injection of rabbit anti-gp330 IgG into rats [19].

Data suggesting that gp330 was the only pathogenic molecule in kidney brushborder membranes was provided by experiments in which rats were immunized against microvillar membrane fractions that had been selectively depleted of gp330 by gel filtration. The rats developed antibrushborder antibodies, but they failed to generate glomerular immune deposits [17]. These data suggested that gp330 was the only—or at least by far the most predominant—antigen of HN.

In these experiments, it was found to be crucial to inhibit proteolysis to avoid degradation of gp330 and generation of fragments of gp330 that were still immunogenic and that could be interpreted as additional pathogenic antigens smaller than gp330. Endogenous proteolysis was a major problem throughout the isolation of gp330 by gel filtration, which resulted in very low yields of gp330. It could be suppressed only by the use of diisopropyl fluorophosphate along with a cocktail of several other inhibitors [17].

Preliminary Characterization of gp330

Gp330 is a glycoprotein, as demonstrated by its ability to bind to lentil lectin [13, 17] and to concanavalin A [18]. It also contains sialic acid, because it can be labeled by the periodate-borotritide method [20]. The stoichiometry of the lectin-binding sugars and sialic acid and the nature of the oligosaccharide chains (O- or N-glycosidic linkages) are not known at present.

Gp330 seemingly is a transmembrane protein, because it is not removed from the membranes by chaotropic agents (urea, KI; unpublished data); also, detergents are required for its solubilization. However, definitive biochemical proof of its transmembrane nature (its insertion into liposomes) is still lacking.

A major part of the gp330 molecule is exposed at the cell surface as shown by immunocytochemistry [17, 18], its accessibility to external radioiodination [17], and its sensitivity to trypsin digestion in intact microvilli [17].

The actual size of gp330 in its native state is not known. It has to be kept in mind that the estimate of its Mr (330,000) was obtained by SDS-PAGE under strongly denaturing conditions [17]. Estimates of molecular size that were obtained by gel filtration in the presence of deoxycholate indicate that it may form larger aggregates (unpublished observations), as observed by others [21].

Localization of gp330 in Normal Glomeruli

The fact that circulating antibodies to a tubular antigen are deposited in the GBM and cause glomerular damage has been explained in several ways. It has been considered that immune complexes containing the pathogenic antigen(s) and the specific antibodies are preformed in the circulation and become trapped in the GBM [4, 12]. Alternatively, an in situ mechanism for the formation of glomerular immune deposits has been proposed [22–24], because when anti-Fx1A IgG was perfused into isolated kidneys under conditions (blood-free salt solution) in which formation of circulating immune complexes was avoided, typical glomerular immune deposits were formed [23, 24]. It was concluded that the HN antigen(s) must be present in the glomerulus; indeed, it subsequently has been detected there by immunocyto-chemistry. Rat anti-Fx1A serum, heterologous rabbit anti-Fx1A IgG, and eluates from the HN-nephritic glomeruli have been used for immunofluores-cence and immunoperoxidase at the light and electron microscopic levels. The immunofluorescent findings demonstrate that the antigen is distributed in a diffuse punctate pattern [23, 25, 26]. Attempts to define the site of its localization at the ultrastructural level have yielded conflicting results—the antigen was variously localized to the GBM, to the surface of all types of glomerular cells, and to the cell membrane at the base of the glomerular epithelium [23, 25, 27, 28]. The reason for these discrepancies probably lies in the variable nature and multispecificity of the antibody preparations used or in the vagaries of the immunoperoxidase procedures [29].

Using a monoclonal anti-gp330 IgG or (with identical results) anti-gp330 IgG that had been affinity-purified on Sepharose 4B coupled to purified gp330, we have observed via immunofluorescence [19] a punctate pattern of distribu-tion of gp330 in glomeruli of both Sprague-Dawley and Lewis rats (a strain that is highly susceptible to the induction of active HN) that closely resembles that seen by previous workers with anti-Fx1A antibodies. Using indirect immunoperoxidase [18, 19] and immunogold [18] techniques at the electron microscopic level, we localized gp330 exclusively to the glomerular epithelial cells, where it was found both intracellularly and at the cell surface. Along the cell surface, it was restricted in its distribution to coated pits that were found along both the sides and base of the foot processes (Figs. 3, 4). Intracel-lularly, it was found in biosynthetic compartments (rough ER, Golgi) and in lysosomal or prelysosomal compartments (multivesicular bodies) as well. A major result of these experiments was the finding that gp330 is concentrated in coated pits located at the base of the foot processes, where they face the GBM [19].

From these morphologic data and supporting biosynthetic and biochemical data [19], we concluded that in the glomerulus gp330, the HN antigen: (1) is a resident epithelial membrane protein produced by the glomerular epithelial cells, and (2) is concentrated at the cell surface in coated pits—structures that are known to play a key role in receptor-mediated endocytosis in many other systems [30, 31]. Subsequent studies (reviewed below) have established

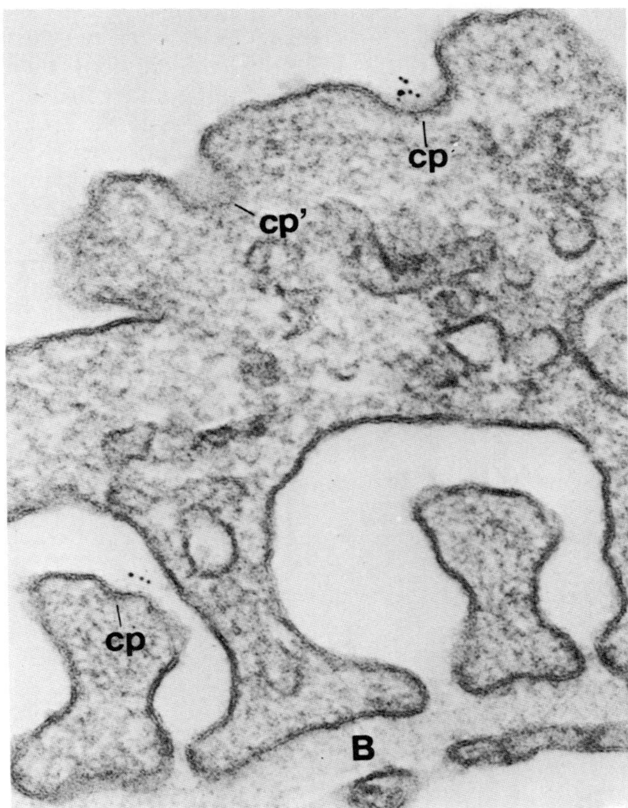

Fig. 3. Immunogold localization of gp330 to coated pits (*cp*) on glomerular epithelial cells using affinity-purified rabbit anti-gp330. Clusters of protein-A are found in two coated pits. *Cp'* indicates a coated pit that is not reactive. *B*, glomerular basement membrane (×52,000).

that gp330 is also concentrated in coated pits in the proximal tubule cell and in a number of other absorptive epithelia as well.

Induction of Passive HN by Anti-gp330 IgG

After having localized gp330 on the cell membranes of glomerular epithelial cells, it was necessary—for verification of its pathogenic role—to show that anti-gp330 IgG was able to form immune complexes in this location. Based on the knowledge that HN could be transferred passively by infusion of anti-Fx1A antibodies [32, 33], we injected rats intravenously with rabbit anti-gp330 IgG [19] and sacrificed them 3 days later. Via immunofluorescence and immunoperoxidase, rabbit IgG was found to be distributed in a granular pattern along the GBM. Via electron microscopy, the rabbit anti-gp330 IgG was detected in the lamina rara externa under the slit diaphragms, and also (interestingly) in coated pits at the base of the foot processes; that is, the same location where the gp330 antigen had been localized previously.

These data suggest that coated pits on the plasmalemma of glomerular epithelial cells play an important role in the formation of immune complexes, in that they may represent the site where the endogenous antigen—the membrane glycoprotein, gp330—and its specific circulating (anti-gp330) antibody meet. It is clear that for the pathogenic anti-gp330 IgG to reach its specific

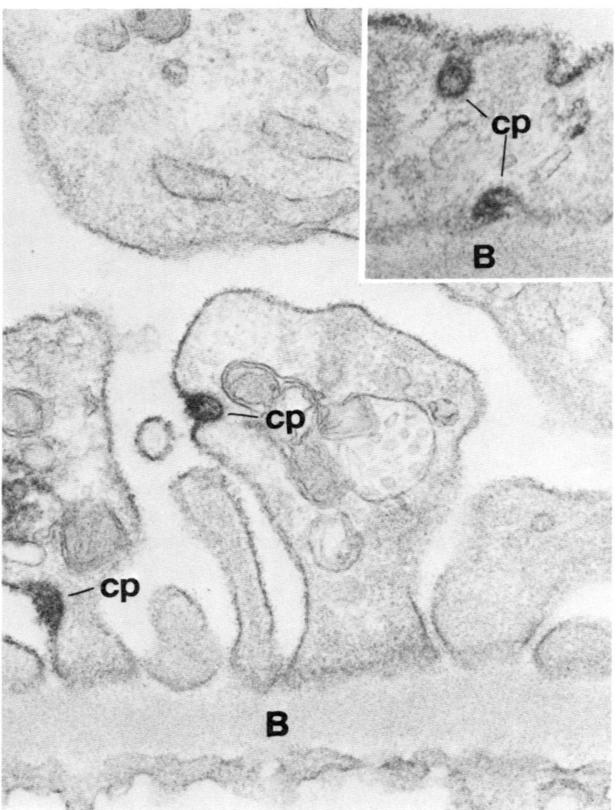

Fig. 4. Indirect immunoperoxidase staining of normal Lewis rat kidney using monoclonal anti-gp330 IgG as first antibodies. Coated pits (*cp*) located on the surface of the glomerular epithelial cells contain an electron-dense reaction product. In the inset, gp330 also is demonstrated in a coated pit (*cp*) located at the base of the foot process abutting the glomerular basement membrane (*B*) (×35,000; inset, ×40,000).

antigen, it must be able to cross the electrostatic barrier [34] that is represented by the GBM [35, 36] to reach the antigen located on the cell membranes of glomerular epithelial cells. In this regard, it is interesting to note that although the monoclonal anti-gp330 IgG (clone D1-55-F2) and polyclonal IgG have given identical results when used for the immunochemical localization of gp330, the monoclonal IgG failed to produce immune deposits when used for the induction of passive HN. This could be due to its charge, the fact that it recognizes an epitope that is not accessible in vivo, or to other (unknown) factors. Recently we determined the charge of this monoclonal IgG and found it had a pI < 5.0 (Berstein, Kerjaschki, and Farquhar, unpublished data). Thus, its anionic nature might prevent it from penetrating the lamina densa of the GBM to any great extent. Experiments carried out with differently charged proteins [37–39], including IgG [38], clearly indicate that cationic species more readily penetrate the lamina densa and bind to the laminae rara externa than anionic species of the same protein.

Distribution of gp330 in the Kidney Proximal Tubule Brushborder: Comparison with Maltase

After having identified gp330 as the pathogenic antigen of HN, we were interested in determining its function. Because it was obtained from kidney microvillar fractions, its properties were compared to known microvillar membrane components that had been defined biochemically by previous workers [40]. It was found to be quite similar in size (300 to 340 kd) to brushborder maltase, which was recently purified to homogeneity [41]. This prompted a comparative immunochemical and immunocytochemical study of maltase and gp330 by using monoclonal antibodies that were specific for gp330 and maltase. It was found [18] that monoclonal antibodies directed against maltase specifically immunoprecipitated a slightly smaller band with an apparent molecular weight of 300 kd by SDS-PAGE; our monoclonal anti-gp330 IgG precipitated selectively the 330 kd band—gp330. Interestingly, both gp330 and maltase (gp300) were precipitated by our polyclonal rabbit antibody that was raised against purified gp330. When maltase (gp300) and gp330 were purified by affinity chromatography (using their specific monoclonal antibodies) and were subjected to cleavage with cyanogen bromide, the two proteins were found to have a similar—but not identical—pattern of peptides. The structural similarity (shared peptides) revealed by peptide mapping undoubtedly explains the cross-reactivity of the polyclonal anti-gp330 IgG with gp330 and maltase (gp300). Indirect data indicated that gp300, indeed, possesses maltase activity, whereas gp330 is not enzymatically active.

After the structural similarity of gp330 and maltase (gp300) had been established, the question arose as to whether these molecules are located at the same sites in the proximal tubule brushborder. To answer this question, monoclonal antibodies were used for immunohistochemical localization of the two antigens [18]. It was found that gp330 is concentrated in coated

invaginations located at the base of the microvilli (referred to as the intermicrovillar microdomain) of the brushborder (Figs. 5, 6), while maltase (gp300)
is restricted to the microvillar membranes and is absent from the coated
invaginations. Gp330 (but not maltase) was also found intracellularly within
endosomes. The restricted localization of gp330 and maltase in the coated
invaginations and microvillar domains, respectively, of the apical plasmalemma was seen only with monoclonal antibodies. This segregation was most
obvious in S1 and S2 segments of proximal tubules and was less strict in
the S3 segments. As might be expected (since it recognizes both gp330 and
maltase), the polyclonal antibody stained both the coated pits and microvilli
[18].

Close inspection of the cytoplasmic side of the coated invaginations where
gp330 is concentrated revealed that they were endowed with an extensive
layer of cage-like material (also observed by earlier investigators) that resembled clathrin-coated pits seen in many other systems [42, 43]. Immunohistochemistry carried out on kidney cortex sections with anticlathrin antibodies
[44] has revealed the presence of an extensive layer of clathrin—the main
coated vesicle protein [43]—around the entire luminal circumference of proximal tubules in a position identical to that of gp330, but on the opposite
side of the membrane. When brushborder membranes were isolated [45] under
conditions that maintain the clathrin coat, and immunocytochemistry was
performed on these fractions, it was found that the segregation of gp330
and maltase (gp300) into the different microdomains was largely preserved
[44].

These data indicate that in the proximal kidney brushborder, gp330 is
colocalized with clathrin. The nature and extent of the clathrin coats in
this location has not been previously appreciated. The question arises, then,
as to what gp330 is doing in this membrane microdomain. Experiments designed to determine the function of gp330 are in progress.

Localization of gp330 in Other Organs

Since HN had been induced by extracts of various organs besides the kidney
[46], and since anti-Fx1A antibodies have revealed the presence of the Fx1A
antigens in several organs via immunofluorescence [47], it was interesting
to map the distribution of gp330—the nephritogenic component of the Fx1A
protein mixture—in other organs and compare it to that in the kidney. For
this purpose, we have screened various epithelia by immunocytochemistry
[48] and by immunoblotting for the presence of gp330 by using monoclonal
anti-gp330 IgG. The gp330 antigen was found to be widely distributed at
the cell surfaces of several other absorptive epithelia, where—as in the case
of the proximal tubule cell—it was restricted to coated pits and endosome-
like structures located at the luminal surfaces of these organs. Coated vesicles
containing gp330 were abundant in the epididymis and yolk sac and were
present (although fewer in number) in hepatocytes, where they were located
along both the sinusoidal and bile canalicular cell surfaces. In epididymis

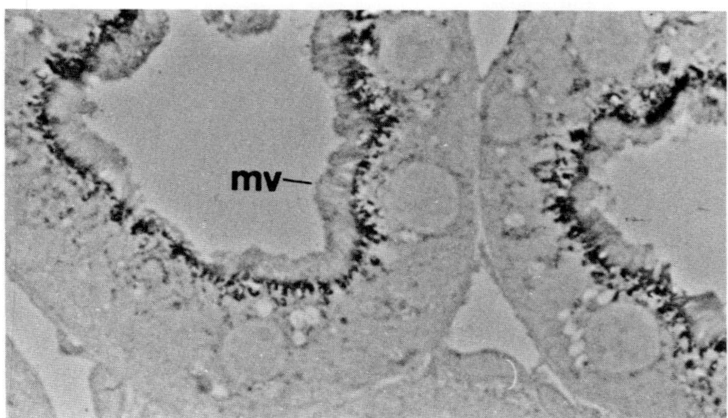

Fig. 5. Indirect immunoperoxidase staining of a 1 μm plastic section from a rat kidney incubated with monoclonal anti-gp330 IgG. Gp330 is concentrated in a zone located at the base of the microvilli, but it is not found in the microvilli (*mv*) themselves (×620).

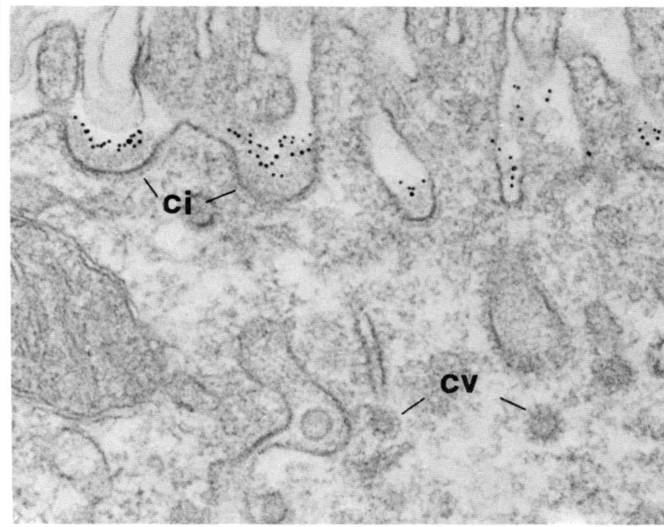

Fig. 6. Localization of gp330 in a rat proximal tubule cell as seen by labeling with protein A-gold. Gold particles are concentrated in coated invaginations (*ci*) on which clathrin-like coats are visible and are located at the base (intermicrovillar microdomains) of the brushborder microvilli. The gold particles are separated from the cell membrane by a thick amorphous layer, presumably constituted by immunoglobulins plus the membrane proteins (×53,000).

and yolk sac, gp330 was also detected in biosynthetic compartments (endoplasmic reticulum and Golgi complex), indicating that it is synthesized by the corresponding epithelia. However, gp330 was not a universal resident of all coated pits in any cell type, and it was not detected in some cell types (fibroblasts or endothelial cells).

From these findings, we conclude that gp330 is a common component of coated pits of epithelia in organs that have an amplified protein absorption capacity. Because of its location in coated pits, which is typical for many receptors [30, 31], we speculate that gp330 may be either a receptor for which the ligand(s) is unknown at present or (alternatively) perhaps a constitutive component of coated pits. The extrarenal presence of gp330 may explain the nephritogenic response elicited by immunization with extracts of other organs [46].

Summary and Conclusions

The data summarized in this review indicate that gp330—a large membrane glycoprotein—is the pathogenic antigen of HN. This glycoprotein is found on both the proximal tubule and glomerular epithelia, where it is concentrated in coated pits at the cell surface. It is also present in several other epithelia (epididymis or yolk sac), where it is found in the same location.

Evidence that gp330 is the pathogenic antigen of HN derives from the following findings: (1) IgG eluted from glomeruli of HN-afflicted rats immunized against crude rat cortical extract (Fx1A) is specific for gp330, (2) active HN is caused by immunization of rats with purified gp330, and (3) passive HN can be induced by either rat or rabbit IgG that is monospecific for gp330. Recent data also indicate that gp330 is detected in the glomerular immune deposits of rats with advanced active HN induced with Fx1A (Kerjaschki and Andres, unpublished data).

The interesting aspect of these findings is that gp330 is a cell surface antigen rather than a basement membrane component. Accordingly, we propose that in this disease, immune deposits are formed by in situ accumulation of anti-gp330 IgG at the sites where the antigen resides. Anti-gp330 binds to its antigen (gp330) in the coated pits located at the base of the foot processes; the complex thus formed is shed into the lamina rara externa of the GBM. Shedding of immune complexes formed on the plasmalemma from cell membrane proteins and antibodies is a well-known phenomenon in lymphocytes [49] and in other situations (virus-infected cells [50] and pulmonary endothelial cells [51]). The major difference between the other systems (where shedding has been documented) and HN is the fact that whereas the former events occur on free cell surfaces, the complexes are formed on the surfaces of epithelial cells in HN, where they are attached firmly to the GBM. This restricts the diffusion and elimination of the shed immune complexes, which results in their trapping and accumulation, rather than their release into the medium or bloodstream.

The physiologic function of gp330 remains unknown. Its association with coated pits and endosomes is similar to that of receptor molecules, such as those for low-density lipoproteins, asialoglycoproteins, and peptide hormones (for a review, see [30, 31]), which are taken up by receptor-mediated endocytosis along with their ligands. Therefore, we speculate that gp330 may be involved in receptor-mediated endocytosis, either as a constitutive component of a class of coated pits or as a receptor for which the ligands are currently unknown; and, also that in the glomerulus, gp330 may play a role in the normal removal of filtration residues that accumulate in the lamina rara externa. Such residues are known to be taken up by the epithelium via endocytosis [52–54].

Further studies are needed to bridge the gap between human membranous glomerulonephritis and the findings in HN. It currently is not clear whether gp330 or related molecules can participate in the formation of immune deposits in human membranous glomerulonephritis (as suggested by the detection of antibrushborder antibodies in some patients with this disease [55, 56]); or, if a similar mechanism of immune deposit formation—involving different cell surface antigens—is operative in humans. In addition to cell surface components, components of the lamina rara externa—especially proteoglycans [36] and Farquhar, Lemkin, and Stow in this Section)—may also serve as points of initiation of immune complex formation by virtue of their electrostatic and steric exclusion properties (see Farquhar, Lemkin, and Stow, this Section) and must be considered as an alternative or additional contributory mechanism in the pathogenesis of membranous glomerulonephritis.

Acknowledgments. This research was supported by Research Grant AM 17724 from the National Institutes of Health.

References

1. HEYMANN W, HACKEL DB, HARWOOD S, WILSON SGF, HUNTER JL: Production of nephrotic syndrome in rats by Freund's adjuvant and rat kidney suspensions. *Proc Soc Exp Biol Med* 100:660–664, 1959
2. ALOUSI MA, POST RA, HEYMANN W: Experimental autoimmune nephrosis in rats. Morphogenesis of the glomerular lesion: Immunohistochemical and electron microscopic studies. *Am J Pathol* 54:47–71, 1969
3. SCHNEEBERGER EE, LEBER PD, KARNOVSKY MJ, MCCLUSKEY RT: Altered functional properties of the renal glomerulus in autologous immune complex nephritis. An ultrastructural tracer study. *J Exp Med* 139:1283–1242, 1974
4. GLASSOCK RJ, EDGINGTON TS, WATSON JI, DIXON FJ: Autologous immune complex nephritis induced with rat renal tubular antigen: II. The pathogenic mechanisms. *J Exp Med* 127:573–587, 1968
5. COUSER WG, WAGONFELD JB, SPARGO BH, LEUW EJ: Glomerular deposition of tumor antigen in membranous nephropathy associated with colonic carcinoma. *Am J Med* 57:962–970, 1974
6. SLUSARCZYK J, MICHALAK T, NARACEWICZ-DENEZER T, KRAWCZYNSKI K, NOWOSLAWSKY A: Membranous glomerulopathy associated with hepatitis core antigen immune complexes in children. *Am J Pathol* 98:29–44, 1980
7. TALAMO TS, BOROCHOVITZ D: Membranous glomerulonephritis associated with the Guillain-Barre syndrome. *Am J Clin Pathol* 78:563–566, 1982
8. EDGINGTON TS, GLASSOCK RJ, DIXON FJ: Autologous immune complex patho-

genesis of experimental allergic glomerulonephritis. *Science* 155:1432–1434, 1967
9. GRUPE WE, KAPLAN MH: A proximal tubular antigen in the pathogenesis of autoimmune nephrosis (*abstract*). *Fed Proc* 26:573, 1967
10. GRUPE WE, KAPLAN MH: Demonstration of an antibody to proximal tubular antigen in the pathogenesis of experimental autoimmune nephrosis in rats. *J Lab Clin Med* 74:400–409, 1969
11. EDGINGTON TS, GLASSOCK RJ, DIXON FJ: Autologous immune complex nephritis induced with renal tubular antigen: I. Identification and isolation of the pathogenic antigen. *J Exp Med* 127:555–572, 1968
12. NARUSE T, FUKASAWA T, HIRAKAWA N, OIKE S, MIYAKAWA Y: The pathogenesis of experimental membranous glomerulonephritis induced with homologous nephritogenic tubular antigen. *J Exp Med* 144:1347–1362, 1976
13. MIETTINEN A, TÖRNROTH T, TIKKANEN I, VIRTANEN I, LINDER E: Heymann nephritis induced by kidney brush border glycoproteins. *Lab Invest* 43:547–555, 1980
14. MAKKER SP: Evidence that the antigen of autologous immune complex glomerulonephritis of rats is a mannose and glucose containing glycoprotein. *Proc Soc Exp Med* 163:95–99, 1980
15. HUBBARD AL, COHN ZA: Externally disposed plasma membrane proteins. I. Enzymatic iodination of mouse L cells. *J Cell Biol* 64:461–483, 1975
16. COLLETT MS, ERIKSON RL: Protein kinase activity associated with the avian sarcoma virus src gene product. *Proc Natl Acad Sci USA* 75:2021–2024, 1978
17. KERJASCHKI D, FARQUHAR MG: The pathogenic antigen of Heymann nephritis is a glycoprotein of the renal proximal tubule brush border. *Proc Natl Acad Sci USA* 79:5557–5561, 1982
18. KERJASCHKI D, NORONHA-BLOB L, SACKTOR B, FARQUHAR MG: Microdomains of distinctive glycoprotein composition in the kidney proximal tubule brush border. *J Cell Biol* 98:1505–1513, 1984
19. KERJASCHKI D, FARQUHAR MG: Immunocytochemical localization of the Heymann nephritis antigen (gp330) in glomerular epithelial cells of normal Lewis rats. *J Exp Med* 157:667–686, 1983
20. KERJASCHKI D, SHARKEY DJ, FARQUHAR MG: Identification and characterization of Podocalyxin—the major sialoprotein of the renal glomerular epithelial cell. *J Cell Biol* 98:1591–1596, 1984
21. SINGH AK, MAKKER SP: The autoantibody reactive glycopeptide gp70 is present in all glycopeptide subunits of gp500, the nephritogenic macromolecule of Heymann nephritis (*abstract*). *Fed Proc* 42:512, 1983
22. COUSER WG, SALANT DJ: In situ immune complex formation and glomerular injury. *Kidney Int* 17:1–11, 1980
23. VAN DAMME BJC, FLEUREN GJ, BAKKER WW, VERNIER RL, HOEDEMAEKER PHJ: Experimental glomerulonephritis in the rat induced by antibodies directed against tubular antigens. V. Fixed glomerular antigens in the pathogenesis of heterologous immune complex glomerulonephritis. *Lab Invest* 38:502–510, 1978
24. COUSER WG, STEINMULLER DR, STILMANT MM, SALANT DJ, LOWENSTEIN LM: Experimental glomerulonephritis in the isolated perfused rat kidney. *J Clin Invest* 62:1275–1287, 1978
25. NEALE TJ, WILSON CB: Glomerular antigens in Heymann nephritis: Reactivity of eluted and circulating antibody. *J Immunol* 128:323–330, 1982
26. BERTANI T, NOLIN L, FOIDART J, VANDERWALLE A, VERROUST P: The effect of puromycin on subepithelial deposits induced by antibodies directed against tubular antigens: A quantitative study. *Europ J Clin Inv* 9:465–472, 1979
27. FLEUREN GJ, GROND J, HOEDEMAEKER PHJ: The pathogenetic role of free

and circulating antibody in autologous immune complex glomerulonephritis. *Clin Exp Immunol* 41:205–217, 1980

28. NEALE TJ, COUSER WG, SALANT DJ, LOWENSTEIN LM, WILSON CB: Specific uptake of Heymann's nephritic kidney eluate by rat kidney: Studies in vivo and in isolated perfused kidneys. *Lab Invest* 46:450–453, 1982

29. COURTOY PJ, PICTON DH, FARQUHAR MG: Resolution and limitations of the immunoperoxidase procedure in the localization of extracellular matrix antigens. *J Histochem Cytochemistry* 31:945–951, 1983

30. GOLDSTEIN JL, ANDERSON RGW, BROWN MS: Coated pits, coated vesicles, and receptor mediated endocytosis. *Nature* 279:679–682, 1979

31. BROWN MS, ANDERSON RGW, GOLDSTEIN JL: Recycling receptors: The round trip itinerary of migrant membrane proteins. *Cell* 32:663–667, 1983

32. SUGISAKI TJ, KLASSEN GA, ANDRES GA, MILGROM F, McCLUSKEY RT: Passive transfer of Heymann's nephritis with serum. *Kidney Int* 3:66–73, 1973

33. BARABAS AZ, LANNIGAN R: Induction of an autologous immune complex glomerulonephritis in the rat by intravenous injection of heterologous anti-rat kidney tubular antibody. I. Production of chronic progressive immune complex glomerulonephritis. *Br J Exp Pathol* 55:47–55, 1974

34. BRENNER BM, HOSTETTER TH, HUMES HD: Glomerular permselectivity barrier function based on discrimination of molecular size and charge. *Am J Physiol* 234:F455–F460, 1978

35. RENNKE HG, COTRAN RS, VENKATACHALAM MA: Role of molecular charge in glomerular permeability. Tracer studies with cationized ferritin. *J Cell Biol* 67:638–644, 1975

36. KANWAR YS, FARQUHAR MG: Isolation of glycosaminoglycans (heparan sulfate) from glomerular basement membranes. *Proc Natl Acad Sci USA* 76:4493–4497, 1979

37. OITE T, BATSFORD SR, MIHATSCH MJ, TAKAMIYA H, VOGT A: Quantitative studies of in situ immune complex glomerulonephritis in the rat induced by planted cationized antigen. *J Exp Med* 155:460–478, 1982

38. ADLER S, WANG H, WARD HJ, COHEN AH, BORDER WA: Electrical charge. Its role in the pathogenesis and prevention of experimental membranous nephropathy in the rabbit. *J Clin Invest* 71:487–499, 1983

39. GALLO GR, CAULIN-GLASER T, LAMM M: Charge of circulating immune complexes as a factor in glomerular basement membrane localization in mice. *J Clin Invest* 67:1305–1313, 1981

40. KENNY AJ, MAROUX S: Topology of microvillar membrane hydrolases of kidney and intestine. *Physiol Rev* 62:91–128, 1932

41. REISS U, SACKTOR B: Kidney brush border membrane maltase: Purification and properties. *Arch Biochem Biophys* 209:342–348, 1981

42. ROTH TF, PORTER KR: Yolk protein uptake in the oocyte of the mosquito *aedes aegypti*. *J Cell Biol* 20:313–332, 1964

43. PEARSE BMF: Coated vesicles from pig brain: Purification and biochemical characterization. *J Mol Biol* 97:93–99, 1975

44. RODMAN JS, KERJASCHKI D, MERISKO E, FARQUHAR MG: Presence of an extensive clathrin coat on the apical plasmalemma of the rat kidney proximal tubule cell. *J Cell Biol* 98:1630–1636, 1984

45. THUNEBERG L, ROSTGAARD J: Isolation of brush border fragments from homogenates of rat and rabbit kidney cortex. *Exp Cell Res* 51:123–140, 1968

46. HEYMANN W, GRUPE WE, HUNTER JLP, CAMMA A, HACKEL DB, CUPPAGE FE, WEINBERG AG: Production of experimental autoimmune nephrosis in rats by heterologous tissues. *Nephron* 7:363–376, 1970

47. MIETTINEN A, LINDER E: Membrane antigens shared by renal proximal tubules and other epithelia associated with absorption and excretion. *Clin Exp Immunol* 23:568–577, 1976
48. DOXSEY SD, KERJASCHKI D, FARQUHAR MG: A large membrane glycoprotein (gp330) is a resident of coated pits of several absorptive epithelia (*abstract*). *J Cell Biol* 99:178, 1983
49. SCHREINER GF, UNANUE ER: Membrane and cytoplasmic changes in B lymphocytes induced by ligand-surface Ig interaction. *Adv Immunol* 24:38–54, 1976
50. OLDSTONE MBA, FUJINAMI RS: Virus persistence and avoidance of immune surveillance. How measles viruses can be induced to persist in cells, escape immune assault and injure tissues, in *Virus Persistence Symposium 33,* edited by MAHY BWJ, MINSON AC, DARBY GR, London, Cambridge University Press, 1982, pp 185–202
51. BARBA LM, CALDWELL PRB, DOWNIE GH, CAMUSSI C, BRENTJENS J, ANDRES G: Lung injury mediated by antibodies to endothelium. I. In the rabbit a repeated interaction of heterologous anti-angiotensin converting enzyme antibody with alveolar endothelium results in resistence to immune injury through antigenic modulation. *J Exp Med* 158:2141–2158, 1983
52. FARQUHAR MG, PALADE GE: Glomerular permeability. II. Ferritin transfer across the glomerular wall in nephrotic rats. *J Exp Med* 114:699–716, 1961
53. CAULFIELD JP, FARQUHAR MG: The permeability of glomerular capillaries of aminonucleoside nephrotic rats to graded dextrans. *J Exp Med* 142:61–83, 1975
54. SHARON Z, SCHWARTZ MM, LEWIS EJ: The glomerular localization and transport of aggregated protamine-heparin complexes. *Lab Invest* 37:43–52, 1977
55. NARUSE T, MIYAKAWA Y, KITAMURA K, SHIBATA S: Membranous glomerulonephritis mediated by renal tubular epithelial antigen-antibody complex. *J Allergy Clin Immunol* 54:311–318, 1974
56. DOUGLAS MFS, RABIDEAU DP, SCHWARTZ MM, LEWIS EJ: Evidence of autologous immune complex nephritis. *N Engl J Med* 26:1326–1329, 1981

Monoclonal Antibodies as Probes of Normal and Abnormal Renal Structure

Chairpersons: Gary E. Striker and Robert C. Atkins
Discussants: Wayne Hancock, John Hunt, Steven R. Holdsworth,
Akira Y. T. Wu, Alfred F. Michael, Pierre Verroust,
Dontscho Kerjaschki, Charles D. Pusey, Donna L. Mendrick, and
Pierre Ronco

With the advent of the technique for monoclonal antibody production by
Kohler and Milstein in 1975, a potent new tool became available to study
kidney disease. Monoclonal antibodies, because of their exquisite specificity,
relative immortality, and their availability in large amounts, have the potential
for use in many areas of the investigation of kidney structure and function.
This workshop highlighted various areas where monoclonal antibodies have
been used and also emphasized some intrinsic difficulties and limitations in
their use.

Atkins considered guidelines to the use of monoclonal antibodies to localize
structures in tissues. He stated that there are specific problems in the recognition of sparse cell surface antigens by monoclonal antibodies within tissues.
First, there is a fixation compromise between adequate morphology and antigen preservation. For each individual antibody it may therefore be necessary
to determine the optimal fixative. In addition, the sensitivity of the detection
technique needs to be taken into account. In many instances indirect immunofluorescence or peroxidase localization is inadequate and a multilayer technique may need to be used. Enzyme predigestion to uncover hidden antigens
may also be necessary. Additional complications become evident when investigating the role of infiltrating leukocytes within renal tissue. These include
differences in antigenic profile between circulating and tissue leukocytes due
to maturation, activation, or local environmental effects. Thus, for example,
a macrophage marker may be present on a circulating monocyte, but not
on a tissue monocyte. Therefore, it is important to ensure in such studies
that the pertinent cell surface antigen is used.

Another problem is the sharing of antigens between leukocytes and tissue
components. For example, the Ia antigen is present on endothelium and
tubules in the human kidney as well as monocytes.

Michael addressed the use of monoclonal antibodies to investigate struc-

---

This narrative is a summary of a Workshop by the same title.

tural components of the kidney. He said that there are a number of issues that need to be considered in the use of monoclonal antibodies to investigate structural macromolecules. The first is that there may be "hidden" epitopes. Second, the ability to isolate and identify various clones depends on the adequacy of the available screening procedures for the characterization of monoclonal antibodies.

Several components of the glomerular basement membrane lend themselves to characterization, including the collagens (Types IV and V), glycoproteins, proteoglycans, anionic plasma proteins, and so on. The field has been enriched by the availability of antibodies derived from EHS sarcoma antigens.

There are a number of techniques that are useful in the evaluation of monoclonal antibodies, including agents such as paraphenylene-diamine, which decrease quenching due to the oxidation of fluorochrome.

A large number of monoclonal antibodies to glomerular antigens have been developed. Some are specific for particular regions within the glomerulus whereas others recognize multiple areas within both the glomerulus and other tissues. They have been useful in the study of the developmental anatomy of the extracellular matrix as well as the localization of different matrix components within the glomerulus. There now is developing an area of investigation into the abnormalities of extracellular matrix that are present in different diseases. One example is that of diabetes mellitus. The findings are relatively complex, but there is an appearance of new antigens as well as an increase in some endogenous proteins and a loss of others. This field of study is new.

Hancock described monoclonal antibodies that were prepared by immunizing mice with whole human glomeruli. It was his objective to attain antibodies to glomerular cell antigens and structural components that could be used to identify glomerular cells in culture, and to delineate changes in patients with glomerulonephritis. Several antibodies were produced and have been reported previously, including an antibody to glomerular cells, to Type IV collagen and to fibronectin. Other monoclonal antibodies defined a new series of human glomerular protein and carbohydrate antigens. The antibodies stained cellular outgrowths of isolated glomeruli cultured in vitro.

Pusey described a mouse monoclonal antibody (MCA) to human glomerular basement membrane (GBM) using standard fusion techniques. The binding of the antibody in a radioimmunoassay for anti-GBM antibody could be inhibited by collagenase-solubilized GBM and sera from patients with Goodpasture syndrome. On Western blotting, the MCA and sera from our patients ($N = 32$) recognized the same 5 major brands (26 to 58 kd) in collagenase-solubilized human GBM. Preincubation with the MCA blocked the subsequent binding of sera, from all 5 patients studied, to these bands. Indirect immunofluorescence, using normal human tissue, revealed that the MCA and antibody eluted from the kidney of a patient with Goodpasture syndrome bound in an identical pattern, giving linear fluorescence on the GBM, certain distal tubule basement membrane (TBM), Bowman capsule, alveolar basement membrane (BM), and choroid plexus BM. Therefore, it is likely that MCA-Pl and human autoantibodies recognize the same (or a very closely related) single autoantigen and that the specificity of the autoimmune response is highly restricted.

Ten young men with Alport syndrome were studied, and it was found that the MCA (and eluted autoantibody) bound weakly to the GBM of six; it failed to bind to four. It therefore appears that there is variability of expression of the Goodpasture antigen in Alport syndrome. Further studies should determine whether this MCA is of value in making the diagnosis, or predicting the prognosis, in Alport syndrome.

Verroust produced monoclonal antibodies against isolated rabbit renal cortical cells. Eleven such clones were found to be directed against the brushborder and five against basolateral membrane or intracytoplasmic constituents. In addition, one was found to recognize cells of the collecting tubule. Antibodies against brushborder were characterized by immunoprecipitation or radiolabeled brushborder vesicles. Seven antigens were identified with molecular weights ranging from 90,000 to over 350,000 daltons. One of these was identified as a leucine-aminopeptidase. When coupled to Sepharose, a mixture of three monoclonal antibrushborder antibodies was able to retain 90% of the isolated cells passed over the column. Less than 10% were retained when an indifferent antibody was coupled to the Sepharose. The effluent from the column with specific antibody to proximal tubular brushborder contained an enriched population of nonproximal tubular cells.

In summary, monoclonal antibodies may be useful in the separation of specific cell types within homogenates of whole kidney.

Kerjaschki isolated and purified two membrane proteins, maltase and gp330, known to be present in the proximal tubule brushborder. They were found to be large glycoproteins of similar molecular weight (300,000 daltons). Monoclonal antibodies raised against these purified proteins were found to localize in unique and distinct regions of the brushborder of the proximal tubule. The antibody to maltase localized on the lateral surfaces of the microvilli by immunoelectron microscopy. The antibody to gp330 localized in the basal segments of the brushborder and the clathrin-coated apical invaginations at the base of the microvilli.

Thus, these two different antigens, which are located at the apical surface of the proximal convoluted tubules, may be useful as markers for their individual geographic domain.

Hunt presented data on monoclonal antibodies to Tamm-Horsfall protein. He has produced six IgG monoclonal antibodies that stain proximal tubules. The antibodies can be used for detection of Tamm-Horsfall protein in serum as well as for its localization within tissues.

Striker stated that the identification of glomerular cells in vitro has depended principally upon morphologic techniques supplemented by investigations of biosynthetic products. When isolated, single glomeruli are explanted in vitro an early population of cells emerge that have a cuboidal appearance. These have been labelled variously but they have most often been thought to represent epithelial cells. Later more elongated cells appear that have been designated as mesangial. Both cell types have been studied for synthesis of extracellular matrix components. The first, cuboidal, cell type synthesizes basement membrane components whereas the latter synthesizes both basement membrane and interstitial matrix components. To identify the cells further, monoclonal antibodies against intermediate elements have been prepared. Examinations of the "epithelial" cell outgrowth revealed that a number of the cells did not contain antibodies against the intermediate filament that is common to epithelial cells in vitro, cytokeratin. Further investigation revealed that these cells contained von Willebrand factor. Thus, some of the cells were found to be endothelial cells. They were studied further and found to synthesize basement membrane components, and to have angiotensin-converting enzyme on their surface. In addition they had platelet-derived growth factor receptors on their surface and responded to this mitogen in vitro.

In summary, monoclonal antibodies have proven to be useful in the identification of different cell types in the outgrowth from isolated human glomeruli in vitro and in the isolation of a new glomerular cell type, endothelial cells.

Atkins discussed the usefulness of monoclonal antibodies as markers for infiltrating leukocytes in renal tissue. Monoclonal antibodies have provided a useful way of quantifying cellular infiltrates in order to define mechanisms of transplant rejection, to enumerate leukocytes in different types of glomerulonephritis (within both the glomeruli and the interstitium), and to study crescent formation. Glomerular neutrophils and macrophages were present in postinfectious and crescentic glomerulonephritis. No T cells were detected. There was a substantial interstitial infiltrate in most forms of glomerulonephritis that consisted of T cells predominantly. The question as to which cells constitute crescents in nephritis has been answered partially by studies using monoclonal antibodies. About 30% of the crescentic cells were macrophages whereas only 8% were epithelial in origin as demonstrated by use of the antiepithelial cell marker. The use of monoclonal antibodies as cell markers provides the means to delineate cell types within renal tissue.

Holdsworth has used monoclonal antibodies to study the involvement of lymphocytes in experimental glomerulonephritis. He studied a preimmunized model of anti-GBM antibody-induced glomerulonephritis in the rat. The late phase proteinuria in this model has been shown to be dependent on the infiltration of macrophages. Helper, suppressor, and T-cell markers were used to enumerate lymphocytes in glomeruli by indirect immunofluorescence.

The apparance of glomerular lymphocytes was correlated with proteinuria, autologous antibody production, and glomerular macrophage accumulation. A transient lymphocyte infiltration (predominantly helper T cells) preceded the peak of macrophage accumulation. Use of the anti-T-cell agent, cyclosporine-A, prevented autologous antibody synthesis and T-cell infiltration. Macrophage accumulation and proteinuria did not occur in cyclosporine-treated animals.

The results suggested a role for T-cell-directed, macrophage-induced injury in glomerulonephritis.

Monoclonal antibody-induced proteinuria was discussed by Mendrick. She showed that glomerular alterations can be induced in the rat by two monoclonal antibodies directed against previously undescribed endogenous glomerular antigens. The antibodies produced glomerular injury independently of complement activation or leukocyte infiltration.

The first monoclonal antibody reacted with an endogenous mesangial matrix component. This monoclonal antibody formed immune complexes in situ that became electron-dense deposits visible within the mesangial matrix.

Podocyte alterations and proteinuria were induced by a monoclonal antibody directed against an 118/107 kd antigen complex present in the glomerular capillary wall and on the cell surface of the proximal tubule brushborder. The amount of glomerular-bound immunoglobulin necessary to induce glomerular lesions with this monoclonal antibody was orders-of-magnitude lower than that required for polyclonal rabbit or mouse anti-rat GBM serum.

Wu demonstrated that a monoclonal antibody could produce proteinuria and proliferative changes in a rabbit experimental model of nephritis. A monoclonal antibody to rabbit glomerular basement membrane induced proteinuria with as little as 2.0 μg of antibody fixed per g of kidney tissue. The mechanism of proteinuria was complement-independent and the hypercellular glomeruli contained neutrophils and perhaps macrophages. It was thought that this monoclonal antibody might recognize the nephrogenic or similar antigen as it masked staining of the basement membrane by a polyclonal nephrotoxic antisera.

Ronco analyzed the antigens common to glomeruli epithelial cells and brushborder (BB), and their potential role. He produced monoclonal antibodies (Mab) to rat brushborder and selected those with both reactivities. These antibodies identified at least two different antigens on both the top brushborder and the glomerulus. The first bound to the brushborder wall, which was stained diffusely. The second bound to the brushborder but also gave a very fine and dotted staining on the glomerulus.

The corresponding antigens were distinct as shown by immunoprecipitation analysis and immunoperoxidase electron microscopy. The first precipitated a protein of approximately 90 kd whereas the second precipitated a protein of higher molecular weight close to 330 kd. The latter comigrated with the material precipitated by Ig eluted from the glomeruli of rats with passive Heymann nephritis as well as with the major band precipitated by our anti-gp330 antiserum. By immunoperoxidase the electron microscopy binding of the second was restricted to the coated pits of the epithelial cells and the base of microvilli of the brushborder whereas the second bound diffusely to epithelial and endothelial cells, and to the entire surface of the microvilli.

In vivo renal binding was studied by immunofluorescence and by paired label methodology. Renal-specific binding of the first was maximum at 4 hr and then decreased rapidly thereafter, whereas the binding of the second remained fairly stable over several days. After injection in vivo, the first induced proteinuria and epithelial cell damage.

These results suggested that at least two antigen-antibody systems are common to brushborder and glomerular epithelial cells, that both can induce epimembranous deposits in vivo, and that the kinetics of deposition and removal are markedly different.

Role of Proteoglycans in Glomerular Function and Pathology

Marilyn Gist Farquhar, Margaret C. Lemkin, and Jennifer L. Stow

Since their detection in the glomerular basement membrane (GBM) 5 years ago [1, 2], proteoglycans have been the subject of considerable interest, experimentation, and speculation. Evidence has been presented suggesting that they are necessary for maintaining the normal permeability properties of the GBM [3]. In addition, they have been implicated as a causative factor of the proteinuria that occurs in several experimental renal diseases (aminonucleoside nephrosis and diabetic glomerular nephropathy) and as a contributory factor in immune complex formation. In this presentation the information obtained thus far on the role of proteoglycans in glomerular function and pathology will be summarized; and, recent results obtained in our laboratory on this topic will be presented.

The Importance of Anionic Glomerular Components in Glomerular Filtration

Among the major advances in glomerular physiology within the last decade that have influenced our thinking about glomerular function and pathology were the demonstrations: (1) that the glomerulus exercises charge selectivity as well as size selectivity during the filtration of macromolecules [4, 5], and (2) that charge selectivity, rather than size selectivity, is lost in certain glomerular diseases that are associated with proteinuria (nephrotoxic serum nephritis [NSN] [5], aminonucleoside nephrosis [5], and human minimal change nephropathy [6]). From the beginning, this charge selectivity was attributed to the presence of fixed negatively charged groups in the glomerular capillary wall [4, 5]. Originally, it was assumed that sialoglycoproteins on the epithelial

This manuscript was presented as part of a symposium on *Recent Advances in the Structure, Biochemistry and Function of the Glomerulus.*

cell surface were the responsible anionic components, because they were the only anionic macromolecules known to be present in the glomerulus and because (at the time) the epithelial slits were believed by many investigators to represent the main structural barrier responsible for retaining plasma proteins in the circulation. More recently, however, with the accumulation of evidence (reviewed in [7, 8]) that the barrier to anionic and neutral macromolecules exists at the level of the lamina rara interna of the GBM, and also with the demonstration [4] that the GBM itself is negatively charged, we turned our attention to searching for negatively charged components in the GBM. It was this search that led to the discovery of proteoglycans—initially in the GBM, and more recently on the endothelial and epithelial cell surfaces.

What are Proteoglycans and How are They Studied?

To evaluate the information obtained thus far on glomerular proteoglycans, some knowledge of the properties of proteoglycans and the analytic methods used in their study may be useful.

The special properties of proteoglycans (summarized in Table 1) [9–11] that are especially important in the context of their role in glomerular function and pathology are: (1) their high net-negative charge (the highest of any known biologic macromolecule), and (2) their high viscosity due to the fact that they form polymeric networks in aqueous solution [10]. Structurally, they consist of a core protein of variable size to which one or more glycosaminoglycan (GAG) side chains (formerly known as acid mucopolysaccharides) is covalently bound (during biosynthesis). The distinguishing features of proteoglycans are their GAG chains, which are made up of disaccharide repeating units (consisting of hexuronic or iduronic acid and glucosamine or galactosamine)—of which chondroitin sulfate, hyaluronic acid, keratan sulfate, heparan sulfate, and heparin are the major types.

Methods are available for the identification of proteoglycans in situ in tissues, for the purification of intact proteoglycan molecules (core protein plus GAG chains), and for the isolation and analysis of the disaccharide (GAG) side chains. It is noteworthy that all, or at least most, of the analytic approaches currently used to identify or to isolate proteoglycans take advantage of their high net-negative charge and rely on the ionic (electrostatic)

Table 1. Properties of glycosaminoglycans (proteoglycans)

High net-negative charge and charge density
    Repel anionic macromolecules
    Bind divalent cations (Ca^{++})
    Bind cationic proteins
Viscous gel-like consistency
    Retard transport of macromolecules
    Retard diffusion of ions
    Resist compression

interaction of these molecules with oppositely charged (cationic) substances.

In tissues, proteoglycans can be detected in situ with various cationic dyes (for example, ruthenium red, alcian blue, safranin, or colloidal iron) or proteins (lysozyme or cationized ferritin). Since the binding of these cationic probes is nonspecific (based on charge interaction alone), the specificity of their binding to proteoglycans and the type of proteoglycan present are established by demonstrating elimination of staining after subjecting the specimen to digestion with specific GAG-degrading enzymes.

For isolation of the entire proteoglycan molecule (core protein with attached GAG chains), radiolabeled tissues are extracted (usually with 4 M guanidine-hydrochloric acid [HCl] in the presence of detergents) and the proteoglycans are purified by ion-exchange chromatography [12]. Their molecular weights are determined by molecular-sieve chromatography rather than by their mobility on SDS-PAGE, because due to their highly anionic and bulky nature, intact proteoglycans do not enter the usual (3 to 15%) SDS gels. Separation of different proteoglycans (for example, keratan sulfate and chondroitin sulfate proteoglycans) sometimes can be achieved at the ion-exchange chromatography step (if the individual proteoglycan types carry a sufficiently different net-negative charge); however, if not, further steps are required, such as separation on cesium chloride gradients or digestion with specific GAG-degrading enzymes.

Often, isolation of the whole proteoglycan is bypassed, and only the polysaccharide (GAG) moieties are isolated for analysis. Since GAG do not exist free in tissues [11], with the exception of hyaluronic acid, analysis of GAG chains gives a reliable indication of the amounts and types of proteoglycans present in tissues. For the isolation of GAG, tissues usually are subjected to pronase or papain digestion (to release glycopeptides); the GAG are then separated from other glycopeptides either by gel filtration or by precipitation with cationic detergents (for example, cetylpyridinium chloride). Individual GAG species then may be identified by cellulose acetate electrophoresis (based on their mobility compared to known GAG standards) or by their susceptibility to digestion with specific GAG-degrading enzymes.

Characterization of Proteoglycans Isolated from the Glomerular Basement Membrane

Proteoglycans were first detected in the rat GBM in situ [13, 1] by use of cationic probes, as described above. Initially, lysozyme [13, 14] and later ruthenium red [15], cationized ferritin [15], alcian blue [16], polyethyleneimine [17], and protamine-heparin complexes [18] all were shown to bind to a regular (60-nm spacing) lattice-like network of anionic sites that is located in the laminae rarae (interna and externa) of the GBM (Fig. 1) and in the mesangial matrix. The anionic sites were composed of heparan sulfate proteoglycans; this was established [1] by the fact that they were removed by digestion with heparitinase or by nitrous acid treatment (procedures that specifically degrade heparan sulfates), but they were not affected by other

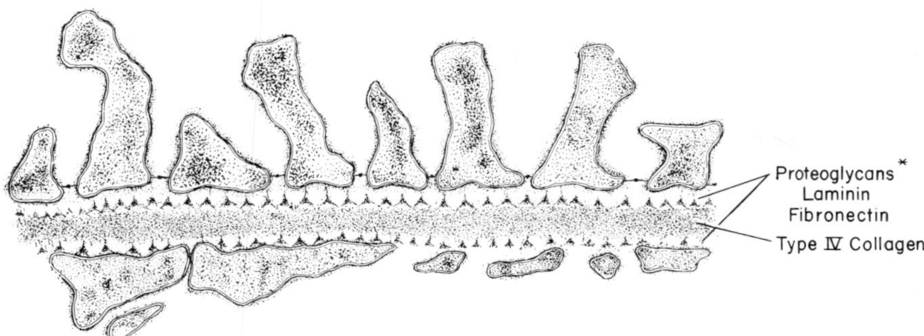

Fig. 1. Schematic representation of the organization of the GBM (based on the results of work reviewed in [7, 8]). The GBM is visualized as consisting of three layers of different composition: the lamina densa or backbone is composed of type IV collagen, whereas the lamina rarae interna and externa on either side have a different composition. Heparan sulfate proteoglycans and the attachment proteins, laminin and fibronectin are located in these outer layers. The heparan sulfate-rich anionic sites are drawn as angular particles (20 nm) with fine filaments (3 nm) extending from their points to connect one particle with another, with the membranes of adjoining epithelial and endothelial cells and with the lamina densa. The anionic sites are depicted as they appear after ruthenium red staining [15]. However, based on studies of cartilage proteoglycans [9], it can be assumed that each particle consists of proteoglycan monomers that collapse during fixation and processing for electron microscopy. It also can be assumed that in their normal hydrated state, they occupy a domain several times that of the collapsed particle. (From [26])

treatments (digestion with neuraminidase or other GAG-degrading enzymes). Subsequently, the presence of proteoglycans in the GBM was confirmed [2] by extraction and analysis of GAG isolated from fractions of purified rat GBM that was prepared by detergent treatment [7, 15]; they were found to constitute $\sim$ 1% of the dry weight of these GBM fractions (which also include mesangial matrix). Analysis of either unlabeled (extracted in bulk) [2] or radiolabeled [19] GAG revealed that they consist mainly ($\sim$ 85%) of heparan sulfate proteoglycans in both the rat [2, 19] and dog [20] GBM fractions. Similar findings were obtained on the rat [21], bovine [22], and human [23] GBM by other investigators. Smaller amounts of other GAG (chondroitin sulfates [19] and hyaluronic acid [2, 19]) also were detected in GBM fractions. Recently, evidence has been obtained showing that chondroitin sulfate proteoglycans are confined to the mesangial matrix [24, 25]. The precise location of hyaluronic acid in the glomerular matrix is presently unknown.

Subsequent isolation and analysis of intact proteoglycans (core proteins plus GAG chains) that were purified from GBM fractions revealed [26] that the heparan sulfate proteoglycans (HSPG) and the chondroitin sulfate proteoglycans (CSPG) have similar properties; both have an Mr of $\sim$ 130,000 and contain four GAG chains (Mr = 26,000). Noteworthy is the fact that

HSPG isolated from the rat GBM have different properties, in terms of their overall size (molecular weight) and the size of their GAG chains, from HSPG isolated from other sources (Table 2). It is particularly of interest that HSPG isolated from GBM fractions are much smaller and have smaller GAG chains than those isolated from the basement membrane-like matrix secreted by the EHS sarcoma [27]—a mouse tumor often used as a source of basement membrane components.

The significance of the discovery of proteoglycans in the GBM and mesangial matrix lies in the fact that—even though they are present in relatively small amounts—due to their high-charge density and viscosity [10, 11], their presence would be expected to greatly modify the permeability properties of this structure (Laurent and Torvard, personal communication).

Functions of Proteoglycans

Proteoglycans are widely distributed on cell surfaces and in the extracellular matrix, where they have been shown to serve many diverse functions [9–11, 28], some of which are listed in Table 3. Any of the these functions could apply to the proteoglycans in the glomerular matrix. For example, based on their ability to interact with collagen and other GBM components (laminin or fibronectin), they may play a role in determining the organization (porosity) of the lamina densa or backbone of the GBM (Fig. 1). Also, given their concentration in the laminae rarae, they may serve as cushions that prevent collapse of the cells onto the lamina densa. Of greatest interest, however, is their potential role in maintaining the barrier function of the GBM by modifying its permeability. This is the only function of proteoglycans in the GBM for which there is currently evidence.

Proteoglycans Affect the Permeability Properties of the GBM

There is now increasing evidence that proteoglycans do play an important role in establishing the permeability properties of the GBM. Much of the

Table 2. Comparative properties of some proteoglycans

	Type	Source	Molecular radius	Size of GAG chains	Reference
Chondroitin sulfate	Cartilage	Rat	2,000,000	20,000 (8)[b]	9
Heparan sulfate	EHS sarcoma	Mouse	750,000[a]	70,000	27
Heparan sulfate	Hepatocyte	Rat	75,000[a]	14,000	28
Heparan sulfate	GBM	Rat	130,000[a]	26,000 (4 to 5)	26

[a] Based on molecular sieve chromatography using cartilage proteoglycan standards.
[b] Number given in parenthesis indicates the number of GAG chains present where this is known.

Table 3. Known functions of proteoglycans

Modify permeability
Cation exchange
Absorb compressive loads (cartilage)
Interact with collagens to affect fibril formation
Facilitate cell-to-substrate attachment by binding to fibronectin, laminin, and cell surface components
Direct morphogenetic movements during embryonic development
Prevent thrombosis (heparin, heparan sulfates)
Modulate binding of hormones and LDL to their receptors (heparin, heparan sulfates)

evidence is still circumstantial and indirect (see below); however, direct evidence was provided by experiments in which the permeability of the GBM to ferritin was determined after removal of GAG chains from proteoglycans via enzymatic digestion [3]. Normally, anionic ferritin and other neutral and anionic macromolecules of Mr > 7 nmol (greater than that of albumin) do not penetrate the GBM to any extent [7, 8]. However, when the kidney was first perfused with heparinase (removes all GAG except keratan sulfates) prior to infusion with native ferritin, this large (12-nm) tracer penetrated the GBM and reached the urinary spaces in large amounts. In kidneys perfused with *Streptomyces* hyaluronidase (which removes hyaluronic acid) or with chondroitinase ABC (removes hyaluronic acid and chondroitins 4- and 6-sulfates plus dermatan sulfate), little or no ferritin penetrated beyond the lamina rara interna of the GBM, as it did in controls. It was concluded that removal of heparan sulfate along with all other GAG—but not hyaluronic acid alone or hyaluronic acid together with chondroitin sulfates—leads to a dramatic increase in the permeability of the GBM to molecules ranging to the size of ferritin. It was later shown [29, 30] that when [^{125}I]BSA (bovine serum albumin) was used as the permeability tracer, increased leakage of protein (detected via autoradiography) occurred after treatment with all three enzymes; this indicated that hyaluronic acid and perhaps chondroitin sulfates also play a role in establishing the restrictive permeability properties of the GBM. Indirect evidence suggesting the involvement of proteoglycans in GBM permeability also was provided by experiments showing that infusion of various polycationic substances (protamine [31, 32], hexadimethrine [33] or poly-l-lysine [32], or polyethyleneimine [34]) into the glomerulus resulted in an increased permeability of the GBM to circulating plasma proteins.

Potential Involvement of Proteoglycans in Glomerular Pathology

Based on the known physiologic functions of proteoglycans, one can readily predict several ways in which glomerular proteoglycans might play a role in the pathogenesis of various glomerular diseases (Table 4). Evidence has already been obtained (see below) connecting alterations in proteoglycans with alterations in glomerular permeability, because changes in the composition or turnover of glomerular proteoglycans have been reported as occurring in several glomerular diseases associated with proteinuria. Beyond a role in modifying permeability, a wide-ranging series of events could be initiated as a result of the propensity of proteoglycans to interact with oppositely charged (cationic) molecules. Due to their exposed nature and high net-negative charge, proteoglycans would be expected to bind, thereby concentrating any cationic molecules in their immediate vicinity. Indeed, binding of tracers ranging in size from relatively small molecules, such as polyethyleneimine (Mr = 1200) and lysozyme (Mr = ~ 14,000), up to that of cationized ferritin (Mr = 480,000) has been demonstrated. Moreover, studies with cationized ferritin show that for binding to occur, cationic molecules do not need to necessarily have a high isoelectric point as long as they have a high surface charge density—because ferritin fractions with isoelectric points of only ~ 7.3 to 7.5 specifically bind to the HSPG-rich anionic sites [15].

Upon discovering GAG in the GBM, we predicted [1] that they could play a role in the pathogenesis of glomerular diseases by binding various cationic molecules present in the circulation—such as cationic antigens, antibodies or immune complexes, or vasoactive amines, cationic drugs, or antibiotics (for example, adriamycin [35]) and toxic substances. Evidence has already been obtained in favor of the preferential involvement of cationic immune complexes [36, 37], antigens [38–40], and antibodies [41] in immune complex formation.

There currently is no direct evidence for the other entries in Table 4; however, based on the known properties of proteoglycans, one can (with some assurance) predict that it is only a matter of time until these are also validated.

Changes in Anionic Sites in the Glomerular Basement Membrane in Glomerular Diseases Associated with Proteinuria

Circumstantial evidence connecting alterations in the anionic sites that are composed of HSPG with alterations in glomerular permeability came from

Table 4. Potential roles of proteoglycans in glomerular diseases

Could modify permeability and lead to proteinuria
Could bind nonspecifically—by electrostatic interaction—antigen-antibody complexes, or antigens or antibodies alone, and lead to immune complex formation
Could trap nonspecifically—by electrostatic interaction—various toxic substances, cationic drugs, or antibiotics and vasoactive amines
Could affect attachment of epithelial and endothelial cells to the GBM
Could affect the porosity of the collagenous proteins, thereby leading to changes in GBM permeability

observations showing that binding of cationic probes to these sites is reduced to glomerular disease in which there is proteinuria associated with a loss of charge selectivity [14, 16, 43, 44].

We obtained this evidence in aminonucleoside-nephrotic rats before we knew the composition of the GBM sites. Using lysozyme as a cationic probe, we found [14] that not only was there a loss of fixed negative charges from epithelial surfaces, as had been known for some time [42], but there also was a loss of charge (based on the reduced binding of lysozyme) from the lamina rara interna and externa of the GBM. Subsequently, Caulfield [16] and Seiler et al [43] reported a reduction in the binding of alcian blue and protamine-heparin complexes (respectively); and, we [44] demonstrated a reduction in the amount of cationized ferritin that bound to the anionic sites in the laminae rarae in aminonucleoside-nephrotic rats. We also found that the ferritin that did bind could be eluted at a lower salt concentration than in normal rats (0.2 instead of 0.3 M KCl). Mynderse et al [45] reported that there was a reduction in the staining for proteoglycans in the GBM of aminonucleoside-nephrotic rats via immunocytochemistry (using antiproteoglycan antibodies raised against HSPG isolated from the EHS sarcoma [27]). Very recently, changes in the anionic sites in the laminae rarae of the human GBM have been described by Vernier et al [46] in patients with congenital nephrotic syndrome. In the latter case, both a reduced binding and a change in the spacing of the proteoglycan lattice was detected by using the cationic probe, polyethyleneimine.

Disturbances in the distribution of the anionic sites in the laminae rarae also have been reported in two experimental glomerular immune complex disease models—the NZB mouse [47] and Heymann nephritis [48].

Thus, there is now circumstantial evidence for an association between a reduction in the charge density of the anionic sites composed of HSPG (based on binding of cationic probes), a loss of charge selectivity, and proteinuria in several pathologic conditions.

Biochemical Data on the Biosynthesis of Proteoglycans in Glomerular Diseases

Increased Proteoglycan Synthesis in Aminonucleoside Nephrosis

At present, the available data on proteoglycan synthesis in this disease model of minimal change nephropathy is somewhat limited; however, the information available suggests that proteoglycan synthesis may be *increased* in aminonucleoside nephrosis. We have obtained data indicating that biosynthesis of GAG (as determined by radiolabeling) is increased in both whole cortex and glomeruli from aminonucleoside-nephrotic rats [49]. As shown in Table 5, 1.7 and 2.3 times more [^{35}S]sulfate and 6.2 and 1.8 times more [^{3}H]glucosamine are incorporated into cortex and glomeruli (respectively) of nephrotic kidneys, in comparison to controls. The ratio of synthesis of HSPG to CSPG was normal or slightly increased. Similar data was obtained

Table 5. Average specific radioactivities in GAG from cortex and glomeruli of nephrotic versus normal kidneys labeled by perfusion[a]

Kidney fraction	Average specific radioactivity in GAG (cpm/100 μg DNA)	
	^{35}S	^{3}H
Normal glomeruli	118,069	15,028
Normal cortex	229,887	65,593
Nephrotic glomeruli	339,240	6500
Nephrotic cortex	655,096	195,861

[a] Kidneys of normal and nephrotic rats were labeled with [^{35}S]sulfate and [^{3}H]glucosamine for 4 hr in a perfusion system [26]. GAG fractions were isolated from cortex and medulla by pronase digestion and gel filtration (as described in [19]). Samples of the labeled cortex and glomeruli were homogenized in 0.5 N PCA, and the DNA content was determined. Data from normal kidneys represent the average of three experiments; data from nephrotic kidneys is the average of two experiments (from [49]).

by Dehnel et al [50], who reported that increased amounts of GAG were synthesized and released into the medium by nephrotic glomeruli incubated in vitro.

These results, which suggest that GAG synthesis is increased in aminonucleoside-nephrotic animals, came as a surprise in view of the evidence obtained with cationic probes (summarized above) demonstrating a *decrease* in the charge density of the GBM anionic sites in this disease. Viewed together, these data suggest that the reduction in charge density of the HSPG in the GBM is *not* due to reduced biosynthesis of proteoglycans; rather, it may be due to either the production of abnormal proteoglycans (a defect in their insertion into the GBM) or an increase in their turnover (degradation). In view of the recent detection of two antigenically distinct populations of HSPG in the rat glomerulus (see below), further studies are required to clarify the relationship between the different proteoglycan populations and pools before the nature of the alterations in proteoglycans in nephrotic animals can be fully understood.

Reduced Proteoglycan Synthesis in Experimental Diabetes

In diabetic animals, a *reduction* (up to 30 to 40%) in the synthesis of GAG and their incorporation into the GBM has been documented by several investigators [51–54]. Information has been obtained by studying the biosynthesis of GAG [51] or of proteoglycans [52] in glomeruli of streptozoticin-diabetic rats, and also in EHS sarcomas transplanted either into streptozoticin-induced diabetic mice [53] or into diabetic mutant mice [54]. Furthermore, comparative analysis of GBM isolated from glomeruli of diabetic and normal patients [23] also indicates that the heparan sulfate content of GBM is reduced in the diabetic patient. Based on these findings, a causative relationship between the reduced HSPG content of the GBM and proteinuria has been proposed [23, 51–54] in this disease.

Proteoglycans as a Contributory Factor in Immune Complex Formation

As already mentioned, there is now considerable evidence that deposition of cationic antigens [38–40], antibodies [41], or immune complexes [36, 37] in the lamina rara externa is favored over negatively charged or neutral molecules of the same type. That deposition of cationic species is favored is understandable because: (1) neutral or anionic macromolecules the size of albumin or larger do not penetrate, to any extent, beyond the lamina rarae of the GBM [7, 8], and (2) the experiments of Rennke et al [4] with cationic ferritins make it clear that even very large molecules (up to 120 Å in size) can cross the lamina densa if they carry a net-positive charge.

The question that arises then is *how* are proteoglycans involved in immune complex deposition? To begin with, based on charge interaction, the proteoglycans can be expected to bind and, thereby, to focally concentrate cationic species that penetrate the lamina densa and arrive in the lamina rara externa. Once bound, they may serve as a nidus for further immunoprecipitation and aggregation of immune complexes.

Beyond these expectations that have been deduced directly from the results of experiments with cationic probes, the physical properties of proteoglycans in solution are such that their presence in connective tissues is known to favor the precipitation of immune complexes [55, 56]. In addition, individual IgG subtypes appear to have specific properties that favor their interaction with proteoglycans. It has been shown [57] that among monoclonal IgG of similar electrophoretic mobility, there are some that specifically interact with acidic polysaccharides (including heparin) and others that do not. The interactions appear to involve electrostatic binding between cationic sites on the Fab region of the IgG molecule and sulfate residues of polysaccharides.

From the above, it should be clear that the potential is great for nonspecific (electrostatic) and physical (precipitation, lattice formation) interactions between IgG and proteoglycans; therefore, this is a significant factor to be taken into account when contemplating the pathogenesis of immune complex diseases.

Are All Glomerular Proteoglycans Associated with the Glomerular Basement Membrane?

Besides their association with extracellular matrices, proteoglycans—especially heparan sulfate proteoglycans—are known to be widely distributed along cell surfaces [9, 11]. To fully understand the role of proteoglycans in glomerular function and pathology, it is important to know how many different proteoglycan populations there are in the glomerulus and how they are distributed—especially which ones are associated with the GBM and with individual cell types.

To obtain information on this topic, we labeled kidneys in vitro with [35S]sulfate and [3H]glucosamine, determined the label present in whole glomeruli [49], and obtained a balance sheet (Table 6) on the amounts of incorporated labels extracted at each step in the preparation of GBM fractions by a modified [15] Meezan procedure [58]. The results were surprising; only 6 to 10% of the total incorporated sulfate (two-thirds of which is incorporated into proteoglycans [49]) was recovered in GBM fractions. The rest were extracted during the various preparative steps, with significant losses occurring during hypotonic lysis (28%), sodium/DNase washes (40%), and deoxycholate treatment (25%)—treatments that effectively disrupt and remove the cells. Very similar findings were obtained after labeling with [3H]glucosamine. It did not seem likely that the losses could be explained entirely by a loss of proteoglycans from the GBM or mesangial matrix, because the HSPG-rich anionic sites are well preserved in isolated GBM [15]. Thus, these results gave us the first clue that a significant amount of the total glomerular proteoglycans might be present in or on glomerular cells (epithelial, endothelial, or mesangial).

Which Glomerular Cell Types Synthesize Proteoglycans?

In principle, all cell types are capable of making proteoglycans. Observations of homogeneous glomerular cell lines maintained in culture [59, 60] indicate that mesangial cells and epithelial cells synthesize proteoglycans; however, there is a difference in the types of proteoglycans that they make—mesangial cells predominantly synthesize CSPG and epithelial cells predominantly synthesize HSPG. Data are not yet available on glomerular endothelial cells. In any case, results obtained on cultured cells do not indicate the relative contributions of the different cell types to the biosynthesis of proteoglycans in the intact glomerulus in situ.

We have obtained information on this topic via quantitative electron microscopic autoradiography [49]. Glomeruli were radiolabeled by perfusion with [35S]sulfate, were fixed and prepared for electron microscopic autoradiography as described [61], and grains located over the GBM (versus those located over

Table 6. Radioactivity extracted
during GBM isolation[a]

	Radioactivity extracted (%)	
Extraction step	^{35}S	^{3}H
Water	28.0	23.0
NaCl/DNase	40.0	33.0
Deoxycholate	25.0	35.0
First wash	0.6	0.9
Second wash	0.2	0.3
Recovered in GBM	6.4	7.4
% recovery	93.0	105.0

[a] Kidneys were labeled with either [^{35}S]sulfate or [^{3}H]glucosamine for 4 hr by perfusion [26]. Glomeruli were isolated and GBM fractions were prepared therefrom (as described in [19]). The percentage (%) of the radioactivity extracted during each step in the isolation of GBM was determined. The percentages given represent the averages of three experiments for ^{35}S, and data from one experiment for ^{3}H. The % radioactivity extracted = [(cpm extracted in a specific step)/(total cpm recovered)] × 100. The starting glomerular preparation contained 93,250 cpm of ^{3}H and an average of 136,870 cpm of ^{35}S. (From [49]).

the three glomerular cell types) were counted. As shown in Table 7, 9.5% of the total grains fell over the GBM, and the rest (~ 90%) were over the cells; 67% of the cell-associated grains were found over the epithelium, 20% were found over the endothelium, and only 5% were found over the mesangial cells. These data indicate that: (1) the bulk of the ^{35}S radioactivity is associated with the cells, and (2) among the glomerular cells, the epithelium accounts for most (~ 80%)[1] of the total cell-associated radioactivity, indicating that this cell type is the major biosynthetic contributor of sulfated macromolecules (including both proteoglycans and sulfated glycoproteins) in the glomerulus. Proteoglycans are known to account for two-thirds of this total [19, 49].

---

[1] This estimate is based on the assumption that the direct counts of grains over the GBM (10%) and cells (90%) probably are too high, because due to radiation spread that limits the resolution (~ 2300 Å) of ^{35}S autoradiography, some of the grains emanating from the GBM would be expected to fall over the adjoining cells. When the data were analyzed further, taking into account radiation spread to obtain a maximum figure for grains emanating from the GBM as opposed to the cells, only 28% of the cell-associated grains fell within 5000 Å (2 HD) of the GBM. Since this figure also would include some grains emanating from the epithelial cell membrane and cytoplasm, 80% is considered to be a reasonable compromise as an estimate of cell-associated label.

Table 7. Percentage of autoradiographic grains over glomerular
components after [^{35}S]sulfate labeling[a]

	>2 HD-GBM[b] (%)	< 2 HD-GBM (%)	Total (%)
Epithelial cells	49.3	17.2	66.5
Endothelial cells	9.8	9.8	19.6
Mesangial cells	2.5	1.9	4.4
GBM	9.5	—	9.5

[a] Kidneys were labeled with [^{35}S]sulfate by perfusion for 4 hr, flushed with
unlabeled medium, and fixed and processed for electron microscopic
autoradiography. Grain counts were made by the simple grain density method
of Salpeter (as described in [61]).

[b] The half-distance (HD) is defined as the distance from the radioactive source
within which 50% of the grains can be expected to fall. For ^{35}S, the HD is
2300 Å under the conditions used.

Detection of Two Antigenically Distinct Types of HSPG in Rat Glomeruli—One Associated with Cell Membranes and the Other with Basement Membranes

Both the extraction data and the autoradiographic data suggested that a
significant fraction of the total glomerular proteoglycans is associated with
the cells, especially the visceral epithelium. The question then arose regarding
the relationship between the proteoglycans in the GBM and those in or on
the cells. To obtain information on this point, we have used two specific
antisera raised against different populations of proteoglycans. One antibody
was raised against a total population of proteoglycans that was purified from
isolated glomeruli; the other was raised against HSPG extracted from rat
liver membranes [28]. Both IgGs specifically recognize only HSPG (by immunoprecipitation) and do not cross-react (by radioimmunoassay) with other
basement membrane components (laminin, type IV collagen, and fibronectin).
The antibodies raised against liver membrane HSPG (anti-LHSPG) via immunoperoxidase immunocytochemistry specifically stain the sinusoidal surface
of hepatocytes, whereas those raised against glomerular proteoglycans (anti-
GHSPG) do not [62, 63].

When applied to kidney cortical tissue, the two antibodies stained different
structures; anti-GHSPG specifically stains basement membranes—not only
the GBM, but all other renal basement membranes as well (that is, tubular
and peritubular capillary basement membranes plus Bowman's capsule) (Figs.
2, 3). On the other hand, anti-LHSPG does not stain basement membranes.
As in the liver, it stains the cell membranes of a number of cell types, including
the glomerular (Fig. 4) and proximal tubule epithelium and the endothelium
of both glomerular (Fig. 4b) and peritubular capillaries. In the glomerulus,

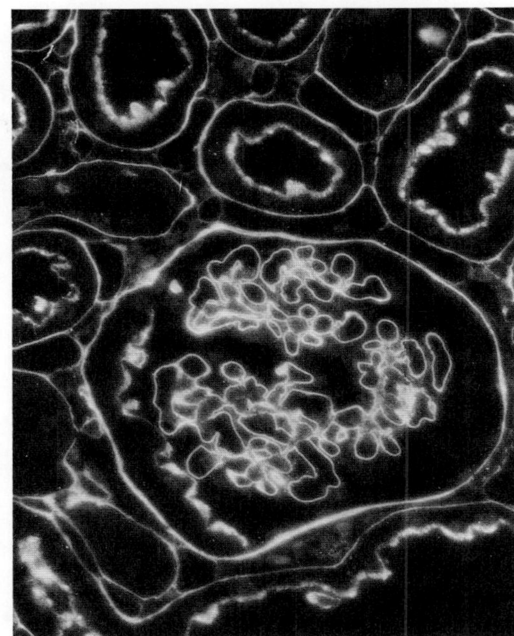

Fig. 2. Immunofluorescence micrograph of kidney cortex demonstrating the localization of heparan sulfate proteoglycans (HSPG) obtained with an antibody (anti-GHSPG) raised against purified glomerular proteoglycans that specifically recognize only HSPG. Staining is seen in all renal basement membranes—the GBM, Bowman's capsule, and the tubular and peritubular capillary basement membranes. The only other renal structures besides basement membranes that stain with these antibodies are the coated invaginations at the base of the brush border in the proximal tubule cell (×650).

the staining is variable, but (generally) staining of the epithelium and endothelium is more prominent than staining of the mesangial cells. Both of these HSPG are produced by the glomerular epithelium; this is indicated by the fact that with both, IgG reaction product often can be detected intracellularly in biosynthetic compartments (rough ER and Golgi) of these cells. The lack of staining of biosynthetic compartments in other cell types could be due to the fact that they do not make proteoglycans, or (more likely) that they are present at such low concentrations that we cannot detect them.

These findings provide the first evidence that—besides those in the GBM—there is a separate population of HSPG associated with the cell membranes of the glomerular endothelium and epithelium. Thus, there are two antigenically distinct types of HSPG in the kidney: one that is membrane-associated and the other that is basement membrane-associated. For a full understanding of the role of proteoglycans in glomerular functions and pathologic processes, it will be essential (in the future) to further characterize these two populations to determine their relationship to one another and their rates of synthesis and turnover in normal and diseased glomeruli.

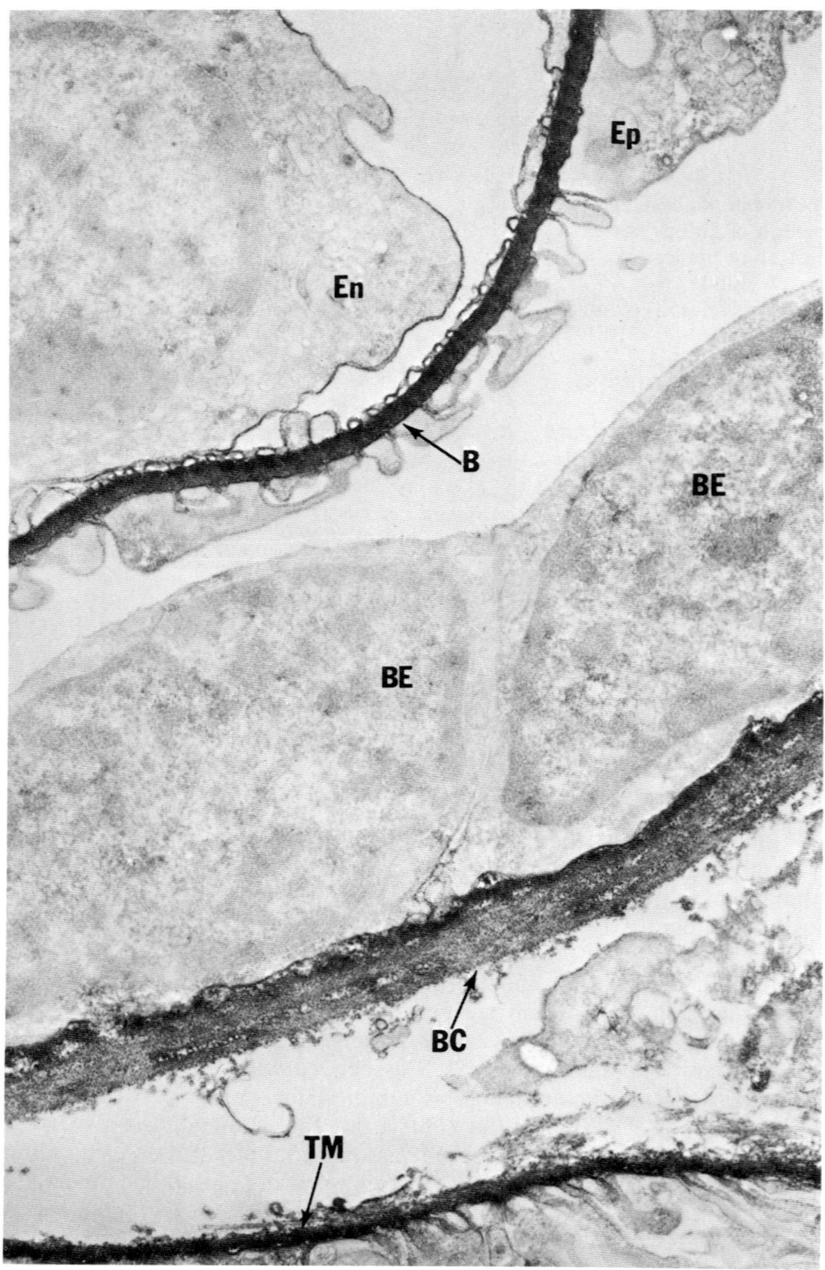

Fig. 3. Electron micrograph of a glomerulus incubated by an indirect immunoperoxidase procedure with the same anti-GHSPG IgG as in Figure 2. The GBM (*B*), the tubular basement membrane (*TM*), and Bowman's capsule (*BC*) are heavily stained. Little or no staining is seen on the surfaces of the visceral epithelium (*Ep*), endothelium (*En*), or epithelium of Bowman's capsule (*BE*) (×19,000).

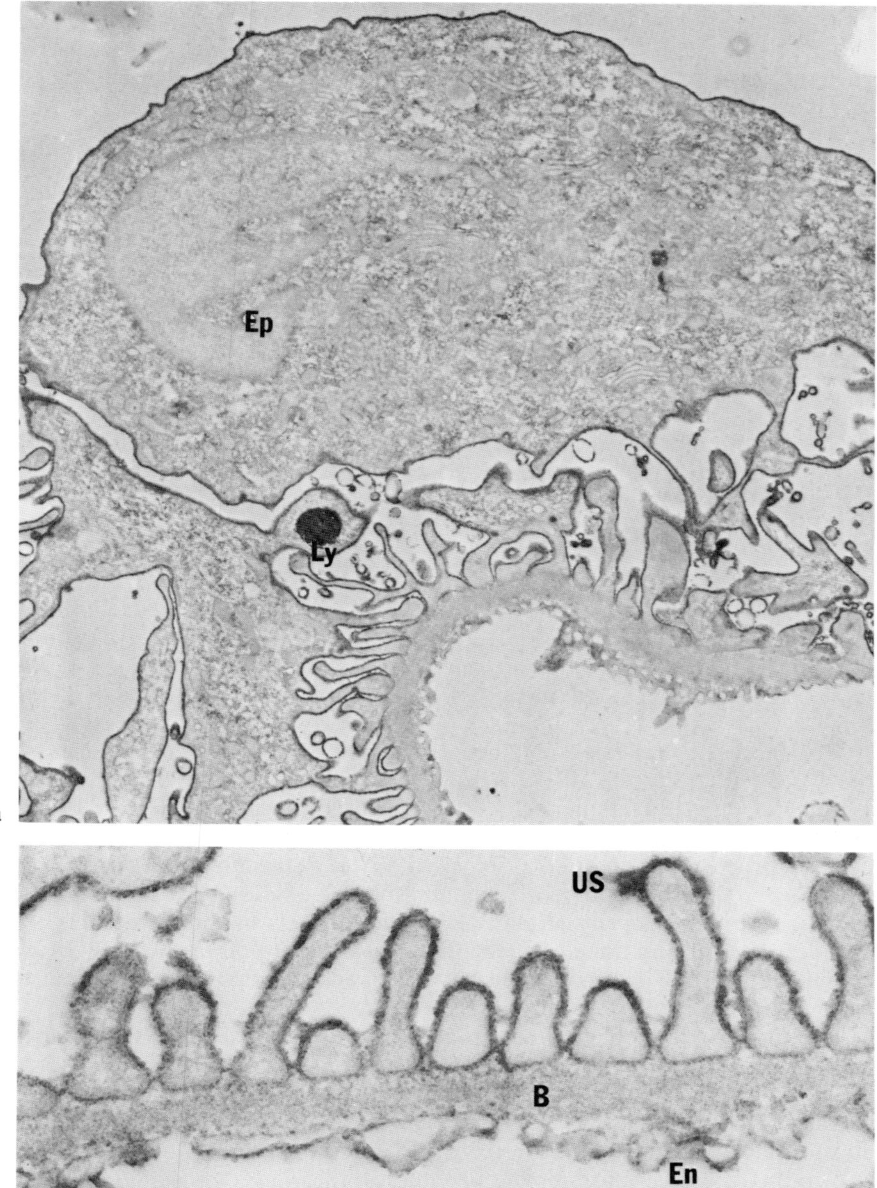

Fig. 4. Immunoperoxidase preparations of glomeruli from kidney tissue incubated with an antibody (anti-LHSPG) raised against heparan sulfate proteoglycans purified from liver membranes. Staining is present on the surfaces of both epithelial (*Ep*) and endothelial (*En*) cells. **a** The surface of the entire glomerular epithelium is outlined by peroxidase reaction product. Reaction product also is seen within a large lysosome (*Ly*) that is present in the epithelial cytoplasm. No staining of the GBM is detected. **b** The foot processes are covered by a layer of reaction product that is thicker on the surfaces exposed to the urinary spaces (*US*) than at their base, where they face the GBM (*B*). A lighter staining of the endothelial membrane (*En*) where it faces the capillary lumen is also seen (**A**, ×10,400; **B**, ×50,000).

Summary and Conclusions

Proteoglycans are highly negatively charged molecules that have been shown to be integral components of the glomerular matrix (the GBM plus mesangial matrix). Two types are present: heparan sulfate proteoglycans (HSPG) and chondroitin sulfate proteoglycans (CSPG). Small amounts of hyaluronic acid also have been detected. The main types present are the HSPG that constitutes 85 to 90% of the total. Their heparan sulfate chains are concentrated in discrete "anionic sites" in the laminae rarae interna and externa and in the mesangial matrix, where they are distributed in a regular, ordered lattice-like array. The CSPG appear to be concentrated in the mesangial matrix; the location of the hyaluronic acid is not yet known. The physical and chemical properties of proteoglycans are such (a polyanionic nature and a high viscosity in solution) that they can be expected to play a major role in determining the permeability properties of the GBM.

Evidence has been obtained demonstrating that the integrity of proteoglycans (especially the HSPG lattice) is essential for maintaining both the size and charge-selective properties of the GBM, because when the GAG chains are removed from the proteoglycans or when their charge is neutralized by infusion of polycations (neutralizes the charge on both proteoglycans and epithelial sialoproteins), anionic proteins that are normally retained at the level of the laminae rarae can cross the lamina densa and appear in the urine.

Evidence also has been obtained that the proteoglycan components of the GBM, especially the HSPG-rich anionic sites, are altered in several glomerular diseases. In aminonucleoside nephrosis, the charge density of the HSPG in the GBM has been found to be reduced (based on binding of cationic probes), but the overall biosynthesis of proteoglycans is increased. In diabetes, the GAG content (heparan sulfate) of the GBM is decreased, and the rates of proteoglycan and GAG biosynthesis in the glomerulus are also decreased. In immune complex diseases, a disruption in the HSPG-rich anionic sites in the laminae rarae has been reported that appears to occur prior to the onset of proteinuria.

Recent work from our laboratory has been presented indicating that besides those in the GBM, a large fraction (90%) of the total glomerular proteoglycans are associated with the glomerular cells. Immunochemical and immunocyto-chemical studies using specific anti-HSPG antibodies indicate that there is an antigenically distinct population of HSPG on the surfaces of the endothelial and epithelial cells. Autoradiographic studies following radiosulfate labeling indicate that the epithelium produces ~ 80% of the total proteoglycans and other sulfated macromolecules synthesized by the glomerulus.

The outstanding property of proteoglycans is their high net-negative charge—a property that is taken advantage of in analytic studies aimed at their identification and purification. Hence, their presence in the GBM and in and on glomerular cells means that proteoglycans constitute another type of polyanion (in addition to epithelial sialoglycoproteins) that comprises the so-called "glomerular polyanion"; this must be considered when contemplating normal glomerular functions and mechanisms of glomerular injury.

Finally, it is clear that the fact that the GBM is exposed directly to circulating molecules, and that cationic molecules of a certain size have access to its deepest layers, renders it particularly vulnerable to immune and toxic injury. This is quite different from the situation in other types of capillaries, in which a continuous or quasicontinuous endothelial layer is interposed between the circulation and the basement membrane [64, 65]. It can be anticipated that while proteoglycans normally serve to maintain the normal charge and size-selective properties of the GBM, these highly interactive molecules—by virtue of their characteristic physical properties—may be expected to initiate, potentiate, and otherwise complicate glomerular injury.

Acknowledgment. This research was supported by a grant (AM17724) from the National Institutes of Health. Dr. Stow was supported by a Fogarty International Fellowship (3 FO5 TWO3268) and Dr. Lemkin was supported by a National Service Award (5 T32 GMO7223).

References

1. KANWAR YS, FARQUHAR MG: Presence of heparan sulfate in the glomerular basement membrane. *Proc Natl Acad Sci USA* 76:1303–1307, 1979
2. KANWAR YS, FARQUHAR MG: Isolation of glycosaminoglycans (heparan sulfate) from the glomerular basement membrane. *Proc Natl Acad Sci USA* 76:4493–4497, 1979
3. KANWAR YS, LINKER A, FARQUHAR MG: Increased permeability of the glomerular basement membrane to ferritin after removal of glycosaminoglycans (heparan sulfate) by enzyme digestion. *J Cell Biol* 86:688–693, 1980
4. RENNKE HG, COTRAN RS, VENKATACHALAM MA: Role of molecular charge in glomerular permeability. Tracer studies with cationized ferritin. *J Cell Biol* 67:638–646, 1975
5. BRENNER, BM, HOSTETTER TH, HUMES HD: Molecular basis of proteinuria of glomerular origin. *N Engl J Med* 298:826–833, 1978
6. BRIDGES CR, MYERS BD, BRENNER BM, DEEN WM: Glomerular charge alterations in human minimal change nephropathy. *Kidney Int* 22:677–684, 1982
7. FARQUHAR MG: The glomerular basement membrane—a selective macromolecular filter, in *The Cell Biology of the Extracellular Matrix,* edited by HAY ED, New York, Plenum Press, 1981, pp 335–378
8. FARQUHAR MG, COURTOY PJ, LEMKIN MD, KANWAR YS: Current knowledge of the functional architecture of the glomerular basement membrane, in *New Trends in Basement Membrane Research,* edited by KUHN K, SCHONE H, TIMPL R, New York, Raven Press, 1982, pp 9–29
9. HASCALL VC, HASCALL GK: Proteoglycans, in *The Cell Biology of the Extracellular Matix,* edited by HAY ED, New York, Plenum Press, 1981, pp 39–63
10. COMPER WD, LAURENT TC: Physiological function of connective tissue polysaccharides. *Physiol Rev* 58:255–315, 1978
11. LINDAHL U, HÖÖK M: Glycosaminoglycans and their binding to biological macromolecules. *Ann Rev Biochem* 47:385–417, 1978
12. YANAGISHITA M, HASCALL VC: Characterization of low buoyant density dermatan sulfate proteoglycans synthesized by rat ovarian granulosa cells in culture. *J Biol Chem* 258:12847–12856, 1983
13. CAULFIELD JP, FARQUHAR MG: Distribution of anionic sites in glomerular base-

ment membranes. Their possible role in filtration and attachment. *Proc Natl Acad Sci USA* 73:1646–1650, 1976

14. CAULFIELD JP, FARQUHAR MG: Loss of anionic sites from the glomerular basement membrane in aminonucleoside nephrosis. *Lab Invest* 39:505–512, 1978

15. KANWAR YS, FARQUHAR MG: Anionic sites in the glomerular basement membrane. In vivo and in vitro localization to the laminae rarae by cationic probes. *J Cell Biol* 81:137–153, 1979

16. CAULFIELD JP: Alterations in the distribution of alcian blue-staining fibrillar anionic sites in the glomerular basement membrane in aminonucleoside nephrosis. *Lab Invest* 40:503–511, 1979

17. SCHURER JW, KALICHARAN D, HOEDEMAEKER PHJ, MOLENAAR I: The use of polyethyleneimine for demonstration of anionic sites in basement membranes and collagen fibrils. *J Histochem Cytochem* 26:688–689, 1978

18. SEILER MW, HOYER JR, KRUEGER TE: Altered localization of protamine-heparin complexes in aminonucleoside nephrosis. *Lab Invest* 43:9–17, 1980

19. LEMKIN MC, FARQUHAR MG: Sulfated and nonsulfated glycosaminoglycans and glycopeptides are synthesized by kidney in vivo and incorporated into glomerular basement membranes. *Proc Natl Acad Sci USA* 78:1726–1730, 1981

20. LINKER A, HOVINGH P, KANWAR YS, FARQUHAR MG: Characterization of heparan sulfate isolated from dog glomerular basement membrane. *Lab Invest* 44:560–565, 1981

21. BROWN, DM, MICHAEL AF, OEGEMA TR: Glycosaminoglycan synthesis by glomeruli in vivo and in vitro. *Biochim Biophys Acta* 674:96–104, 1981

22. PARTHASARATHY N, SPIRO RG: Characterization of the glycosaminoglycan component of the renal glomerular basement membrane and its relationship to the peptide portion. *J Biol Chem* 256:507–513, 1981

23. PARTHASARATHY N, SPIRO RG: Effect of diabetes on the glycosaminoglycan component of the human glomerular basement membrane. *Diabetes* 31:738–741, 1982

24. KANWAR YS, JAKUBOWSKI ML, ROSENZWEIG LJ: Distribution of sulfated glycosaminoglycans in the glomerular basement membrane and mesangial matrix. *Eur J Cell Biol* 31:290–295, 1983

25. KLEIN DJ, OEGEMA TR, EISENSTEIN R, FURCHT L, MICHAEL AF, BROWN DM: Renal localization of heparan sulfate proteoglycan by immunohistochemistry. *Am J Pathol* 111:323–330, 1983

26. KANWAR YS, HASCALL VC, FARQUHAR MG: Partial characterization of newly synthesized proteoglycans isolated from the glomerular basement membrane. *J Cell Biol* 90:527–532, 1981

27. HASSELL JR, ROBEY PG, BARRACH HJ, WILCZEK J, RENNARD SI, MARTIN GR: Isolation of a heparan sulfate-containing proteoglycan from basement membrane. *Proc Natl Acad Sci USA* 77:4494–4498, 1980

28. OLDBERG A, KJELLEN L, HOOK M: Cell surface heparan sulfate. Isolation and characterization of a proteoglycan from rat liver membranes. *J Biol Chem* 254:8508–8510, 1979

29. KANWAR YS, FARQUHAR MG: Role of glycosaminoglycans in the permeability of glomerular basement membrane. *Fed Proc* 30:334, 1980

30. ROSENZWEIG LJ, KANWAR YS: Removal of sulfated (heparan sulfate) or nonsulfated (hyaluronic acid) glycosaminoglycans results in increased permeability of the glomerular basement membrane to ^{125}I bovine serum albumin. *Lab Invest* 47:177–184, 1982

31. KELLEY VE, CAVALLO T: Glomerular permeability. Transfer of native ferritin in glomeruli with decreased anionic sites. *Lab Invest* 39:547–553, 1978

32. VEHASKARI VM, ROOT ER, GERMUTH FG JR, ROBSON AM: Glomerular charge

and urinary protein excretion: Effects of systemic and intrarenal polycation infusion in the rat. *Kidney Int* 22:127–135, 1982

33. HUNSICKER LW, SHEARER TP, SHAFFER SJ: Acute reversible proteinuria induced by infusion of the polycation hexadimethrine. *Kidney Int* 20:7–17, 1981

34. BARNES JL, RADNIK RA, GILCHRIST EP, VENKATACHALAM MA: Size and charge selective permeability defects induced in glomerular basement membrane by a polycation. *Kidney Int* 25:11–19, 1984

35. MENOZZI M, ARCAMONE F: Binding of adriamycin to sulfated mucopolysaccharides. *Biochem Biophys Res Comm* 80:313–318, 1978

36. GALLO GR, CAULIN-GLASER T, LAMM ME: Charge of circulating immune complexes as a factor in glomerular basement membrane localization in mice. *J Clin Invest* 67:1305–1313, 1981

37. CAULIN-GLASER T, GALLO GR, LAMM ME: Nondissociating cationic immune complexes can deposit in glomerular basement membrane. *J Exp Med* 158:1561–1572, 1983

38. OITE T, BATSFORD SR, MIHATSCH MJ, TAKAMIYA H, VOGT A: Quantitative studies of in situ immune complex glomerulonephritis in the rat induced by planted, cationized antigen. *J Exp Med* 155:460–474, 1982

39. VOGT A, ROHRBACH R, SHIMIZU F, TAKAMIYA H, BATSFORD S: Interaction of cationized antigen with rat glomerular basement membrane: In situ immune complex formation. *Kidney Int* 22:27–35, 1982

40. ADLER S, WANG H, WARD HJ, COHEN AH, BORDER WA: Electrical charge. Its role in the pathogenesis and prevention of experimental membranous nephropathy in the rabbit. *J Clin Invest* 71:487–499, 1983

41. GAUTHIER VJ, MANNIK M, STRIKER GE: Effect of cationized antibodies in preformed immune complexes on deposition and persistence in renal glomeruli. *J Exp Med* 156:766–777, 1982

42. MICHAEL AF, BLAU E, VERNIER RL: Glomerular polyanion. Alteration in aminonucleoside nephrosis. *Lab Invest* 23:649–657, 1970

43. SEILER MW, HOYER JR, KRUEGER TE: Altered localization of protamine-heparin complexes in aminonucleoside nephrosis. *Lab Invest* 43:9–17, 1980

44. FARQUHAR MG, KANWAR YS: Functional organization of the glomerulus: Presence of glycosaminoglycans (proteoglycans) in the glomerular basement membrane, in *Immune Mechanisms in Renal Diseases,* edited by CUMMINGS NG, MICHAEL AF, WILSON CB, New York, Plenum Press, 1982, pp 1–45

45. MYNDERSE LA, HASSELL JR, KLEINMAN HK, MARTIN GR, MARTINEZ-HERNANDEZ A: Loss of heparan sulfate proteoglycan from glomerular basement membrane of nephrotic rats. *Lab Invest* 48:292–320, 1983

46. VERNIER RL, KLEIN DJ, SISSON SP, MAHAN JD, OEGEMA TR, BROWN DM: Heparan sulfate-rich anionic sites in the human glomerular basement membrane. Decreased concentration in congenital nephrotic syndrome. *N Engl J Med* 309:1001–1009, 1983

47. MELNICK GF, LADOULIS CT, CAVALLO T: Decreased anionic groups and increased permeability precedes deposition of immune complexes in the glomerular capillary wall. *Am J Pathol* 105:114–1120, 1981

48. SCHNEEBERGER EE, STAVRAKIS G, MCCARTHY K: Alterations in glomerular anionic sites in autologous immune complex nephritis. *Lab Invest* 49:445–452, 1983

49. LEMKIN MC: The biosynthesis of sulfated and non-sulfated glycosaminoglycans (GAG) and glycopeptides by rat kidney and their incorporation into the glomerular basement membrane (GBM). Doctoral Thesis, Yale University, 1982

50. DEHNEL PJ, KLEIN DJ, OEGEMA TR, MICHAEL AF, BROWN DM: Glomerular

^{35}S-glycosaminoglycan (GAG) metabolism in aminonucleoside-induced (PAN) nephrotic syndrome in rats (*abstract*). *Kidney Int* 23:181, 1983

51. BROWN DM, KLEIN DJ, MICHAEL AF, OEGEMA TR: ^{35}S-Glycosaminoglycan and ^{35}S-glycopeptide metabolism by diabetic glomeruli and aorta. *Diabetes* 31:418–425, 1982

52. KANWAR YS, ROSENZWEIG LJ, LINKER A, JAKUBOWSKI ML: Decreased *de novo* synthesis of glomerular proteoglycans in diabetes: Biochemical and autoradiographic evidence. *Proc Natl Acad Sci USA* 80:2272–2275, 1983

53. ROHRBACH DH, HASSELL JR, KLEINMAN HK, MARTIN GR: Alterations in the basement membrane (heparan sulfate) proteoglycan in diabetic mice. *Diabetes* 31:185–188, 1982

54. ROHRBACH DH, WAGNER CW, STAR VL, MARTIN GR, BROWN KS: Reduced synthesis of basement membrane heparan sulfate proteoglycan in streptozotocin-induced diabetic mice. *J Biol Chem* 258:11672–11677, 1983

55. HELLSING K: Immune reactions in polysaccharide media. The effect of hyaluronate, chondroitin sulfate and chondroitin sulfate-protein complex on the precipitin reaction. *Biochem J* 112:475–481, 1969

56. HELLSING K: Immune reactions in polysaccharide media. Investigation on complex-formation between some polysaccharides, albumin and immunoglobulin G. *Biochem J* 112:483–487, 1969

57. LEVY DE, HORNER AA, SOLOMON A: Immunoglobulin-sulfated polysaccharide interactions. *J Exp Med* 153:883–896, 1981

58. MEEZAN E, BRENDEL K, HJELLE JT, CARLSON EC: A versatile method for the isolation of ultrastructurally and chemically pure basement membranes without sonication, in *Biology and Chemistry of Basement Membranes,* edited by KEFALIDES NA, New York, Academic Press, 1978, pp 31–42.

59. FOIDART JM, FOIDART JB, MAHIEU PR: Synthesis of collagen and fibronectin by glomerular cells in culture. *Renal Physiol* 3:183–192, 1980

60. STRIKER GE, KILLEN PD, FARIN FM: Human glomerular cells *in vitro:* Isolation and characterization. *Transplant Proc* 12:88–99, 1980

61. FARQUHAR MG, REID JA, DANIELL L: Intracellular transport and packaging of prolactin. A quantitative electron microscope autoradiography study of mammotrophs dissociated from rat pituitaries. *Endocrinology* 102:296–311, 1978

62. STOW JL, HOOK M, FARQUHAR MG: Localization of heparan sulfate proteoglycans (HSPG) on the plasmalemma and in intracellular compartments of hepatocytes and renal glomerular and tubular cells. *J Cell Biol* 98(No 5, Pt 2): 1a, 1983

63. STOW JL, KJELLEN L, HOOK M, FARQUHAR MG: Heparan sulfate proteoglycans (HSPG) are concentrated on the sinusoidal domain of hepatocytes. *J Cell Biol* (submitted, 1984)

64. PALADE GE, SIMIONESCU M, SIMIONESCU N: Structural aspects of the permeability of the microvascular endothelium. *Acta Physiol Scand* 463(Suppl):11–32, 1979

65. SIMIONESCU N, SIMIONESCU M, PALADE GE: Differentiated microdomains on the luminal surface of the capillary endothelium. *J Cell Biol* 90:605–621, 1982

Glomerular Arachidonic Acid Metabolism in Nephrotoxic Serum Nephritis

Michael J. Dunn, Elias A. Lianos, and John E. Stork

Nephrotoxic serum nephritis (NSN) is a reproducible model of acute, immune renal disease that is induced by the intravenous injection of rabbit antisera directed against rat glomerular basement membrane (GBM) antigen [1]. This model is characterized by glomerular cellular proliferation, proteinuria, reductions of the renal plasma flow (RPF) and glomerular filtration rate (GFR), and progressive renal insufficiency [2–5]. Many cellular and humoral mediators have been implicated in the pathophysiology and pathology of the disease. Since glomeruli have cyclo-oxygenase and lipoxygenase enzymes that synthesize prostaglandins, thromboxane, and 12-hydroxyeicosatetraenoic acid (12-HETE), we evaluated the importance of these biologically active eicosanoids in NSN.

Methods

Nephrotoxic serum nephritis (NSN) was induced in male Sprague-Dawley rats weighing approximately 250 g, using the single intravenous administration of 1 ml of rabbit antirat glomerular basement membrane (GBM) antiserum [6]. Antiglomerular basement membrane (anti-GBM) antiserum was produced in rabbits immunized with rat particulate GBM that was prepared from frozen rat kidneys (Pelfreez Biologicals, Rogers, Arkansas). The rabbit antisera was complement-inactivated at 56°C for 30 min and was absorbed with rat peripheral blood cells. Evaluation of the glomerular disease by light, immunofluorescence, and electron microscopy showed endothelial denudation from the GBM and linear deposition of immunoglobulin and complement along the basement membrane. There also was mild mesangial proliferation and focal mononuclear cellular infiltration on day 14 of the disease. Glomeruli

---

This manuscript was presented as part of the Symposium on *Prostaglandins and the Kidney*.

were isolated for the glomerular biochemical experiments by using minced cortical tissue and sequential sieving [6]. The minced cortical tissue with a paste-like consistency was pressed through a 106-μm metal sieve, and the large tubular fragments were separated from glomeruli. The glomerular paste was removed from the bottom surface of the 106-μm sieve and was resuspended in buffer and passed through a 75-μm sieve. Glomeruli were harvested from the upper surface of the 75-μm sieve and were resuspended in buffer. The purity of the glomerular preparation that was determined microscopically by counting all identifiable particles, including glomeruli and tubular fragments, was 93 to 95%.

Isolated glomeruli were incubated in modified Earle's balanced salt solution that contained 0.01 mg/ml gelatin, 25 mM HEPES buffer, pH 7.4, and 5 μg/ml arachidonic acid. Incubations were for 30 to 45 min at 37°C without agitation. At the end of the incubation period, the glomerular suspension was centrifuged and the supernatant solution was removed for prostaglandin assay. The wet weight of the glomeruli was determined. In experiments assessing the conversion of radiolabeled arachidonic acid to lipoxygenase metabolites, we used octatritiated arachidonic acid, 500 to 600 $\times$ 10^3 cpm (New England Nuclear), in the incubation media. The enzymic and nonenzymic conversion of tritiated arachidonate to tritiated lipoxygenase products was determined by using the lipoxygenase inhibitor nordihydroguaiaretic acid (Sigma) in a concentration of 33 μM. After incubation for 45 min at 37°C, the glomerular suspensions were acidified with 0.1 hydrochloric acid (HC1) to pH 3.5, extracted triply with ethyl acetate and dried under nitrogen. The samples were reconstituted in hexane and analyzed using high-performance liquid chromatography (HPLC) [7].

Incubation media were assayed for prostaglandins and thromboxane without organic solvent extraction. The PGE_2 antisera was purchased from Institut Pasteur, thromboxane B_2 antisera was a gift from Dr. William Campbell, Dallas, Texas, and the antisera for $PGF_2\alpha$ and 6-keto-$PGF_1\alpha$ were prepared in our laboratory. The sensitivities and cross-reactivities of these four radioimmunoassays have been previously described [8]. The antisera for 12-HETE was generously donated by Dr. Lawrence Levine, Brandeis, Massachusetts.

The effects of NSN on GFR and renal plasma flow (RPF), and the effects of inhibitors of thromboxane synthetase and arachidonate cyclo-oxygenase, were determined by using inulin clearance (C_{In}) as a measure of GFR and para-aminohippuric acid (PAH) clearance (C_{PAH}) as a measure of RPF. In our initial studies, inulin and PAH were mixed to final concentrations of 5 and 0.2%, respectively; and, 1.5 ml of this solution was infused intravenously as a priming load followed by constant infusion at 3 ml/hr. Approximately 60 min of constant infusion were allowed before initiation and determination of the clearances. Blood samples of 50 to 70 μl were obtained from the tail vein at the midpoint of each clearance period, and urine was obtained in preweighed vessels via bladder catheterization. Plasma and urine inulin and PAH were determined by methods previously described and modified for microliter samples [6]. In the experiments assessing chronic administration of thromboxane synthetase inhibitors, as well as cyclo-oxygenase inhibition on day 14 of the disease, we used ^{3}H-inulin and ^{14}C-PAH. Comparison of the chemical techniques to the radiolabeled techniques revealed excellent agreement. The clearance of PAH by using ^{3}H-PAH was corrected for renal extraction, since we determined renal venous ^{3}H-PAH at the end of the experiment.

Results

Within 24 hr of administration of anti-GBM antibodies, rats developed significant proteinuria ranging from 50 to 150 mg/24 hr. The acute heterologous response in NSN is shown in Figure 1. C_{In} and, to a lesser extent, C_{PAH} decreased within 2 hr and showed some spontaneous recovery at 3 hr. At the nadir of C_{PAH} and C_{IN} glomerular thromboxane synthesis (measured as TxB_2, which is the stable hydrolysis product of TxA_2) was increased substantially and increased further to greater than 10-fold by 3 hr. There were concomitant increases in the vasodilatory eicosanoids, PGE_2 and PGI_2, especially at 3 hr. To assess the pathophysiologic significance of these biochemical alterations, we inhibited glomerular thromboxane A_2 synthesis with either OKY-1581 or UK-38485, both of which are chemically dissimilar inhibitors of thromboxane synthetase. OKY-1581 decreased glomerular TxB_2 synthesis from 1029 ± 104 to 23 ± 2 pg/mg of glomerular weight per 45 min. UK-38485 had similar effects, reducing glomerular TxB_2 from 612 ± 81 to 17 ± 2 pg/mg of glomerular wet weight per 45 min. These inhibitors of TxA_2 production prevented the decrements of C_{In} and C_{PAH} at 2 and 3 hr after

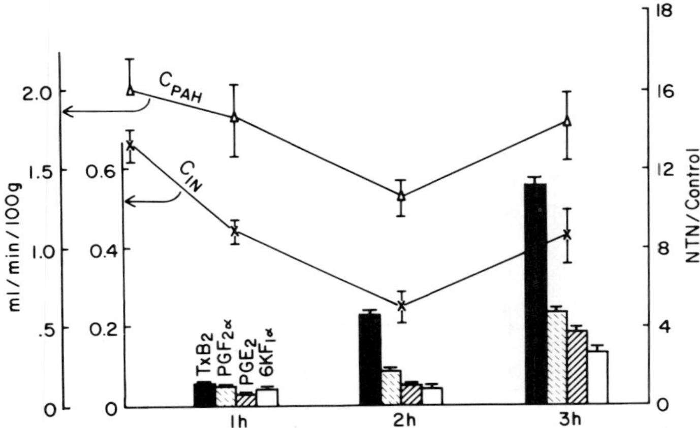

Fig. 1. Acute changes in C_{In} and C_{PAH} (*left ordinates*) and changes of glomerular prostaglandin synthesis expressed as fold increments compared with simultaneous controls (*right ordinate*). PG synthesis in control glomeruli, in pg/mg glomerular weight per 45 min ($N = 12$), were: $TxB_2 = 79 \pm 2$; $PGE_{2\alpha} = 1,199 \pm 28$; $PGE_2 = 550 \pm 81$; 6-keto-$PGF_{1\alpha} = 46 \pm 3$. (Reproduced with permission from [6])

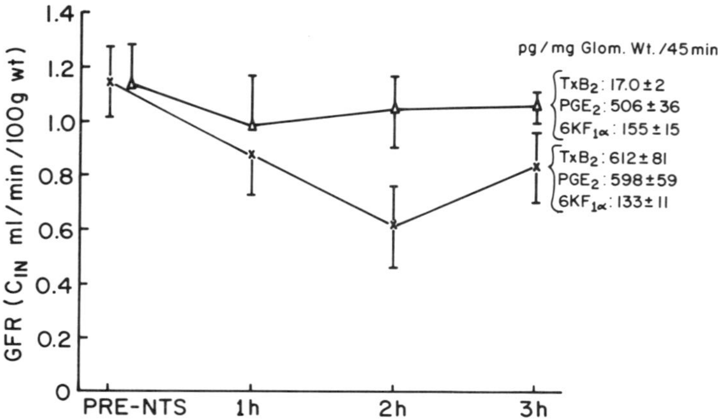

Fig. 2. Modification of NTS-induced changes in GFR by UK-38485 (X) NTS ($N = 4$). ($\triangle$) UK-38485 plus NTS ($N = 4$). At infusion rates of 400 μg/hr, UK-38485 inhibited glomerular TxB_2 synthesis and preserved GFR at 2 and 3 hr. Synthesis of PGE_2 and 6-keto-$PGF_{1\alpha}$ were unaltered. (Reproduced with permission from [6])

the induction of NSN (Fig. 2). The inhibitors of TxA_2 synthetase had no effect on renal hemodynamics in control animals. Low doses of OKY-1581, which fully inhibited platelet TxA_2 synthesis, had no effect on either glomerular TxA_2 production rates or on renal hemodynamics.

In the next series of experiments, we set out to evaluate the biochemical and physiologic alterations of NSN at the peak of the heterologous phase (1 to 2 days), and later in the autologous phase (14 days) of NSN. At 24 to 48 hr after injection of NSN antisera, glomerular TxA_2 is increased 10-fold to 654 ± 183 pg/mg glomeruli per 45 min, compared to control values of 41 ± 17. Although these changes persisted until day 14, the fold increment of TxB_2 decreased to 5-fold. Prostaglandin E_2 synthesis increased dramatically at both 1 to 2 days and 14 days after the induction of NSN; it ranged from 1100 ± 167 (day 1) to 1300 ± 285 (day 14) pg/mg of glomerular weight, compared to control values of 120 ± 25. Table 1 summarizes these

Table 1. The effects of NSAID on renal function in NSN

	GFR (ml/min)	RPF (ml/min)	Glomerular PGE₂/TxB₂ (pg/mg)
Controls	2.6 ± 0.2	7.8 ± 0.9	118 ± 26 / 41 ± 17
NSN Day 1	1.9 ± 0.2[a]	10.0 ± 1.0	1107 ± 167[a]/654 ± 183[a]
NSN Day 14	2.3 ± 0.3	12.1 ± 1.5[a]	1324 ± 285[a]/185 ± 35[a]
NSN + NSAID	0.9 ± 0.1[a]	5.8 ± 0.6[a]	46 ± 10 / 52 ± 17

Abbreviations: NSAID, Nonsteroidal anti-inflammatory drugs [9]; GFR, inulin clearance; RPF, PAH clearance.

[a] $P < 0.05$ vs. controls.

changes as well as the measurements of GFR and RPF in the controls, the rats with NSN on days 1 and 14, and rats with NSN who had received cyclo-oxygenase inhibitors (nonsteroidal anti-inflammatory drugs [NSAID]). There were substantial increments of RPF on days 1 and 14, and a reduction of GFR on day 1 with improvement by day 14. The hemodynamic importance of glomerular PGE_2 synthesis was demonstrated by the deleterious effects of cyclo-oxygenase inhibition with either indomethacin or meclofenamate, 3 mg/kg over 20 min intravenously. Inhibition of prostaglandin synthesis with these drugs was accompanied by a precipitous decline of both GFR and RPF to values less than 50% of the preinfusion baseline.

Nonsteroidal anti-inflammatory drugs (such as indomethacin or meclofenamate) inhibit cyclo-oxygenase, thereby inhibiting the formation of all prostaglandins and thromboxane. The physiologic results shown in Table 1 are accompanied by reductions not only of vasodilatory prostaglandins, but also of vasoconstrictor thromboxane A_2. To separately evaluate the importance of glomerular TxA_2, we used intravenous infusions of UK-38485 or 24-hr oral treatment with OKY-1581. Inhibition of thromboxane synthesis, which was documented by greater than 95% reductions of glomerular TxB_2, did not alter GFR or RPF on either day 1 or day 14 of NSN. Since endoperoxides may accumulate during thromboxane synthetase inhibition and may mimic the action of TxA_2, we studied the effects of the TxA_2 receptor blocker EP-092. Inhibition of thromboxane synthetase with UK-38485, followed by thromboxane receptor antagonism with EP-092, also had no beneficial effects for raising GFR or altering RPF.

The synthesis of lipoxygenase products of arachidonic acid was also assessed in NSN by using tritiated arachidonic acid. The percent conversion of tritiated arachidonic acid to tritiated 12-HETE was $1.95 \pm 0.2\%$ in control glomeruli and $14.2 \pm 2\%$ in nephritic glomeruli on day 2 of NSN. We could detect no tritiated 5-HETE synthesis that indicated the absence of the 5-lipoxygenase pathway. Enhanced tritiated 12-HETE synthesis from tritiated arachidonate substrate was detectable as early as 3 to 5 hr; and, it persisted to days 7 and 14 when synthetic rates were two to four times that of the control glomeruli [7]. To obtain more unequivocal evidence of increased 12-HETE synthesis in NSN, we used HPLC-UV detection and radioimmunoassay of 12-HETE in additional experiments. These results confirmed the radiometric HPLC results; namely, that we detected enhanced glomerular 12-HETE synthesis as early as 3 to 5 hr following the administration of nephrotoxic serum, with a peak at day 2 (10-fold enhancement of 12-HETE production) and increments on day 7 and day 14 to approximately twice of the control synthetic rates [7].

Discussion

In the acute phase of NSN, the dramatic increases of glomerular thromboxane A_2 synthesis have clear hemodynamic actions. The increased glomerular TxA_2, measured by radioimmunoassay of TxB_2, could be of glomerular (mesangial and epithelial) or leukocytic origin. It seems unlikely that platelets account for the increased TxA_2 synthesis, not only because they are minimally involved in the acute phase of NSN, but also because doses of OKY-1581 that eliminated platelet thromboxane synthesis did not affect the glomerular production rate of TxB_2 [7]. Since thromboxane is a potent autacoid that acts locally, it may be unimportant whether the high glomerular thromboxane synthesis is from endogenous glomerular cells or is invading leukocytes and macrophages. The experiments with the thromboxane synthesis inhibitors show that the acute effect of nephrotoxic serum, to reduce C_{PAH} and C_{In} at 2 and 3 hr of NSN, can be attributed to the actions of thromboxane both on the renal arterioles and perhaps on the glomerular mesangial cells [10]. An intraglomerular action of thromboxane on the mesangium would be consistent with previous measurements that show a decrease in the glomerular ultrafiltration coefficient in NSN [3, 4].

Contrary to our original hypothesis, thromboxane did not exert important hemodynamic intrarenal actions on days 1 and 2 and day 14 of NSN. Despite a greater than 95% inhibition of glomerular TxA_2 synthesis with either OKY-1581 or UK-38485, we could not show improvement of the C_{In}. The C_{PAH} also did not increase, but it should be noted that C_{PAH} was supranormal on day 2 and 14 of the disease. We also assessed the possibility that thromboxane synthetase inhibition might be followed by an accumulation of endoperoxides, with subsequent endoperoxide occupancy of TxA_2 receptors. The experiments with the TxA_2 receptor antagonist EP-092 eliminated this possibility, and they further enhanced our conclusion that thromboxane did not play an important part in the renal changes at this stage of the disease. However, increases of glomerular PGE_2 synthesis did exert important vasodilatory actions in NSN, particularly by day 14. Cyclo-oxygenase inhibition with either indomethacin or meclofenamate reduced PGE_2 synthesis by 95% and substantially reduced RPF and GFR. These actions of PGE_2 may reflect not only afferent and efferent arteriolar vasodilatory effects, but also mesangial relaxant effects of PGE_2 [10]. Until recently, PGE_2 was considered to be a renal vasoconstrictor in the rat, unlike its vasodilatory actions in other species. However, excellent evidence has been presented that this is a dose-dependent effect of PGE_2, and also that low doses of PGE_2 as well as PGI_2 infused into the rat kidney produce vasodilatation [11, 12]. Higher doses may lead to vasoconstriction because of the action of PGE_2 and PGI_2 to stimulate renin [11, 12]. The subsequent vasoconstriction is angiotensin-dependent, and it can be abolished with angiotensin receptor antagonists [13].

12-hydroxyeicosatetraenoic acid has chemotactic and chemokinetic properties that may be important in glomerulonephritis [14, 15]. Glomerular epithelial and mesangial cells synthesize 12-HETE and are potential sources of the increased synthesis in NSN [16, 17]. Less likely sources of the increased glomerular 12-HETE include platelets and leukocytes, but the 12-HETE alterations were not paralleled by similar changes of platelet involvement in the glomeruli; the absence of 5-HETE synthesis makes polymorphonuclear leukocytes an unlikely source, since these cells have active 5- and 12-lipoxygenases. The significance of the enhanced 12-HETE synthesis in glomeruli in NSN remains to be explored, particularly through the use of 12-lipoxygenase inhibitors. Macrophages and leukocyte migration and adherence to glomerular endothelium and basement membrane may be partially mediated by 12-HETE. It is conceivable that inhibition of 12-lipoxygenase would be accompanied by reduced glomerular damage and reduction of the proteinuria.

Acknowledgments. This work was supported by the National Institutes of Health (HL22563) and by National Research Service Awards to Dr. E. A. Lianos (AM06634) and Dr. J. E. Stork (AM07470). Ono Pharmaceuticals, Osaka, Japan provided the OKY-1581 and Pfizer, Incorporated, Groton, Connecticut, supplied the UK-38485. Dr. R. L. Jones, Edinburgh, Scotland kindly donated the EP-092.

References

1. UNANUE ER, DIXON FJ: Experimental glomerulonephritis: immunological events and pathogenetic mechanisms. *Adv Immunol* 6:1–10, 1967
2. ALLISON MEM, WILSON CB, GOTTSCHALK CW: Pathophysiology of experimental glomerulonephritis in rats. *J Clin Invest* 53:1402–1423, 1974
3. BLANTZ RC, WILSON CB: Acute effects of antiglomerular basement membrane antibody on the process of glomerular filtration in the rat. *J Clin Invest* 58:899–911, 1976
4. MADDOX DA, BENNETT CM, DEEN WM, GLASSOCK RJ, KNUTSON D, DAUGHARTY TM, BRENNER BM: Determinants of glomerular filtration in experimental glomerulonephritis in the rat. *J Clin Invest* 55:305–318, 1975
5. BLANTZ RC, TUCKER BJ, WILSON CB: The acute effects of antiglomerular basement membrane antibody upon glomerular filtration in the rat. The influence of dose and complement depletion. *J Clin Invest* 61:910–921, 1978
6. LIANOS EA, ANDRES GA, DUNN MJ: Glomerular prostaglandin and thromboxane synthesis in rat nephrotoxic serum nephritis. *J Clin Invest* 72:1439–1448, 1983
7. LIANOS EA, DUNN MJ: Glomerular biosynthesis of hydroxyeicosatetraenoic acids in nephrotoxic serum nephritis. *Trans Assoc Am Phys* XCVI:444–450, 1983
8. BECK TR, HASSID A, DUNN MJ: The effect of arginine vasopressin and its analogues on the synthesis of PGE_2 by rat renal medullary interstitial cells in culture. *J Pharmacol Exp Ther* 215:15–19, 1980
9. STORK JE, DUNN MJ: Immune glomerulonephritis in the rat: renal function, thromboxane $A_2(TxA_2)$ and PGE_2 (*abstract*). *Clin Res* 32:565A, 1984.
10. SCHARSCHMIDT LA, LIANOS EA, DUNN MJ: Arachidonate metabolites and the control of glomerular function. *Fed Proc* 42:3058–3063, 1983
11. SAKR HM, DUNHAM EW: Mechanism of arachidonic acid-induced vasoconstriction in the intact rat kidney. Possible involvement of thromboxane A_2. *J Pharmacol Exp Ther* 221:614–622, 1982
12. JACKSON EK, HEIDEMANN HT, BRANCH RA, GERKENS JF: Low dose intrarenal infusions of PGE_2, PGI_2 and 6-keto-PGE_1 vasodilate the in vivo rat kidney. *Circ Res* 51:67–72, 1982
13. SCHOR N, BRENNER BM: Possible mechanism of prostaglandin-induced renal vasoconstriction in the rat. *Hypertension* 3(Suppl II):II-81–II-85, 1981
14. STENSON WF, PARKER CW: Monohydroxyeicosatetraenoic acids (HETEs) induce degranulation of human neutrophils. *J Immunol* 124:2100–2104, 1980
15. GOETZL EJ, PICKETT WC: The human PMN leukocyte chemotactic activity of complex hydroxy-eicosatetraenoic acids (HETEs). *J Immunol* 125:1789–1791, 1980

16. JIM K, HASSID A, SUN F, DUNN MJ: Lipoxygenase activity in rat kidney glomeruli, glomerular epithelial cells and cortical tubules. *J Biol Chem* 257:10294–10299, 1982
17. SRAER J, RIGAUD M, BENS M, RABINOVITCH H, ARDAILLOU R: Metabolism of arachidonic acid via the lipoxygenase pathway in human and murine glomeruli. *J Biol Chem* 258:4325–4330, 1983

Effects of Dexamethasone on Cultured Mesangial Cell Function During Phagocytosis

Laurent Baud, Joelle Perez, Diego Pujol, and Raymond Ardaillou

Recent experimental evidence supports the view that the mesangial cells of the renal glomerulus possess a phagocytic function. Using heat-aggregated antiperoxidase immunoglobulins, Mancilla-Jimenez et al [1] showed that rat mesangial cells could incorporate this material following its administration in vivo. Previous in vitro studies from our laboratory [2] also have established that a high percentage of rat-cultured mesangial cells phagocytized serum-treated zymosan (STZ). Phagocytosis was associated with the production of reactive oxygen species [2, 3], particularly superoxide anion (O_2^-) and hydrogen peroxide (H_2O_2). This oxidative burst appeared to be dependent on stimulation of the lipoxygenase pathway [2], but not of the cyclo-oxygenase pathway [4]. It has been demonstrated that corticosteroids modified many functions of the phagocytic cells (polymorphonuclear leukocytes and macrophages). These drugs inhibit phospholipase activity and prostaglandin production [5, 6] via the synthesis and release of a second messenger, macrocortin or lipomodulin. They also produce a decrease in reactive oxygen formation [7, 8] and in lysosomal enzyme release [7, 9]. Finally, they regulate the phagocytic capability of the cells [9–11] and modify the function of complement component C3b and Fc receptors [11, 12]. These properties of corticosteroids could be mediated either by steroid-receptor interaction followed by modulation of RNA and protein synthesis or by direct effect on the plasma membrane [13]. Although corticosteroids are used widely in high doses for the treatment of human and experimental glomerulonephritis [14], their role in glomerular cell functions has been sparsely documented. It has only been shown that ³H-dexamethasone bound specifically to rabbit glomeruli [15] and that in vivo administration to rats of this glucocorticoid altered the glomerular concentration of cyclic AMP [16]. The aim of this present study was to investigate the effects of dexamethasone on the biochemical events associated with phagocytosis in mesangial cells and to determine the mechanism of these effects.

This manuscript was presented as part of a Symposium on *Recent Advances in the Structure, Biochemistry and Function of the Glomerulus.*

Methods

Cell Cultures

Cultured glomerular mesangial and epithelial cells were obtained from primary cultures of glomeruli that were isolated from rat renal cortex according to the slightly modified method of Foidart et al [17]. Glomeruli were prepared from the renal cortices of Sprague-Dawley rats that weighed 100 to 150 g by sieving techniques and differential centrifugations [18]. The final preparation was checked for purity by light microscopy. It contained decapsulated glomeruli with virtually no afferent or efferent arterioles. Isolated glomeruli were then cultured at 37°C in plastic flasks containing 5 ml of RPMI medium (Flow Laboratories, Irvine, UK), which was supplemented with 10% decomplemented fetal bovine serum and buffered with 20 mM N-2 hydroxyethyl-piperazine-N'-2 ethanesulphonic acid (Hepes), pH 7.2. Under such conditions, mesangial cells grow rapidly with a maximum of cell division on day 14, when epithelial cells can no longer be detected. The phagocytic activity and the associated biochemical events were studied with mesangial cells on day 14 or later. To confirm that mesangial cells were not contaminated by macrophages or monocytes of extrarenal origin, the nonspecific esterase stain was used with dissociated mesangial cells and with rat peritoneal macrophages obtained for control purposes. Cultured mesangial cells were not esterase-positive, whereas rat peritoneal macrophages—studied either immediately after collection or after 2 weeks of culture under the same conditions as those used for mesangial cells—stained markedly in the presence of the reagents that were specific for esterase. Moreover, it has been shown that glomeruli of normal rats contain fewer than 0.1 esterase-positive cells per tuft [19]. Macrophage contamination was also excluded on the basis of several other arguments as reported previously [2].

The effects of steroids on phagocytosis by cultured mesangial cells, and its associated biochemical events, were studied after addition to the culture medium of dexamethasone (Sigma, St. Louis, Missouri) at final concentrations between 10 pmoles and 1 μmole per liter for 0.5 to 48 hr before each experiment. Dexamethasone was dissolved in absolute ethanol (1 M). Appropriate concentrations were obtained by further dilutions in the RPMI medium. When necessary, a new antiglucocorticoid compound, RU 38486 (Roussel-Uclaf, Paris, France), was also added to the culture medium at final concentrations between 0.1 and 5.0 μM. This drug is a potent competitor for dexamethasone binding sites, and it possesses almost no agonist activity up to 5 μM [20]. To know whether the effect of dexamethasone was genomic, we also used actinomycin D (an inhibitor of RNA synthesis) and cycloheximide (an inhibitor of protein synthesis [Sigma]). The cells were cultured for 6 hr in the presence of 0.2 μg/ml actinomycin D or 0.1 μg/ml cycloheximide.

Phagocytosis and its associated biochemical events were studied with dissociated mesangial cells scraped off their flasks. The flasks were washed twice with 3 ml of Dulbecco's solution, and then were exposed for 2 min at room temperature to the same solution containing 2.5 mM EDTA (disodium salt).

This medium was removed, and the flasks were kept for 15 min at 37°C. Then 3 ml of Dulbecco's solution were added to the flasks and the cells were scraped away by using a rubber policeman. The suspension obtained was filtered through a 50-μm sieve and was centrifuged at 120 $\times$ g for 10 min. The supernatant was discarded, and the pellet was suspended in Krebs-Ringer phosphate (KRP) solution.

Preparation of Opsonized Particles

Zymosan A (Sigma) was boiled for 30 min, washed twice with 0.16 M sodium chloride (NaCl), and incubated at a concentration of 10 mg/ml with fresh rat serum for 30 min at 37°C. After centrifugation and washing, the resulting preparation of STZ was resuspended in KRP, pH 7.4, containing 0.8 mM $CaCl_2$ and was used at a final concentration of 1000 μg/ml.

Determination of Prostaglandin E_2 Synthesis by Mesangial Cells

Approximately 100,000 cells were incubated at 37°C for 30 min with or without 1000 μg/ml STZ in 0.6 ml of KRP solution. Radioimmunoassay of prostaglandin (PGE_2) was carried out according to Dray et al [21]. Anti-PGE_2 antiserum was purchased from Institut Pasteur (Paris); this antibody cross-reacts only slightly with other prostaglandins and can be considered to be as specific [21]. Prostaglandin E_2 was a gift from Dr. J. Pike (Upjohn Co, Kalamazoo, Michigan) and [^{3}H]PGE_2 was purchased from the Radio-chemical Centre (Amersham, UK). PGE_2 was assayed directly in the supernatant at three increasing dilutions. We have shown in a previous study [22] that prior extraction was not necessary for assay in the protein-free medium. The PGE_2 synthesis was expressed as ng/30 min/100,000 cells.

Determination of Hydrogen Peroxide (H_2O_2) Production by Mesangial Cells

Duplicate or triplicate reaction mixtures containing approximately 100,000 mesangial cells were incubated with or without STZ, and also in the presence of 0.28 mM phenol red sodium salt (Sigma) and 50 μg/ml type II horseradish peroxidase (Sigma) in 0.6 ml of 10 mM potassium phosphate buffer, pH 7.0 (containing 5.5 mM dextrose and 140 mM NaCl [23]). The incubation was stopped by centrifugation at 3000 $\times$ g for 3 min at 4°C. The supernatants were collected and the pH was adjusted to 12.5 by addition of 20 μl 3 M NaOH. Absorbance was read at 610 nmoles with a Model 25 Beckman spectrophotometer against a blank that contained the same reagents except for the cells. Standard curves of absorbance against H_2O_2 concentration (1 to 20 μM) were obtained and the results were expressed as nanomoles of H_2O_2 generated per 100,000 cells.

Phagocytosis Assay

To quantitate the amount of zymosan that was bound to or incorporated in the mesangial cells, the particles of zymosan were labeled with ^{125}I via the ammonium persulfate method [24] and then were opsonized as described above. Approximately 150,000 cells were incubated at 37°C for 30 min in the presence of 1000 μg/ml STZ (0.12 μCi/mg) in 0.3 ml of KRP solution that was supplemented with 5% (v/v) decomplemented fetal bovine serum— to minimize background binding of labeled zymosan to cell-free wells [25]. At the end of the incubation, 0.5 ml of ice-cold KRP was added, and this total volume was layered on ice-cold Ficoll (Pharmacia, Uppsala, Sweden) sodium diatrizoate (Sigma) gradient (specific gravity equal to 1.095 g/cm^3) [26]. After centrifugation (400 $\times$ g, 10 min, 4°C), the free particles of STZ appeared in the pellet and the mesangial cells in the upper phase, as demonstrated in parallel studies with ^{3}H-thymidine-labeled cells. [125]I present in these fractions was counted in a crystal-type scintillation detector (Searle model 1185). Results were expressed either as percentages of values obtained under control conditions or as the average number of STZ particles per cell. To calculate the latter value, we used the specific activity of STZ (0.12 μCi/mg) and the weight of zymosan particles (1μg = 37,500 particles).

Results

Hydrogen Peroxide and Prostaglandin E_2 Production by Mesangial Cells Preincubated with Dexamethasone

Pretreatment of mesangial cells for 48 hr by increasing concentrations of dexamethasone had no effect on basal production of H_2O_2 and PGE_2, whereas it produced a marked decrease in the synthesis of these two compounds during exposure to 1 mg/ml of STZ for 30 min (Fig. 1). Maximum inhibition was obtained with 1 μM dexamethasone. The H_2O_2 production decreased from 6.45 $\pm$ 0.28 ($\pm$ SEM) to 0.86 $\pm$ 0.09 nmoles/10^5 cells/30 min. The 50% inhibitory concentration (IC_{50}) of dexamethasone was 32 nM. The PGE_2 synthesis also decreased from 2.89 $\pm$ 0.19 to 0.96 $\pm$ 0.40 ng/10^5 cells/30 min, with an IC_{50} for dexamethasone of 0.63 nM. Thus, similar relative effects were obtained at lower doses of dexamethasone for PGE_2 than for H_2O_2 production. To know whether this inhibitory effect of dexamethasone was genomic, we have studied the influence of the time period of preincubation of the drug with the cells. Dexamethasone did not produce any effect after short incubation periods (0.5 to 1 hr). A statistically significant inhibition of H_2O_2 and PGE_2 synthesis, both under basal conditions and after stimulation in the presence of STZ, was observed from 3-hr incubation times (Fig. 2). The inhibitory effect increased progressively until 24 hr of exposure to the steroid; and, it remained unchanged for incubation periods between 24 to 72 hr. Maximum inhibitions for phagocytizing cells were 84.2 $\pm$ 3.5% for H_2O_2 release and 92.5 $\pm$ 0.3% for PGE_2 synthesis. Thus, pretreatment of

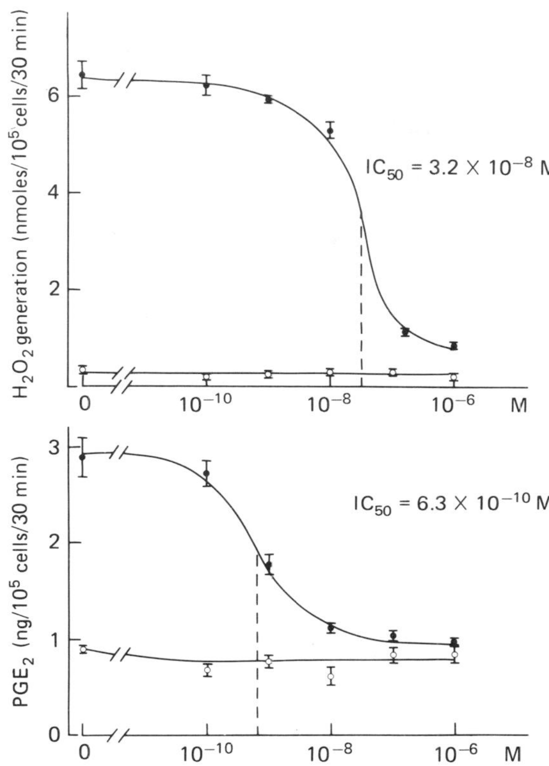

Fig. 1. Hydrogen peroxide (H_2O_2) (*upper part*) and PGE_2 (*lower part*) synthesis by mesangial cells incubated with (*closed circles*) or without (*open circles*) serum-treated zymosan (1 mg/ml) as a function of the concentration of dexamethasone used for preincubation of the cells during 48 hr. The *dotted lines* indicate the concentrations corresponding to 50% inhibitions (IC_{50}).

the cells by 1 μmole dexamethasone for 72 hr completely inhibited the PGE_2 response to STZ stimulation.

The effect of drugs that inhibit protein synthesis was also studied to better analyze the mechanism of action of dexamethasone. Treatment for 6 hr by actinomycin D at 0.2 μg/ml inhibited H_2O_2 production per se via the mesangial cells due to the general toxic effect of this drug. Basal production of H_2O_2 changed from 6.10 ± 0.30 to 4.12 ± 0.23 with actinomycin D, and 6.40 ± 0.15 with cycloheximide (nmoles/10^5 cells/30 min). Addition of 1 μM dexamethasone—which produced 51% inhibition for untreated cells (2.97 ± 0.24 nmoles/10^5 cells/30 min)—produced only 28% inhibition for cells treated with cycloheximide (4.57 ± 0.76 nmoles/10^5 cells/30 min) and 18% inhibition for those cells treated with actinomycin D (3.36 ± 0.26 nmoles/10^5 cells/30 min).

The ability of a new antiglucocorticoid, RU 38486, was also tested; it was considered as a potent competitor for dexamethasone receptors to counteract the inhibitory effect of dexamethasone. This compound at 5 μM did not possess any agonist activity on both H_2O_2 and PGE_2 synthesis. However, at this same concentration, it completely reversed the inhibitory effect of 0.1 μM dexamethasone (Table 1).

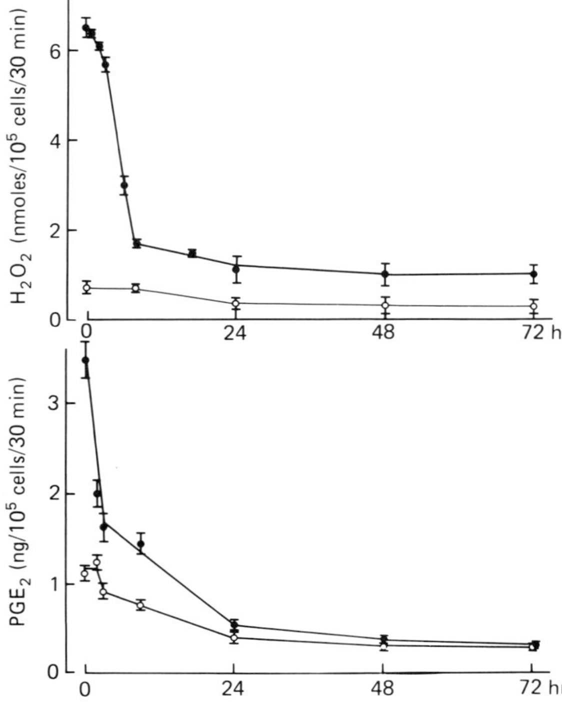

Fig. 2. Hydrogen peroxide (H_2O_2) (*upper part*) and PGE_2 (*lower part*) synthesis by mesangial cells incubated with (*closed circles*) or without (*open circles*) serum-treated zymosan (1 mg/ml) as a function of the time of preincubation of the cells with 1 μM dexamethasone.

Table 1. Effects of an antiglucocorticoid—RU 38486—on the phagocytic capability of cultured mesangial cells and on H_2O_2 and PGE_2 production by these cells during phagocytosis[a]

Drugs tested	H_2O_2 formation (nmoles/10^5 cells/30 min)	PGE_2 synthesis (ng/10^5 cells/30 min)	Phagocytosis (particles of STZ/cell)
None	6.18 ± 0.16 (100)	3.25 ± 0.12 (100)	2.01 ± 0.18 (100)
RU 38486 (5 μmoles)	6.14 ± 0.14 (99.4)	2.91 ± 0.35 (89.6)	1.99 ± 0.15 (98.7)
Dexamethasone (0.1 μmoles)	3.47 ± 0.31^b (56.1)	1.83 ± 0.11^b (56.3)	0.95 ± 0.07^b (47.1)
RU 38486 (5 μmoles) + Dexamethasone (0.1 μmoles)	6.62 ± 0.52 (107.2)	2.98 ± 0.35 (91.8)	2.01 ± 0.29 (99.8)

[a] Dexamethasone and/or RU 38486 were added to the incubation medium of mesangial cells 24 hr before the experiments. The H_2O_2 formation, PGE_2 synthesis, and quantitative phagocytosis were measured after incubation of mesangial cells for 30 min with 1 mg/ml STZ. Results are means $\pm$ SEM of 6 to 12 individual values. Values in parentheses represent percentages of control. Student's t test for unpaired values was used to compare the results obtained under control conditions and in the presence of drugs.

[b] $P < 0.05$.

^{125}I-STZ Uptake by Mesangial Cells Preincubated with Dexamethasone

Pretreatment of mesangial cells for 48 hr by increasing doses of dexamethasone produced a decrease in the phagocytic capability of the cells. Quantitative phagocytosis was reduced at 37% of control value after incubation with 1 μM dexamethasone. No effect of dexamethasone at 1 μM could be observed after a 30-min incubation. Inhibition of phagocytosis was clear-cut after 3 hr of exposure to dexamethasone. The inhibitory effect was maximum at 48 hr (Fig. 3). Control phagocytosis corresponded to an association of 2.01 $\pm$ 0.18 ^{125}I STZ particles per cell. Incubation of the cells with RU 38486 at 5 μM for 48 hr did not modify the phagocytic capability of the cells, whereas the inhibitory effect of 0.1 μM dexamethasone was completely suppressed by the simultaneous addition of 5 μM RU 38486 (Table 1).

Discussion

These results indicate that dexamethasone, which is considered to be a potent glucocorticoid drug, inhibits both H_2O_2 formation and PGE_2 synthesis by

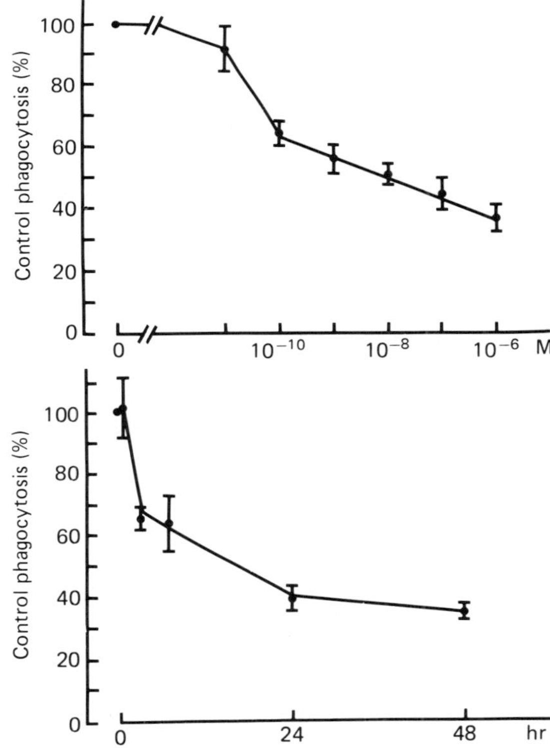

Fig. 3. Percentage of control phagocytosis in the presence of serum-treated zymosan (1 mg/ml) as a function of the concentration of dexamethasone used for preincubation of the cells during 48 hr (*upper part*) or of the time of preincubation of the cells with 1 μM dexamethasone (*lower part*). Phagocytosis was estimated from the amount of ^{125}I serum-treated zymosan associated to the cells.

mesangial cells during phagocytosis. These effects occur at concentrations of dexamethasone that are lower than 1 μM, which corresponds to the plasma concentrations of the synthetic steroids currently achieved for therapeutic purposes [27]. The inhibitory effect of glucocorticoids on reactive oxygen release by human polymorphonuclear leukocytes exposed to STZ has been reported by Goldstein et al [28]; they observed a decrease in superoxide anion production by these cells during phagocytosis after incubation for 30 min with hydrocortisone or methylprednisolone at 500 μM. The short period of incubation and the high concentration used suggest, in this case, a pharmacologic and direct effect of the drugs on the cell membrane. On the contrary, the H_2O_2 release from human monocytes induced by phorbol myristate acetate (PMA) was nearly abolished by preincubation of the cells for at least 72 hr with 0.3 μM hydrocortisone. Shorter periods of exposure to hydrocortisone were without effect on H_2O_2 release [29]. Similar results were observed with macrophages [30]. The necessity of a lag time for the effect of glucocorticoids on reactive oxygen production by stimulated cells suggested that the drug acted through receptor-mediated modulation of RNA and protein synthesis. Such a mechanism of action is also very likely to explain the results observed in this present study for the following reasons: (1) a lag period longer than 1 hr was necessary to observe an effect of dexamethasone, (2) when present in a 10- to 50-fold excess, RU 38486 completely counteracted the inhibitory effect of the glucocorticoid (the necessity of such an excess to get a maximum effect of this antagonist has been reported already [31]), and (3) inhibitors of RNA and protein synthesis blocked the steroid-induced responses. However, as observed by other investigators [6, 32], actinomycin D produced a decrease in the basal activity of the cells due to its own toxicity. Viewed together, these different results suggest that dexamethasone induces the synthesis by mesangial cells of a protein capable of inhibiting H_2O_2 generation during phagocytosis. Since dexamethasone also affected PGE_2 synthesis by the mesangial cells during phagocytosis, the same dexamethasone-induced protein could be at the origin of the inhibition of both H_2O_2 and PGE_2 formation. This protein is likely to be macrocortin-lipomodulin, which is considered to be a potent inhibitor of phospholipase activity [5, 6, 32]. Reactive oxygen production by stimulated human neutrophils requires phospholipase activity [33], probably as the preliminary step for stimulation of the lipoxygenase pathway. Inhibition of phospholipase would result in a decrease in arachidonic acid release from membrane phospholipids; thus, it would affect the lipoxygenase pathway and the associated reactive oxygen production through two main reactions: (1) the transformation of hydroperoxy-intermediates [HPETE] of arachidonic acid into the hydroxyderivatives [HETE] [2], and (2) the activation of O_2^--generating NADPH oxidase by metabolites of the lipoxygenase pathway [34, 35]. Alternatively, dexamethasone could control the synthesis of another protein directly inhibiting the synthesis of an enzyme responsible for reactive oxygen production.

Another conclusion from this study is that dexamethasone, at concentrations lower than 1 μM also inhibits the phagocytic capability of the mesangial cells in a dose-dependent manner. Such a role for glucocorticoids has already been shown with other phagocytic cells. Hydrocortisone produced a reduction in phagocytosis by polymorphonuclear leukocytes of healthy subjects exposed to STZ [36]; and, dexamethasone inhibited yeast phagocytosis by murine macrophages [10]. The latter results, contrary to the former, were obtained only when dexamethasone (at 1 μM at least) had been added to the cultured medium 1 day before the phagocytosis assay. Similarly, no or little effect of hydrocortisone on phagocytosis by human monocytes was observed for short periods of incubation [37]. The necessity of a lag period also was observed in this present study, which suggests a genomic effect of dexamethasone for the inhibition of phagocytosis as well as for that of H_2O_2 and PGE_2 synthesis. This conclusion is confirmed by the inhibitory effect of RU 38486 on the dexamethasone-induced reduction in phagocytosis. This antagonist, when added in a 50-fold excess, completely abolished the effect of 1 μM dexamethasone. It had been shown in a previous report [2] that H_2O_2 generation by mesangial cells that were exposed to STZ was dependent on the coating of the particle by a thermolabile serum protein, which suggests a role for C3b receptor-mediated phagocytosis in stimulation of reactive oxygen production. It cannot be entirely excluded that the effect of dexamethasone on phagocytosis may be due to a decrease in the binding capacity of these C3b receptors, although this property of glucocorticoids probably implies a direct mechanism. Indeed, the effect of glucocorticoids on the IgG and C3b receptors of human neutrophils and monocytes was immediate, and, it occurred only at high doses (100 μM) of these drugs [11, 12]. These characteristics probably correspond to a nongenomic effect and are opposed to those observed in the present study. Finally, the most likely hypothesis is the induction by dexamethasone of a single protein that primarily inhibits phospholipase activity and, as a consequence, the phagocytic process. This would be in agreement with the findings of Garcia Gil et al [38], who reported that inhibitors of phospholipase activity both reduced arachidonic acid generation and phagocytosis.

These results suggest that the same dexamethasone-induced protein reduces H_2O_2 and PGE_2 production, as well as phagocytosis, as a consequence of inhibition of phospholipase activity. However, the inhibitory effect of dexamethasone on phagocytosis by mesangial cells cannot completely explain its role on H_2O_2 production for the following reasons: (1) dexamethasone also produced a decrease in H_2O_2 generation under basal conditions in the absence of any phagocytic stimulus (Fig. 2), and (2) as shown previously [2], the H_2O_2 production by mesangial cells exposed to STZ partly depended on the phagocytosis, since cytochalasin B (a blocker of phagocytosis) only partially inhibited this production. It remains to be determined whether the same inhibitory effects of dexamethasone occur after in vivo administration, and whether they play a role in the therapeutic properties of the drug.

References

1. Mancilla-Jimenez R, Bellon B, Kuhn J, Belair MF, Rouchon M, Druet P, Bariety J: Phagocytosis of heat-aggregated immunoglobulins by mesangial

cells. An immunoperoxidase and acid phosphatase study. *Lab Invest* 46:243–253, 1982

2. BAUD L, HAGEGE J, SRAER J, RONDEAU E, PEREZ J, ARDAILLOU R: Reactive oxygen production by cultured rat glomerular mesangial cells during phagocytosis is associated with stimulation of lipoxygenase activity. *J Exp Med* 158:1836–1852, 1983

3. SEDOR JR, ABBOUD HE: Histamine modulates superoxide anion production in cultured rat mesangial cells (*abstract*). *Kidney Int* 25:218, 1984

4. SCHLONDORFF D, SATRIANO JA, HAGEGE J, PEREZ J, BAUD L: Effect of platelet activating factor and serum-treated zymosan on PGE_2 synthesis, arachidonic acid release and contraction of cultured rat mesangial cells. *J Clin Invest* (in press, 1984)

5. BLACKWELL GJ, CARNUCCIO R, DiROSA M, FLOWER RJ, PARENTE L, PERSICO P: Macrocortin: a polypeptide causing the antiphospholipase effect of glucocorticoids. *Nature* 287:147–149, 1980

6. HIRATA F, SCHIFFMANN E, VENKATASUBRAMANIAN K, SALOMON D, AXELROD J: A phospholipase A_2 inhibitory protein in rabbit neutrophils induced by glucocorticoids. *Proc Natl Acad Sci USA* 77:2533–2536, 1980

7. GOLDSTEIN IM, ROOS D, WEISSMANN G, KAPLAN HB: Influence of corticosteroids on human polymorphonuclear leukocyte function in vitro. Reduction of lysosomal enzyme release and superoxide production. *Inflammation* 1:305–315, 1976

8. LEHMEYER JE, JOHNSTON RB JR: Effect of anti-inflammatory drugs and agents that elevate intracellular cyclic AMP on the release of toxic oxygen metabolites by phagocytes: studies in a model of tissue-bound IgG. *Clin Immunol Immunopathol* 9:482–490, 1978

9. SMITH RJ: Phagocytic release of lysosomal enzymes from guinea pig neutrophils. Regulation by corticosteroids, autonomic neurohormones and cyclic nucleotides. *Biochem Pharmacol* 26:2001–2009, 1977

10. GRASSO RJ, WEST LA, GUAY RC JR, KLEIN TW: Inhibition of yeast phagocytosis by dexamethasone in macrophage cultures: reversibility of the effect and enhanced suppression in cultures of stimulated macrophages. *J Immunopharmacol* 4:265–278, 1982–1983

11. FORSLID J, HED J: In vitro effect of hydrocortisone on the attachment and ingestion phases of immunoglobulin G- and complement component 3b- mediated phagocytosis by human neutrophils. *Infect Immunol* 38:811–816, 1982

12. SCHREIBER AD, PARSONS J, McDERMOTT P, COOPER RA: Effect of corticosteroids on the human monocyte IgG and complement receptors. *J Clin Invest* 56:1189–1197, 1975

13. DUVAL D, DURANT S, HOMO-DELARCHE F: Non-genomic effects of steroids. Interactions of steroid molecules with membrane structures and functions. *Biochim Biophys Acta* 737:409–442, 1983

14. BOREL Y, LEWIS RM, ANDRE-SCHWARTZ J, STOLLAR BD, DIENER E: Treatment of lupus nephritis in adult $(NZB + NZW)F_1$ mice by cortisone-facilitated tolerance to nucleic acid antigens. *J Clin Invest* 61:276–286, 1978

15. FARMAN N, VANDEWALLE A, BONVALET JP: Autoradiographic study of aldosterone and dexamethasone binding in isolated glomeruli of rabbit kidney. *Am J Physiol* 243:F235–F242, 1982

16. ABBOUD HE, SHAH SV, DOUSA TP: Effects of dexamethasone on cyclic nucleotide accumulation in glomeruli. *J Lab Clin Med* 94:708–717, 1979

17. FOIDART JB, DECHENNE CA, MAHIEU P, CREUTZ CE, DE MEY J: Tissue culture

of normal rat glomeruli. Isolation and morphological characterization of two homogeneous cell lines. *Invest Cell Pathol* 2:15–26, 1979

18. SRAER J, SRAER JD, CHANSEL D, JUEPPNER H, HESCH RD, ARDAILLOU R: Evidence for glomerular receptors for parathyroid hormone. *Am J Physiol* 235:F96–F103, 1978

19. STERZEL RB, EHRICH JH, LUCIA H, THOMSON D, KASHGARIAN M: Mesangial disposal of glomerular immune deposits in acute malarial glomerulonephritis of rats. *Lab Invest* 46:109–214, 1982

20. MOGUILEWSKY M, PHILIBERT D: RU 38486: Potent antiglucocorticoid activity correlated with strong binding to the cytosolic glucocorticoid receptor followed by an impaired activation. *J Steroid Biochem* (in press, 1984)

21. DRAY F, CHARBONNEL B, MACLOUF J: Radioimmunoassay of prostaglandins F_α, E_1 and E_2 in human plasma. *Eur J Clin Invest* 5:311–318, 1975

22. SRAER J, SRAER JD, CHANSEL D, RUSSO-MARIE F, KOUZNETZOVA B, ARDAILLOU R: Prostaglandin synthesis by isolated rat renal glomeruli. *Mol Cell Endocrinol* 16:29–37, 1979

23. PICK E, KEISARI Y: A simple colorimetric method for the measurement of hydrogen peroxide produced by cells in culture. *J Immunol Methods* 38:161–170, 1980

24. WEBB LS, KEELE BB JR, JOHNSTON RB JR: Inhibition of phagocytosis-associated chemiluminescence by superoxide dismutase. *Infect Immun* 9:1051–1056, 1974

25. BESTERMAN JM, AIRHART JA, LOW RB: Macrophage phagocytosis: analysis of particle binding and internalization. *Am J Physiol* 242:C339–C346, 1982

26. INGRAHAM LM, WEENING RS, CLARKE MF, BOXER LA, BAEHNER RL: Relation of respiratory burst and arachidonate metabolism during phagocytosis by guinea pig alveolar macrophages. *J Lab Clin Med* 99:908–916, 1982

27. STUBBS SS: Corticosteroids and bioavailability. *Transplant Proc* 7:11–19, 1975

28. GOLDSTEIN IM, MALMSTEN CL, KAPLAN HB, JINDAHL H, SAMUELSSON B, WEISSMANN G: Thromboxane generation by stimulated human granulocytes: inhibition by glucocorticoids and superoxide dismutase (*abstract*). *Clin Res* 25:518A, 1977

29. NAKAGAWARA A, DESANTIS NM, NOGUEIRA N, NATHAN CF: Lymphokines enhance the capacity of human monocytes to secrete reactive oxygen intermediates. *J Clin Invest* 70:1042–1048, 1982

30. MASUR H, MURRAY HW, JONES TC: Effect of hydrocortisone on macrophage response to lymphokine. *Infect Immunol* 35:709–774, 1982

31. DUVAL D, DURANT S, HOMO-DELARCHE F: Effect of antiglucocorticoids on dexamethasone-induced inhibition of uridine incorporation and cell lysis in isolated mouse thymocytes. *J Steroid Biochem* 20:283–287, 1984

32. RUSSO-MARIE F, PAING M, DUVAL D: Involvement of glucocorticoid receptors in steroid-induced inhibition of prostaglandin secretion. *J Biol Chem* 254:8498–8504, 1979

33. STOCKER R, RICHTER C: Involvement of calcium, calmodulin and phospholipase A in the alteration of membrane dynamics and superoxide production of human neutrophils stimulated by phorbol myristate acetate. *FEBS Lett* 147:243–246, 1982

34. PICK E, BROMBERG Y: Quo vadis macrophage activation. Role of phospholipids in the elicitation of the oxidative burst in macrophages. *Transplant Proc* 14:570–574, 1982

35. BROMBERG Y, PICK E: Unsaturated fatty acids as second messengers of superoxide generation by macrophages. *Cell Immunol* 79:240–252, 1983

36. HEINE KJ, COTTON SHALLCROSS J JR, TRACHTENBERG LS, GALLAND RB, POLK JC Jr: A reassessment of the influence of steroids on neutrophil phagocytosis. *Am Surg* 49:221–224, 1983
37. RINEHART JJ, BALCERZAC SP, SAGONE AL, LO BUGLIO AF: Effects of corticosteroids on human monocyte function. *J Clin Invest* 54:1337–1343, 1974
38. GARCIA GIL M, ALONSO F, ALVAREZ CHIVA V, SANCHEZ CRESPO M, MAHO JM: Phospholipid turnover during phagocytosis in human polymorphonuclear leukocytes. *Biochem J* 206:67–72, 1982

Diseases of the Kidneys

Primary Glomerular Diseases

Poststreptococcal Glomerulonephritis

Bernardo Rodríguez-Iturbe

Glomerulonephritis following poststreptococcal infection (PSGN) is a well-defined clinical entity. I shall review some aspects of the bacteriology, pathogenesis, host response, and natural history of the disease in the light of recent evidence.

Nephritogenic Streptococci

Group A streptococcal infections may be associated with rheumatic fever or acute glomerulonephritis, but only rarely with both in the same host. The concept of nephritogenic types of streptococci is based on this observation [1–3]. Streptococcus M types 1, 2, 4, 12, 18, 25, 49, 55, 57, and 60 have been isolated from patients who developed nephritis and are therefore considered to be responsible for the disease [4]. Nontypable group A beta-hemolytic streptococci have also been cultured from patients with glomerulonephritis, presumably representing unclassified nephritogenic strains.

It is unusual to develop a second attack of poststreptococcal glomerulonephritis. Therefore, it is probable that the disease is induced by an antigen that provides long-lasting immunity; a feature that is shared by all of the streptococci with nephritogenic potential.

The identity of the nephritogenic fractions of the bacteria is controversial. Two general possibilities have been suggested [5]: first, that the nephritogenic antigen is a specific component of some streptococci, and second, that the streptococcal infection itself triggers an autoantigenic reactivity in the host organism. Alternatively, autoantigenic reactivity can play a secondary, but by no means trivial, role in modifying the natural history of the disease. The lack of a suitable animal model for PSGN has made it difficult to clarify the issues in the pathogenesis.

This manuscript was presented in a Symposium on *Tropical Nephrology*.

The streptococcal M protein has been traditionally considered to be the relevant antigenic fraction for reasons of specificity and pathogenicity [6, 7]. Acid-extracted M protein type 1 forms complexes with fibrinogen that localize in the glomerulus [8, 9], and nephritis may be induced with injections of M protein and M protein-fibrinogen complexes [10, 11]. In addition, M protein may be antigenically cross-reactive with the glomerular basement membrane [12], which suggests another mechanism in which M protein could be implicated. However, more recent evidence appears to indicate that the nephritogenic fraction is different from M protein. Tresser et al [13, 14] showed that serum from convalescing patients contained antibody that, when labeled with fluorescein, could be used to stain early biopsy specimens of patients with PSGN, thereby identifying free antigenic sites. This finding was independent of the M type of the original infection and therefore indicated a non-M antigen at the glomerular level [14].

At the present time, three streptococcal fractions are under study as potential triggers for nephritis. The first was described by the New York Medical College group [13, 15–17]. They obtained it after disruption of nephritogenic streptococci and found that it had the ability to preabsorb the suspected specific antibody of convalescent sera. This conclusion was based on its ability to block the staining capacity of late sera when applied to early biopsy specimens. This antigen has a molecular weight between 40,000 and 50,000 daltons [16, 17]. Antibody titers to this antigen have been found in patients with PSGN but also in 10 to 74% of normal individuals [16, 17]. More recently, it has been suggested that this material may act as a "planted" antigen for an in situ immune reaction in the glomerular basement membrane [18].

The second fraction, a protein unique to nephritogenic strains, was identified from cultures of streptococci by Villareal et al [19]. They detected this in 56% of the renal biopsy specimens taken from patients with acute PSGN, but not in biopsy tissue from patients with rheumatic fever or glomerulonephritis of different etiologies. From 93 to 96% of the patients with glomerulonephritis have serum antibody levels against this fraction, as do 5 to 15% of the patients with rheumatic fever and 13 to 20% of normal individuals [20].

The third fraction was identified by Vogt et al [21], who studied cultures from nephritogenic streptococci looking for cationic proteins that might penetrate more easily the glomerular basement membrane barrier. It was reasoned that cationic proteins would not be properly rejected by the overall negative charge of that structure [22, 23]. Cationic antigens separated by chromatofocusing with a pH range of 8 to 11 were identified in culture supernatants of nephritogenic streptococci. Antibodies raised against these proteins enabled them to demonstrate the existence of these cationic antigens in 8 of 18 renal biopsy specimens taken from patients with acute PSGN; on the other hand, these antigens were undetected in biopsy specimens from other patients with IgG-positive glomerulonephritis who were not poststreptococcal. Serum antibodies to these antigens were detected in all 18 patients with acute PSGN [21].

In addition to the streptococcal fractions just mentioned, the possibility exists that the streptococcus may trigger an autologous immune complex disease by inducing an antigenic modification of a normal component of the organism. McIntosh et al [24, 25] raised this question and were able to induce cryoglobulinemia and nephritis in animals injected with autologous IgG, provided that this material was sialic acid-depleted with streptococcal neuraminidase. Davis, Baig, and Ayoub [26] reported that streptococci of the so-called nephritogenic M types were frequently neuraminidase producers. Potter et al [27] could not detect neuraminidase production in streptococci isolated from patients with acute PSGN; but contrary to their findings, we have detected neuraminidase activity in culture supernatants of 16 out of 20 bacterial strains isolated from our patients [28]. It is possible that the discrepancy is due to the fact that neuraminidase-producing strains cease frequently their enzyme production after repeated subculturing (Mosquera J, et al, unpublished observations). More significant, however, is the fact that Potter et al [27] could show neuraminidase production in streptococci isolated from patients with rheumatic fever [27]; this finding would appear to separate nephritogenicity from neuraminidase production in group A streptococci.

At the present time, it is difficult to assess the relative importance of the antigenic fractions and mechanisms just discussed in the development of acute poststreptococcal glomerulonephritis.

Pathogenesis

The evidence indicates that acute PSGN is an immune complex disease: 90% of the patients with acute PSGN have elevated levels of IgG and IgM; 93% have depressed complement levels; and two-thirds of the patients have detectable cryoglobulins in the first 2 weeks of the disease [5]. Circulating immune complexes, as measured by Clq binding activity (ClqBA), can be detected in the serum of two-thirds of the patients in the first week of the disease and in about 20% of the patients after week 4 of the disease [29–32]. Circulating immune complexes have been reported to correlate with the severity of the disease and with the demonstration of renal immune deposits [33, 34], but we have not detected a correlation between the ClqBA and the intensity of the clinical manifestations [29].

The responsible antigen may be met by antibody circulation or, as it has been suggested more recently [18], at the glomerular level where the antigen could be planted. Cationic antigens, which penetrate more easily the anionic barrier of the glomerular basement membrane, would appear to be likely candidates for triggering an in situ immune reaction [35, 36].

A role for antiglobulins has been postulated in the pathogenesis of acute PSGN. If indeed streptococcal neuraminidase were able to remove sialic acid from immunoglobulins, they could become autoantigenic. In fact, circulating anti-immunoglobulins have been detected in almost 50% of the patients [5], and glomerular fixed antiglobulins were detected in 19 of 22 renal biopsy specimens from patients with the disease [37]. Furthermore, IgG eluted from the kidney of a patient who died in the acute stage showed anti-IgG reactivity

[38]. Moreover, patients with acute PSGN, tested with the skin-window technique, react to normal human IgG with lymphocyte migration to the skin in a manner similar to that observed in recognition reaction to challenge with antigens to which the patients had previous exposure [39].

Finally, thiobarbituric acid-reactive material, presumably free sialic acid, was detected in the serum of 28 of 39 patients with acute PSGN, 8 of which had, in addition, detectable neuraminidase activity [40]. However, Potter et al [27] studied serum samples from 6 patients with acute PSGN and 6 patients with rheumatic fever and could not detect neuraminidase activity; 2 patients with acute PSGN and 2 patients with rheumatic fever were found to have increased levels of sialic acid.

In summary, the role of antiglobulins in acute PSGN is undefined. It may represent an irrelevant epiphenomenon or it may have importance in modulating the intermediate and long-term course of the disease.

Epidemiology

It is generally agreed that the number of cases of poststreptococcal glomerulonephritis has diminished significantly in the United States, Central Europe, and Great Britain in the last 20 to 30 years [41]. However, PSGN continues to have high incidence in other areas of the world as indicated by reports of the disease in Alaska [42], Africa [33], the Caribbean [43], and South America [44].

The disease strikes all ages, but 60% of the cases are children 2 to 12 years old, and as many as 10% of the patients in large series are older than 40 years of age [45]. Clinical acute PSGN is more frequent in males; in our experience, 60% of the patients are males. However, the higher male incidence is not observed when subclinical as well as clinical cases are taken into account [46].

The site of streptococcal infection is usually the upper respiratory tract or the skin and more rarely the middle ear [47]. Airborne droplets are responsible for the spread of streptococcal pharyngitis [48]. Few systemic symptoms or, alternatively, fever and cervical lymphadenopathy may accompany this infection.

Streptococcal M types 49, 55, 57, and 60 are frequently isolated from the skin of patients with impetigo who develop glomerulonephritis [49]. Frequently, the same bacteria can be demonstrated in the throat and the skin, and in those instances the skin infection precedes that of the throat [50]. Streptococcal pyodermitis usually presents as vesicular lesions that later may become pustular. Regional adenopathy is present in 9 out of 10 patients [51]; and elevated white cell count in about half [52]. Fever, chills, and malaise are rare, however.

There is a latent period of 1 to 2 weeks after the throat infections and of 3 to 6 weeks after the skin infections. Albuminuria and microscopic hematuria may be found in the interval between infection and nephritis. These findings can be detected in about half the cases with streptococcal upper respiratory infections and are more likely to occur in the patients who later on develop nephritis [47].

The risk of developing nephritis after infection with nephritogenic streptococcus has been estimated to be about 15% [49], and infection with M type 49 carries a risk of about 5% if present in the throat and five times higher if present in the skin [50].

Poststreptococcal nephritis appears in the form of both sporadic cases and epidemic outbreaks [53]. Epidemics tend to occur in closed communities [54, 55] or in highly populated rural or city areas in which poor hygiene is a common denominator [43, 44]. In certain communities, epidemics have had a tendency to appear in periodic outbreaks separated by 5 to 7 years [43, 44]. There is no adequate explanation for this. A close correlation between the endemic incidence and the incidence of epidemic cases has been noted in areas within a city [56]. Malnutrition, anemia, and intestinal parasites have a high incidence in communities in which epidemics of PSGN occur [56].

From the epidemiologic point of view, it is important to recognize that acute PSGN may be entirely asymptomatic. Furthermore, subclinical disease is more frequent than symptomatic disease. Sagel et al [57] followed patients at the outpatient clinic after upper respiratory tract infections and found that subclinical disease was 19 times more common than was overt acute nephritis. The subclinical/clinical disease ratio was 1.5 in the Red Lake epidemic of 1966 [58]. The subclinical/clinical acute PSGN ratio in families in Trinidad may be as low as 0.03 [59]. In our prospective family studies [46], this ratio was found to be 4:0, which is in agreement with the study of Dodge et al [60] who found a ratio of 5:3.

The factors responsible for the milder clinical picture in some patients are unknown, and there are no studies on long-term follow-up of patients with subclinical disease.

Genetic Considerations

It is well recognized that cases of acute PSGN may occur in siblings of patients with the disease. Dodge, Spargo, and Travis [60] reported a 20% incidence of subclinical and clinical nephritis in siblings of index cases. We have studied prospectively 22 families of index cases with acute PSGN, comprising a total of 141 first-degree relatives [46]. There was no epidemic when the study was conducted, and it was found that 72 siblings at risk developed nephritis; therefore, the attack rate for siblings in affected families in nonepidemic conditions is 37.8%. This value is higher than the attack rate of the population at risk in epidemics, for Anthony et al [58] found nephritis and/ or urinary abnormalities in 28.3% and 4.5% of the children at risk with skin infection and throat infection, respectively, during the Red Lake epidemic. Inasmuch as the attack rate in families of children with sporadic acute PSGN is higher, a familial susceptibility to the disease was postulated [46]. An analysis, with correction for incomplete selection in the sibships, showed a proportion of 0.260 ± 0.016, which is an excellent fit for the expected ratio in single autosomal-recessive inheritance [61]. Clearly, this intriguing finding awaits confirmation by a more definite genetic proof.

Several studies have analyzed HLA antigens in glomerulonephritis, although it is well recognized that inheritance characteristics in the disease are multifactorial. Read et al [62] found that the HLA antigen distribution in acute PSGN is similar to that found in the general population. This is in contrast with studies in rheumatic fever, which have reported a decreased incidence of HLA-A3 [63], an increased incidence of BW25 [64], and a linkage disequilibrium of HLA-B5 [62]. Our own investigations [65] tested HLA-A, B, C, and D antigens in families with affected and nonaffected children. Some antigens (CW1 and DR3) showed deviation from the expected $1:1$ ratio in affected siblings in backcross families. In addition, we compared the frequency of 61 HLA antigens in 42 unrelated acute PSGN patients and 109 controls and found that HLA-DRW4 is more frequent among the former. At the present time, no firm conclusions can be drawn as to definite associations—or the lack of them—between HLA antigens and nephritis.

Prognosis

The early mortality of acute PSGN is 0.5 to 0.8% [5]. As to the long-term prognosis, reports on sporadic cases of PSGN indicate that progression to chronicity is rare [66, 67], but known to occur [68].

Early reports on epidemics suggest that almost all patients recover, but the follow-up periods were relatively short [69]. A study done 10 years after the Red Lake epidemic found no difference in the incidence of hematuria and biopsy changes between the patients and control children [70]. In 1954, Baldwin et al [71] found evidence of chronic renal disease in more than 50% of the patients followed 2 to 15 years after the episode of acute PSGN. Reports from other groups [72–75] differ with respect to the incidence of chronicity, but, in general, they continue to indicate that progression to chronicity is a rare event.

As reviewed in a recent publication [5], part of the disagreement might be due to the methods used to investigate progression to chronicity and to the fact that the patients in the various series are not strictly comparable. With respect to the latter, the prognosis is probably better in children than in adults, and epidemic cases may have a milder disease than do sporadic cases. With respect to the methods of evaluating the long-term course of the disease, it is recognized that the incidence of histologic changes, in particular, glomerular sclerosis, is much higher than the incidence of clinical or renal function abnormalities [56, 71], but these lesions may be residual [74] or they may represent progressive disease [75]. In reviewing all the studies with significant follow-up periods, one must reach the conclusion that, whatever the incidence of histologic damage and renal function abnormalities, uremia is rare after a decade of follow-up. The combined series suggest that terminal renal failure has developed in about 1% of the patients followed by various research groups [5].

Acknowledgments. This work was supported by CONICIT grant No. SAL-001 (Venezuela) and a grant From the Asociación de Amigos del Riñón (Maracaibo).

References

1. BERNSTEIN SH, STOLLERMAN M: A study of the association of group A streptococci with acute glomerulonephritis. *Ann Intern Med* 52:1026–1034, 1960
2. BISNO AL, PEARCE IA, WALL HP, MOODY MD, STOLLERMAN G: Contrasting epidemiology of acute rheumatic fever and acute glomerulonephritis: Nature of the antecedent streptococcal infection. *N Engl J Med* 283:561–565, 1970
3. RAMMELKAMP CH, WEAVER RS: Acute glomerulonephritis: The significance of variations in the incidence of disease. *J Clin Invest* 32:345–358, 1953
4. RODRIGUEZ-ITURBE B, CASTILLO L, VALBUENA R, CUENCA L: Acute poststreptococcal glomerulonephritis: A review of recent developments. *Paediatrician* 8:307–324, 1979
5. RODRIGUEZ-ITURBE B: Epidemic poststreptococcal glomerulonephritis. *Kidney Int* 25:129–136, 1984
6. KELLY DK, WINN JF: Renal lesions produced by group A type 12 streptococci. *Science* 127:1337, 1958
7. VOSTI KL, JOHNSON RH, DILLON MF: Further characterization of purified fractions of M protein from a strain of group A, type 12 streptococcus. *J Immunol* 107:104–114, 1971
8. KANTOR FS: Fibrinogen precipitation by streptococcal M protein: II. Renal lesions induced by intravenous infections of M protein into mice and rats. *J Exp Med* 121:861–879, 1965
9. KAPLAN MH: Localization of streptococcal antigens in tissues: I. Histologic distribution and persistence of M protein types 1, 5, 12, and 19 in tissues of the mouse. *J Exp Med* 107:341–368, 1958
10. HUMAIR L, POTTER EV, KWAAN HC: The role of fibrinogen in renal disease: I. Productions of experimental lesions in mice. *J Lab Clin Med* 74:60–71, 1969
11. HUMAIR L, KWAAN HC, POTTER EV: The role of fibrinogen in renal disease: II. Effects of anticoagulants and urokinase on experimental lesions in mice. *J Lab Clin Med* 74:72–78, 1969
12. MARKOWITZ AS, LANGE CF: Streptococcal related glomerulonephritis: I. Isolation, immunochemistry and comparative chemistry of soluble fractions from type 12 nephritogenic streptococci and human glomeruli. *J Immunol* 94:565–573, 1964
13. TRESSER G, SEMAR M, MCVICAR M, FRANKLIN M, TY A, SAGEL I, LANGE K: Antigenic streptococcal components in acute glomerulonephritis. *Science* 163:676–677, 1969
14. TRESSER G, SEMAR M, SAGEL I, TY A, STERZEL RB, SCHAERF R, LANGE K: Independence of the nephritogenicity of group A streptococci from their M types. *Clin Exp Immunol* 9:57–62, 1971
15. LANGE K, AHMED U, KLEINBERGER H, TRESSER G: A hitherto unknown streptococcal antigen and its probable relation to acute poststreptococcal glomerulonephritis. *Clin Nephrol* 5:207–215, 1976
16. YOSHISAWA N, TRESSER G, IWASAKI M, TAKAHSHI K: Further characterization of a streptococcal antigen in acute glomerulonephritis, in *Basic Concepts of Streptococci and Streptococcal Diseases,* edited by HOLM SH, CHRISTENSEN P, Surrey, England, Reedbooks Ltd., 1982, pp 257–259
17. LANGE K, CRONIN W, SELIGSON G: Endostreptosin: Its characteristics and clinical significance, in *Basic Concepts of Streptococci and Streptococcal Diseases,* edited by

by HOLM SH, CHRISTENSEN P, Surrey, England, Reedbooks Ltd., 1982, p 260
18. LANGE K, SELIGSON G, CRONIN W: Evidence for the in-situ origin of poststreptococcal glomerulonephritis: Glomerular localization of endostreptosin and clinical significance of subsequent antibody response. *Clin Nephrol* 19:3–10, 1983
19. VILLAREAL H JR, FISCHETTI VA, VAN DE RIJN I, ZABRISKIE JB: The occurrence of a protein in the extracellular products of streptococci isolated from patients with acute glomerulonephritis. *J Exp Med* 149:459–472, 1979
20. OHKUNI H, FRIEDMAN J, VAN DE RIJN I, FISCHETTI VA, ZABRISKIE JB: Serological studies on streptococcal nephritis patients with an extracellular protein associated with nephritogenic streptococci, in *Basic Concepts of Streptococci and Streptococcal Diseases,* edited by HOLM SH, CHRISTENSEN P, Surrey, England, Reedbooks Ltd., 1982, pp 263–265
21. VOGT A, BATSFORD S, RODRIGUEZ-ITURBE B, GARCIA R: Cationic antigens in poststreptococcal glomerulonephritis. *Clin Nephrol* 20:271–279, 1983
22. VOGT A, ROHRBACK R, SHIMIZU F, TAKAMIYA H, BATSFORD S: Interaction of cationized antigen with rat glomerular basement membrane: In situ immune complex formation. *Kidney Int* 22:27–35, 1982
23. RENKE GH, COTRAN RS, VENKATACHALAM MA: Role of molecular charge in glomerular permeability: Tracer studies with cationized ferritins. *J Cell Biol* 67:638–646, 1975
24. MCINTOSH RM, KULVINSKAS C, KAUFMAN DB: Alterations of the chemical composition of human immunoglobulin G by streptococcus pyogenes. *J Med Microbiol* 4:535–538, 1971
25. MCINTOSH RM, KAUFMAN DB, MCINTOSH JR, GRISWOLD W: Glomerular lesions produced in rabbits by autologous serum and autologous IgG modified by treatment with a culture of hemolytic streptococcus. *J Med Microbiol* 5:1–7, 1972
26. DAVIES L, BAIG MM, AYOUB EM: Properties of extracellular neuraminidase produced by group A streptococcus. *Infect Immunol* 24:780–786, 1979
27. POTTER EV, SHAUGHNESSY MA, POON-KING T, EARLE DP: Streptococcal neuraminidase in acute glomerulonephritis. *Infect Immunol* 38:1196–1202, 1982
28. MOSQUERA J, RODRIGUEZ-ITURBE B: Extracellular neuraminidase production of streptococci associated with acute nephritis. *Clin Nephrol* 21:21–28, 1984
29. RODRIGUEZ-ITURBE B, CARR RI, GARCIA R, RABIDEAU D, RUBIO L, MCINTOSH RM: Circulating immune complexes and serum immunoglobulins in acute poststreptococcal glomerulonephritis: Evidence for circulating immune complex pathogenesis. *Clin Nephrol* 13:1–5, 1980
30. MOHAMMED I, ANSELL BM, HOLBOROW EJ, BRICSON ADM: Circulating immune complexes in subacute infective endocarditis and poststreptococcal glomerulonephritis. *J Clin Pathol* 30:308–311, 1977
31. OOI YM, VALLOTA EH, WEST CD: Serum immune complexes in membranoproliferative and other glomerulonephritis. *Kidney Int* 11:275–283, 1977
32. VAN DE RIJN I, FILLIT H, BRANDEIS WE, REID H, POON-KING T, MCCARTHY M, DAY NK, ZABRISKIE JB: Serial studies on circulating immune complexes in poststreptococcal sequelae. *Clin Exp Immunol* 34:318–325, 1978
33. ONYEWOTU II, MEE J: Circulating immune complexes and complement levels in relation to the clinical presentation of Nigerian children with acute poststreptococcal glomerulonephritis. *J Clin Pathol* 31:817–822, 1978
34. COHEN SL, FISHER C, NOWBRAY JF, HOPP A, BURTON-KEE J: Circulating and deposited immune complexes in renal disease and their clinical correlation. *J Clin Pathol* 32:1135–1139, 1979
35. BATSFORD SR, TAKAMIYA H, VOGT A: A model of in-situ immune complex

glomerulonephritis in the rat employing cationized ferritin. *Clin Nephrol* 14:211–216, 1980

36. OITE T, BATSFORD SR, MIHATSCH MJ, TAKAMIYA H, VOGT A: Quantitative studies of in-situ immune complex glomerulonephritis in the rat induced by planted, cationized antigen. *J Exp Med* 155:460–474, 1982

37. MCINTOSH RM, GARCIA R, RUBIO L, RABIDEAU D, RODRIGUEZ-ITURBE B: Evidence for an autologous immune complex pathogenic mechanism in acute poststreptococcal glomerulonephritis. *Kidney Int* 14:501–510, 1978

38. RODRIGUEZ-ITURBE B, RABIDEAU D, GARCIA R, RUBIO L, MCINTOSH RM: Characterization of the glomerular antibody in acute poststreptococcal glomerulonephritis. *Ann Intern Med* 92:478–481, 1980

39. RODRIGUEZ-ITURBE B, SILVA-BEAUPERTHUY V, PARRA G, RUBIO L, GARCIA R: Skin window immune response to normal human IgG in patients with rheumatoid arthritis and acute poststreptococcal glomerulonephritis. *Am J Clin Pathol* 76:270–275, 1981

40. RODRIGUEZ-ITURBE B, KATIYAR VN, COELLO J: Neuraminidase activity and free sialic acid levels in the serum of patients with acute poststreptococcal glomerulonephritis. *N Engl J Med* 304:1506–1510, 1981

41. MCCARTY M: The streptococcus and human disease. *Am J Med* 65:717–718, 1978

42. MARGOLIS HS, LUM MKW, BENDER JR, ELLIOT SR, FITZGERALD M, HARPSTER AP: Acute glomerulonephritis and streptococcal skin lesions in Eskimo children. *Am J Dis Child* 134:681–685, 1980

43. POON-KING T, MOHAMMED I, COX R, POTTER E, SIMON N, SIEGEL A, EARLE DP: Recurrent epidemic nephritis in South Trinidad. *N Engl J Med* 277:728–733, 1967

44. RODRIGUEZ-ITURBE B, GARCIA R, RUBIO L: Glomerulonefritis poststreptococcica: Aspectos controversiales de investigación reciente; la enfermedad en Venezuela. *Acta Cientif Venez* 28:245–248, 1977

45. SCHWARTZ WB, KASSIER JP: Clinical aspects of acute poststreptococcal glomerulonephritis, in *Disease of the Kidney* (2nd ed), edited by STRAUSS MB, WELT LG, Boston, Little, Brown and Co., 1971, p 419

46. RODRIGUEZ-ITURBE B, RUBIO L, GARCIA R: Attack rate of poststreptococcal nephritis in families: A prospective study. *Lancet* 1:401–403, 1981

47. NISSENSON ASR, BARAFF LJ, FINE RN, KNUTSON DW: Poststreptococcal acute glomerulonephritis: Fact and controversy. *Ann Intern Med* 91:76–85, 1979

48. WANNAMAKER LW: The epidemiology of streptococcal infections, in *Streptococcal Infections,* edited by MCCARTHY M, New York, Columbia University Press, 1954, pp 157–175

49. WANNAMAKER LW: Differences between streptococcal infections of the throat and of the skin. *N Engl J Med* 282:78–85, 1979

50. ANTHONY BF, KAPLAN E, WANNAMAKER LW, BRIESE FW, CHAPMAN SS: Attack rates of acute nephritis after type 49 streptococcal infection of the skin and of the respiratory tract. *J Clin Invest* 48:1697–1704, 1969

51. DILLON HC: Impetigo contagiosa: Suppurative and non-suppurative complications: I. Clinical, bacteriologic and epidemiologic characteristics of impetigo. *Am J Dis Child* 115:530–541, 1968

52. BURNETT JW: Management of pyogenic cutaneous infections. *N Engl J Med* 266:164–169, 1962

53. STETSON CA, RAMMELKAMP CH, DRAUSE RM, KOHEN RJ, PERRY WD: Epidemic acute nephritis: Studies on etiology, natural history and prevention. *Medicine (Baltimore)* 34:431–450, 1955

54. REINSTEIN CR: Epidemic nephritis at Red Lake, Minnesota. *J Pediatr* 47:25–33, 1965
55. ZIMMERMAN R, CROSS M, MILLER DR, SCIPLE GW: A streptococcal epidemic in an isolated civilian population with institution of mass prophilaxis. *J Pediatr* 69:40–45, 1966
56. RODRIGUEZ-ITURBE B, GARCIA R, RUBIO L, CUENCA L, TRESSER G, LANGE K: Epidemic glomerulonephritis in Maracaibo: Evidence for progression to chronicity. *Clin Nephrol* 5:197–206, 1976
57. SAGEL I, TRESSER G, TY A, YOSHISAWA N, KLEINBERGER H, YUCEOGLU M, WASSERMAN E, LANGE K: Occurrence and nature of glomerular lesions after group A streptococcal infection in children. *Ann Intern Med* 79:492–499, 1973
58. ANTHONY BF, KAPLAN EL, CHAPMAN SS, QUIE PG, WANNAMAKER LW: Epidemic acute nephritis with reappearance of type 49 streptococcus. *Lancet* 2:787–789, 1967
59. SHARRET AR, POON-KING T, POTTER EN, FINKLEA JF, EARLE DP: Subclinical nephritis in South Trinidad. *Am J Epidemiol* 94:231–245, 1971
60. DODGE WF, SPARGO BF, TRAVIS LB: Occurrence of acute glomerulonephritis in sibling contacts of children with sporadic acute glomerulonephritis. *Pediatrics* 40:1028–1030, 1967
61. RODRIGUEZ-ITURBE B, MORENO-FUENMAYOR H, RUBIO L, GARCIA R, LAYRISSE Z: Mendelian recessive ratios in acute poststreptococcal glomerulonephritis. *Experientia* 38:918–919, 1982
62. READ SE, POON-KING T, REID HFM, ZABRISKIE JB: HLA and group A streptococcal sequelae, in *Streptococcal Diseases and the Immune Response,* edited by READ SE, ZABRISKIE JB, New York, Academic Press, 1980, pp 347–353
63. FALK JA, FLEISHMAN JL, ZABRISKIE JB, FALK RE: A study of HL-A antigen phenotype in rheumatic fever and rheumatic heart disease patients. *Tissue Antigens* 3:173–178, 1973
64. LEIRISALO M, LAIFINEN O, TIILIKAIEN A: HLA phenotypes in patients with rheumatic fever, rheumatic heart disease, and *Yersinia* arthritis. *J Rheumatol* 4(Suppl 3):78–83, 1977
65. LAYRISSE Z, RODRIGUEZ-ITURBE B, GARCIA R, RODRIGUEZ A, TIWARI J: Family studies of the HLA system in acute poststreptococcal glomerulonephritis. *Hum Immunol* 7:177–185, 1983
66. DODGE WF, SPARGO BH, TRAVIS LB, SRIVASTAVA RN, CARVAJAL H, DE BENKELAER MD, LONGLEY MP, MENCHACA JA: Poststreptococcal glomerulonephritis: A prospective study in children. *N Engl J Med* 286:273–278, 1972
67. HINGLAIS N, GARCIA-TORRES R, KLEINKNECHT D: Long-term prognosis in acute glomerulonephritis. *Am J Med* 56:52–60, 1974
68. SCHACHT RG, GLUCK MC, GALLO GR, BALDWIN DS: Progression to uremia after remission of acute poststreptococcal glomerulonephritis. *N Engl J Med* 295:977–981, 1976
69. STETSON CA, RAMMELKAMP CH, KRAUSE RA, KOHEN RJ, PERRY WA: Epidemic acute nephritis: Studies on etiology, natural history and prevention. *Medicine* 34:431–450, 1955
70. PERLMAN LV, HERDMAN RC, KLEIMAN H, VERNIER RL: Poststreptococcal glomerulonephritis: A ten year follow-up on epidemic. *JAMA* 194:175–182, 1965
71. BALDWIN DS, MELVIN C, GLUCK MC, SCHACHT RG, GALLO G: The long-term course of poststreptococcal glomerulonephritis. *Ann Intern Med* 80:342–358, 1974
72. POTTER EV, LIPSCHULTZ SA, ABIDH S, POON-KING T, EARLE DP: Twelve to

seventeen-year follow-up of patients with poststreptococcal acute glomerulonephritis in Trinidad. *N Engl J Med* 307:725–729, 1982
73. LIEN JKW, MATHEW TH, MEADOWS R: Acute poststreptococcal glomerulonephritis in adults: A long-term study. *Q J Med* 189:99–111, 1979
74. TRAVIS LB, DODGE WF, BEATHARD GA, SPARGO BH, LORENTZ WB, CARVAJAL HT, BERGER M: Acute glomerulonephritis in children: A review of the natural history with emphasis on prognosis. *Clin Nephrol* 1:169–181, 1979
75. GARCIA R, RUBIO L, RODRIGUEZ-ITURBE B: Long-term prognosis of epidemic poststreptococcal glomerulonephritis in Maracaibo: Follow-up studies 11–12 years after the acute episode. *Clin Nephrol* 15:291–298, 1981

Minimal Change Disease, Mesangial Proliferative Glomerulonephritis and Focal Sclerosis: Individual Entities or a Spectrum of Disease?

Chairpersons: Renée Habib and Jacob Churg
Discussants: Jay Bernstein, J. Stewart Cameron, Arthur H. Cohen, Marie-France Gagnadoux, and Edmund J. Lewis

The wide utilization of renal biopsy and the introduction of electron microscopic (EM) and immunohistologic (IF) methods have allowed better definition of the clinicopathologic conditions associated with the nephrotic syndrome [1–4]. Two major categories of facts can be differentiated. In the first one, diffuse glomerular lesions, either secondary to specific diseases or apparently "primary," such as membranous or membranoproliferative glomerulonephritis (GN) are responsible for the increased permeability of the glomerular capillaries. In most of these, there is evidence that immunologic mechanisms play a role in the injury of the glomerular capillary. In the second one, usually referred to as the idiopathic nephrotic syndrome (INS), the mechanism of glomerular capillary alteration is unknown. In the majority of patients with INS, light microscopic (LM) studies have shown that the glomeruli are normal and EM studies have demonstrated swelling of the podocytes with loss of foot processes. The terms "minimal change disease" or "minimal change nephrotic syndrome" (MCNS) are widely used for this condition. However, other patterns have been identified: namely, focal glomerular sclerosis (FGS) and diffuse mesangial proliferation (DMP; sometimes called mesangial proliferative GN). In addition, immunofluorescence (IF) microscopy has revealed that in some cases of INS (whether they show MCNS, FGS, or DMP by LM), various amounts of Ig and particularly IgM with or without C3 could be found diffusely in the mesangial areas. This immunopathologic feature has given birth to a so-called entity: IgM nephropathy.

This narrative is a summary of a Workshop by the same title.

The clinical significance of these findings in INS has been studied extensively both prospectively and retrospectively. It appears from all investigations that these morphologic features have prognostic value. The differences in response to corticosteroids and subsequent clinical course of each of these clinicopathologic conditions have led some to suggest they are individual entities, whereas others have proposed that they are a group of diseases that share a common pathogenesis and differ only in the severity of expression. There is still considerable controversy about the exact relationship among these four patterns and the discussants presented their own data for or against a unifying concept. Our complete lack of understanding of the pathogenesis of the minimal change lesion hampered any firm conclusion.

Minimal Change Nephrotic Syndrome (MCNS)

Studies of the idiopathic nephrotic syndrome (INS) by the International Study of Kidney Diseases in Children (ISKDC) have shown that 93% of children with MCNS responded with complete remission within 8 weeks during the initial course of steroid therapy, and that they usually have a good prognosis [5]. The response rate improved to 98% within a year. An analysis of the histopathologic subcategories of MCNS demonstrated that patients with biopsy specimens showing mild mesangial hypercellularity and focal tubular changes had significantly higher rates of nonresponse (about 15%) than did those with MCNS as a whole (7%) and nil disease (5%). Those differences disappeared with continued therapy, however, and there remained no significant differences among the subgroups after 52 weeks [6, 7]. There were also no differences among the histopathologic subgroups in the rates of early relapse (relapse during the first 8 weeks of treatment after an initial response), frequent relapse (2 or more relapses within 6 months of the initial response), late nonresponse (failure to respond to steroid therapy within 8 weeks during a relapse after initial response), and death. Followup studies of late nonresponders showed 6 of 33 patients to have persistent proteinuria (four patients), chronic renal failure (two patients), and delayed responsiveness during relapse. Late nonresponsiveness may therefore identify a subgroup of initial responders at increased risk of unfavorable outcome [8, 9]. Early nonresponsiveness (initial nonresponse and early relapse) also identified a subgroup at risk (25%) of dying, despite later patterns of response in those patients.

For Bernstein, late nonresponsiveness and perhaps late development of FSGS and chronic renal failure are not predicted by the initial histopathologic pattern of glomerular injury, and their apparently random occurrence suggests that differences in late responsiveness and the late development of FSGS with progressive disease are due to quantitative variations in the same disease process rather than to different disease processes. An important indicator of outcome in MCNS is the type of response to steroid therapy.

Focal Segmental Glomerular Sclerosis (FSGS)

The two morphologic features that characterize the sclerosed segmental lesion of FSGS are the presence of large intracapillary deposits of hyaline material that, by IF, fix IgM and C3 antisera and degenerative podocytic changes. By LM the podocytes are separated from the basement membrane by a clear halo around the affected capillary loops; and, by EM, they are detached from the capillary basement membrane with a filling of the resulting space by a cloudy acellular material composed of very thin and irregular layers of newly formed basement membrane. The uninvolved glomeruli, apart from diffuse fusion of foot processes, may show varying degrees of mesangial hypercellularity.

FSGS is a lesion that can be seen as a superimposed feature in all kinds of glomerular diseases as well as in other conditions of nonglomerular origin. Although nonspecific, the lesion of FSGS, when found in the setting of an INS, is an important finding regarding prognosis even if few glomeruli and capillary loops are affected. The observation that FSGS may be found early in the course of the disease and that, in contrast to MCNS, most of the patients have poorly selective proteinuria, hematuria, resistance to steroid therapy, and a significant propensity for progression to renal failure favors the concept that such patients are affected by a distinct clinicopathologic entity.

In fact, this sharp contrast between MCNS and FSGS is only partly true and there is an almost complete spectrum of patients ranging from a completely corticosteroid-sensitive patient with MCNS to a relentlessly progressive patient with severe FSGS [10–16]. Other arguments speak in favor of a unifying concept. It is clear from the recurrence of proteinuria first, and sclerosing lesions second, in patients with allografts and recurrent glomerular lesions and from long-term proteinuria induced by puromycin in rats that the segmental sclerosing lesion can arise in association with proteinuria and perhaps as a result of it. Work with remnant kidneys suggests further that segmental sclerosing lesions can follow glomerular hyperperfusion and proteinuria, and perhaps provide a clue for the first time as to why the juxtaglomerular glomeruli are peculiarly vulnerable to the lesion since their hemodynamics differ from superficial nephrons. All of this is supported by the appearance of proteinuria and segmental sclerosing lesions in the scarred kidneys of children with reflux nephropathy.

The detailed pathogenesis of the segmental sclerosing lesion is unknown. Some workers suggest that the mesangial prominence and sclerosis seen in the affected segments leads to segmental collapse of the glomerulus [17]. Others, impressed with the prominent and early changes in the podocytes, have proposed that the primary defect is damage to the podocyte [18, 19].

The hypothesis that the lesion of FSGS might represent only an irreversible lesion of the podocytes, the cause of which remains to be determined, would explain the finding of this lesion in all sorts of glomerular or nonglomerular diseases. In the setting of INS it would therefore be nothing more than a complicating feature of MCNS; a hypothesis that is supported by the finding of identical ultrastructural changes of the supposedly unaffected glomeruli in FSGS [20].

For Cameron, the accumulated evidence of the nonspecificity of the FSGS lesions, the fact that FSGS may appear in MCNS patients with continued proteinuria in both native kidneys and allografts, the corticosteroid responsiveness and relapsing course in a proportion of patients with FSGS, the interchange over time of both structural and behavioral aspects of both groups of patients, all suggest to him that the two lesions most likely represent different aspects of the same condition and that proteinuria may play a yet undefined role in the induction of the FSGS lesion.

Diffuse Mesangial Proliferation (Mesangial Proliferative GN)

Diffuse mesangial proliferation (DMP) (this term seems preferable to that of mesangial proliferative GN, which implies a distinct type of glomerular disease) accounts for fewer than 5% of patients with the nephrotic syndrome. It is characterized histologically by the presence of diffuse mesangial hypercellularity with increased mesangial matrix but without other changes. Immunofluorescence examination is usually negative, although in some cases mesangial deposits of IgM and C3 are seen and have been postulated to be of pathogenetic importance (see IgM nephropathy). According to the WHO Committee for Nomenclature [21] the lower limit for the diagnosis of DMP should be more than 3 cells per mesangial zone. However, some workers have included all cases of mesangial proliferation regardless of its degree in that category. The striking differences in the reported outcome and response to therapy are probably related to differences in morphologic categorization. Garin et al [22] have shown well that nephrotic patients with marked mesangial proliferation were more severely affected than those with moderate mesangial proliferation. Knowing these limitations, most data [22–30] show that patients with INS and mesangial hypercellularity, with or without immune deposits, have a poorer initial response to therapy and therefore a poorer outcome than those with normal glomerular cellularity. These differences seem more likely to be related to a more severe form of INS rather than to a separate entity. Evidence for the close relationship between DMP and MCNS is based on several facts: (a) By EM, apart from the increase in mesangial cells, the findings are identical to those described in MCNS whether the patient responds to steroid therapy or not; (b) by IF, negativity in some cases and the presence of mild amounts of Ig and/or C3 either in mesangial areas or as peripheral capillary streaks in some others, have both been reported in MCNS and DMP; (c) in repeated biopsies, patients with MCNS may evolve to DMP and the reverse is also true; (d) finally, lesions of FSGS may complicate both conditions. It is, however, interesting to note that the likelihood to develop FSGS is greater in patients with DMP than in those with MCNS [23, 24]. Furthermore, progression to renal failure seems to occur much more rapidly in patients in whom FSGS is superimposed on DMP than when this lesion is associated with MCNS. Similarly, such patients seem more prone to recur their NS after grafting.

IgM Mesangial Nephropathy

IgM nephropathy is a glomerular lesion defined by its immunopathologic feature: the presence of IgM as the sole or dominant immunoglobulin in glomerular mesangial regions in a diffuse and generalized distribution. The light microscopic manifestations are those of mild to slightly more extensive expension of mesangial regions, sometimes associated with increased cellularity. Thus, it appears that IgM mesangial nephropathy cannot be equated with the mesangial proliferative form of INS. Ultrastructural examination discloses the presence of typical electron-dense mesangial deposits in approximately 50% of the biopsy specimens.

A commonly emphasized clinical presentation of IgM nephropathy is heavy proteinuria, most often in the nephrotic range. However, asymptomatic proteinuria or hematuria, or heavy proteinuria with hematuria have also been presenting manifestations [28, 31–34]. Since the reports of Cohen, Border, and Glassock [32] and Bhasin et al [29], there has been considerable debate on both the existence of this entity as well as the prognostic significance of mesangial IgM in patients with the nephrotic syndrome. Furthermore, the relationship of this form of glomerular injury to MCNS, FSGS, and DMP has been the focus of much controversy and speculation.

The central question to the controversy is whether diffuse and generalized mesangial IgM deposits in glomeruli from patients with nephrotic syndrome are a marker for the likelihood of a poor response to steroids (dependent or resistant) or of progression to renal failure, especially in comparison to patients with minimal change disease (lipoid nephrosis). While there is some evidence that deposited IgM and C3 may represent immune complexes [35] and that circulating immune complex deposits have been observed in such patients [32], it is likely that they represent an epiphenomenon and may not be pathologically significant; their presence in glomeruli may well be an indication of altered mesangial function [36].

In Cohen's experience [32, 33] with 24 affected and treated patients, none achieved a sustained remission with adequate prednisone therapy, 54% were steroid-dependent and/or had multiple relapses, and 46% were steroid-resistant. Of the steroid-dependent patients, 21 achieved a sustained remission with cyclophosphamide. Of the refractory patients, 5% had a decline in renal function and, on subsequent renal biopsy, had segmental glomerular sclerosis. The response to steroids is similar to that noted in several other published series [37–39]. In addition, there is greater likelihood of poor response and progression in patients who have hematuria associated with nephrotic range proteinuria at presentation or onset.

While these results are not accepted universally [40–45], institutional, patient population, and geographic variations may be factors that are not consistently considered in all studies, whether or not they show a difference from minimal change disease patients. Furthermore, the lack of significant differences in some series may be due to the fact that some patients with minimal change disease, especially children, who undergo renal biopsy tend to have more atypical courses, and comparison of IgM positive and negative groups would, therefore, tend to blunt or obscure any differences with the uncomplicated minimal change disease patients.

Immunofluorescence Findings in INS

In fact, the only way of evaluating the significance of IgM deposits in INS is to correlate this finding with all the variants of the disease including those cases complicated by FSGS, excluding the well-recognized presence of IgM in regions of segmental glomerular sclerosis.

Gagnadoux, in this workshop, has reported her findings in a group of 163 patients (95 MCNS, 5 DMP, 53 FSGS, and 10 FSGS with mesangial hypercellularity). She compared the response to steroid therapy and outcome of 85 patients with immune deposits (of which 53 contained IgM) to the same parameters in 78 patients without immune deposits. Of the 92 patients with MCNS or DMP the percentage of response was 64% in patients with deposits vs. 73.5% in those without. Of the 59 patients with FSGS ± DMP the percentage of response was 24% in patients with deposits vs. 18.5% in those without. As far as outcome is concerned among the 91 patients with MCNS or DMP, it was favorable in 87% of the patients with deposits vs. 86% of the patients without. Of the 59 patients with FSGS ± DMP the outcome was favorable in 66.6% of the patients with deposits vs. 68.5% of those without. The figures were comparable since only those patients with IgM deposits were considered. She concluded that the presence of diffuse immune deposits is correlated neither with a poor response to steroids nor a poor outcome. These findings are similar to those published recently by Ji-Yun et al [45].

Transplantation in Idiopathic Nephrotic Syndrome (INS)

It has been suggested [42, 43] that the criteria for evidence of recurrence of the disease should be: (1) a past history in the recipient of INS associated with any of the morphologic variants of this clinical entity; that is, MCNS, DMP FSGS, or IgM nephropathy; (2) the rapid recurrence of massive proteinuria following transplantation; and (3) the demonstration in the graft of any of the patterns observed in patients with INS, including MCNS.

The incidence of recurrence is difficult to assess because, to date, most descriptions of this event have dealt with isolated cases. In the series of patients in which all of the patients transplanted are available for analysis the rate of recurrence varies from 75% to 5.6% [46, 48–56]. The findings are also variable as far as the consequences of recurrence on graft function are concerned. Another feature of interest is the fact that in some patients the disease recurred in two successive transplants [47–53, 55, 57, 58].

A comparison of recurring and nonrecurring patients shows that risk factors for recurrence, at least among children, are: (a) age at onset (older children being at greater risk of recurrence), (b) duration of original disease (most of the recurring patients progress to end-stage kidney failure in less than 3 years), (c) diffuse mesangial proliferation on initial biopsy [46].

In this workshop, Lewis reported on his observations taken from two patients with a past history of INS with FSGS who had an immediate recurrence of the NS following renal transplantation. In each case renal biopsy was performed early in the course of the recurrent NS. In the available material he observed: (1) that not all glomeruli manifested abnormal morphology; only about one-third of the glomeruli showed significant alteration of the visceral epithelial cells, a change he called epitheliosis and considered as the earliest lesion of recurrent NS associated with FSGS. In addition, he was able to demonstrate the presence of T cells in these areas; (2) based on the evidence that only some proximal convoluted tubules showed protein reabsorption droplets, he concluded that only a small proportion of glomeruli manifested abnormal permeability; (3) he therefore likened the lesions observed in recurrent INS to those in MCNS where there is diffuse foot process fusion [59].

As far as the pathogenesis of the recurrent lesion is concerned he concluded that rapid recurrence would seem to suggest that a circulating factor that increases glomerular permeability may be operative. However, the morphologic abnormalities suggest that some secondary insult (alone or in combination with a circulating factor) may be required to explain the limited, random, and focal distribution of the lesion. Lewis believes that recurrent FSGS does not appear as the result of an effect of chronic proteinuria upon glomerular elements; instead, the scarring lesion appears to be the result of a primary segmental lesion involving the visceral epithelial cells.

Conclusion

For many investigators, the term lipoid nephrosis is still synonymous with MCNS while FSGS, DMP, and IgM nephropathy are considered as separate entities. It has become apparent, over the years, however, that there was a definite clinical overlap among these different patterns, and most of the discussants seemed to agree on this unifying concept. Although each of these histologic variants is important because they are prognostic indicators, it seems illogical to consider them as individual entities only because response to therapy and long-term outcome are different. At a clinical level, the initial response to corticosteroid treatment of the nephrotic patient is more important than the appearance of the renal biopsy in the early determination of likely outcome. It therefore appears that INS, which would better be called lipoid nephrosis, is a disease with variable histologic expressions, the nature of which remain to be explained. These various patterns probably share a common pathogenesis although this issue was not discussed.

The best evidence for such a concept is given by the results of transplantation and the immediate recurrence of massive proteinuria in approximately 30% of patients affected with INS, whatever the initial pattern on biopsy during the original disease. This rapid recurrence is clear evidence that INS is not a disease of the kidneys and that it is related to an as yet unknown circulating factor that increases glomerular permeability and induces proteinuria. If this theory is correct, it may be hypothesized that this factor is responsible for the initial disease; then, because of the irreversibility of the podocytic changes, the development of FSGS leads progressively to complete loss of nephrons and finally to chronic renal failure. If the circulating factor is still present at the time of transplantation, it is further responsible for recurrent disease in the grafted kidney. This group of patients with recurrent disease is important because with appropriate studies, they will provide the answer to the pathogenesis of lipoid nephrosis and its morphologic variants.

References

1. CHURG J, HABIB R, WHITE RHR: Pathology of the nephrotic syndrome in children: A report for the International Study of Kidney Diseases in children. *Lancet* 1:1299–1302, 1970
2. HABIB R, KLEINKNECHT C: The primary nephrotic syndrome in childhood. Classification and clinicopathologic study of 406 cases. *Pathol Ann* 417–474, 1971
3. INTERNATIONAL STUDY OF KIDNEY DISEASE IN CHILDREN: Nephrotic syndrome in children: Prediction of histopathology from clinical and laboratory characteristics at time of diagnosis. *Kidney Int* 13:159–165, 1978
4. HABIB R, LEVY M, GUBLER MC: Clinicopathologic correlations in the nephrotic syndrome. *Paediatrician* 8:325–348, 1979
5. A REPORT OF THE INTERNATIONAL STUDY OF KIDNEY DISEASES IN CHILDREN: The primary nephrotic syndrome in children. Identification of patients with MCNS from initial response to prednisone. *J Paediatr* 98:561–564, 1981
6. A REPORT OF THE INTERNATIONAL STUDY OF KIDNEY DISEASES IN CHILDREN: Primary nephrotic syndrome in children: clinical significance of histopathologic variants of minimal change and of diffuse mesangial hypercellularity. *Kidney Int* 20:765–771, 1981
7. BERNSTEIN J, EDELMANN CM: Minimal change nephrotic syndrome. Histopathology and steroid responsiveness. *Arch Dis Child* 57:816–817, 1982
8. TRAININ EB, GOMEZ-LEON G: Development of renal insufficiency after long standing steroid responsive nephrotic syndrome. *Int J Pediatr Nephrol* 3:55–58, 1982
9. NASH MA, BAKARE MA, D'AGATI V, PIRANI CL: Late development of chronic renal failure in steroid responsive nephrotic syndrome. *J Pediatr* 101:411–413, 1982
10. HABIB R: Focal glomerular sclerosis. *Kidney Int* 4:355–361, 1973
11. GUBLER MC, BROYER M, HABIB R: Signification des lésions de sclérose/hyalinose segmentaire et focale dans la néphrose, in *Proc VIth Int Congr Nephrol*, Montréal, Basel, Karger, 1978, pp 437–445

12. CAMERON JS, TURNER DR, OGG CS, CHANTLER C, WILLIAMS DG: The long-term prognosis of patients with focal segmental glomerusclerosis. *Clin Nephrol* 10:213–218, 1978

13. CAMERON JS: The problem of focal segmental glomerulosclerosis, in *Progress in Glomerulonephritis,* edited by KINCAID-SMITH P, D'APICE AJF, AND ATKINS RC, New York, John Wiley, 1979, pp. 209–228

14. MONGEAU JG, CORNEILLE L, ROBITAILLE P, O'REGAN S, PELLETIER M: Primary nephrosis in childhood associated with focal glomerular sclerosis: Is long term prognosis that severe? *Kidney Int* 20:743–746, 1981

15. ARBUS GS, POUCELL S, BACHEGIE GS, BAUMAL R: Focal segmental glomerulosclerosis with idiopathic nephrotic syndrome: 3 types of clinical response. *J Pediat* 101:40–45, 1982

16. TEJANI A, NICASTRI AD, SEN D, CHEN CK, BUTT KMH: Long-term evaluation of children with nephrotic syndrome and focal segmental glomerular sclerosis. *Nephron* 35:225–231, 1983

17. GROND J, SCHILTHUIS MS, KOUDSTAAL J, ELEMA JD: Mesangial function and glomerular sclerosis in rats after unilateral nephrectomy. *Kidney Int* 22:338–343, 1982

18. GRISHMAN E, CHURG J: Focal glomerular sclerosis in nephrotic patients: an electron microscopic study of glomerular podocytes. *Kidney Int* 7:111–122, 1975

19. COHEN AH, MAMPASO F, ZAMBONI L: Glomerular podocyte degeneration in human renal disease: an ultrastructural study. *Lab Invest* 37:30–42, 1977

20. HOSHIKAWA N, CAMERON AH, WHITE RHR: Ultrastructure of the non sclerotic glomeruli in childhood nephrotic syndrome. *J Pathol* 136:133–148, 1982

21. CHURG J, SOBIN LH: *Renal Disease. Classification and Atlas of Glomerular Disease.* Igaku Shoin, Tokyo, New York, 1982

22. GARIN EH, DONNELLY WH, GEARY D, RICHARD GA: Nephrotic syndrome and diffuse mesangial proliferative glomerulonephritis in children. *Am J Dis Child* 137:109–113, 1983

23. WALDHERR R, GUBLER MC, LEVY M, BROYER M, HABIB R: The significance of pure diffuse mesangial proliferation in idiopathic nephrotic syndrome. *Clin Nephrol* 10:171–179, 1978

24. SCHEONEMAN MJ, BENNETT G, GREIFER I: The natural history of focal segmental glomerulosclerosis with and without mesangial hypercellularity in children. *Clin Nephrol* 9:45–54, 1978

25. MURPHY WM, JUKKOLA AF, ROY S: Nephrotic syndrome with mesangial cell proliferation in children. A distinct entity? *Am J Clin Pathol* 72:42–47, 1979

26. BROWN E, UPADHYAYA K, HAYSLETT JP, KASHGARIAN M, SIEGEL NJ: The clinical course of mesangial proliferative glomerulonephritis. *Medicine* 58:295–303, 1979

27. A REPORT OF THE SOUTHWEST PEDIATRIC NEPHROLOGY STUDY GROUP: Childhood nephrotic syndrome associated with diffuse mesangial hypercellularity. *Kidney Int* 24:87–94, 1983

28. LAWLER W, WILLIAMS G, TARPEY P, MALLICK NP: IgM associated primary diffuse mesangial proliferative glomerulonephritis. *J Clin Pathol* 33:1029–1038, 1980

29. BHASIN HK, ABUELO JG, RAMAKRISHNA N, ESPARZA A: Mesangial proliferative glomerulonephritis. *Lab Invest* 39:21–29, 1978

30. VANGELISTA A, FRASCA G, BIAGINI G, BONOMINI V: Long-term study of mesangial proliferative glomerulonephritis with IgM deposits. *Proc EDTA* 18:503–507, 1981

31. HELIN H, MUSTONEN J, PASTERNACK A, ANTONEN J: IgM associated glomerulonephritis. *Nephron* 31:11–16, 1982

32. COHEN AH, BORDER WA, GLASSOCK RJ: Nephrotic syndrome with glomerular mesangial IgM deposits. *Lab Invest* 38:610–619, 1978

33. COHEN AH, BORDER WA: Mesangial proliferative glomerulonephritis *Sem Nephrol* 2:228–240, 1982

34. PARDO V, BERIAN MG, LEVY DF, STRAUSS J: Benign primary hematuria: clinicopathologic study of 65 patients. *Am J Med* 67: 817–822, 1979

35. CAVALLO T, JOHNSON MP: Immunopathologic study of minimal change glomerular disease with mesangial IgM deposits. *Nephron* 27:281–284, 1981

36. MICHAEL AF, KEANE WF, RAIJ L, VERNIER RL, MAUER SM: The glomerular mesangium. *Kidney Int* 17:141–154, 1980

37. TEJANI A, NICASTRI AD: Mesangial IgM nephropathy. *Nephron* 35:1–5, 1983

38. JENNETTE JC: Evolution of mesangial IgM nephropathy into focal segmental glomerulonephrosis. *Am J Nephrol* 1:222, 1981

39. KOBAYASHI Y, SHIGEMATSU H, TATENO S, HIKI Y: Nephrotic syndrome with diffuse mesangial IgM deposits. *Acta Pathol Jpn* 32:307–317, 1982

40. MANPASO F, GONZALO A, TERNEL J, LOSADA M, GALLEGO N, ORTUNO J, BELLAS C: Mesangial deposits of IgM in patients with the nephrotic syndrome. *Clin Nephrol* 16:230–234, 1981

41. VILCHES AR, TURNER DR, CAMERON JS, OGG CS, CHANTLER C, WILLIAMS DG: Significance of mesangial IgM deposition in "Minimal Change" Nephrotic syndrome. *Lab Invest* 46:10–15, 1982

42. PAPADOPOULO ZL, JENIS EH, TINA LU, NOVELLO AC, JOSE PA, CALCAGNO PL: Chronic relapsing minimal change nephrotic syndrome with or without mesangial deposits: long-term follow-up. *Int J Ped Nephrol* 3:179–186, 1982

43. ALLEN WR, TRAVIS LB, CAVALLO T, BROUHARD BH, CUNNINGHAM RJ: Immune deposits and mesangial hypercellularity in minimal change nephrotic syndrome: clinical relevance. *J Pediatr* 100:188–191, 1982

44. PARDO V, RIESGO I, ZILLERUELO G, STRAUSS J: The clinical significance of mesangial IgM deposits and mesangial hypercellularity in minimal change nephrotic syndrome. *Am J Kidney Dis* 3:264–269, 1984

45. JI-YUN Y, MELVIN T, SIBLEY R, MICHAEL AF: No evidence for a specific role of IgM in mesangial proliferation of idiopathic nephrotic syndrome. *Kidney Int* 25:100–106, 1984

46. HABIB R, HEBERT D, GAGNADOUX MF, BROYER M: Transplantation in idiopatic nephrosis. *Transplant Proc* 14:489–495, 1982

47. LEWIS EJ: Recurrent focal sclerosis after renal transplantation. *Kidney Int* 22:315–323, 1982

48. HOYER JR, RAIJ L, VERNIER RLJ, SIMMONS RL, NAJARIAN JS, MICHAEL AF: Recurrence of idiopathic nephrotic syndrome after renal transplantation. *Cancer* 2:343–348, 1972

49. HAMBURGER J, CROSNIER J, NOEL LH: Recurrent glomerulonephritis after renal transplantation. *Ann Rev Med* 29:67–72, 1978

50. MALEKZADEH MH, HEUSER ET, ETTENGER RB, PENNISI AJ, UITTENBOGAART CH, WARSHAW BL, FINE RN: Focal glomerulosclerosis and renal transplantation. *J Pediatr* 95:249–254, 1979

51. CHEIGH JS, SOLIMAN M, MOURADIAN J, TAPIA L, RIGGIO RR, STUBENBORD W, STENZEL KH, RUBIN AL: Focal segmental glomerulosclerosis in kidney transplants. *Transpl Proc* 13:125–127, 1981

52. MAIZEL SE, SIBLEY RK, HORSTMAN JP, KJELLSTRAND CM, SIMMONS RL: Incidence and significance of recurrent focal segmental glomerulosclerosis in renal allograft recipients. *Transplantation* 32:512–516, 1981

53. PAPADOPOULO ZL, HELFRICH GB, TURNER ME, SHAHINFAR S, CURRIER CB,

Jose PA, Calcagno PL: Recurrence of focal segmental glomerulosclerosis in children following renal transplantation. *Trans Am Soc Artif Intern Organs* 27:325–328, 1981

54. Pinto J, Lacerda G, Cameron JS, Turner DR, Bewick M, Ogg CS: Recurrence of focal segmental glomerulosclerosis in renal allografts. *Transplantation* 32:83–89, 1981
55. Morzycka M, Crocker BP, Seigler HF, Tischer CC: Evaluation of recurrent glomerulonephritis in kidney allografts. *Am J Med* 72:588–598, 1982
56. Axelsen RA, Seymour AE, Mathew TH, Fischer G, Pascoe V: Recurrent focal glomerulosclerosis in renal transplants. *Clin Nephrol* 21:110–114, 1984
57. Chandra M, Lewy JE, Mouradian J, Susin M, Hoyer JR: Recurrent nephrotic syndrome with three successive renal allografts. *Am J Nephrol* 1:110–114, 1981
58. Case Records of the MGH, Case No 20, 1976. *N Engl J Med* 294:1108–1115, 1976
59. Grishman E, Churg J: Focal glomerular sclerosis in nephrotic patients: An electron microscopic study of glomerular podocytes. *Kidney Int* 7:111–122, 1975

Pathogenetic Mechanisms of IgA Nephropathy from Studies of Experimental Models

Andrew J. Woodroffe and Jane D. Lomax-Smith

This article reviews the animal models of mesangial IgA deposition that have been published in recent years, and it examines their relevance to our understanding of the pathogenesis of human IgA nephropathy (Table 1).

Passive Models of Mesangial IgA Deposition

Ward et al showed some years ago that intravenous (i.v.)-aggregated IgA is taken up by the mesangium in mice, and that it persists there longer than aggregated IgG [1]. This observation has since been confirmed by Egido et al [2], and it has been ascribed to a markedly reduced catabolism by the kidney of IgA versus IgG aggregates.

Table 1. Experimental models of IgA nephropathy

Passive	
Aggregated IgA i.v.	mice
IgA/DNP-BSA immune complex i.v.	mice
Active immunization	
Oral ovalbumin, bovine gamma globulin,	
horse spleen ferritin	mice
Parenteral dextrans	mice
Spontaneous models	
Aleutian disease	mink
Hepatosplenic schistosomiasis and/or partial	
ligation of the portal vein	mice
Bile duct ligation	rats
Carbon tetrachloride-induced cirrhosis	rats

This manuscript was presented as part of a Symposium on *IgA Nephropathy*.

Intravenously administered IgA class antigen-antibody complexes (IC) are similarly taken up by the mesangium in mice—a precondition being that the IgA is polymeric [3]. In this study, IgA anti-DNP (MOPC-315 ascitic fluid) was complexed to DNP-BSA and was used to induce mesangial deposits. The IgA was localized to the mesangium and capillary lumen of all glomeruli and it was accompanied by smaller amounts of C3. Histologic changes were focal mesangial expansion and the presence of intraluminal PAS-positive material, with no increase in mesangial cells or neutrophilic infiltration. Hematuria, 2 hours after injection and lasting 4 to 6 hours, occurred in about 50% of the mice. Antigen-antibody complexes prepared with larger amounts of antibody (3 or 4 mg) and between 3- and 7-fold antigen excess were most likely to cause hematuria. No deposits occurred when the IC were prepared with monomeric IgA antibody.

Rifai et al also described mesangial IgA and C3 deposition in mice that made dinitrophenyl/bovine serum albumin (IgA/DNP-BSA) IC in vivo [3]. Of particular interest was the fact that mice with high levels of circulating IgA antibody developed a mild endothelial- and mesangial-proliferative glomerulonephritis after injection of the antigen. The deposits were shown to clear gradually over 96 hours. Depletion of C3 had no effect on the mesangial deposition of IgA IC.

The conclusions from these very elegant studies are that mesangial IgA IC can be deposited under conditions of either antibody or antigen excess, and that the amounts of antibody and antigen in the circulation are more important than the antigen:antibody ratio. The analogies with human IgA nephropathy are obvious and totally consistent with the concept of mediation by mucosally derived antigen-polymeric IgA IC. These studies and others give some guide to the factors determining the mesangial localization of immune deposits. It is suggested that IC of high molecular weight [4], neutral charge [5], and high antibody avidity [4, 6–8] have a predilection for the mesangium. In contrast, capillary wall deposits occur with IC of low molecular weight, positive charge, and low antibody avidity.

Active Immunization

Emancipator et al have shown that mesangial IgA deposits can be induced in mice by the oral administration of various foreign proteins [9]. Ovalbumin, bovine gamma globulin (BGG), and horse spleen ferritin were used as antigens and were administered in drinking water for 14 weeks. A mucosal and specific IgA response was observed. The mesangial deposits in these mice were shown to contain J-chain and the relevant antigen evidence for their mucosal origin. However, none of the animals had C3 deposits, histologic glomerular changes, or hematuria. Secretory component could not be detected in the deposits.

This "oral serum sickness" model conclusively shows that antigens presented mucosally can generate IgA IC and mesangial deposits. The better results with an "antigen-binding" immunofluorescence technique for the identification of antigen suggest that the mesangial IC are in antibody excess. This could reflect continued deposition of free antibody from the circulation. The absence of both C3 deposits and glomerular injury imply some differences from the human disease. However, the authors have subsequently been able to induce a true "nephritis" in these mice with associated IgG, IgM, and C3 deposits, by a final IV injection of antigen [10].

Immunization with dextrans also results in mesangial IgA deposition in mice; the selectively IgA response apparently is determined by the nature of the antigen [11].

The dextrans were administered intraperitoneally and then intravenously over a period of 10 weeks. This model is associated with C3 deposition and histologic glomerular disease; the mesangial distribution of the deposits was subsequently correlated with the charge of the dextran molecules—neutral or polyanionic [12]. The model is of particular interest in two respects: (1) an in situ mechanism for the mesangial deposits is possible (but not proven), and (2) carbohydrates are suggested as possible antigens in immune complex glomerulonephritis.

"Spontaneous Models"

Mesangial IgA deposits are seen in mink with Aleutian disease. Raised serum IgA concentrations, glomerular AD viral antigens, and eluted anti-AD viral antibodies have been described in this disease [13]. Mice with hepatosplenic schistosomiasis and/or partial ligation of the portal vein also have mesangial IgA deposits [14]. Similar findings have been reported in rats after bile duct ligation [15, 16], but (in this case) the IgA and C3 deposits are accompanied by secretory component as well. In the latter situation, and in the rat model of carbon tetrachloride (CCl_4)-induced cirrhosis [17], the glomerular deposits are thought to result from impairment of the normal handling of polymeric IgA- and IgA-containing IC.

Our observations with the cirrhotic model [17] are described as follows. After 5 weeks, all CCl_4-treated rats showed cirrhosis; proteinuria and hematuria were not detected. Light microscopic examination showed mildly enlarged glomeruli with no diffuse or segmental lesions. Electron microscopic examination showed thickening of glomerular basement membranes with increased mesangial matrix and mesangial dense deposits, which occasionally extended into contiguous capillary loops. The mesangial expansion and quantity of deposit in cirrhotic rats increased with the duration of the experiment. Immunofluorescence microscopy of all glomeruli from cirrhotic rats revealed deposits of IgA, C3, and (to a lesser extent) IgG and IgM. These deposits were mainly mesangial, but occasionally extended onto capillary walls. Deposits were present as early as 5 weeks, but were maximal in rats killed at 20 and 40 weeks. Serum concentrations of all immunoglobulin classes were elevated in cirrhotic rats. In particular, levels of IgA and IgM showed a 3-fold increase, compared with controls; this was demonstrated at 5 weeks. Circulating IC were demonstrated in cirrhotic rats by solid phase Clq radioimmunoassay (37.0 ± 25.4 μg aggregated rat IgG/ml versus < 10 μg/ml for controls).

These "hepatic" examples clearly underline the central role of the liver in the normal clearance of polymeric IgA- and IgA-class IC, at least in the above species; the situation in humans is less well defined [18]. In mice, it has been shown that IgA antibodies (either naturally occurring or passively administered) are able to transport bacterial antigens into bile [19]. This is a property that is not shared by IgG or IgM, and the authors emphasize the role of circulating polymeric IgA in the elimination of bacterial macromolecular products [19]. It is not known whether the same mechanism is operative in humans, but there is certainly a high prevalence of mesangial IgA deposits in patients with alcoholic liver disease; these patients also have increased serum concentrations of IC and IgA polymers and of antibodies to common bacterial antigens [20].

Mediation of Injury

IgA aggregates or IC can fix complement (via the alternate pathway [21]) and may initiate glomerular injury through this mechanism. Certainly, some additional factor is required, since mesangial IgA deposits can be present with no morphologic abnormality. Activation of the local coagulation process with glomerular sclerosis has been invoked by some investigators as being important in this regard [22]; however, other mechanisms may also contribute, for example, degradation of the glomerular basement membrane (GBM) by proteases released from mesangial cells [23], or disturbed prostaglandin synthesis by mesangial cells with resultant abnormalities in the intraglomerular circulation [24]. More experimental work is needed in these areas.

Natural History

Relatively little experimental attention has been paid to the turnover and duration of mesangial IgA deposits. However, one study with mice showed that the deposits can clear within 4 days [3]; in the human kidney transplant model, IgA deposits in donor kidneys have been shown to disappear in as little as 2 weeks when transplanted into non-IgA nephropathy recipients [25]. This last observation is of fundamental importance, and it should provide encouragement to those of us who are interested in testing new forms of treatment for the disease.

Therapeutic Considerations

Based on what we know of the pathogenetic mechanisms, the following approaches to treatment could be considered: removal of antigen, decreased production of IgA, increased clearance of IgA IC, and interference with the mediation of glomerular injury. We have evaluated some of these in the CCl_4-cirrhotic rat model of IgA nephropathy; specifically, neomycin (to alter gut flora), phenytoin (to lower serum IgA concentrations), *d*-penicillamine (to dissociate circulating IC), dapsone (for its efficacy in the IgA-related disease, dermatitis herpetiformis), and PGE_1 (which has been shown to have a beneficial effect in murine lupus and in experimental serum sickness). The details of these experiments were presented at the 1st International Milano Meeting of Nephrology [26] and are reviewed briefly here.

Male D/A rats (180 to 220 g) were given subcutaneous injections of 0.05 ml CCl_4 (diluted 1:3 in olive oil)/100 g body twice weekly for 3 months [27]. Control animals were injected with the same volume of olive oil. A controlled trial was conducted with the various therapeutic agents:

a. Neomycin—25 mg in 0.25 ml PBS per day intragastrically;
b. Phenytoin—1 mg in 0.2 ml propylene glycol per day intragastrically;
c. *d*-Penicillamine—2 mg in 0.2 ml 10% ethanol-PBS per day subcutaneously;
d. Dapsone—4 mg in 0.2 ml propylene glycol per day intragastrically;
e. PGE_1 (15 [S]-15 methyl PGE_1)—225 μg or 150 μg in 0.1 ml 10% ethanol-PBS per day subcutaneously.

These agents were given for 3 months concurrently with CCl_4. A subgroup of rats given CCl_4 alone for 3 months was then treated with PGE_1 (150 μg/d) for 2 months; the CCl_4 was continued during this time. Control rats were given each of the five therapeutic agents or their diluents alone for 3 months.

After 2 months, all CCl_4-treated rats (and none of the controls) had cirrhosis. At 3 months, all cirrhotic rats had prominent mesangial deposits of IgA that usually were associated with smaller amounts of IgG, IgM, and C3. None of the control rats had staining for IgA, IgG, or C3. Serial serum studies showed a progressive increase in IgA, IgM, and IgG concentrations. The effect of the various therapeutic agents was as follows:

a. Neomycin—All nine treated rats had mesangial IgA deposits. Mean serum IgA and IgG concentrations were reduced in this group.
b. Phenytoin—All six treated rats had mesangial IgA deposits. Mean serum IgA concentrations were reduced in this group.
c. *d*-Penicillamine—All nine treated rats had mesangial IgA deposits. Mean serum IgA and IgG concentrations were reduced in this group.
d. Dapsone—All 13 treated rats had mesangial IgA deposits. Mean serum immunoglobulin concentrations were not altered.
e. PGE_1:

   Only 4 of 10 rats given 225 μg/d PGE_1 survived for 3 months. Of these, only one had cirrhosis and none had mesangial IgA deposits. Mean serum IgA concentrations were reduced in this group.
   11 of 15 rats given 150 μg/d PGE_1 survived to 3 months. Of these, only three had cirrhosis. IgA deposits were present in only one of these three rats. Mean serum IgA concentrations were reduced in this group.

6 of 6 rats started on PGE_1 (150 $\mu g/d$) after 3 months CCl_4 treatment survived to 5 months. All had cirrhosis and persisting mesangial IgA deposits. Mean serum immunoglobulin concentrations were not altered.

In conclusion, PGE_1 was the only therapeutic agent that reduced the mesangial deposits; however, it also was cytoprotective against liver injury and had no effect on the kidney once cirrhosis had been established.

Obviously, other forms of treatment now need to be considered and tested in a similar fashion. There are advantages in using an experimental model for such purposes, at least in the first instance.

Extrapolations

These must be made with caution in view of the differences in IgA metabolism between species [18]. However, we would judge that the experimental evidence confirms the role of IgA-class IC in IgA nephropathy with mucosally presented antigens and polymeric IgA. In the absence of any clinically apparent increase in antigen exposure, such patients must be presumed to have a primary defect in IgA immunoregulation or clearance. Rational advances in treatment require further understanding of these defects and of the mediators responsible for the glomerular injury.

References

1. WARD DM, SPIEGELBERG HL, WILSON CB: Persistence of IgA aggregates in the glomerular mesangium in mice (abst). *Kidney Int* 16:801, 1979
2. EGIDO J, SANCHO J, RIVERA F, SANCHEZ-CRESPO M: Handling of soluble IgA aggregates by the mononuclear phagocytic system in mice. A comparison with IgG aggregates. *Immunology* 46:1–7, 1982
3. RIFAI A, SMALL PA, TEAGUE PO, AYOUB EM: Experimental IgA Nephropathy. *J Exp Med* 150:1161–1173, 1979
4. GERMUTH FG, RODRIGUEZ E: Classification of human immune complex deposit glomerular disease, in *Immunopathology of the Renal Glomerulus,* Boston, Little Brown & Co, 1973, pp 57–161
5. GALLO GR, CAULIN-GLASER T, EMANCIPATOR SN, LAMM ME: Nephritogenicity and differential distribution of glomerular immune complexes related to immunogen charge. *Lab Invest* 48:353–362, 1983
6. KOYAMA A, NIWA Y, SHIGEMATSU H, TANIYUCHI M, TADA T: Studies on passive serum sickness II. Factors determining the localization of antigen-antibody complexes in the murine renal glomerulus. *Lab Invest* 38:253–262, 1978
7. DEVEY ME, STEWART MW: The induction of chronic antigen-antibody disease in selectively bred mice producing either high or low affinity antibody to protein antigens. *Immunology* 41:303–311, 1980
8. ISKANDAR SS, JENNETTE JC: Influence of antibody avidity on glomerular immune complex localization. *Am J Pathol* 112:155–159, 1983
9. EMANCIPATOR SN, GALLO GR, LAMM ME: Experimental IgA nephropathy induced by oral immunization. *J Exp Med* 157:572–582, 1983

10. LAMM M: The secretory immune system in experimental IgA nephropathy, in *Contributions to Nephrology,* edited by BERLYNE GM, GIOVANNETTI S, THOMAS S, Basel, Karger (in press, 1984)

11. ISAACS K, MILLER F, LANE B: Experimental model for IgA nephropathy. *Clin Immunol Immunopathol* 20:419–426, 1981

12. ISAACS KL, MILLER F: Antigen size and charge in immune complex glomerulonephritis. *Am J Pathol* 111:298–306, 1983

13. PORTIS JL, COE JE: Deposition of IgA in renal glomeruli of mink affected with Aleutian Disease. *Am J Pathol* 96:227–236, 1979

14. VAN MARCK EAE, DEELDER AM, GIGASE PLJ: Effect of partial portal vein ligation on immune glomerular deposits in Schistosoma mansoni infected mice. *Br J Exp Pathol* 58:412–417, 1977

15. MELVIN T, BURKE B, MICHAEL AF, KIM Y: Experimental IgA nephropathy in bile duct ligated rats. *Clin Immunol Immunopathol* 27:369–377, 1983

16. EMANCIPATOR SN, GALLO GR, RAZABONI R, LAMM ME: Experimental cholestasis promotes the deposition of glomerular IgA immune complexes. *Am J Pathol* 113:19–26, 1983

17. GORMLY AA, SMITH PS, SEYMOUR AE, CLARKSON AR, WOODROFFE AJ: IgA glomerular deposits in experimental cirrhosis. *Am J Pathol* 104:50–54, 1981

18. DELACROIX DL, FURTADO-BARREIRA G, DE HEMPTINNE B, GOUDSWAARD, J, DIVE C, VAERMAN JP: The liver in the IgA secretory immune system. Dogs, but not rats and rabbits, are suitable models for human studies. *Hepatology* 3:980–988, 1983

19. RUSSELL MW, BROWN TA, CLAFLIN JL, SCHROER K, MESTECKY J: Immunoglobulin A-mediated hepatobiliary transport constitutes a natural pathway for disposing of bacterial antigens. *Infect Immun* 42:1041–1048, 1983

20. WOODROFFE AJ: IgA, glomerulonephritis and liver disease. *Aust NZ J Med* 11:109–111, 1981

21. PFAFFENBACH G, LAMM ME, GIGLI I: Activation of the guinea pig alternative complement pathway by mouse IgA immune complexes. *J Exp Med* 155:231–247, 1982

22. SHIGEMATSU H, KOBAYASHI Y, TATENO S, HIKI Y, KUWAO S: Glomerular tissue injury in IgA nephritis. *Acta Pathol Jpn* 33:367–380, 1983

23. LOVETT DH, RYAN JL, KASHGARIAN M, STERZEL RB: Lysosomal enzymes in glomerular cells of the rat. *Am J Pathol* 107:161–166, 1982

24. SCHARSCHMIDT LA, DUNN MJ: Prostaglandin synthesis by rat glomerular mesangial cells in culture—effects of angiotensin II and arginine vasopressin. *J Clin Invest* 71:1756–1764, 1983

25. SILVA FG, CHANDER P, PIRANI CL, HARDY MA: Disappearance of glomerular mesangial IgA deposits after renal allograft transplantation. *Transplantation* 33:241–246, 1982

26. WOODROFFE AJ, GORMLY AA, CLARKSON AR, SEYMOUR AE, LOMAX-SMITH JD: Experimental cirrhosis and deposition of glomerular IgA immune-complexes, in *Contributions to Nephrology,* edited by BERLYNE GM, GIOVANNETTI S, THOMAS S, Basel, Karger (in press, 1984)

27. SAKAGUCHI H, DACHS S, MANTNER W, GRISHMAN E, CHURG J: Renal glomerular lesions after administration of carbon tetrachloride and ethionine. *Lab Invest* 13:1418–1426, 1964

Immunologic Aspects of IgA Nephropathy in Humans

Jesus Egido, Jaime Sancho, R. Blasco, L. Lozano, and Luis Hernando

In 1968 Berger and Hinglais [1] described the presence of IgA and IgG deposits in the mesangium of a group of patients with hematuria and proteinuria. The initial cautious acceptance of their work soon became enthusiastic with the appearance of an enormous number of papers dedicated to the clinical and histologic aspects of the disorder. These studies confirmed the existence and the world-wide distribution of this common glomerulonephritis, now termed *IgA nephropathy*. The constant presence of IgA in the glomerular mesangium and the frequent finding of elevated serum IgA concentrations have focused attention on the role of IgA in the pathogenesis of this disease. In the last 5 years, the number of publications devoted to the immunopathogenetic aspects of IgA nephropathy has been substantial. Reviews concerning this topic have been published [2–6], and in this paper we will deal with recent developments concerning the pathogenesis of this disease in man.

IgA Nephropathy as an Immune Complex Disease

The granular pattern of the IgA deposited in the glomerular mesangium, the occasional detection of IgA deposits in the skin and muscle vessels [7, 8], and the recurrence of IgA in renal allografts [9] suggested an immune complex disease. Preliminary attempts to demonstrate immune complexes in patients with IgA nephropathy were largely unsuccessful owing, at least in part, to the absence of good methods to detect specific IgA immune complexes (reviewed in Ref. 2). Our group showed initially the presence of such complexes in these patients by sucrose density gradient ultracentrifugation at physiologic and acid pH values [10]. However, the practical limitation of this laborious assay was evident. In the last years, several authors have

---

This manuscript was presented as part of a Symposium on *IgA Nephropathy*.

adopted other techniques to solve this difficulty. The percentages of IgA immune complexes found by different techniques range from 31% to 68% of the patients studied [11–15]. Their frequency increased up to 90% when sequential examinations were performed, which is in favor of the intermittence of their appearance. Several groups, including ours, have found a significant correlation between the bouts of macroscopic hematuria, or the persistence of microhematuria, and the presence of IgA immune complexes in the circulation [11, 13, 15]. Furthermore, the recurrence of IgA deposits in the grafted kidney was correlated with these circulating complexes [12].

Limited studies of the size of IgA complexes in patients with IgA nephropathy have been carried out in a small number of patients. Most authors agree that they are small (7–13S) or intermediate (13–17S) in size [13, 15, 16]. This stands in marked contrast with the larger complexes in patients with Henoch-Schönlein purpura [17, 18], a disease with some common links with IgA nephropathy [19]. As a note of caution, different assays detect immune complexes of a different size [15]. Furthermore, the repetitive examination of IgA immune complexes in patients at different periods of time show some changes in the complex size [15]. Thus, it is conceivable that the size of serum immune complexes depends also on the time of sampling. The results from elution studies on kidneys obtained from autopsy examinations of patients with alcoholic cirrhosis and IgA nephropathy showed that the deposited complexes were mostly intermediate in size [20]. In the recently described model of IgA nephropathy in mice, the mesangial localization of IgA was most prominent when complexes were formed in antibody excess [21]. It is possible that, besides the size, other characteristics of the IgA could be important in the development of the nephritis. In that experimental model, polymeric IgA was observed to be critical for the renal deposition of complexes and induction of nephritic histologic changes. Immune complexes formed either in vivo or in vitro with monomeric IgA failed to induce glomerulonephritis [21]. This is in accordance with the finding of polymeric IgA in the mesangium in patients with IgA nephropathy [19, 22–24]. We have recently developed a simple method for determining specific polymeric IgA immune complexes; it is based on the binding of this immunoglobulin to the secretory component [25]. In a group of 31 patients with IgA nephropathy, we found a closer correlation between hematuria and polymeric IgA immune complexes than with monomeric IgA [26]. Furthermore, polymeric IgA immune complexes were found more commonly at the initial stages of the disease, in which, at least in some patients, the bouts of macroscopic hematuria, for unknown reasons, are more frequent. In this sense, peripheral blood and tonsil lymphocytes from these patients produce, after polyclonal stimulation, significantly more polymeric IgA than those of normal subjects [27, 28].

The nature and origin of the IgA deposited in the renal mesangium in patients with IgA nephropathy have not been fully determined. Because this disease often follows infections of the upper respiratory tract, it seemed probable that the source of that IgA was in the external secretions. However, several studies have failed to reveal glomerular localization of a secretory piece in IgA nephropathy [29, 30]. Since around 90% of serum IgA belongs to the IgA1 subclass, while IgA from the external secretions is equally represented by IgA1 and IgA2, some authors studied the subclasses of the IgA deposited in the mesangium in an attempt to establish the mucosal origin of this IgA. The preliminary results afforded conflicting data, probably caused by the use of polyclonal or monoclonal antisera. Thus, André et al [31], using polyclonal antisera, found that glomerular IgA deposits consist predominantly of IgA2. By contrast, Conley, Cooper, and Michael [32], using monoclonal antibodies, have shown predominantly IgA1. Recently, other authors [14, 23, 24, 33], also using monoclonal antibodies, have confirmed that the glomerular IgA in this disease is mostly IgA1 and polymeric. This latter characteristic was demonstrated by its ability to bind the secretory component [24] and by the size after elution from kidney biopsy samples [23]. Furthermore, one of these authors [24] has also shown that circulating immune complexes contained IgA1 as determined by an anti-IgA inhibition binding assay. All these results are in agreement with our early findings on the presence of polymeric IgA in the mesangium determined by its ability to bind the secretory component [19], findings that were later confirmed by others by the same technique [22–24] or by the presence of a J chain [33, 34]. Recent data support the idea that polymeric IgA has an equal distribution between the IgA1 and IgA2 subclasses [35] and that, in order to know about the polymeric nature of mesangial IgA, it is probably more appropriate to use its ability to bind the secretory component or to look for the J chain (excluding the presence of IgM, which also shows these two characteristics) than to study the IgA subclasses. The reasons why IgA1 predominates over IgA2 in the glomerular mesangium of patients with IgA nephropathy are not known, but the possibility of problems related to technique in some cases cannot be completely discarded. Thus, the destruction of the epitope on IgA2 but not on IgA1 in certain staining conditions (for example, with the indirect peroxidase method) has been recently demonstrated [36]. An alternative explanation would be the existence of a specific abnormality of IgA1 in patients with IgA nephropathy, because the synthesis of IgA1 and IgA2 seems regulated by different and unidentified factors [37].

The intermittency in the finding of circulating immune complexes in IgA nephropathy could be due to episodic formation or a transient defect in their blood clearance. In this sense, a reduction in the ability of the mononuclear phagocyte system to cope with circulating complexes has been considered of great importance in the pathogenesis of glomerulonephritis in man. Soluble immune complexes, as opposed to those formed with particulate antigens, are eliminated chiefly by the liver. Those composed of IgA also have some differences in their clearance with respect to those composed of IgG. Thus, IgA immune aggregates (akin to immune complexes) injected into mice are cleared from the circulation more slowly than are IgG immune aggregates, and their catabolism by the liver cells and macrophages is also less [38]. Polymeric IgA immune complexes are removed by the liver through the secretory component of the hepatocytes, at least in rodents [39]. Our group has demonstrated recently that both polymeric and monomeric IgA complexes are also eliminated through the Fcα receptors of the hepatocytes and Kupffer cells [40]. All these studies are in agreement with the high prevalence of IgA deposits in the glomerular mesangium of patients with alcoholic cirrhosis, probably owing to a decrease in the hepatic clearance of immune complexes [20]. In fact, this has been clearly demonstrated in mice with experimental cirrhosis of the liver [41] (see Woodroffe, this volume). Furthermore, in an experimental model of IgA nephropathy induced by dextran, a defective hepatocyte handling of soluble IgA immune aggregates was considered an important step for the appearance of IgA deposits in the mesangium [42].

Although there are no available in vivo techniques to measure the clearance of soluble IgA immune complexes in man, it has been observed that in patients with IgA nephropathy there is a delay in the elimination of physiologic polymeric IgA immune complexes after they ingest a large amount of protein [43]. For unknown reasons, the splenic component of reticulophagocytic function (measured by the clearance of altered radiolabeled autologous erythrocytes) is also impaired in most patients with IgA nephropathy [44]. Sato et al also have also found a depressed phagocytic activity of polymorphonuclear leukocytes in these patients [45]. Taking into account the suppressor effects of polymeric IgA on the chemotaxis and phagocytosis of polymorphonuclear cells [46], the temporal increase of serum concentrations of polymeric IgA observed in these patients could contribute to the slow clearance and long persistence in the circulation of IgA immune complexes, with their subsequent deposition in the glomerular mesangium. Thus, a good correlation between the serum concentrations of polymeric IgA and the presence of circulating IgA complexes has been found [15].

The high percentage of patients with IgA nephropathy presenting with IgG immune complexes, and to a lesser degree IgM immune complexes, in the blood and probably in the mesangium is surprising. Although the IgG immune complexes were considered nephritogenic in children with Henoch-Schönlein purpura [17], other groups have not found any relation between these immune complexes and the presence of hematuria in patients with IgA nephropathy [15, 16]. Woodroffe et al [16], using a solid-phase C1q radioimmunoassay, showed that immune complexes in these patients contained IgA or IgG, or both, and that IgM was less common. Some authors have not found rheumatoid factors, using latex test [16, 47]; however, it would not be surprising if IgA rheumatoid factors did exist. The presence of a polymeric IgA rheumatoid factor has been found in patients with Sjögren's syndrome [48], a disease with involvement of the external secretions, and even in some patients with infectious endocarditis [49]. Recently, we have isolated anti-idiotypic antibodies to anti-BSA (mostly of IgA class) in the sera of two patients with IgA nephropathy. This could suggest that, at least in some patients, the anti-anti-idiotype antibodies participate in immune complex formation in vivo, thus competing with dietary BSA or other antigens for binding sites on the anti-BSA antibody. This could probably explain the decrease in IgA immune complexes after the ingestion of a large amount of protein [43]. Although the meaning of this is not known, it is important to note that idiotype-anti-idiotype immune complexes have been found in the glomerular mesangium of an experimental nephritis [50].

As in other types of glomerulonephritis, final confirmation of immune complex mediation in IgA nephropathy rests on the detection of an antigen. The possibility that antigens are masked by antibody in excess must be considered. The IgA may participate in complexes as either antigen or as antibody. No circulating antibody to IgA has been found in the serum of these patients [47] although the tests employed were not fully adequate for this purpose. Eluates from three kidney needle-biopsy samples failed to bind to normal renal sections in vitro [47]. In contrast, an eluate from a nephrectomy specimen of one patient with IgA nephropathy reacted weakly with the mesangium of a normal human kidney [47]. This observation suggested the possibility that IgA was reacting with either the mesangium or an antigen sequestered within the mesangium, an analogy to the experimental mesangial glomerulonephritis described by Mauer et al [51]. However, there have been no other reports confirming these data. In recent work, Tomino et al [52] demonstrated that most antibodies obtained from open renal biopsy specimens of 15 patients with IgA nephropathy specifically recombined with autologous tissues, although only one third of them combined with allogeneic renal specimens with IgA nephropathy, and none did so with specimens of patients with other glomerular diseases or normal kidneys. More interesting was the finding that the eluted IgA antibodies did react with tonsillar cells from the same patients [53], which supports the theory that some antigens localized in the upper respiratory tract could be involved in this nephropathy. This is in agreement with the frequent appearance of macroscopic hematuria following local infections and after tonsillectomy in these patients.

The existence of high serum antibody titers to respiratory pathogens (*Mycoplasma pneumoniae,* herpes virus, influenza), to gut flora (certain *E. coli* serotypes), and to common dietary antigens such as bovine serum albumin, ovalbumin, casein, and others [16, 43] suggests that many common exogenous antigens, entering through the mucosal system, might be involved in the pathogenesis of this disease. These facts, together with the occasional association of this nephropathy with celiac disease, dermatitis herpetiformis, mucin-secretion adenocarcinomas, and Yersinia enteritides, could suggest a defect in antigen exclusion at the mucosal level, which would permit an increased antigen entry [2]. Since no gastrointestinal involvement exists in the large majority of patients with IgA nephropathy and no quantitative increase in the percent of IgA secreting cells was observed in intestinal biopsy specimens [54], the abnormality must reside in the immune regulation of IgA in other sites of the mucosal system.

Immune Cell Abnormalities

In the last few years, some groups have studied the cellular bases that could explain the existence of high serum levels of IgA in around 50% of patients with IgA nephropathy. In this respect, peripheral blood lymphocytes have, spontaneously or after polyclonal stimulation, an increase in the synthesis of IgA [55–57], although some authors did not confirm these results [58]. These patients also present an increased ratio of OKT4$^+$ (helper T cells) to OKT8$^+$ (suppressor/cytotoxic T cells ratio) owing to an absolute increase in T4$^+$ cells [57] or a reduction in T8$^+$ cells [56, 59]. T cells obtained from these patients were significantly more efficient than T cells from controls in providing IgA-helper activity for normal allogeneic B cells [57, 60]. Although a decrease in the activity of IgA specific suppressor cells was initially shown [55], the use of higher doses of concanavalin A demonstrated a significantly lower IgA suppression in patients than in controls, probably indicating a subtle or secondary involvement of IgA suppressor cells [57].

The existence of a B cell abnormality as a primary phenomenon in this disease is supported by the following data. Some authors have observed that the number of IgA-bearing lymphocytes is markedly increased in peripheral blood [28, 61] and in the tonsils of these patients [28, 62]. Probably more important is the augmented production of polymeric IgA by peripheral blood lymphocytes after polyclonal stimulation [27]. Since the number of T cells with surface membrane receptors of IgA (T_α cells) is increased in mice with IgA-secreting myelomas, a phenomenon closely linked to the high serum concentrations of polymeric IgA [63], the increase in the number of T_α and B_α cells found in these patients [60, 64] could be explained in this way. We have also recently observed that the addition of serum from patients with IgA nephropathy to lymphocyte cultures of normal subjects induced a significant increase in the production of IgA when compared with that induced by control serum, probably owing to an increase in the number of Fc_α receptors specific for IgA. However, the cell expression of these receptors was not increased in patients with IgA nephropathy following incubation with mouse myeloma IgA (MOPC 315), probably indicating that they were already expressed in vivo on the cells of these patients [65]. Whether the increase in the number of T_α and B_α cells in patients with IgA nephropathy is the fundamental abnormality or is due to the increase in serum levels of polymeric IgA is still not clear.

The immunologic studies performed in healthy relatives of patients with IgA nephropathy are also in favor of a B cell abnormality. Thus, there is an increase of IgA-bearing lymphocytes in blood [66], and around 60% of 25 healthy relatives of patients with IgA nephropathy studied by us [67, 68] present an increased production of polymeric IgA by circulating lymphocytes. However, most of these persons have subtle derangements in the generation of IgA-suppressor T cells and a normal OKT4$^+$/OKT8$^+$ cell ratio. The lesser percentage of relatives having high serum levels of polymeric IgA in relation to those who synthesized a large amount of polymeric IgA is in favor of a good clearance of this immunoglobulin by the liver in these persons.

On the basis that no family member studied throughout 2 years presented microhematuria [68], the relation between the cellular abnormalities found in the patients' relatives and the appearance of IgA nephropathy is uncertain, and it does not seem that they can by themselves explain the pathogenesis of this disease. It is possible that the persistence of high serum levels of polymeric IgA could be an important factor. The absence of IgA immune complexes seen in relatives, as well as their high prevalence in patients, suggests that in predisposed persons other factors (genetic or not) are required for the development of IgA nephropathy.

In certain diseases, such as systemic lupus erythematosus, characterized by B cell hyperactivity, hypergammaglobulinemia and autoantibodies against a number of self-determinants [69] frequently occur, but these are not found in most patients with IgA nephropathy. Nevertheless, the existence of a cold reactive antinuclear factor that is predominantly of the IgM class in a large proportion of patients [70], the occasional association with scleritis [71], and the presence of antibodies against some self-determinants of serum immunoglobulins (see the preceding) suggest that some autoimmune mechanism may be involved in the development of IgA nephropathy.

It is possible that IgA polymers in the circulation, with a special affinity for the renal mesangium, result from a selective overproduction by highly active B cells. The proliferation of one or several polymeric IgA-producing clones is indirectly suggested by the study of tonsil lymphocytes from patients with IgA nephropathy [28]. A restriction of glomerular IgA to a unique light chain isotope, either kappa (one patient) or lambda (three patients), whereas serum IgA was polyclonal, has been shown in a study of 45 patients with IgA nephropathy [72]. Recently, the charge of renal eluted IgA was found not to be different from normal IgA [73].

Stachura et al have found that IgA-producing lymphoid cells were detected in the renal interstitium of patients with IgA nephropathy, especially those showing glomerular crescents [74]. The local role of these cells, if these data are confirmed, remains speculative at the moment.

Immunogenetic Aspects

The possible association between the HLA system and IgA nephropathy was suspected because some patients' relatives were found to have IgA nephropathy. Tolkoff-Rubin et al [75] and Sabatier et al [76] were the first to fully describe the development of IgA nephropathy in two pairs of HLA identical siblings who shared the HLA Bw35 antigen. A relation between this antigen and IgA nephropathy has been documented by several groups, mostly in France and occasionally in Australia and the USA [3] (Table 1). In a recent review of a larger number of patients, the frequence of the HLA-Bw 35 was found to be increased 2.0 to 2.5 times in patients with IgA nephropathy when compared with a control group, but the difference was not significant [27]. This is in agreement with other reports from different geographic areas, which failed to detect a higher incidence of that antigen (Table 1). In fact, in Spain, where IgA nephropathy occurs at least as frequently as it does in France, no association could be found with any HLA-A, B, C, or DR antigens [78].

The initial data of Berthoux et al [79], based on 50 patients with IgA nephropathy and suggesting a poor prognosis for those having the HLA Bw 35, has been enlarged by other French groups. A total of 293 patients has now been studied [77]. The frequency of this antigen in patients with chronic renal failure was 35.4%, compared with 22% in the whole group of patients. Although this antigen has also been associated with (1) segmental sclerosis, (2) progressive disease, and (3) the presence of IgG immune complexes, we have not been able to confirm these observations [15].

Table 1. HLA antigens and IgA nephropathy

Authors	No. of patients studied	HLA antigen with significant prevalence	Country
McDonald et al (1976)	13	Bw 35	Australia
Dupont et al (1977)	30	Bw 35	France
Noel et al (1978)	45	Bw 35	France
Berthoux et al (1978)	43	Bw 35	France
Brettle et al (1978)	17	Cw 1	England
Nagy et al (1979)	24	None	Hungary
Richman et al (1979)	17	B 12	USA
Komori et al (1979)	37	DEn	Japan
Savi et al (1979)	23	None	Italy
Fauchet et al (1980)	40	DR 4	France
Hors et al (1980)	30	DR 4	France
Pardo et al (1980)	21	Bw 35	USA
Mouzon-Cambon et al (1980)	14	None	France
Arnaiz-Villena et al (1981)	27	None	Spain
Egido et al (1981)	40	None	Spain
Kasahara et al (1982)	104	DR 4	Japan
Kashiwabara et al (1982)	42	DR 4	Japan
Hiki et al (1982)	103	DR 4	Japan

Other groups have occasionally noted an increased frequency of HLA-B12, -Cw 1, and -DEn in these patients (Table 1). The finding in France and Japan of an increased incidence of HLA-DR4 seems interesting. Furthermore, an IgA nephropathy developed in two siblings who shared the DR4 antigen but who were otherwise unrelated in terms of HLA-A, B, and C [80]. The significance of the presence of this antigen in patients with IgA nephropathy is not clear. In fact, contradictory results have been found by the Japanese authors. Thus, Hiki et al [81] found that the frequence of the HLA-DR antigens in patients with a stable clinical course was 90.5% whereas it was 36% in patients with progressive renal failure. In contrast, for Kashiwabara et al [82], the frequency of these antigens was 57.1% in patients with normal renal function, 87.5% in those with decreased renal function, and 100% in dialysis patients.

The absence of unanimous results concerning the frequence and significance of HLA antigens could be due to ethnic differences, the generally small numbers of patients studied, and probably the weak association of this nephropathy with the HLA antigens of classes I and II. We have recently described IgA abnormalities in patients and healthy relatives unrelated to any HLA antigens [83]. Furthermore, the description of new families with several members affected [80, 83], the finding of an increase in IgA-bearing peripheral blood lymphocytes [66], the presence of a cold-reacting antinuclear factor [70], and the increased synthesis of polymeric IgA by peripheral blood lymphocytes in some patients' relatives, as commented above, are all in favor of some immunogenetic aspects in this nephropathy. It is possible that, together with or aside from the genes in the HLA complex, other genes controlling antigen nonspecific functions and environmental factors are necessary to the appearance of the disease [84].

The necessary brevity of this text does not permit comments on the immunologic relation between primary IgA nephropathy and other IgA-related nephrites as seen in Henoch-Schönlein purpura and alcoholic liver disease. Also, the occasional association of IgA nephropathy with several entities such as celiac disease, dermatitis herpetiformis, epithelial tumors, ankylosing spondilitis, and other secondary forms, may provide new insight concerning the pathogenesis of the primary IgA nephropathy. Some of these aspects have been discussed in recent reviews [2, 3].

Acknowledgments. Most of our work on IgA nephropathy has been made possible by grants from Fondo de Investigaciones Sanitarias de la Seguridad Social (FIS).

References

1. BERGER J, HINGLAIS N: Les dépôts intercapillaires d'IgA-IgG. *J Urol Nephrol* 74:694–695, 1968
2. WOODROFFE AJ, CLARKSON AR, SEYMOUR AE, LOMAX-SMITH JD: Mesangial IgA nephritis. *Springer Semin Immunopathol* 5:321–332, 1982
3. EGIDO J, SANCHO J, BLASCO R, HERNANDO L: Immunopathogenetic aspects of IgA nephropathy. *Adv Nephrol* 12:103–137, 1983
4. EGIDO J, SANCHO J, BLASCO R, HERNANDO L: Le rôle de l'IgA polymerique dans la pathogenie de la nephropathie à IgA. *Nephrologie* 4:99–101, 1983
5. CLARKSON AR, WOODROFFE AJ, BANNISTER KM, LOMAX-SMITH JD, AARONS I: The syndrome of IgA nephropathy. *Clin Nephrol* 21:7–14, 1984
6. KINCAID-SMITH P, NICHOLLS K: Mesangial IgA nephropathy. *Am J Kidney Dis* 3:90–102, 1983
7. BAART DE LA FAILLE-KUYPER EH, KATER L, KNIGTEN RH, KOOIKER CJ, WAGENAAR SS, VAN DER ZUUWEN P, DORHOUT MEES EJ: Occurrence of vascular IgA deposits in clinical normal skin of patients with renal disease. *Kidney Int* 9:424–429, 1976
8. TOMINO Y, NOMOTO Y, ENDOH M, SAKAI H: Deposition of IgA-dominant immune complexes in muscular vessels from patients with IgA nephropathy. *Acta Pathol Jpn* 31:361–365, 1981
9. BERGER J, YANEVA H, NABARRA B, BARBANEL C: Recurrence of mesangial deposition of IgA after renal transplantation. *Kidney Int* 7:232–241, 1975
10. LÓPEZ-TRASCASA M, EGIDO J, SANCHO J, HERNANDO L: IgA glomerulonephritis (Berger's disease): Evidence of high serum levels of polymeric IgA. *Clin Exp Immunol* 42:247–254, 1980
11. COPPO R, BASOLO B, MARTINA G, ROLLINO C, DE MARCHI M, GIACCHINO F, MAZZUCCO G, MESSINA M, PICCOLI G: Circulating immune complexes containing IgA, IgG and IgM in patients with primary IgA nephropathy and with Henoch-Schönlein nephritis: Correlation with clinical and histologic signs of activity. *Clin Nephrol* 18:230–239, 1982
12. LESAVRE P, DIGEON M, BACH JF: Analysis of circulating IgA and detection of immune complexes in primary IgA nephropathy. *Clin Exp Immunol* 48:61–69, 1982
13. VALENTIJN RM, KAUFFMANN RH, BRUTEL DE LA RIVIERE G, DAHA MR, VAN ES LA: Presence of circulating macromolecular IgA in patients with hematuria due to primary IgA nephropathy. *Am J Med* 74:375–381, 1983

14. HALL RP, STACHURA I, CASON J, WHITESIDE TL, LAWLEY TL: IgA-containing circulating immune complexes in patients with IgA nephropathy. *Am J Med* 74:56–63, 1983

15. EGIDO J, SANCHO J, RIVERA F, HERNANDO L: The role of IgA and IgG immune complexes in IgA nephropathy. *Nephron* 36:59–66, 1984

16. WOODROFFE AJ, GORMLY AA, MCKENZIE DE, WOOTON AM, THOMPSON AJ, SEYMOUR AE, CLARCKSON AR: Immunologic studies in IgA nephropathy. *Kidney Int* 18:366–374, 1980

17. LEVINSKY RJ, BARRAT TM: IgA immune complexes in Henoch-Schönlein purpura. *Lancet* 2:1100–1103, 1979

18. KAUFFMAN RM, HERMANN WA, MEYER CJLM, DAHA MR, VAN ES LA: Circulating IgA immune complexes in Henoch-Schönlein purpura. *Am J Med* 69:859–866, 1980

19. EGIDO J, SANCHO J, MAMPASO F, LÓPEZ-TRASCASA M, SÁNCHEZ-CRESPO M, BLASCO R, HERNANDO L: A possible common pathogenesis of the mesangial IgA glomerulonephritis in patients with Berger's disease and Schönlein-Henoch syndrome. *Proc EDTA* 17:660–666, 1980

20. SANCHO J, EGIDO J, SÁNCHEZ-CRESPO M, BLASCO R: Detection of monomeric and polymeric IgA containing immune complexes in serum and kidney from patients with alcoholic liver disease. *Clin Exp Immunol* 47:327–335, 1982

21. RIFAI A, SMALL PA, TEAGUE PO, AYURB EM: Experimental IgA nephropathy. *J Exp Med* 150:1161–1173, 1979

22. BENE MC, FAURE G, DUHEILLE J: IgA nephropathy characterization of the polymeric nature of mesangial deposits by in vitro binding of free secretory component. *Clin Exp Immunol* 47:527–534, 1982

23. TOMINO Y, SAKAI M, MIURA M, ENDOH M, NOMOTO Y: Detection of polymeric IgA in glomeruli from patients with IgA nephropathy. *Clin Exp Immunol* 49:419–425, 1982

24. VALENTIJN RM, RADL I, HAAIMAN JJ, DAHA MR, VAN ES LA: Circulating macromolecular IgA-1 and mesangial secretory component-binding IgA-1 in primary IgA nephropathy (abst). *Kidney Int* 24:408, 1983

25. SANCHO J, EGIDO J, GONZALEZ E: A simplified method for determining polymeric IgA-containing immune complexes. *J Immunol Method* 60:305–317, 1983

26. EGIDO J, SANCHO J, HERNANDO P, GONZALEZ J, HERNANDO L: The presence of specific IgA immune complexes in IgA nephropathy. *Contrib Nephrol* 40 (in press), 1984

27. EGIDO J, BLASCO R, SANCHO J, LOZANO L, SÁNCHEZ-CRESPO M, HERNANDO L: Increased rates of polymeric IgA synthesis by circulating lymphoid cells in IgA mesangial glomerulonephritis. *Clin Exp Immunol* 47:309–316, 1982

28. EGIDO J, BLASCO R, LOZANO L, SANCHO J: Immunological abnormalities in tonsils of patients with IgA nephropathy: Inversion in the percentage of IgA versus IgG-bearing lymphocytes and increased polymeric IgA synthesis. *Clin Exp Immunol* 57:101–106, 1984

29. DOBRIN RS, KNUDSON FE, MICHAEL AF: The secretory immune system and renal disease. *Clin Exp Immunol* 21:318–328, 1975

30. LOMAX-SMITH JD, ZABROWARNY LA, HOWARTH GS, SEYMOUR AE, WOODROFFE AJ: The immunochemical characterization of mesangial IgA deposits. *Am J Patholol* 113:359–364, 1983

31. ANDRÉ C, BERTHOUX C, ANDRE F, GUILLON J, GENIN C, SABATIER JC: Prevalence of IgA₂ deposits in IgA nephropathy: A clue for their pathogenesis. *N Engl J Med* 303:1343–1346, 1980

32. CONLEY ME, COOPER MD, MICHAEL AF: Selective deposition of immunoglobu-

lin A$_1$ in immunoglobulin A nephropathy, anaphylactoid purpura nephritis and systemic lupus erythematosus. *J Clin Invest* 66:1432–1436, 1980

33. MURAKAMI T, FURUSE A, HATTORI S, KOBAYASHI K, MATSUDA I: Glomerular IgM and IgA$_2$ deposits in IgA nephropathies. *Nephron* 35:120–123, 1983

34. DOMINI V, CASANOVA S, ZIMI N, ZUCCHELLI P: The presence of J-chain in mesangial immune deposits of IgA nephropathy. *Proc EDTA* 19:655–661, 1982

35. DELACROIX DL, LIROUX E, VAERMAN JP: High proportion of polymeric IgA in young infant's sera and independence between IgA-size and IgA-subclass distributions. *J Clin Immunol* 3:53–58, 1983

36. HAAIJMAN JJ, DEEN C, KROSE CJM, ZIJLSTRA JJ, COOLEN J, RADL J: Monoclonal antibodies in immunocytology: A jungle full of pitfalls. *Immunol Today* 5:56–58, 1984

37. CONLEY ME, KOOPMAN WJ: Serum IgA1 and IgA2 in normal adults and patients with systemic lupus erythematosus and hepatic disease. *Clin Immunol Immunopathol* 26:390–397, 1983

38. EGIDO J, SANCHO J, RIVERA F, SÁNCHEZ-CRESPO M: Handling of soluble IgA aggregates by the mononuclear phagocytic system in mice: A comparison with IgG aggregates. *Immunology* 46:1–7, 1982

39. PEPPARD J, ORLANS E, PAYNE AWR, ANDREW E: The elimination of circulating complexes containing polymeric IgA by excretion in the bile. *Immunology* 42:83–89, 1981

40. SANCHO J, GONZALEZ E, RIVERA F, ESCANERO JF, EGIDO J: Hepatic and kidney uptake of soluble monomeric and polymeric IgA aggregates. *Immunology*, in press

41. SANCHO J, GONZALEZ E, EGIDO J: Handling of IgA immune aggregates by liver cells. *Contrib Nephrol*, in press

42. SANCHO J, GONZALEZ E, GONZALEZ J, BLASCO R, LOZANO L, EGIDO J: Defective hepatocyte handling of soluble IgA aggregates in experimental IgA nephropathy (abst). *Abstracts of IXth Int Congress Nephrol, Los Angeles, June,* 1984

43. SANCHO J, EGIDO J, RIVERA F, HERNANDO L: Immune complexes in IgA nephropathy: Presence of antibodies against diet antigens and delayed clearance of specific polymeric IgA immune complexes. *Clin Exp Immunol* 54:104–111, 1983

44. LAWRENCE S, PUSSELL BA, CHARLESWORTH JA: Mesangial IgA nephropathy: Detection of defective reticulophagocytic function in vivo. *Clin Nephrol* 16:280–283, 1983

45. SATO M, KINUGASA E, IDEURA T, KOSHIKAWA S: Phagocytic activity of polymorphonuclear leukocytes in patients with IgA nephropathy. *Clin Nephrol* 19:166–171, 1983

46. EGIDO J, SANCHO J, LORENTE F, FONTAN G: Inhibition of neutrophil migration by serum from patients with IgA nephropathy. *Clin Exp Immunol* 49:709–716, 1982

47. LOWANCE DC, MULLINS JD, MCPHAUL JJ JR: IgA associated glomerulonephritis. *Int Rev Exp Pathol* 17:143–172, 1977

48. ELKON KB, DELACROIX DL, GHARAVI AE, VAERMAN JP, HUGHES GRV: Immunoglobulin A and polymeric IgA rheumatoid factors in systemic sicca syndrome: Partial characterization. *J Immunol* 129:576–581, 1982

49. ELKON KB, INMAN RD, CULHANE L, CHRISTINAL CL: Induction of polymeric IgA rheumatoid factor in infective endocarditis. *Am J Med* 75:785–789, 1983

50. GOLDMAN M, ROSE LM, HOCHMANN A, LAMBERT PH: Deposition of idiotype-anti-idiotype immune complexes in renal glomeruli after polyclonal B cell activation. *J Exp Med* 155:1385–1399, 1982

51. MAUER SM, SUTHERLAND DER, HOWARD RJ, FISH AJ, NAJARIAN JS, MI-

CHAEL AF: The glomerular mesangium: III. Acute immune mesangial injury, a new model of glomerulonephritis. *J Exp Med* 137:553–570, 1973

52. TOMINO Y, ENDOH M, NOMOTO Y, SAKAI H: Specificity of eluted antibodies from renal tissues of patients with IgA nephropathy. *Am J Kidney Dis* 1:276–280, 1982

53. TOMINO Y, SAKAI H, ENDOH M, SUGA T, MIURA M, KANESHIGE H, NOMOTO Y: Cross-reactivity of IgA antibodies between renal mesangial areas and nuclei of tonsillar cells in patients with IgA nephropathy. *Clin Exp Immunol* 51:605–610, 1983

54. WESTBERG NG, BAKLIEN K, SCHMEKEL B, GILLBERG R, BRANDTZAEG P: Quantitation of immunoglobulin-producing cells in small intestinal mucosa of patients with IgA nephropathy. *Clin Immunol Immunopathol* 26:442–445, 1983

55. SAKAI H, NOMOTO Y, ARIMORI S: Decrease of IgA-specific suppressor T activity in patients with IgA nephropathy. *Clin Exp Immunol* 38:243–248, 1979

56. BANNISTER KM, DREW PA, CLARKSON AR, WOODROFFE AJ: Immunoregulation in glomerulonephritis, Henoch-Schönlein purpura and lupus nephritis. *Clin Exp Immunol* 54:384–390, 1983

57. EGIDO J, BLASCO R, SANCHO J, LOZANO L: T cell dysfunctions in IgA nephropathy: Specific abnormalities in the regulation of IgA synthesis. *Clin Immunol Immunopathol* 26:201–212, 1983

58. COSIO FG, LAM S, FOLANI AO, CONLEY ME, MICHAEL AF: Immune regulation of immunoglobulin production in IgA-nephropathy. *Clin Immunol Immunopathol* 23:430–436, 1982

59. CHATENOUD L, BACH MA: Abnormalities of T cell subsets in glomerulonephritis and systemic lupus erythematosus. *Kidney Int* 20:267–274, 1982

60. SAKAI H, ENDOH M, TOMINO Y, NOMOTO Y: Increase of IgA specific helper Tα cells in patients with IgA nephropathy. *Clin Exp Immunol* 50:77–82, 1982

61. NOMOTO Y, SAKAI H, ARIMORI S: Increase of IgA bearing lymphocytes in peripheral blood from patients with IgA nephropathy. *Am J Clin Pathol* 71:158–160, 1979

62. BENE MC, FAURE G, HURAULT DE LIGNEY B, KESSLER M, DUHEILLE J: Immunoglobulin A nephropathy: Quantitative immunomorphometry of the tonsillar plasma cells evidences an inversion of the immunoglobulin A versus immunoglobulin G secreting cell balance. *J Clin Invest* 71:1342–1347, 1983

63. HOOVER RG, DIECKGRAEFE BK, LYNCH RG: T cells with Fc receptors for IgA: Induction of Tα cells in vivo and in vitro by purified IgA. *J Immunol* 127:1560–1565, 1981

64. ENDOH M, SAKAI H, SUGA T, MIURA M, TOMINO Y, NOMOTO Y: Increase of peripheral blood B cell with Fc receptor for IgA in patients with IgA nephropathy. *Scand J Immunol* 17:437–441, 1983

65. ADACHI M, YODOI J, MASUDA T, TAKATSUKI K, UCHINO H: Altered expression of lymphocyte Fcα receptor in selective IgA deficiency and IgA nephropathy. *J Immunol* 131:1246–1251, 1983

66. SAKAI H, NOMOTO Y, ARIMORI S, KOMORI K, INOUYE H, TSUJI K: Increase of IgA-bearing peripheral blood lymphocytes in families of patients with IgA nephropathy. *Am J Clin Pathol* 72:452–456, 1979

67. EGIDO J, BLASCO R, SANCHO J: Immunoregulation abnormalities in patients with IgA nephropathy. *Ann NY Acad Sci* 409:816–817, 1983

68. EGIDO J, BLASCO R, SANCHO J, HERNANDO L: Immunological abnormalities in healthy relatives of patients with IgA nephropathy. *Am J Nephrol,* in press

69. FAUCI AS: Immunoregulation in autoimmunity. *J Allergy Clin Immunol* 66:5–15, 1980

70. NOMOTO Y, SAKAI H: Cold reacting antinuclear factor in sera from patients with IgA nephropathy. *J Lab Clin Med* 94:76–87, 1979
71. NOMOTO Y, SAKAI H, ENDOH M, TOMINO Y: Scleritis and IgA nephropathy. *Arch Intern Med* 140:783–785, 1980
72. DROZ D, NOEL LH, BARBANEL CI, LEIBOWITCH J: Glomerulonéphrite à dépôts intercapillaires d'IgA lors d'une gammapathie monoclonale benigne. *Nov Press Med* 10:3652–3653, 1981
73. MONTERO R: Oral presentation. *Milano Meeting on IgA mesangial glomerulonephritis, 1983*
74. STACHURA I, SINGH G, WHITESIDE TL: Immune abnormalities in IgA nephropathy (Berger's disease). *Clin Immunol Immunopathol* 20:373–388, 1981
75. TOLKOFF-RUBIN NE, COSINI AB, FULLER T, RUBIN RH, COLVIN RB: IgA nephropathy in HLA-identical siblings. *Transplantation* 26:430–433, 1978
76. SABATIER JC, GENIN C, ASSENAT H, COLON S, DUCRET F, BERTHOUX FC: Mesangial IgA glomerulonephritis in HLA identical brothers. *Clin Nephrol* 11:35–39, 1979
77. BERTHOUX FC, GENIN C, LE PETIT JC, LAURENT B: Immunogenetique des glomerulonephrites intercapillaires a depots d IgA. *Nephrologie* 4:283–287, 1983
78. EGIDO J, RIVERA F, SANCHO J, MORENO M, KREISLER M, HERNANDO L: Estudio del sistema HLA y factores de riesgo para la insuficiencia renal en la glomerulonefritis mesangial IgA. *Nefrologia* 1:21–27, 1981
79. BERTHOUX FC, GENIN C, GAGNE A, LE PETIT JC, SABATIER JC: HLA Bw 35 antigen and mesangial IgA glomerulonephritis a poor prognosis marker. *Proc EDTA* 16:551–555, 1979
80. MONTOLIU J, DARNELL A, TORRAS A, ERCILLA G, VALLES M, REVERT L: Familial IgA nephropathy. *Arch Intern Med* 140:1374–1375, 1980
81. HIKI Y, KOBAYASHI Y, TATENO S, SADA M, KASHIWAGI N: Strong association of HLA-DR4 with benign IgA nephropathy. *Nephron* 32:222–226, 1982
82. KASHIWABARA H, SHISHIDO H, TOMURA S, TUCHIDA H, MIYAJIMA T: Strong association between IgA nephropathy and HLA-DR4 antigen. *Kidney Int* 22:377–382, 1982
83. EGIDO J, BLASCO R, SANCHO J, LOZANO L, GUTIERREZ MILLET V: Immunological studies in a familial IgA nephropathy. *Clin Exp Immunol* 54:532–538, 1983
84. BIOZZI G, SIQUEIRA M, STIFFEL C, IBAÑEZ OM, MOUTON D, FERREIRA VCA: Genetic selections for relevant immunological functions, in *"Immunology 80" Progress in Immunology IV*, edited by FOUGERAU M, DAUSSET J, London, Academic Press, 1980, pp 432–457.

Clinicopathologic Correlations in IgA Nephropathy

Raja Sinniah and Gordon Ku

IgA nephropathy has been recognized as a distinct form of primary glomerulo-nephritis since its first description by Berger in 1968 [1, 2]. Its characteristic feature is the diffuse glomerular deposition of immunoglobulin A as the predominant protein. There is no associated systemic disease, and the condition excludes systemic lupus erythematosus [3], Henoch Schönlein purpura [4, 5], cirrhosis [6, 7], and cancer [8]. The typical distribution of IgA in the mesangium distinguishes this disease from, for example, resolving poststreptococcal glomerulonephritis. The predominance of IgA in the glomerular mesangium suggests an association between IgA and the development of glomerulo-nephritis, although direct evidence has not yet been found for a role of IgA immune complexes in the pathogenesis of this type of glomerulonephritis.

It is the most common type of adult primary glomerulonephritis in France [3, 9, 10], Italy [11], Japan [12], Singapore [13], and Australia [4], accounting for 20 to 40% of the reported cases, though lower incidences ranging from 1.5 to 10.0% have been reported from Britain, the United States, and Canada [14–17].

Reported here is a prospective study of the pathology of IgA nephropathy and its clinical correlations. It is based on immunopathologic studies of renal biopsy samples sent to the Department of Pathology, National University of Singapore.

Methods

The study was conducted on all patients who underwent renal biopsy in Singapore and were felt to have idiopathic glomerulonephritis by the physicians on the nephrology team. There was no evidence of systemic disease,

---

This manuscript was presented as part of a Symposium on *IgA Nephropathy*.

and systemic lupus erythematosus, Henoch Schönlein purpura, cirrhosis, and cancer were excluded by complete clinical, radiologic, and serologic investigations as described previously [18]. All biopsy specimens contained at least five glomeruli.

For light microscopy examination, all of the specimens were fixed in Bouin's solution, embedded in paraffin, and sectioned at 2 μm. The sections were stained with hematoxylin and eosin (H & E), periodic acid Schiff (PAS), periodic acid silver-methenanine (PASM), Masson's trichrome, and Martius scarlet blue (MSB) stains. For electron microscopy examination, the specimens were fixed in 4% glutaraldehyde, post-fixed in 1% Dalton's chrome-osmium fixative, and embedded in Araldite. Thin sections cut at 60 to 90 μm were stained with uranyl acetate and lead citrate. The sections were examined and photographed in a Hitachi HS-8 or Philips electron microscope.

The techniques for immunofluorescence microscopy have been described previously [18]. All specimens were stained with rabbit antisera to human IgG, M, A, D, E, IgA secretory piece (IgA-SC), C3, Clq, C4, fibrin, HBsAg, and albumin. The intensity and distribution of immunofluorescence was recorded semiquantitatively as negative (0), mild (1+), moderate (2+), and heavy (3+).

Results

Immunopathology

IgA was found as the predominant immunoglobulin in the glomerular mesangium of 268 (32.6%) of 822 patients with idiopathic glomerulonephritis whose biopsy specimens were examined by immunofluorescence microscopy. IgA of grades 2+ to 3+ was found in 225 patients (84%), whereas the intensity of fluorescence for other immunoglobulins such as C3 and fibrin was not as marked. In the 33 patients (12.3%) with IgG of grades 2+ to 3+ intensity, the fluorescence of the immunoglobulin did not exceed that of IgA. The constant site of deposition was the mesangium. Localization of IgA and other immunoglobulins to the mesangium alone within all glomeruli (Fig. 1) was found in 183 patients (68.3%). In 85 patients (31.7%), IgA and other proteins were found both in the mesangium and in some of the peripheral capillary loops in a paramesangial-subendothelial position. IgA was found as casts in the tubule lumen in approximately 50% of patients, and less frequently as tubular epithelial secretions.

A variety of immunoglobulins was found in association with the glomerular deposition of IgA in the 268 patients (Table 1). IgA was found unassociated with other immunoglobulins in 117 patients (43.7%); an IgA-IgG combination was seen in 128 (47.7%); an IgA-IgM combination was seen less frequently in 23 patients (8.6%). Clq and C4 were present as weak, scattered specks in 10 patients (3.7%), and all were accompanied by IgM and/or IgG deposits. IgA-SC and HBsAg were absent consistently. Deposits of glomerular fibrinogen were detected in 193 patients (72%) and were always present in those groups where mesangial IgA was found in combination with other immunoglobulins.

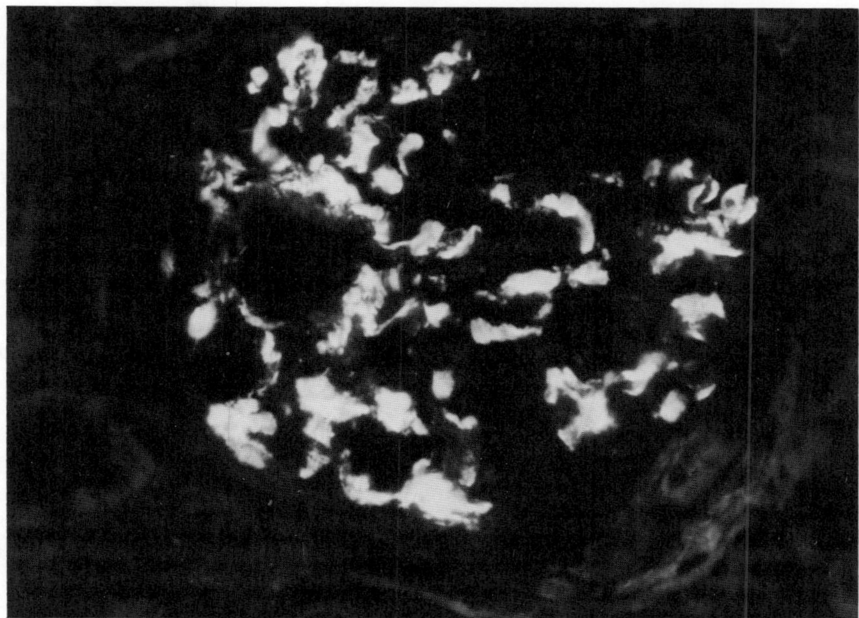

Fig. 1. Immunofluorescence microscopy showing heavy deposition of IgA in the typical mesangial distribution in a patient with Berger's disease. (×350)

Glomerular Morphology

A wide range of glomerular lesions was subdivided into five basic groups or grades according to the WHO criteria for the classification of glomerular

Table 1. Mesangial deposits of immunoglobulins and complements in IgA nephropathy[a]

Combinations of immunoglobulins and C3	Positive findings		Clq/C4 (No. of patients)
	No. of patients	%	
A	27	10.1 $\left.\right\}$ 43.7	
A, C3	90	33.6	
A, M, C3	23	8.6	4
A, G	16	6.0	
A, G, C3	67	25.0 $\left.\right\}$ 47.7	2
A, G, M	3	1.1	
A, G, M, C3	42	15.6	4
Total	268	100.0	10 (3.7%)

[a] IgA casts were found in lumen (50%) and tubular epithelial cells (10%) of the biopsy samples. *Note:* Determinations for IgA-SC and HBsAg were negative.

diseases [19]: *Group 1* had minimal lesions that appeared "normal" on light microscopy. There were 10 patients (3.7%) in this group. *Group 2* had minor changes, with widening of the mesangium and increased cellularity of groups of up to 3 cells per area in the periphery of glomeruli. There were 80 patients (29.9%) in this group. *Group 3* had focal and segmental glomerulonephritis with less than 50% of the glomeruli showing localized or segmental sclerosis and mesangial cell proliferation. The remaining glomeruli showed minor changes. This type of lesion was found in 29.5% of the patients; 64 patients (23.9%) exhibited focal sclerosis ± hyalinosis, and 15 (5.6%) showed focal and segmental proliferative glomerulonephritis. *Group 4* had diffuse mesangial cell proliferation which varied in the degree of hypercellularity and was irregular in distribution. There were 97 patients (36.2%) in this group, subdivided into mild, moderate, and marked mesangial cell hyperplasia. *Group 5* had diffuse sclerosing glomerulonephritis with involvement of more than 80% of the glomeruli. This was an uncommon finding (0.7%) on initial biopsy.

In approximately one third of the patients, mesangial deposits were detected with PAS, MSB, and Masson trichrome stains. The frequent superimposed glomerular lesions (Table 2) were segmental or global sclerosis (or both), hyalinosis, and capsular adhesions. Segmental crescents were observed in 17.3% of the patients and were associated more commonly with mesangial proliferative glomerulonephritis (Fig. 2).

Tubulointerstitial lesions consisting of focal interstitial edema and lymphocytic cell infiltrates were found in 40% of the patients. The severity of tubulointerstitial fibrosis and tubular atrophy reflected the severity of the glomerular lesions.

Arteriolosclerosis and arteriosclerosis were seen more frequently in patients with diffuse mesangial proliferation and superimposed lesions of glomerular sclerosis, and in patients with diffuse sclerosing glomerulonephritis.

Electron Microscopy

Electron microscopic examination of the glomeruli of 120 patients with mesangial IgA nephropathy (Berger's disease) with minor change, focal lesions and diffuse mesangial cell proliferation showed constant deposition of electron-dense material in the mesangium (Fig. 3). Approximately a third of them (36%) showed paramesangial-subendothelial extensions, but more frequently (50%) with diffuse mesangial cell proliferation; only a few (7%) showed occasional subepithelial deposits in the peripheral capillary loops [13]. In IgA nephropathy, the immunoproteins appear to gain access from the capillary lumen to the mesangium via endothelial fenestrae. The deposits appear to be transported into the deeper mesangium by imbibition or diffusion, and there they directly or indirectly stimulate mesangial cell hyperplasia with increased production of mesangial matrix. The amount of deposits did not correlate directly with the degree of mesangial hypercellularity. The mesangial matrix was more dense in patients with diffuse mesangial cell proliferation and minor change with superimposed lesions than it was in patients with minimal/minor change alone.

Table 2. Correlation of glomerular morphology and clinical disease in IgA nephropathy[a]

Clinical disease	No. of patients	Minimal lesion		Minor change		Focal GN					Diffuse mesangial proliferation							Diffuse sclerosing GN		
		N	%	N	%	N	%	With crescents	With TIC	With AS	N	%	With segmental sclerosis	With crescents	%	With TIC	With AS	N	%	With AS + TIC
Asymptomatic recurrent proteinuria	12	4	33.3	4	33.3	2	16.7		2		2	16.7	2	2	16.6					
Asymptomatic recurrent microhematuria with proteinuria	123	3	2.4	43	35.0	39	31.7	8	8		38	30.9	32	19	15.4	12				
Symptomatic microhematuria and proteinuria, recurrent	20	1	5.0	5	25.0	7	35.0		1		7	35.0	6	3	15.0	1				
Macroscopic hematuria	46	1	2.2	15	32.6	13	28.3	7	4	2	17	36.9	12	5	10.9	7	2			
Acute nephritis	24	0	0	4	16.7	5	20.8	1	2		15	62.5	11	7	29.2	5	3			
Nephrotic syndrome	28	1	3.6	7	25.0	5	17.8				15	53.6	14	8	28.6	8	4			
Hypertension	11	0		2	18.2	5	45.5				3	27.3	1	2	18.2	1	1	1	9.0	1
Hypokalemic "nephritis"	3	0				3	100.0													
Rapidly progressive GN	1																	1	100.0	1
Total	268	10	3.7%	80	29.9%	79	29.5%				97	36.2%						2	0.7%	

[a] Abbreviations are defined as follows: TIC = tubulointerstitial change; AS = arteriolosclerosis; GN = glomerulonephritis.

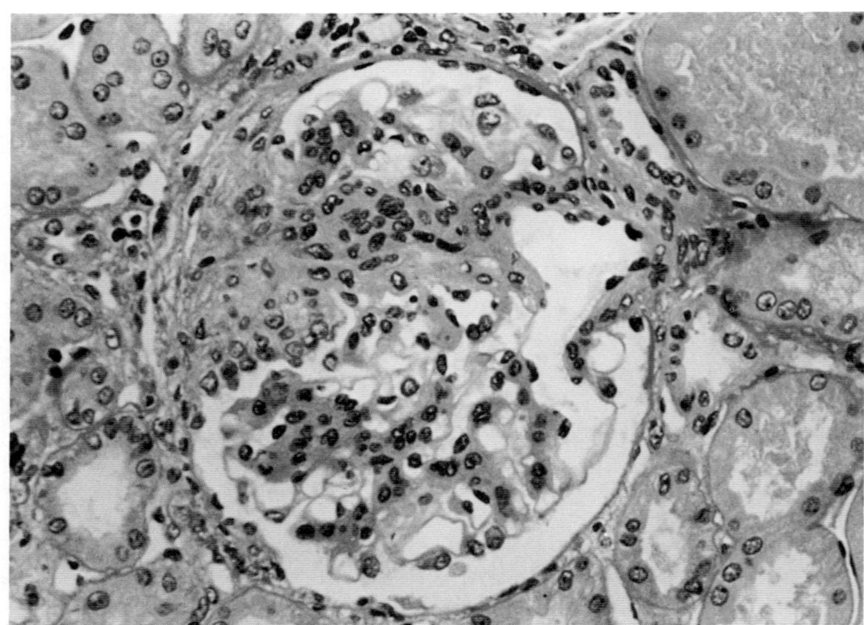

Fig. 2. Diffuse mesangial cell hyperplasia with a segmental crescent and adhesions. (H & E stain; ×400)

Capillary loop changes were found frequently; focal thickening was seen in about 60% of patients in all groups, but more frequently in diffuse mesangial cell proliferation. Focal and segmental areas of mesangial interposition with the formation of a double contour were noted along the peripheral capillary loops in 34% of all patients with chronic disease. Obliteration and broadening of foot processes were seen frequently (77%), especially in patients with the nephrotic syndrome and other clinical states with an associated protein-uria. Polymorphonuclear neutrophils were seen in the capillary lumen in 25% of patients. Clumps of platelets also were seen in the capillary lumens in 20% of the patients. There was evidence of mesangiolysis, which may reflect irreversible progression to mesangial sclerosis, and finally glomerular obsolescence [20]. The mesangial cells showed no definite capacity to phagocytize the electron-dense deposits [20–22].

Clinical Data

The mean age of the 268 Singapore patients with IgA nephropathy was 22.9 ± SD 12.8 yrs; range, 3 to 64 yr). Males outnumbered females by a ratio of 2.3:1 (187 males; 81 females), but this was due to a high selection of patients with asymptomatic microscopic hematuria-proteinuria, or recurrent proteinuria discovered during the regular medical examination of male Army inductees (Table 3). There was no significant age or sex difference in the other clinical groups.

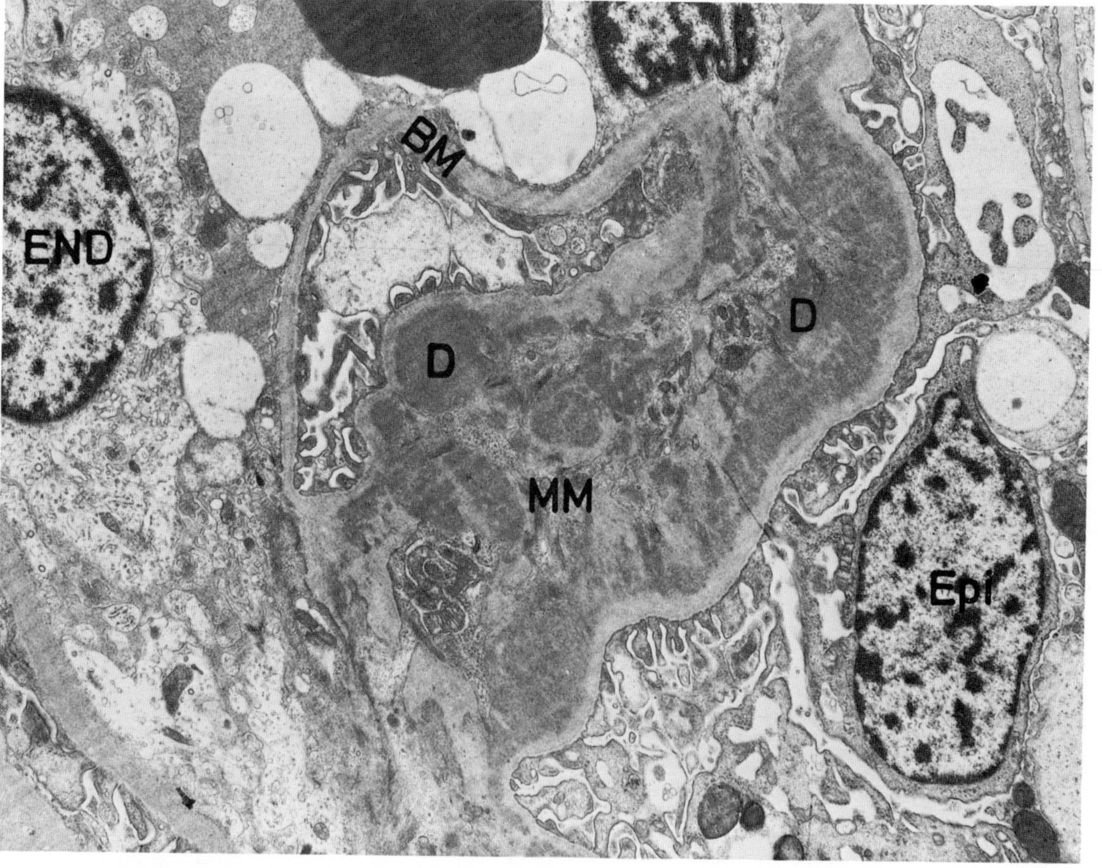

Fig. 3. Electron micrograph of a portion of the glomerulus showing heavy deposition of electron-dense material in the mesangium. *END* denotes endothelial cell; *Epi*, epithelial cell; *MM*, mesangial matrix; *BM*, basement membrane; *D*, dense deposits. (×9720)

Table 3. Clinical data in patients with idiopathic mesangial IgA nephropathy

Clinical disease	No. of patients	%	Sex		Age, yr		Mode of discovery		
			Male	Female	Mean ± SD	Range	Initial symptoms	No. of patients	%
Asymptomatic recurrent proteinuria	12	4.5	12	0	20.6 ± 2.5	17 to 24	None: Regular army medical exam	12	100.0
Asymptomatic recurrent microhematuria with proteinuria	123	45.9	104	19	20.5 ± 6.3	14 to 64	None: Regular army medical exam	99	80.5
							Other regular medical exam	21	
							During pregnancy	3	
Symptomatic microhematuria with proteinuria	20	7.5	12	8	28.0 ± 7.6	15 to 42	Loin pain, ankle/ periorbital edema, fever, upper respiratory infection	3	15.0[a]
Macroscopic hematuria	46	17.2	23	23	24.3 ± 8.1	11 to 50	Painless	25	54.3
							Loin pain, dysuria, fever	21	
							Upper respiratory infection	14	30.4[a]

Acute nephritis	24	8.9	10	14	24.7 ± 8.6	14 to 41	Fever, loin pain, periorbital edema, macro/microhematuria	24	100.0
							Upper respiratory infection	10	41.7[a]
Nephrotic syndrome	28	10.4	16	12	23.0 ± 11.0	3 to 49	Edema	28	100.0
							Associated macro/microhematuria	10	35.7
							Upper respiratory infection	3	10.7[a]
Hypertension	11	4.1	7	4	30.7 ± 4.2	25 to 40	Regular medical exam	3	
							During pregnancy	2	
							Headaches, dyspnea	2	
Hypokalemic "nephritis"	3	1.1	2	1	29.3 ± 17.1	21 to 49	Muscle weakness	3	
Rapidly progressive nephritis	1	0.4	1	0	37.5		Fever, vomiting, hypertension, uremia	1	
Total	268	100.0	187	81	22.9 12.8	3 to 64			

[a] Percentage of patients with upper respiratory tract infection.

An earlier study conducted in the Singapore Army showed asymptomatic recurrent proteinuria or microscopic hematuria-proteinuria in 2.1% of all recruits (1,410 of 67,695 recruits). Mesangial IgA as the predominant immunoglobulin was found in 56.2% of 96 patients with microscopic hematuria, and in 34.3% of 35 patients with proteinuria [18, 23].

Though the most common clinical presentation was asymptomatic microscopic hematuria (123 patients; 45.9%), IgA nephropathy had protean clinical manifestations. The most frequent symptomatic clinical presentations were gross hematuria (46 patients; 17.2%), nephrotic syndrome (28 patients; 10.4%), and acute nephritis (24 patients; 9%). Hypertension was infrequent as the initial presentation; three patients were seen with potassium-losing nephropathy and mesangial IgA deposits. Investigation for Bartter syndrome with renin and aldosterone estimations was negative. One patient presented clinically with rapidly progressive glomerulonephritis, and biopsy examination showed a diffuse sclerosing glomerulonephritis with mesangial IgA deposits in the nonsclerotic glomeruli.

Upper Respiratory Tract Infections

A history of an upper respiratory tract infection was found in 30 of 133 patients (22.5%) with symptomatic IgA nephropathy (Table 3). The highest incidences were observed in patients with clinical acute nephritis (41.7%) and macroscopic hematuria (30.4%) as the presenting syndromes. A raised antistreptolysin 0 titer of greater than 200 Todd units was found in the blood of 27 of 120 patients (22.5%) tested for this factor. The patients belonged to the various clinical groups, and no significant difference was found between them. Throat swab cultures from 44 patients grew a β-hemolytic streptococcus in only ten (22.8%). There was no consistent pattern to implicate this organism as a cause of the disease, but it was clearly an associated factor sometimes [13].

The serum IgA concentration has been found to be elevated in 12.5 to 38% of patients with IgA nephropathy [13, 24, 25], whereas a slight or no significant increase has been reported by others [12, 16, 26]. This disparity may be due to patient selection or chance. There was not a significant correlation between the IgA concentration and the occurrence of the disease [13].

Correlation Between Glomerular Morphology and Clinical Disease

In the asymptomatic microscopic hematuria-proteinuria and recurrent proteinuria groups, the more frequent lesions were minor change, and focal and segmental glomerulonephritis (Table 2). Minor change including minimal lesion accounted for 66.6% of the patients with recurrent proteinuria and for 37.4% of the patients with recurrent asymptomatic microscopic hematuria. Diffuse mesangial cell proliferation was seen in 15 of 24 patients (62.5%) with acute nephritis and in 15 of the 28 patients (53.6%) with the nephrotic syndrome, with the lowest incidence being observed in asymptomatic recurrent proteinuria. Of the 11 patients with hypertension, five (45.5%) had focal segmental glomerulonephritis, three had diffuse mesangial cell proliferation, and one had diffuse sclerosing glomerulonephritis. The one patient admitted with rapidly progressive glomerulonephritis had a diffuse sclerosing glomerular lesion with extensive tubulointerstitial fibrosis and atrophy, with both arteriolosclerosis and arteriosclerosis. Three patients with generalized weakness were found to have a potassium-losing nephropathy with focal glomerulonephritis and mesangial IgA deposits. There was no significant difference in the types of glomerular lesions between the patients with microscopic recurrent hematuria and macroscopic hematuria, with or without symptoms.

Superimposed glomerular lesions of segmental crescents, adhesions, and sclerotic areas were present in both focal glomerulonephritis and diffuse mesangial cell proliferative glomerulonephritis. These superimposed lesions were more commonly found in diffuse mesangial proliferative glomerulonephritis. Crescents were present in 16 of 79 patients (20.3%) with focal glomerulonephritis, and in 46 of the 97 patients (47.4%) with diffuse mesangial cell proliferation. In approximately 40% of the patients, the crescents occupied over 50% of the glomerular circumference. Crescents were also seen more frequently in patients presenting with acute nephritis and the nephrotic syndrome than in patients with less severe clinical disease of asymptomatic and symptomatic recurrent proteinuria and microscopic hematuria. There was a much lower incidence (10.9%) of crescent formation in patients presenting with macroscopic hematuria.

Tubulointerstitial lesions of focal interstitial edema and focal lymphocytic cell infiltrates were found in 94 of the patients (35%), and in all clinical syndromes. The severity of the interstitial fibrosis and tubular atrophy reflected the severity of the glomerular morphology and the clinical syndrome. Vascular narrowing with arteriolosclerosis also reflected a more severe glomerular lesion.

Correlation Between the Onset of Symptoms and Time of Biopsy

In biopsy examinations done within one year of the onset of symptoms, the more frequent lesion was minor change (Table 4); focal lesions, diffuse mesangial cell proliferation, and diffuse sclerosing glomerulonephritis were seen more frequently in biopsy specimens taken three years after the clinical onset of disease. Patients with symptomatic disease of more than one year's duration tended to show diffuse mesangial cell proliferation ($P < 0.01$). In patients with asymptomatic disease with recurrent proteinuria and microscopic hematuria discovered on regular medical examination, the most frequent lesion was minor change (41.7%). As the onset of the disease was difficult to determine in these groups of patients, focal and diffuse types of glomerular lesions may represent later stages of the disease.

Correlation of Creatinine Clearance with Glomerular Pathology

The creatinine clearance is a good measure of the glomerular filtration function of the kidneys. It is a useful and relatively simple test, for it involves only

Table 4. Relationship of glomerular pathology to time of biopsy in IgA nephropathy

| Time of biopsy | No. of patients | Minor change | | Focal segmental GN[a] | | | | Diffuse mesangial cell proliferation | | | Diffuse sclerosing GN[a] | |
		N	%	N	%	With segmental sclerosis	With segmental proliferation	N	%	With superimposed lesions	N	%
Asymptomatic disease	132	55	41.7	37	28.0	28	9	40	30.3	36		
Symptomatic disease												
Less than 1 year	71	32	45.1	21	29.5	16	5	18	25.4	12		
1 to 3 yr	37	7	18.9	8	21.6	7	1	22	59.5	16		
3 to 6 yr	14	0	0	4	28.6	4	0	8	57.1	6	2	14.3
Over 6 yr	14	1	7.1	6	42.9	4	2	7	50.0	4		

[a] GN refers to glomerulonephritis; $x^2 = 27.5$ at six degrees of freedom ($P < 0.01$).

the collection of a 24-hr urine sample and 5 ml of the patient's blood. The correlation between the creatinine clearance and glomerular pathology was determined in 33 patients with IgA nephropathy. The normal value was accepted as a clearance of over 70 ml/min. An abnormal clearance of 40 to 69 ml/min was classified as mild; 20 to 39 ml/min, as moderate; and over 20 ml/min, as severe dysfunction.

In the 20 patients with a normal creatinine clearance (Table 5), the most frequent glomerular lesion was minor change, observed in 9 of the 20 patients (45%). In the 13 patients with an abnormal clearance, minor change was not found. The major lesion was diffuse mesangial cell proliferation occurring in seven of the patients (77.8%) with mild, and in three of the patients (100%) with moderate dysfunction. Superimposed glomerular lesions of sclerosis ($\pm$ hyalinosis) and crescent formation were also seen in these latter groups of patients. In the one patient with severe renal dysfunction, the biopsy specimen showed diffuse sclerosing glomerulonephritis.

There was no correlation between the intensity of the mesangial IgA deposits (and accompanying immunoproteins IgG and IgM) and the type of glomerular lesion. There was also no correlation between the pattern of mesangial immunoprotein deposits and the creatinine clearance. On electron microscopic examination of the glomeruli, mesangial dense deposits were found constantly in all of the patients, with paramesangial-subendothelial extensions in twelve (36.4%). Subendothelial deposits were present in all of the patients with moderate to severe renal dysfunction as determined by the creatinine clearance.

There was a correlation between the degree of tubulointerstitial change and the severity of the glomerular lesions, indicative of a progressive renal parenchymal disease in this disorder.

Correlation of Proteinuria with Glomerular Pathology

An attempt was made to correlate the degree of proteinuria with the glomerular and tubulointerstitial changes in patients with IgA nephropathy who presented with recurrent microscopic hematuria and associated proteinuria. The normal range of proteinuria was accepted as less than 0.19 g per 24 hr. In mild proteinuria, the daily loss was 0.2 to 0.99 g; in moderate proteinuria, 1.0 to 2.49 g; and in severe proteinuria, more than 2.5 g. There were 65 patients in this study, and the results are shown in Table 6. The predominant glomerular lesion in the patients with proteinuria within the normal range was minor change, observed in seven (77.8%). In patients with moderate to severe proteinuria, the predominant lesion was diffuse mesangial cell proliferation ($P < 0.05$), with frequently associated superimposed glomerular lesions of sclerosis. This was seen in 45.4% (5) and 83.3% (5), respectively, of the patients in these two groups. The tubulointerstitial changes reflected the severity of the glomerular lesions, and thereby indicated the presence of progressive renal parenchymal damage in IgA nephropathy.

There was no correlation between the intensity of mesangial IgA deposits (and accompanying immunoproteins IgG and IgM) and the degree of proteinuria. There also was no correlation with the severity of the glomerular lesions

Table 5. Correlation of creatinine clearance with glomerular pathology in IgA nephropathy (33 patients)[a]

Creatinine clearance ml/min	Total No. of patients	Minor change			Focal GN				Diffuse mesangial proliferation						Diffuse sclerosing GN		Mes. + subend. EDD	
		N	%	TIC	N	%	Cr	TIC	N	%	Cr	Scl	TIC	AS	N	TIC and AS	N	%
Normal (>70ml)	20	9	45	2	3	15	1	2	8	40	3	7	5				5	25
Abnormal																		
a. Mild (40–69ml)	9				2	22.2	1		7	77.8	3	7	7	1			3	33
b. Moderate (20–39ml)	3								3	100	1	3	3	1			3	100
c. Severe (<20ml)	1														1	1	1	100

[a] Abbreviations: TIC, tubulointerstitial change; Cr, crescent; Scl, sclerosis; AS, arteriosclerosis; Mes. + subend. EDD = mesangial with subendothelial electron dense deposits.

Table 6. Correlation of proteinuria with renal pathology in IgA nephropathy with recurrent microhematuria (65 patients)[a]

Degree of proteinuria g/24 hr	No. of patients	Minor change			Focal GN				Diffuse mesangial proliferation						Mes. + Subend. EDD	
		N	%	TIC	N	%	Cr	TIC	N	%	Cr	Scl	TIC	AS	N	%
Normal (0.0 to 0.19g)	9	7	77.8	2	2	22.2										
Mild (0.2 to 0.99g)	39	18	46.2	4	8	20.5	2		13	33.3	7	10	4		13	33.3
Moderate (1.0 to 2.49g)	11	3	27.3		3	27.3	1	1	5[c]	45.4	2	4	2		11[b]	100
Severe (2.5g and over)	6				1	16.7			5[c]	83.3	3	5	5	2	5[b]	83.3

[a] Abbreviations: TIC, tubulointerstitial change; Cr, crescent; Scl, sclerosis; AS, arteriosclerosis; Mes. + Subend. EDD, mesangial with subendothelial electron dense deposits.

[b] Correlation between moderate to severe proteinuria and mes. + Subend. EDD was significant ($P < 0.01$).

[c] Correlation between moderate to severe proteinuria and diffuse mesangial proliferation was significant ($P < 0.05$).

and immunoprotein deposits. On electron microscopic examination, dense deposits were observed in the glomerular mesangium of all the patients; paramesangial-subendothelial extensions were noted along capillary loops in 83 to 100% of the patients with moderate to severe degrees of proteinuria ($P < 0.01$).

Minor Change Nephrotic Syndrome with Mesangial IgA Deposits

There were eight patients with nephrotic syndrome who showed minor change glomerular lesions on light microscopy and diffuse mesangial IgA deposits on immunofluorescence microscopy. Clinical follow-up data on and observations in response to prednisolone therapy were available in six patients (Table 7). Five of the patients were started on a regimen of steroids and followed for periods of 1 to 5 years. Remission of the nephrotic syndrome was observed in two patients with combined prednisolone, persantin, and cyclophosphamide treatment. Two patients had frequent relapses, one had a partial remission, and a poor response to steroid therapy was noted in one.

Progressive IgA Renal Disease

The disease is a chronic one, with signs and symptoms changing little with time. Microhematuria may be intermittent, waxing and waning over long periods. The percentage of patients who progress to renal failure has varied from 0 to 20%, with several workers reporting a favorable prognosis [15, 27]. The highest percentage of renal failure was reported by van der Peet et al [28], supported by Droz [10], who reported 18.1% of 182 patients progressing to terminal renal failure during a follow-up period between one and 32 years.

There was a fairly good correlation between the activity and severity of

Table 7. Minor change nephrotic syndrome with mesangial IgA deposits

Patient no.	Age (yrs)	Sex	Therapy	Response	Followup (yrs)
1	19	M	(a) Prednisolone	Poor	5
			(b) Prednisolone, cyclophosphamide	Relapses	
2	28	M	Prednisolone	Poor	2
3	27	M	Prednisolone	Relapses	2
4	46	F	Prednisolone, persantin	Remission	2
5	15	M	Prednisolone	Partial remission	2
6	29	M	Prednisolone, cyclophosphamide, persantin	Remission	1

the lesions and prognosis. Patients with mild lesions had a benign course or showed evidence of active disease without deterioration of renal function, whereas patients with more severe lesions of grades 4 or 5 and who were followed for more than one year developed end-stage renal failure [18, 29]. Co-deposition of IgG and/or IgM in humans appeared to correlate with more severe disease [4, 15, 18]. Hyalinized glomeruli, adhesions, fibrocellular crescents, and tubular degeneration with interstitial fibrosis were unfavorable prognostic signs.

Discussion

IgA nephropathy is a widespread disease, and is the most common type of primary glomerulonephritis in many countries, including Singapore (32.6% of cases). In the initial description of IgA nephropathy in France [1, 9, 30, 31], investigators found a consistent combination of IgA with IgG and C3, but not IgM. Studies from other countries have shown a higher incidence of associated IgM [12, 14, 15], and an IgA-IgG combination was found in approximately 50% of patients (13, 32, 33), with IgA alone in approximately 40% of patients. Since IgA is the only constant immunoglobulin, the appropriate term is mesangial IgA nephropathy. Most workers have failed to find IgA-SC in the glomerular mesangium [13–15, 26]. Several studies have shown the deposits of IgA to be subclass IgA-1 [34, 35], whereas others have observed IgA-2 [36, 37]. This difference may be due to the types of antisera used or to different techniques. A possible geographic variation in the antibody response cannot be excluded completely until further work is done. There was no correlation between the intensity of IgA and accompanying deposits of immunoproteins and the type of glomerular lesion or clinical manifestation of disease. Early complement components Clq and C4 were either absent or were found infrequently and in weak scattered specks, and always in the presence of IgM or IgG. The activation of C3 via the alternative pathway is well established [12, 13, 15, 16, 38], and properdin has been demonstrated in the deposits [15, 39].

The glomerular morphology was reported initially as a focal type of glomerulonephritis that affected only part of a glomerulus [2, 9, 10], but others have observed a variable glomerular morphology [4, 13–15, 29, 40]. The basic glomerular lesions were minimal and minor change, focal glomerulonephritis, diffuse mesangial proliferative glomerulonephritis, and diffuse sclerosing glomerulonephritis. Superimposed lesions of sclerosis, adhesions, and crescents were more frequent in proliferative glomerular lesions. The glomerular lesions were related to the stage, duration, and severity of the disease, with a higher incidence of diffuse mesangial cell proliferation with sclerosis, and tubulointerstitial fibrosis where the biopsies were performed at the later stages, and also in more severe diseases like acute nephritis and the nephrotic syndrome.

The mean age of the patients (22.9 ± [SD] 12.8 yr) agreed with the age distribution reported by others [4, 12]. The age of onset of hematuria in children with IgA was 4 to 14 yrs [27]. The higher incidence of IgA nephropathy in males has been due to the performance of regular medical examinations on male army recruits [13, 18, 23], and no sex difference was observed in the patients with symptomatic disease. However, others have reported a definite male predominance [17]. Initially, Berger [2] reported that his patients showed microhematuria with slight or no proteinuria, and no nephrotic syndrome. Subsequent reports showed varied clinical expression of the disease [10, 13, 15, 40]. The higher incidence of the nephrotic syndrome in Singapore than in other centers [16, 26, 33, 41] may reflect more severe involvement in our patients. Though no infective agent was identified, upper respiratory infections precipitated or exacerbated the disease.

There was a good correlation between the creatinine clearance and the type of glomerular lesion. There was an abnormal clearance in patients with diffuse mesangial cell proliferation, and with superimposed glomerular lesions of sclerosis and crescent formation. A similarly good correlation was observed between the degree of proteinuria and the type of glomerular lesion. There was heavier proteinuria in patients with diffuse mesangial cell proliferation and associated glomerulosclerosis than that found in patients with minor change. The distribution pattern of IgA and immunoprotein mesangial deposits was not significant, but observations on electron microscopy showed that paramesangial-subendothelial extensions of the mesangial deposits were indicative of a more severe renal disease than pure mesangial deposits. Mesangiolysis also appeared to precede the development of glomerular sclerosis. These findings could be useful indicators of the severity of the renal lesion and prognosis.

The group of patients with minor change nephrotic syndrome and mesangial IgA deposits may represent either a variant of IgA nephropathy, or the development of IgA nephropathy superimposed upon minimal change disease (lipoid nephrosis). Incidental mesangial IgA deposits were found as a predominant immunoglobulin in 4% of 200 consecutive control autopsies in Singapore (42), and it is possible that IgA might be present in the mesangium of these minor change nephrotic syndrome patients as an incidental finding. However, unlike "classical" lipoid nephrosis, the majority of patients had frequent relapses and remission was obtained in some only with combined prednisolone, cyclophosphamide, and persantin therapy. It is advisable to obtain data from more patients, with longer follow-up to resolve this problem of one or two co-existent lesions in minor change nephrotic syndrome with mesangial IgA deposits.

Though the enigma of IgA nephropathy has yet to be solved, we have made considerable progress in a better understanding of this widespread disease(s). We owe much to Dr. Berger for having defined this immunopathological lesion, one that is now attracting much attention from nephrologists in many countries.

Acknowledgments. This work was supported by grants from the National University of Singapore, The Ministry of Health and the P.B. Davar Memorial Fund.

References

1. BERGER J, HINGLAIS N: Les depots intercapillaires d'IgA-IgG. *J Urol Nephrol* 74:694–695, 1968
2. BERGER J: IgA glomerular deposits in renal disease. *Transplant Proc* 1:934–944, 1969
3. SINNIAH R, FENG PH: Lupus nephritis: Correlation between light, electron microscopic and immunofluorescent findings and renal function. *Clin Nephrol* 6:340–351, 1976
4. CLARKSON AR, SEYMOUR AE, THOMPSON AJ, HAYNES WDG, CHAN YL, JACKSON B: IgA nephropathy: A syndrome of uniform morphology, diverse clinical features, and uncertain prognosis. *Clin Nephrol* 8:459–471, 1977
5. SINNIAH R, FENG PH, CHEN BTM: Henoch-Schönlein syndrome: A clinical and morphological study of renal biopsies. *Clin Nephrol* 9:219–228, 1978
6. CALLARD P, FELDMANN G, PRANDI P, BELAIR MF, MAUDET C, WEISS Y, DRUET P, BENHAMOU JP, BARIETY J: Immune complex type glomerulonephritis in cirrhosis of the liver. *Am J Pathol* 80:329–337, 1975
7. BERGER J, YANEVA H, NABARRA B: Glomerular changes in patients with cirrhosis of the liver, in *Advances in Nephrology,* edited by HAMBURGER J, CROSNIER J, MAXWELL H, Chicago, Year Book Medical, 1978, p 3
8. SINNIAH R: Mucin secreting cancer with mesangial IgA deposits. *Pathology* 14:303–308, 1982
9. MOREL-MAROGER L, LEATHEM A, RICHET G: Glomerular abnormalities in non-systemic diseases: Relationship between findings by light microscopy and immunofluorescence in 433 renal biopsy specimens. *Am J Med* 53:170–184, 1972
10. DROZ D: Natural history of primary glomerulonephritis with mesangial deposits of IgA. *Contrib Nephrol* 2:150–157, 1976
11. DI BELGIOJOSO GB, TARANTINO A, CIVATI G, LIMIDO D, MINETTI L: Glomerulonefrite A Depositi Intercapillari Di IgA-IgG. *Studio Clinico E Morfologico Di 63 Casi Rincera Clin Lab* 3:30–62, 1973
12. SHIRAI T, TOMINO Y, SATO M, YOSHIKI T, ITOH T: IgA nephropathy: clinicopathology and immunopathology. *Contrib Nephrol* 9:88–100, 1978
13. SINNIAH R, JAVIER AR, KU G: The pathology of mesangial IgA nephritis with clinical correlation. *Histopathology* 5:469–490, 1981.
14. LOWANCE DC, MULLINS JD, MCPHAUL JJ JR: Immunoglobulin A (IgA) associated GN. *Kidney Int* 3:167–176, 1973
15. MCCOY RC, ABRAMOWSKY CR, TISHER CC: IgA nephropathy. *Am J Pathol* 76:123–144, 1974
16. SISSONS JGP, WOODROW DF, CURTIS JR, EVANS DJ, GOWER PE, SLOPER JC, PETERS DK: Isolated glomerulonephritis with mesangial IgA deposits. *Br Med J* 3:611–614, 1975
17. BURKHOLDER PM, ZIMMERMAN SW, MOORTHY AV: A clinicopathologic study of the natural history of mesangial IgA nephropathy, in *Glomerulonephritis: Progression and Regression,* edited by YOSHITOSHI Y, UEDA Y, Baltimore, University Park Press, 1978, p 143
18. SINNIAH R, PWEE HS, LIM CH: Glomerular lesions in asymptomatic microscopic haematuria discovered on routine medical examination. *Clin Nephrol* 5:216–228, 1976
19. CHURG J, SOBIN LH: *WHO Classification and Atlas of Glomerular Diseases.* Tokyo, New York, Igaku-Shoin, 1982
20. SINNIAH R, CHURG J: Effect of IgA deposits on the glomerular mesangium in Berger's disease. *Ultrastruct Pathol* 4:9–22, 1983

21. VERNIER RL, MAUER SM, FISH AF, MICHAEL AF: The mesangial cell in glomerulonephritis. *Adv Nephrol* 1:31–46, 1971
22. ELEMA JD, HOYER JR, VERNIER RL: The glomerular mesangium: Uptake and transport of intravenously injected colloidal carbon in rats. *Kidney Int* 9:395–406, 1976
23. SINNIAH R, LAW CH, PWEE HS: Glomerular lesions in patients with asymptomatic persistent and orthostatic proteinuria discovered on routine medical examination. *Clin Nephrol* 7:1–14, 1977
24. NEWKIRK MM, KLEIN MH, KATZ A, FISHER MM, UNDERDOWN BJ: Estimation of polymeric IgA in human serum: An assay based on binding of radiolabelled human secretory component with applications in the study of IgA neophropathy, IgA monoclonal gammopathy, and liver disease. *J Immunol* 130:1176–1181, 1983
25. SAKAI O, KITAJIMA T, KAWAMMA K, UEDA Y: Clinicopathological studies on IgA glomerulonephritis, in *Glomerulonephritis, Proceedings of the International Symposium on Glomerulonephritis,* edited by YOSHITOSHI Y, UEDA Y, Tokyo, University of Tokyo Press, 1979, p 167
26. BERGER J, YANEVA H, NABARRA B, BARBANEL C: Recurrence of mesangial deposition of IgA after renal transplantation. *Kidney Int* 7:232–241, 1975
27. MCENERY PT, MCADAMS AJ, WEST CD: Glomerular morphology, natural history and treatment of children with IgA-IgG mesangial nephropathy, in *Glomerulonephritis: Morphology, Natural History and Treatment,* edited by KINCAID-SMITH P, MATHEW TH, BECKER EL, New York, John Wiley & Sons, 1973, p 305
28. VAN DER PEET J, ARISZ L, BRENTJENS JRH: The clinical course of IgA nephropathy in adults. *Clin Nephrol* 8:335–340, 1977
29. KURT LEE SM, RAO VM, FRANKLIN WA, SCHIFFER MS, ARONSON AJ, SPARGO BH, KATZ AI: IgA nephropathy: Morphologic predictors of progressive renal disease. *Human Pathol* 13:314–322, 1982
30. DRUET P, BARIETY J, BERNARD D, LAGRUE G: Les glomerulopathies primitives a depots mesangiaux d'IgA et d'IgG: Etude clinique et morphologique de 52 cas. *Presse Med* 78:583–587, 1970
31. LEVY M, BEAUFILS H, GUBLER MC, HABIB R: Idiopathic recurrent macroscopic haematuria and mesangial IgA-IgG deposits in children (Berger's disease). *Clin Nephrol* 1:63–69, 1973
32. BARIETY J, DRUET PH: Resultats de L'immunohistochemic de 589 biopsies renales (Transplantes exclus). *Ann Med Intern* 122:63–69, 1971
33. WOODROFFE AJ, THOMSON NM, MEADOWS R, LAWRENCE JR: IgA-associated glomerulonephritis. *Aust NZ J Med* 5:97–100, 1975
34. CONLEY ME, COOPER MD, MICHAEL AF: Selective deposition of immunoglobulin A-1 in immunoglobulin A nephropathy, anaphylactoid purpura nephritis, and systemic lupus erythematosus. *J Clin Invest* 66:1432–1436, 1980
35. TOMINO Y, ENDOH M, NOMOTO Y, SAKAI H: Immunoglobulin A1 in IgA nephropathy. *N Engl J Med* 305:1159–1160, 1981
36. ANDRE C, BERTHOUX FC, ANDRE F, GILLOU J, GENIN C, SABATIER JC: Prevalence of IgA2 deposits in IgA nephropathies: A clue to their pathogenesis. *N Engl J Med* 303:1343–1346, 1980
37. BENE MC, FAURE G, LEVY M, DUHEILLE J: Identification de la sous-classe IgA1 et/ou IgA2 des depots mesangiaux d'IgA. *Nouv Presse Med* 11:2639–2640, 1982
38. GÖTZE O, MÜLLER-EBERHARD HJ: The C3-activator system: An alternate pathway of complement activation. *J Exp Med* 134:90–108, 1971
39. EVANS DJ, WILLIAMS DG, PETERS DK, SISSONS JGP, BOULTON-JONES JM, OGG

CS, Cameron JS, Hoffbrand BI: Glomerular deposition of properdin in Henoch-Schönlein syndrome and idiopathic focal nephritis. *Br Med J* 3:326–328, 1973

40. LEVY M, BEAUFILS H, GUBLER MC, HABIB R: Idiopathic recurrent macroscopic hematuria and mesangial IgA-IgG deposits in children (Berger's disease). *Clin Nephrol* 1:63–69, 1973

41. FINLAYSON G, ALEXANDER R, JUNCOS L, SCHLEIN E, TEAGUE P, WALDMAN R, CADE R: Immunoglobulin A glomerulonephritis: A clinicopathologic study. *Lab Invest* 32:140–148, 1975

42. SINNIAH R: Occurrence of mesangial IgA and IgM deposits in a control necropsy population. *J. Clin Pathol* 36:276–279, 1983.

Natural History and Treatment of Idiopathic IgA Nephropathy

Giuseppe D'Amico

IgA nephropathy appears to be a ubiquitous disorder, but its geographical distribution is irregular [1, 2]. In some countries (the USA, Britain, and Holland), it seems to be uncommon (5% of all glomerular diseases [3–10]. It is very common in other countries [11–32], including Southern Europe (France, Italy and Spain), Asia (Japan and Singapore) and Australia; its incidence ranges from 20 to 25% in Southern Europe and Australia to 30 to 40% in Japan. At the moment, it is difficult to say whether these divergent estimates reflect real differences in the occurrence of the disease in the various areas or reflect differences in the indications for renal biopsy among investigators, patient populations, or the frequency and extent of immunohistochemic investigations of renal biopsy material in the different countries. In Japan, where the disease is reported most frequently, a periodic screening of urine in a healthy population of different age groups and a subsequent study of those with urinary abnormalities are an accepted routine: this policy allows for an early discovery of all cases of IgA mesangial nephropathy in whom asymptomatic urinary abnormalities are the only presenting clinical syndrome [33]. In a recent retrospective analysis of all renal biopsy examinations performed in Northeast Scotland [34], where the principal reason for biopsy in 55% of them was an asymptomatic isolated microscopic hematuria, IgA mesangial nephropathy represented 21.8% of all primary glomerular disease. This figure is similar to that reported in Southern Europe, and higher than that previously reported from Britain [19].

The disease occurs at all ages [3–32], but it is most common in the second and third decades of life (Fig. 1). It affects males more frequently than females [1, 2]. The male:female ratio varies from country to country. It is less than 2:1 in Japan, based on a multicenter survey of 2,675 patients [33]. It is 2.4:1.0 in our 374 patients [2] and in the 244 patients of Droz et al [35]. And it is higher than 3:1 (up to 6:1) in the majority of reports from Northern Europe and the USA [3, 4, 6, 7, 9, 10, 26, 36, 37].

This manuscript was presented as part of a Symposium on *IgA Nephropathy*.

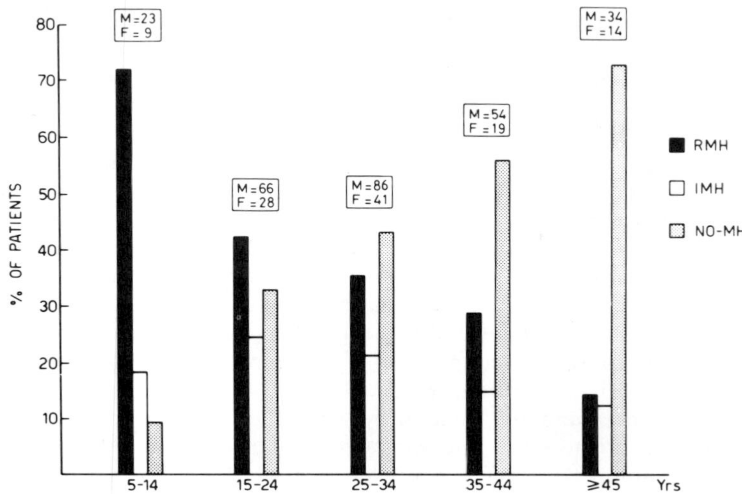

Fig. 1. Sex and number of patients, and relative incidence (%) of the three types of hematuria, in the various age groups. *RMH* refers to recurrent macroscopic hematuria; *IMH,* isolated episode of macroscopic hematuria; *No-MH,* no known history of macroscopic hematuria.

A higher prevalence among white patients, in comparison with blacks, is reported in the USA, even though this is based on very small numbers of patients [7, 8]. Some studies report its occurrence in members of the same family [9, 17, 26, 38–40], but this appears to be an uncommon finding in all the largest surveys.

The clinical signs at the time of diagnostic study are varied. One of the following three types of hematuria can be observed or reported by the patients:

1. *Asymptomatic microscopic hematuria (No-MH), with usually mild proteinuria.* Asymptomatic microscopic hematuria is often casually discovered during an occasional urinalysis. These patients have no history of previous episodes of macroscopic hematuria or other signs of renal disease. The microscopic hematuria is persistent, sometimes intermittent, and its extent appears to vary over time, as shown when the Addis count is used to monitor the presence of red cells in the urinary sediment. During the subsequent follow-up examinations, the appearance of an episode of gross hematuria is an exceptional phenomenon (3 out of 165 patients, in our experience).

2. *Isolated episode of macroscopic hematuria (IMH).* Some patients experience an isolated episode of macroscopic hematuria, which marks the apparent clinical onset of the disease and probably coincides with its true onset. The gross hematuria is not associated at presentation with the other signs that characterize the acute nephritic syndrome (elevation of BUN, arterial hypertension, massive proteinuria), except in a minority of patients (from 1 to 9% in different surveys [1]). The hematuric syndrome may be associated closely with an episode of pharyngitis or other infectious events involving the mucosal system, and may be accompanied by loin pain and fever. The

interval between the precipitating infectious event and the appearance of gross hematuria is characteristically very short (24 to 48 hours). The duration of macroscopic hematuria varies from a few hours to many days. In a few patients, the episode of gross hematuria is associated not only with a nephritic syndrome, but also with an acute oliguric renal failure, which is usually reversible. During the subsequent follow-up examinations of urine, there is a persistent, often intermittent microscopic hematuria, with a proteinuria, which is usually mild and without presence of casts.

3. *Recurrent macroscopic hematuria (RMH)*. Some patients have recurring episodes of macroscopic hematuria. The recurrence is often associated closely with the same type of infectious events just described, or less frequently with a physical strenuous effort; in our experience, infections were localized in the respiratory tract in 77% of these patients, in the urinary tract in 8%, in the gastrointestinal tract in 4%, in others areas in 11%. The number of recurrences and the interval between the different episodes are variable. In our experience, the interval ranged from a few months to many years, and the number of recurrences ranged from 1 to 15 (1 in 15 patients, 2 in 46 patients, between 3 and 5 in 32 patients, between 6 and 15 in 8 patients). In patients with many recurrences, the interval between the different episodes tends to become longer with time.

The relative incidence of these three clinical syndromes is dependent on the age of the patients. Figure 1, which summarizes our data on 374 patients [2], shows that with increasing patient age at the apparent onset of the disease, the relative incidence of RMH progressively decreases, whereas the disease is increasingly found, often casually, in patients without any previous history of gross hematuria (No-MH). The incidence of IMH as the presenting syndrome appears to be much less age-dependent, even though it also tends to become less frequent in oldest patients. Data from the literature (for review, see Ref. 1) confirm the high incidence of RMH (80 to 95% of patients) as the characterizing clinical syndrome in all pediatric surveys [41–45] and show also that in adult populations of patients who do not differ in their mean age the relative incidence of this syndrome varies greatly [1, 2]. As has been pointed out in discussing the variable reported incidence of the disease, this difference can be due to the criteria used to select which patients will undergo biopsy examination. In particular, it can be due to the different attitudes concerning the diagnosis of patients with mild asymptomatic microscopic hematuria and proteinuria. However, this variable incidence in the different geographical areas can reflect true differences in the clinical presentation of the disease as well.

Proteinuria is usually mild in IgA mesangial nephropathy. At the time of diagnostic study, it was less than 1 g (per 24 hr) in 64.2% of our patients, between 1.1 and 2 g in 21.9%, between 2 and 3 g in 7%, and greater than 3 g only in 6.9% [2].

Clinically evident nephrotic syndrome is infrequent either at presentation or during the follow-up examinations [1], even though the percentages reported have ranged from less than 10 to up to 24% by some investigators from different geographical areas, and in particular from the USA [4–6, 19, 24, 36, 37, 46]. In patients without renal insufficiency, proteinuria is rather selective [17, 47]. In most reports, abnormally high levels of serum IgA are found in one-third to one-half of the patients [1]. Lower percentages (8% and 15%, respectively) have been reported in two pediatric populations [41, 44]. Levels over 350 mg/dl were found in 38% of our patients [2]. Serum complement factors are in the normal range. Circulating cryoglobulins are absent, according to the majority of investigators, including ourselves. An abnormally high incidence of hyperuricemia has been described [17, 48].

Determination of circulating immune complexes (CICs), especially of IgA-containing CICs, can give useful information, as will be discussed elsewhere in this volume.

Natural History and Outcome

For some time, the disease has been recognized as a distinct form of primary glomerular disease on the basis of its immunohistologic features (diffuse mesangial deposition of immunoglobulins, predominantly IgA, on immunofluorescence microscopy). But it is only in the last 10 to 15 years that a study on a sufficiently large cohort of patients has been made possible through the use of immunohistologic tests. Furthermore, it is impossible to establish, even approximately, the true onset of the disease in the No-MH subgroup of patients (those who have asymptomatic microscopic hematuria and proteinuria and no history of previous macroscopic hematuria). Therefore, the natural history of the disease and its outcome are still defined incompletely. However, a few long-term studies have become available in the last few years, and they indicate several features of the disease: (a) Idiopathic IgA mesangial nephropathy is a relentlessly chronic disease; even though a few cases of rather prolonged regression of all clinical signs have occasionally been found, disappearance of IgA deposition on immunofluorescence with histologic healing has never been described to our knowledge. (b) There is more and more evidence for progression to renal failure in an increasing number of patients, even though considerable debate still exists about the overall incidence of renal insufficiency and the average rate of its progression to end-stage. (c) The most frequent clinical course is an indolent, slowly progressive one, eventually leading to chronic renal failure after quite a long term, but the rapidity of the progression appears to vary greatly. The majority of investigators have described a few patients who develop end-stage renal failure very soon after the first incidental discovery of urinary abnormalities or the first episode of gross hematuria.

Figure 2 shows the actuarial curve of progression to the start of maintenance dialysis in 365 of the 374 patients studied by us in Milan [49]. They had had the disease at least 1 year (1 to 46 years) since its apparent onset (average follow-up, 7.79 ± 6.19 years; median, 6.16 years), and 15.3% and 33.8% of them received maintenance dialysis for 10 and 20 years, respectively, after the apparent onset. Similar survival rates have recently been reported in France by Droz and Noel [50] and in Spain by Egido et al [19]. Considering that the true onset can considerably antedate the apparent onset from which

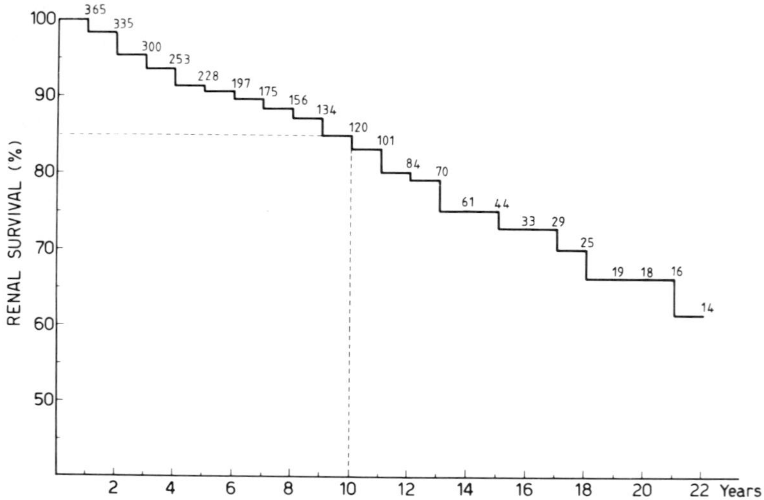

Fig. 2. Renal survival curve in 365 patients. The curve was calculated according to Kaplan and Meier [73].

survival is calculated, at least in the subgroup of patients in whom no episodes of gross hematuria mark the start of the disease, we can estimate that renal survival in idiopathic IgA mesangial nephropathy is higher than 90% at 10 years and 75% at 20 years.

The clinical course of the disease is usually characterized by very few clinical signs. For years, microscopic hematuria and proteinuria, usually mild, may be the only sign in patients who do not present a history of recurrent macroscopic hematuria. The same occasional infectious diseases that precipitate the new episodes of gross hematuria in the RMH subgroup of patients may cause a transitory increase in the number of urinary red cells in the No-MH subgroup of patients.

The amount of proteinuria tends to remain rather stable. However, some occasional transitory exacerbations occur in a few patients, sometimes associated with a recurrent episode of macroscopic hematuria or with an increase in the amount of microscopic hematuria. These exacerbations are sometimes linked to one of the aforementioned infectious events that precipitate the episodes of gross hematuria, but they occur often without any recognizable cause. In some patients they are the first sign of a progressive course. High blood pressure develops frequently during the clinical course, often before the serum creatinine concentration increases to pathologic levels. In our experience [2], at the time of biopsy examination, after an average period of 3.66 ± 5.04 years (range, 0 to 43 years) from the apparent onset of the disease, 135 of 374 patients (36.1%) showed arterial hypertension, with no different incidence in males and females. At the same time, only 91 of 374 patients (24.3%) presented serum creatinine concentrations greater than 1.4 mg/dl ($>$ 3 mg/dl in 17). At the latest observation, at the end of 1983, after an average post-biopsy follow-up of 5.05 ± 3.66 years (median, 4.08 years), 50 more patients out of 292 with a post-biopsy follow-up of at least 1 year showed arterial hypertension; 47 of them had a serum creatinine concentration greater than 1.4 mg/dl and 21 were receiving maintenance dialysis.

In a smaller group of patients, however, we demonstrated [51] that the incidence of high blood pressure at different degrees of renal insufficiency is not higher than it is in other types of primary glomerulonephritis such as membranous or membranoproliferative glomerulonephritis and that it is lower than it is in focal glomerulosclerosis. In a few patients, hypertension has an accelerated course, leading to rapid deterioration of renal function. The incidence of malignant hypertension appears to vary in the different reports: it is very low in our experience and increases to 7% in the study of Clarkson et al [13] and to 10% in that of Rambausek et al [26]. A very rapid decline in renal function, with the clinical syndrome of acute renal failure, may develop during the course of the disease, even without the previous or concomitant appearance of malignant hypertension. We observed two such patients in whom serum creatinine reached the levels of 7.5 and 13 mg/dl, respectively. The first one showed this abrupt deterioration after more than one year of a clinical course characterized by two episodes of macroscopic hematuria with normal renal function. In the second, the acute syndrome developed after only two months of a history of gross hematuria and mild edema. No precipitating events could be shown in either patient. Renal biopsy examination at that time revealed the presence of cellular circumferential crescents in 50% and 67% of glomeruli, respectively. Similar patients with crescents in the majority of glomeruli have been described by others [13, 45, 52, 53].

Serum IgA concentrations do not change much during follow-up; patients with initially high concentrations usually continue with their increased concentration, and those with initially normal levels show no tendency to develop an abnormal elevation. After repeated long-term monitoring (1 to 8 years) of serum IgA concentrations in 66 patients, we observed at the latest determination an abnormal increase in only 3 of 35 patients with an initially normal concentration (< 350 mg/dl), and a decrease to normal in only 6 of 31 with initially high concentrations (> 350 mg/dl). Pregnancy is usually well tolerated by patients and does not result in deterioration of renal function or a rise in blood pressure [17, 18, 54]. IgA mesangial nephropathy recurs very frequently after transplantation within 1 to 4 years [18, 55–57]. So far, the clinical course of the recurrent disease appears to be mild, light proteinuria and microscopic hematuria usually being the only clinical manifestation. In contrast, transplantation of donor kidneys with mesangial IgA deposits into patients with previous non-IgA-related disease results in disappearance of the deposits [58–60].

Clinical and Histologic Prognostic Markers

Because IgA mesangial nephropathy is a disease with a variable rate of progression and is, at least in some countries, one of the most frequent causes of chronic renal failure requiring maintenance dialysis and transplantation, it is obviously of paramount importance to single out at the time of diagnostic study which clinical or histologic parameters are the most useful as prognostic indexes. Data reported in the past were disappointing, possibly because of the small number of prolonged post-biopsy follow-up studies on sufficiently large populations. However, the analysis of some larger cohorts of patients has recently brought to light some significant clinicopathologic correlations and some reliable prognostic indexes.

We chose two different approaches to this problem: (a) We compared the renal survival curves from the apparent onset in 365 of our 374 patients with at least one year of overall follow-up (to study the importance of age, sex, and type of hematuria for survival), and from the time of biopsy in 292 patients with at least one year of post-biopsy follow-up (to study the importance of some other clinical and histologic parameters for survival). (b) We compared two populations who had a normal serum creatinine at the time of biopsy but a different outcome (normal or abnormal serum creatinine) within five years of the post-biopsy follow-up [49]. The results of our statistical analysis, summarized in Table 1, allow the following conclusions:

Table 1. Clinical, histologic, and immunohistologic markers of poor prognosis in idiopathic IgA nephropathy

Parameters	Increased risk[a]	Actual development of renal insufficiency[b]
Clinical parameters		
Older age at onset	Yes ($P < 0.04$)	No ($P = 0.058$)
Male sex	No	No ($P = 0.073$)
Absence of episodes of macroscopic hematuria	Yes ($P < 0.002$)	Yes ($P < 0.04$)
Heavy proteinuria (>1 g per 24 hrs)	Yes ($P < 0.001$)	No
High levels of serum IgA (>350 mg/dl)	No	No
Arterial hypertension	Yes ($P < 0.0001$)	Yes ($P < 0.0002$)
Histologic parameters		
Diffuse and global mesangial proliferation	Yes ($P < 0.0001$)	No ($P = 0.082$)
Extracapillary proliferation	Yes ($P < 0.04$)	No
Global glomerular sclerosis	Yes ($P < 0.0001$)	Yes ($P < 0.0008$)
Segmental glomerular sclerosis	Yes ($P < 0.0005$)	Yes ($P < 0.003$)
Segmental thickening of glomerular capillary walls	Yes ($P < 0.0005$)	—
Interstitial sclerosis	Yes ($P < 0.0001$)	Yes ($P < 0.02$)
Arteriolar hyalinosis	No ($P = 0.076$)	No
Immunohistologic parameters		
Parietal extension of deposits at IF	Yes ($P < 0.002$)	No ($P = 0.078$)
Presence of IgM, C3, C4, or fibrinogen at IF	No	No

[a] Increased risk was determined by the log-rank test on renal survival curves [74]. This group of patients ($N = 292$) were those who had at least one year of post-biopsy follow-up.

[b] This refers to development of renal insufficiency within 5 years from the time of biopsy (determined by contingency table analysis) ($N = 92$ patients with normal serum creatinine concentration at biopsy.)

1. The rate of progression to renal failure was not necessarily time-dependent. Even in the group of patients in whom an episode of macroscopic hematuria was reported, which very likely heralded the true onset of the disease, those who had more severe lesions at the time of biopsy and a more rapid development of renal insufficiency did not have a significantly longer duration of the prebiopsy follow-up. Similar results have been reported by others [4, 6, 19, 45].

2. The relative risk of developing renal failure significantly increased in certain patients: (a) those who were older at onset (1.77 in patients aged $\geq$ 40 yr, vs. 1.18 in those aged 25 to 39 yr, vs. 0.49 in those aged 5 to 24 yr); (b) those who had a proteinuria greater than 1 g per 24 hr at the time of biopsy (1.95 vs. 0.44); (c) those who had a high blood pressure at the time of biopsy (2.00 vs. 0.41); (d) those who did not report a history of recurrent macroscopic hematuria (1.69 vs. 0.91 for isolated episodes of macroscopic hematuria and 0.40 for recurrent macroscopic hematuria). Other investigators have also recently reported some correlation between severity of lesions or progression to renal failure and age at onset [19, 26, 35], proteinuria at biopsy [4, 6, 13, 19, 21, 26, 35, 45–47], arterial hypertension at biopsy [3, 6, 7, 10, 19, 21, 26, 29, 50], and absence of recurrent macroscopic hematuria [9, 13, 19, 26, 29, 35, 36, 47].

In our patients who had isolated episodes of macroscopic hematuria (IMH), the relative risk of progression to renal failure was significantly higher than it was for those with RMH, and the renal survival curve was intermediate between those of the RMH subgroup and of the No-MH subgroup (Fig. 3), in spite of the fact that some patients now classified in the IMH subgroup

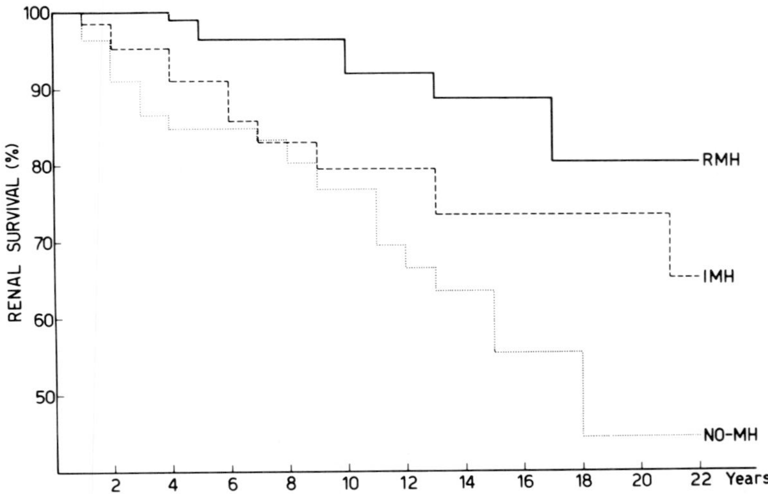

Fig. 3. Renal survival curves of the patients with the three different types of hematuria. *RMH* refers to recurrent macroscopic hematuria; *IMH,* to isolated episode of macroscopic hematuria; *No-MH,* to no known history of macroscopic hematuria.

will possibly experience new episodes of gross hematuria in the future and therefore belong to the RMH subgroup. Since the true onset of the disease could be established with comparable accuracy in both subgroups presenting with macroscopic hematuria (RMH and IMH), our data suggest that the probability of developing renal failure in IgA nephropathy is inversely proportional to the number of episodes of macroscopic hematuria—the opposite of what one would expect. A discontinuous effect of the injuring mechanism, limited to the clinical exacerbations, in RMH, as opposed to a continuous one in No-MH and in IMH, could explain this phenomenon.

Since patients with RMH are in general younger than those with IMH or with No-MH, we adjusted the renal survival curves to reflect age (stratification by age groups). For the three subgroups with different types of hematuria, we found, in contrast with the results of Droz et al [35], that the risk of developing renal failure was still significantly lower in patients with RMH (0.40 vs. 1.05 in those with IMH and 1.45 in those with No-MH; $P = 0.002$).

Furthermore, we studied the effect of age on progression to renal failure separately in the subgroup of patients with RMH, in whom the true onset of the disease could be ascertained with good approximation: again, the older patients had a higher risk of progression (3.48 in patients aged $\geq$ 40 yr vs. 0.26 in patients aged 5 to 24 yr). This disproves the assumption that older patients seem to have a more rapid progression only because the disease is discovered in a later stage.

In contrast with the results of others [26, 35, 36, 45], we could not find any significant difference in the severity of lesions or rate of progression to renal failure in males as compared to females. As reported also by other investigators [6, 13, 19, 21, 29, 35, 37], the serum IgA concentration did not show any value as a prognostic marker.

3. The relative risk of developing renal failure significantly increased (Table 1) in patients who showed certain features at the time of biopsy. One feature was a severe and diffuse mesangial proliferation (2.47 vs. 0.67 of those with focal and segmental proliferation, and 0.00 of those with minimal histologic lesions). Another feature was some degree of extracapillary proliferation (1.42 vs. 0.77), segmental thickening of peripheral capillary wall (2.39 vs. 0.80). Other features were severe global glomerular sclerosis (4.06 in those with > 30% of obsolescent glomeruli, vs. 1.64 in those with 16 to 30%, vs. 0.17 in those with 0 to 15%); segmental glomerular sclerosis (1.35 vs. 0.22); and interstitial sclerosis (1.45 vs. 0.07).

On the contrary, the increase in the relative risk of renal failure in patients with arteriolar hyalinosis (1.34 vs. 0.80) did not reach statistical significance ($P = 0.08$).

None of our 80 patients without obsolescent glomeruli and only one of the 89 patients without interstitial sclerosis developed renal failure within the average 5.05 $\pm$ 3.66 years of post-biopsy follow-up. As already stated by others [3, 6, 13, 19, 21, 26, 29], the degree of glomerular and interstitial sclerosis is the predominant factor in conditioning progression to renal failure in this glomerulonephritis. Some investigators have also stressed the prognostic significance of extracapillary proliferation [7, 21], of vascular lesions [19, 21, 26], and of lesions of the glomerular capillary wall [25, 28, 47].

Even when adjusted for global glomerular sclerosis, interstitial sclerosis significantly affected the relative risk of renal failure (1.13 vs. 0.18; $P = 0.02$), suggesting a partially independent effect. A similar independent effect in increasing the relative risk of renal failure, when data were adjusted for global glomerular sclerosis, showed diffuse mesangial proliferation (1.43, vs. 0.75 of patients with focal segmental proliferation, vs. 0.00 of patients with minimal histologic lesions; $P = 0.014$) and proteinuria greater than 1 g per 24 hours (1.27 vs. 0.66; $P = 0.027$), but not extracapillary proliferation (1.17 vs. 0.87; $P = 0.31$).

4. The relative risk of developing renal failure significantly increased (Table 1) in patients who showed at the time of biopsy an immunohistologic pattern characterized by the extension of immunofluorescent deposits to the peripheral capillary walls (1.61 vs. 0.68), whereas no prognostic significance could be found for the presence of the different immunoreactants (IgG, IgM, C3, C4, C1q, fibrinogen) in concomitance with IgA. The relative risk of renal failure in patients with the mesangial plus parietal pattern of deposition significantly increased even when data were adjusted for global glomerular sclerosis (1.49 vs. 0.68; $P = 0.005$).

Treatment

There is no proven therapy for IgA nephropathy. Long-term immunosuppression treatment does not seem to confer any benefit, although controlled trials have not been reported so far and are probably not warranted in view of the extended natural history. Only in two special subgroups of patients has the use of these drugs been advocated, and their trial is justified in our opinion: (1) The first of these are the patients with a rapidly progressive course and an acutely appearing renal failure, associated with the presence of circumferential crescents in more than 60% of glomeruli. In two such patients, we obtained a marked improvement of renal insufficiency with the use of steroids (including i.v. pulses) and cyclophosphamide; (2) The second consists of the very few patients with the peculiar syndrome that is characterized by proteinuria in the nephrotic range and is associated with minimal mesangial lesions and the immunohistologic features typical of IgA nephropathy. This syndrome has been described anecdotally by some investigators [61–63] and confirmed by many others at the recent Milano Workshop on IgA nephropathy [64, 65]. Patients seem to respond to corticosteroid therapy, with a complete disappearance of proteinuria, even though a multiple relapsing steroid-sensitive course has been described in the majority of the reported cases. Because upper respiratory tract infections seem to trigger clinical exacerbations in many cases, some French authors [66, 67] performed tonsillectomy and eradication of infected dental foci in IgA nephropathy and reported the consequent reduction of the recurrences of gross hematuria, of the amount of proteinuria, and of the serum levels of IgA. We could not show any beneficial effect of these surgical procedures on the progression to renal failure. Tonsillectomy was performed in 83 out of the 244 patients whose total follow-up period was at least 5 years (in 28 patients before, and in 55 after the clinical onset of the disease). The rate of progression to renal failure at the end of this period of follow-up was not significantly different ($P = 0.28$) in patients without tonsillectomy (9.7%), in those whose tonsils were removed before the clinical onset (10.7%), or in those whose tonsils were removed after the clinical onset (7.3%).

We recommend antibiotic treatment for identified infections during exacerbations of disease, but in our opinion neither long-term administration of these drugs nor tonsillectomy or other active intervention to remove septic foci is warranted. Neither would phenytoin seem warranted. After the first report [68] indicating that phenytoin was capable of decreasing serum IgA, especially polymeric IgA levels, and thereby reducing the number of episodes of macroscopic hematuria and, in some patients, decreasing the amount of IgA deposits, a recent trial [69] failed to show any significant influence of this treatment on the clinical and histologic course. This finding seems in accordance with another recent study demonstrating that the drug is ineffective in reducing concentrations of IgA-containing CICs [70].

Recent experiments have demonstrated that in all renal diseases hemodynamic factors contribute to the progression of glomerular sclerosis, a progression that is aggravated by arterial hypertension and high-protein intake [71, 72]. These findings serve to point out the importance of an adequate treatment of high blood pressure and of specific dietary restrictions to delay the progression of renal impairment in IgA nephropathy.

In spite of the disappointing results of all therapeutic remedies so far, we think that our increasing awareness of the pathogenetic mechanisms responsible for this disease can lead us to more successful approaches in a very near future. As is discussed elsewhere in this section (Egido et al), a defect in the regulation of IgA production caused by an abnormally activated, mucosal immune system seems to be responsible for the accumulation of IgA-containing CICs in the blood, with their subsequent deposition at the glomerular mesangial level to give mesangial overload and glomerular injury. The increased IgA production by B lymphocytes seems to be due to the overactivity of T helper cells, uninhibited by adequate suppressor T cells activity, at the mucosal level. If this pathogenetic mechanism is confirmed, two types of therapeutic approaches appear to be promising and worth trying: (1) selective pharmacologic block of T_α cells or IgA-producing B cells by more specific immunosuppressive agents or mononuclear antibodies; (2) removal of IgA CICs through periodic selective plasma exchange with immunoadsorbants, so that chronic mesangial overload can be partially avoided.

Acknowledgments. Our experience presented here is the result of a close collaboration with two other groups working in Milan, Minetti and colleagues at Ca' Granda Hospital and Ponticelli and colleagues at Policlinico Hospital. The study was supported by Consiglio Nazionale delle Ricerche (Rome), grants 82.01303.04 and 83.02898.04.

We also thank E. Marrubini and G. Duca of the Medical Statistics and Biometry Institute of the University of Milan for performing the statistical analysis.

References

1. D'AMICO G: Idiopathic mesangial IgA nephropathy, in *Glomerular Injury 300 years after Morgagni,* edited by BERTANI T, REMUZZI G, Milan, Wichtig, 1983, p 205

2. COLASANTI G, BANFI G, BARBIANO DI BELGIOIOSO G, BERTOLI S, FOGAZZI G, RAGNI A, PONTICELLI C, MINETTI L, D'AMICO G: Idiopathic IgA mesangial nephropathy: Clinical features. *Contrib Nephrol,* in press

3. BURKHOLDER PM, ZIMMERMAN SW, MOORTHY AV: A clinicopathologic study of the natural history of mesangial IgA nephropathy, in *Glomerulonephritis,* edited by YOSHITOSHI Y, UEDA Y, Baltimore, University Park Press, 1979, p 143

4. CROKER BP, DAWSON DV, SANFILIPPO F: IgA nephropathy: Correlation of clinical and histologic features. *Lab Invest* 48:19–24, 1983

5. FEINER HD, CABILI S, BALDWIN DS, SCHACHT RG, GALLO GR: Intrarenal vascular sclerosis in IgA nephropathy. *Clin Nephrol* 18:183–192, 1982

6. HOOD SA, VELOSA JA, HOLLEY KE, DONADIO JV: IgA-IgG nephropathy: Predictive indices of progressive disease. *Clin Nephrol* 16:55–62, 1981

7. LEE SMK, RAO MV, FRANKLIN WA, SCHIFFER MS, ARONSON AJ, SPARGO BH, KATZ AI: IgA nephropathy: Morphologic predictors of progressive renal disease. *Human Pathol* 13:314–322, 1982

8. McCOY RC, ABRAMOWSKY CR, TISHER CC: IgA nephropathy. *Am J Pathol* 76:123–140, 1974

9. SISSONS JGP, WOODROFFE DF, CURTIS JR: Isolated glomerulonephritis with mesangial IgA deposits. *Br Med J* 3:611–614, 1975

10. VAN DER PEET J, ARISZ L, BRENTJENS JRH, MARRINK J, HOEDEMAEKER PJ: The clinical course of IgA nephropathy in adults. *Clin Nephrol* 8:335–340, 1977

11. BERGER J, HINGLAIS N: Les Dépôts intercapillaires d'IgA-IgG. *J Urol Nephrol* 74:694–695, 1968

12. BERGER J, YANEVA H, CROSNIER J: La glomérulonéphrite à dépôts mésangiaux d'IgA: Une cause fréquente d'insuffisance rénale terminale. *Nouv Presse Med* 9:215–221, 1980

13. CLARKSON AR, SEYMOUR AE, THOMPSON AJ, HAYNES WDG, CHAN YL, JACKSON B: IgA nephropathy: A syndrome of uniform morphology, diverse clinical features and uncertain prognosis. *Clin Nephrol* 8:459–471, 1977

14. COPPO R, BASOLO B, MARTINA G, ROLLINO C, DE MARCHI M, GIACCHINO F, MAZZUCCO G, MESSINA M, PICCOLI G: Circulating immune complexes containing IgA, IgG and IgM in patients with primary IgA nephropathy and with Henoch-Schönlein nephritis: Correlation with clinical and histological signs of activity. *Clin Nephrol* 18:230–239, 1982

15. COVARSI A, FLORES R, BARCELO P, SANTAULARIA JM, BALLARIN J, DEL RIO G: Glomerulonephritis por depòsitos mesangiales de IgA (enfermedad de Berger): Parametros evolutivos. *Nefrologia* 1:15–19, 1981

16. D'AMICO G, FERRARIO F, COLASANTI G, RAGNI A, BESTETTI BOSISIO M: IgA mesangial nephropathy (Berger's disease) with rapid decline in renal function. *Clin Nephrol* 16:251–257, 1981

17. DE WERRA P, MOREL-MAROGER L, LEROUX-ROBERT C, RICHET G: Glomérulites a dépôts d'IgA diffus dans le mésangium: Etude de 96 cas chez l'adulte. *Schweiz Med Wochenschr* 103:761–768, 1973
18. DROZ D: Natural history of primary glomerulonephritis with mesangial deposits of IgA. *Contrib Nephrol* 2:150–156, 1976
19. EGIDO J, RIVIERA HERNANDEZ F, SANCHO J, MORENO M, HERNANDO L: Estudio del sistema HLA y factores de riesgo para la insuficiencia renal en la glomerulonephrithis mesangial IgA. *Nefrologia* 1:21–27, 1981
20. FRASCÀ GM, VANGELISTA A, BIAGINI G, BONOMINI V: Immunological tubulo-interstitial deposits in IgA nephropathy. *Kidney Int* 22:184–191, 1982
21. GUTIERREZ-MILLET V, NAVAS PALACIOS JJ, PRIETO C, RUILOPE LM, USERA G, BARRIENTOS A, ALCAZAR JM, PEREZ AJ, JARILLO MD, RODICIO JL: Glomerulonephrithis mesangial IgA idiopatica: Estudio clinico e immunopatologico de 40 casos y revision de la literatura. *Nefrologia* 2:21–34, 1982
22. HIKI Y, KOBAYASHI Y, TATENO S, SADA M, KASHIWAGI N: Strong association of HLA-DR4 with benign IgA nephropathy. *Nephron* 32:222–226, 1982
23. IMBASCIATI E, COLASANTI G, BARBIANO DI BELGIOIOSO G, BANFI G, DURANTE A, RAGNI A, PONTICELLI C, MINETTI L, D'AMICO G: Long term follow-up of IgA mesangial deposits glomerulonephritis. *Proc EDTA,* 1977, p 472
24. NAKAMOTO Y, ASANO Y, DOHI K, FUJIOKA M, IIDA H, KIBE Y, HATTORI N, TAKEUCHI J: Primary IgA glomerulonephritis and Schönlein-Henoch purpura nephritis: Clinicopathological and immunohistological characteristics. *Q J Med* 47:495–516, 1978
25. NG WL, CHAN CW, YEUNG CK, HUA SP: The pathology of primary IgA glomerulonephritis: A renal biopsy study. *Pathology* 13:137–143, 1981
26. RAMBAUSEK M, SEELING HP, ANDRASSY K, WALDHERR R, KEHRY I, LENHARD V, RITZ E: Mesangial IgA Glomerulonephritis: Neue Aspekte zur Diagnose, Klinik und Prognose. *Dtsch Med Wochenschr* 108:125–130, 1983
27. SAKAI O, KITAJIMA T, KAWAMURA K, UEDA Y: Clinicopathological studies on IgA glomerulonephritis, in *Glomerulonephritis: Proceedings of the International Symposium on Glomerulonephritis; Progression and Regression,* edited by YOSHITOSHI Y, UEDA Y, Baltimore, University Park Press, 1979, p 167
28. SHIGEMATSU H, KOBAYASHI Y, TATENO S, HIKI Y, KUVAO S: Ultrastructural glomerular loop abnormalities in IgA nephritis. *Nephron* 30:1–7, 1982
29. SHIRAI T, TOMINO Y, SATO M, YOSHIKI T, ITOH T: IgA nephropathy: Clinicopathology and immunopathology. *Contrib Nephrol* 9:88–100, 1978
30. SINNIAH R, JAVIER AR, KU G: The pathology of mesangial IgA nephritis with clinical correlation. *Histopathology* 5:469–490, 1981
31. UEDA Y, SAKAI O, YAMAGATA M, KITAJIMA T, KAWAMURA K: IgA glomerulonephritis in Japan. *Contrib Nephrol* 4:36–47, 1977
32. YOKOSKA H, NAGASE M, MAEDA T, KOIDE K: Mesangial IgA glomerulonephritis: Clinicopathological study of 85 cases. *Contrib Nephrol* 9:101–110, 1978
33. KITAJIMA T, MURAKAMI M, SAKAI O: Clinicopathological features in the Japanese patients with IgA nephropathy. *Jpn J Med* 22:219–222, 1983
34. POWER DA, MURHEAD N, SIMPSON JG, HORNE CHW, NICHOLLS AJ, CATTO GRD, EDWARD N: Asymptomatic hematuria and IgA nephropathy: Results of a retrospective renal biopsy study (*abstract*). *Kidney Int* 22:219, 1982
35. DROZ D, KRAMAR A, NAWAR T, NOEL LH: Primary IgA nephropathy: Prognostic factors. *Contrib Nephrol,* in press
36. GÄRTNER HV, HÖNLEIN F, TRAUB U, BOHLE A: IgA-nephropathy (IgA-IgG-

nephropathy/IgA-nephritis): A Disease Entity? *Virchows Arch [Pathol Anat]* 385:1–27, 1979

37. SCHMECKEL B, SVALANDER C, BUCHT H, WESTBERG NG: Mesangial IgA glomerulo-nephritis in adults. *Acta Med Scand* 210:363–372, 1981
38. MONTOLIU J, DARNELL A, TORRAS A, ERCILLA G, VALLES M: Familial IgA nephropathy: Report of two cases and brief review of the literature. *Arch Intern Med* 140:1374–1375, 1980
39. SABATIER JC, GENIN C, ASSENAT H, COLON S, DUCRET F, BERTOUX FC: Mesangial IgA glomerulonephritis in HLA-identical brothers. *Clin Nephrol* 11:35–38, 1978
40. TOLKOFF-RUBIN NE, COSIMI B, RUBIN RH, COLVIN RB: IgA nephropathy in HLA identical siblings. *Transplantation* 26:430–433, 1978
41. KHER KK, MAKKER SP, MOORTHY B: IgA nephropathy (Berger's disease): A clinicopathologic study in children. *Int J Pediatr Nephrol* 4:11–18, 1983
42. LEVY M, BEAUFILS H, GUBLER MC, HABIB R: Idiopathic recurrent macroscopic hematuria and mesangial IgA-IgG deposits in children (Berger's disease). *Clin Nephrol* 1:63–69, 1972
43. LINNÉ T, APERIA A, BROBERGER O, BERGSTRAND A, BOHMAN SO, RECOLA S: Course of renal function in IgA glomerulonephritis in children and adolescents. *Acta Pediatr Scand* 71:735–743, 1982
44. MICHALK D, WALDHERR R, SEELING HP, WEBER HP, SHARER K: Idiopathic mesangial IgA glomerulonephritis in childhood. *Eur J Pediatr* 134:13–22, 1980
45. SOUTHWEST PEDIATRIC NEPHROLOGY STUDY GROUP: A multicentric study of IgA nephropathy in children, *Kidney Int* 22:643–652, 1982
46. KATZ A, WALKER JF, LANDY PJ: IgA nephritis with nephrotic range proteinuria. *Clin Nephrol* 20:67–71, 1983
47. BEUKHOF JR, OCKHUIZEN T, FLEUREN GJ, HAAS M, DONGA J, DONKER AMJ, HOEDEMAEKER PJ, VAN DER HEM GK: The relation between proteinuria and morphology in IgA nephropathy. *Contrib Nephrol,* in press
48. DE FERRARI ME, RADAELLI L, BARBIANO DI BELGIOSO G, BERTOLI S, MINETTI L: Alterazioni del metabolismo dell'acido urico nella malattia di Berger, in *Nefrologia, Dialisi, Trapianto,* edited by BRANCACCIO D, LUPO A, OLDRIZZI C, RUGIU C, VALVO E, Milano, Wichtig, 1982, p 395
49. D'AMICO G, BARBIANO DI BELGIOIOSO G, IMBASCIATI E, FOGAZZI G, RADAELLI L, FERRARIO F, FELLIN G, PONTICELLI C, MINETTI L: Idiopathic IgA mesangial nephropathy: Natural history. *Contrib Nephrol,* in press
50. DROZ D, NOEL LH: Ré-evaluation du prognostic des glomérulonephritides a dépôts intracapillaires d'IgA. *Seminaires de Nephrologie Pediatrique,* Paris, May 1983, p 26
51. VENDEMIA F, FORNASIERI A, VELIS O, BARONI M, SCARDUELLI B, D'AMICO G: Different prevalence rates of hypertension in various renoparenchimal diseases, in *Secondary Forms of Hypertension,* edited by BLAUFOX MD, BIANCHI C, New York, Grune and Stratton, 1980, p 89
52. MARTINI A, MAGRINI U, SCELSI M, CAPELLI V, BARBERIS L: Chronic mesangioproliferative IgA glomerulonephritis complicated by a rapidly progressive course in a 14-year-old boy. *Nephron* 29:164–166, 1981
53. ESPARZA AR, ABUELO JG, MATARESE RA, ENDRENY RG, CARVAHLO JS, ALLEGRA SR: Rapidly progressive IgA nephropathy (abst). *Kidney Int* 23:122, 1983
54. SURIAN M, IMBASCIATI E, COSCI P, BANFI G, BARBIANO DI BELGIOIOSO G, BRANCACCIO D, MINETTI L, PONTICELLI C: Glomerular disease and pregnancy:

A study of 123 pregnancies in patients with primary and secondary glomerular diseases. *Nephron* 36:101–105, 1984

55. BERGER J, YANEVA H, NABARRA B, BARBANEL C: Recurrence of mesangial deposition of IgA after renal transplantation. *Kidney Int* 7:232–241, 1975

56. MATHEWS TH, DC, HOBB JB, KINCAID-SMITH P: Glomerular lesions after renal transplantation. *Am J Med* 59:177–190, 1975

57. CAMERON JS, TURNER DR: Recurrent glomerulonephritis in allografted kidneys. *Clin Nephrol* 7:47–54, 1977

58. LIMAS C, SPECTOR D, WRIGHT JR: Histologic changes in preserved cadaveric renal transplants. *Am J Pathol* 88:403–428, 1977

59. SANFILIPPO F, CROKER BP, BOLLINGER RR: Fate of four cadaveric donor renal allografts with mesangial IgA deposits. *Transplantation* 33:370–376, 1982

60. SILVA FG, CHANDER P, PIRANI CL: Disappearance of glomerular mesangial IgA deposits after renal allograft transplantation. *Transplantation* 33:214–216, 1982

61. SAINT-ANDRE JP, SINARD CL, SPIESSERR, HOUSSIN A: Syndrome néphrotique de l'enfant a lésion glomérulaires minimes, avec dépôts mesangiaux d'IgA. *Nouv Presse Med* 9:531–532, 1980

62. MUSTONEN J, PASTERNACK A, RANTALA I: The nephrotic syndrome in IgA glomerulonephritis: Response to corticosteroid therapy. *Clin Nephrol* 20:172–176, 1983

63. ABREO K, WEN SF: A case of IgA nephropathy with an unusual response to corticosteroid and immunosuppressive therapy. *Am J Kidney Dis* 3:54–57, 1983

64. HOGG RJ, SILVA FG: IgA nephropathy: Natural history and prognostic indices in children. *Contrib Nephrol,* in press

65. D'AMICO G, MINETTI L, PONTICELLI C: IgA mesangial nephropathy: Discussion of session III. *Contrib Nephrol,* in press

66. LAGRUE G, SANDREUX T, LAURENT J, HIRBEC G: Is there a treatment of mesangial IgA glomerulonephritis? *Clin Nephrol* 16:161, 1981

67. VIALTEL P, DECHELETTE E, HACHACHE T, COLOMB H, CORDONNIER D, ROUX O, DUMAS G, ACCOYER B: Role de l'amygdalectomie sur l'évolution des symptomes de la glomérulonephrite a dépôts mésangiaux d'IgA, in *Seminaires d'Uro-Nephrologie,* edited by KÜSS R, LEGRAIN M, Paris, Masson, 1981, p 173

68. LOPEZ-TRASCASA M, EGIDO J, SANCHO J, HERNANDO L: Evidence of high polymeric IgA levels in serum of patients with Berger's disease and its modifications with phenytoin treatment. *Proc EDTA,* 1979, p 513

69. CLARKSON AR, SEYMOUR AE, WOODROFFE AJ, MCKENZIE PE, CHAN YL, WOOTTON AM: Controlled trial on phenytoin therapy in IgA nephropathy. *Clin Nephrol* 13:215–218, 1980

70. COPPO R, BASOLO B, BULZOMÌ MR, PICCOLI G: Ineffectiveness of phenytoin treatment on IgA-containing circulating immune complexes in IgA nephropathy. *Nephron* 36:275–276, 1984

71. BRENNER BM, MEYER TW, HOSTETTER TH: Dietary protein intake and the progressive nature of kidney disease: The role of haemodynamically mediated glomerular injury in the pathogenesis of progressive glomerular sclerosis in aging, renal ablation and intrinsic renal disease. *N Engl J Med* 307:652–659, 1982

72. NEUGARTEN J, FEINER HD, SCHACHT RG, GALLO GR, BALDWIN DS: Aggravation of experimental glomerulonephritis by superimposed clip hypertension. *Kidney Int* 22:257–263, 1982

73. KAPLAN EL, MEIER P: Nonparametric estimation from incomplete observations. *J Am Stat Assoc* 53:457–481, 1958

74. PETO R, PIKE MC, ARMITAGE P, BRESLOW NE, COX DR, HOWARD SV, MANTEL N, MCPHERSON K, PETO J, SMITH PG: Design and analysis of randomized clinical trials requiring prolonged observation of each patient: II. Analysis and examples. *Br J Cancer* 35:1–39, 1977

Acute Renal Failure

Principles of Acute Renal Failure

Michael Steinhausen and Niranjan Parekh

The term *acute renal failure* (ARF) denotes a dramatic clinical situation in which both kidneys stop their excretory function within a very short period of time. The loss of renal function is reflected by oligoanuria and a steady rise in the concentration of urea and creatinine in plasma. The major causes of ARF are either ischemia or toxic insult of the kidneys. Typically, ARF is induced by an acute circulatory shock with oligoanuria persisting for days, even after stabilization of systemic blood pressure. If the patient is treated by dialysis, there is a good chance for complete restitution of kidney function within weeks.

The pathophysiologic mechanisms of ARF have been investigated extensively in the last few decades, and the literature on ARF has been summarized and reviewed many times [1–6]. It is recognized that a number of functional changes are involved in ARF, but the relative importance of these individual changes is controversial. Analysis of the morphologic changes during ARF also gives fruitful information on operative mechanisms. The structural data, however, must be combined with the corresponding functional data to allow for the most meaningful interpretations. Therefore, in this presentation, structural and functional correlates will be discussed together.

A variety of experimental models have been used to study ARF. In experimental animals, ischemic renal damage can be produced by temporary occlusion of one or both renal arteries. One hour of temporary ischemia in rats will cause damage of tubular cells and anuria, but the changes, both structural and functional, are reversible within a few weeks. Similar results can be obtained by a continuous infusion of constrictor levels of norepinephrine into the renal artery to give interrupted renal circulation [7, 8]. Unilateral ischemic ARF avoids uremia, electrolyte imbalance, and mortality, but it causes a compensatory hypertrophy of the contralateral kidney. Also the recovery of renal function in the unilateral model is much slower and less

---

This manuscript was presented as part of a Symposium on *Acute Renal Failure: Structure-Function Relationships.*

complete than in the bilateral model. Other models of ARF use toxic agents such as mercuric chloride (to which tubular cells are very susceptible). The severity of damage can be regulated by varying the doses of the applied toxins. Intramuscular injection of glycerol in dehydrated rats is also used to produce experimental ARF. This model is considered analogous to the clinical "crush syndrome" that is encountered after excessive muscle destruction and is accompanied by myoglobinuria. Pathogenetic factors in the glycerol model are complex. Since increased myoglobin alone will not produce ARF [9], other toxic substances that are released from damaged muscle cells must be involved. Furthermore, the elevated sympathetic tone resulting from pain during muscle disintegration can produce renal ischemia and may contribute to renal damage.

ARF is a process rather than a state. It begins with cellular damage initiated by the primary insult, and it continues until renal function and structure have essentially recovered. Although the time courses of injury and recovery overlap and are variable, ARF may be grossly divided into three phases: pathogenetic phase, manifestation phase, and recovery phase. In the first of these, there is a progressive disintegration and necrosis of tubular cells. Renal inulin clearance is reduced, and oliguria often prevails. In the manifestation phase, there is oligoanuria with severely reduced clearances of creatinine and inulin. These last up to a few days depending on the degree of renal damage. During this phase, additional adverse effects of the initial insult are unlikely, but the regenerative process has made little progress. In the recovery phase, there is an increasing urine production, followed by a gradually increasing concentrating ability of the kidney and eventual normalization of renal function. It should be noted that too mild an insult would not lead to a manifestation of ARF and excessive initial renal damage would not allow for recovery, and thus would not be ARF.

Mechanisms of ARF

Physiologic and morphologic studies suggest that there are four major possible pathogenic mechanisms for ARF. We will consider each of these in turn.

Renal Vasoconstriction

Persisting renal vasoconstriction has been proposed as a mechanism of ARF. A rise in renal vascular resistance would decrease renal blood flow (RBF) and glomerular filtration rate (GFR). Moreover, if the increase in resistance is predominantly confined to the preglomerular vessels, then the effective filtration pressure and filtration fraction would fall and filtration might even stop.

In the ischemic ARF model, the impaired renal circulation is evidenced by the patchy appearance of the kidney surface immediately after the renal artery constriction is released [10]. There are also areas of no flow, which have been demonstrated in renal sections after an intraarterial injection of carbon particles [11] or silicon rubber [12]. This impaired renal circulation is due to a compression of renal vessels by cells that swell during the ischemia. In less than an hour, renal circulation appears to become homogeneous. In the study of ARF, however, measurement of RBF is a major methodologic problem. Renal clearance of paraaminohippurate (PAH), a convenient index for the calculation of RBF in normal kidneys, is not valid for diseased kidneys [13]. Arendshorst, Finn, and Gottschalk [14], however, succeeded in measuring RBF in the rat with an electromagnetic flowmeter. Within the first few hours after renal ischemia, they found a 50% reduction in total kidney blood flow. The glomerular pressures in these kidneys, however, were normal. Daugharty et al [15], using a micropuncture technique, had previously shown normal glomerular pressure also during the first hours of ARF in the face of a 50% reduction in single glomerular plasma flow. Normal glomerular pressures in this early phase were confirmed later by Tanner and Sophasan [16].

We studied renal circulation 1 to 3 days after unilateral ischemia. Cortical blood flow in peritubular capillaries measured by high frequency cinematography was 75% of control [17]. We later confirmed these results for both outer and inner cortex by using the hydrogen clearance technique [18]. On the other hand, the blood flow in the papillary vasa recta measured by the kymographic technique was actually slightly above the control value [19]. Total kidney blood flow measured by cannulating the renal vein [13] or by using an electromagnetic flowmeter [19] was reduced by 10 to 20%. Also, glomerular pressures in these kidneys were practically normal [16, 20]. Arendshorst, Finn, and Gottschalk [14] measured the reduced RBF at 1 day after unilateral ischemia. They then increased the flow above normal by an i.v. infusion of plasma, but found that the increased blood flow did not improve renal function. In contrast to the unilateral model, a normal RBF was found 1 day after bilateral ischemia [21, 22]. This difference probably occurs because the bilateral models avoid a compensatory redistribution of flow between the two kidneys. A normal blood flow during the manifestation phase has also been reported for the bilateral models using glycerol and mercuric chloride [21]. Accordingly, renal vasoconstriction does not appear to be an important mechanism in the manifestation phase of ARF.

Reduced Glomerular Permeability

A reduced GFR caused by a decreased glomerular hydraulic conductivity (K_f) has been proposed as a pathogenetic mechanism in ARF. This hypothesis is based on ultrastructural glomerular changes found in different models of ARF [23, 24]. Also, the K_f values calculated from micropuncture data have been shown to be reduced [24, 25]. Oken [4], however, has pointed out that because of the complex relation between permeability and filtration, large changes in permeability may have only a small effect on filtration. The nephron GFR, measured by collecting tubular fluid from proximal convolutions, was found to be close to normal for a number of models of ARF [16, 25–28]. This is difficult to reconcile with a substantial effect of a permeability change on GFR. On day 1 after temporary ischemia, we measured nephron GFR with an optical method by tracing a bolus of fluorescent-labeled dextran in the proximal convolutions [20]. We found a 40% reduction in nephron GFR after ischemia, but this reduction could be explained by an increase in tubular pressure. Therefore, a glomerular permeability change seems to have little or no effect in ARF.

Tubular Obstruction

The mechanisms of ARF are now thought to be located more at the tubular level than at the vascular level. That tubular obstruction causes the loss of renal function and the anuria is perhaps the oldest concept in this area; it was proposed by Pontfick [29] in 1875. In histologic examinations of sections of kidneys from anuric patients who died after hemolytic episodes, he found that the nephrons and collecting ducts were filled with precipitates of chromoproteins. Tubular obstruction has also been shown for other models of ARF. However, except for the glycerol model, the obstructive material is not filtered protein, but rather originates largely from damaged proximal tubular epithelium. During the pathogenic (early) phase of ischemic ARF, exfoliated brushborder microvilli are found in the tubular lumen. Cell swelling may also cause the tubular lumen to be narrowed. During the manifestation phase, casts of compact cell debris and hyalin cylinders are abundant in Henle's loops and collecting ducts. Histologic techniques make it easy to demonstrate tubular obstruction, but it is difficult to estimate how many nephrons are involved. Furthermore, to evaluate the role of obstruction in ARF one must know whether obstruction is the cause or an effect of anuria.

The influence that tubular obstruction by protein precipitates would have on renal function was studied in early investigations [30, 31]. Systemically infused myoglobin, which is not toxic and which is filtered to a considerable extent, precipitated in distal nephron segments of hydropenic animals, and in so doing, it reduced urine flow. Using intravital microscopy we observed renal papillae of golden hamsters after myoglobin infusion [9]. Collecting ducts in these kidneys were obstructed by large amounts of myoglobin, but the precipitates could be flushed out slowly if the animals were allowed to have wet food prior to the experiments. Removal of the obstruction was accelerated by inducing osmotic diuresis, and urine flow was soon recovered. Following these observations we mistakenly considered tubular obstruction to be of little importance for anuria. Later, Tanner (during his visit in our laboratory) conducted experiments that showed that tubular obstruction from cell debris (unlike that from myoglobin precipitates) cannot be washed out. In these experiments, the proximal convolutions of the kidney, either a few hours or 2 to 3 days after ischemia, were infused with an equilibrium solution at rates of 15 or 50 nl/min, and the pressure in these convolutions was monitored. During the tubular infusion, the pressure increased to nonphysiologic values (100 mm Hg or more), but still it was not usually possible to flush out the obstruction [32]. Similar results were also obtained following renal ischemia of 2 hours in *Tupaia belangeri,* a primitive primate [8]. (Interesting and unresolved is the question of why the *Tupaia* kidney has a twofold higher ischemic tolerance than the rat.) Neugarten, Aynedjian, and Bank [33] used the same technique recently to demonstrate tubular obstruction in toxic gentamycin-induced ARF. These results demonstrate the potential ability of obstruction to cause anuria in ARF.

Increased pressure in proximal tubules is considered a crucial test for the importance of obstruction in ARF. However, in most experimental models of ARF, the pressure in proximal convolutions was heterogenous rather than homogeneously elevated. In the ischemic model, the pressures were almost homogeneously elevated during the early pathogenic phase [14, 16]. In a recent study [20] we investigated the role of tubular obstruction and tubular leakage (see the following section) during the manifestation phase of ischemic ARF. On day 1 after ischemia, pressure in early proximal convolutions was increased by 3 mm Hg because of the increased flow resistance in the proximal tubules. Pressures in late proximal convolutions, however, were subnormal, and, therefore, more distal obstructions were nonfunctional at this time. The apparent importance of latent obstruction increased by day 3 as pressure in the proximal tubules increased to 10 mm Hg above normal. A key role for obstruction on renal function was also observed during the regeneration phase of ARF (Parekh et al, manuscript in preparation). By day 10 after temporary ischemia, inulin clearance had increased to 10 to 20% of the control value. At this time about 20% of the superficial nephrons had normal pressure and flow in both the proximal and distal convolutions, whereas the remaining nephrons had proximal tubular pressures that were close to stop-flow pressure and indeed had practically no flow.

Tubular Leakage

The proximal tubules normally reabsorb about three fourths of the filtered fluid and a large amount of the filtered solutes. Therefore, it is quite conceivable that leakage in these tubules could permit a complete rediffusion of the filtrate. A wide-spread necrosis in proximal epithelium, which is observed during the manifestation phase in different models of ARF [3, 4], would be consistent with an increase in leakiness. On the other hand, active sodium transport, which is required for fluid reabsorption, appears to be back to normal by the time of the manifestation phase. Oxygen consumption in kidney slices, an index of active transport, was found to be about 70% of normal in several models of ARF [34–37]. On day 1 after temporary renal ischemia we found that renal oxygen uptake in vivo was 55% of the control value [18]. This amount of energy expenditure would be sufficient for active reabsorption of 65% of the filtrate in these kidneys [20].

Tubular leakage was first shown by Bank et al [28] in mercuric chloride-induced ARF. He found that intratubular inulin and lissamine green diffused out of the proximal tubules. Since then a number of investigations have shown significant tubular leakage for inulin and other molecules in various experimental models of ARF, as well as in human ARF [10, 38–40].

Studies on ischemic ARF indicate an apparent correlation between necrosis of proximal tubular epithelium and leakage. Within the first few hours after ischemia, epithelial cells are altered, but not necrotic. The high pressure that is measured in proximal tubules at this time strongly suggests that there is no tubular leakage. One day later, however, necrosis and leakage are maximal. At this time (day 1 after ischemia), we found that filtration in superficial nephrons is 65% of control, but the filtrate rediffuses almost completely in the first half of the proximal convoluted tubule [20]. By day 3, necrotic cells are still present, but the integrity of the tubular epithelium seems to be largely restored by newly generated daughter cells. A significant reduction in leakage at this time is indicated by high pressure, slow flow, and the accumulation of systemically injected fluorescent dextran (mol wt, 3000 daltons) in many superficial proximal convolutions. This phenomenon was also observed in obstructed tubules on day 10.

Conclusions

Our conclusions are based primarily on the processes observed following unilateral ischemia in rats, but they also appear to apply with only small modifications to other models of ARF and to clinical ARF in humans.

During the pathogenic phase, glomerular filtration is reduced owing to tubular obstruction by sloughed brush border and owing to narrowing of the tubular lumen by swollen cells. Cell swelling may also compromise RBF via vascular compression at this time.

During the early manifestation phase of ARF, glomerular filtration increases slowly, and the filtrate provides a flow in the leaky proximal tubules. This flow, although slow, probably facilitates a gradual accumulation in the more distal nephron segments of compact cell debris from damaged proximal tubules and precipitates from the filtrate. In the course of the manifestation phase, leaky tubular sites are gradually mended by daughter cells, but the nephrons are obstructed by firm tubular cylinders in more distal segments. Finally, the recovery phase starts with the clearing of obstruction in a few nephrons, and ends when all nephrons are free.

Future Directions

If we now direct our attention toward the problems that remain unresolved, then the first question must be: Can we influence the processes of ARF for therapeutic effects? For example, is it possible to enhance cell regeneration or to accelerate degradation and removal of tubular obstruction (compare with Ref. 41)? Other questions would include: What are the vascular changes during the hypoxic and early pathogenic phases of ARF? Does altered responsiveness of renal vessels to pressure changes and vasoactive substances [42] have some influence on development of ARF?

We have recently developed a renal microcirculation model that may allow some of these questions to be answered. We are using the split hydronephrotic kidney [43]. With this preparation, we can clearly observe all levels of renal microcirculation, we can precisely control tissue conditions, and we can make controlled applications of numerous drugs. Early investigations have already shown that different arterial segments have different responses to vasoactive substances such as norepinephrine and angiotensin. Very preliminary experiments have suggested some alterations in vascular responsiveness following temporary ischemia. Upcoming studies can explore this and possible therapeutic interventions. A better understanding of the alterations in the renal microcirculation may provide new ways to approach ARF.

Acknowledgments. Parts of this work were supported by German Research Foundation (SFB 90).

References

1. FLAMENBAUM W: Pathophysiology of acute renal failure. *Arch Intern Med* 131:911–928, 1973
2. STEIN JH, LIFSCHITZ MD, BARNES LD: Current concepts on the pathophysiology of acute renal failure. *Am J Physiol* 234:F171–F181, 1978
3. LEVINSKY NG, ALEXANDER EA, VENKATACHALAM MA: Acute renal failure, in *The Kidney* (2nd ed), edited by BRENNER BM, RECTOR FC, Philadelphia, WB Saunders, 1981, pp 1181–1236
4. OKEN DE: Pathogenetic mechanisms in acute renal failure, in *Toxicology of the Kidney,* edited by HOOK JB, New York, Raven Press, 1981, pp 117–134
5. STEINHAUSEN M, PAREKH N, ZIMMERHACKL B: Pathophysiology of acute renal failure, in *Acute Renal Failure,* edited by SEYBOLD D, GESSLER U, Basel, Karger, 1982, pp 9–22
6. SOLEZ K (ed.) *Acute Renal Failure: Correlation between Morphology and Function.* New York, Basel, Marcel Dekker, 1984
7. COX JW, BAEHLER RW, SHARMA H, O'DORSIO T, OSGOOD RW, STEIN JH, FERRIS TF: Studies on the mechanism of oliguria in a model of unilateral acute renal failure. *J Clin Invest* 53:1546–1558, 1974
8. STEINHAUSEN M, THEDERAN H, NOLINSKI D, DALLENBACH FD, SCHWAIER A: Further evidence of tubular blockage after acute ischemic renal failure in Tupaia belangeri and rats. *Virchows Arch [Pathol Anat]* 381:13–34, 1978
9. STEINHAUSEN M: In vivo Beobachtung an der Nierenpapille von Goldhamstern nach intravenoeser Lissamingruen-Injektion. *Pfluegers Arch* 279:195–213, 1964
10. EISENBACH GM, STEINHAUSEN M: Micropuncture studies after temporary ischemia of rat kidneys. *Pfluegers Arch* 343:11–25, 1973
11. SUMMERS WK, JAMISON RL: The no-reflow phenomenon in renal ischemia. *Lab Invest* 25:635–643, 1971
12. FLORES J, DiBONA DR, BECK CH, LEAF A: The role of cell swelling in ischemic renal damage and the protective effect of hypertonic solute. *J Clin Invest* 51:118–126, 1972
13. EISENBACH GM, KITZLINGER B, STEINHAUSEN M: Renal blood flow after temporary ischemia of rat kidneys: Renal venous outflow and clearance techniques. *Pfluegers Arch* 347:223–234, 1974
14. ARENDSHORST WJ, FINN WF, GOTTSCHALK CW: Pathogenesis of acute renal failure following temporary renal ischemia in the rat. *Circ Res* 37:558–568, 1975

15. DAUGHARTY TM, UEKI IF, MERCER PF, BRENNER BM: Dynamic of glomerular ultrafiltration in the rat: V. Response to ischemic injury. *J Clin Invest* 53:105–116, 1974

16. TANNER GA, SOPHASAN S: Kidney pressure after temporary renal artery occlusion in the rat. *Am J Physiol* 230:1173–1181, 1976

17. STEINHAUSEN M, EISENBACH GM, BOETTCHER W: High-frequency microcinematographic measurements on peritubular blood flow under control conditions and after temporary ischemia of rat kidneys. *Pfluegers Arch* 339:273–288, 1973

18. PAREKH N, VEITH U: Renal hemodynamics and oxygen consumption during postischemic acute renal failure in the rat. *Kidney Int* 19:306–316, 1981

19. BOETTCHER W, STEINHAUSEN M: Microcirculation of the renal papilla of rats under control conditions and after temporary ischemia. *Kidney Int* 10(Suppl 6):S74–S80, 1976

20. PAREKH N, ESSLINGER HU, STEINHAUSEN M: Glomerular filtration and tubular reabsorption during anuria in postischemic acute renal failure. *Kidney Int* 25:33–41, 1984

21. CHURCHILL S, ZARLENGO MD, CARVALHO JS, GOTTLIEB MN, OKEN DE: Normal renocortical blood flow in experimental acute renal failure. *Kidney Int* 11:246–255, 1977

22. FREGA NS, DIBONA DR, GUERTLER B, LEAF A: Ischemic renal injury. *Kidney Int* 10(Suppl 6):S17–S25, 1976

23. AVASTHI PS, EVAN AP, HAY D: Glomerular endothelial cells in urenyl nitrate-induced acute renal failure in rats. *J Clin Invest* 65:121–127, 1980

24. WILLIAMS RH, THOMAS CE, NAVAR LG, EVAN AP: Hemodynamic and single nephron function during the maintenance phase of ischemic acute renal failure in the dog. *Kidney Int* 19:503–515, 1981

25. BLANTZ RC: Mechanism of acute renal failure after uranyl nitrate. *J Clin Invest* 55:621–635, 1975

26. TANNER GA, SLOAN KL, SOPHASAN S: Effects of renal artery occlusion on kidney function in the rat. *Kidney Int* 4:377–389, 1973

27. STEIN JH, GOTTSCHALK J, OSGOOD RW, FERRIS TF: Pathophysiology of a nephrotoxic model of acute renal failure. *Kidney Int* 8:27–41, 1975

28. BANK N, MUTZ BF, AYNEDJIAN HS: The role of "leakage" of tubular fluid in anuria due to mercury poisoning. *J Clin Invest* 46:695–704, 1967

29. PONFICK: Experimentelle Beitraege zur Lehre von der Transfusion. *Arch Pathol Anat Physiol* 62:273–335, 1875

30. SHIMAMINE T: Experimentelle Untersuchunger ueber die pathogenetische Bedeutung der "Chromoproteinurie" fuer die Entstehung der "Chromoproteinniere." *Beitr Path Anat* 116:330–368, 1956

31. JAENIKE JR: Micropuncture study of methemoglobin-induced acute renal failure in the rat. *J Lab Clin Med* 73:459–468, 1969

32. TANNER GA, STEINHAUSEN M: Tubular obstruction in ischemia-induced acute renal failure in the rat. *Kidney Int* 10(Suppl 6):S65–S73, 1976

33. NEUGARTEN J, AYNEDJIAN HS, BANK N: Role of tubular obstruction in acute renal failure due to gentamycin. *Kidney Int* 24:330–335, 1983

34. REIMER KA, JENNINGS RB: Alterations in renal cortex following ischemic injury: II. PAH uptake, O_2-consumption, and water content in slices of cortex after ischemia or autolysis. *Lab Invest* 25:185–195, 1971

35. MERGNER WJ, SMITH MW, TRUMP BF: Studies on the pathogenesis of ischemic cell injury: XI P/O ratio and acceptor control. *Virchows Arch* [*Cell Pathol*] 26:17–26, 1977

36. HOHENEGGER M, KRAMAR R: Energy metabolism of the mouse kidney following

mercury poisoning: Relation to acute renal insufficiency, in *Donausymposium fuer Nephrologie,* edited by WATSCHINGER B, Friedberg, Hessen, Verlag C Bindernagel, 1977, pp 152–154

37. PREUSS HG: Tubular function in experimental acute tubular necrosis in rats. *Kidney Int* 10(Suppl 6):S51–S57, 1976
38. THIEL G, WILSON DR, ARCE ML, OKEN DE: Glycerol-induced hemoglobinuric acute renal failure in the rat. *Nephron* 4:276–297, 1967
39. STEINHAUSEN M, EISENBACH GM, HELMSTAEDTER V: Concentration of lissamine green in proximal tubules of antidiuretic and mercury poisoned rats and the permeability of these tubules. *Pfluegers Arch* 311:1–15, 1969
40. MYERS BD, CHUI F, HILBERMAN M, MICHAELS AS: Transtubular leakage of glomerular filtrate in human acute renal failure. *Am J Physiol* 6:F319–F325, 1979
41. TOBAK FG, TEEGARDEN DE, HAVENER LJ: Amino acid-mediated stimulation of renal phospholipid biosynthesis after acute tubular necrosis. *Kidney Int* 15:542–547, 1979
42. MATTHYS E, PATTON MK, OSGOOD RW, VENKATACHALAM MA, STEIN JH: Alterations in vascular function and morphology in acute ischemic renal failure. *Kidney Int* 23:717–724, 1983
43. STEINHAUSEN M, SNOEI H, PAREKH N, BAKER R, JOHNSON P: Hydronephrosis: A new model to visualize vas afferens, efferens, and glomerular network. *Kidney Int* 23:794–806, 1983

Pathology of Acute Renal Failure

Ruth E. Bulger and Dennis C. Dobyan

Experimental acute renal failure induced by ischemia or the administration of toxic agents is characterized by a progression of well-defined events. Initially, the epithelial cells lining the proximal tubule (the principal site of damage along the nephron) exhibit varying degrees of sublethal cell injury that can ultimately culminate in cellular necrosis. This often results in the sloughing of lethally injured cells or cellular debris into tubular lumens, with subsequent denudation of the tubular basement membranes and cast formation in the distal nephron. Most early studies assessing structural injury to the kidney were largely descriptive in nature. However, the current use of more sophisticated methods of morphometric analysis has significantly improved our ability not only to quantitatively evaluate the extent of cellular damage, but also to correlate this injury with the concomitant functional state. Positive correlations between structural alterations and functional impairment in experimental acute renal failure now have been demonstrated by numerous investigators. For example, in a recent study, Solez and Finckh [1] made an excellent attempt to relate structure and function in human acute renal failure despite the prevalent viewpoint that less correlation occurs in the human situation than in experimental models.

In this article, we will attempt to select from a vast literature and to present an overview of some of the salient new developments in the following areas: (1) the steps and possible mechanisms in tubule cell injury and necrosis, (2) the use of pharmacologic agents to ameliorate cell injury, (3) the selective susceptibility of nephron segments to experimental injury, and (4) the possible role of the renal corpuscle in the pathogenesis of experimentally induced acute renal failure. However, it should be noted that the development of renal dysfunction in the various models appears to be multifactorial; hence, it is unlikely that any one mechanism will provide a suitable explanation for the myriad of observations that have been reported in the literature.

This manuscript was presented as part of a Symposium on *Acute Renal Failure: Structure-Function Relationships*.

Because the important roles of obstruction and renin-induced vasoconstriction are being discussed by other contributors to this volume, they will not be considered in this review.

Steps and Possible Mechanisms in Renal Cell Injury

An understanding of the cellular and molecular events that occur after a cell is subjected to an injurious stimulus is essential if we are to devise manipulations for controlling or preventing irreparable damage to the kidney. Most cells exhibit a characteristic spectrum of changes following an ischemic or toxic insult, and such alterations are frequently related to primary or secondary redistributions of ions. Interruptions in normal homeostasis generally are reversible; but, if allowed to persist, they will cause the cell to become irreversibly injured, resulting in necrosis. It appears that increased levels of cytosolic calcium may be the final common pathway leading to cell death [2–5]. Trump et al [6, 7] have described seven stages of cellular injury. The first four stages are considered to be reversible, while the remaining three describe the development of irreversible cell injury. The rate at which cells progress through these stages depends on the type of insult and the susceptibility of the particular cell to the injurious stimulus. For the purpose of this discussion, we will consider the stages of injury normally following an ischemic episode [5].

Cells in stage 1 are considered to be functionally and morphologically normal. (To distinguish what is proposed to be happening at a biochemical level from what can be seen morphologically, the latter will be italicized in this discussion.) Following an ischemic insult, the cell progresses to stage 1A. Cellular oxygen tension decreases, which is accompanied by a rapid decline in mitochondrial phosphorylation and cellular adenosine triphosphate (ATP) levels [8, 9]. With a diminished ATP supply, there is stimulation of anaerobic glycolysis and a *decrease in available glycogen stores*. The resultant increases in lactate, as well as hydrogen ion accumulation, lead to a decrease in cytosolic pH with subsequent *clumping of the nuclear chromatin*. The decreased ATP also leads to impairment in cell ion pumping systems and causes the beginning of redistributions of ions such as sodium, potassium, and calcium.

Stage 2 is considered to be a reversible phase. The intracellular redistribution of ions and water leads to *swelling of the lumens of the endoplasmic reticulum* and to ion accumulation within the mitochondrial compartment (Fig. 1) [10, 11]. The accumulation of intracellular calcium appears to effect normal microtubule and microfilament function, causing *changes in cell shape* (Fig. 2) [12, 13]. Perpetuation of decreased energy stores effects impairment of protein synthesis and cellular ion transport.

Stage 3, which is also reversible, is characterized by *intracristal swelling of mitochondria* and *dilatation of the endoplasmic reticulum,* which are consequences of continued ion shifts. The increases in cellular sodium and water and the decreases in potassium are associated with a *swollen cell sap,* a loss

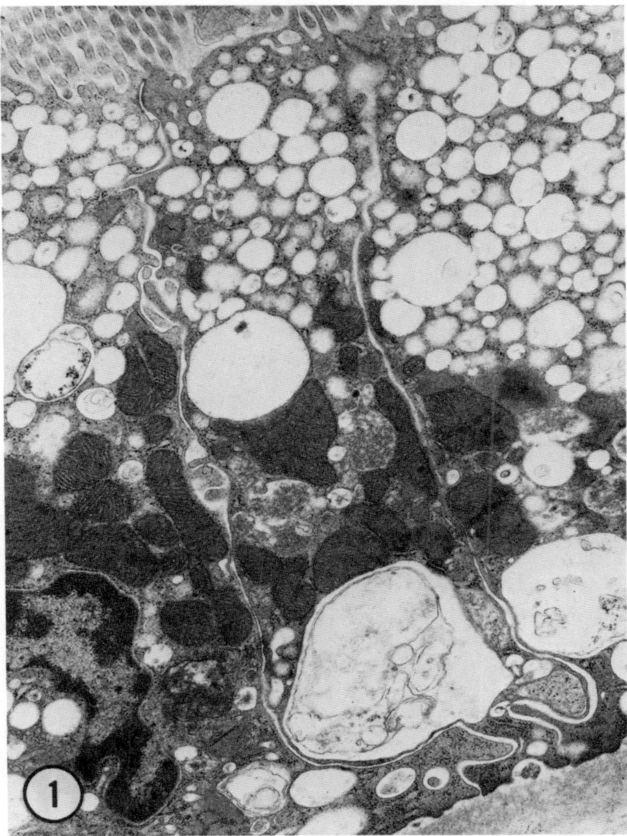

Fig. 1. Electron micrograph of an injured proximal tubule from a dog that was subjected to a 40 min intrarenal infusion of norepinephrine. Note the increased vesiculation in the apical cytoplasm, the simplified cell shape, and the rounding of the mitochondria with slight intracristal swelling. (x15,000)

in both free and bound polysomes (now present as monosomes), and cessation of protein synthesis.

Stage 4 is a transition phase in which cell death begins. Some mitochondria at this point begin to show *swelling of their inner matrical compartments*, and they also contain *small dense aggregates* of what is presumed to be reversibly denatured matrix proteins. The continued increase in cytoplasmic calcium results in phospholipase activation, a breakdown of phospholipids, and the accumulation of free fatty acids.

The remaining stages are typified by irreversible cellular injury. In stage 5, there is *high-amplitude swelling of all mitochondria,* and *large flocculent densities* appear within the mitochondrial matrix (Fig. 2, 3). Controversy exists regarding the nature of these accumulations. Collan, McDowell, and

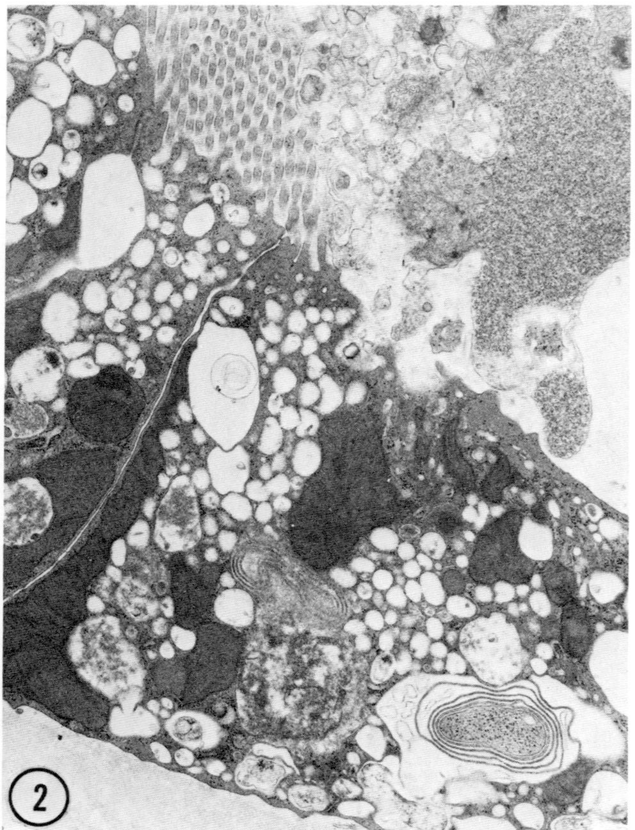

Fig. 2. A further progression of injury in this same model showing swelling of the endoplasmic reticulum, the presence of membrane whorls in the cytoplasm, and the loss of apical microvilli in the cells lining this proximal tubule. Necrotic debris can be seen within the lumen. (x12,000)

Trump [14] believed them to be proteinaceous, because they could be digested with pronase, while Jennings and Ganote [15] believed them to be lipid in composition. During stage 5, there is a marked increase in membrane permeability with a diffusion of enzymes, lipids, and other cell factors. *Large membrane discontinuities* are seen and *chromatin digestion* occurs. *Necrosis* with digestion of cellular constituents characterizes stage 6. *Karyolysis, lysosomal disruption, and changes in the staining properties* of cellular components also are apparent at this time. The final degradation of the cell and the *appearance of myelin figures* and total absence of enzymatic activity signals (the final) stage 7.

The progression to cell death, as described above, appears to involve at least two mechanisms [3, 5]. The first mechanism, which is independent of

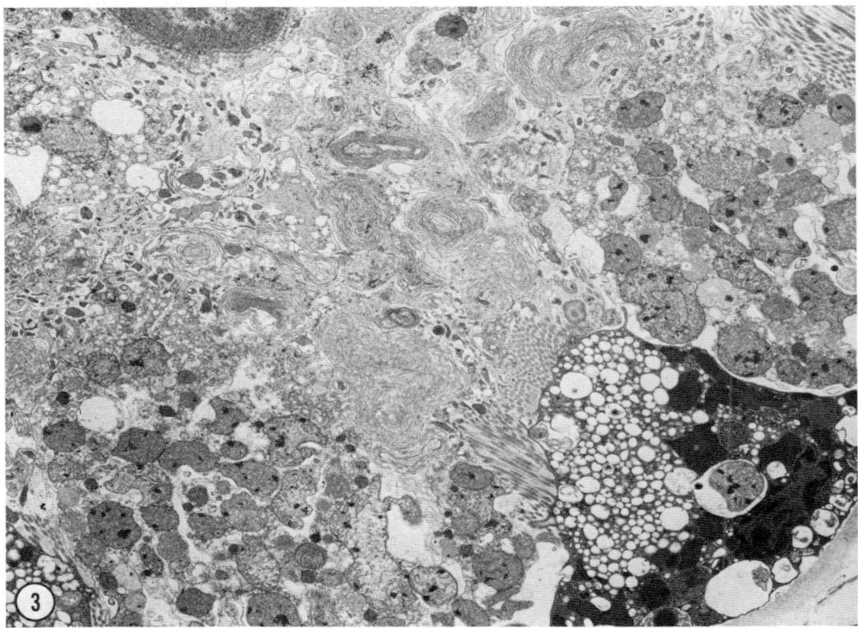

Fig. 3. Necrotic debris fills the lumen of the proximal tubule. Note the extensive membrane whorls. One injured proximal tubule cell is seen in the lower right portion. (x6250)

extracellular calcium ions, involves disruption in the integrity of the plasma membrane either by ischemia or by direct cell membrane damage. The second step is a functional consequence of an injurious stimulus, and it most likely involves the influx of extracellular calcium down its steep concentration gradient into the cell. Since calcium ions are normally maintained at a low cytosolic level (10^{-6} M) by the presence of a relatively impermeable cell membrane or by calcium translocation systems within these membranes, the rapid influx of calcium into the injured cell initiates by some mechanism the final common pathway for cell death. In this respect, Shanne et al [3] examined primary cultures of rat hepatocytes that were treated in the presence or absence of extracellular calcium with 10 different membrane-active toxins. They showed that in the presence, but not in the absence, of extracellular calcium, more than 50% of the cells were killed with each toxin used.

It appears that the increased cytosolic calcium may, in some manner, initiate many of the catabolic processes that effect the transition from a reversible type of injury to an irreversible one that inevitably leads to necrosis. The exact mechanism by which calcium effects cellular injury remains speculative. Calcium ions could lead to the activation of endogenous calcium-dependent phospholipases. Such a mechanism could cause degradation of membrane phospholipids and the accumulation of toxic lipid metabolites, as well as perpetuation of further membrane damage [16, 17]. Smith et al [18] demonstrated that mitochondrial phospholipids decrease soon after an ischemic injury. In this respect, mitochondria normally function as a control system for regulating intracellular calcium content by active sequestration of excess cytosolic calcium. Such excessive uptake of calcium by mitochondria takes precedence over oxidative phosphorylation—in essence, uncoupling this process [19]. Furthermore, the sequestered calcium can also alter inner mitochondrial membrane function by activating membrane phospholipases [18]. Elevated cytosolic calcium can effect changes in the cytoskeleton [20, 21]. One of the earliest structural changes noted in experimental models of acute renal failure is the alteration in the brush border and apical cell membranes [22–24]. Whether this is the result of a direct effect on the cell membrane or a consequence of a calcium-related change in the cytoskeleton is uncertain.

Amelioration of Renal Cell Injury

Recent studies center on the use of pharmacologic interventions to prevent or ameliorate the progression of cellular injury in experimental renal failure. Because calcium has been suggested to play an important role in the pathogenesis of irreversible cell injury, it is not surprising that agents blocking the movement of calcium into cells are currently under investigation. Calcium channel blockers, such as verapamil or nifedipene, have been used in attempts to prevent calcium entry in experimentally induced renal cell injury. Burke, Arnold, and Schrier [25] administered verapamil 30 min prior to and for 2 hr after intrarenal infusion of norepinephrine; they observed a beneficial effect on both functional and biochemical parameters in this model of ischemic renal injury. In agreement with these studies are the observations of Dobyan et al [26], who have shown a decrease in injury to the proximal tubules when verapamil was given after norepinephrine infusion. Weinberg, Hunt, and Humes [27] subjected isolated proximal tubule-rich suspensions from rabbit kidneys to 30 min of ischemia, with and without verapamil added to the incubation medium; they showed that after 60 min of recovery, verapamil limited calcium overload and improved adenosine triphosphate within the cells.

Several investigators have also shown that verapamil pretreatment affords protection, as assessed by preservation of the glomerular filtration rate (GFR) in both norepinephrine [28] and renal artery clamping [29] models of acute renal failure. In these same studies, however, it was noted that if verapamil was administered after norepinephrine infusion or after renal artery clamping, no protection was observed. Malis et al [28] postulated that verapamil acted by attenuating the vasoactive effects of norepinephrine.

The question of whether the ameliorative effects of verapamil in ischemic models of renal cell injury result from direct effects on slow calcium channels by blocking calcium entry or result from indirect effects on the renal vasculature remains a topic of considerable debate. Gordon and Ferris [30] showed that neither verapamil nor methoxyverapamil influenced the net influx of calcium across renal tubules in vitro. In this respect, Borle [31] also found a negative effect of verapamil on calcium fluxes, and he questioned if kidney cells did in fact have voltage-dependent calcium channels.

It is well established that the ATP content of the renal cortex falls to half its normal level within 30 sec after an ischemic insult in a variety of animal species [32–36]. ATP is degraded to adenosine diphosphate (ADP) and finally to adenosine monophosphate (AMP), which in turn is either dephosphorylated to adenosine or deaminated to inosine. The subsequent loss of small diffusible substances from the cell may be an additional crucial step in the development of irreversible cell injury.

The infusion of solutions containing ATP and magnesium chloride ($MgCl_2$) has been shown to have a beneficial effect in restoring ATP levels in hemorrhagic shock [37]. Siegel et al [38] reported attenuation of ischemic renal cell injury when ATP-$MgCl_2$ was administered immediately after or as long as 8 to 24 hr after the initial insult. The infusion of ATP-$MgCl_2$ appears to preserve sublethally injured cells, restore cellular morphology, and improve both glomerular and tubular function in ischemic renal failure [34, 38–40]. Furthermore, Siegel et al [34] used nuclear magnetic resonance to show an accelerated recovery of tissue ATP levels after ischemia and ATP-$MgCl_2$ infusion. Finally, Andrews and Coffey [41] flushed rat kidneys with ATP-$MgCl_2$ 1 hr prior to renal artery clamping in the rat, and they showed more substantial protection from normothermic ischemia when compared to tissues treated with those solutions currently being used for storage of kidneys prior to transplantation.

Cell work has been shown to accelerate anoxic cell injury in the medullary ascending thick segment in isolated, perfused rat kidneys [42]. The administration of ouabain to such a preparation abolishes the anoxic lesion caused by hypoxia or infusion of potassium cyanide [43]. Siegel et al [44] also have shown attenuation of structural and functional alterations to the proximal tubules with prior ouabain treatment in a renal artery clamping model in the dog.

The accelerated degradation of membrane phospholipids has been suggested to be an important event that results in irreversible injury in liver, myocardium, and kidney [16, 45, 46]. Several recent studies have shown that the anesthetic amine, chlorpromazine, prevents the degradation of membrane phospholipids and the rise in tissue calcium in ischemic and toxic myocardial and liver cell injury [3, 16, 47]. Chlorpromazine also has been shown to afford partial protection against the renal structural and functional impairment that is seen in a model of mercuric chloride-induced acute renal failure in rats [48]. The mechanism by which chlorpromazine provides its protection is uncertain. However, it is interesting to note that two important actions of this agent are to block calcium fluxes and to inhibit phospholipases [49].

Significant changes in membrane phospholipids are currently being reported in various models of acute renal failure. Matthys, Patel, and Venkatachalam [50] examined an ischemic model of renal cell injury and noted a defect in membrane phospholipid metabolism with a breakdown in structural phospholipids. The administration of the potent aminoglycoside, gentamicin, results in an increase in phosphatidylinositol and phosphotidic acid as early as 15 min after a single dose of this agent, and at a time when there is no evidence of necrosis [51]. It is interesting to note that in diabetic rats, which are resistant to gentamicin-induced acute renal failure, there is altered phosphatidylinositol metabolism [52].

Another possible source of membrane damage after an ischemic or toxic insult is the generation of activated oxygen species such as O_2^-, H_2O_2, and OH^-. These reactive free radicals can induce lipid peroxidation and subsequent membrane damage [53], suggesting that agents that are potent scavengers of free radicals may be important in ameliorating renal cell injury. For example, glutathione protects cells from oxidative injury caused by electrophilic compounds and free radicals. Perfusion of the isolated rat kidney with glucose, a regimen that depletes cellular glutathione, resulted in deterioration in renal function and degeneration of the medullary ascending thick segment of the nephron [42, 43, 54]. The investigators also showed that these changes could easily be ameliorated by adding amino acid supplements or glutathione to the perfusate.

With the administration of acetaminophen, Mitchell et al [55] showed a dose-dependent, acute renal necrosis in male Fischer rats. In this study, it was observed that acetaminophen caused a marked depletion of target organ glutathione and resulted in the binding of large amounts of the metabolite of this drug to renal protein. Pretreatment with cobalt chloride, which is an inhibitor of hepatic and renal drug metabolism, resulted in a decrease both in irreversible binding of metabolite and in glutathione. This was associated with concomitant protection against tissue damage. Finally, glutathione has also been suggested to be involved in the protection against interstitial nephritis caused by radiomimetic agents that act by increasing the formation of free radicals [56].

Sites of Cell Injury Along the Nephron

The exact location along the nephron where injury and necrosis are induced varies with the experimental model. The patterns of injury seen with several agents were well described in the classic paper of Oliver, MacDowell, and Tracy [57]. Although in some models, the reason for the site of preferential injury is understood, the understanding is less well defined in many models. A discussion of these factors is beyond the scope of this review.

The most common site of injury is in the proximal pars recta in the outer stripe of the medulla. Models that induce prominent necrosis in this region include mercuric chloride (Fig. 4) [58, 59], uranyl nitrate [60–62], cis-platinum [63], renal arterial occlusion [23, 24, 64, 65], and hemorrhagic shock [66, 67]. When the dose of the toxic agent or the time of the ischemic insult is increased in many of these models, the injury extends to include the pars recta in the medullary ray and the proximal convolutions of the cortex (Fig. 5). Casts in the distal nephron are frequently described. Several

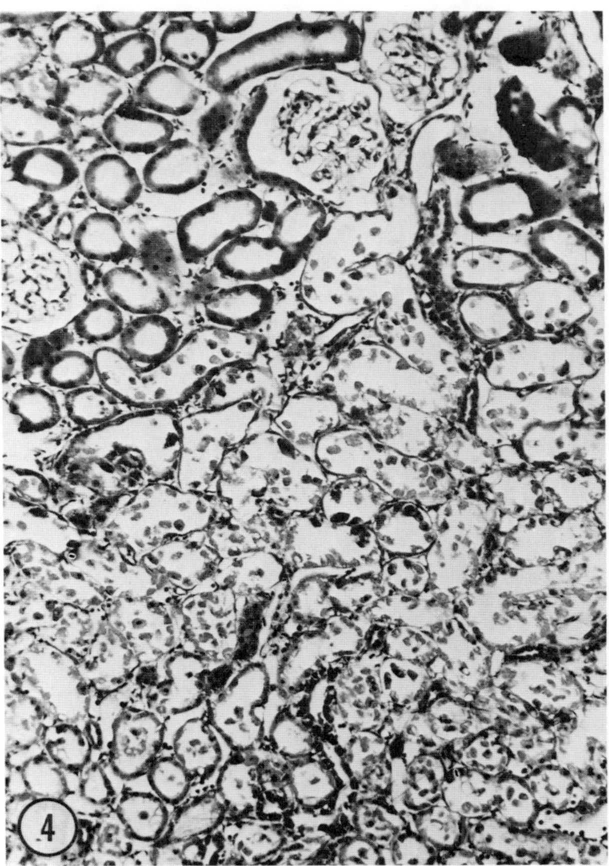

Fig. 4. Light micrograph from a rat given 2 mg/kg of mercuric chloride. Note the necrotic debris present within the outer stripe region of the outer medulla (*bottom half*). The proximal tubules in the cortex appear to be more normal (*upper half*). (Hematoxylin and eosin; x120)

of these agents, such as cis-platinum and uranyl nitrate, cause progressive lesions that culminate in cyst formation [68, 69].

Human ischemia [57] and norepinephrine-induced acute renal failure (Fig. 6) [26] have a patchy distribution of cell necrosis that involves both proximal convoluted tubules and proximal pars recta tubules with cast formation. Aminoglycosides such as gentamicin involve the proximal tubule S1 and S2 regions (Fig. 7) [70]. Tubular necrosis produced by cephaloradine is preferentially located in the S2 region of the proximal tubule [71].

Recently, when Brezis et al [42, 43, 54] used a model of isolated perfused kidneys, they demonstrated preferential lesions in the ascending thick limb of Henle's loop in a variety of situations.

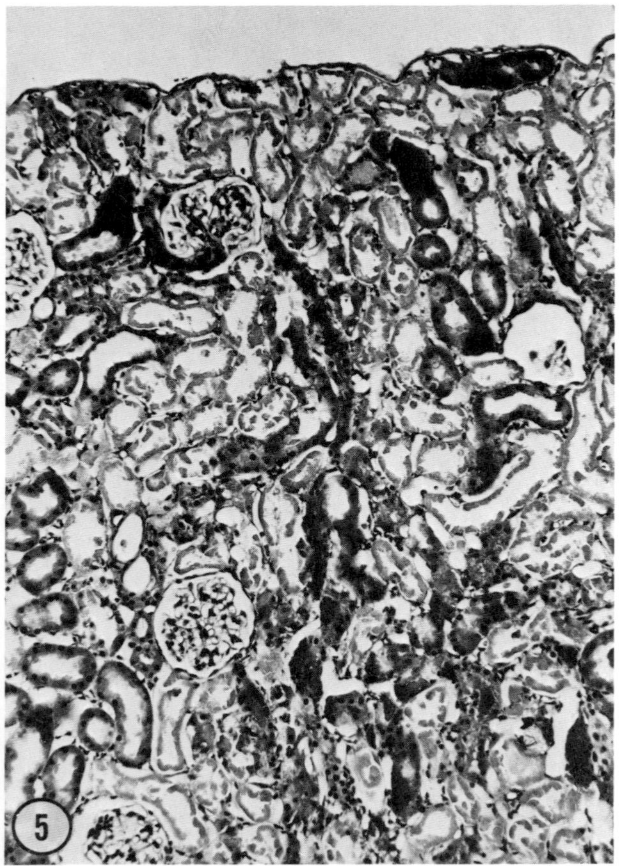

Fig. 5. Light micrograph from a rat kidney showing a more extensive degree of proximal tubule injury resulting from the administration of mercuric chloride. The injury now extends up the medullary ray and into the proximal convolutions. (Hematoxylin and eosin; x120)

Role of the Renal Corpuscle in Initiation and Maintenance of Acute Renal Failure

An area of investigation that has been generating intense interest and controversy due to the variation in reported results is the manner in which structural changes in the renal corpuscle may influence glomerular filtration; particularly, as these alterations relate to the initiation and maintenance of acute

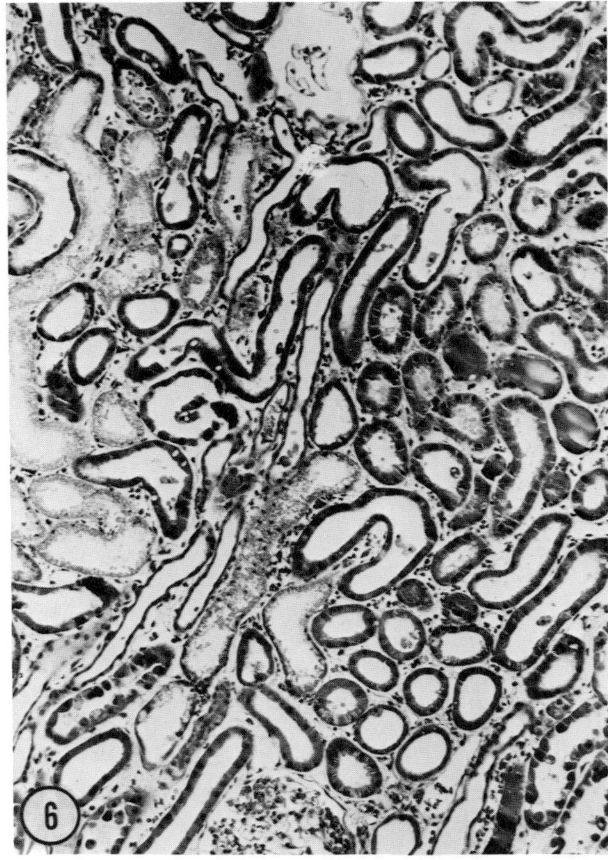

Fig. 6. Light micrograph showing proximal tubule necrosis in the kidney of a dog subjected to intrarenal norepinephrine infusion. Both the proximal convoluted and the pars recta segments show evidence of injury. (Hematoxylin and eosin; x120)

renal failure. A decrease in the glomerular capillary ultrafiltration coefficient (Kf) (the product of the effective hydraulic permeability of the capillary wall and the surface area available for filtration) has been reported by Blantz [72] in uranyl nitrate-induced acute renal failure, by Schor et al [73] with aminoglycoside-treated animals, by Baylis, Rennke, and Brenner [74] after gentamicin administration, and by Williams et al [75] in ischemic acute renal failure. Blantz [72] also showed that pretreatment with angiotensin-converting enzyme inhibitors or plasma volume expansion inhibited the decrease in Kf seen after uranyl nitrate fadmination. These observations have prompted investigators to try and identify a concomitant anatomic alteration to explain the decrease in Kf in these various models.

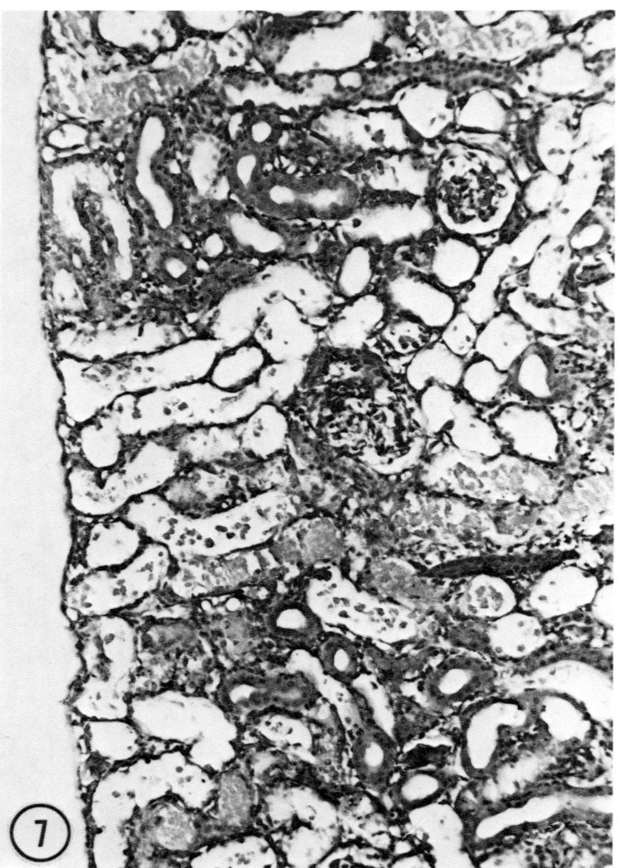

Fig. 7. Light micrograph showing necrotic proximal convoluted tubules in the kidney of a rat that was administered gentamicin. (Hematoxylin and eosin; x120)

Changes in Epithelial Cells (Podocytes)

Cox et al [76] described widespread *smudging* and *fusion* of glomerular podocytes in an irreversible model of acute renal failure in dogs that was caused by the intrarenal infusion of norepinephrine for 2 hr. Similar changes, more focal in nature, were reported by Stein et al [60] 48 hr after uranyl nitrate injection. Flamenbaum, Langlinais, and Merrill [81], who also studied a uranyl nitrate model of acute renal failure, failed to identify any changes in the glomerular podocytes at 6 hr, but they described altered trabeculae and pedicels at 24 and 48 hr. More recently, flattening and spreading of podocyte cell bodies, major processes, and pedicels have been noted in the rat and rabbit kidneys after renal artery occlusion, as well as in the glomeruli of humans with ischemic acute renal failure [77–80]. Similar changes can be produced by dehydration alone or by administration of angiotensin II or vasopressin in vitro [80]. Partial protection from these podocyte alterations has been noted in the renal clamp model in the rabbit after mannitol infusion and with clonidine, but not with captopril administration [79–81].

Other investigators have failed to observe similar changes. Myers, Langlinais, and Merrill [81] could not detect any glomerular abnormalities in ischemic acute renal failure in humans. Dobyan, Nagle, and Bulger [67] reported no changes after 110 min of sustained hypovolemia. Cronin et al [82] infused norepinephrine intrarenally for 40 min and observed normal glomeruli at 3 and 24 hr in all but two animals (those demonstrating infarcts). Baylis, Rennke, and Brenner [74] gave gentamicin at a dose of 4 or 40 mg/kg/d for 10 days and failed to see any glomerular changes. Similar results were obtained in norepinephrine-induced acute renal failure in dogs and rats [83, 84]. Some minor changes in the glomerular podocyte trabeculae and pedicels were noted by Bulger, Cronin, and Dobyan [85] 48 hr after a 2-hr intrarenal infusion of norepinephrine and by Baehler et al [86] after mercuric chloride administration due to the minimal nature of these lesions; the latter authors concluded that these mild changes in the glomerular podocytes could not be the primary pathophysiologic mechanism causing the decreased GFR. In addition, Bulger, Gorman, and Dobyan (unpublished observations) have not seen significant changes at 3 hr after mercuric chloride administration to rats. More recently, Zager et al [87] studied the effect of pre-existing glomerular injury or nephrotic syndrome on the subsequent course of a 30-min ischemic insult, and they failed to find support for the hypothesis that foot process fusion is important in the pathophysiology of acute renal failure.

Andrews and Coffey [41] recently noted that glomerular podocytes contain abundant actin filaments in the foot processes or pedicels. They proposed that a relaxation of actin could lead to narrowing of the foot processes that would have the potential to regulate GFR and to alter the number of slits available for filtration.

Much interest has recently been directed at studying only the glomerular capillaries, in particular their lining endothelium. In 1970, Clarkson et al [88] found marked intravascular accumulation of fibrin and platelets in patients with ischemic acute renal failure. Hornych, Beaufils, and Richet [89] described glomerular capillary narrowing during angiotensin II infusion. Dach and Kurtzman [90] reported amorphous particulate matter in the glomeruli soon after the administration of glycerol.

The development of a method of freeze-cracking specimens for scanning electron-microscopic observation has made the study of endothelial surfaces more practical [91]. The normal structure of the epithelium lining the glomerular capillaries has been described by several investigators [92–94]. A decrease in the size and density of endothelial fenestrae has been noted in acute renal failure induced by uranyl nitrate [95], by aminoglycosides such as gentamicin [96], by ischemia [75], by glycerol [97], and in human acute renal failure

[79]. Evan et al [98] have also described similar changes in spontaneously hypertensive rats before and after their blood pressure increased and in alloxan-induced diabetes [99]. These investigators have proposed that the decreased endothelial fenestral size and density provides the anatomic basis for the altered glomerular capillary ultrafiltration coefficient.

Not all investigators have been able to substantiate similar changes in capillary fenestrae. Baylis, Rennke, and Brenner [74], Schor et al [73], and Bulger et al [94] failed to detect any changes in fenestral size or area in gentamicin-induced acute renal failure. Similarly, no changes in the glomerular fenestrae were noted after puromycin administration [100], in ischemic acute renal failure in rats [79], or after mercuric chloride injection [94]. In addition, similar areas to those reported as abnormal have been noted in normal tissue [93]. Hence, the role of the glomerular capillary endothelial fenestrae in decreased Kf remains in question.

Role of the Mesangium

An exciting new hypothesis implicates the role of the intraglomerular mesangial cells in either the shunting of blood within the glomerulus or the decrease in the glomerular capillary filtration surface. The contractile activities of mesangial cells were noted in 1969 by Burnick [101]. Becker [102] postulated that these cells could reduce the overall size of the glomerular tuft or their overall surface area. Ausiello et al [103] demonstrated that cultured glomerular cells of mesangial origin could contract in response to angiotensin II or vasopressin. Specific angiotensin II receptors have been localized on mesangial cells [104–105]. Since Schor et al [73] have reported that arginine vasopressin and angiotensin II effect a decrease in glomerular ultrafiltration coefficient, these hormones may be regulators of intraglomerular blood flow by their action on mesangial cells. These authors also have suggested that dibutyryl cyclic AMP, parathyroid hormone, and prostaglandins PGI and PGE might appear to act through angiotensin. Changes in the number of angiotensin II receptor sites appear to have important pathophysiologic consequences as well. Ballermann et al [106] showed a decreased number of angiotensin II receptor sites in isolated glomeruli from streptozoticin-induced diabetic rats. Since Kreisberg [107] has demonstrated that mesangial cells in culture do not contract without insulin, this might be correlated with the protection seen in acute renal failure in streptozoticin-induced diabetic rats. We feel that additional work is necessary to test whether or not the lowering of the Kf is affected through the mesangial cells.

References

1. SOLEZ K, FINCKH ES: Is there a correlation between morphologic and functional changes in human acute renal failure? Data of Finckh, Jeremy, Whyte reexamined

twenty years later, in *Acute Renal Failure. Correlations Between Morphology and Function,* edited by SOLEZ K, WHELTON A, New York, Marcel Dekker, Inc, 1984, pp 3–12

2. FARBER JL: Biology of disease. Membrane injury and calcium homeostasis in the pathogenesis of coagulative necrosis. *Lab Invest* 47:114–123, 1982

3. SCHANNE FA, KANE AB, YOUNG EE, FARBER JL: Calcium dependence of toxic cell death: A final common pathway. *Science* 206:700–702, 1979

4. TRUMP BF, JONES RT, BEREZESKY IK, PHELPS PC, LAIHO KU: Role of calcium in cell injury. *Fed Proc* 37:403, 1978

5. TRUMP BF, BEREZESKY IK, LAIHO KV, OSORNIO AR, MERGNER WJ, SMITH MW: The role of calcium in cell injury. A review. Scanning Electron Microscopy II, AMF O'Hare, Chicago, SEM Inc, 1980

6. TRUMP BF, LAIHO KA, MERGNER WJ, ARSTILA AU: Studies on the subcellular pathophysiology of acute lethal cell injury. *Beitr Path Bd* 152:243–271, 1974

7. TRUMP BF, STRUM JM, BULGER RE: Studies on the pathogenesis of ischemic cell injury. I. Relation between ion and water shifts and cell ultrastructure in rat kidney slices during swelling at 0–4 degrees C. *Virch Arch B Cell Pathol* 16:1–34, 1974

8. MERGNER WJ, SMITH MW, SAHAPHONG S, TRUMP BF: Studies on the pathogenesis of ischemic cell injury. VI. Accumulation of calcium by isolated mitochondria of ischemic rat kidney cortex. *Virch Arch B Cell Pathol* 26:1–16, 1977

9. MERGNER WJ, SMITH MW, TRUMP BF: Studies on the pathogenesis of ischemic cell injury. XI. P/O ratio and acceptor control. *Virch Arch B Cell Pathol* 26:17–26, 1977

10. LAIHO KU, SHELBURNE JD, TRUMP BF: Observations on cell volume, ultrastructure, mitochondrial conformation and vital-dye uptake in Ehrlich ascites tumor cells: Effects of inhibiting energy production and function of the plasma membrane. *Am J Pathol* 65:203–230, 1971

11. LAIHO KU, TRUMP BF: Studies on the pathogenesis of cell injury. Effects of inhibitors of metabolism and membrane function on the mitochondria of Ehrlich ascites tumor cells. *Lab Invest* 32:163–182, 1975

12. TRUMP BF, PENTTILA A, BEREZESKY IK: Studies on cell surface conformation following injury. I. Scanning and transmission electron microscopy of cell surface changes following p-chloromercuribenzene sulfonic acid (PCMBS)-induced injury of Ehrlich ascites tumor cells. *Virch Arch B Cell Path* 29:281–296, 1979

13. TRUMP BF, PENTTILA A, BEREZESKY IK: Studies on cell surface conformation following injury. II. Scanning and transmission electron microscopy of cell surface changes following anoxic injury in Ehrlich ascites tumor cells. *Virch Arch B Cell Pathol* 29:297–307, 1979

14. COLLAN Y, MCDOWELL E, TRUMP BF: Studies on the pathogenesis of ischemic cell injury. VI. Mitochondrial flocculent densities in autolysis. *Virch Arch B Cell Pathol* 35:189–199, 1981

15. JENNINGS RB, GANOTE CE: Mitochondrial structure and function in acute myocardial ischemic injury. *Circ Res* 38(Suppl I):I80–I91, 1976

16. CHIEN KR, PFAU RG, FARBER JL: Ischemic myocardial cell injury. Prevention by chlorpromazine of an accelerated phospholipid degradation and associated membrane dysfunction. *Am J Pathol* 97:505–529, 1979

17. FRANSON R, WAITE M: Relation between calcium requirement, substrate charge, and rabbit polymorphonuclear leukocyte phospholipase A2 activity. *Biochemistry* 17:4029–4033, 1978

18. SMITH MW, COLLAN Y, KAHNG MW, TRUMP BF: Changes in mitochondrial

lipids of rat kidney during ischemia. *Biochim Biophys Acta* 618:192–201, 1980

19. CHANCE B: The energy-linked reaction of calcium with mitochondria. *J Biol Chem* 240:2729–2748, 1965

20. SCHLIWA M: The role of divalent cations in the regulation of microtubule assembly. In vivo studies on microtubules of the heliozan axopodium using the ionophore A23187. *J Cell Biol* 70:527–540, 1976

21. TRUMP BF, PHELPS PC, SHAMSUDDIN AM, HARRIS CC: Cell surface changes in premalignant and malignant lesions of the colon. *Lab Invest* 40:289, 1979

22. REIMER KA, GANOTE CE, JENNINGS RB: Alterations in renal cortex following ischemic injury. III. Ultrastructure of proximal tubules after ischemia or autolysis. *Lab Invest* 26:347–363, 1972

23. VENKATACHALAM MA, BERNARD DB, DONOHOE JF, LEVINSKY NG: Ischemic damage and repair in the rat proximal tubule. Differences among the S1, S2 and S3 segments. *Kidney Int* 14:31–49, 1978

24. VENKATACHALAM MA, JONES DB, RENNKE HG, SANDSTROM D, PATEL Y: Mechanism of proximal tubule brush border loss and regeneration following mild renal ischemia. *Lab Invest* 45:355–365, 1981

25. BURKE TJ, ARNOLD PE, SCHRIER RW: A role for intracellular calcium in the pathogenesis of norepinephrine-induced acute renal failure (*abstract*). *Clin Res* 29:457A, 1981

26. DOBYAN DC, BURKE T, CRONIN R, SCHRIER R, BULGER RE: The morphology of norepinephrine (NE)-induced acute renal failure (ARF) in the dog (*abstract*). Proc. IXth International Congress of Nephrology, Los Angeles, 1984

27. WEINBERG JM, HUNT D, HUMES HD: Effects of verapamil on in vitro ischemic injury to isolated rabbit proximal tubules (*abstract*). *Kidney Int* 25:239, 1984

28. MALIS CD, CHEUNG JY, LEAF A, BONVENTRE JV: Effects of verapamil in models of ischemic acute renal failure in the rat. *Am J Physiol* 245:F735–F742, 1983

29. GOLDFARB D, IAINA A, SERBAN I, GAVENDO S, KAPULER S, ELIAHOU HE: Beneficial effect of verapamil in ischemic acute renal failure in the rat (41576). *Prox Soc Exp Biol Med* 172:389–392, 1983

30. GORDON EE, FERRIS RK: Stimulation of renal gluconeogenesis by verapamil and D-600. *Biochem Pharmacol* 26:1089–1091, 1977

31. BORLE AB: Calcium transport by kidney cells, in *Calcium and Phosphate Transport Across Biomembranes,* edited by BRONNER F, PETERLIK M, New York, Academic Press, 1981, pp 193–198

32. HEMS DA, BROSNAN JT: Effects of ischemia on content of metabolites in rat liver and kidney in vivo. *Biochem J* 120:105–111, 1970

33. KESSLER RH: Effects of ischemia on the concentration of adenine nucleotides in the kidney of anesthetized dogs. *Proc Soc Exp Biol Med* 134:1091–1095, 1970

34. SIEGEL NJ, AVISON MJ, REILLY HF, ALGER JR, SHULMAN RG: Enhanced recovery of renal ATP with postischemic infusion of ATP-MgCl$_2$ determined by ^{31}P-NMR. *Am J Physiol* 245:F530–F534, 1983

35. HUMES HD, WEINBERG JM: Cellular energetics in acute renal failure, in *Acute Renal Failure,* edited by BRENNER BM, LAZARUS JM, Philadelphia, WB Saunders & Co, 1983, pp 47–98

36. BONVENTRE JV: Cellular response to ischemia, in *Acute Renal Failure. Correlations Between Morphology and Function,* edited by SOLEZ K, WHELTON A, New York, Marcel Dekker, Inc, 1984, pp 195–220

37. CHAUDRY IH, SAYEED MM, BAUE AE: The effect of adenosine triphosphate-magnesium chloride administration in shock. *Surgery* 75:220–227, 1974

38. SIEGEL NJ, GLAZIER WB, CHAUDRY IH, GAUDIO KM, LYTTON B, BAUE AE, KASHGARIAN M: Enhanced recovery from acute renal failure by the post-ischemic infusion of adenine nucleotides and magnesium chloride in rats. *Kidney Int* 17:338–349, 1980
39. GAUDIO KM, TAYLOR MR, CHAUDRY IH, KASHGARIAN M, SIEGEL NJ: Accelerated recovery of single nephron function by the postischemic infusion of ATP-MgCl₂. *Kidney Int* 22:13–20, 1982
40. GAUDIO KM, ARDITO TA, REILLY HF, KASHGARIAN M, SIEGEL NJ: Accelerated cellular recovery after an ischemic renal injury. *Am J Pathol* 112:338–346, 1983
41. ANDREWS PM, COFFEY AK: Protection of kidneys from acute renal failure resulting from normothermic ischemia. *Lab Invest* 49:87–98, 1983
42. BREZIS M, SILVA P, EPSTEIN FH, ROSEN S: Selective vulnerability of the thick ascending limb to anoxia (*abstract*). *Clin Res* 31:549A, 1983
43. ROSEN S, BREZIS M, SILVA P, EPSTEIN FH: Cell work accelerates anoxic cell injury. Implications for acute renal failure (*abstract*). *Kidney Int* 25:237, 1984
44. SIEGEL M, RICE J, BARNES J, OSGOOD R, STEIN J: Protective effect of mini dose of ouabain in ischemic renal failure in the dog (*abstract*). *Clin Res* 31:518A, 1983
45. CHIEN KR, ABRAMS J, SERRONI A, MARTIN JT, FARBER JL: Accelerated phospholipid degradation and associated membrane dysfunction in irreversible ischemic liver cell injury. *J Biol Chem* 253:4809–4817, 1978
46. FARBER JL, YOUNG EE: Accelerated phospholipid degradation in anoxic rat hepatocytes. *Arch Biochem Biophys* 211:312–320, 1981
47. CHIEN KR, ABRAMS J, PFAU RG, FARBER JL: Prevention by chlorpromazine of ischemic liver cell death. *Am J Pathol* 88:539–558, 1977
48. DOBYAN DC, BULGER RE: Partial protection by chlorpromazine in mercuric chloride-induced acute renal failure in rats. *Kidney Int* 25:229, 1984
49. KUNZE H, NAHAS N, TRAYNOR JR, WURL M: Effects of local anesthetics on phospholipases. *Biochem Biophys Acta* 441:93–102, 1976
50. MATTHYS E, PATEL Y, VENKATACHALAM M: Membrane phospholipid defect in ischemic renal damage (*abstract*). *Kidney Int* 21:220, 1982
51. KNAUSS TC, WEINBERG JM, HUMES HD: Alterations in renal cortical phospholipid content induced by gentamicin: time course, specificity, and subcellular localization. *Am J Physiol* 244:F535–F546, 1983
52. KALOYANIDES GJ, WANG M, GAUVEA W, KELLEY J, ALPERT H, VAAMONDE CA: Altered phosphatidyl inositol (PI) metabolism in diabetic (D) rats confers resistance to gentamicin-induced acute renal failure (G-ARF) (*abstract*). *Kidney Int* 12:531A, 1981
53. FREEMAN BA, CRAPO JD: Free radicals and tissue injury. *Lab Invest* 47:412–426, 1982
54. BREZIS M, ROSEN S, SILVA P, EPSTEIN FH: Effect of glutathione (GSH) depletion on structure and function of the isolated perfused kidney (*abstract*). *Clin Res* 30:538A, 1982
55. MITCHELL JR, McMURTY RJ, STATHAM CN, NELSON SD: Molecular basis for several drug-induced nephropathies. *Am J Med* 62:518–526, 1977
56. HARMON WE, COHEN HJ, SCHNEEBERGER EE, GRUPE WE: Chronic renal failure in children treated with methyl CCNU. *N Engl J Med* 300:1200–1203, 1979
57. OLIVER J, MacDOWELL M, TRACY A: The pathogenesis of acute renal failure associated with traumatic and toxic injury: Renal ischemia, nephrotoxic damage and the ischemuric episode. *J Clin Invest* 30:1307–1439, 1951

58. CUPPAGE FE, TATE A: Repair of the nephron following injury with mercuric chloride. *Am J Pathol* 51:405–430, 1967
59. GRITZKA TL, TRUMP BF: Renal tubular lesions caused by mercuric chloride. *Am J Pathol* 52:1225–1278, 1968
60. STEIN JH, GOTTSCHALL J, OSGOOD RW, FERRIS TF: Pathophysiology of a nephrotoxic model of acute renal failure. *Kidney Int* 8:27–41, 1975
61. FLAMENBAUM W, HAMBURGER RJ, HUDDLESTON ML, KAUFMAN J, MCNEIL JS, SCHWARTZ JH, NAGLE R: The initiation phase of experimental acute renal failure: An evaluation of uranyl nitrate-induced acute renal failure in the rat. *Kidney Int* 10:S115–S122, 1976
62. HALEY DP: Morphologic changes in uranyl nitrate induced acute renal failure in saline- and water-drinking rats. *Lab Invest* 46:196–208, 1982
63. DOBYAN DC, LEVI J, JACOBS C, KOSEK J, WEINER MW: Mechanism of cis-platinum nephrotoxicity: II. Morphological observations. *J Pharmacol Exp Ther* 213:551–556, 1980
64. GLAUMANN B, GLAUMANN H, BEREZESKY IK, TRUMP BF: II. Morphological changes of the pars convoluta (P1 & P2) of the proximal tubule of the rat kidney made ischemic in vivo. *Virch Arch B Cell Pathol* 19:281–302, 1975
65. GLAUMANN B, TRUMP BF: Studies on the pathogenesis of ischemic cell injury: III. Morphological changes of the proximal pars recta tubules (P3) of the rat kidney made ischemic in vivo. *Virch Arch B Cell Pathol* 19:303–323, 1975
66. KREISBERG JI, BULGER RE, TRUMP BF, NAGLE RB: Effects of transient hypotension on the structure and function of rat kidney. *Virch Arch B Cell Path* 22:121–133, 1976
67. DOBYAN DC, NAGLE RB, BULGER RE: Acute tubular necrosis in the rat kidney following sustained hypotension. Physiologic and morphologic observations. *Lab Invest* 37:411–422, 1977
68. DOBYAN DC, HILL D, LEWIS T, BULGER RE: Cyst formation in rat kidney induced by cis-platinum administration. *Lab Invest* 45:260–268, 1981
69. HALEY DP, BULGER RE, DOBYAN DC: The long term effects of uranyl nitrate on the structure and function of the rat kidney. *Virch Arch B Cell Pathol* 41:181–192, 1982
70. KOSEK JC, MAZZE RI, COUSINS MJ: Nephrotoxicity of gentamicin. *Lab Invest* 30:48–57, 1974
71. SILVERBLATT F, TURCK M, BULGER R: Nephrotoxicity due to cephaloridine: A light and electron microscopic study in rabbits. *J Infect Dis* 122:33–44, 1970
72. BLANTZ RC: The mechanism of acute renal failure after uranyl nitrate. *J Clin Invest* 55:621–635, 1975
73. SCHOR N, ICHIKAWA I, RENNKE HG, TROY JL, BRENNER BM: Pathophysiology of altered glomerular function in aminoglycoside-treated rats. *Kidney Int* 19:288–296, 1981
74. BAYLIS C, RENNKE HR, BRENNER BM: Mechanisms of the defect in glomerular ultrafiltration associated with gentamicin administration. *Kidney Int* 1:344–353, 1977
75. WILLIAMS RH, THOMAS CE, NAVAR LG, EVAN AP: Hemodynamic and single nephron function during the maintenance phase of ischemic acute renal failure in the dog. *Kidney Int* 19:503–515, 1981
76. COX JW, BAEHLER RW, SHARMA H, O'DORISIO T, OSGOOD RW, STEIN JH, FERRIS TF: Studies on the mechanism of oliguria in a model of unilateral acute renal failure. *J Clin Invest* 53:1546–1558, 1974
77. BARNES JL, OSGOOD RW, REINECK HJ, STEIN JH: Glomerular alterations in an ischemic model of acute renal failure. *Lab Invest* 45:378–386, 1981

78. SOLEZ K, MOREL-MAROGER L, SRAER J-D: The morphology of "acute tubular necrosis" in man: Analysis of 57 renal biopsies and a comparison with the glycerol model. *Medicine* 58:362–376, 1979
79. SOLEZ K, RACUSEN LC, WHELTON A: Glomerular epithelial cell changes in early postischemic acute renal failure in rabbits and man. *Am J Pathol* 103:163–173, 1981
80. RACUSEN LC, PROZIALECK DH, SOLEZ K: Glomerular epithelial cell changes after ischemia or dehydration. Possible role of angiotensin II. *Am J Pathol* 114:157–163, 1984
81. MYERS WD, LANGLINAIS P, MERRILL RH: Glomerular alterations by scanning electron microscopy in acute renal insufficiency in man (*abstract*). *Kidney Int* 12:531A, 1977
82. CRONIN RE, DE TORRENTE A, MILLER PD, BULGER RE, BURKE TJ, SCHRIER RW: Pathogenic mechanisms in early norepinephrine-induced acute renal failure: Functional and histological correlates of protection. *Kidney Int* 14:115–125, 1978
83. TAGUMA Y, SASAKI Y, KYOGOKU Y, ARAHAWA M, SHIOJI R, FURUYAMA T, YOSHINAGA K: Morphological changes in an early phase of norepinephrine-induced acute renal failure in unilaterally nephrectomized dogs. *J Lab Clin Med* 96:616–632, 1980
84. CONGER JD, ROBINETTE JB, GUGGENHEIM SJ: Effect of acetylcholine on the early phase of reversible norepinephrine-induced acute renal failure. *Kidney Int* 19:399–409, 1981
85. BULGER RE, CRONIN RE, DOBYAN DC: Glomerular architectural changes after a two hour infusion of norepinephrine. *Am J Anat* 159:379–384, 1980
86. BAEHLER RW, KOTCHEN TA, BURKE JA, GALLA JH, BHATHENA D: Considerations of the pathophysiology of mercuric chloride-induced acute renal failure. *J Lab Clin Med* 90:330–340, 1977
87. ZAGER RA, BALTES LA, SHARMA HM, COUSER WG: Glomerulopathy does not increase renal susceptibility to acute ischemic injury. *Am J Physiol* 246:F272–F281, 1984
88. CLARKSON AR, MACDONALD MK, FUSTER V, CASH JD, ROBSON JS: Glomerular coagulation in acute ischemic renal failure. *Q J Med* 39:585–600, 1970
89. HORNYCH H, BEAUFILS M, RICHET G: The effect of exogenous angiotensin on superficial and deep glomeruli in the rat kidney. *Kidney Int* 2:336–343, 1972
90. DACH JL, KURTZMAN NA: A scanning electron microscopic study of the glycerol model of acute renal failure. *Lab Invest* 34:406–414, 1976
91. TOKUNAGA J, EDANAGA M, FUJITA T, ADACHI K: Freeze cracking of scanning electron microscope specimens. A study of the kidney and spleen. *Arch Histol Jap* 37:165–182, 1974
92. FUJITA T, TOKUNAGA J, EDANAGA M: Scanning electron microscopy of the glomerular filtration membrane in the rat kidney. *Cell Tissue Res* 166:299–314, 1976
93. PURCELL DJ II, EKNOYAN G, DOBYAN DC, BULGER RE: Normal glomerular endothelial morphology (*abstract*). *Kidney Int* 21:204, 1982
94. BULGER RE, EKNOYAN G, PURCELL DJ II, DOBYAN DC: Endothelial characteristics of glomerular capillaries in normal, mercuric chloride-induced and gentamicin-induced acute renal failure in the rat. *J Clin Invest* 72:128–141, 1983
95. AVASTHI PS, EVAN AP, HAY D: Glomerular endothelial cells in uranyl nitrate-induced acute renal failure in rats. *J Clin Invest* 65:121–127, 1980
96. LUFT FC, EVAN AP: Comparative effects of tobramycin and gentamicin on glomerular ultrastructure. *J Infect Dis* 142:910–914, 1980

97. GATTONE VH II, EVAN AP, MONG SA, CONNORS BA, ARONOFF GR, LUFT FC: The morphology of the renal microvasculature in glycerol- and gentamicin-induced acute renal failure. *J Lab Clin Med* 101:183–195, 1983

98. EVAN AP, LUFT FC, GATTONE V, CONNORS BA, McCARRON DA, WILLIS LR: The glomerular filtration barrier in the spontaneously hypertensive rat. *Hypertension* 3(Suppl I):I-154–I-161, 1981

99. EVAN AP, MONG SA, CONNORS BA, LUFT FC: Scanning electron microscopic changes in the filtration barrier of insulin treated and untreated alloxan diabetic rats (*abstract*). *Clin Res* 29:461, 1981

100. OLSON JL, RENNKE HG, VENKATACHALAM MA: Alterations in the charge and size selectivity barrier of the glomerular filter in aminonucleoside nephrosis in rats. *Lab Invest* 44:271–279, 1981

101. BURNICK MB: Contractile activity of human glomeruli in culture. *Nephron* 6:1–10, 1969

102. BECKER CG: Demonstration of actomyosin in mesangial cells of renal glomerulus. *Am J Pathol* 66:97–110, 1972

103. AUSIELLO DA, KREISBERG JI, ROY C, KARNOVSKY MJ: Contraction of cultured rat glomerular cells of apparent mesangial origin after stimulation with angiotensin II and arginine vasopressin. *J Clin Invest* 65:754–760, 1980

104. SRAER JD, SRAER J, ARDAILLOU R, MIMOUNE O: Evidence for renal glomerular receptors for angiotensin II. *Kidney Int* 6:241–246, 1974

105. BROWN GP, DOUGLAS JG, KRONTIRIS-LITOWITZ J: Properties of angiotensin II receptors of isolated rat glomeruli: Factors influencing binding affinity and comparative binding of angiotensin analogs. *Endocrinology* 106:1923–1929, 1980

106. BALLERMANN BJ, DZAU VJ, SKORECKI KL, BRENNER BM: Altered glomerular angiotensin II (AII) receptor modulation in untreated diabetic rats (*abstract*). *Kidney Int* 23:272, 1983

107. KREISBERG JI: Contractile properties of the glomerular mesangium. *Fed Proc* 42:3053–3057, 1983

Experimental Acute Renal Failure: Pathophysiology and Methods of Protection

Terrance A. Fried and Jay H. Stein

Four main pathophysiologic mechanisms have been proposed to explain the decrease in creatinine and/or inulin clearance noted with nephrotoxic and ischemic acute renal failure: hemodynamic alterations, alterations in the glomerular capillary permeability, tubular obstruction, and tubular backleak. In the following pages, we will briefly review these four mechanisms, drawing mainly upon the experimental ischemic model of acute renal failure for illustrative purposes. In addition, we will consider some of the protective maneuvers that have attempted to reverse or prevent these functional alterations.

Hemodynamics

Acute renal failure has been associated with variable decrements in renal blood flow in humans as well as in experimental animals. For instance, Hollenberg et al [1] measured the total renal blood flow (RBF) in 20 patients with acute oliguric renal failure of different etiologies. These results were compared with those obtained in 36 normal patients being assessed as kidney transplant donors. They noted that the RBF was reduced to approximately one-third of normal [1]. Additional studies have confirmed these findings [2, 3].

Experimental acute renal failure following mercuric chloride, uranyl nitrate, glycerol, and ischemic insults are each associated with a marked decrement in RBF. Specifically, both temporary renal artery occlusion and intrarenal norepinephrine in the rat are associated with the subsequent fall in RBF to approximately 50% of normal [4, 5]. Similarly, intrarenal norepinephrine in the dog is followed by a marked drop in RBF, which only slowly returns to control levels [6]. A number of mechanisms have been proposed to explain this decrease in RBF. Franklin and Merrill [7] suggested in 1960 that intersti-

This manuscript was presented as part of a Symposium on *Acute Renal Failure: Structure-Function Relationships.*

tial edema may cause extrinsic compression of the renal arterioles, which leads to an increase in the renal vascular resistance and a decrease in RBF. Experimental support for this hypothesis has not been found. Flores et al [8] suggested an alternative hypothesis—that ischemia may lead to endothelial swelling and that this, in turn, results in an increase in renal vascular resistance and (thereby) a fall in RBF. One would predict from this theory that there should be a progressive fall in RBF with time, which is, however, not what is experimentally found. In addition, subsequent studies from the same laboratory did not confirm this hypothesis [9].

Alternatively, an increase in renal vascular resistance and a decrease in RBF may be a result of either humoral or neural alterations in response to the insult. Conceivably, the increase in renal vascular resistance may be a consequence of alterations in the adrenergic nervous system. This could be mediated either through the renal nerves or possibly via circulating catecholamines. Exogenous norepinephrine certainly can cause acute renal failure, and this may merely represent an exaggeration of the endogenously released catechols following an ischemic or nephrotoxic insult. Further, the *Tupaia belangeri* (tree shrew) has been shown to develop acute renal failure following psychic stress alone [10]. When a male of this species is introduced to another male, a fight for dominance ensues. If the subordinate is removed from the victor's cage and is placed in a neighboring cage that allows visual, but not physical contact, he remains in a state that indicates persistent activation of the sympathetic nervous system. Within 2 to 16 days, the subordinate lapses into a coma and dies. Renal failure and uremia are important contributors to his demise.

Additional support for a role of the renal nerves in the pathophysiology of acute renal failure is suggested by the use of denervation as a therapeutic maneuver. Although initially meeting with some success [11], this effort has not been substantiated by others [12]. Similarly, cadaver kidney transplantation is frequently associated with acute renal failure despite the absence of intact renal nerves.

Vasoactive compounds released in response to ischemia and/or nephrotoxins could be responsible for the increase in renal vascular resistance. Thromboxane, vasopressin, norepinephrine, and angiotensin each have been suggested as possible mediators. Thromboxane levels increase in association with ureteral obstruction [13], glycerol injection [14], and glomerulonephritis [15]. However, direct measurement has not been reported in other nephrotoxic or ischemic injuries.

Vasopressin given systemically is associated with a marked increase in the renal vascular resistance [16]; therefore, it has been suggested as a possible mediator of the increase in renal vascular resistance associated with acute renal failure. Vasopressin also has been implicated as a vasoconstrictor substance in glycerol-induced acute renal failure, as well as following renal artery clamping [17, 18]. Too few studies, however, have been performed to state anything definitive on its role in acute renal failure. Indeed, experimental acute renal failure can be readily induced in rats with hereditary diabetes insipidus, suggesting that antidiuretic hormone (ADH) at least is not necessary for acute renal failure to occur [19].

Lastly, the renin-angiotensin system has been proposed as a pathogenic mediator in acute renal failure. Plasma renin activity as well as plasma angiotensin levels are increased during the oliguric phase of acute renal failure in both humans and experimental animals. Goormaghtigh, in 1945 [20], suggested that a substance produced in the juxtaglomerular apparatus and, perhaps, in the preglomerular vessels may be important in the etiology of acute renal failure. Indeed, Weber et al [21] and Thurau et al [22] have shown increased levels of renin in juxtaglomerular apparatuses that were microdissected from animals with acute renal failure. An increase in renin or angiotensin in association with acute renal failure, of course, does not prove a causative relationship. Initial enthusiasm supporting this relationship followed reports that chronic saline loading, which is a maneuver associated with a decrease in renal plasma renin levels, was protective in various models of acute renal failure. Indeed, chronic saline loading is protective against glycerol-, uranyl nitrate-, and mercuric chloride-induced acute renal failure [23, 24]. However, it has not been shown to be protective in ischemic acute renal failure [25, 26]. Additionally, neither renin nor angiotensin immunization have been conclusively shown to be effective in any model of acute renal failure, including those that respond to saline loading [27, 28]. Furthermore, the protective effect of chronic saline loading in glycerol- and mercuric chloride-induced acute renal failure can be separated from the effect on renal renin levels; that is, by using either diuretics or a two-kidney Goldblatt model, one can show protection with saline loading despite concomitant increases in the renal renin to very high levels. In summary, the renin-angiotensin system is activated in most models of acute renal failure, especially those associated with oliguria. However, the role that this activation plays in the reduction of glomerular filtration remains to be determined.

. Indeed, the role that both an increase in renal vascular resistance and a decrease in RBF play in the decrement in glomerular filtration rate (GFR) is also not clear. In most cases of renal failure, the inulin clearance is decreased considerably more than the RBF. Furthermore, in a number of circumstances, one can increase the RBF without altering the inulin clearance. Arendshorst et al [29] showed this in the rat. They volume-expanded their animals 24 hr following a 60-min renal artery occlusion. With this regimen, the RBF was increased to supernormal levels without altering the GFR. Similarly, Cox et al [30] volume-expanded dogs 24 hr following norepinephrine-induced renal failure. They were able to increase the RBF to supernormal levels without measurably altering the GFR.

An increase in total RBF may not be associated with an increase in flow in some critical area of the kidney. It is conceivable that important areas remain poorly perfused despite supernormal total flow rates. One possible candidate for such an area is the inner stripe of the outer medulla. The blood supply to this area is low and the vasculature is fragile [31]. Following ischemia, the capillaries in this region are dilated and the region is congested with red blood cells. Karlberg et al [32] have shown, by using the ^{86}Rb extraction method, that the blood flow to this area is approximately 10 to 20% that of normal immediately following ischemia. They argue that since the medullary blood flow under normal circumstances represents only approximately 10% of the total blood flow, even a 90% decrease in this area may go undetected. The vasa recta in this region supply nutrients to the loops of Henle and, possibly, also to the pars recta regions, both of which are severely damaged following ischemia [31, 33]. It is unclear from these studies if this medullary ischemia/congestion plays any etiologic role in the decrement of inulin/creatinine clearance (C_{cn}) associated with acute renal failure. Thiel would favor a secondary phenomenon. He suggests that dilated, proximal straight tubules cause pressure collapse of the ascending vasa recta of the inner stripe of the outer medulla [33]. Mason, however, suggests that the damaged vasculature in this area may play a more causative role in the pathogenesis of ischemic acute renal failure [33]. Investigation into this interesting phenomenon obviously must be continued.

Glomerular Permeability

A second mechanism by which the GFR may decrease following nephrotoxic or ischemic injury to the kidney is by an alteration in the glomerular capillary permeability; that is, a decrease in the ultrafiltration coefficient (K_f), which is a measurement of the permeability of the glomerular capillary membrane, may result in a decrease in the GFR. The K_f is the product of two terms: the hydraulic permeability of the glomerular capillary membrane (L_p) and the capillary surface area (A) through which filtration occurs. A decrease in either of these two terms will decrease K_f and possibly filtration. Unfortunately, these two terms cannot be individually measured; therefore, the contribution of each to K_f is never really known. Direct measurements of K_f have been performed in uranyl nitrate- [34] and gentamicin-induced acute renal failure [35], and they have revealed a decrease in both models. These decreases have been associated with morphologic changes in the glomerular membrane as well. There is evidence both for and against a role of K_f in ischemic acute renal failure. Williams et al [36] measured K_f in six dogs following temporary renal artery occlusion and found an approximate 50% decrease in K_f. Similarly, Cox et al [30] have suggested from indirect observations that the K_f may be decreased in norepinephrine-induced acute renal failure. More recently, Savin [37] has reported in vitro evidence that the glomerular ultrafiltration coefficient in dogs is decreased 24 hr following an ischemic episode. However, not all investigators have found a decrease in K_f following ischemia. Daugharty et al [38] directly estimated K_f, and found it to be normal following partial renal artery occlusion. Similarly, indirect evidence from Arendshorst et al [29] would suggest that the glomerular K_f, if decreased, most probably plays only a minor role in the renal functional impairment. They noted that 24 hr following renal artery occlusion, volume expansion was associated with a definite increase in glomerular filtration, which was evidenced by a dilation of the proximal tubules and by a marked increase in the proximal tubular hydrostatic pressure. Similarly, reports of both normal and abnormal glomerular morphology have been reported [39, 40] in ischemic models of acute renal failure.

In summary, alterations in the permeability of the glomerular capillary membrane appears to play a role following certain cellular insults. However, the magnitude of this role is limited; acute renal failure will ensue only in combination with other mechanisms.

Obstruction

Ponfick, in 1875 [41], suggested that casts may cause tubular obstruction and, in this way, may be important in the pathophysiology of acute renal failure. Indeed, obstruction appears to play a definite role in the reduction of GFR following most experimental models of acute renal failure. This is particularly true for ischemic acute renal failure, although a contributory role for casts and obstruction also has been suggested in mercuric chloride [42], gentamicin [43], and myohemoglobinuric [44] acute renal failure. Dibona [45], in a reconsideration of an earlier study, noted a strong correlation between cast formation and the blood urea nitrogen (BUN) concentration. Cushner et al [46], studying the glycerol model, noted markedly elevated proximal tubular pressure following volume expansion at 18 to 24 hr. They additionally noted a strong inverse correlation between the number of casts and the inulin clearance (C_{in}). Richards and DiBona [47] also found a significant correlation between the number of casts and serum creatinine in the gylcerol model of acute renal failure. Similarly, in a separate study, Solez [12] noted a significant correlation between cast formation and serum creatinine in the pedicle clamp model of acute renal failure.

The evidence for a functional role of casts and/or obstruction in the pathophysiology of acute renal failure comes mainly from morphologic and micropuncture studies. Donohoe et al [48] evaluated the effect of 15, 25, and 60 min of renal artery occlusion in the rat with light and electron microscopy. Fifteen min of ischemia was associated with minimal or no morphologic or functional changes. The early reflow period following 25 min of ischemia was associated with interiorization of microvilli into the cytoplasm of the proximal convoluted and straight tubules. Cells of the proximal straight tubules became necrotic, and cellular debris appeared in the tubular lumen. An occasional straight tubule showed evidence of obstruction. Following 60 min of ischemia, which is a frequently employed occlusion period, almost all of the tubules showed evidence of intratubular obstruction. Shortly after reflow, almost all proximal straight tubules were occluded with membrane-bound blebs, and most of the proximal convoluted tubules were dilated. After 24 hr, the thin limbs of Henle, the distal tubules, and the collecting ducts were filled with casts. These findings confirmed and extended the earlier work of Tanner and Sophasan [49]. They had also noted proximal tubular dilatation and obstruction in the early reflow period and the presence of distal cast formation at 24 hr. In addition, these authors quantitated the fraction of nephrons containing casts. They microdissected distal tubules and found that over 80% of the dissected tubules contained hyaline casts.

Micropuncture data obtained in the early and late reflow periods of ischemic acute renal failure also support an important role for casts and obstruction. Tanner and Sophasan [49] performed micropuncture in the rat following 60 min of ischemia. They found the proximal tubular pressures to be markedly elevated in the early reflow period to values approximately 3-fold that of normal. At 24 hr the proximal tubular pressures were still elevated, but they were only about 50% higher than the baseline preischemic values. Arendshorst et al [50] reported similar findings. They noted that the proximal and distal tubules 1 to 3 hr after a 60 min renal artery occlusion in the rat were filled with fluid and were markedly dilated. The tubular pressures were heterogeneous, but were greatly elevated with proximal tubular pressures of 31 mm Hg and distal tubular pressures of 16 mm Hg (control pressures were 11.5 and 5.3 mm Hg, respectively). Twenty-four hr after reflow, the proximal tubular pressures were no longer elevated; indeed, they were significantly decreased (9.2 mm Hg). Following acute volume expansion, however, the proximal tubular pressure was noted to be significantly elevated (18.2 mm Hg), but no change in the GFR occurred. This suggests that obstruction persists and may be playing an important role during this time period. Confirmatory evidence for this was reported by Tanner and Steinhausen [51], who measured the proximal tubular pressure of individual nephrons undergoing microperfusion. They investigated two time frames: shortly after renal artery clamp release and 2 to 3 days following release. The baseline proximal tubular pressures 1 to 7 hr following reflow were approximately three times that of normal, but they had decreased to approximately 50% greater than normal at 2 to 3 days. Pressures greater than 100 mm Hg, and at times greater than 150 mm Hg, were obtained when these proximal tubules were microperfused. During these perfusions, they noted that a maximal pressure would be reached, and that this was followed by a gradual decrease in intratubular pressure despite continued perfusion. This suggested to them that the maximal pressure obtained had dislodged the intratubular material (casts), and thereby released the obstruction that led to the subsequent decrease in the intratubular pressure. From these experiments, the magnitude of the obstruction is certainly emphasized.

Additional support for intratubular obstruction playing an important role in the pathophysiology of ischemic acute renal failure comes from a comparison of measurements of single nephron glomerular filtration rate (SNGFR) and total kidney glomerular filtration rates. Tanner, Sloan, and Sophasan [52] noted that the mean SNGFR measured by proximal tubular free-flow collections was 22 nl/min following 60 min of ischemia, as compared with 30 nl/min in normal kidneys. This represents an approximate one-third decrease. However, the whole kidney GFR was decreased by 90%. They concluded that the difference between whole kidney and single-nephron values was a result of the release of intratubular obstruction during SNGFR determination (that is, the decrease in the proximal tubular pressure and the resulting increase in effective filtration pressure). Although appealing and certainly supportive for a role of obstruction in the marked decrease in glomerular filtration following ischemia, additional explanations also may be invoked to explain these findings. Mason et al [53] have recently reported that SNGFR measured in superficial nephrons following renal ischemia may not be representative of deeper nephrons. They note that superficial nephrons are at least partly protected by the ambient oxygen concentration during the ischemia, and that deeper nephrons that are not exposed to air are more severely affected. Significant amounts of backleak also could account for the discrepancy between SNGFR and total kidney GFR.

In summary, obstruction most likely plays a major role in the pathophysiology of acute renal failure. This role is most marked during the early initiation phase although it contributes to the drop in SNGFR and total GFR during the later maintenance phase as well.

Backleak

In 1929, Richards [54], studying the effect of mercuric chloride in the frog, noted that there was leakage of fluid through the damaged tubular epithelium. He was the first to suggest that tubular backleak may play a functional role in acute renal failure. Backleak represents a fourth mechanism by which the measured C_{cr} or C_{in} may be reduced in acute renal failure. This mechanism does not actually entail a decrease in glomerular filtration—rather, the measured clearance is decreased due to a loss through the tubular epithelium of the marker used to quantitate glomerular filtration. That is, inulin or creatinine actually may be filtered, but because of the loss through the damaged tubule, it does not appear in the urine; therefore, the measured total kidney filtration rate is decreased.

A quantitation of the amount of backleak has been performed in many different models of acute renal failure. The method most widely employed for this measurement is the injection of labeled inulin into individual proximal tubules and the subsequent measurement of its appearance in the urine from the ipsilateral and the contralateral kidneys. If no backleak occurs, such as in the normal kidney, the degree of marker recovery from the ipsilateral kidney should be 95 to 100%. However, if there is significant backleak, then one would expect a percentage of the marker that "backleaks" to appear in the urine of the opposite kidney.

Evidence has accumulated to suggest that backleak may play a role in experimental acute renal failure due to mercuric chloride, uranyl nitrate, and ischemia. Backleak following uranyl nitrate has been assessed, and it appears to play a significant role [55]. Mercuric chloride has also been shown to be associated with measurable amounts of backleak, with only 45.5% of the amount recovered appearing from the ipsilateral kidney and 54.5% being recovered from the contralateral kidney [56]. Ischemic acute renal failure has received the most attention. Donohoe et al [48] measured the amount of ^{14}C-inulin recovered from both kidneys after injecting it into proximal tubules of one kidney. They reported that following 25 min of renal artery occlusion, 78.6% of the marker was found in the urine of the kidney into which it was injected, whereas 10.8% was excreted by the opposite kidney. However, following 60 min of ischemia, the degree of backleak was considerably more impressive with only 38.5% of the injected marker being recovered from the ipsilateral kidney and 34.9% being recovered from the contralateral kidney. Tanner, Sloan, and Sophasan [52], using a similar protocol, found that after 1 hr of renal artery ischemia, 36.4% was recovered from the urine of the ischemic kidney and 27.3% was recovered from the contralateral non-ischemic kidney. Similarly, Eisenbach and Steinhausen [57] recovered between 42 and 50% of the injected inulin from the contralateral kidney. Daugharty et al [38], on the other hand, using a slightly different model of ischemic acute renal failure—that of partial rather than complete renal artery occlusion—could not demonstrate any significant backleak.

It should be noted, however, that the validity of the microinjection method for determining backleak has been questioned. Microinjection of inulin into tubules may elevate the intratubular pressure, thereby increasing the amount of backleak. This problem has been addressed by Donohoe et al [48]. In addition to the microinjection of inulin mentioned above, they also injected animals intravenously with horseradish peroxidase, thus avoiding any possible alteration in intratubular pressure. This protein (molecular wt, 40,000) is filtered at the glomerulus; and, in control animals, there is no leakage through the tubular cells. In the ischemic kidneys, however, the horseradish peroxidase was noted to diffuse through the tubular epithelium of both the proximal convoluted and proximal straight tubules.

Myers et al [58] have investigated the amount of backleak present in human acute renal failure. They infused inulin and dextran-40 (Einstein-Stokes 20 to 40 Å) into 10 postoperative cardiac surgery patients who had developed acute renal failure. They collected the urine from these patients and compared the fractional clearance profile of dextran molecules of different sizes with that from a set of control patients. They noted that in 7 of the 10 patients, the sieving coefficient of the dextran was greater than 1. The only possible explanation for this is that there was backleakage of inulin leading to an underestimation of C_{in}. Their calculations indicated that up to 50% of the filtered inulin was lost by tubular backleak.

In summary, tubular backleak, especially in association with tubular obstruction, probably plays a role in the reduction of measured GFR in acute renal failure. The magnitude of this abnormality varies from model to model; therefore, the functional role of backleak in acute renal failure should not be generalized.

In addition to the primary alterations that tubular obstruction and backleak cause, they also may decrease the GFR by secondarily increasing the renal vascular resistance and, hence, decreasing RBF. This was first proposed by Schnermann et al [59]. Their basic premise is that acute renal failure is associated with a decrease in solute reabsorption proximal to the distal tubule. This is sensed by the macula densa as an increase in glomerular filtration, leading to afferent arteriolar vasoconstriction. This theory requires that two conditions are met: (1) the tubuloglomerular feedback system must be intact in acute renal failure, and (2), an increase in solute must reach the macula densa. Both of these have been shown to occur, at least in some settings. Mason et al [60] has shown that the tubuloglomerular feedback system is intact in mercuric chloride, uranyl nitrate, methemoglobin, and ischemic acute renal failure. They have also shown that the sodium content of tubular fluid in the early distal tubule is markedly elevated following ischemia, suggesting that the second condition is also met [61]. Hanley [62] has also reported data derived from isolated perfused tubular experiments showing that there is a marked defect in the reabsorption of filtrate in all tubular segments investigated between the glomerulus and the macula densa. The tubuloglomerular feedback system also may be activated in response to proximal tubular obstruction. In otherwise normal kidneys, the placement of an oil block in single proximal tubules leads to afferent vasoconstriction 24 hr later [63]. This also seems to be mediated by the macula densa [64].

The decrement in GFR that is measured following experimental acute renal failure is not explained simply. There are multiple interacting events that, in concert, lead to functional impairment. Although any one mechanism may predominate in a single model or during a single time frame, many mechanisms appear to be of importance.

Protective Maneuvers

Numerous attempts have been undertaken to protect or enhance the recovery from experimental acute renal failure. Most of these have met with only limited success. However, the usefulness of these studies is not merely in the amount of protection they might bring about, but also in the insight into the pathophysiology of acute renal failure that they may offer. We will address some of the more recently devised maneuvers that have been designed to counteract some of the basic biochemical or cellular events that are important mediators of cell death.

Hemodynamic

Due to the enormous amount of attention that this mechanism has received, one might correctly suspect that a fair number of studies have been undertaken to prevent or reverse the hemodynamic alterations that occur following the induction of acute renal failure. As mentioned previously, the RBF can be returned to normal 24 hr following ischemia, but this does not alter the course of the renal failure [30]. Perhaps, one must return the blood flow to normal at an earlier time or prevent the decrease in RBF from occurring altogether. Attempts along these lines have been made. Because of the data suggesting that the renin-angiotensin system may be involved in the increase in renal vascular resistance following the induction of acute renal failure, many attempts have been designed to interrupt this system. From 3 to 4 weeks of saline loading with or without deoxycorticosterone acetate (DOCA) treatment leads to a marked decrease in the renal renin content. If the renin-angiotensin system were involved, then one would expect this might lead to significant protection. Indeed, this is the case for mercuric chloride-, uranyl nitrate-, and glycerol-induced acute renal failure. However, ischemic acute renal failure does not seem to be protected by this maneuver, with most of the studies suggesting no benefit from saline and/or DOCA pretreatment [25, 26, 65]. Any interpretation of the mechanism for the protection offered by saline loading is further complicated when a more direct inhibition of the renin-angiotensin system is undertaken. Antibodies to renin, as well as to angiotensin, do not appear to offer protection; similarly, specific antagonists do not appear to be protective. Additional studies alluded to above, which have investigated the relationship between renin levels and protection, also have been performed by using the two-kidney Goldblatt model. These animals have a silver clip placed on one of their kidneys. Over a short time period, this is associated with a marked increase in renin production by the clipped kidney and a marked decrease by the unclipped kidney. If the renin level were important in the pathophysiology of acute renal failure, one would expect the unclipped kidney to be protected or at least the clipped kidney to be more severely affected. However, no significant difference between the two kidneys following glycerol or uranyl nitrate has been shown [65, 66]. These data, together with the immunization/antagonist data, suggest that saline loading may be offering its protection through a mechanism other than the inhibition of the renin-angiotensin system. Alternatively, the renin-angiotensin immunization and the angiotensin antagonists were not reaching a local site of angiotensin production; therefore, no amelioration of acute renal failure occurred.

In addition to the above methods for reversing or preventing the hemodynamic alteration of acute renal failure, other approaches also have been undertaken. Both bradykinin and acetylcholine are vasodilators that have been successfully used in norepinephrine-induced acute renal failure [6]. The mechanism for their protection is also not entirely clear, although it may be at least partly due to a decrease in the renal vascular resistance. Similar doses of these agents have been tried in the renal artery clamp model without success [67]. The prostaglandins, PGE_2 and PGI_2, have also been tried with some success. Casey et al [68] noted that both PGE_2 and PGI_2 could protect the kidneys histologically from renal ischemia, although no functional protection was evident in their studies. Recently, Neumayer et al [69] reported preliminary results employing PGI_2 with some success. Lifschitz, in our laboratory (personal communication), also has data to suggest a protective effect of PGI_2 in ischemic acute renal failure in the rat. Although it is far from clear that the protection by the prostaglandins is through an alteration in renal hemodynamics, it is certainly a possibility. Other models of acute renal failure, such as glycerol and norepinephrine, also have responded favorably to prostaglandin infusions [70, 71].

Obstruction

It is difficult to devise maneuvers that will specifically prevent tubular obstruction from occurring. The difficulty is partly due to the fact that tubular necrosis and cast formation go hand-in-hand under most circumstances. In most of the interventions that have resulted in a decrease in cast formation, there is also a significant decrement in the amount of necrosis that is present.

This is understandable if one considers that cast formation and secondary obstruction can, by themselves, lead to a feedback decrease in RBF (afferent arteriolar vasoconstriction) and to further ischemia, necrosis, and cast formation. In a recent investigation of the gylcerol model of acute renal failure in our laboratory, we found that chronic Ringer's infusion could indeed differentiate these two components [46]. The protection of C_{in} at 18 to 24 hr was associated with a prevention or decrease in the number of casts despite similar degrees of necrosis; that is, there was an inverse correlation between the number of casts present and the C_{in}, whereas no such correlation was observed between cell necrosis and C_{in}. It is also interesting to speculate that part of the protection by saline loading in the nephrotoxic models of acute renal failure derives from the prevention or washing out of casts. This could lead directly to more filtration by decreasing the intratubular hydrostatic pressure, as well as indirectly by decreasing the amount of ischemia through a prevention or decrease in the amount of feedback vasoconstriction. Further studies into the mechanism of cast formation and more direct attempts to alter this formation are needed.

Cellular Events

The intracellular events that lead to cell injury and death following ischemia remain to be fully elucidated. Most of the attention in this area has centered on the consequences of a reduction in high-energy compounds. Shortly after ischemia begins, the adenosine triphosphate and adenosine diphosphate levels drop sharply. As ischemia continues, adenosine monophosphate and adenosine levels fall as well, making a replenishment following reinstitution of flow more difficult. The consequences of decreased energy supply are multiple, and they include a decrease in the ability of the cell to regulate intracellular sodium and calcium concentrations. The loss of intracellular sodium homeostasis leads to increases in cytosolic sodium and cell swelling. This, in turn, may lead to organelle dysfunction and to further cellular dysfunction. Similarly, the cell loses its ability to extrude calcium from the cytosol. This increase in cytosolic calcium may result in a number of additional disruptions, including further dysfunction of the mitochondrial energy machine as well as activation of different enzyme systems within the cell that may themselves be disruptive.

A number of studies have addressed these issues in an attempt to modify ischemic injury. Our laboratory has investigated the effect of a combination of Collins solution with low doses of ouabain infused through the renal artery during temporary renal artery occlusion in the dog [72]. The rationale for using this combination is that the ouabain, by partially inhibiting the Na-K-ATPase, will decrease the cellular metabolic rate. An inhibition of this enzyme system under normal circumstances should result in cell swelling due to the movement of sodium from the extracellular environment down its concentration gradient into the cell. However, it was reasoned that cell swelling could be prevented if the sodium gradient was prevented by replacement of the normal high-sodium, low-potassium concentration of extracellular fluid with Collins solution, which has an electrolyte makeup similar to that of intracellular fluid (low-sodium, high-potassium). This combination was associated with an approximate 3-fold increase in C_{in} when compared with animals receiving Collins or saline infusion alone.

A more direct attempt at increasing the high-energy compounds has been with the infusions of adenosine triphosphate and/or its precursors. Both inosine and adenosine have been shown to offer some protection [73]. However, direct adenosine triphosphate administration has not seemed to be as effective; on the other hand, if adenosine triphosphate (ATP), adenosine diphosphate (ADP), or adenosine monophosphate (AMP) are combined with mercuric chloride ($MgCl_2$), they offer considerable protection [74, 75]. The protection offered by ATP-$MgCl_2$ is quite impressive, with essentially normal morphology being maintained. Although it has been suggested that the ATP-$MgCl_2$ supplies the needed high-energy requirement of the cell, the mechanism of this protection is still somewhat speculative.

Besides preservation of high-energy compounds, attempts have been made to limit the amount of damage by preventing the intracellular buildup of calcium. Verapamil, which is a calcium channel blocker, has been used in both norepinephrine and renal artery occlusion models of acute renal failure. Indeed, verapamil appears to be protective against norepinephrine-induced acute renal failure [76] and, perhaps, against temporary renal artery occlusion as well [77]. Malis et al [78], however, were unable to show any protection in a pedicle clamp model. They suggested that the protection offered from norepinephrine was due to the vasodilatory effect of verapamil, rather than to the inhibition of calcium transport. On a cellular level, Weinberg et al [79] have shown that verapamil can protect isolated proximal tubule cells in cell culture from ischemia. Similarly, Wilson et al [80] dissected individual proximal tubules, medullary thick ascending limb, and cortical collecting ducts from rabbit kidneys and placed them in culture for 7 days. At that point, they subjected them to 45 min of ischemia (nitrogen atmosphere). They noted that removal of calcium from the culture media significantly reduced the amount of cell death, thereby suggesting that calcium is an important mediator of cell death following ischemia. Additional studies are needed to further define both the role of calcium in ischemic acute renal failure and the mechanism of the possible protective effect of calcium channel blockers.

Besides attempts to maintain higher concentrations of adenosine triphosphate in the cell and to block the effect of high intracellular calcium concentrations, attempts at maintaining cellular integrity have used free-radical scavengers [81], DMSO [82], and other maneuvers. These investigations hold a considerable amount of promise, and further attempts to prevent or lessen the amount of damage to cells and intracellular processes need to be pursued.

Summary

In conclusion, the pathophysiology of acute renal failure continues to be only partially understood. There are a number of mechanisms that are operative, many of which are no doubt inter-related. A better understanding of these mechanisms will lead to more rational approaches to the treatment and prevention of acute renal failure. In this respect, the most promise seems to lie in a further investigation of the intracellular events that occur during the early stages of acute renal failure.

References

1. HOLLENBERG NK, EPSTEIN M, ROSEN SM, BASCH RI, OKEN DE, MERRILL JP: Acute oliguric renal failure in man. *Medicine* 47:455–474, 1968
2. REUBI FC, GOSSWEILER N, GURTLER R: Renal circulation in man studied by means of dye-dilution method. *Circulation* 33:426–442, 1966
3. EPSTEIN M, SCHNEIDER NS, BEFELER B: Effect of intrarenal furosemide on renal function and intrarenal hemodynamics in acute renal failure. *Am J Med* 58:510–516, 1975
4. FINN WF, CHEVALIER RL: Recovery from post-ischemic acute renal failure in the rat. *Kidney Int* 16:113–123, 1979
5. CONGER JD, ROBINETTE JB, GUGGENHEIM SJ: Effect of acetylcholine on the early phase of reversible norepinephrine induced acute renal failure. *Kidney Int* 19:399–409, 1981
6. PATAK RV, FADEM SZ, LIFSCHITZ MD, STEIN JH: Study of factors which modify the development of norepinephrine induced acute renal failure in the dog. *Kidney Int* 15:227–237, 1979
7. FRANKLIN SS, MERRILL JP: Acute renal failure. *N Engl J Med* 262:761–767, 1960
8. FLORES J, DIBONA DR, BECK CH, LEAF A: The role of cell swelling in ischemic renal damage and the protective effect of hypertonic solute. *J Clin Invest* 51:118–126, 1972
9. FREGA NS, DIBONA DR, GUERTLER B, LEAF A: Ischemic renal injury. *Kidney Int* 10:S17–S25, 1976
10. HOLST D: Renal failure as the cause of death in *Tupaia belangeri* exposed to persistent social stress. *J Comp Physiol* 78:236–273, 1972
11. FEKETE A, TARABA I, VISY M: Splanchnicotomy affords protection against acute renal failure in dogs. *ACTA Physiol Acad Sci Hung* 26:245–249, 1965
12. SOLEZ K, D'AGUSTINI RJ, STAWOWY BA, FREEDMAN MT, SCOTT WW, SIEGELMAN SS, HEPTINSTALL RH: Beneficial effect of propranolol in a histologically appropriate model of postischemic acute renal failure. *Am J Pathol* 88:163–192, 1977
13. OKEGAWA T, JONAS PE, DESCHRYVER K, KAWASAKI A, NEEDLEMAN P: Metabolic and cellular alterations underlying the exaggerated renal prostaglandin and thromboxane synthesis in ureter obstruction in rabbits. *J Clin Invest* 71:81–90, 1983
14. BENABE JE, KLAHR S, HOFFMAN MK, MORRISON AR: Production of thromboxane A_2 by the kidney in glycerol induced acute renal failure in the rabbit. *Prostaglandins* 19:333–347, 1980
15. LIANOS EA, ANDRES GA, DUNN MJ: Glomerular prostaglandin and thromboxane synthesis in rat nephrotoxic serum nephrites. *J Clin Invest* 72:1439–1448, 1983
16. SZCZEPANSKA-SADOWSKA E: Thermodynamic effects of a moderate increase of the plasma vasopressin level in conscious dogs. *Pflügers Arch* 338:313–322, 1973
17. HOFBAUER KG, KONRADS A, BAUEREISS K, MOEHRING B, MOEHRING J, GROSS

F: Vasopressin and renin in glycerol induced acute renal failure in the rat. *Circ Res* 41:424–428, 1977

18. IAINA A, ORNDORFF M, GAVENDO S, SOLOMON S: ADH effects in development of ischemic acute renal failure. *Proc Soc Exp Bio Med* 163:206–211, 1980

19. WILSON DR, THIEL G, ARCE ML, OKEN DE: The role of the concentration mechanism in the development of acute renal failure: Micropuncture studies using diabetes insipidus rats. *Nephron* 6:128–139, 1969

20. GOORMAGHTIGH N: Vascular and circulatory changes in renal cortex in the anuric crush syndrome. *Proc Soc Exp Bio Med* 59:303–305, 1945

21. WEBER P, HELD E, UHLICH E, EIGLER JOC: Reaction constants of renin in juxtaglomerular apparatus and plasma renin activity after renal ischemia and hemorrhage. *Kidney Int* 7:331–341, 1975

22. THURAU K, VOGT C, DAHLHEIM H: Renin activity in the juxtaglomerular apparatus of the rat kidney during postischemia acute renal failure. *Kidney Int* 10:S177–S182, 1976

23. McDONALD FD, THIEL G, WILSON DR, DiBONA GF, OKEN DE: The prevention of acute renal failure by long term saline loading. *Proc Soc Exp Bio Med* 131:610–614, 1969

24. BIDANI A, CHURCHILL P, FLEISCHMANN L: Sodium-chloride induced protection in nephrotoxic acute renal failure: Independence from renin. *Kidney Int* 16:481–490, 1979

25. PLOTH DW, THOMAS CE, ROY RN, RUDOLPH JG: Ischemic acute renal failure in DOCA-salt loaded and Goldblatt hypertensive rats. *J Lab Clin Med* 92:1009–1018, 1978

26. KRAMER HJ, NEUMARK A, SCHMIDT S, KLINGMULLER D, GLANZER K: Renal functional and metabolic studies on the role of preventive measures in experimental acute renal failure. *Clin Exp Dialysis Apheresis* 7:77–99, 1983

27. MATTHEWS PG, MORGAN TO, JOHNSTON CI: The renin-angiotensin system in acute renal failure. *Clin Sci Mol Med* 47:79–88, 1974

28. FLAMENBAUM W, KOTCHEN TA, OKEN DE: Effect of renin immunization on mercuric chloride and glycerol induced renal failure. *Kidney Int* 1:406–412, 1972

29. ARENDSHORST WJ, FINN WF, GOTTSCHALK CW: Pathogenesis of acute renal failure following temporary renal ischemia in the rat. *Circ Res* 37:558–568, 1975

30. COX JW, BUEHLER RW, CHARMA H, O'DORISIO F, OSGOOD RW, STEIN JH, FERRIS TF: Studies on the mechanism of oliguria in a model of unilateral acute renal failure. *J Clin Invest* 53:1546–1558, 1976

31. KRIZ W: Structural organization of renal medullary circulation. *Nephron* 31:290–295, 1982

32. KARLBERG L, KALLSKOG O, NORLEN BJ, WOLGAST M: Postischemic renal failure. *Acta Physiol Scand* 115:1–10, 1982

33. THIEL G, DE ROUGEMONT D, KRIZ W, MASON J, TORHORST J, WOLGAST M: The role of reduced medullary perfusion in the genesis of acute ischemic renal failure. *Nephron* 31:321–323, 1982

34. BLANTZ RC: The mechanism of acute renal failure after uranyl nitrate. *J Clin Invest* 55:621–635, 1975

35. BAYLIS C, RENNKE HR, BRENNER BM: Mechanisms of the defect in glomerular ultrafiltration associated with gentamicin administration. *Kidney Int* 12:344–353, 1977

36. WILLIAMS RH, THOMAS CE, NAVAR LG, EVAN AP: Hemodynamic and single nephron function during maintenance phase of acute renal failure in the dog. *Kidney Int* 19:503–515, 1981

37. SAVIN VJ, PATAK RV, MARR G, HERMRECK AS, RIDGE SM, LAKE K: Glomerular ultrafiltration coefficient after ischemic renal injury in dogs. *Circ Res* 53:439–447, 1983
38. DAUGHARTY TM, UEKI IF, MERCER PF, BRENNER BM: Dynamics of glomerular ultrafiltration in the rat: Response to ischemic injury. *J Clin Invest* 53:105–116, 1974
39. BARNES JL, OSGOOD RW, REINECK HJ, STEIN JH: Glomerular alterations in an ischemic model of acute renal failure. *Lab Invest* 45:378–386, 1981
40. JONES DB: Ultrastructure of human acute renal failure. *Lab Invest* 46:254–264, 1982
41. PONFICK K: Experimentelle beitrage zur lehre von der Transfusion. *Arch Path Anat Physiol Klin Med* 62:273–335, 1875
42. HOSTETTER TH, WILKES BM, BRENNER BM: Mechanisms of impaired filtration in acute renal failure, in *Acute Renal Failure,* edited by BRENNER BM, STEIN JH, New York Churchill Livingstone, 1980, pp 52–78
43. BAYLIS C, RENNKE HG, BRENNER BM: Mechanisms of the defect in glomerular ultrafiltration associated with gentamicin administration. *Kidney Int* 12:344–353, 1977
44. FINCKH ES: Experimental acute tubular necrosis following subcutaneous injection of glycerol. *J Path Bact* 73:69–85, 1957
45. DIBONA G: Light microscopic structural-functional correlatures in acute renal failure, in *Acute Renal Failure,* edited by SOLEZ K, WHELTON A, New York, Marcel Dekker, Inc, 1984
46. CUSHNER H, BARNES J, REINECK HJ, STEIN JH: Studies on the role of volume depletion in the pathophysiology of glycerol induced acute renal failure (*abstract*). *Kidney Int* 25:228, 1984
47. RICHARDS CJ, DIBONA GF: Acute renal failure: Structural-functional correlation. *Proc Soc Exp Bio Med* 146:880–884, 1974
48. DONOHOE JF, VENKATACHALAM MA, BERNARD DB, LEVINSKY NG: Tubular leakage and obstruction in acute ischemic renal failure. *Kidney Int* 13:208–222, 1978
49. TANNER GA, SOPHASAN S: Kidney pressures after temporary artery occlusion in the rat. *Am J Physiol* 230:1173–1181, 1976
50. ARENDSHORST WJ, FINN WF, GOTTSCHALK CW, LUCAS HK: Micropuncture study of acute renal failure following temporary renal ischemia in the rat. *Kidney Int* 10:S100–S105, 1976
51. TANNER GA, STEINHAUSEN M: Tubular obstruction in ischemia induced acute renal failure in the rat. *Kidney Int* 10:S65–S73, 1976
52. TANNER GA, SLOAN KL, SOPHASAN S: Effects of renal artery occlusion on kidney function in the rat. *Kidney Int* 4:377–389, 1973
53. MASON J, WELSCH J, TAKABATAKE T: Disparity between surface and deep nephron function early after renal ischemia. *Kidney Int* 24:27–36, 1983
54. RICHARDS AN: Direct observations of change in function of the renal tubule caused by certain poisons. *Trans Assoc Am Phys* 44:64–76, 1929
55. STEIN JH, GOTTSCHALL J, OSGOOD RW, FERRIS TF: Pathophysiology of a nephrotoxic model of acute renal failure. *Kidney Int* 8:27–41, 1975
56. STEINHAUSEN M, EISENBACH GM, HELMSTADTER V: Concentration of lissamine green in proximal tubules of antidiuretic and mercury poisoned rats and the permeability of these tubules. *Pflügers Arch* 311:1–15, 1969
57. EISENBACH GM, STEINHAUSEN M: Micropuncture studies after temporary ischemia of rat kidneys. *Pflügers Arch* 343:11–25, 1973

58. MYERS BD, CHUI F, HILBERMAN M, MICHAELS AS: Transtubular leakage of glomerular filtrate in human acute renal failure. *Am J Physiol* 237:F319–F325, 1979
59. SCHNERMANN J, NAGEL W, THURAU K: Die fruhdistale natrium konzentration in Rattennieren nach renaler ischamie and hemorrhagischer hypotension. *Pflügers Arch* 287:296–310, 1966
60. MASON J, TAKABATAKE T, OLBRICH TC, THURAU K: The early phase of experimental acute renal failure. III. Tubuloglomerular feedback. *Pflügers Arch* 373:69–76, 1978
61. MASON J, GUTSCHE HU, MOORE L, MULLER-SUUR R: The early phase of experimental acute renal failure. IV. The diluting ability of the short loops of Henle. *Pflügers Arch* 379:11–18, 1979
62. HANLEY MJ: Isolated nephron segments in a rabbit model of ischemic acute renal failure. *Am J Physiol* 239:F17–F23, 1980
63. TANNER GA: Effects of kidney tubule obstruction on glomerular function in rats. *Am J Physiol* 237:F379–F385, 1979
64. TANNER GA, YUM MN: Effects of chronic tubular obstruction in necturus kidney. *Am J Physiol* 234:F112–F116, 1978
65. MASON J, KAIN H, SHIIGAI T, WELSCH J: Early phase of experimental acute renal failure. *Pflügers Arch* 380:233–243, 1979
66. CHURCHILL PC, BIDANI A, FLEISCHMANN L: Mercuric chloride induced acute renal failure in the Goldblatt rat. *J Lab Clin Med* 91:660–665, 1978
67. LEWIS RM, PATTON MK, OSGOOD RW, STEIN JH: Evaluation of renal blood flow, urine flow, the effects of mannitol, furosemide, bradykinin in acute renal failure induced by renal artery occlusion in the dog (*abstract*). *Clin Res* 30:541A, 1982
68. CASEY KF, MACHIEDO GW, LYONS MH, SLOTMAN GJ, NOVAK RT: Alteration of post-ischemic renal pathology by prostaglandin infusion. *J Surg Res* 29:1–10, 1980
69. NEUMAYER HH, WAGNER K, SCHUDROWITSCH L, PREUSCHOF L, STANCE H, SCHULTZE G, MOLZAHN M: Beneficial effect of prostaglandin I_2 in postischemic acute renal failure (*abstract*). *Kidney Int* 25:235, 1984
70. WERB R, CLARK WF, LINDSAY RM, JONES EOP, TURNBULL DI, LINTON AL: Protective effect of prostaglandin (PGE_2) in glycerol induced acute renal failure. *Clin Sci Mol Med* 55:505–507, 1978
71. MAUK RH, PATAK RV, FADEM SZ, LIFSCHITZ MD, STEIN JH: Effect of prostaglandin E administration in a nephrotoxic and vasconstrictor model of acute renal failure. *Kidney Int* 12:122–130, 1977
72. SIEGEL M, RICE J, BARNES J, OSGOOD R, STEIN J: Protective effect of mini dose ouabain in ischemic renal failure in the dog (*abstract*). *Clin Res* 31:518A, 1983
73. MARBERGER M, GUNTHER R, ALKEN P, RUMPF W, RANC M: Inosine: alternative or adjunct to regional hypothermia in the prevention of post ischemic renal failure? *Eur Urol* 6:95–102, 1980
74. GAUDIO KM, TAYLOR MR, CHAUDRY IH, KASHGARIAN M, SIEGEL NJ: Accelerated recovery of single nephron function by the postischemic infusion of ATP-$MgCP_2$. *Kidney Int* 22:13–20, 1982
75. SIEGEL NJ, GLAZIER WB, CHAUDRY IH, GAUDIO KM, LYTTON B, BAUE AE, KASHGARIAN M: Enhanced recovery from acute renal failure by the postischemic infusion of adenine nucleotides and magnesium chloride in rats. *Kidney Int* 17:338–349, 1980
76. BURKE TJ, ARNOLD PE, GROSSFELD PD, SCHRIER RW: Effect of calcium mem-

brane inhibition on norepinephrine induced acute renal failure, in *Acute Renal Failure,* edited by ELIAHOU HE, London, John Libbey, 1982, pp 239–240

77. GOLDFARB D, IAINA A, SERBAN I, GAVENDO S, KAPULER S, ELIAHOU HE: Beneficial effect of verapamil on ischemic acute renal failure in the rat. *Proc Soc Exp Bio Med* 172:389–392, 1982

78. MALIS CD, CHEUNG JY, LEAF A, BONVENTRE JV: Effects of verapamil in models of ischemic acute renal failure in the rat. *Am J Physiol* 245:F735–F742, 1983

79. WEINBERG JM, HUNT D, HUMES HD: Effects of verapamil on in-vitro ischemic injury to isolated rabbit proximal tubules (*abstract*). *Kidney Int* 25:239, 1984

80. WILSON PD, SCHRIER RW: Protection against ischemic cell death in cultured rabbit nephron segments (*abstract*). *Clin Res* 32:68A, 1984

81. PALLER MS, HOIDAL JR, FERRIS TF: Oxygen free radicals in ischemia acute renal failure in the rat (*abstract*). *Kidney Int* 25:236, 1984

82. KEDAR I, COHEN J, JACOB ET, RAVID M: Alleviation of experimental ischemic renal failure by dimethyl sulfoxide. *Nephron* 29:55–58, 1981

Control of Renal Regeneration After Acute Tubular Necrosis

F. Gary Toback

In the predialysis era, death from acute renal failure was usually caused by hyperkalemia and volume overload. Today, despite the effectiveness of measures now used for diagnosing and treating these complications, the mortality for acute renal failure remains high, especially when the syndrome appears after surgery or trauma. Although many patients die with, and not of, renal failure, mortality often exceeds 60% [1, 2]. Thus, the conventional dialysis and management strategies used in caring for these patients are clearly inadequate.

When acute renal failure is associated with structural damage, recovery depends on repair and replacement of injured and necrotic tubular cells [3, 4]. An understanding of the mechanisms by which cells repair the injury and regenerate would permit a more rational approach to treatment. The purpose of this presentation is to delineate specific factors that could contribute to repair of the injured nephron following acute tubular necrosis. It is hoped that future studies will uncover the factors controlling renal regeneration and lead to the development of innovative therapeutic modalities of treating this too often fatal disorder.

Enhancement of Renal Regeneration by Amino Acids, Adenine Nucleotides, and Thyroxin

A major principle underlying the treatment of acute renal failure is that the kidney lesion can heal by itself. Efforts in the past were directed at providing supportive care so that the kidney could fully utilize its regenerative capacity. Renal regeneration and repair, however, are anabolic processes that

This manuscript was presented as part of a Symposium on *Acute Renal Failure: Structure-Function Relationships*.

must be carried out in a setting of systemic catabolism. That complete restoration of renal function can occur despite reduced caloric intake, retention of toxins and nitrogen, acidosis, electrolyte imbalance, and anemia demonstrates the extraordinary capacity of renal cells to regenerate. Thus, the need is great for precise delineation of the conditions that will ensure optimal renal cell growth in this systemic environment.

Hypercatabolism during acute renal failure often aggravates nitrogen retention and results in the loss of lean body mass. It is difficult to provide a sufficient supply of protein and nonprotein calories because anorexia, nausea, and vomiting prevent adequate oral intake and because the loss of renal excretory capacity severely limits the volume of nutrient-containing solutions that can be infused. These clinical observations suggest that the rate of renal regeneration may be suboptimal, because hypercatabolism increases the demand for calories and nutrients whereas the adverse effects of the syndrome on renal excretory and gastrointestinal function decrease their supply.

Amino Acids

Some attempts have been made to reverse the catabolic state. The provision of calories as a hypertonic glucose solution has long been used for its protein-sparing effect [5]. The administration of essential amino acids given orally by Berlyne et al [6] and intravenously by Wilmore and Dudrick [7], resulted in reduction of the blood urea nitrogen concentration, achievement of positive nitrogen balance, and improvement of uremic symptoms. The provision of α-keto analogues of essential amino acids to patients with chronic renal failure has had similar beneficial effects [8]. The importance of the nonessential amino acids has been stressed by Pennisi, Wang, and Kopple [9], who reported that mixtures of essential and nonessential amino acids were superior to essential amino acids alone for maintaining the nutritional status of uremic animals.

In 1973, Abel et al assessed the effect of amino acid treatment in 53 adult patients with postsurgical acute renal failure [10]. A double-blind prospective trial was used for comparing the efficacy of a solution containing amino acids and hypertonic glucose with an isocaloric, isovolemic glucose infusion. The most dramatic result of the study was that amino acid treatment increased survival after the acute renal failure episode. Of the 28 patients treated with amino acids, 75% survived as compared to 44% of the 25 patients given glucose alone. Amino acid treatment was most effective in patients requiring dialysis and in those who developed complications such as pneumonia, generalized sepsis, or gastrointestinal hemorrhage. Kidney function was studied in nondialyzed and dialyzed patients up to the time the procedure was initiated. In patients treated with amino acids, the serum creatinine concentration reached its highest value on day 2 of treatment and then declined. In contrast, the creatinine concentration continued to rise until day 7 in patients treated with the control solution.

Thus, infusion of essential L-amino acids improved survival from the acute renal failure syndrome, especially in those postoperative patients requiring dialysis and in whom hypercatabolic complications were observed. The recovery of renal function also appeared to be more rapid.

The mechanism by which amino acids improve survival in patients with acute renal failure is unknown. Studies in humans do not permit direct assessment of either repair or replacement of injured renal tissue, leaving it unresolved as to whether amino acid infusions act directly on the kidney to speed cellular regeneration. To address this question, investigators have studied the effect of amino acids on the course of acute renal failure in animal models.

Membrane metabolism was assessed in rats recovering from nephrotoxic and ischemic renal failure because organelles and surface membranes must be produced by regenerating cells to restore normal renal structure and function [11, 12]. Renal phospholipid and protein biosynthesis was examined because cellular membranes are composed largely of these macromolecules. The results indicated that amino acid infusions act directly on the rat kidney to stimulate phosphatidylcholine biosynthesis of new membrane formation in regenerating cells [13]. They enhanced the cellular uptake of the phospholipid precursor choline and increased the V_{max} of two reactions of the Kennedy pathway of phosphatidylcholine biosynthesis [14]. Renal protein synthesis was also increased, and the cellular deficit in the concentration of at least one essential amino acid, leucine, was corrected [15]. This enhancement of phosphatidylcholine and protein synthesis was superimposed on the increased rates that occur during renal regeneration in untreated animals. Apparently, synthesis of these macromolecules is suboptimal in the absence of exogenous amino acids. In addition, there was amelioration of renal functional insufficiency, which was also observed by Abel et al in humans [10]. Finally, amino acid infusion did not increase mortality.

These results in animal models suggest a course to follow for patients with acute renal failure, that infused amino acids could act directly on the kidney to speed repair of the injury. This therapeutic maneuver may also preserve lean body mass and permit a more effective defense against infection for nonrenal tissues.

The beneficial effects of this suggested therapeutic regimen [10, 16] have not been observed consistently [17–19]. At present, it is not possible to identify the patients who are most likely to respond, but two groups who do not respond are the very seriously ill and those with mild acute renal failure. Until better clinical criteria are available, workers have suggested that treatment be given to the patients who require dialysis [20, 21]. The exact composition of the dosage that will maximally accelerate recovery from acute renal failure awaits a better understanding of the different factors and mechanisms that mediate repair and recovery of the injured tissue.

Adenine Nucleotides

Another successful approach to enhancing the repair of nephrons following experimental acute renal injury appears to be the infusion of adenosine triphosphate (ATP) combined with stoichiometric amounts of magnesium chloride [22]. This approach is based on the observation that ischemia depletes tissue of adenine nucleotides and that if this process reaches a critical level cell injury and death may ensue. Chaudry et al found that an i.v. administration of an ATP and magnesium chloride solution replenished the reduced intracellular levels of ATP in kidney as well as liver after hemorrhagic shock [23]. These findings led to a series of experiments by Siegel et al to assess the effect of ATP and magnesium chloride in three animal models of kidney injury: ischemic injury (bilateral renal artery occlusion), toxic injury (potassium dichromate), and obstructive injury [24]. The provision of ATP and magnesium chloride after initiation of the kidney injury enhanced recovery of both glomerular and tubular function. Amelioration of intratubular obstruction and backleak of tubular fluid were observed, as well as was the restoration of structural integrity of the nephron. It is proposed that the adverse cellular consequences of ischemia mediated by a reduction in renal cell ATP content are reversed by the infusion of ATP and magnesium chloride. Recently, the infusion has been shown by NMR spectroscopy to specifically accelerate the return of tissue ATP content to normal following an ischemic insult [25]. This action would appear to reverse the metabolic consequences of ischemia and permit the survival of sublethally injured cells.

Although the efficacy of this mode of treatment has not yet been evaluated in humans, its provision to the perfusate of canine kidneys did improve preservation and function after transplantation [26].

Thyroxin

Several observations suggest that the administration of thyroxin (T_4) could have a beneficial effect on recovery from acute renal failure. This hormone is known to enhance kidney growth, stimulate protein synthesis and uptake of nutrient molecules in renal tubular cells, and increase the activity of sodium-potassium-ATPase activity in kidney cortex [24, 27, 28]. Accelerated recovery of several tubular enzyme activities has also been observed in rats treated with thyroxin following the induction of acute tubular necrosis by mercuric chloride [29]. In addition, in rats with acute renal failure induced by potassium dichromate, thyroxin treatment resulted in improved glomerular and tubular function, and it accelerated recovery comparable to that observed following an infusion of ATP and magnesium chloride [30]. There are no reports, however, of a controlled trial of thyroxin treatment of patients with acute renal failure.

Growth Control in Renal Epithelial Cells

Regeneration after Acute Tubular Necrosis

In considering other factors that promote kidney regeneration after acute tubular necrosis, it is useful to begin with an examination of the recovery process following mercuric chloride induction of acute renal failure in the rat. This model, which has been described in detail by Cuppage and Tate, provides a reversible syndrome for study [31]. Following an i.v. injection of mercury at 1 mg/kg of body wt, the rat kidney underwent changes that simulated the syndrome of nonoliguric acute tubular necrosis in humans. On day 1 there were increases in the blood urea nitrogen (BUN) concentration and in the excretion of sodium in the urine [11, 31]. Glucosuria and proteinuria appeared, food intake decreased, and the animal lost weight. On day 3, the BUN reached a maximum and body weight a minimum. By day 5, the BUN returned to the control value whereas body weight and food intake were still increasing.

These physiological alterations were associated with necrosis of proximal tubular cells, which was nearly complete on day 1 and was limited to the inner cortex [32]. Figure 1 depicts the denuded tubular basement membrane, the partially damaged non-necrotic cells at the edge of the wound, and the necrotic cell debris, which may act to obstruct the flow of tubular fluid down the nephron. Epithelial cells at both ends of the necrotic segment of the nephron and other surviving isolated cells along its denuded surface appear to be responsible for regenerating the tubular epithelial lining [33]. Proliferation of these cells with subsequent sliding along the undamaged basement membrane appears to permit rapid restitution of the tubular structure. The intact basement membrane plays an important role in the healing process, at least in part, by providing a structural framework for the proliferating cells. The sliding movement of the growing cells at the edge of the wound

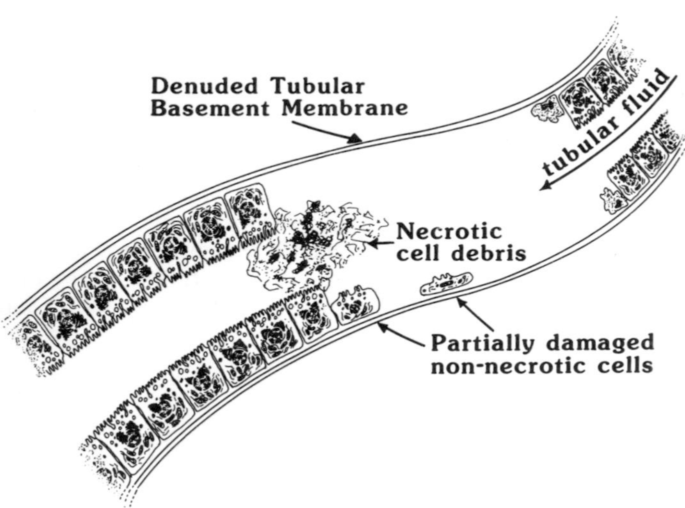

Fig. 1. Longitudinal section of an injured nephron following mercuric chloride-induced acute tubular necrosis. Non-necrotic cells at the edges of the wound and along the denuded tubular basement membrane proliferate and migrate to reepithelialize the nephron.

is similar to repair processes in other epithelia. These observations suggest that local as well as systemic factors could play a regulatory role in mediating the regeneration process. By day 3, squamoid or cuboidal epithelial cells containing a few projections of luminal brush border replaced the necrotic cells [33, 34]. Most tubules were relined with new cells by day 5. The squamoid cells that participate in this stage of regeneration gradually developed into cells of normal size and acquired surface structures and organelles characteristic of mature cells. Although the reepithelialization of the nephron was complete by day 5, turnover of epithelial cells persisted at a high rate so that the structural and biochemical aspects of regeneration were not complete until day 28 [11, 31, 34].

The rapid proliferation of tubular epithelial cells was associated with enhanced synthesis of protein, nucleic acids, and phospholipid by day 2 of the syndrome [11, 33, 35, 36]. Thus, the unknown anabolic mechanisms that initiate and maintain the regeneration process appear to operate in a metabolic milieu characterized by systemic catabolism. There is a decrease in the availability of calories and nutrients at a time when the demand for them by the regenerating cells is increased, and there is accumulation of the end products of tissue metabolism, which are probably toxic [1]. The stimulus to renal growth in regenerating cells can apparently overcome the unfavorable effects of catabolism and the azotemic environment that ordinarily inhibits growth of other cells. These findings also suggest that systemic factors may oppose rather than enhance the regeneration process and raise the possibility that local factors could play a role.

An observation that supports a role for local factors in regeneration is one made more than 30 years ago by Oliver, MacDowell, and Tracy [3, 4] and subsequently confirmed by others [31, 34, 37]. These workers found that focal proliferation of tubular epithelial cells occurs at sites along the nephron where growth is most exuberant. These papillary collections of epithelial cells sometimes project into the tubular lumen or into the interstitium. This finding suggests that excessive growth-stimulatory activity results in these focal proliferations of epithelial cells.

Renal Compensatory Growth After Uninephrectomy

A study of factors that have been proposed as mediators of compensatory kidney growth after uninephrectomy [38] could provide the basis for delineating mechanisms that control regeneration after acute renal failure. Currently, the stimulus for compensatory renal growth is thought to be a humoral substance(s) originating from the kidney or another organ [39]. It is proposed that this substance (or substances) could initiate renal growth directly or perhaps antagonize a specific growth inhibitor. Alternatively, compensatory growth may result from a decrease in the plasma concentration of a tissue-specific growth inhibitor (chalone) made by renal cells, an effect that releases the chronic inhibition of kidney growth and thereby restores renal mass toward normal [40, 41]. The existence of a humoral factor that directly stimulates kidney growth has been suggested by the observation that serum from uninephrectomized rats stimulates renal growth when it is injected into normal rats, as measured by increased tritiated thymidine uptake by kidney but not by liver cells [42–44]. The existence of such a factor has also been suggested by studies of parabiotic animals [45, 46], tissue culture systems [47], and isolated perfused kidneys [48]. The factor is probably continuously produced after a reduction of renal mass, and its presence appears to be required to maintain compensatory growth [49].

The nature of this humoral growth factor is unknown; however, it appears unable to pass through the placental barrier [50], although it may possibly enter the urine [51, 52]. The factor is probably not of neural or immunologic origin because human transplanted kidneys, which are denervated, undergo compensatory growth in patients subjected to maximal chemical immunosuppression [53, 54] and thymectomy [55].

Renal Epithelial Cells in Culture

Several determinants of cell proliferation have been defined by studies of renal epithelial cells in culture. In epithelial cells of the established BSC-1 line derived from African green monkey kidney, a number of factors contribute to growth control. These include growth factors and hormones in normal serum and their receptors on the cell surface, growth inhibitors produced by the cells, and low molecular weight nutrients [56–58]. Specific growth stimulatory molecules contained in serum include vasopressin [59] and epidermal growth factor (EGF) [56, 60]. The latter polypeptide has a mol wt of 6,045 daltons, is synthesized primarily in the submaxillary and submandibular glands, and appears in the urine of humans and animals. Although this substance is a powerful mitogen for renal epithelial cells in culture [56], its contribution to renal growth in vivo is as yet unknown.

The growth of BSC-1 cells in culture is also regulated by the cellular production of several inhibitors. These include lactate, ammonium ion, and a glycoprotein that has a mol wt of 24,000 daltons [58]. The inhibitor protein, which has been purified and characterized by Holley et al, is active at very low concentrations (2 ng/ml) on epithelial cells grown in culture, impedes exit of cells from the G_0/G_1 (resting) phase of the cell cycle, acts in a reversible manner, and can be overcome by the stimulatory action of serum or EGF [61]. Injection of the inhibitor protein into nodules of human mammary carcinoma cells growing in nude mice results in decreased incorporation of tritiated thymidine into DNA in the cancer cells [62].

Evidence that molecules produced by kidney epithelial cells contribute to growth control has been obtained in recent studies of factors that mediate increased renal growth during potassium depletion nephropathy [63]. Cultures of BSC-1 cells were used to study this phenomenon because their growth was accelerated in medium containing a reduced potassium concentration [64]. The increased multiplication of these kidney cells was associated with the appearance of growth-stimulatory activity in the culture medium [65]. Thus, the cells apparently transduced the information inherent in a reduction of the extracellular potassium concentration into endogenous growth-promoting activity. Addition of the purified growth inhibitor protein to the culture antagonized the growth-stimulatory activity in the medium. These findings suggest that kidney epithelial cells can regulate their proliferation by producing molecules with opposite effects on growth.

Growth-inhibitory and -stimulatory molecules appear to exert their effect, at least in part, by acting on the determinants of net sodium flux. In monkey kidney epithelial cells of the BSC-1 line, and in many other types of cells, an increase in sodium entry across the plasma membrane appears to be a critical early event during mitogenesis [66–70]. The growth-inhibitor protein secreted by BSC-1 cells can inhibit the increase in net sodium flux during mitogenic stimulation in a reversible manner [71].

In summary, these observations suggest that proliferation of kidney epithelial cells in culture, and possibly in vivo, is regulated by the interplay of opposing growth-promoting and growth-inhibitory factors, some of which are made by the cells.

Growth of Malignant Cells

A consideration of the differences between normal and malignant cells offers another approach to understanding the mechanisms that could regulate renal regeneration.

A distinguishing characteristic of cells that have undergone malignant transformation is that they require a smaller amount of exogenous growth factors to achieve maximal growth in culture than do their normal counterparts [72]. Cultures of viral-transformed fibroblasts, for example, require much less serum for optimal growth and multiplication than do cells that are not transformed [73]. Since normal growth is apparently controlled by the interaction of different hormones, growth factors, and inhibitors, it is possible that transformation confers on the cell its capacity to achieve maximal growth in the presence of subnormal amounts of growth-stimulatory factors. Accumulated recent evidence also suggests that malignant transformation of normal cells could be mediated by the synthesis and release of specific growth-promoting molecules by the cells, for which they have functional receptors on their surface [74]. This secretion of a hormone-like substance by cells, to which they can respond, is termed "autocrine" stimulation [75, 76]. This offers one explanation for the reduced need of malignant cells for exogenous growth factors. Endogenous production of growth factors by transformed cells would decrease their requirement for an exogenous supply of substances with similar activity. A class of molecules called transforming growth factors which exhibit this activity has been described [77]. These polypeptides have a molecular weight of 6,000 to 20,000 daltons, are acid-stable, and have been isolated from several non-neoplastic tissues, including kidney [78].

Control of Renal Regeneration: An Hypothesis

Growth-stimulatory and -inhibitory factors of cellular origin, which appear to control the growth of renal epithelial cells in culture and are postulated

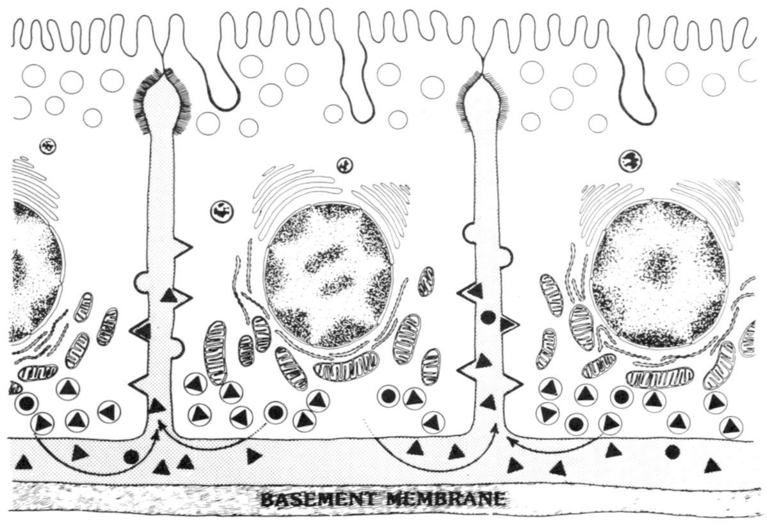

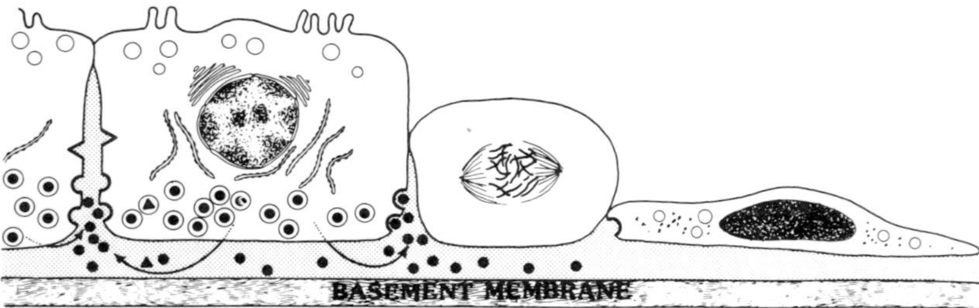

Fig. 2. Schema of growth regulation in normal and regenerating kidney epithelial cells. **Top** *Normal cells.* Normal cells synthesize both growth-inhibitory (▲) and stimulatory (●) polypeptides, which are depicted as zymogens in the cytoplasm. Release of the active molecule into the extracellular space permits subsequent binding to its designated receptor on the surface of the cell that produced it or to a neighboring cell. It is proposed that the very low growth rate in normal renal tissue is mediated, at least in part, by the predominance of growth-inhibitory molecules. The thickened curved and angular regions of the plasma membrane indicate receptor sites for growth-promoting and -inhibitory molecules, respectively. **Bottom** *Regenerating cells.* Cells at the edge of an injured segment of the nephron are shown during early renal regeneration following acute tubular necrosis. Migrating squamoid, dividing, and non-necrotic epithelial cells are seen. It is suggested that exuberant proliferation is, at least in part, the result of synthesis and secretion of growth-stimulatory molecules by the regenerating cells.

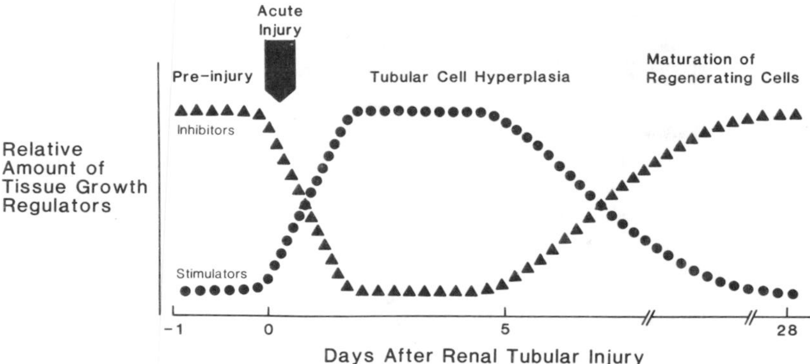

Fig. 3. Regulation of renal regeneration after acute tubular necrosis by growth-inhibitory and -stimulatory molecules produced by the cells. Local control of repair of the injured nephron is proposed in addition to the contribution of hormones, growth factors, and nutrients in the plasma. Prior to injury, the low mitotic index in the tissue is mediated by the predominance of growth-inhibitory molecules. Following injury, tubular cell proliferation could be mediated by increased production of growth-stimulatory molecules, whereas the formation of inhibitors is reduced. With time, the integrity of the epithelial lining of the nephron is reestablished, and the production of growth-regulatory molecules by the cells returns to control levels.

to play a role in malignant transformation, could take part in mediating regeneration of the injured nephron following acute tubular necrosis in concert with hormones, growth factors, and nutrients in the blood.

A proposed role for growth-regulating factors made by the cells must be in accord with the observation that normal renal tissue is characterized by a very low mitotic index (0.1%) [79]. This is presented in schematic form in the top panel of Figure 2, which shows that renal tubular epithelial cells can produce growth-inhibitory and growth-stimulatory molecules in a zymogen or precursor form in the cytoplasm. As the cells depicted are in a nongrowing state, there is marked predominance of growth-inhibitory molecules. The release of these polypeptides into the interstitial space permits their subsequent binding to receptors on the surface of the cells that produced them or neighboring cells. Unlike endocrine secretions, these molecules are postulated to act locally and need not enter the peritubular capillary blood for delivery to a distant site to exert their effect.

A schema for growth regulation in regenerating renal tissue is shown in the bottom panel of Figure 2. It is proposed that the surviving cells at the edge of the wound secrete their own growth-promoting factors in large amounts and display receptors for them on the cell surface. Thus, cells at the edge of the wound, or non-necrotic or embryonic rest cells along the tubular basement membrane, could undergo rapid growth mediated by the production of endogenous growth-stimulatory factors, for which the cells have receptors and to which they can respond (Fig. 3). This internal production of growth-promoting polypeptides could serve as a stimulus for continued cell division, thereby releasing the cells from some of their normal endogenous and exogenous physiologic growth-inhibitory controls. Presumably, when the integrity of the injured nephron is reestablished, autocrine secretions would be greatly reduced, or cell surface receptors would become less numerous or responsive to the growth-stimulatory factors, or both. The production of growth-inhibitory molecules that was suppressed during the onset of the regeneration process would again become dominant, and new or more functional receptors for these molecules would appear on the cell surface, as depicted in Figure 3.

It is possible that the reparative burst of growth exhibited by regenerating kidney epithelial cells is mediated by the same mechanisms that operated in the kidney during normal embryogenesis. Thus, during tissue regeneration and normal development, growth-inhibitory molecules could limit cell proliferation and thereby establish the setting for normal organ function.

References

1. TOBACK FG: Amino acid treatment of acute renal failue, in *Contemporary Issues in Nephrology,* edited by BRENNER BM, STEIN JH. New York, Churchill Livingstone, 1980, vol. 6, pp. 202–228
2. BUTKUS DE: Persistent high mortality in acute renal failure: Are we asking the right questions? *Arch Intern Med* 143:209–212, 1983
3. OLIVER J, MACDOWELL M, TRACY A: The pathogenesis of acute renal failure associated with traumatic and toxic injury: Renal ischemia, nephrotoxic damage and the ischemuric episode. *J Clin Invest* 30:1307–1439, 1951
4. OLIVER J: Correlations of structure and mechanisms of recovery in acute tubular necrosis. *Am J Med* 15:535–559, 1953
5. GAMBLE JL: Physiological information from studies on the life-raft ration. *Harvey Lect* 42:247–273, 1946–1947
6. BERLYNE GM, BAZZARD FJ, BOOTH EM, JANABI K, SHAW KB: The dietary treatment of acute renal failure. *Q J Med* 36:59–83, 1967
7. WILMORE DW, DUDRICK SJ: Treatment of acute renal failure with intravenous essential L-amino acids. *Arch Surg* 99:669–673, 1969
8. WALSER M, COULTER AW, DIGHE S, CRANTZ FR: The effect of ketoanalogues of essential amino acids in severe chronic uremia. *J Clin Invest* 52:678–690, 1973
9. PENNISI AJ, WANG M, KOPPLE JD: Effects of protein and amino acid diets in chronically uremic and control rats. *Kidney Int* 13:472–479, 1978
10. ABEL RM, BECK CH JR, ABBOTT WM, RYAN JA JR, BARNETT GO, FISCHER JE: Improved survival from acute renal failure after treatment with intravenous essential L-amino acids and glucose: Results of a prospective, double-blind study. *N Engl J Med* 288:695–699, 1973
11. TOBACK FG, HAVENER LJ, DODD RC, SPARGO BH: Phospholipid metabolism during renal regeneration after acute tubular necrosis. *Am J Physiol* 232:E216–E222, 1977
12. SIEGEL MB, LOWENSTEIN LM, LEVINSKY NG: Choline uptake into renal phospholipids following renal ischemia in rats. *Circ Res* 44:62–67, 1979

13. TOBACK FG: Amino acid enhancement of renal regeneration after acute tubular necrosis. *Kidney Int* 12:193–198, 1977
14. TOBACK FG, TEEGARDEN DE, HAVENER LJ: Amino acid-mediated stimulation of renal phospholipid biosynthesis after acute tubular necrosis. *Kidney Int* 15:542–547, 1979
15. TOBACK FG, DODD RC, MAIER ER, HAVENER LJ: Amino acid administration enhances renal protein metabolism after acute tubular necrosis. *Nephron* 33:238–243, 1983
16. BAEK S-M, MAKABALI GG, BRYAN-BROWN CW, KUSEK J, SHOEMAKER WC: The influence of parenteral nutrition on the course of acute renal failure. *Surg Gynecol Obstet* 141:405–408, 1975
17. LEONARD CD, LUKE RG, SIEGEL RR: Parenteral essential amino acids in acute renal failure. *Urology* 6:154–157, 1975
18. OKEN DE, SPRINKEL FM, KIRSCHBAUM BB, LANDWEHR DM: Amino acid therapy in the treatment of experimental acute renal failure in the rat. *Kidney Int* 17:14–23, 1980
19. FEINSTEIN EI, BLUMENKRANTZ MJ, HEALY M, KOFFLER A, SILBERMAN H, MASSRY SG, KOPPLE JD: Clinical and metabolic responses to parenteral nutrition in acute renal failure: A controlled double-blind study. *Medicine* 60:124–137, 1981
20. LEE HA: The role of intravenous nutrition in the management of acute renal failure. *S Afr Med J* 50:1703–1705, 1976
21. NG RCK, SUKI WN: Treatment of acute renal failure, in *Contemporary Issues in Nephrology,* edited by BRENNER BM, STEIN JH. New York, Churchill Livingstone, 1980, vol. 6, pp. 229–273
22. SIEGEL NJ, GLAZIER WB, CHAUDRY IH, GAUDIO KM, LYTTON B, BAUE AE, KASHGARIAN M: Enhanced recovery from acute renal failure by the postischemic infusion of adenine nucleotides and magnesium chloride in rats. *Kidney Int* 17:338–349, 1980
23. CHAUDRY IH, PLANER GJ, SAYEED MM, BAUE AE: Depletion and restoration of tissue ATP in hemorrhagic shock. *Arch Surg* 108:208–211, 1974
24. SIEGEL NJ: Amino acids and adenine nucleotides in acute renal failure, in *Acute Renal Failure,* edited by BRENNER BM, LAZARUS JM. Philadelphia, Saunders, 1983, pp. 741–752
25. SIEGEL NJ, AVISON MJ, REILLY HF, ALGER JR, SHULMAN RG: Enhanced recovery of renal ATP with postischemic infusion of ATP-MgCl$_2$ determined by ^{31}P-NMR. *Am J Physiol* 245:F530–F534, 1983
26. LYTTON B, VAISBORT VR, GLAZIER WB, CHAUDRY IH, BAUE AE: Improved renal function using ATP-MgCl$_2$ in preservation of canine kidneys subjected to warm ischemia. *Transplantation* 31:187–189, 1981
27. KATZ AI, LINDHEIMER MD: Renal sodium- and potassium-activated adenosine triphosphatase and sodium reabsorption in the hypothyroid rat. *J Clin Invest* 52:796–804, 1973
28. LO CS, EDELMAN IS: Effect of triiodothyronine on the synthesis and degradation of renal cortical (Na$^+$ + K$^+$)-adenosine triphosphatase. *J Biol Chem* 251:7834–7840, 1976
29. SCHULTE-WEISSERMANN H, STRAUB E, FUNKE PJ: Influence of L-thyroxine upon enzymatic activity in the renal tubular epithelium of the rat under normal conditions and in mercury-induced lesions: I. Histochemical studies of alkaline phosphatase, acid phosphatase, adenosine-triphosphatase and leucine-aminopeptidase. *Virchows Arch [Cell Pathol]* 23:163–173, 1977

30. SIEGEL NJ, REILLY H, HENDLER F: Amelioration of toxic acute renal failure by treatment with thyroxin (*abstract*). *Pediatr Res* 15:699, 1981
31. CUPPAGE FE, TATE A: Repair of the nephron following injury with mercuric chloride. *Am J Pathol* 51:405–429, 1967
32. GANOTE CE, REIMER KA, JENNINGS RB: Acute mercuric chloride nephrotoxicity: An electron microscopic and metabolic study. *Lab Invest* 31:633–647, 1974
33. CUPPAGE FE, CUNNINGHAM N, TATE A: Nucleic acid synthesis in the regenerating nephron following injury with mercuric chloride. *Lab Invest* 21:449–457, 1969
34. HAAGSMA BH, POUND AW: Mercuric chloride-induced tubulonecrosis in the rat kidney: The recovery phase. *Br J Exp Pathol* 61:229–241, 1980
35. CUPPAGE FE, CHIGA M, TATE A: Cell cycle studies in the regenerating rat nephron following injury with mercuric chloride. *Lab Invest* 26:122–126, 1972
36. NICHOLLS DM, NG K: Regeneration of renal proximal tubules after mercuric chloride injury is accompanied by increased binding of aminoacyl-transfer ribonucleic acid. *Biochem J* 160:357–365, 1976
37. SIEGEL FL, BULGER RE: Scanning and transmission electron microscopy of mercuric chloride-induced acute tubular necrosis in rat kidney. *Virchows Arch [Cell Pathol]* 18:243–262, 1975
38. MALT RA: Compensatory growth of the kidney. *N Engl J Med* 280:1446–1459, 1969
39. MALT RA: Humoral factors in regulation of compensatory renal hypertrophy. *Kidney Int* 23:611–615, 1983
40. BULLOUGH WS: Mitotic and functional homeostasis: A speculative review. *Cancer Res* 25:1683–1727, 1965
41. CHOPRA DP: Regulation of mitosis in the embryonic kidney (Xenopus laevis) by kidney growth inhibitor (chalone). *Natl Cancer Inst Monogr* 38:189–196, 1973
42. LOWENSTEIN LM, STERN A: Serum factor in renal compensatory hyperplasia. *Science* 142:1479–1480, 1963
43. VICHI FL, EARLE DP: Renal hypertrophy factor in serum of nephrectomized rats, with observations on species specificity. *Proc Soc Exp Biol Med* 135:38–41, 1970
44. PREUSS HG, GOLDIN H: A renotropic system in rats. *J Clin Invest* 57:94–101, 1976
45. KURNICK NB, LINDSAY PA: Compensatory renal hypertrophy in parabiotic mice. *Lab Invest* 19:45–48, 1968
46. VAN VROONHOVEN TJ, SOLER-MONTESINOS L, MALT RA: Humoral regulation of renal mass. *Surgery* 72:300–305, 1972
47. YAMAMOTO N, KANETAKE H, YAMADA J: In vitro evidence from tissue cultures to prove existence of rabbit and human renotropic growth factor. *Kidney Int* 23:632–634, 1983
48. SHAMES D, MURPHY JJ, BERKOWITZ H: Evidence for a humoral factor in unilaterally nephrectomized dogs stimulating renal growth in isolated canine kidneys. *Surgery* 79:573–576, 1976
49. SILBER S, MALVIN RL: Compensatory and obligatory renal growth in rats. *Am J Physiol* 226:114–117, 1974
50. GOSS RJ: Effects of maternal nephrectomy on foetal kidneys. *Nature* 198:1108–1109, 1963
51. MORRIS GCR: Growth of rats' kidneys after unilateral ureterocaval anastomosis. *J Physiol* 258:755–767, 1976
52. HARRIS RH, HISE MK, BEST CF: Renotropic factors in urine. *Kidney Int* 23:616–623, 1983

53. Krohn AG, Ogden DA, Holmes JH: Renal function in 29 healthy adults before and after nephrectomy. *JAMA* 196:322–324, 1966
54. Flanigan WJ, Burns RO, Takacs FJ, Merrill JP: Serial studies of glomerular filtration rate and renal plasma flow in kidney transplant donors, identical twins, and allograft recipients. *Am J Surg* 116:788–794, 1968
55. Bump S, Malt RA: Preservation of compensatory renal growth in thymectomized mice. *Transplantation* 8:750–751, 1969
56. Holley RW, Armour R, Baldwin JH, Brown KD, Yeh Y-C: Density-dependent regulation of growth of BSC-1 cells in cell culture: Control of growth by serum factors. *Proc Natl Acad Sci USA* 74:5046–5050, 1977
57. Holley RW, Armour R, Baldwin JH: Density-dependent regulation of growth of BSC-1 cells in cell culture: Control of growth by low molecular weight nutrients. *Proc Natl Acad Sci USA* 75:339–341, 1978
58. Holley RW, Armour R, Baldwin JH: Density-dependent regulation of growth of BSC-1 cells in cell culture: Growth inhibitors formed by the cells. *Proc Natl Acad Sci USA* 75:1864–1866, 1978
59. Walsh-Reitz MM, Toback FG: Vasopressin stimulates growth of renal epithelial cells in culture. *Am J Physiol* 245:C365–C370, 1983
60. Carpenter G, Cohen S: Epidermal growth factor. *Annu Rev Biochem* 48:193–216, 1979
61. Holley RW, Böhlen P, Fava R, Baldwin JH, Kleeman G, Armour R: Purification of kidney epithelial cell growth inhibitors. *Proc Natl Acad Sci USA* 77:5989–5992, 1980
62. Holley RW, Armour R, Baldwin JH, Greenfield S: Activity of a kidney epithelial cell growth inhibitor on lung and mammary cells. *Cell Biol Int Rep* 7:141–147, 1983
63. Aithal HN, Walsh-Reitz MM, Toback FG: Appearance of a cytosolic protein that stimulates glyceraldehyde-3-phosphate dehydrogenase activity during initiation of renal epithelial cell growth. *Proc Natl Acad Sci USA* 80:2941–2945, 1983
64. Walsh-Reitz MM, Toback FG: Kidney epithelial cell growth is stimulated by lowering extracellular potassium concentration. *Am J Physiol* 244:C429–C432, 1983
65. Mordan LJ, Toback FG: Growth of kidney epithelial cells in culture: Evidence for autocrine control. *Am J Physiol* 246:C351–C354, 1984
66. Cone CD Jr, Tongier M Jr: Contact inhibition of division: Involvement of the electrical transmembrane potential. *J Cell Physiol* 82:373–386, 1973
67. Rozengurt E, Heppel LA: Serum rapidly stimulates ouabain-sensitive ^{86}Rb$^+$ influx in quiescent 3T3 cells. *Proc Natl Acad Sci USA* 72:4492–4495, 1975
68. Johnson JD, Epel D, Paul M: Intracellular pH and activation of sea urchin eggs after fertilization. *Nature* 262:661–664, 1976
69. Koch KS, Leffert HL: Increased sodium ion influx is necessary to initiate rat hepatocyte proliferation. *Cell* 18:153–163, 1979
70. Toback FG: Induction of growth in kidney epithelial cells in culture by Na$^+$. *Proc Natl Acad Sci USA* 77:6654–6656, 1980
71. Walsh-Reitz MM, Toback FG, Holley RW: Cell growth and net Na$^+$ flux are inhibited by a protein produced by kidney epithelial cells in culture. *Proc Natl Acad Sci USA* 81:793–796, 1984
72. Holley RW: Control of growth of mammalian cells in cell culture. *Nature* 258:487–490, 1975
73. Holley RW, Kiernan JA: "Contact inhibition" of cell division in 3T3 cells. *Proc Natl Acad Sci USA* 60:300–304, 1968

74. NILSEN-HAMILTON M, HAMILTON RT: Secreted proteins, intercellular communication, and the mitogenic response. *Cell Biol Int Rep* 6:815–836, 1982
75. TODARO GJ, DE LARCO JE: Growth factors produced by sarcoma virus-transformed cells. *Cancer Res* 38:4147–4154, 1978
76. SPORN MB, TODARO GJ: Autocrine secretion and malignant transformation of cells. *N Engl J Med* 303:878–880, 1980
77. ROBERTS AB, ANZANO MA, LAMB LC, SMITH JM, SPORN MB: Transforming growth factors: Isolation of polypeptides from virally and chemically transformed cells by acid-ethanol extraction. *Proc Natl Acad Sci USA* 77:3494–3498, 1980
78. ROBERTS AB, ANZANO MA, LAMB LC, SMITH JM, SPORN MB: New class of transforming growth factors potentiated by epidermal growth factor: Isolation from non-neoplastic tissues. *Proc Natl Acad Sci USA* 78:5339–5343, 1981
79. MCCREIGHT CE, SULKIN NM: Compensatory renal hyperplasia following experimental surgical deletions of the kidney complement. *Am J Anat* 110:199–202, 1962

Contribution of Proteases to Hypercatabolism in Acute Renal Failure

August Heidland and Walter H. Hörl

Most patients with acute renal failure (ARF) are severely catabolic, particularly if multiple trauma, major surgery, septicemia, shock, and acute pancreatitis are the underlying causes. The blood urea nitrogen (BUN) concentration may increase by more than 30 mg/dl a day, and the nitrogen balance is negative [1–3]. Urea nitrogen appearance (UNA) as an indicator of net protein degradation rises to about 12 g a day and may exceed 40 g a day in occasional patients [4]. The concentration of most essential and nonessential amino acids in blood serum and striated muscle is decreased [2, 5]. Disturbances of carbohydrate metabolism are in part due to insulin resistance [6] and hyperglucagonemia [7]. As a consequence of malnutrition, enhanced catabolism, overhydration, and capillary leakage, there is a drop in the concentration of various plasma proteins (total protein, albumin, transferrin, and so forth), and symptoms of marked wasting of skeletal muscle develop. Frequently, many organ systems fail. These failures are characterized by impaired function of the central nervous system, adult respiratory distress syndrome (ARDS), pancreopathy, liver damage, and intestinal malfunctions [8]. Despite extensive supportive therapy by prophylactic daily dialysis, aggressive antibiotic therapy, supply of a high caloric diet with essential and nonessential amino acids, the prognosis of catabolic ARF is extremely bad [4]. Most patients die from severe complications such as pneumonia, ARDS, peritonitis, septicemia, gastrointestinal bleeding, and cardiocirculatoric failure.

The pathogenesis of the hypercatabolic state is poorly understood. Numerous factors, such as infection, malnutrition, hormonal disorders, bleeding complications, and immobilization, seem to be involved. In severe cases, inadequate protein synthesis is not the single cause of altered protein metabolism. There is growing evidence that the protein breakdown, too, is enhanced [9, 10]. This report aims to discuss a potential role of proteases in the pathogenesis of the hypercatabolic state in patients with ARF and in rats with acute uremia.

This manuscript was presented as part of a Symposium on *Nutritional Aspects of Renal Disease.*

Methods

Patients

Our investigations were performed in patients (age, 22 to 72 years) with renal trauma ($N = 18$) or with drug-induced renal failure ($N = 5$). All of them were treated by hemodialysis [11, 12]. Parenteral nutrition was achieved by supplying glucose and essential and nonessential amino acids. In 8 ARF patients with complicating adult respiratory distress syndrome, artificial ventilation was necessary.

Animal Studies

In male Wistar unilever rats (220 to 250 g in body wt) acute uremia was induced either by bilateral nephrectomy (BN) or by bilateral ureter ligation (BUL). Following these operations, all rats were deprived of food and water. Before nephrectomy, 25 rats were pretreated by furosemide (2 mg/day orally) and a potassium-poor diet for 3 days to prevent hyperpotassemia in the anuric state. The effects of uremia or sham operation, respectively, on the particular parameters were studied 48 hours and, in some animals, also 70 hours after operation.

Assays

To reveal changes in the plasma proteolytic enzyme systems, we assayed some key components of them by using chromogenic peptide substrates (CPS assays [14]). Plasma prekallikrein (PKK) as an indicator of contact phase proteins was assayed by using dextran sulfate as a PKK activator and substrate S-2302. For the determination of plasminogen substrate, S-2251 was used. In rat experiments, instead of streptokinase (proposed for men), urokinase (Medac, Hamburg) was used as an activator of plasminogen. The C3 levels in rats were determined by radial immunodiffusion using citrate plasma. Partigen plates (Behring, Marburg) with 10 ml of a 1% (wt/vol) agarose solution and a 1% (vol/vol) antiserum (goat antirat C3, Cappel Lab., USA) content were used.

In uremic patients and normal controls, free proteolytic activities in plasma, dialysate, and urine fractions were measured as previously described using phosphorylase kinase (obtained from rabbit skeletal muscle) and azocasein as substrates [12, 13]. Furthermore, the proteolytic activity of bronchoalveolar lavage (BAL) fluid was determined in the patients with ARDS (which appeared in the course of ARF) and in acute uremic rats. This was done by using substrate A-2288 to determine the broad spectrum serine proteases (trypsin, thrombin, cathepsin B, kallikrein, plasmin, and so on).

The lysosomal activity of polymorphonuclear (PMN) neutrophils in blood smears from normal subjects and patients with acute and chronic renal failure was evaluated by the cytochemical test of Klessen [15]. Plasma levels of elastase α_1 protease inhibitor (E-α_1PI) complex were determined by a highly sensitive enzyme-linked immunoassay [16]. Plasma concentrations of α_2 macroglobulin (α_2M) and α_1 protease inhibitor (α_1PI) in men were evaluated by a radial immunodiffusion technique using standardized immunodiffusion plates (Behringwerke, Marburg, FRG). The inhibitory activity of α_1PI was estimated by the addition of increasing amounts of trypsin to 0.1 ml of plasma using azocasein as a substrate [12].

Morphologic studies of lungs obtained from normal and acute uremic rats were performed by light and electron microscopy [17].

Results and Discussion

Role of Proteases in Human Catabolic Renal Failure

Key Components of Proteolytic Enzyme Systems in Plasma

In 10 patients with postoperative ARF, marked alterations in some key components of plasma proteolytic enzyme systems were found. As compared with normal values, the plasminogen level showed a decrease from 106.6 $\pm$ 4.2% to 88 $\pm$ 13.1% ($P < 0.05$) using a photometric method; when estimating plasminogen immunologically, a drop from 101 $\pm$ 4.5% to 69 $\pm$ 12% ($P < 0.05$) was observed. The mean antithrombin III level fell to 72 $\pm$ 5% ($P < 0.05$), while the PKK was reduced to 74 $\pm$ 6% ($P < 0.05$). As recently published, these parameters show a progressive decline in cases of septicemia and polytrauma with a fatal outcome [18].

Several factors, including plasma dilution, may be responsible for the observed alterations. Furthermore, proteolytic processes such as blood coagulation, fibrinolysis, and kinin generation should also be considered.

Occurrence of Small Peptide Fractions in Serum of Patients with Post-Traumatic ARF

Estimation of protein concentration (by the Lowry method) in serum supernatant obtained after TCA precipitation from post-traumatic ARF patients showed a 6- to 7-fold rise as compared with controls (1.65 $\pm$ 0.11, vs. control of 0.24 $\pm$ 0.02 mg/ml; $P < 0.001$) [12]. In serum ultrafiltrate, the concentrations averaged 2.17 $\pm$ 0.15 mg/ml (vs. control of 0.34 $\pm$ 0.02 mg/ml; $P < 0.001$). In 5 patients with drug- or uric acid-induced ARF, the protein concentration in serum supernatant (after TCA precipitation) was 0.53 $\pm$ 0.69 mg/ml, and in serum ultrafiltrate it was 0.55 $\pm$ 0.046 mg/ml. These much lower concentrations indicate that the increases of low-molecular-weight proteins in post-traumatic ARF patients are not solely caused by retention of plasma proteins which are normally excreted or metabolized by the kidney. It is assumed that proteolytic enzymes may be involved in the formation of small peptides or protein degradation products observed in post-traumatic acute renal failure patients [12].

Altered Granulocyte Lysosomal Function in Uremia

Using the cytochemical test of Klessen [15], we found that the blood smears of ARF patients showed a marked reduction in lysosomal activity of PMN neutrophiles as compared to normal persons [11, 19]. Degradation of erythrocytes and plasma around the PMN neutrophiles, visualized by halo formation, was significantly reduced in ARF. This phenomenon was observed irrespective of the cause of ARF. Similar results have also been observed in patients with severe uremic intoxication resulting from chronic renal failure but without signs of active infection [11].

Neutrophil granulocytes contain a broad variety of proteolytic enzymes including the neutral protease elastase, cathepsin G, and collagenase, as well as the acidic cathepsins B and D. Furthermore, they are rich in hydralases, glycosidases, myeloperoxidase, and superoxide radicals [20–23]. These enzymes or substances are released into the extracellular fluid space during cell death, phagocytosis, or exposure to antigen antibody complexes, complement components, and endotoxins, respectively. The reduced lysosomal function of granulocytes in the blood smears of patients with ARF as stated in our studies may be due to either a reduced formation or an enhanced release of these substances into the circulation.

Elevated Plasma Elastase α_1 Protease Inhibitor Complex in ARF Patients

Determination of plasma E-α_1PI complex in ARF patients showed an increase to 204.9 $\pm$ 31.8 ng/liter as compared with normal values (97.5 $\pm$ 3.9 ng/liter) ($P < 0.05$). This rise in the level of E-α_1PI complex was not related to the cause of ARF (septicemia, acute pancreatitis, shock, rupture of an aortic aneurysm, or dye-induced renal failure).

According to these findings, the reduced lysosomal activity of PMN neutrophiles in blood smears seem to be due to the release of elastase into the circulation. Probably there is a concomitant release of other leukocyte proteinases, such as cathepsin G, B, D, and collagenase, as well as myeloperoxidase and superoxide radicals (H_2O_2). An extraordinary increase of plasma E-α_1PI complex has been reported in septicemia [24], particularly that with a lethal course [25].

Decrease of Antiproteolytic Activity in Uremic Men

Endogenous proteolytic activity is controlled by numerous antiproteases: They include inhibitors of blood enzyme systems such as clotting (antithrombin III, referred to as ATIII), kallikrein (C1-inhibitor, or C1-INA), fibrinolysis (α_2 plasmin inhibitor, or α_2PI), and the complement system (C1-INA). Plasma inhibitors primarily directed against lysosomal proteinases are α_2 macroglobulin (α_2M), α_1 protease inhibitor (α_1PI), α_1 antichymotrypsin (α_1AC), β-collagenase inhibitor, and inter-α-trypsin inhibitor [26, 27]. All these inhibitors account for more than 10% of the plasma proteins. Ninety percent of the plasmatic antiproteolytic activity is due to α_1PI and α_2M.

In patients with post-traumatic ARF, the concentration of α_1PI increases markedly, whereas the concentration of α_2M may be depressed [12]. However, the concentrations of these inhibitors, determined immunologically, show no relationship to their biological activity, which may be markedly different. The first data on plasma protease inhibitory activity in uremic patients were published by Hörl et al [12]. In these studies, a significant drop of the plasmatic antitrypsin activity was found. Especially in patients with post-traumatic ARF and, to a smaller degree, in patients on regular hemodialysis treatment, the plasmatic antitrypsin activity was reduced. This suggests that despite an enhanced serum concentration of α_1PI in patients with post-traumatic ARF, there exists a protease-antiprotease imbalance.

Enhanced Protease Activity in Post-Traumatic ARF Proved by In Vitro Tests

For the evaluation of free proteolytic activity in plasma from patients with ARF, phosphorylase kinase obtained from rabbit skeletal muscle was used as a substrate. This key enzyme of glycogen metabolism, localized in the sarcoplasm as well as in muscle membranes, is extremely sensitive to proteolytic attack. Phosphorylase kinase has a mol wt of 1,340,000 daltons and consists of the subunits alpha, beta, and gamma [28]. Plasma ultrafiltrates obtained from healthy persons and patients on routine dialysis therapy had no effect on degradation of this enzyme within 24 hours. In contrast, plasma ultrafiltrates obtained from patients with post-traumatic ARF were highly proteolytic. Particularly, the α and γ chains were susceptible to proteolytic degradation [12, 29]. In a similar manner, incubation of urine fractions of patients with post-traumatic ARF resulted in the degradation of phosphorylase kinase [13]. In contrast to plasma ultrafiltrates, all subunits (alpha, beta, and gamma) were digested simultaneously. This digestion pattern suggests that different enzymes (probably of renal origin) are involved in the degradation of this enzyme.

Using a broad spectrum serine protease substrate, we were able to demonstrate free proteolytic activity in bronchoalveolar lavage (BAL) fluid in 6 out of 8 patients with postoperative ARF complicated by ARDS (Fig. 1). The highest proteolytic activity was observed in one patient with a pseudomonas-induced infection of the lung. As is known, pseudomonas bacteria contain large amounts of serine proteases [30]. There is growing evidence that proteases and oxidants released from PMN neutrophiles and macrophages (and probably bacteria), as well as complement activation, play a key role in the pathogenesis of ARDS [31–36].

From our results, it may be concluded that in patients with post-traumatic ARF (and concomitant ARDS) free proteolytic activity is released in plasma,

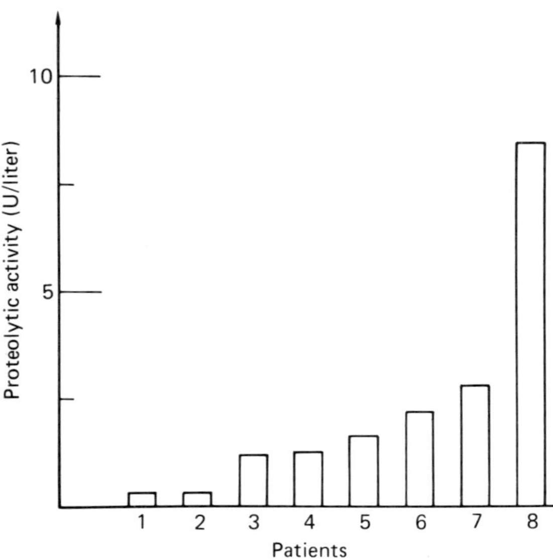

Fig. 1. Proteolytic activity of various serine proteases in bronchoalveolar lavage (BAL) fluid in eight patients with postoperative ARF and complicating adult respiratory distress syndrome (ARDS).

urine, and BAL fluid. The first data about an enhanced proteolytic activity in plasma of hypercatabolic states were presented by Richet and Ardaillou [37].

In relation to our results, the data of Clowes et al [38] should be mentioned. Using a bioassay, these authors compared the proteolytic activity of plasma obtained from post-traumatic or septic patients with that of normal persons. In patients, they found a rise of the proteolytic activity up to $190 \pm 8\%$. By ultrafiltration and chromatography, they identified the proteolysis-inducing factor as being a peptide with a mol wt of approximately 4,772 daltons. During fever, leukocytic pyrogen (interleukin 1) may be a candidate for stimulation of muscle protein degradation via enhanced prostaglandin E_2 release [39].

Release of Proteases During Hemodialysis Treatment

Hemodialysis therapy has been reported to be a catabolic event. It has been shown that glucose in the dialysate, as well as continuous amino acid infusion, is ineffective in preventing this catabolic state [40]. The pathogenesis of hemodialysis-induced protein catabolism remains unclear. One possibility could be the release of granulocyte proteinases after hemodialysis therapy is started. Craddock et al [41] have demonstrated that the hemodialysis-induced leukopenia and pulmonary vascular leukostasis may result from complement activation by the dialyzer cellophane or the cuprophane membranes. By determining the plasma E-α_1PI complex during hemodialysis treatment, we observed a tremendous rise, with maximum levels after 3 to 5 hours. In some patients, a 10-fold increase was observed. It is of interest that diabetic patients in particular revealed the highest rises of E-α_1PI complex [19, 42, 43].

Granulocyte elastase could be released during hemodialysis because of the contact of the blood with the blood lines and the dialyzer (cuprophane) membrane. Such contact may result in a so-called frustrated phagocytosis followed with an extracellular release of lysosomal proteinases. Furthermore, the hemodialysis-induced complement (C5a) activation may be of importance.

An unexpected finding was the observation that the impaired trypsin inhibitory capacity or uremic plasma improves during hemodialysis treatment. Probably, the removal of unspecific, as yet unidentified, proteolytic (azocasein hydrolyzing) activity during hemodialysis might be the underlying mechanism [42].

Investigations Performed in Rats with Experimental Uremia

The clinical course of patients with ARF is complicated by numerous factors, such as rhabdomyolysis, infection, shock, and so on. Any of these factors may influence the protease-antiprotease balance. Therefore, it is extremely difficult to evaluate the "specific" role of uremic intoxication in the pathogenesis of the hypercatabolic state.

For this reason, male Wistar rats were used as a test model of uremia, which was induced either by bilateral nephrectomy (BN) or by bilateral ureter ligation (BUL). Forty-eight hours after BN, the mean BUN level was 275 $\pm$ 65 and that of creatinine was 9.1 $\pm$ 1.3 mg/dl. Seventy hours after BN, a further increase of BUN to 382.5 $\pm$ 54.6 and of creatinine to 12.1 $\pm$ 2.4 mg/dl was stated. Forty-eight hours after BUL, an increase of BUN to 284.3 $\pm$ 58.8 and creatinine to 8.9 $\pm$ 1.4 mg/dl was noted. Pretreatment of the animals by furosemide and a potassium-poor diet for 3 days was followed by a drop of plasma potassium to 5.4 $\pm$ 0.24 mval/liter 48 hours after BN as compared to 10.02 $\pm$ 0.49 mval/liter in the untreated animals. Seventy hours after BN, potassium averaged 5.9 $\pm$ 0.33 mval/liter in the diuretic-treated animals as compared to 11:13 $\pm$ 0.68 mval/liter in untreated uremic rats.

Key Components of Proteolytic Enzyme Systems in Acute Uremic Rats

Forty-eight hours after BN, plasma plasminogen concentration decreased by 40% (Table 1). A similar drop was observed 48 hours after BUL. In contrast, no change was noted in the plasminogen concentration of sham-operated animals. Plasma prekallikrein (PKK) was decreased by 68% 48 hours after BN. After 70 hours, the decrease was less pronounced (50%). Plasma C3 complement rose significantly in sham-operated rats (128 $\pm$ 2.6%),

Table 1. Key components of plasma proteolytic enzyme systems[a]

	Controls	Sham operated	Acute uremia 48 hrs after nephrectomy	P
Prekallikrein (%)	100.0 ± 3.3	93.1 ± 3.9	31.9 ± 2.4	<0.0005
	$(N = 20)$	$(N = 20)$	$(N = 45)$	
Plasminogen (%)	100.0 ± 1.08	99.53 ± 1.57	59.94 ± 2.63	<0.0005
	$(N = 54)$	$(N = 14)$	$(N = 8)$	
C3 complement (%)	100.0 ± 3.19	128.2 ± 2.63	74.60 ± 4.28	<0.001
	$(N = 14)$	$(N = 14)$	$(N = 12)$	

[a] Values are the means $\pm$ SEM; they are expressed as the percentage of values obtained with a standard plasma pool from healthy controls.

whereas it decreased by 25% of the normal controls in uremic rats (48 hours after BN). The activity of the broad spectrum serine proteases in serum was unchanged in the acute uremic animals.

Proteolytic Activity in Various Organs of Acute Uremic Rats

Determination of broad spectrum serine proteases in BAL fluid showed a striking rise in the BN rats as compared to sham-operated controls (Fig. 2). This increase was less pronounced 70 hours after operation. In the furosemide pretreated animals with normal serum potassium, the rise of total serine protease was identical to that of the uremic rats without diuretic pretreatment.

Assessment of the cells in BAL fluid in sham-operated rats showed only a small number of macrophages and lymphocytes. A striking rise in the cell count (5 to 10 times) was observed 48 hours after BN. There was a clear preponderance of alveolar macrophages and desquamated alveolocytes. Occasionally, erythrocytes were found.

Light and electron microscopic examination of uremic lung tissue (obtained 48 hours after BN or BUL) revealed similar abnormalities as observed in patients in the early stages of ARDS. These alterations were characterized by edema formation in the interstitial and alveolar space and an infiltration by mononuclear cells. The electron microscopic findings suggest a partial degradation of elastic fibers, collagen, and proteoglycans. Desquamation of type II alveolocytes also was observed. Intraalveolocyte multilaminated bodies were irregular, indicating an abnormal surfactant production [17]. This observation is consistent with earlier investigations performed on lungs of dogs with experimental uremia [44]. The destruction of elastic fibers, collagen, and proteoglycans in the interstitial space of uremic lungs is probably caused by macrophage- and leukocyte-derived proteolytic enzymes and oxidants.

Enhanced Proteolysis in Rat Skeletal Muscle in Uremia

In acute and chronic uremia, there is an increased muscle catabolism. An accelerated release of various amino acids (alanine, phenylalanine, tyrosine,

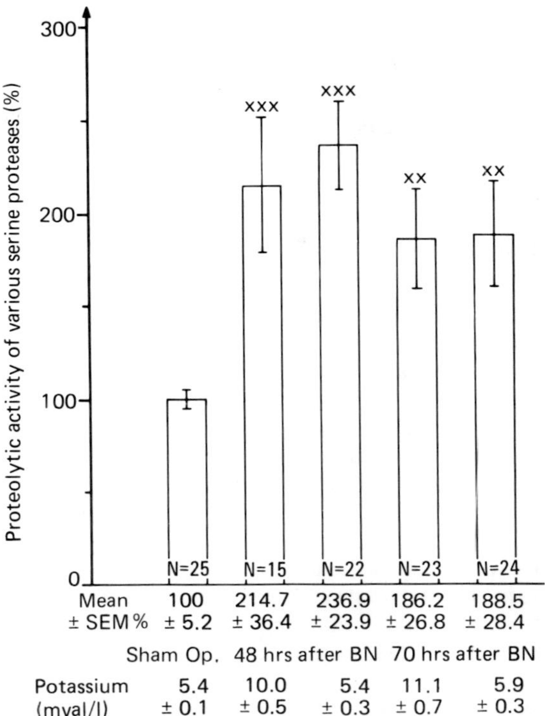

Fig. 2. Enhanced proteolytic activity of various serine proteases in bronchoalveolar lavage (BAL) fluid of acute uremic rats (48 and 70 hrs after bilateral nephrectomy). Serum potassium does not influence the test results. xx, $P < 0.0025$; xxx, $P < 0.0005$.

glutamine, and glutamate) has been observed [45, 46]. In the perfused posterior hemicorpus of BN rats, an enhanced protein degradation was shown, whereas protein synthesis was unchanged [47]. Despite the accelerated protein catabolism in striated muscle, the activities of cathepsin B_1 and D, as well as alkaline protease, did not differ from controls [47]. However, enhanced proteolytic enzyme activity might be demonstrable in other assay systems.

According to recent investigations, it is possible that prostaglandins play a role in the muscle wasting of hypercatabolic states. In rat soleus muscle, Rodemann and Goldberg [48] demonstrated a stimulation of protein degradation by arachidonic acid and PGE_2. Tissue injury and fever increase the levels of PGE_2. The in vitro administration of indomethacin, as well as an inhibitor of thiol proteases, prevented the accelerated degradation in rat skeletal muscle [48]. After rhabdomyolysis, there was a tremendous release of proteolytic enzymes from the damaged muscle [49]. Homogenization of striated muscle activates the complement system [50]. The potential role of prostaglandins needs further study.

Proteolysis in Uremic Liver

Earlier investigations in isolated perfused livers of acute uremic rats have shown an enhanced proteolysis and accelerated amino acid utilization [51]. Therefore, a stimulation of proteases in the liver needs to be investigated in the acute uremic rat.

Conclusion

All the aforementioned data support the existence of a catabolic dysfunction both in clinical and experimental uremia. Among other factors (enhanced concentration of glucagon [7], as well as corticosteroids [52] and insulin resistance [6]), proteases released from blood cells, lungs, liver, striated muscle (in rhabdomyolysis), and damaged kidney cortex may contribute to an accelerated protein catabolism. The imbalance of the protease-antiprotease system suggests the introduction of active antiproteolytic agents into the treatment of these pathologic states. Our own observation of an in vitro suppression of enhanced proteolysis by the administration of α_2M seems to support the usefulness of such a procedure [53]. As long as α_2M is not available, the value of its treatment has to be confirmed by the administration of fresh frozen plasma containing α_2M in a large number of patients. Also the search for other active antiproteolytic agents is required.

Acknowledgments. This contribution is dedicated to Prof. Dr. W. Siegenthaler on the occasion of his sixtieth birthday.

References

1. KOPPLE JD: Metabolic and endocrine abnormalities: C. Nitrogen metabolism, in *Clinical Aspects of Uremia and Dialysis,* edited by MASSRY SG, SELLERS A, Springfield, Charles C. Thomas, 1976, pp 241–273.
2. KOPPLE JD, JONES M, FUKUDA S, SWENDSEID ME: Amino acid and protein metabolism in renal failure. *Am J Clin Nutr* 31:1532–1540, 1978
3. GIORDANO C, DE SANTO NG, SENATORE R: Effects of catabolic stress in acute and chronic renal failure. *Am J Clin Nutr* 31:1561–1571, 1978
4. FEINSTEIN EI, BLUMENKRANTZ MJ, HEALEY M, KOFFLER A, SILBERMAN H, MASSRY SG, KOPPLE JD: Clinical and metabolic responses to parenteral nutrition in acute renal failure. *Medicine* 60:124–137, 1981
5. FÜRST P, ALVESTRAND A, BERGSTRÖM J: Effects of nutrition and catabolic stress on intracellular amino acids pools in uremia. *Am J Clin Nutr* 33:1387–1395, 1980
6. DEFRONZO RA, ALVESTRAND A: Glucose intolerance in uremia: Site and mechanism. *Am J Clin Nutr* 33:1438–1445, 1980
7. BILBREY GL, FALOONA GR, WHITE MG, KNOCHEL JP: Hyperglucagonemia of renal failure. *J Clin Invest* 53:841–847, 1974
8. BELL RC, COALSON JJ, SMITH JD, JOHANSON WG: Multiple organ system failure

and infection in adult respiratory distress syndrome. *Ann Intern Med* 99:293–298, 1983

9. LONG CL, JEEVANANDAM M, KIM BM, KINNEY JM: Whole body protein synthesis and catabolism in septic man. *Am J Clin Nutr* 30:1340–1344, 1977

10. BIRKHAHN RH, LONG LC, FITKIN D, JEEVANANDAM M, BLAKEMORE WS: Whole-body protein metabolism due to trauma in man as estimated by L-(^{15}N) alanine. *Am J Physiol* 241:E64–E71, 1981

11. HEIDLAND A, HÖRL WH, HELLER N, HEINE H, NEUMANN S, SCHAEFER RM, HEIDBREDER E: Granulocyte lysosomal factors and plasma elastase in uremia: A potential factor of catabolism. *Klin Wochenschr* 62:218–224, 1984

12. HÖRL WH, STEPINSKI J, GANTERT C, HÖRL M, HEIDLAND A: Evidence for the participation of proteases on protein catabolism during hypercatabolic renal failure. *Klin Wochenschr* 59:751–759, 1981

13. HÖRL WH, STEPINSKI J, SCHAEFER RM, HEIDLAND A: Role of proteases in hypercatabolic patients with renal failure. *Kidney Int* 24 (Suppl) 16:16–37, 1983

14. FRIBERGER P: Chromogenic peptide substrates: Their use for the assays of factors in the fibrinolytic and the plasma kallikrein-kinin systems. *Scand J Clin Lab Invest* 42 (Suppl 162):1–298, 1982

15. KLESSEN C: On testing the activity of proteases from human polymorphonuclear neutrophiles on blood smears. *J Biochem Cytochem* 26:759–760, 1978

16. NEUMANN S, HENNRICH N, GUNZER G, LANG H: Enzyme-linked immunoassay for human granulocyte elastase in complex with α_1-proteinase inhibitor. *Adv Exp Med Biol* 167:379–390, 1984

17. HEIDLAND A, HEINE H, HAUNSCHILD J, WEIPERT J, HEIDBREDER E, HÖRL WH: Uremic pneumonitis: Evidence for participation of proteolytic enzymes. *Contrib Nephrol,* in press

18. AASEN AO, KIERULF P, VAAGE J, GODAL HC, AUNE S: Determination of components of the plasma proteolytic enzyme systems gives information of prognostic value in patients with multiple trauma. *Adv Exp Med Biol* 156B:1037–1047, 1983

19. HEIDLAND A, HÖRL WH, HELLER N, HEINE H, NEUMANN S, HEIDBREDER E: Proteolytic enzymes and catabolism: Enhanced release of granulocyte proteinases in uremic intoxication and during hemodialysis. *Kidney Int* 24 (Suppl) 16:27–36, 1983

20. OHLSSON K, OLSSON J: The neutral proteases of human granulocytes: Isolation and partial characterization of two granulocyte collagenases. *Eur J Biochem* 36:473–481, 1973

21. JANOFF A, BLONDIN J, SANDHAUS RA, MOSSER A, MALEMUD CJ: Human neutrophil elastase: In vitro effects on natural substrates suggest important physiological and pathological action, in *Proteases and Biological Control,* edited by REICH E, Cold Spring Harbor, Cold Spring Harbor Laboratory, 1975, pp 603–630

22. BAGGIOLINI M: The neutrophil, in *Handbook of Inflammation,* edited by WEISSMANN G, Amsterdam, Elsevier/North Holland Biomedical Press, 1979, vol 2

23. HAVEMANN K, GRAMSE M: Physiology and pathophysiology of neutral proteinases of human granulocytes. *Adv Exp Med Biol* 167:1–20, 1984

24. EGBRING R, SCHMIDT W, FUCHS G, HAVEMANN K: Demonstration of granulocyte proteases in plasma of patients with acute leukemia and septicemia with coagulation defects. *Blood* 49:219–231, 1977

25. JOCHUM M, DUSWALD KH, NEUMANN S, WITTE J, FRITZ H: Proteinases and their inhibitors in septicemia: Basic concepts and clinical implications. *Adv Exp Med Biol* 167:391–404, 1984

26. LAURELL CB, JEPPSSON JO: Protease inhibitors in plasma, in *The Plasma Proteins,* edited by PUTZNAM FW, New York, San Francisco, London Academic Press, 1975, pp 229–264

27. FRITZ H: Proteinase inhibitors in severe inflammatory processes (septic shock and experimental endotoxaemia): Biochemical, pathophysiological and therapeutic aspects, in *Protein Degradation in Health and Disease* (Ciba Foundation Symposium 75), Amsterdam, Excerpta Medica, 1980, pp 351–379

28. COHEN P: The subunit structure of rabbit skeletal muscle phosphorylase kinase and the molecular basis of its activation reactions. *Eur J Biochem* 34:1–14, 1973

29. HÖRL WH, HEIDLAND A: Enhanced proteolytic activity: Cause of protein catabolism in acute renal failure. *Am J Clin Nutr* 33:1423–1427, 1980

30. MORIHARA K, TSUZUKI H: Production of protease and elastase by Pseudomonas aeruginosa strains isolated from patients. *Infect Immunol* 15:679–685, 1977

31. HOSEA SW, HAMMER CH, FRANK M: The role of complement in the respiratory distress syndrome. *Clin Res* 26:397A, 1978

32. LOE CT, FEIN AM, LIPPMANN M, HOLTZMAN H, KIMBAL P, WEINBAUM G: Elastolytic activity in pulmonary lavage fluid from patients with adult respiratory distress syndrome. *N Engl J Med* 304:192–196, 1981

33. REILLY CF, TRAVIS J: The degradation of human lung elastin by neutrophil proteinases. *Biochem Biophys Acta* 621:147–157, 1980

34. HAMMERSCHMIDT DE, WEAVER LJ, HUDSON LD, CRADDOCK PR, JACOB HS: Association of complement activation and elevated plasma-C5a with adult respiratory distress syndrome. *Lancet* 3:947–949, 1980

35. COCHRANE CG, SPRAGG RG, REVAK SD: Studies on the pathogenesis of the adult respiratory distress syndrome: Evidence of oxidant activity in bronchoalveolar lavage fluid. *J Clin Invest* 71:754–761, 1983

36. MARTIN WJ, GADEK JE, HUNNINGHAKE GW, CRYSTAL RG: Oxidant injury of lung parenchyma cells. *J Clin Invest* 68:1277–1294, 1981

37. RICHET G, ARDAILLOU R: L'activité tripeptidasique due plasma au cours des affections severes contribution a l'étude de l'hypercatabolisme protidique. *Presse Medicale* 30:1229–1232, 1959

38. CLOWES GHA, GEORGE BC, VILLEE CA JR, SARAVIS CA: Muscle proteolysis induced by a circulating peptide in septic and traumatized patients. *N Engl J Med* 308:545–552, 1983

39. BARACOS V, RODEMANN HP, DINARELLO CHA, GOLDBERG AL: Stimulation of muscle protein degradation and prostaglandin E_2 release by leukocytic pyrogen (interleukin −1): A mechanism for the increased degradation of muscle proteins during fever. *N Engl J Med* 308:553–558, 1983

40. FARRELL P, HONE P: Dialysis-induced catabolism. *Am J Clin Nutr* 33:1417–1422, 1980

41. CRADDOCK PR, FEHR J, DALMASSO AP, BRIGHAM KL, JACOB HS: Hemodialysis leukopenia: Pulmonary vascular leukostasis resulting from complement activation by dialyzer cellophane membranes. *J Clin Invest* 59:879–888, 1977

42. HÖRL WH, JOCHUM M, HEIDLAND A, FRITZ H: Release of granulocyte proteinases during hemodialysis. *Am J Nephrol* 3:213–217, 1983

43. HÖRL WH, HEIDLAND A: Evidence for the participation of granulocyte proteinases in intradialytic catabolism. *Clin Nephrol,* in press

44. ORLOWSKI T, AJEWSKI Z, WASIUTYNSKI A: Uremic lung syndrome, in *Renal Insufficiency,* edited by HEIDLAND A, HENNEMANN H, KULT J, Stuttgart, Georg Thieme Verlag, 1976, pp 225–229

45. GARBER AJ: Skeletal muscle protein and amino acid metabolism in experimental

chronic uremia in the rat: Accelerated alanine and glutamine formation and release. *J Clin Invest* 62:623–632, 1978

46. HARTER HR, KARL KE, KLAHR S, KIPNIS DM: Effects of reduced renal mass and dietary protein intake on amino acid release and glucose uptake by rat muscle in vitro. *J Clin Invest* 64:513–523, 1979

47. FLÜGEL-LINK RM, SALUSKY JB, JONES MR, KOPPLE JD: Protein and amino acid metabolism in posterior hemicorpus of acutely uremic rats. *Am J Physiol* 244 (Endocrinol Metab 7):E615–E623, 1983

48. RODEMANN HP, GOLDBERG AL: Arachidonic acid, prostaglandin E_2 and F_{2a} influence rates of protein turnover in skeletal and cardiac muscle. *J Biol Chem* 257:1632–1638, 1982

49. MASSRY SG: Rhabdomyolysis: A clinical entity for the study of role of proteases. *Adv Exp Med Biol* 167:581–586, 1984

50. HEIDEMAN M, KAIJSER B, GELIN LE: Complement activation by homogenized muscle tissue. *J Surg Res* 25:518–525, 1978

51. MAIER KP, HOPPE-SEYLER G, TALKE H, FRÖHLICH J, SCHOLLMEYER P, GEROK W: Enzymatic and metabolic studies on carbohydrate and amino acid metabolism in rat liver during acute uremia. *Eur J Clin Invest* 3:201–207, 1971

52. DULAWA J, KOKOT F, GRZESZCZAK F: Der Einfluß von Naloxone auf den Cortisol- und Aldosteronspiegel im Blutplasma bei Kranken mit akutem Nierenversagen. *Dtsch Gesundh Wesen* 38:1517–1520, 1983

53. HÖRL WH, GANTERT C, AUER IO, HEIDLAND A: In vitro inhibition of protein catabolism by $alpha_2$-macroglobulin in plasma from a patient with posttraumatic acute renal failure. *Am J Nephrol* 2:32–35, 1982

Cellular Mechanisms of Protection in Nephrotoxic and Ischemic Acute Renal Failure

H. David Humes, Deborah A. Hunt, Mary J. Clark, Michael P. White, and Joel M. Weinberg

It is becoming increasingly clear that the final common pathogenetic pathway for the development of both ischemic and nephrotoxic acute renal failure is renal tubular cell injury [1, 2]. Acute renal failure developing from either ischemic or nephrotoxic insults occurs from tubular cell injury that produces only segmental necrosis in renal tubules, so that a patchy distribution of frankly necrotic lesions appears to be the rule rather than the exception in the pathology of acute renal failure [3]. The segmental, patchy renal tubular cell necrosis initiates a variety of factors responsible at the nephron level for excretory failure of the kidney. Ultimately, the understanding of the pathogenesis of acute tubular necrosis resides in the understanding of the biochemical alterations responsible for the loss of renal tubular cell injury; in recent years these biochemical events have become areas of increased investigation [1, 2]. As these biochemical events initiating renal cell injury become better understood, rational approaches to prevent renal cell injury can be tested. In this regard, the cellular mechanisms of several protective maneuvers in both nephrotoxic and ischemic acute renal failure have been recently investigated in our laboratory.

Aminoglycoside Nephrotoxicity

Growing evidence suggests that nephrotoxins and ischemia exert their primary detrimental effects on cells by disturbing the membrane phase of the cell [1, 2]. Both plasma membranes and intracellular organellar membranes are potential sites of damage. In this regard, aminoglycoside-induced plasma and subcellular membrane damage appear to be critical pathogenetic pathways in aminoglycoside nephrotoxicity [4]. The divalent cations calcium and mag-

This manuscript was presented as part of a Symposium on *New Frontiers in the Prevention of Acute Renal Failure.*

nesium are known to competitively inhibit a large number of aminoglycoside-membrane interactions [5–12] so that calcium prevents both the neurotoxic and ototoxic effects of these antibiotics acutely in vitro. Calcium may play a similar role in aminoglycoside-induced acute renal failure.

To test this possibility in vivo, a study was conducted in which rats were given a 4% calcium-supplemented diet to increase the delivery of calcium to the kidney [13] and single daily s.c. injections of gentamicin (100 mg/kg) for 10 days [14]. These rats were compared with a simultaneously studied group of rats receiving identical gentamicin dosages and normal diets. The study showed that calcium supplementation ameliorated gentamicin-induced acute renal failure. After ten doses of gentamicin, blood urea nitrogen (BUN) values in the group on a normal diet averaged 213 mg/dl as compared to 25 mg/dl in animals on a calcium-supplemented diet. This progressive decline in renal excretory function, as measured by BUN in animals on a normal diet, was accompanied by simultaneous declines in renal cortical mitochondrial function and elevations in renal cortex and mitochondrial calcium content, which are quantitative indices of the degree of renal tubular cell injury. Oral calcium loading markedly attenuated these gentamicin-induced biochemical derangements within the renal cortex.

The mechanism for this protective effect of calcium may relate to the action of calcium to competitively inhibit the critical gentamicin-renal membrane interactions that lead to cell injury. In this regard, multiple binding sites for the aminoglocoside antibiotics have been characterized in a variety of membranes [15–19]. For developing toxicity, the high affinity site is most critical and has been recently identified as the acidic phospholipids of the membrane. This binding reaction is therefore due to a charge interaction between the polycationic aminoglycoside antibiotics and the anionic head groups of the acidic phospholipids. Calcium was found to be a competitive inhibitor both of ^{125}I-gentamicin's binding to isolated renal brush border membranes (the initial site of interaction between gentamicin and renal tubule cells, with a composite inhibition constant, K_i, of 12 μM) and of ^{125}I-gentamicin binding to phosphatidic acid (an important membrane acidic phospholipid, with a K_i of 170 μM) [14]. Dietary calcium supplementation, however, did not alter either peak renal cortical gentamicin concentrations or the time course to achieve peak levels compared with animals receiving gentamicin and normal diets, suggesting that the mechanism of calcium protection may not be related only to an inhibition of gentamicin binding to and uptake along the plasma membrane of the renal tubular cell. Thus, calcium is an effective competitive inhibitor of gentamicin renal membrane binding interactions, and oral calcium loading significantly protects against the later stages of gentamicin nephrotoxicity, perhaps by the action of calcium to inhibit detrimental effects of gentamicin at critical subcellular membrane sites of the renal proximal tubule cell.

Another possible factor that may contribute to this protective effect may be related to phosphate. A recent study has shown that dietary calcium supplementation produces phosphate depletion and serum phosphate reductions [20]. Since cellular calcium overload, occurring in part as calcium phosphate, is an important determinant of the time course and degree of cell injury [21], declines in serum and cellular phosphate may lessen the amount of cellular calcium overload and, thus, the degree of cell injury produced by a toxic or ischemic event. Certainly, phosphate loading has been shown to potentiate acute renal failure [22]. Future studies will undoubtedly shed further insight into the role of calcium and phosphate in potentiating or ameliorating this form of nephrotoxic acute renal failure.

Ischemic Renal Tubule Cell Injury

Efficacy of a number of maneuvers in ameliorating the degree of renal tubular cell injury and the degree of excretory failure after an ischemic insult has been recently reported [23–25]. Although in vivo efficacy of these various interventions is ultimately the desired goal of any protective maneuver, the complex interplay of hemodynamic and cellular events makes it extremely difficult to determine from in vivo studies alone either the precise sites of action of protective agents or their mechanisms of protective action at the cellular level. Such information is vital for the further understanding of renal tubular cell injury and of the pathogenesis of acute renal failure and further design of yet more effective protective maneuvers. To better examine the mechanisms of protective maneuvers at the renal tubule cell level, we have developed a preparation of isolated suspensions of rabbit proximal renal tubule segments that allows well-controlled direct measurements and experimental manipulation of cellular parameters of ischemic injury. The use of these suspensions also provides insight into the potential of maneuvers for direct efficacy at the renal tubular cell level and into the cellular mechanisms of action of maneuvers to ameliorate experimental acute renal failure in vivo.

Two agents, verapamil and ATP, have been recently assessed with this system. Suspensions enriched in separated rabbit renal proximal tubules were prepared for these studies by collagenase treatment of slices of rabbit renal cortex followed by purification by centrifugation with Percoll. For final studies, tubules were suspended in a physiological bicarbonate buffered solution containing metabolic substrates equilibrated with 95% oxygen and 5% carbon dioxide. To quantify the degree of cell viability or the degree of cell injury in response to an ischemic stress, we assessed a variety of critical biochemical cellular parameters in these preparations, which are summarized in Table 1. The mitochondrial function of these isolated tubule segments was assessed by measuring tubule oxygen consumption polarographically with a Clark electrode both in basal and uncoupled carbonyl cyanide M-chloro-phenyl-hydrazone (CCClP) states of respiration. Cell injury will result in a decline in the rate of both basal and uncoupled oxygen consumption. The plasma membrane function of this preparation was assessed by measuring tubule cell electrolyte concentrations, primarily potassium and calcium, as measured by atomic absorption spectrophotometry on tubules rapidly separated from their suspending medium by centrifugation through bromododecane. Cell injury will result in a fall in tubule potassium concentrations because of potassium leak through damaged plasma membranes and declines in sodium-

Table 1. Biomedical parameters of cell injury

Functional parameters	Response to injury
1. Mitochondrial function	
Basal O_2 consumption	Decrease
Uncoupled O_2 consumption	Decrease
2. Plasma membrane function	
Cellular potassium	Decrease
Cellular calcium	Increase
3. Adenine nucleotide metabolism	
ATP levels	Decrease
AMP levels	Increase

potassium ATPase activity. Tubule calcium concentrations will increase in response to injury because of cellular calcium overload. Finally, tubule cell adenine nucleotide concentrations were measured by HPLC either on samples of tubule suspensions added directly to 10% trichloroacetic acid (TCA) or rapidly separated from their medium by centrifugation through bromododecane into TCA. With renal cell injury, ATP levels will decline and AMP levels will increase.

To produce hypoxic cell injury, tubule suspensions were gassed with 95% nitrogen and 5% carbon dioxide. After 15 or 30 minutes, tubules were regassed with 95% oxygen and 5% carbon dioxide and allowed to recover for 60 minutes. Both oxygenated control and hypoxic preparations were studied with and without the experimental agents verapamil or ATP. Studies have also been done on the effect of ATP on hypoxic injury to renal tubules at cell densities approximating those present in vivo, thus simulating in vivo ischemia with similar general results.

Calcium Channel Blockers (Verapamil)

Calcium has been implicated as a critical pathogenetic mediator of ischemic cell injury [26]. The precise mechanism (or mechanisms) by which alterations in cellular calcium most critically influence cell viability remains to be agreed upon; however, several potentially important intracellular sites of action and mechanisms of action at these sites have been identified for a number of tissues. Major sites of deleterious calcium action in the cell include the plasma membrane, the mitochondria, the endoplasmic reticulum, and the cytoskeleton. Mechanisms by which calcium promotes injury prominently include activation of membrane-bound and free phospholipases, alterations of membrane permeability properties as a result of both direct effects on permeability pathways, activation of membrane phospholipases, and effects on intracellular contractile and cytoskeletal structures. In this regard, the calcium-channel-blocker verapamil has been demonstrated to prevent ischemic acute renal failure in the norepinephine model of ischemic acute renal failure. The mechanism of protection may relate to an alteration of the vasoconstrictive ischemic effects of norepinephrine or a direct cellular effect to diminish the progression from sublethal to lethal cell injury [23, 24].

In studies of hypoxic damage to the suspension of renal tubules, the most prominent effect of 250 μm of verapamil was to maintain significantly higher tubule cell potassium levels in control tubules as well as in tubules recovering from both mild and severe hypoxia [27]. Severely hypoxic tubules appeared to have slightly better preservation of all adenine nucleotide levels and respiratory rates with verapamil treatment, but these effects were small. Verapamil-treated tubules had lower total calcium levels under all control and hypoxia conditions compared to untreated tubules. However, a reversible rise in tubule calcium was observed as the hypoxic insult became more severe and it occurred in spite of the presence of verapamil.

Dose-response studies demonstrated that the effects similar to those seen at 250 μm of verapamil were present at 125 μm; but a dose of 12.5 μm was without effect. Thus, these experiments demonstrate that verapamil has direct effects on subcellular processes contributing to cell injury. However, the high levels required for these effects probably are not readily obtainable in vivo. The effects of verapamil to ameliorate ischemic acute renal failure in vivo may thus be more related to a hemodynamic rather than to direct cellular effects of this agent.

Adenine Nucleotides

Treatment with exogenous ATP and other adenine nucleotides, either systemically after an acute ischemic insult or intrarenally after ischemia, has been shown to ameliorate the resulting renal tubular cell injury and ischemic acute renal failure [25]. In vivo studies using nuclear magnetic resonance (NMR) have demonstrated increases in renal cell ATP [28] in association with these beneficial effects. It remains unclear whether this protection is due to a direct action of exogenous adenine nucleotides at the renal tubular cell level on its adenine nucleotide metabolism or to other effects of such treatment on renal tubular cell integrity or hemodynamic changes occurring during and after ischemia.

To test the direct effects of exogenous ATP on renal tubule metabolism, studies have used preparations of proximal tubule segments incubated with 250 μM exogenous ATP. This treatment resulted in a twofold increase in tubule cell ATP levels [29]. This increase persisted for at least 90 minutes under control conditions. Tubule cell AMP and ADP levels also significantly increased after the administration of exogenous ATP, but to a slightly lesser extent than the ATP levels. Measurement of incubation medium nucleotide levels demonstrated that the ATP was rapidly degraded and was largely gone within 15 minutes of its addition. ADP transistently appeared in the medium at moderate levels. High levels of AMP appeared in the medium and were sustained for at least 15 to 30 minutes. By 60 minutes after ATP addition, when tubule cell ATP levels were at their peak, less than 10% of the added ATP was present in the medium as nucleotide, predominantly as AMP. The remainder could be accounted for by medium nucleosides, mainly hypoxanthine and inosine. The efficacies of various nucleotides and nucleosides to raise tubule cell ATP levels were also assessed. ATP, AMP, and adenosine all produced significant dose-dependent increases in tubule cell ATP levels. Inosine did not. A dose of 250 μM ATP was significantly more effective in raising tubule cell ATP levels than equimolar doses of AMP or adenosine. AMP was significantly more effective than adenosine.

The influence of exogenous ATP on metabolic indices of tubule cell viability was assessed in tubule preparations exposed to 15 or 30 minutes of hypoxia and then allowed to recover with reoxygenation for an additional 60 minutes. Similar results, although over a different time-frame, have been seen in tubules exposed to in vitro ischemia. ATP was added to the tubule preparations simultaneously with the initiation of hypoxia. Tubule cell ATP levels fell to extremely low levels after 15 and 30 minutes of hypoxia. Slightly higher levels were seen at the end of hypoxia in the ATP-treated preparations compared to control preparations, but the difference did not reach statistical significance. Tubule cell ATP levels recovered to near control levels with 60-minute reoxygenation after 15 minutes of hypoxia but recovered poorly after 30 minutes of hypoxia. Posthypoxic recovery of tubule cell ATP levels was substantially enhanced by exogenous ATP in tubules exposed to 15 minutes of hypoxic stress, but less so after 30 minutes of hypoxia. Tubule potassium concentrations both at the end of the hypoxic period and after the reoxygenation period were not consistently affected by ATP treatment. Tubule cell calcium levels were higher in ATP-treated tubules than in untreated tubules under control, hypoxic, and posthypoxic conditions, suggesting that changes of intracellular ATP levels occur after cellular calcium compartmentation. Tubule respiratory rates measured at the end of the reoxygenated recovery periods were slightly higher with ATP treatment.

Summary

These findings demonstrate that exogenously administered adenine nucleotides, at levels previously shown to ameliorate in vivo ischemic renal tubular cell injury, directly influence in a major way intracellular adenine nucleotide metabolism in renal tubular cells, so that a substantial increase in the size of the tubule adenine nucleotide pool occurs. The use of exogenous ATP appears to have a modest protective effect on renal tubule cell viability in response to mild to moderate hypoxic injury.

These three examples demonstrate the manner in which the understanding of critical cellular derangements during developing nephrotoxic and ischemic renal injury may lead to effective protective maneuvers to ameliorate the degree of renal excretory failure. Furthermore, the latter two studies demonstrate the versatility of the in vitro proximal tubule segment preparation for directly assessing pathogenetic factors critical in renal tubular cell injury and maneuvers for ameliorating cell injury.

References

1. HUMES HD, WEINBERG JM: Alterations in renal tubular cell metabolism during acute renal failure. *Mineral Electrolyte Metab* 9:290–305, 1983
2. HUMES HD, WEINBERG JM: Cellular energetics in acute renal failure, in *Acute Renal Failure,* edited by BRENNER BM, LAZARUS JM, Philadelphia, WB Saunders, 1983, pp 47–98
3. KREISBERG JI, MATTHYS E, VENKATACHALAM MA: Morphologic factors in acute renal failure, in *Acute Renal Failure,* edited by BRENNER BM, LAZARUS JM, Philadelphia, WB Saunders, 1983, pp 21–46
4. HUMES HD, WEINBERG JM, KNAUSS TC: Clinical and pathophysiologic aspects of aminoglycoside nephrotoxicity. *Am J Kidney Dis* 2:5–29, 1982
5. LODHI S, WEINER ND, SCHACHT J: Interactions of neomycin and calcium in synaptosomal membranes and polyphosphoninositide monolayers. *Biochem Biophys Acta* 426:781–785, 1976
6. HANCOCK REW: Aminoglycoside uptake and mode of action, with special reference to streptomycin and gentamicin: I. Antagonists and mutants. *J Antimicrob Chemother* 8:249–276, 1981
7. ADAMS HR, DURRETT LR: Gentamicin blockade of slow Ca^{++} channels in atrial myocardium of guinea pigs. *J Clin Invest* 62:241–247, 1978
8. PITTINGER C, ADAMSON R: Antibiotic blockage of neuromuscular function. *Ann Rev Pharmacol* 12:169–184, 1972
9. HUMES HD, WEINBERG JM: Effect of gentamicin on ADH-induced hydroosmotic water flow in the toad urinary bladder. *J Lab Clin Med* 101:472–478, 1983
10. WEINBERG JM, HUMES HD: Mechanisms of gentamicin-induced dysfunction of renal cortical mitochondria: I. Effects on mitochondrial respiration. *Arch Biochem Biophys* 205:222–231, 1980
11. WEINBERG JM, HARDING PG, HUMES HD: Mechanisms of gentamicin-induced dysfunction of renal cortical mitochondria: II. Effects of mitochondrial monovalent cation transport. *Arch Biochem Biophys* 205:232–239, 1980
12. SASTRASINH M, WEINBERG JM, HUNES HD: Effect of gentamicin on calcium uptake by renal mitochondria. *Life Sci* 30:2309–2315, 1982
13. BENNETT WM, ELLIOTT CW, HOUGHTON DC, GILBERT DN, DeFEHR J, McCARRON DA: Reduction of experimental gentamicin nephrotoxicity in rats by dietary calcium loading. *Antimicrob Agents Chemother* 22:508–512, 1982
14. HUMES HD, SASTRASINH M, WEINBERG J: Calcium is a competitive inhibitor of gentamicin-renal membrane binding interactions and dietary calcium supplementation protects against gentamicin nephrotoxicity. *J Clin Invest* 73:134–147, 1984
15. SASTRASINH M, KNAUSS T, WEINBERG J, HUMES HD: Identification of the aminoglycoside binding site of renal brush border membranes. *J Pharmacol Exp Ther* 222:350–359, 1982
16. SCHACHT J: Isolation of an aminoglycoside receptor from guinea pig inner ear tissues and kidney. *Arch Otorhinolaryngol* 224:129–134, 1979
17. JUST M, HABERMANN E: The renal handling of polybasic drugs: II. In vitro studies with brush border and lysosomal preparations. *Naunyn Schmiedebergs Arch Pharmacol* 300:67–76, 1977
18. LIPSKY JJ, CHENG BS, LIETMAN PS: Gentamicin uptake by renal tubule brush border membrane vesicles. *J Pharmacol Exp Ther* 215:390–393, 1980
19. ANNIKO MD, SJOBACK JW, SCHACHT J: Gentamicin binding to the isolated crista ampullaris of the guinea pig. *Res Commun Chem Pathol Pharmacol* 37:333–342, 1982

20. CHEN SB, EBY B, LAU K: Mechanism for the salutory effects of high diet calcium on blood pressure in spontaneous hypertensive rats (*abstract*). *Kidney Int* 23:167, 1983
21. FARBER JL: The role of calcium in cell death. *Life Sci* 29:1289–1296, 1981
22. ZAGER RA, JOHANNES GA, SHARMA HM: Hyperphosphatemia: A factor that provokes severe experimental acute renal failure. *J Lab Clin Med* 100:230–237, 1982
23. MALIS CD, CHEUNG JY, ALEXANDER L, BONVENTRE J: Effects of verapamil in models of ischemic acute renal failure in the rat. *Am J Physiol* 245 14:F735–F742, 1983
24. BURKE TJ, ARNOLD PE, SCHRIER RW: A role for intracellular calcium in the pathogenesis of neorepinephrine-induced acute renal failure (*abstract*). *Clin Res* 29:457, 1981
25. SIEGEL NJ, GLAZIER WB, CHAUDRY IH, GAUDIO KM, LYTTON B, BAUE AE, and KASHGARIAN M: Enhanced recovery from acute renal failure by the post-ischemic infusion of adenine nucleotides and magnesium chloride in rats. *Kidney Int* 17:338, 1980
26. WEINBERG JM: Calcium as a mediator of renal tubule cell injury. *Semin Nephrol,* in press.
27. WEINBERG JM, HUNT D, HUMES HD: Effects of verapamil on in vitro ischemic injury to isolated rabbit proximal tubules. *Kidney Int* 25:239, 1984
28. SIEGEL NJ, AVISON MJ, REILLY W, SHULMAN RG: Accelerated recovery of cellular ATP by the postischemic infusion of ATPMgCl$_2$ (*abstract*). *Clin Res* 31:441, 1983
29. WEINBERG JM, CLARK M, HUMES HD: Effects of exogenous ATP on tubule cell ATP levels. *Clin Res,* in press

Clonidine, Propranolol, and the Prevention of Acute Renal Failure

Kim Solez, Lorraine C. Racusen, and Andrew Whelton

In the mid-1970s there was a strong suspicion that the renin-angiotensin system played an important pathophysiologic role in acute renal failure by sustaining arteriolar vasoconstriction. Specific inhibitors of angiotensin generation or action had not been shown to prevent acute renal failure, but it was felt that these agents might have limited ability to reach the intrarenal site of production of angiotensin. On the other hand, the antihypertensive beta-blocking agent propranolol was known to block renin release by the kidney effectively, and had been suggested as a specific probe for the study of the role of renin in hypertensive states. Iaina, Solomon, and Eliahou [1] and Solez et al [2] showed that propranolol treatment greatly lessened the severity of postischemic acute renal failure in the rat and rabbit, respectively.

Acute renal failure produced by an hour of pedicle clamping in the rabbit seemed to be a particularly good model for human disease, since unlike many other models [3, 4], it was characterized by oliguria in the maintenance phase (Fig. 1) and by subtle histologic changes similar to those in human acute tubular necrosis [2, 5]. In the rabbit, propranolol was most effective in dehydrated or sodium-depleted (high-renin) animals and had no significant effect in saline-loaded (low-renin) animals, suggesting that the drug acted by interfering with renin release. The beneficial action of propranolol was associated with significantly higher renal blood flow in the immediate post-ischemic period (Fig. 2).

There were conflicting data concerning propranolol's action on the denervated kidney. In postischemic acute renal failure in the rabbit, renal denervation using phenol eliminated propranolol's beneficial effect, suggesting that propranolol exerted its protection via its action as a beta-adrenergic nerve blocker. Phenol denervation also appeared to increase the severity of the renal failure, perhaps as a consequence of phenol-induced arterial damage

This manuscript was presented as part of a Symposium on *New Frontiers in the Prevention of Acute Renal Failure.*

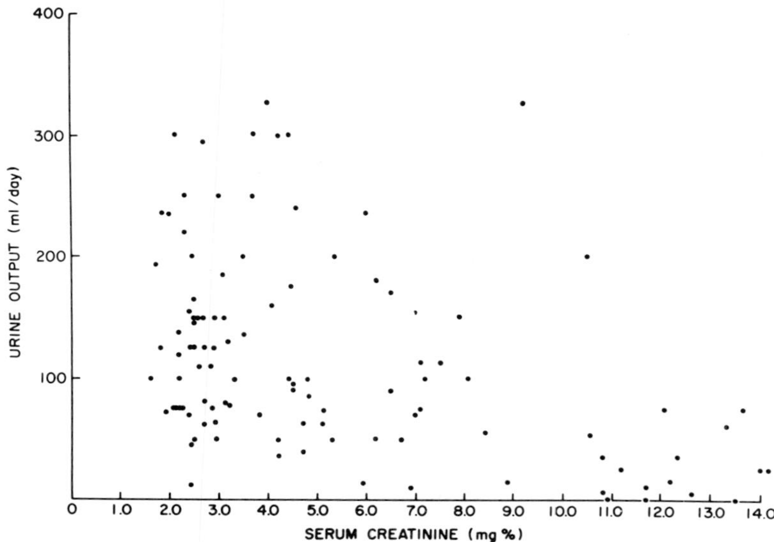

Fig. 1. Plot of average daily urine volume for the 2 days following the ischemic insult versus serum creatinine at 2 days in rabbits with acute renal failure produced by 1 hour of renal pedicle clamping and contralateral nephrectomy. There was a significant inverse correlation between the two parameters (r = 0.41; P < .001). About one third of the rabbits with a serum creatinine greater than 5 mg/dl had urine outputs in the oliguric range [2]. Many other animal models of acute renal failure are characterized by polyuria or normal urine output [3, 4]. (Reprinted with permission of *Am J Pathol* [2].)

[2]. In the autotransplanted (and therefore denervated), ischemically damaged rat kidney, however, although propranolol appeared to slightly lessen renal failure, the difference between propranolol and vehicle-treated animals was not significant statistically [6]. Stowe et al showed that both normal *dl*-propranolol and *d*-propranolol, which does not act as a beta-blocker or inhibit renin release, protected the autotransplanted dog kidney from ischemic acute renal failure [7]. They attributed the effect to the membrane-stabilizing effects of propranolol.

Reasoning that further information about the possible role of the renin-angiotensin system in postischemic acute renal failure could be obtained by studying another renin-blocking anti-hypertensive agent, Solez et al began studies of clonidine treatment in acute renal failure [8, 9]. In addition to blocking renin release, clonidine is also an alpha adrenergic agonist and causes a water diuresis either by inhibiting vasopressin release [10] or by blunting the kidney's response to vasopressin [11, 12]. Clonidine lessened postischemic acute renal failure significantly in dehydrated or vasopressin-treated rabbits but not in animals with normal vasopressin levels. The fact that clonidine was highly effective in vasopressin-pretreated animals, which would not be

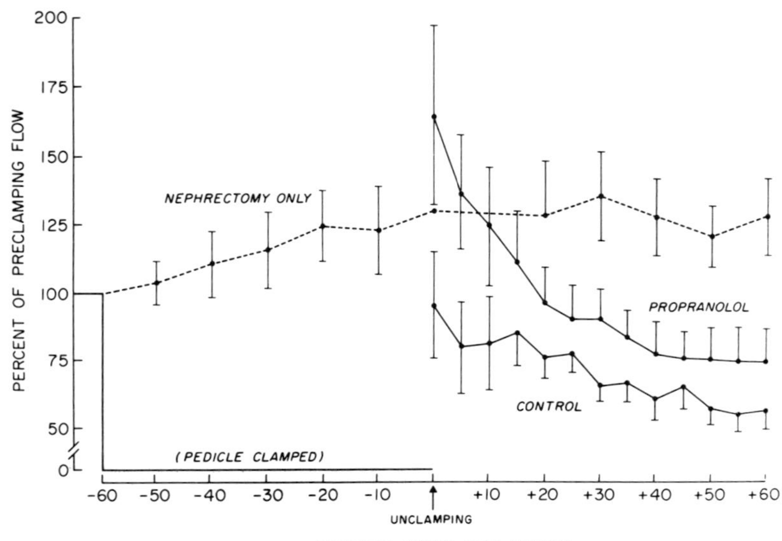

Fig. 2. Renal blood flow (mean ± SEM) over time in propranolol-treated or untreated animals subjected to 1 hour of pedicle clamping and in nephrectomy controls. Propranolol clearly improved renal blood flow in the postischemic period [2]. In contrast, in studies not depicted here, clonidine treatment did *not* improve blood flow even though it provided comparable functional and histologic protection [8]. (Reprinted with permission of *Am J Pathol* [2].)

expected to have a stimulated renin-angiotensin system, suggested that it was clonidine's action on vasopressin rather than its ability to block renin release that was beneficial. Blunting the renal response to vasopressin would be expected to help prevent formation of obstructive tubular casts by increasing tubular fluid flow. Other agents that blunt the kidney's response to vasopressin—demeclocycline and lithium—were protective also [8]. The functional protection afforded by clonidine was associated with a lessening of outer medullary microvascular damage, demonstrated by colloidal carbon labeling (Fig. 3) [8]. Clonidine-treated animals had fewer, shorter, and thinner hyaline casts by microdissection and a reduction in the formation of obstructive tubular casts demonstrated by microradiography [9]. Clonidine pretreatment also lessened glomerular podocyte abnormalities, demonstrated by scanning electron microscopy [13, 14].

Whether clonidine's protective effect can be generalized to other types of acute renal failure remains uncertain. We were unable to demonstrate a beneficial effect of this agent in tobramycin-induced acute renal failure [15]. Eknoyan, Bulger, and Dobyan subsequently demonstrated that clonidine protects against mercuric chloride-induced acute renal failure [16]. Clonidine-pretreated animals maintained a normal urine flow and fractional excretion of sodium; they had a significantly higher glomerular filtration rate than

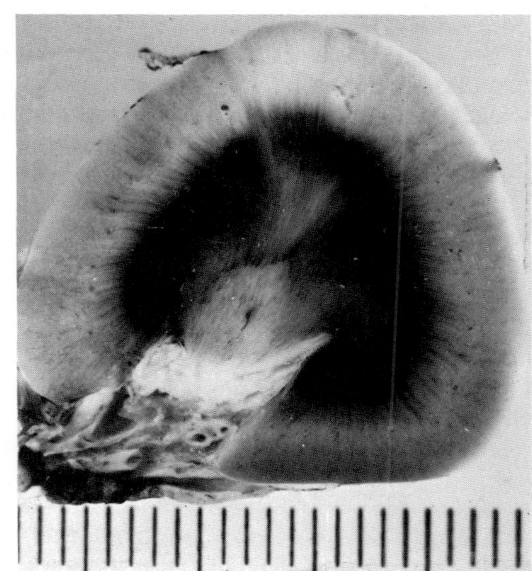

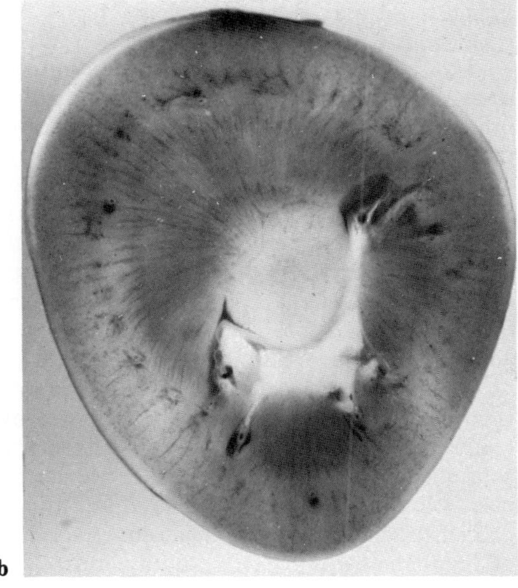

Fig. 3. a Cut section from a representative kidney from a vasopressin-pretreated animal that was given i.v. colloidal carbon immediately after a 1-hour period of renal pedicle occlusion, and was sacrificed 2 hours later. Note the heavy deposition of carbon in the inner stripe of the outer medulla indicating microvascular damage in this region (magnification, ×3.0). **b** Cut section from a representative kidney from an animal identical to that in view A except that clonidine (30 μ/kg) rather than vehicle was given 30 min after placing of the pedicle clamp. There is almost no carbon deposition (magnification, ×3.0). (Reprinted with permission of *Kidney Int* [8])

non-pretreated animals, and they had less proximal tubular cell injury. Eknoyan et al postulated that it was clonidine's alleviation of outer medullary vascular damage [8] that may account for its beneficial effect.

Regardless of the mechanisms by which propranolol and clonidine lessen the severity of acute renal failure, the studies that have been performed with these agents are important for several reasons:

First, propranolol and clonidine are antihypertensive drugs that have been widely used clinically for more than a decade. If they are as effective in man as they are in animals at protecting against acute renal failure, they may be safer for human use than newer protective agents with which there is less clinical experience, such as MgATP, superoxide dismutase, and calcium channel blockers. Clonidine's protective effect may be separable from its hemodynamic (hypotensive) effect and could be due to one of the many other effects of the drug that have been identified [17]. It would be of considerable interest to test whether lower doses of clonidine than those that have been used thus far, or nonhypotensive analogues, are effective in preventing acute renal failure.

Second, these studies demonstrate that the mix of factors responsible for acute renal failure may be quite different depending on certain antecedent circumstances, such as the state of hydration or the intravascular volume. Propranolol and clonidine appear to be most effective in preventing acute renal failure in the dehydrated or volume-depleted state.

Third, these studies show that a number of treatments that do not in themselves significantly alter the severity of renal failure in the pedicle-clamping ischemic model—such as administration of saline water, indomethacin, or heparin—eliminate clonidine's protective effect [18]. Clearly, in considering any protective regimen in man one must take into account the clinical setting and the other pharmacologic agents the patient is receiving.

Fourth, compounds such as clonidine that may cause hypotension or reduce renal blood flow are unlikely to be helpful in sick individuals with *established* acute renal failure because they would be expected to worsen or prolong the renal failure, or lead to other serious sequellae. Agents that protect against acute renal failure may provide no benefit or be deleterious in the treatment of established acute renal failure. Similarly, agents potentially useful in the treatment of acute renal failure may not protect against it. The controlled clinical trial of Abel et al [19] suggested that amino acid hyperalimentation solutions may be a useful treatment for established acute renal failure. However, we and others have found that amino acids given at the time of toxic or ischemic renal injury in animals actually increase the eventual severity of renal failure and the resulting mortality [15, 20, 21]. This nephrotoxic effect of amino acid mixtures may be due, in part, to their content of the amino acid lysine, which is capable of producing acute renal failure on its own, apparently by causing initial tubular obstruction with subsequent arteriolar vasoconstriction [20, 22]. Thus, these studies emphasize that *protection* against acute renal failure and *treatment* of acute renal failure are entirely separate issues.

Studies are currently underway to determine whether clonidine and propranolol will prevent the nephrotoxic effects of the remarkable new immunosuppressive agent cyclosporine [23]. It is of interest to draw some parallels between cyclosporine and aminoglycoside nephrotoxicity.

The mechanisms of nephrotoxicity of the aminoglycosides and the means of preventing it have been intensely investigated over the past ten years. Despite the adverse renal side effects of these drugs, they are such effective antibiotics in seriously ill patients that their usage has not declined significantly even in the face of competition from the new "third generation" cyclosporines and penicillins. About four million courses of aminoglycoside therapy are given each year in the U.S. Many clinical risk factors for aminoglycoside nephrotoxicity have been identified [24–26]. The risk factors—age, female sex, and treatment with other nephrotoxins—are difficult to influence. Other factors, such as dose, duration of therapy, and avoidance of dehydration, can be influenced with a resulting lessening of nephrotoxicity.

Although the mechanisms of aminoglycoside- and cyclosporine-induced acute renal failure are almost certainly different, ongoing research has shown that attention to the "three D's" of dose, duration, and dehydration are also important in lessening the adverse renal effects of cyclosporine. If it could be shown that with the addition of a drug like clonidine or propranolol, cyclosporine nephrotoxicity could be eliminated altogether, this would indeed be a major breakthrough.

Acknowledgments. These studies were supported in part by Grants AM26809 and HL07835 from the National Institutes of Health. Dr. Solez is the recipient of Research Career Development Award AM00835.

References

1. IAINA A, SOLOMON S, ELIAHOU HE: Reduction in severity of acute renal failure in rats by beta-adrenergic blockade. *Lancet* 2:157–159, 1975
2. SOLEZ K, D'AGOSTINI RJ, STAWOWY L, FREEDMAN MT, SCOTT WW JR, SIEGELMAN SS, HEPTINSTALL RH: Beneficial effect of propranolol in a histologically appropriate model of postischemic acute renal failure. *Am J Pathol* 88:163–185, 1977
3. MASON J, OLBRICHT C, TAKABATAKE T, THURAU K: The early phase of experimental acute renal failure: I. Intratubular pressure and obstruction. *Pflüegers Arch* 370:155–163, 1977
4. FINCKH ES: The failure of experimental renal tubulonecrosis to produce oliguria in the rat. *Aust Ann Med* 9:203–210, 1960
5. SOLEZ K, MOREL-MAROGER L, SRAER J-D: Morphology of "acute tubular necrosis" in man: Analysis of 57 renal biopsies and comparison with the glycerol model. *Medicine* 58:362–376, 1979
6. SOLEZ K, FRESHWATER MF, SU TC: The effect of propranolol on postischemic acute renal failure in the rat. *Transplantation* 24:148–151, 1977
7. STOWE N, EMMA J, MAGNUSSON M, LEONING S, YARIMIZU S, OCON J, KHAIRALIAH P, STRAFFRON R: Protective effect of propranolol in the treatment of ischemically damaged canine kidneys prior to transplantation. *Surgery* 84:265–270, 1978
8. SOLEZ K, IDEURA T, SILVIA CB, HAMILTON B, SAITO H: Clonidine after renal ischemia to lessen acute renal failure and microvascular damage. *Kidney Int* 18:309–322, 1980

9. IDEURA T, SOLEZ K, HEPTINSTALL RH: The effect of clonidine on tubular obstruction in postischemic acute renal failure in the rabbit demonstrated by microradiography and microdissection. *Am J Pathol* 98:123–139, 1980

10. HUMPHREYS MH, REID IA: Suppression of antidiuretic hormone secretion by clonidine in the anesthetized dog. *Kidney Int* 7:405–412, 1975

11. OLSEN UB: Clonidine-induced increase in renal prostaglandin activity and water diuresis in conscious dogs. *Eur J Pharmacol* 36:95–101, 1976

12. GULLNER HG: Lack of suppression of vasopressin plasma levels by catapres. *Pharmacol Res Commun* 11:39–44, 1979

13. SOLEZ K, RACUSEN LC, WHELTON A: Glomerular epithelial cell changes in early postischemic acute renal failure in rabbits and man. *Am J Pathol* 103:163–173, 1981

14. RACUSEN LC, SOLEZ K: Podocyte changes in postischemic acute renal failure, in *Acute Renal Failure: Correlations Between Morphology and Function,* edited by SOLEZ K, WHELTON A, New York, Marcel Dekker, 1984, pp 135–145

15. SOLEZ K, STOUT R, BENDUSH B, SILVIA CB, WHELTON A: Adverse effect of amino acid solutions in aminoglycoside-induced acute renal failure in rabbits and rats, in *Acute Renal Failure,* edited by ELIAHOU HE, London, John Libbey, 1982, pp 241–247

16. EKNOYAN G, BULGER RE, DOBYAN DC: Mercuric chloride-induced acute renal failure in the rat: I. Correlation of functional and morphologic changes and their modification by clonidine. *Lab Invest* 46:613–620, 1982

17. HAYDUK K, BOCK KD (Eds): *Central Blood Pressure Regulation: The Role of Alpha 2-Receptor Stimulation* (Clonidine Workshop, Essen, FRG, December 3–4, 1982). Darmstadt, Steinkopff, 1983

18. SOLEZ K: Pathogenesis of acute renal failure. *Int Rev Exp Pathol* 24:277–333, 1983

19. ABEL RM, BECK CH JR, ABBOTT WM, RYAN JA JR, BARNETT GO, FISHER JE: Improved survival from acute renal failure after treatment with intravenous essential l-amino acids and glucose: Results of a prospective, double blind study. *N Engl J Med* 288:695–699, 1973

20. MALIS CD, RACUSEN LC, SOLEZ K, WHELTON A: Nephrotoxicity of lysine and of a single dose of aminoglycoside in rats given lysine. *J Lab Clin Med,* in press

21. ZAGER RA, VENKATACHALAM MA: Potentiation of ischemic renal injury by amino acid infusion. *Kidney Int* 24:620–625, 1983

22. Racusen LC, Finn WF, Whelton A, Solez K: Micropuncture and renal blood flow studies in lysine-induced acute renal failure. (abstract). *Kidney Int* 25:237, 1984

23. CANADIAN MULTICENTRE TRANSPLANT STUDY GROUP: A randomized clinical trial of cyclosporine in cadaveric renal transplantation. *N Engl J Med* 309:809–815, 1983

24. WHELTON A, SOLEZ K: Aminoglycoside nephrotoxicity: A tale of two transports. *J Lab Clin Med* 99:148–155, 1982

25. KOURILSKY O, SOLEZ K, MOREL-MAROGER L, WHELTON A, DUHOUX P, SRAER J-D: The pathology of acute renal failure due to interstitial nephritis in man with comments on the role of interstitial inflammation and sex in gentamicin nephrotoxicity. *Medicine* 61:258–268, 1982

26. MOORE RD, SMITH CR, LIPSKY JL, MELLITS ED, LIETMAN PS: Risk factors for nephrotoxicity in patients treated with aminoglycosides. *Ann Intern Med* 100:352–357, 1984

The Role of Calcium Channel Blockers

Thomas J. Burke, Patricia E. Arnold, and Robert W. Schrier

Mannitol, furosemide, dopamine, prostaglandins, and bradykinin have been shown to be variably successful in preventing the functional defect in some models of acute renal failure [1–3]. Some of these compounds have also proven to be protective in certain clinical situations. Recently, calcium channel blockers (CCBs) have been included in this group, but their usefulness in preventing acute renal failure presently appears to be restricted to the ischemic models only; that is, either the norepinephrine model or the mechanical occlusion model [4, 5]. Since we believe that interest in these results will further stimulate experimental studies and since the mechanism by which CCBs exert their protective effect is not well understood, we will discuss our hypothesis of: (1) the pathogenesis of ischemic renal injury, and (2) the possible mechanism(s) by which CCB administration prevents acute renal failure.

Common Causes of Acute Renal Failure

Acute renal failure describes a reversible clinical problem in which a rising serum creatinine concentration signals vascular and cellular dysfunction and a failure of the normal renal processes of filtration, reabsorption, and secretion. The transient nature of this failure can be limited to days or weeks, and it frequently necessitates dialysis therapy; however, complete or nearly complete recovery of renal function is observed eventually. By contrast, in the absence of such recovery, chronic renal failure ensues.

From an initiation standpoint, it is clear that the majority of acute renal failure clinically seen is the result of two distinct renal insults: (1) inadequate oxygen delivery, or (2) toxic responses to drugs. The former ischemic, anoxic, or hypoxic conditions arise from diverse etiologies that include—but are

This manuscript was presented as part of a Symposium on *New Frontiers in the Prevention of Acute Renal Failure.*

not restricted to—certain surgical procedures, hypotension, or trauma. The toxic form of acute renal failure, which usually is reversible on cessation of drug administration, can occur during the administration of drugs such as cyclosporin or aminoglycosides [6].

Historic Perspective

Efforts in our laboratory during the 1970s were directed at uncovering the pathogenetic factors responsible for initiating and maintaining renal dysfunction, which characterizes acute renal failure induced by renal ischemia. During that period, work in our laboratory [7–10] as well as in those of other investigators [11–13] demonstrated that during the early hours of reflow after intrarenal norepinephrine-induced renal ischemia, renal blood flow (RBF) recovered toward normal at a slow rate. Attempts to effect a more rapid recovery of RBF through the use of volume expansion or vasodilators (with the obvious goal of improving tissue oxygenation) were not always accompanied by a parallel and proportionate improvement in the glomerular filtration rate (GFR). However, because occasional success was observed (especially with compounds that concomitantly increased solute excretion), we extended our studies to examine the novel class of compounds classified as CCB. These drugs also induce renal vasodilation and cause a modest solute diuresis [14].

Preischemic Infusion of Verapamil

Although it was anticipated, based on our studies in normal dogs [14], that an infusion of verapamil before ischemia would increase RBF, the recovery of GFR that we observed was dramatic and unexpected. Specifically, in dogs pretreated with verapamil (5 μg/kg/min) for 30 min prior to norepinephrine, GFR was nearly normal at 24 hr after ischemia; therefore, acute renal failure had been prevented. By contrast, in the absence of verapamil, untreated dogs had very low GFR at 24 hr after the ischemic insult. More impressive, perhaps, were the associated observations that many tubular functions were also protected from ischemic injury as assessed by a more normal fractional sodium excretion, an improved ability to concentrate urine, an increased clearance (secretion) of para-aminohippurate (PAH), and improved renal morphology.

Postischemic Infusion of Verapamil and Nifedipine

Intrigued by these results, which were first reported in preliminary form at this Congress in Athens in 1981 [15], we have extended our studies to include experiments in which verapamil (or nifedipine, another CCB) is infused after, rather than before, norepinephrine. It is clear that initiating a continuous intrarenal infusion of verapamil immediately after ischemia results in a recovery of GFR to about 50% of normal after 1 hr of reflow. If the infusion is stopped after 1 hr of reflow, the improvement in GFR is not sustained; and, at 24 hr, GFR is again as low as it is in studies in which no CCB infusions are employed. However, if the intrarenal infusion is given for 2 continuous hours and GFR is measured at 24 hr, 50% recovery of GFR is observed. A continuous 2-hr infusion of nifedipine (2 μg/kg/min), also begun immediately after ischemia, exerts a similar effect on GFR at 24 hr (Fig. 1).

Role of Increased Renal Blood Flow

Because CCBs are renal vasodilators [14], we considered the possibility that their protective effect was partly due to a rapid recovery in the rate of post-ischemic RBF, which (as stated above) normally recovers quite slowly after norepinephrine. However, although RBF, in fact, was increased markedly shortly after ischemia in the verapamil post-treatment group and was somewhat less increased in the group in which verapamil was given before norepinephrine, this vascular effect does not appear to be the sole reason for the beneficial effects of CCBs. It has been convincingly shown that after ischemia, either a vasodilator-induced or a spontaneous increase in RBF [2, 7–13, 16–18] can be associated with no apparent functional protection. Conversely, an appreciable number of studies demonstrate substantial recovery of GFR, even when RBF recovery continues to be delayed (Fig. 2).

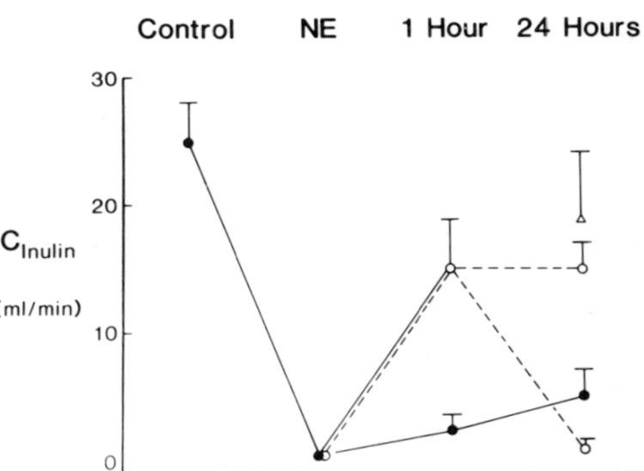

Fig. 1. Inulin clearance (C_{Inulin}) is reduced at 1 and 24 hr after renal ischemia induced by norepinephrine (NE) alone (●——●). An intrarenal verapamil infusion (5 μg/kg/min) begun immediately after halting the NE infusion results in a rapid increase in GFR at 1 hr (○——○). If the infusion is continued for 1 additional hr, GFR at 24 hr averages 50% that of normal values. Nifedipine (2 μg/kg/min) infused for 2 hr also improves GFR at 24 hr (△). If the verapamil infusion is halted after 1 hr, GFR protection at 24 hr does not occur (○·····○).

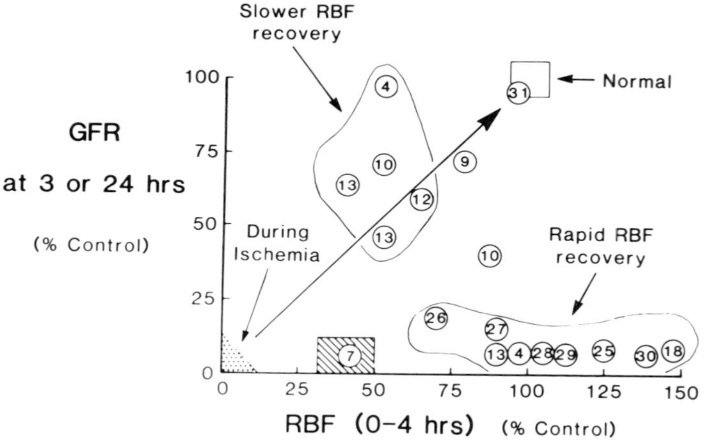

Fig. 2. Comparison of GFR recovery at 3 or 24 hr postischemia induced by renal artery occlusion or norepinephrine, as related to the level of RBF during 0 to 4 hr of reflow. The *hatched box* represents RBF in the norepinephrine model during 1 to 3 hr of reflow; under these conditions, GFR at 3 or 24 hr is very low. As can be seen by the *circled numbers,* spontaneous or vasodilator-induced improvement in RBF to normal or above does not always result in recovery of GFR at either 3 or 24 hr. In contrast, slower recovery of RBF at 0 to 4 hr of reflow often results in substantial improvement of GFR at 24 hr. The *circled numbers* refer to references cited in this study (4, 7, 9, 10, 12, 13, 18, 25–31). Duplicate numbers represent more than one experimental study by the same authors. (See original studies for details of timing and method of creating ischemia, the species used, and when and how GFR and RBF were measured. This survey is only representative.)

Role of Calcium in Ischemic Injury

Since the rate of RBF recovery does not appear to totally explain the impressive reversal of acute renal failure after CCB administration, we have examined the role of verapamil and nifedipine in altering the natural history of abnormal cellular calcium handling following ischemia and reflow. Abnormal calcium handling by ischemic tissue is reflected in a pathologic tissue calcification, and it is thought to reflect a continuous leak of calcium from extracellular to intracellular fluid. The increased cytosolic calcium arises from both structural membrane injury and a loss of active calcium transport mechanisms due to impaired mitochondrial respiration. Large amounts of calcium also are found in mitochondria from ischemic tissue at 24 hr, but not in mitochondria from tissue treated with CCBs. Since mitochondria are capable of buffering against changes in cytosolic calcium, we examined the effect of CCBs on mitochondrial calcium content and on mitochondrial respiration.

In our norepinephrine studies, we did not observe any measurable increase in mitochondrial calcium content during ischemia prior to reflow or at 1 hr of reflow. However, mitochondrial respiration was below normal during ischemia and at 1 hr. The lack of mitochondrial calcium overload at 1 hr, even in the presence of depressed respiration, was initially interpreted as indicating that calcium overload early in ischemic injury is not pathogenetic and that calcium overload seen at 24 hr is simply an index of cell death.

Admittedly, the studies with verapamil, although intriguing, did not offer a mechanism for the protective effect of this drug. However, we have performed additional studies that bear on the role of calcium in ischemic renal cell injury, and we believe these studies help to explain our results. These experiments in the bilateral renal pedicle clamp model (50 min) in the rat demonstrated an increase in mitochondrial calcium at 1 hr postischemia; further progressive increases also were seen after 3 to 4 hr and at 6, 12, 18, and 24 hr of reflow [19, 20]. After 1 hr of reflow, mitochondrial respiration was below normal, but was above the very low mitochondrial respiratory rates seen during ischemia. At 3 hr of reflow, mitochondrial respiration had improved to values very close to normal, even though mitochondrial calcium was steadily increasing. There are two key interpretations of our data that must be emphasized. The first is that the subnormal mitochondrial respiration seen in both the norepinephrine and renal clamp models at 1 hr of reflow does not appear to be due to calcium overload; rather, it may represent an intermediate step in the progressive recovery from ischemic injury.

The second point concerns the measurable mitochondrial calcium overload in the renal clamp model at 1 hr, as contrasted with the norepinephrine model. Although there are obvious species differences to consider, another more fundamental physiologic contrast is apparent between these two models. Renal blood flow recovers slowly in the norepinephrine model, whereas in the renal clamp model, RBF recovers quickly—sometimes within minutes to supranormal levels [16–18]. Nevertheless, after 24 hr of reflow, both groups have similarly impaired mitochondrial function and similarly increased levels of mitochondrial calcium (four to six times that of normal). Therefore, although at 24 hr, the severity of renal morphologic, mitochondrial, and functional injury is similar, this state of injury occurs in the NE model over a different, somewhat slower, time course than it does in the renal clamp model (in which RBF recovery is quite rapid). A corollary of these observations is that only modest evidence of necrosis is observed in the norepinephrine model up to 3 hr of reflow, but necrosis is seen as early as 1 hr in the renal clamp model. Based on these observations, we have proposed: (1) that much of the acute tubular necrosis of ischemic injury occurs during the period of reflow, and (2) that the "rate of injury" is slower in the norepinephrine model compared to the mechanical occlusion model.

Theory of Mechanisms in Ischemic Cell Injury

These observations and our interpretation that rapid RBF recovery (and presumably better oxygen delivery) often is associated with severe early evidence of injury seem to be somewhat paradoxic. Although it is generally assumed that improving oxygen delivery after ischemia is a worthwhile resuscitative effort, recent evidence suggests that in previously ischemic tissue, "normal" oxygen delivery may be "too high," resulting in accelerated production of oxygen-free radicals [21]. A similar excess production of free radicals could occur during reflow, if the ischemic insult had resulted in reduced cellular concentrations of free-radical scavengers. Therefore, rapid reoxygenation of previously ischemic renal tissues—especially those exposed to long periods of warm ischemia—might actually contribute to, rather than protect from, the development of reperfusion necrosis.

In addition, the load of calcium presented to ischemically injured renal tissue is also increased when RBF recovers quickly. Therefore, the evidence of cell necrosis, tubular obstruction, and mitochondrial calcium overload seen at 1 hr in the clamp, but not in the norepinephrine model, apparently correlates with the rate of RBF recovery. This observation may also explain the differences observed in the verapamil pretreatment and post-treatment studies. Verapamil given before norepinephrine induces a modest, but substantial, recovery of RBF to 75% or more of normal within the first reflow hour; functional recovery is very good at 24 hr. By contrast, verapamil after norepinephrine increases RBF to 150% of normal during the 2-hr infusion. The GFR, which only recovers to about 50% of normal at 24 hr, may be compromised either by an increased oxygen-free radical formation or by an excessive calcium delivery to renal tissue that cannot be totally protected by the concentrations of CCBs infused in these studies. The former explanation is more likely, since no increase in renal mitochondrial and tissue calcium is seen in dogs treated after norepinephrine with verapamil or nifedipine; and, the large extracellular-to-intracellular calcium gradient may not be influenced significantly by such differences in RBF.

Mitochondrial and Ischemic Cell Injury

We have observed that during the first 3 to 4 hr of reflow in the rat clamp model, re-energized mitochondria apparently are capable of defending the cytosol against high calcium levels; this buffering capacity, which may be effective in maintaining cytosolic calcium levels close to normal, is accompanied by progressive mitochondrial calcium accumulation. However, mitochondrial calcium content after 3 to 4 hr of reflow appears to reach a level after which further increases are accompanied by a reciprocal deterioration in both mitochondrial respiratory function and calcium buffering ability. This evidence of early mitochondrial functional recovery and the subsequent reversal of the recovery process implies that during the first 3 to 4 hr of reflow after 50 min of warm ischemia induced by renal artery occlusion, lethal cell injury has not yet occurred, and that CCB administration might prevent or arrest the progression to acute renal failure. Shorter periods of warm ischemia usually result in a milder form of acute tubular necrosis and acute renal failure; the usefulness and timing of CCB administration in these models has yet to be explored.

It should be noted that if there was simply a recycling of intracellular calcium from nonmitochondrial to mitochondrial loci during reflow and there was no leak from extracellular fluid into the cell, then mitochondrial calcium would plateau at some level. However, the continuous rise in mitochondrial calcium content over 24 hr suggests a role for ischemia-induced membrane damage, possibly via generation of oxygen-free radicals. Whatever the mechanism, membrane damage during the reflow period would permit a continuous leak of calcium into the cytosol. The failure of mitochondria to buffer calcium effectively while progressively accumulating calcium between 4 to 24 hr strongly suggests a passive equilibration between mitochondrial and cytosolic compartments. Such an equilibration may not only involve an increase in cytosolic calcium concentration, but also damage of the inner mitochondrial membrane.

In Vitro Studies

Verapamil, in the dose used in our studies when infused before or after ischemia, may arrest the early increase in membrane leak of calcium, thus attenuating the necessity for mitochondrial buffering efforts. Mitochondrial respiration and energy production then could be devoted more toward cell repair and energy-dependent regulation of cellular ionic composition. This theory has not been rigorously tested; it does, however, provide researchers with a testable working model, and some experiments in our laboratory are currently in progress to more fully evaluate this hypothesis. In one of these studies, removal of calcium from the incubation medium for the first 2 hr after a 45-min anoxic insult to cultured rabbit tubules substantially improves cellular survival [22]. These acute in vitro experiments involving only tubule epithelium are important adjuncts to whole kidney and to intact animal experiments, because the suggestion that verapamil's protective effect in vivo is due solely to its vascular effect (improved glomerular hemodynamics and/ or more rapid recovery of RBF and oxygen delivery) is not tenable under these conditions.

Nephrotoxic Acute Renal Failure

This discussion has not addressed nephrotoxic-induced acute renal failure; in fact, preliminary results suggest that CCBs do not appear to exert functional protection in models of toxic acute renal failure. The cellular calcium overload seen in aminoglycoside models occurs very late, and no evidence of early cellular calcium overload is observed. In fact, recent reports suggest that some factor associated with increased oral intake of calcium actually is protective against aminoglycoside nephrotoxicity [23].

Summary

In summary, CCBs protect against ischemic acute renal failure and reduce the morphologic and functional indexes of cell injury. The usefulness of

CCBs in preventing, minimizing, or reversing acute renal failure is likely to be more apparent under conditions of ischemic injury than of nephrotoxic injury. With these considerations, it is not surprising that reports have begun to appear concerning the beneficial effect of verapamil in preserving isolated human kidney function or in preventing ischemic injury [24]. One can expect to soon see the results of studies of the effectiveness of CCBs in preventing post-transplant acute tubular necrosis.

References

1. LEVINSKY NG, BERNARD DB, JOHNSON PA: Mannitol and loop diuretics in acute renal failure, in *Acute Renal Failure*, edited by BRENNER BM, LAZARUS JM, Philadelphia, WB Saunders & Co, 1983, pp 712–722
2. PALLER MS, ANDERSON RJ: Use of vasoactive agents in the therapy of acute renal failure, in *Acute Renal Failure*, edited by BRENNER BM, LAZARUS JM, Philadelphia, WB Saunders & Co, 1983, pp 723–740
3. SCHRIER RW, CRONIN RE, MILLER PD, DE TORRENTE A, BURKE TJ, BULGER R: Role of solute excretion in prevention of norepinephrine-induced acute renal failure. *Yale J Biol Med* 51:355–359, 1978
4. BURKE TJ, ARNOLD PE, GROSSFELD PD, SCHRIER RW: Effect of calcium membrane inhibition on norepinephrine-induced acute renal failure, in *Acute Renal Failure*, edited by ELIAHOU HE, London, John Libbey, 1982, pp 39–240
5. GOLDFARB D, IAINA A, SERBAN I, GAVENDO S, KAPULER S, ELIAHOU HE: Beneficial effect of verapamil in ischemic acute renal failure in the rat. *Proc Exp Biol Med* 172:389–392, 1983
6. BENEDETTI RG, HEILMAN JH, GABOW PA: Nephrotoxicity following single dose mithramycin therapy. *Am J Nephrol* 3:277–278, 1983
7. CRONIN RE, DE TORRENTE A, MILLER PD, BULGER RE, BURKE TJ, SCHRIER RW: Pathogenetic mechanisms in early norepinephrine-induced acute renal failure: Functional and histological correlates of protection. *Kidney Int* 14:115–125, 1978
8. DE TORRENTE A, MILLER PD, CRONIN RE, PAULSON PE, ERICKSON AL, SCHRIER RW: Effects of furosemide and acetylcholine in norepinephrine-induced acute renal failure. *Am J Physiol* 235:F131–F136, 1978
9. BURKE TJ, CRONIN RE, DUCHIN KL, PETERSON LN, SCHRIER RW: Ischemia and tubule obstruction during acute renal failure in dogs: Mannitol in protection. *Am J Physiol* 238:F305–F314, 1980
10. BURKE TJ, ARNOLD PE, SCHRIER RW: Prevention of ischemic acute renal failure with impermeant solutes. *Am J Physiol* 244:F646–F649, 1983
11. COX JW, BACHLER RW, SCHARMA H, O'DORISIO T, OSGOOD RW, STEIN JH, FERRIS TF: Studies on the mechanism of oliguria in a model of unilateral acute renal failure. *J Clin Invest* 53:1546–1558, 1974
12. MAUK RH, PATAK RV, FADEM SZ, LIFSCHITZ MD, STEIN JH: Effect of prostaglandin E administration in a nephrotoxic and a vasoconstrictor model of acute renal failure. *Kidney Int* 12:122–130, 1977
13. PATAK RV, FADEM SZ, LIFSCHITZ MD, STEIN JH: Studies of factors which modify the development of norepinephrine-induced acute renal failure in the dog. *Kidney Int* 45:227–237, 1979
14. MCCROREY HL, BERL T, BURKE TJ, DE TORRENTE A, SCHRIER RW: Effect of calcium transport inhibitors on renal hemodynamics and electrolyte excretion in the dog, in *Hormonal Regulation of Sodium Excretion*, edited by LICHARDUS

B, SCHRIER RW, PONCE J, New York, Elsevier/North Holland Biomedical Press, 1980, pp 133–170
15. SCHRIER RW, BURKE TJ, CONGER JD, ARNOLD PE: Newer aspects of acute renal failure. *Proc 8th Int Cong Nephrol,* Athens, 1981, pp 63–69
16. ARENDSHORST WJ, FINN WF, GOTTSCHALK CW: Pathogenesis of acute renal failure following temporary renal ischemia in the rat. *Circ Res* 37:558–568, 1975
17. FREGA NS, DIBONA DR, LEAF A: The protection of renal function from ischemic injury in the rat. *Pflügers Arch* 381:159–164, 1979
18. WILLIAMS RH, THOMAS CE, NAVAR LG, EVAN AP: Hemodynamic and single nephron function during maintenance phase of ischemic acute renal failure in the dog. *Kidney Int* 19:503–515, 1981
19. WILSON DR, ARNOLD P, BURKE T, SCHRIER R: Sequential changes in mitochondrial function in ischemic acute renal failure in the rat. *Kidney Int* 25:519–526, 1984
20. ARNOLD P, LUMLERTGUL D, BURKE T, SCHRIER R: Effect of in vitro versus in vivo mitochondrial calcium accumulation on Mito function in ischemic acute renal failure (*abstract*). *Kidney Int* 25:227, 1984
21. MEERSON FZ, KAGAN VE, KOZLOV Y-P, BELKINA LM, ARKHIPENKO YV: The role of lipid peroxidation in pathogenesis of ischemic damage and the antioxidant protection of the heart. *Basic Res Cardiol* 77:465–485, 1982
22. WILSON PD, SCHRIER RW: Protection against ischemic death in cultured rabbit nephron segments (*abstract*). *Clin Res* 32:68A, 1984
23. HUMES HD, SASTRASINH M, WEINBERG JM: Calcium is a competitive inhibitor of gentamicin-renal membrane binding interactions and dietary calcium supplementation protects against gentamicin nephrotoxicity. *J Clin Invest* 73:134–147, 1984
24. ATUK NO, RUDOLF L, MIHINDU J, VAUGHAN D, TURNER S, WHITE C: Effect of verapamil on preservation of renal function after ischemia (*abstract*). *Kidney Int* 25:339, 1984
25. LEWIS RM, PALLON MK, OSGOOD RW, STEIN JH: Evaluation of renal blood flow, urine flow, and the effects of mannitol, furosemide and bradykinin in acute renal failure induced by renal artery occlusion in the dog (*abstract*). *Clin Res* 30:541A, 1982
26. RILEY AL, ALEXANDER EA, MIGDAL S, LEVINSKY NG: The effect of ischemia on renal blood flow in the dog. *Kidney Int* 7:27–34, 1975
27. WAIT RB, WHITE G, DAVIS JH: Beneficial effect of verapamil on post ischemic renal failure. *Surgery* 94:276–282, 1983
28. CONGER JD, ROBINETTE JB, GUGGENHEIM SJ: Effect of acetylcholine on the early phase of reversible norepinephrine-induced acute renal failure. *Kidney Int* 19:399–409, 1981
29. DONAHOE JF, VENKATACHALAM MA, BERNARD DB, LEVINSKY NG: Tubular leakage and obstruction after renal ischemia: Structural-functional correlations. *Kidney Int* 13:208–222, 1978
30. VENKATACHALAM MA, BERNARD DB, DONAHOE JF, LEVINSKY NG: Ischemic damage and repair in the rat proximal tubule: Differences among the S1, S2 and S3 segments. *Kidney Int* 14:31–49, 1978
31. BURKE TJ, ARNOLD PE, SCHRIER RW: Impairment of mitochondrial respiration and calcium kinetics in ischemic acute renal failure: Prevention by impermeant solute and Ca^{2+} membrane blocker (*abstract*). *Kidney Int* 21:215, 1981

Adenine Nucleotides in the Prevention of Ischemic Acute Renal Failure

NORMAN J. SIEGEL, KAREN M. GAUDIO, AND MICHAEL KASHGARIAN

Over the past 25 years, a great deal of attention has been focused on the pathophysiology of acute renal failure (ARF). Most investigators have been concerned with those factors that initiate and maintain the oliguric phase of experimental ARF. A number of hypotheses have emerged, and these include tubular obstruction, passive back diffusion of tubule fluid, primary diminution in glomerular filtration, a role for intrarenal angiotensin, vascular damage resulting in no reflow, and changes in cortical blood flow distribution and renal vascular resistance, as well as in cytosolic calcium and mitochondrial function. The relative contribution of a number of these different factors in several animal models has already been reviewed [1, 2]. Despite a long-standing interest in the pathogenetic mechanisms of the initiation and maintenance of ARF and the more recent interest in the anatomic and physiologic processes of recovery, there has been very little information about agents that might modify or enhance the recovery process. A number of manipulations *prior to* or *during* the initiation of ARF will limit or modify the degree of functional impairment. Early observations had suggested that renin-depletion during the initiation of ARF would modify the degree of functional impairment. Subsequent observations have shown that mannitol infusion, chronic salt loading with or without DOCA, loop-acting diuretics, and infusion of prostaglandin E have a protective effect when infused prior to the initiation or during the maintenance of ARF. The common characteristic of these agents is the ability to produce a brisk solute diuresis. In fact, Thiel et al have demonstrated that the protective effect of chonic salt loading correlates best with the degree of solute diuresis rather than with suppression of renal renin levels [3]. Likewise, Wilson et al have shown that the high flow rates of dilute urine will not protect against glycerol-induced ARF [4]. With only a few exceptions, agents administered after the acute injury have generally

***

This manuscript was presented as part of a Symposium on *New Frontiers in the Prevention of Acute Renal Failure.*

been ineffective. Tiller and Mudge [5] have reviewed those measures that are effective in preventing ARF, as well as those that may be used in the treatment of firmly established ARF. These investigators have concluded that once this disorder is established, underlying pathophysiologic mechanisms appear *not* to be influenced by currently available pharmacologic intervention. In this context, studies from our laboratory have established the relatively unique therapeutic efficacy of adenine nucleotide combined with mercuric chloride [6–8].

Over the past several years the importance of the role of cellular energy metabolism in ARF has begun to emerge. The adenine nucleotide system is of central importance to the energy metabolism of most cells. In each cell, this system is composed of adenosine triphosphate (ATP), adenosine diphosphate (ADP), adenosine monophosphate (AMP), inorganic phosphate (Pi), and magnesium ions. Hydrolysis of the high-energy phosphate bond of ATP provides energy for vital cell functions including carbohydrate metabolism, muscle contraction, protein synthesis, lipogenesis, and maintenance of cell structure. It also provides energy for the membrane-bound Na-K-ATPase pump, which maintains cell volume by regulating sodium and water transport across the membrane. An inevitable consequence of tissue ischemia is the cessation of cellular respiration and oxidative phosphorylation. Consequently, renal ischemia causes a depletion of tissue levels of ATP, ADP, and AMP. Fernando et al showed that one hour of unilateral renal ischemia followed by contralateral nephrectomy causes a significant decrease in tissue ATP levels [9]. These investigators proposed that the rate at which the post-ischemic kidney can resynthesize ATP after circulation is restored is dependent on the concentration of ATP precursors and the decrease in precursor concentration that occurs during renal ischemia results in diminished resynthesis of ATP following the injury. Buhl, Kemp, and Kemp suggested that the loss of intracellular purine precursors of ATP during ischemia was due to the deamination of AMP to IMP by the enzyme 5′-nucleotidase, which transformed the precursors from impermeable nucleotides to permeable nucleotides [10]. Collins et al showed that unilateral renal ischemia resulted in a rapid decrease in tissue ATP, which was due to dephosphorylation of ATP to ADP and AMP, followed by a slower decrease in total adenine nucleotide concentrations and that total adenine nucleotide concentrations were less than 40% of control values following 60 minutes of ischemia [11]. Thus, the depleted adenine nucleotide pool may lead to a decrease in energy production in renal tissue below a critical level, resulting in cell injury and death. The decrease in tissue adenine nucleotide concentrations may also be related to direct alterations in the cell membrane. Failure of energy production by the adenine nucleotide system results in mitochondrial and nuclear dysfunction, disruption of endoplasmic reticulum, and loss of lysosomal membrane. It has been observed that sodium and potassium transport by cell membranes was diminished during shock, leading to an absence of cell volume regulation and intracellular swelling. It has also been observed that following ischemic renal injury, there is cell swelling; this has been proposed as a significant pathophysiologic event.

Recently, Venkatachalam et al reviewed the role of high-energy phosphate compounds in maintaining cell integrity [12]. The development of irreparable plasma membrane defects may allow cells to leak precursors necessary for the repletion of high-energy phosphates, and the influx of extracellular ionized calcium may irreversibly damage mitochondria and lead to cell death. Thus, it becomes apparent that depletion of cell energy and membrane degradation are clearly interrelated events following ARF. On the other hand, it has been argued that ATP depletion does not play a significant role in the ischemic injury of tissues, because (a) ATP levels can be reduced without evidence of cellular or functional damage and (b) ATP levels recover to 50% of control valves in irreversibly damaged renal tissue. This view may be overly simplistic in that the level of ATP, itself, may be less important than the duration of a sustained reduction of cellular ATP levels or the rate of regeneration of cellular nucleotides following an acute renal injury. In this regard, a recent study is of particular interest. In it, Andrews and Coffey demonstrated that functional and morphologic parameters were indistinguishable from controls when $ATP-MgCl_2$ and sucrose were added to a phosphate-buffered flushing solution prior to 60 minutes of warm ischemia [13]. Thus, it seems reasonable to suggest that maneuvers that may enhance the recovery of cellular energy following ARF may be beneficial in preserving sublethally injured cells and in promoting recovery from an acute renal insult.

In 1974, Chaudry, Sayeed, and Baue showed that the i.v. administration of $ATP-MgCl_2$ reduced the mortality rate of rats subjected to hemorrhagic shock [14]. To determine if adenine nucleotides with magnesium chloride would be effective *after* the induction of ARF, we carried out a series of studies in our laboratory. We found that this combination is effective in three different types of ARF [15] (refer to Fig. 1 of Ref. 15). Detailed investigations have been completed predominantly in the ischemic model of ARF, and the adenine nucleotide with $MgCl_2$ has been given *after* the induction of the ischemic injury.

A postischemic infusion of adenine nucleotides combined with magnesium chloride resulted in enhanced recovery of whole kidney inulin clearance (WKC_{In}), increased renal blood flow (RBF), normalized fractional sodium excretion, and improved urinary osmolarity 24 hours after the acute renal insult as compared to rats receiving normal saline or either ATP or magnesium chloride alone [6]. Rats given dopamine or phenoxybenzamine maintained a low WKC_{In} despite an improved RBF, indicating that the functional improvement was not due to the vasoactive effect of the adenine nucleotide-$MgCl_2$ complex. Also, rats treated with $ATP-MgCl_2$ had improved WKC_{In} despite ischemic periods of 30, 45, or 60 minutes, and the degree of improvement was directly related to the quantity of $ATP-MgCl_2$ administered. Accelerated recovery of WKC_{In} also occurred when the infusion of $ATP-MgCl_2$ was delayed 8 hours or 24 hours after the ischemic insult, and the salutary effect was sustained in that the treated rats recovered to normal levels of WKC_{In} significantly sooner than the control animals in each model of ARF [15].

To characterize the pattern of recovery of nephron function following an ischemic insult, we determined the WKC_{In} and the superficial single nephron inulin clearance (SNC_{In}) at 1, 3, and 7 days after the ischemic injury [7]. The initial enhancement of WKC_{In} was sustained in rats treated with ATP-$MgCl_2$: these animals achieved 64% recovery by day 1, 87% by day 3, and 92% by day 7. In contrast, animals given normal saline had only a 29% recovery of WKC_{In} on day 1, 67% on day 3, and 76% on day 7. In ATP-$MgCl_2$-treated animals, SNC_{In} attained control values by day 1 as compared to low values in normal-saline-treated rats. To further evaluate the discrepancy between WKC_{In} and SNC_{In}, we studied the effect of ATP-$MgCl_2$ on the backleak of tubular fluid. Following the microinjection of ^3H-methoxy-inulin into early proximal tubules, inulin recovery was significantly less in normal-saline-treated rats than it was in ATP-$MgCl_2$-treated animals, indicating significant backleak of tubular fluid in normal saline animals. To define the site of tubular backleak, we measured the SNC_{In} from a proximal and distal convolution within the same nephron. In normal-saline-treated rats, there was a significant decrease in SNC_{In} between these sites whereas there was no significant change in this parameter in either the ATP-$MgCl_2$ rats or the control animals, suggesting that the disparity between the recovery of WKC_{In} and SNC_{In} was due, at least in part, to an increased tubular permeability to inulin occurring beyond the early proximal tubule (S_1) segment [7].

Since cellular damage is known to continue to occur for 8 to 24 hours after an ischemic renal insult, we evaluated the effect of ATP-$MgCl_2$ on physiologic and morphologic parameters at 2, 6, and 24 hours after 45 minutes of renal ischemia to determine if the beneficial effect of this agent was related to an attenuation of the initial insult or an augmentation of the process of repair and recovery from the injury [8]. The impact of ATP-$MgCl_2$ on intratubular obstruction, tubular integrity, and morphologic alterations of the tubular epithelial cells was determined at each time interval. The degree of cell swelling and necrosis was quantified using a histomorphometric scoring system (HMS) [8] (see Table 1).

Table 1. Effect of ATP-$MgCl_2$ on ischemic ARF acute renal failure

Time after ischemic insult	Intratubular obstruction (proximal tubular pressure) (mm Hg)	Tubular integrity (% recovery of microinjected inulin)	Morphologic damage (HMS score of 96)	
			Necrosis	Swelling
At 2 hours				
Saline	23 ± 1	32 ± 9	8 ± 4	41 ± 2
ATP-$MgCl_2$	21 ± 1	40 ± 9	7 ± 4	65 ± 6^a
At 6 hours				
Saline	20 ± 0.5	29 ± 9	25 ± 4	31 ± 6
ATP-$MgCl_2$	18 ± 1	55 ± 5^a	15 ± 2^a	33 ± 5
At 24 hours				
Saline	22 ± 0.5	72 ± 7	18 ± 8	65 ± 9
ATP-$MgCl_2$	17 ± 0.5^a	92 ± 3^a	0.8 ± 0.1^a	18 ± 2^a
Nonischemic control	13 ± 0.5	98 ± 2	0	0

[a] $P < 0.01$, ATP-$MgCl_2$ vs. saline rats.

Two hours after the ischemic insult, both groups of rats demonstrated increased permeability to inulin and significantly elevated proximal tubular pressures. Two populations of tubules were identified in the experimental animals: a subgroup of totally obstructed tubules with markedly elevated pressure (greater than 20 mm Hg) and another group of tubules with either normal or only modestly increased intratubular pressure (10 to 15 mm Hg). The degree of cellular necrosis was similar for both treatment groups, whereas the percentage of tubules with swelling was significantly greater in ATP-$MgCl_2$ rats. Since the physiologic and morphologic aspects of ARF were similar in both groups of rats at this time interval, it seems unlikely that ATP-$MgCl_2$ served only to mitigate the severity of the initial injury (see Table 1).

By 6 hours, ATP-$MgCl_2$ animals had significantly less tubular backleak as compared with saline rats. In animals given ATP-$MgCl_2$, only 25% of the tubules had pressures of 20 mm Hg or more as compared to 60% of the tubules in rats treated with normal saline. The degree of cellular necrosis was significantly less in ATP-$MgCl_2$-treated animals, but the amount of cell swelling was similar in both groups. By this time interval, animals infused with ATP-$MgCl_2$ had early evidence of cellular recovery, but the rats given saline continued to exhibit ongoing ischemic damage (see Table 1).

By 24 hours, rats treated with ATP-$MgCl_2$ had reestablished tubular integrity, whereas saline rats still had significant backleak. Animals treated with ATP-$MgCl_2$ continued to have lower mean proximal tubular pressures. The reduced intratubular pressure in the animals receiving ATP-$MgCl_2$ was the result of the disappearance of the subpopulation of totally obstructed tubules. In contrast, 50% of the tubules in rats given saline continued to have proximal tubular pressures greater than 20 mm Hg. There continued to be a marked difference in the cellular damage as assessed by the HMS between the two experimental groups. Animals given ATP-$MgCl_2$ had an HMS for necrosis and swelling that was reduced significantly. In contrast, saline-treated animals still demonstrated significant cellular alterations.

This sequence of studies establishes several important points: (1) The administration of ATP-$MgCl_2$ *after* the induction of an ischemic renal injury will enhance the recovery of glomerular and tubular function. (2) This salutary effect is mediated via those components of ARF that are felt to contribute to an ischemic injury, that is, intratubular obstruction and backleak of tubular fluid. (3) The initial improvements in WKC_{In} and SNC_{In} are sustained and result in an accelerated return to normal renal function. (4) This beneficial effect is not the result of simply an attenuation of the severity of the ischemic insult. It seems likely that the beneficial effect of ATP-$MgCl_2$ is related to an augmentation of the cellular and metabolic processes that are required for preservation of sublethally injured cells and for the restoration and repair of damaged epithelium following ischemic ARF.

Based on these studies, our next objective was to determine the effect of a postischemic infusion of ATP-$MgCl_2$ on tissue nucleotide levels. In collaboration with Shulman and Avison, we succeeded in combining micropuncture techniques and nuclear magnetic resonance (NMR) technology to obtain ^{31}P-NMR spectra on rat kidneys in vivo [16]. The left kidney is placed in a specially designed plastic (Lucite™) micropuncture cup, which contains a radiofrequency coil. The animals are then put in a TMR-32 spectrometer with 20-cm bore operating at 80.2 MHz for protons and 32.5 MHz for phosphorus 31. In control animals, distinct ^{31}P-NMR peaks corresponding to α, β, and γ phosphate of ATP, sugar phosphate (SP), and inorganic phosphate (Pi) were observed with a good signal-to-noise ratio. Animals and ^{31}P-NMR spectra were stable for 4 to 6 hours. Rats were subjected to 45 minutes of bilateral renal artery ischemia, and ^{31}P-NMR spectra were collected every 7 minutes. Animals received either ATP-MgCl$_2$ or saline immediately following the ischemic interval. In each animal, spectra were obtained prior to, during, and after the ischemic insult, and thus, each animal served as its own control. In these initial studies of ischemic injury, we observed that during renal artery occlusion, the β-ATP peak (the only peak that is unique to ATP) declined appreciably within 10 minutes and fell to less than 10% of baseline values after 45 minutes [16]. Concomitantly, Pi peak intensity increased, and tissue pH fell significantly, by approximately 0.4 pH units. After release of the renal artery, the β-ATP peak returned to low levels within 30 minutes and remained at 50% of baseline values for 3 to 4 hours. Pi levels fell progressively over the same period, and tissue pH increased. In the animals treated with ATP-MgCl$_2$, the decline in tissue ATP levels during the ischemic insult was the same as that observed in the rats given saline. During the ATP-MgCl$_2$ infusion, the β-ATP peak was 50% of control values just as had been seen in the saline animals. Thus, the infused ATP, within the vasculature of the kidney, made little direct contribution to the NMR signal. However, the infusion of 25 μmoles of ATP-MgCl$_2$ resulted in a marked and significant acceleration in the rate of recovery of tissue ATP. By 120 minutes after the ischemic injury, the mean recovery of ATP was 89 $\pm$ 2%, which is clearly significantly different from that found in rats given saline (65 $\pm$ 2%). Since the tubular alterations were similar in both groups at 2 hours, these studies suggest that repair of tissue nucleotides precedes morphologic recovery after ARF.

These investigations establish several important points: (1) ^{31}P-NMR spectroscopy can be used for the study of kidneys in vivo. (2) The magnitude of changes in cellular ATP, Pi, and pH that occur in ARF are easily within the realm of measurement with NMR. (3) Our preparation is stable and will allow a continuous assessment of alterations in cellular pH and high-energy phosphate. And (4) the observation that ATP-MgCl$_2$ can significantly accelerate the recovery of tissue ATP levels provides a biochemical benchmark for the beneficial effect of this complex on renal function.

References

1. STEIN JH, LIFSCHITZ MD, BARNES LD: Current concepts on the pathophysiology of acute renal failure. *Am J Physiol* 234:F171–F181, 1978
2. CONGER JD, SCHREIER RW: Renal hemodynamics in acute renal failure. *Ann Rev Physiol* 42:603–610, 1980
3. THIEL G, BRUNNER F, WUNDERLICH P, HUGUENIN M, BIENKO B, TORHORST

J, Peters-Haefeli L, Kirchertz EJ, Peters G: Protection of rat kidneys against $HgCl_2$-induced acute renal failure by induction of high urine flow without renin suppression. *Kidney Int* 10:S191–S200, 1976
4. WILSON DR, THIEL G, ARCE ML, OKEN DE: The role of concentrating mechanism in the development of acute renal failure: Micropuncture studies using diabetes insipidus rats. *Nephron* 6:128–139, 1969
5. TILLER DJ, MUDGE GH: Pharmacologic agents used in the management of acute renal failure. *Kidney Int* 18:700–711, 1980
6. SIEGEL NJ, GLAZIER WB, CHAUDRY IH, GAUDIO KM, LYTTON B, BAUE AE, KASHGARIAN M: Enhanced recovery from acute renal failure by the postischemic infusion of adenine nucleotides and magnesium chloride in rats. *Kidney Int* 17:338–349, 1980
7. GAUDIO KM, TAYLOR MR, CHAUDRY IH, KASHGARIAN M, SIEGEL NJ: Accelerated recovery of single nephron function by the postischemic infusion of ATP-$MgCl_2$. *Kidney Int* 22:13–20, 1982
8. GAUDIO KM, ARDITO TA, REILLY HF, KASHGARIAN M, SIEGEL NJ: Accelerated cellular recovery after an ischemic renal injury. *Am J Pathol* 112:338–346, 1983
9. FERNANDO AR, GRIFFITHS JR, O'DONOGHUE EPN, WARD JP, ARMSTRONG DMG, HENDRY WF, PERRETT D, WICKHAM JEA: Enhanced preservation of the ischemic kidney with inosine. *Lancet* 1:555–557, 1976
10. BUHL MR, KEMP E, KEMP G: Inosine in preservation of rabbit kidneys for transplantation. *Transplant Proc* 9:1603–1606, 1977
11. COLLINS GM, TAFT P, GREEN RD, RUPRECHT R, HALASZ NA: Adenine nucleotide levels in preserved and ischemically injured canine kidneys. *World J Surg* 1:237–243, 1977
12. VENKATACHALAM MA, KREISBERG JI, STEIN JH, LIFSCHITZ MD: Salvage of ischemic cells by impermeant solute and adenosine triphosphate. *Lab Invest* 49:1–3, 1983
13. ANDREWS PM, COFFEY AK: Protection of kidneys from acute renal failure resulting from normothermic ischemia. *Lab Invest* 49:87–98, 1983
14. CHAUDRY IH, SAYEED MM, BAUE AE: The effect of adenosine triphosphate-$MgCl_2$ administration in shock. *Surgery* 75:220–227, 1974
15. SIEGEL NJ: Amino acids and adenine nucleotides in acute renal failure, in *Acute Renal Failure*, edited by BRENNER BM, LAZARUS JM, MYERS BD, Philadelphia, WB Saunders & Co, 1983, pp 741–752
16. SIEGEL NJ, AVISON MJ, REILLY HF, ALGER JR, SHULMAN RG: Enhanced recovery of renal ATP with postischemic infusion of ATP-$MgCl_2$ determined by ^{31}P-NMR. *Am J Physiol* 245:F530–534, 1983

Mechanisms of Drug Nephrotoxicity

William M. Bennett

The growing list of drugs developed and released by the pharmaceutical industry has been paralleled by an increased awareness of their potential for acute and chronic renal adverse reactions. Major advances in the understanding of how these drugs and environmental chemicals produce renal cell injury, and in turn how this cellular damage is translated into clinical renal dysfunction, has elucidated mechanisms that may be increasingly applicable to nondrug-related renal diseases.

Defining Nephrotoxicity

In recent years, it has become clear that most clinical presentations of renal disease can be mimicked by nephrotoxins. In addition to acute and chronic renal insufficiency, various fluid electrolyte and acid-base disturbances can follow drug administration. Drug-associated proteinuria or nephrotic syndrome may occur on an immunologic basis or may be due to direct toxic effects on the glomerulus. In some instances, the offending toxin is the same one that in other clinical or experimental situations produces typical acute tubular necrosis. The variety of renal lesions associated with mercury toxicity illustrates this point. This overview is restricted to considerations of some commonly used drugs that produce tubular damage and renal failure clinically.

The clinical diagnosis of drug nephrotoxicity usually is delayed until enough damage is present to produce alterations in glomerular filtration rate (GFR). The GFR usually is assessed indirectly by the clinician via measurement of elevations of serum creatinine or more precisely by a decrease in creatinine clearance (C_{cr}). This operational definition may greatly underesti-

---

This manuscript was presented as part of a Symposium on *Nephrotoxicity and Drugs.*

mate toxic effects that do not acutely alter these relatively insensitive markers of renal function. Moreover, the serum creatinine concentration, a value that is most often used as the marker of renal function, may not become elevated above the normal range until the GFR falls to 30 to 50% of normal values because of the nonlinear relationship of serum creatinine to GFR. For example, it is well known that excessive use of combination analgesics usually containing phenacetin may produce renal papillary necrosis, which is clinically silent until the disease is far advanced. It should be kept in mind that because many nephrotoxins primarily injure renal tubular cells, the remarkable reserve and compensatory capacity of uninjured nephrons may mask nephron injury until a considerable amount of kidney tissue is irreparably lost. Various experimental studies have used more sensitive markers of cell injury, such as enzymuria and tubular proteinuria, as markers of nephrotoxicity. Epidemiologic investigations of workers exposed to occupational hazards such as lead, cadmium, and mercury have correlated heavy exposure with these markers [1]. Possibly because of the difficulty in collecting urine samples, these tests have not yet achieved widespread acceptance in clinical medicine. Desperately needed is a simple, convenient marker of tubular injury that ideally can be measured in a venous blood sample. This situation contrasts with the clinical diagnosis of liver injury, in which many sensitive enzyme markers of injury are routinely available.

Until some new diagnostic test is available for clinical use, nephrotoxicity will continue to be defined by indirect measurements of GFR, such as the serum creatinine concentration. It is imperative that new drugs with nephrotoxic potential in preclinical testing are not considered safe until long-term experience provides evidence that cumulative renal damage does not result from long-term, low-dose, or repeated exposures. This caveat probably is applicable to cyclosporine, cis-platin, and aminoglycoside antibiotics in which the serum creatinine concentration may be dissociated from histologic and functional markers of ongoing renal injury [2–5]. For example, it does not necessarily follow that because serum creatinine concentration returns to normal when cyclosporine dosage is reduced, interstitial fibrosis (which will ultimately cause renal transplant failure) is prevented. Hydration and solute diuresis may modify the overt rises in serum creatinine concentration that follow cis-platin chemotherapy; however, repeated courses of therapy may lead to chronic renal insufficiency [6]. In experimental animals receiving continuous gentamicin therapy, GFR returns toward normal values despite pathologic and functional evidence of ongoing tubular injury [7, 8]. Chronic tubulointerstitial nephropathy was recently documented in patients with cystic fibrosis who had received multiple courses of aminoglycosides without apparent acute nephrotoxicity [3].

Mechanisms of Renal Tubular Cell Damage by Specific Drugs

The toxic mechanisms of all the drugs that cause nephrotoxicity is long and cannot be covered in detail here. Examples have been chosen to illustrate specific mechanisms for which some data now exist. Unfortunately, the mechanisms involved in the toxicity of many commonly used compounds have not been well studied. This overview will not discuss immunologic mechanisms involved in renal damage associated with drugs. This has been recently summarized [9, 10]. Drugs such as nonsteroidal anti-inflammatory agents (NSAID) and angiotensin-converting enzyme inhibitors may cause renal dysfunction under certain clinical circumstances by altering renal hemodynamics. These subjects have also been covered in detail elsewhere [10, 11].

Aminoglycoside Antibiotics

There has been intense interest in the mechanism of aminoglycoside antibiotic nephrotoxicity in the past several years due to the continuing problem of clinically important decreases in renal function during therapy using these widely used drugs [12]. Aminoglycosides are sugars in glycoside linkage with side chains containing amino groups [13]. With molecular weights of approximately 500 daltons, they undergo glomerular filtration; and, a large fraction of the filtered drug is excreted unchanged in the urine. In fact, the clearance of aminoglycosides is equal or only slightly less than the clearance of inulin [14].

Gentamicin and, presumably, other aminoglycosides are accumulated by proximal tubular cells and cause patchy tubular necrosis by precise mechanisms that are as yet unclear. In the rat, microinjection and micropuncture studies have suggested that lumenal uptake occurs [15, 16, 18] after binding to a brush border membrane receptor [17]. After attachment and pinocytosis, tritiated gentamicin is incorporated rapidly into lysosomes [18]. Lysosomal swelling with accumulation of membranous whorled material can be visualized in tissue sections prior to declines in GFR. Aminoglycosides as water-soluble cationic compounds inhibit lysosomal phospholipases that lead to an acquired phospholipidosis [19]. Lysosomal membranes may become stabilized and impermeable to osmotically active particles, resulting eventually in rupture and possibly in cell necrosis [20, 21]. Other lysosomal hydrolases such as proteolytic enzymes may be inhibited, thus interfering with renal metabolism of endogenous intracellular proteins as well as exogenous low molecular weight proteins [22].

Interference with mitochondrial-oxidative phosphorylation by aminoglycosides may compromise tubular cell transport function, leading to loss of cell membrane integrity and to cell necrosis [23]. In vitro exposure of cortical mitochondria to gentamicin results in inhibition of state 3 and dinitrophenol-uncoupled respiration while stimulating state 4 respiration. Gentamicin probably displaces magnesium from sites at the inner mitochondrial membrane, where the divalent cation regulates sodium and potassium permeability [24]. Because of binding and redistribution during isolation and preparation of mitochondria for in vitro study, it is difficult to be sure that these abnormalities are similar to those seen with in vivo treatment. Rats treated with gentamicin show only a depression of state 3 and dinitrophenol-uncoupled respiration, raising the question of whether aminoglycosides really interact with mito-chondria in situ prior to the onset of lethal cell injury [25]. The presence of definite abnormalities prior to other morphologic or functional evidence of cell necrosis does imply an important role for impairment of cell energetics in the pathogenesis of cell injury. Changes in mitochondrial function correlate with a decrease in kidney adenosine triphosphate content at a time when morphologic studies show only focal loss of brush border and increased num-bers of secondary lysosomes [23]. Although cell debris is noted at this time in some tubular lumens, obstructing casts are not present [23]. Gentamicin limits mitochondrial uptake of calcium [26], as well as competitively displacing calcium from brush border membrane phospholipid binding sites [17]. It is of interest that dietary calcium has been reported to inhibit gentamicin-renal brush border binding reactions and to modify gentamicin nephrotoxicity [27, 28]. With increased dietary calcium, mitochondrial calcium was decreased and respiratory function was improved compared to control animals receiving toxic doses of gentamicin [27].

Aminoglycosides can cause a reversible decline in membrane-bound Na-K-ATPase after a single large dose [29]. However, with repeated doses, declines in enzyme activity may be related to generalized membrane deteriora-tion related to other intracellular events [30]. Aminoglycoside effects on mem-brane phospholipids may be critically related to dysfunction of Na-K-ATPase, which is an enzymatic regulator of the cation gradients essential for cell survival [31]. Renal wasting of the intracellular cations, potassium and magne-sium, may precede or occur independently of alterations in GFR also as a result of drug effects on Na-K-ATPase [32–34].

The pathogenetic sequence that leads to acute renal failure due to aminogly-coside-induced nephrotoxic tubular injury is unclear. In rats with superficial glomeruli that are accessible to micropuncture, there was a similar decline in glomerular capillary ultrafiltration coefficient (K_f) with both toxic and nontoxic doses of gentamicin [35]. Furthermore, no evidence of backleak of glomerular filtrate was noted with microinjected inulin [35]. It is doubtful that these glomerular effects play more than an adjunctive role in causing clinical renal failure. There may be early decreases in renal blood flow (RBF) in sodium-depleted animals prior to any change in GFR [36]. Swollen blebs of brush border membrane, which are debris from damaged tubular cells, likely cause tubular obstruction by forming casts in gentamicin-induced acute renal failure. Neugarten et al have recently shown that severe gentamicin nephrotoxicity is associated with a heterogeneous renal lesion in which varying degrees of tubular obstruction contribute to the reduction in whole kidney GFR [37].

Amphotericin B

Amphotericin B is an amphoteric polyene antibiotic with a molecular weight of 960 that has predictable cumulative nephrotoxicity [38]. Necrosis of both proximal and distal tubular epithelial cells with calcium deposits has been noted in patients [39]. The drug binds avidly to cell membranes, leading to increased permeability to ions and small molecules that are changing electrical properties of transporting epithelia [40, 41]. The tubular cell lysosomal membrane may be a particular target [41]. Renal vasoconstriction may play an important adjunctive role in reducing oxygen supply [42] to cells, with an increased oxygen demand for transport due to enhanced cell sodium entry [43].

Cephalosporins

Cephalosporin antibiotics rarely are nephrotoxic in humans. Cephaloridine, which is no longer used clinically, was associated with acute renal failure when given in doses of more than 4 to 6 g/d [44]. However, studies on the mechanisms of nephrotoxicity have provided a conceptual framework on which to base further modifications of the molecule to achieve a higher therapeutic index. Cephalosporins are actively accumulated in the proximal tubular cells by the organic acid transport system [45]. Drug transport requires intact cell metabolism, and it is inhibited by probenecid [46]. The nephrotoxicity is believed to be secondary to high intracellular drug concentrations with congeners that do not diffuse well inside the cell into the tubular lumen [47]. Recent studies with cephaloglycin, which is nephrotoxic in rabbits, have suggested that the reactivity of the B-lactam ring itself is an important determinant of nephrotoxicity independent of cytochrome P-450 mixed-function oxidases [48]. Inhibitory effects of cephalosporins on mitochondrial respiration in vitro have been described, but the structural characteristic that renders some cephalosporins nephrotoxic is unknown [49, 50].

Cis-platinum

Cis-platin is an effective cancer chemotherapeutic agent that has as its major adverse effect a cumulative dose-related nephrotoxicity [51]. Patients develop both tubular dysfunction and reversible decreases in GFR. With high total doses, recovery of renal function is incomplete [51, 52]. The major site of cis-platin nephrotoxicity is the proximal tubule, where necrosis occurs primarily in the S_3 segment [52]. Cis-platin, like other heavy metals such as mercury, is known to react with sulfhydryl groups. Thus, it is likely that cis-platin nephrotoxicity is related to intracellular platinum binding to cortical sulfhydryl (SH) groups that are necessary for key cellular enzyme functions, particularly membrane transport [53, 54]. Levi et al demonstrated a marked fall in renal protein-bound SH groups in rats that was temporally related to renal accumulation of platinum, but prior to any fall in GFR [55]. Mitochondrial and cytosolic fractions showed the largest decreases in SH groups and the highest platinum concentrations. Histologic damage was maximal in the outer medulla, where platinum concentrations were highest [55]. Nonprotein-bound SH groups and tissue glutathione rose after cis-platin [55]. The drug had no reactivity in vitro with cysteine. Since the glycerol model of experimental acute renal failure does not reduce renal SH groups when corrected for an increase in kidney weight, it is suggestive that the cis-platin effect on these moieties is specific [54, 55]. In vitro active uptake of cis-platin by renal cortical slices has been demonstrated. This uptake could not be inhibited by ouabain or probenecid, but it could be reduced by the organic base, triethanolamine [56]. However, probenecid may modify nephrotoxicity in vivo [57]. Clearance studies in humans that show clearances of free platinum greater than inulin also suggest net tubular secretion [56].

Despite evidence of tubular injury, falls in GFR can be modified by hydration, solute diuresis, or mannitol diuresis [58]. Compounds that provide SH groups such as reduced glutathione, thiosulfate, and thiourea have been reported to reduce experimental cis-platin nephrotoxicity [58–62]. Heavy metal chelators have been variably effective as modifiers of toxicity [63]. Superoxide dismutase, presumably by preventing the formation of superoxide radicals, reduces cis-platin nephrotoxicity in rats [64]. Renal tubular magnesium wasting, which is a frequent consequence of cis-platin treatment, may be observed even in the absence of decreases in GFR [51]; sometimes, hypokalemia is observed [51]. Both abnormalities may be ameliorated by increasing magnesium reabsorption with amiloride [65]. Although these pharmacologic maneuvers provide possible clues to the cellular mechanisms of cis-platin-induced tubular damage, they are at best indirect. For example, reduced glutathione may inactivate peroxides and free radicals, as well as providing SH groups [53]. Further studies are indicated to better define the precise cause of cell injury.

Micropuncture studies in rats have demonstrated that backleak of glomerular filtrate plays a major role in the pathophysiology of cis-platin-induced acute renal failure. Superficial single-nephron GFR (SNGFR) was preserved relative to whole kidney GFR. However, SNGFR could not be returned to control values by volume expansion, implying a distinct effect of cis-platin on GFR [66]. Safirstein et al also had previously found a greater fall in whole kidney GFR than in superficial SNGFR, suggesting tubular backleak [67].

Acetaminophen and Toxic Drug Metabolites

The commonly used drug acetaminophen may cause direct proximal renal tubular necrosis in overdose situations, usually in association with the more widely appreciated centrilobular hepatic necrosis [68]. The pathophysiologic mechanisms of renal tubular necrosis are also thought to be similar to acetaminophen-induced hepatic necrosis [69, 70]. The drug is converted to a chemically active arylating metabolite by the cytochrone P-450-NADPH-dependent enzyme system. This metabolite covalently binds to cellular macromolecules. The binding and subsequent cell necrosis are correlated with a reduction of the protective glutathione, which is bound by the reactive metabolite N-acetyl imidoquinone [71]. Of interest is the enhanced ability of acetaminophen to deplete sulfhydryl groups and increase toxicity when animals are exposed to polybrominated biphenyls, which are environmental toxicants [72]. Para-aminophenol, which is a metabolite of phenacetin and acetaminophen, produces proximal tubular necrosis via oxidation by an NADPH-independent mechanism to a reactive metabolite without any papillary toxicity [73]. The role of renal metabolism in the activation of nephrotoxic agents is likely to take on more clinical importance as new knowledge of the kidneys' substantial role in these processes increases.

Chronic tubulointerstitial damage and renal failure may result from excessive use of analgesic compounds that usually contain mixtures of several ingredients. Phenacetin, which is rapidly metabolized by the liver to acetaminophen, has been implicated as the major offending agent in causing the initial renal lesion of renal papillary necrosis [74]. However, the site and type of this renal lesion is distinct from the proximal tubular necrosis described above. The combination of ingredients in the ingested drugs may have synergistic nephrotoxicity [75]. Major metabolites other than acetaminophen are polar compounds such as glucuronides or sulfates, which are excreted quantitatively in the urine. In addition to the small amount of lipid-soluble unchanged phenacetin, which has a urine-to-plasma concentration ratio of 1, acetaminophen has a higher ratio as it becomes concentrated in tubular fluid and cells [76]. Covalent binding of acetaminophen to renal tissue proteins is greater in the papilla than in the cortex, suggesting that there is an enzyme system responsible for generating reactive metabolites that are distinct from the NADPH-dependent cytochrome mixed-function oxidase system, which is virtually nonexistent in the papilla [77]. Acetaminophen is metabolically co-oxidized by peroxidases in the kidney papilla concurrently with prostaglandin intermediates by the hydroxyperoxidase activity of prostaglandin H synthase [76, 77]. Reduced glutathione activity is decreased in the papilla compared to the cortex; thus, it provides less protection from oxidant challenges.

Salicylate achieves a concentration in the renal papilla that is greater than plasma or renal cortex. The salicylate volume of distribution is greater than inulin, presumably due to cellular uptake. Salicylate interferes with the hexose monophosphate shunt production of NADPH, which further decreases the concentration of reduced glutathione in the papilla [75]. Aspirin may also reduce RBF by inhibition of arachidonic acid cyclo-oxygenases. Ischemia probably potentiates the cytotoxic effects of acetaminophen or phenacetin metabolites [78].

Cyclosporine

Cyclosporine is a new, exciting immunosuppressive drug that can prolong allograft survival without depressing the bone marrow. Its major adverse effect is dose-related nephrotoxicity. Cyclosporine is a lipophilic drug with a molecular weight of 1202 daltons. It is highly metabolized in the liver. Its renal excretion is low, and its handling by the kidney is presently unstudied.

Although clinical aspects of cyclosporine nephrotoxicity have recently been summarized, the mechanism of toxicity is poorly understood [79]. There is no suitable animal model in which cyclosporine administration reliably produces renal failure. With large oral doses in the rat, enzymuria, mild renal dysfunction, and proximal tubular vacuolization have been described [80]. Increased numbers of lysosomes and cytosegresomes with rare cell necrosis suggest a direct toxic effect of the drug; however, studies in other species, including humans, have shown a paucity of morphologic changes. In some experimental and clinical studies, vascular changes that are prominent in small blood vessels represent a major target for the drug's nephrotoxic action [81]. Cyclosporine has little effect in vitro or in vivo on rat renal cortical or hepatic mitochondria [82]. It is possible that some aspect of hepatic drug metabolism of cyclosporine is important in subsequent nephrotoxicity, since inducers of hepatic mixed-function oxidase drug-metabolizing enzymes may reduce renal dysfunction [83]. Chronic nephrotoxicity due to prolonged cyclosporine immunosuppression may produce tubulointerstitial fibrosis [5]. The clinical significance of this effect on long-term allograft survival awaits further experience.

Summary

Drugs causing nephrotoxicity are an increasing cause of morbidity in clinical medicine. This overview summarizes some cellular mechanisms of renal toxicity by using specific drugs as examples. Aminoglycosides, amphotericin B, and cephalosporins are the antibiotics reviewed. The renal effects of cis-platinum and cyclosporine are also covered. Acetaminophen is used to illustrate the important subject of metabolic activation of xenobiotics. The role of the kidney in drug metabolism is being widely recognized. Both cortical and medullary enzyme systems may produce reactive metabolites that can bind covalently to cell macromolecules. This produces necrosis when there is depletion of the intracellular sulfhydryl groups that protect against oxidant stress.

Acknowledgments. These studies were supported, in part, by grants from Nephrology Research Associates and the Blaine Bramble Foundation.

References

1. WEDEEN RP: Occupational renal disease. *Am J Kidney Dis* 3:241–252, 1984
2. WARD JM, FAURIE KA: The nephrotoxic effects of cis-diammine-dichloro platinum (11) (NSC-119875) in male F344 rats. *Toxicol Appl Pharmacol* 38:535–547, 1976
3. ABRAMOWSKY CR, SWINEHART GL: The nephropathy of cystic fibrosis: A human model of chronic nephrotoxicity. *Human Pathol* 13:934–939, 1982

4. GILBERT DN, HOUGHTON DC, BENNETT WM, PLAMP CE, PEGER K, PORTER GA: Reversibility of gentamicin nephrotoxicity in rats: Recovery during continued drug administration. *Proc Soc Exp Biol Med* 160:99–103, 1979

5. MORAN M, NEWTON L, PERLROTH M, MYERS B: Cyclosporin nephrotoxicity in man (*abstract*). *Kidney Int* 25:346, 1984

6. DENTINO M, LUFT FC, YUM MN, WILLIAM SD, EINHORN LH: Long-term effect of cis-diamminedichloride platinum (CDDP) on renal function and structure in man. *Cancer* 41:1274–1281, 1978

7. ELLIOTT WC, HOUGHTON DC, GILBERT DN, DeFEHR J, BENNETT WM: Gentamicin nephrotoxicity. I. Degree and permanence of acquired insensitivity. *J Lab Clin Med* 100:501–512, 1982

8. HOUGHTON DC, GILBERT DN, BENNETT WM: Resistance to experimental gentamicin nephrotoxicity: A state of asynchronous acute tubular necrosis. *Proc Interscience Conf on Antimicrob Agents Chemother* 23:191, 1984

9. FILLASTRE JP, MERY JP, DRUET P: Drug-induced glomerulonephritis, in *Acute Renal Failure Correlations Between Morphology and Function,* edited by SOLEZ K, WHELTON A, New York, Marcel Dekker, Inc, 1984, pp 389–407

10. CLIVE DM, STOFF JS: Renal syndromes associated with non-steroidal anti-inflammatory drugs. *N Engl J Med* 310:563–572, 1984

11. BLYTHE W: Captopril and renal autoregulation. *N Engl J Med* 308:390, 1983

12. BENNETT WM: Aminoglycoside nephrotoxicity. *Nephron* 35:73–77, 1983

13. HUMES HD, WEINBERG JM, KNAUSS TC: Clinical and pathophysiologic aspects of aminoglycoside nephrotoxicity. *Am J Kidney Dis* 2:1–29, 1982

14. GYSELYNCK AM, FORREY A, CUTLER R: Pharmacokinetics of gentamicin: Distribution, plasma and renal clearance. *J Infect Dis* 124:570–576, 1971

15. PASTORIZA-MUNOZ E, BOWMAN RL, KALOYANIDES GJ: Renal tubular transport of gentamicin in the rat. Kidney Int 16:440–450, 1979

16. SENEKJIAN HO, KNIGHT TF, WEINMAN EJ: Micropuncture study of the renal handling of gentamicin in the rat. Kidney Int 19:416–423, 1981

17. SASTRASINH M, KNAUSS TC, WEINBERG JM, HUMES HD: Identification of the aminoglycoside binding site of renal brush border membranes. *J Pharmacol Exp Ther* 222:350–359, 1982

18. SILVERBLATT FJ, KUEHN C: Autoradiography of gentamicin uptake by the rat proximal tubule cell. *Kidney Int* 15:335–345, 1979

19. FELDMAN S, WANG MY, KALOYANIDES GJ: Aminoglycosides induce a phospholipidosis in the renal cortex of the rat: An early manifestation of nephrotoxicity. *J Pharmacol Exp Ther* 220:514–520, 1982

20. POWELL JH, REIDENBERG MM: In vitro response of rat and human kidney lysosomes to aminoglycosides. *Biochem Pharmacol* 31:3447–3453, 1982

21. POWELL JH, REIDENBERG MM: Further studies of the response of kidney lysosomes to aminoglycosides and other cations. *Biochem Pharmacol* 32:3213–3220, 1983

22. COJOCEL C, SMITH JH, MAITA K, SLEIGHT SD, HOOK JB: Renal protein degradation: A biochemical target of specific nephrotoxicants. *Fund Appl Toxicol* 3:278–284, 1983

23. SIMMONS C, BOGUSKY R, HUMES HD: Inhibitory effects of gentamicin on renal cortical mitochondrial oxidative phosphorylation. *J Pharmacol Exp Ther* 214:709–715, 1980

24. WEINBERG J, HARDING P, HUMES HD: Mechanism of gentamicin-induced dysfunction of renal cortical mitochondria. II. Effects of mitochondrial monovalent cation transport. *Arch Biochem Biophys* 205:232–239, 1980

25. HUMES HD, WEINBERG JM: Alterations of renal tubular cell metabolism in acute renal failure. *Min Electrolyte Metab* 9:290–305, 1983
26. SASTRASINH M, WEINBERG JM, HUMES HD: Effect of gentamicin on calcium uptake by renal mitochondria. *Life Sci* 30:2309–2315, 1982
27. HUMES HD, SASTRASINH M, WEINBERG JM: Calcium is a competitive inhibitor of gentamicin-renal membrane binding interactions and dietery calcium supplementation protects against gentamicin nephrotoxicity. *J Clin Invest* 73:134–137, 1984
28. QUARUM ML, HOUGHTON DC, GILBERT DN, MCCARRON DA, BENNETT WM: Increasing dietary calcium moderates experimental gentamicin nephrotoxicity. *J Lab Clin Med* 103:104–114, 1984
29. WILLIAMS PD, HOLOHAN PD, ROSS CR: Gentamicin nephrotoxicity. I. Acute biochemical correlates in the rat. *Toxicol Appl Pharmacol* 61:234–242, 1981
30. CRONIN R, NIX K, FERGUSON E, SOUTHERN PM, HENRICH WL: Renal cortex ion composition and Na-K-ATPase activity in early gentamicin nephrotoxicity. *Am J Physiol* 242:F477–F483, 1982
31. QUEENER SF, LUFT FC, HAMEL FG: Effect of gentamicin treatment on adenylate cyclase and Na$^+$, K$^+$-ATPase activities in renal tissues of rats. *Antimicrob Agents Chemother* 24:815–818, 1983
32. CRONIN RE, BULGER RE, SOUTHERN P, HENRICH WL: Natural history of aminoglycoside nephrotoxicity in the dog. *J Lab Clin Med* 95:463–474, 1980
33. BENNETT WM, MCDOUGALL J, POTOCNIK S, WRIGHT RD, WHITWORTH JA: Renal handling and acute urinary electrolyte effects of aminoglycoside antibiotics: Use of a solitary renal autotransplant in the conscious sheep. *Life Sci* 32:205–212, 1983
34. FINTON CK, BJORKLAND S, ZALOGA GP, UDDIN DE, CHERNOW B: Gentamicin-induced hypomagnesemia. *Am Surg* 49:576–578, 1983
35. BAYLIS C, RENNKE HR, BRENNER BM: Mechanisms of the defect in glomerular ultrafiltration associated with gentamicin administration. *Kidney Int* 12:344–353, 1977
36. KLOTMAN PE, YARGER WE: Reduction of renal blood flow and proximal bicarbonate reabsorption in rats by gentamicin. *Kidney Int* 24:638–643, 1983
37. NEUGARTEN J, AYNEDJIAN HS, BANK N: Role of tubular obstruction in acute renal failure due to gentamicin. *Kidney Int* 24:330–335, 1983
38. BUTLER WT, HILL GJ, SZWED CF, KNIGHT V: Amphotericin B renal toxicity in the dog. *J Pharmacol Exp Ther* 143:47–56, 1964
39. BUTLER WT, BENNETT JE, ALLING DW, WESTLAKE PT, UTZ JP, HILL GJ: Nephrotoxicity of amphotericin B: Early and late effects in 81 patients. *Ann Int Med* 61:175–187, 1964
40. ANDREOLI TE: On the anatomy of amphotericin B-cholesterol pores in lipid bilayer membranes. *Kidney Int* 4:337–345, 1973
41. WEISSMANN G, PRAS M, HIRSCHHORN R: A common mechanism for the fungicidal and nephrotoxic effects of amphotericin B (*abstract*). *J Clin Invest* 45:1084, 1966
42. BHATHENA DB, BULLOCK WE, NUTTALL CE, LUKE RG: The effects of amphotericin B therapy on the intrarenal vasculature and renal tubules in man. *Clin Nephrol* 9:103–110, 1978
43. SPOKES K, BREZIS M, SILVA P, EPSTEIN FH, ROSEN S: Transport dependent cell injury: A mechanism for amphotericin nephrotoxicity (*abstract*). *Proc Am Soc Nephrol* 1983, p 101A
44. CHILD KJ, DODDS MG: Nephron transport and renal tubular effects on cephaloridine in animals. *Br J Pharmacol Chemother* 30:354–370, 1967

45. Tune BM, Fernholt M, Schwartz A: Mechanism of cephaloridine transport in the kidney. *J Pharmacol Exp Ther* 191:311–317, 1974
46. Tune BM: Effect of organic acid transport inhibitors on renal cortical uptake and proximal tubular toxicity of cephaloridine. *J Pharmacol Exp Ther* 181:250–256, 1972
47. Tune BM: Relationship between the transport and toxicity of cephalosporins in the kidney. *J Infect Dis* 132:189–194, 1975
48. Browning MC, Tune BM: Reactivity and binding of b-lactam antibiotics in rabbit renal cortex. *J Pharmacol Exp Ther* 226:640–644, 1983
49. Tune BM, Fravert D: Mechanisms of cephalosporin nephrotoxicity: A comparison of cephaloridine and cephaloglycin. *Kidney Int* 18:591–600, 1980
50. Tune BM, Wu KY, Fravert D, Holtzman D: Effect of cephaloridine on respiration by renal cortical mitochondria. *J Pharmacol Exp Ther* 210:98–100, 1979
51. Blachley JD, Hill JB: Renal and electrolyte disturbances associated with cisplatin. *Ann Intern Med* 95:628–632, 1981
52. Gonzalez-Vitale JC, Hayes DM, Cvitkovic E, Sternberg SS: The renal pathology in clinical trials of cis-platinum (11) diamminedichloride. *Cancer* 39:1362–1371, 1977
53. Leyland-Jones B, Morrow C, Tate S, Urmacher C, Gordon C, Young CW: Cis-diamminedichlore platinum (11) nephrotoxicity and its relationship to renal q-glutamyltranspeptidase and glutathione. *Cancer Res* 43:6072–6076, 1983
54. Weiner MW, Jacobs C: Mechanism of cisplatin nephrotoxicity. *Fed Proc* 42:2974–2978, 1983
55. Levi J, Jacobs C, Kalman S, McTigue M, Weiner M: Mechanism of cisplatinum nephrotoxicity. I. Effects of sulfhydryl groups in rat kidney. *J Pharmacol Exp Ther* 213:545–550, 1980
56. Jacobs C, Kalman SM, Tretton M, Weiner M: Renal handling of cis-diamminedichlore platinum (II). *Cancer Treat Rep* 64:1223–1226, 1980
57. Ross DA, Gayle GR: Reduction of the renal toxicity of cis-dichlorodiammine platinum (II) by probenecid. *Cancer Treat Rep* 63:781–787, 1979
58. Ozols RF, Corden BJ, Jacob J, Wesley MN, Ostchega Y, Young RC: High-dose cisplatin in hypertonic saline. *Ann Intern Med* 100:19–24, 1984
59. Zunino F, Tofanetti O, Besati A, Cavalletti E, Savi G: Protective effect of reduced glutathione against cis-dichlorodiammine platinum (II)-induced nephrotoxicity and lethal toxicity. *Tumori* 69:105–111, 1983
60. Borch R, Pleasants ME: Inhibition of cis-platinum nephrotoxicity by diethyldithiocarbamate rescue in a rat model. *Proc Natl Acad Sci USA* 76:6611–6614, 1979
61. Elliott WC, Newcom SR, Houghton DC, Baines-Hunter J, Bennett WM: Cis-diamminedichloroplatinum (II) nephrotoxicity: Tubular function after rescue with sodium diethyldithiocarbamate in rats. *Cancer Res* 43:3759–3762, 1983
62. Howell SB, Taetle R: Effect of sodium thiosulfate on cis-dichloroammine platinum (II) toxicity and anti-tumor activity in L-1210 leukemia. *Cancer Treat Rep* 64:611–616, 1980
63. Graziano J: The effect of heavy metal chelators on the renal accumulation of platinum after cis-diammine-platinum II administration to the rat. *Br J Pharmacol* 73:649–654, 1981
64. McGinness JE, Proctor PH, Demopoulos HB, Hokanson JA, Kirkpatrick DS: Amelioration of cis-platinum nephrotoxicity by orgotein (superoxide dismutase). *Physiol Chem Phys* 10:267–277, 1978

65. JUREIDINI KF, HOGG RJ, RICE MS, TOOGOOD IRG, BARRATT L: Prevention of cis-platinum nephrotoxicity with amiloride (*abstract*). *Proc Asian Pacific Soc Nephrology* 2:41, 1983

66. CHOPRA S, KAUFMAN JS, JONES TW, HONG WK, GEHR MK, HAMBURGER RJ, FLAMENBAUM W, TRUMP BJ: Cis-diamminedichloroplatinum-induced acute renal failure in the rat. *Kidney Int* 21:54–162, 1982

67. SAFIRSTEIN R, MILTER P, DIKMAN S, LYMAN N, SHAPIRO C: Cisplatin nephrotoxicity in rats: Defect in papillary hypertonicity. *Am J Physiol* 241:175–185, 1981

68. NEWTON JF, BAILIE MB, HOOK JB: Acetaminophen nephrotoxicity in the rat. Renal metabolic activation *in vitro*. *Toxicol Appl Pharmacol* 70:433–444, 1983

69. MCMURTY RJ, SNODGRASS WR, MITCHELL JR: Renal necrosis, glutathione depletion and covalent binding after acetaminophen. *Toxicol Appl Pharmacol* 46:87–100, 1978

70. HINSON JA, POHL LR, MONKS TJ, GILLETTE JR: Acetaminophen-induced hepatotoxicity—Mini review. *Life Sci* 29:107–116, 1981

71. MUDGE GH: Analgesic nephropathy renal drug distribution and metabolism, in *Nephrotoxic Mechanisms of Drugs and Environmental Toxins,* edited by PORTER GA, New York, Plenum Press, 1982, pp 209–225

72. HOOK JB, SERBIA VC: Potentiation of the action of nephrotoxic agents by environmental contaminants, in *Nephrotoxic Mechanisms of Drugs and Environmental Toxins,* edited by PORTER GA, New York, Plenum Press, 1982, pp 345–356

73. DAVIS JM, EMSLIC KR, SWECT RS, WALKER LL, NAUGHTON RJ, SKINNER SL, TANGE JD: Early functional and morphological changes in renal tubular necrosis due to p-aminophenol. *Kidney Int* 24:740–747, 1983

74. SHELLEY JH: Pharmacological mechanisms of analgesic nephropathy. *Kidney Int* 13:15–26, 1978

75. BLEUMLE LW, GOLDBERG M: Renal accumulation of salicylate and phenacetin: Possible mechanisms in the nephropathy of analgesic abuse. *J Clin Invest* 49:2507–2514, 1968

76. MOHANDAS J, DUGGAN GG, HORVATH JS, TILLER DJ: Regional differences in peroxidatic activation of paracetamol (acetaminophen) mediated by cytochrome P-450 and prostaglandin endoperoxide synthetase in rabbit kidney. *Res Commun Chem Path Pharmacol* 34:69–80, 1981

77. ZENSER TV, COHEN SM, MATTAMMAL MB, DAVIS B: Prostaglandin H synthase: An enzymatic mechanism of renal urinary tract carcinogenesis and chemical nephrotoxicity (*abstract*). *Kidney Int* 25:338, 1984

78. MITTMAN N, SCHLONDORFF D: Inhibition of medullary prostaglandin synthesis may contribute to analgesic nephropathy (*abstract*). *Kidney Int* 25:240, 1984

79. BENNETT WM, PULLIAM JP: Cyclosporine nephrotoxicity. *Ann Intern Med* 99:851–854, 1983

80. WHITING PH, THOMSON AW, BLAIR JT, SIMPSON JG: Experimental cyclosporin A nephrotoxicity. *Br J Exp Pathol* 63:88–94, 1982

81. SHULMAN H, STRIKER G, DEEG HJ, KENNEDY M, STORB R, THOMAS ED: Nephrotoxicity of cyclosporin A after allogeneic marrow transplantation: Glomerular thromboses and tubular injury. *N Engl J Med* 301:1392–1395, 1981

82. KIRWAN PD, BAXTER CR, DUGGIN G: Giant mitochondria, renal transplant biopsy and cyclosporin A. *Lancet* 2:146–147, 1981

83. CUNNINGHAM C, BURKE MD, WHITING PH, SIMPSON JG, WHEATLEY DN: Ketaconazole, cyclosporin and the kidney. *Lancet* 2:1464, 1982

Nephrotoxicity of Nonsteroidal Anti-Inflammatory Drugs

William L. Henrich

Nonsteroidal anti-inflammatory drugs (NSAIDs) have been established as valuable therapeutic agents in modern clinical practice. These drugs have become increasingly popular because of their proven effectiveness in a broad range of common clinical disorders, such as arthritis, overuse injuries such as tendonitis, orthopedic injuries, and dysmenorrhea. Coupled with this increase in use has been a growing recognition that these drugs are capable of causing an acute reduction in renal function. In fact, NSAID-related acute renal failure is now reported to rank behind aminoglycoside antibiotics as a cause of nephrotoxic acute renal failure.

Several of the important clinical effects that these agents may induce in patients depend on their capacity for inhibiting renal prostaglandin synthesis. Renal prostaglandin synthesis and metabolism is reviewed elsewhere in this volume. This review concentrates on the physiologic consequences of prostaglandin inhibition for the kidney and the clinical syndromes of nephrotoxicity.

Physiologic Effects of Prostaglandins: Studies Based on Prostaglandin Inhibition

It should be noted that renal prostaglandin synthesis is dramatically enhanced by a number of biochemical and physical stimuli; it is believed that these stimuli share the effect of increasing phospholipase A_2 activity, which leads to a release of arachidonic acid. The increased availability of arachidonic acid leads to the further synthesis of prostaglandins and thromboxanes within seconds to minutes. Several of the most important stimuli of endogenous prostaglandin synthesis and release are provided in Table 1. The physical

This manuscript was presented as part of a Symposium on *Nephrotoxicity and Drugs.*

Table 1. Stimuli of prostaglandin synthesis
in the kidney

Physical factors	Circulating factors
Renal ischemia	Angiotensin
Renal nerve stimulation	Bradykinin
Ureteral obstruction	Catecholamines
	Vasopression

factors listed in this table may induce prostaglandin synthesis and release
via angiotensin or their circulating mediators [1–11].

Table 2 provides a partial list of the available NSAIDs that have been
used experimentally and clinically to inhibit the cyclo-oxygenase step of the
prostaglandin synthesis cascade. Acetylsalicylic acid acetylates the cyclo-oxygenase enzyme and irreversibly inhibits its action; new enzyme must be
synthesized to overcome this effect—a process that may take days in the
kidney [12, 13]. The other NSAIDs listed in Table 2 reversibly inhibit cyclo-
oxygenase and have effects that depend on the individual drug half-life and
binding properties. The rationale underlying the use of NSAIDs to probe
physiologic prostaglandin actions assumes that inhibition of prostaglandin
synthesis blocks their basal physiologic effects. It is important that prostaglandin concentration is measured in these studies, since different stimuli to prostaglandin synthesis may be sufficient to overcome the effects of cyclo-oxygenase
inhibition. It is also worthwhile to note that in most prostaglandin inhibition
studies, prostaglandin levels are still detectable; therefore, conclusions regarding prostaglandin-independent effects may be overstated. Finally, NSAIDs
have enzymatic effects other than cyclo-oxygenase inhibition that may interfere with precise interpretation. Notable among these effects is phosphodiesterase inhibition—an effect that leads to an increase in cyclic AMP accumulation
[14]. This effect is particularly troublesome in studies of prostaglandins and
renin release, since cyclic AMP may induce renin release [15]. Despite these
caveats, the use of cyclo-oxygenase inhibitors has been helpful in delineating
the roles of prostaglandins in normal renal physiology, as discussed below.

Effects of NSAIDs on Renal Blood Flow, Glomerular Filtration Rate, and Acute Renal Failure

In euvolemic patients with normal basal function, prostaglandin synthesis
inhibition with NSAIDs induces little or no change in renal function [16,
17]. However, volume depletion unmasks a potentially important physiologic
role for prostaglandins in preserving renal function under hypovolemic conditions. In one recent study of 10 healthy subjects by Muther and Bennett
[18], sodium restriction alone had no effects on renal function, but it was
associated with an increase in plasma renin activity and urinary prostaglandin
E excretion. The administration of aspirin during sodium restriction decreased
urinary prostaglandin E excretion and decreased both creatinine and inulin

Table 2. Families of nonsteroidal anti-inflammatory drugs

Carboxylic acids	Enolic acids
Salicyclic acids and esters	Pryazolones
Aspirin	Oxypenbutazone
Diflunisal	Phenylbutazone
Benorylate	Apazone
Acetic acid	Feprazone
Phenylacetic acids	Prioxicam
Diclofenac	Sudoxicam
Alclofenac	Isoxicam
Fenclofenac	CP-14,304
Carbocyclic and heterocyclic acetic acids	
Indomethacin	
Sulindac	
Tolmetin	
Zomepirac	
Proprionic acids	
Ibuprofen	
Naproxen	
Flurbiprofen	
Fenbufen	
Benoxaprofen	
Fenoprofen	
Indoprofen	
Ketoprofen	
Pirprofen	
Fenamic acids	
Flufenamic	
Mefenamic	
Meclofenamic	
Niflumic	

clearances; para-aminohippuric acid (PAH) clearance was unaffected. Thus, the addition of cyclo-oxygenase inhibitors under conditions producing higher angiotensin levels and volume depletion uncovered a role for prostaglandins in maintenance of renal functional integrity. Of interest is a recent preliminary communication [19] implying that patients taking NSAIDs chronically may develop mild renal insufficiency in the absence of overt volume depletion. This observation is deserving of further study.

A number of in vivo studies have enhanced our understanding of the interplay of factors that modify renal hemodynamics. Renal prostaglandins (notably PGE_2 and PGI_2) are acknowledged to be potent renal vasodilators [20–23]. When infused directly into the kidney, renal blood flow (RBF) promptly increases and renal vascular resistance declines. If a renal vasoconstrictive stimulus is applied to the kidney (for example, norepinephrine infusion, angiotensin II infusion, or exogenous renal nerve stimulation), the synthesis and release of prostaglandins sharply increase. This increase in prostaglandin release counterbalances the vasoconstrictive stimulus, resulting in preservation of RBF. If the vasoconstrictive stimulus is reapplied after prostaglandin synthesis inhibition, the result is unopposed vasoconstriction and a sharp decrease in RBF. Similar conditions apply to clinical situations in which angiotensin II levels are increased, including acute reductions of cardiac output [24], hemorrhage [10], endotoxemia [25], and cirrhosis [26].

Several studies suggest a tonic vasodilatory role for prostaglandins. Zia et al have correlated plasma renin activity and 24-hr urinary prostaglandin E excretion in cirrhotic patients with ascites [27]. The administration of indomethacin to cirrhotic patients with ascites effected sharp decrements in the glomerular filtration rate (GFR) and effective renal plasma flow (Fig. 1) [28, 29]. Boyer et al have demonstrated that a fall in creatinine clearance (C_{cr}) and renal plasma flow (RPF) caused by indomethacin that is seen in cirrhotic patients was reversed by an infusion of exogenous prostaglandins [29]. Similarly, indomethacin treatment has resulted in a documented decline in urinary prostaglandin excretion concomitant with a reversible decrease in renal function in congestive heart failure [30] and nephrotic syndrome [31]. Thus, under conditions in which prostaglandin synthesis would be expected to increase (that is, volume depletion or high angiotensin II states), prostaglandins may be demonstrated to play an important role in maintenance of RBF and GFR. Under euvolemic, normoreninemic circumstances, no adverse renal effect of NSAIDs are usually demonstrable.

A role for thromboxane has been postulated in the renal vasoconstrictive state that accompanies urinary tract obstruction [32, 33]. In one recent study, imidazole (an inhibitor of thromboxane synthesis), but not indomethacin, clearly improved inulin and PAH clearance in canine kidneys obstructed for 24 hr [34]. This model of urinary tract obstruction provides the most convincing evidence of a role for thromboxane in control of renal hemodynam-

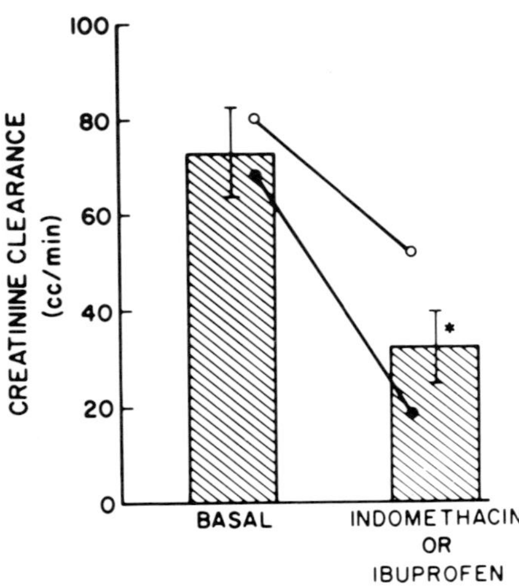

Fig. 1. Influence of indomethacin on GFR in cirrhotic patients. (○, Urine Na < 10 mEq/d; ●, Na < 1 mEq/d; $P < 0.001$; $N = 12$). From [28]

ics. One hypothesis, which has received experimental support, is that bradykinin and angiotensin cause the hydronephrotic kidney to produce thromboxane A_2—a metabolite of arachidonic acid that normally is not synthesized by rabbit kidney [35]. Local production of thromboxane A_2 may cause vasoconstriction that is reversible with a thromboxane synthesis inhibitor [35].

Renal prostaglandins may also influence the development of acute renal failure through their effects on RBF. Mauk et al [36] could not demonstrate a protective effect of prostaglandin E administration on kidney function in a model of renal failure induced by the nephrotoxin, uranyl nitrate. By contrast, the administration of prostaglandin E prior to intra-arterial norepinephrine was associated with significantly greater preservation of GFR. Patak et al [37] suggested this protective effect derived from the increase in osmolar excretion secondary to PGE_2 infusion. Prostaglandin E_2 infusions have been noted to protect against the acute renal failure seen in other experimental models of acute renal failure, such as glycerol [38]. Conversely, the inhibition of prostaglandin synthesis may enhance the incidence and severity of glycerol and gentamicin-induced acute renal failure [39].

Prostaglandins and NSAIDs: Effects on Renin Release

In the past decade, considerable experimental evidence demonstrated that prostaglandins are involved in several pathways to renin release. The infusion of arachidonic acid of PGI_2 into the renal artery results in a marked increase in renin secretion [40, 41]. Of the major known pathways to renin release, prostaglandins have been most convincingly shown to be of critical importance in the renal baroreceptor pathway [42], macula densa pathway [43], and renal nerve pathway [44] to renin release. Controversy surrounds the role of prostaglandins in influencing sympathetic nervous system input to renin release. On the one hand, studies by Campbell et al [15], Suzuki et al [45], Feurstein and Feurstein [46], and Romero et al [47] suggest that this pathway is prostaglandin-dependent. Conversely, a body of other studies suggests that this modulator of renin release is prostaglandin-independent [48–52]. A recent preliminary report performed in vitro to obviate the systemic effect of circulating beta agonists suggests that beta-sympathetic effects on renin release are prostaglandin-independent [53]. Whether prostaglandins and other agonists for renin secretion stimulate renin release via the same cyclic AMP-dependent mechanism as sympathetic agonists is presently unknown. The clinical relevance of the prostaglandin-renin release relationship is supported by the observation of decreased urinary prostaglandin excretion in patients with hyporeninemic hypoaldosteronism [54]. Similarly, sporadic reports of hyperkalemia following indomethacin treatment have appeared [55]. This is most likely a highly unusual complication of indomethacin and other NSAIDs—given the infrequency of these reports.

Effects of Prostaglandins and NSAIDs on Renal Sodium Excretion

The effects of prostaglandins on renal sodium handling have been the subject of intense investigation and controversy. The hemodynamic effects of prostaglandins have significant influence on medullary tonicity, which is a major determinant of sodium reabsorption. The least ambiguous studies suggesting a direct tubular prostaglandin effect are studies showing that PGE_2 further increases sodium excretion (in the presence of acetylcholine) without changing RBF [56]. The administration of a prostaglandin synthesis inhibitor often induces sodium retention, even if GFR remains stable [57]. Clearance studies in humans have suggested that the medullary segment of the thick ascendig limb and the distal diluting segments of the nephron are likely to be involved [58, 59]. Isolated, perfused tubule experiments have demonstrated that prostaglandins inhibit chloride reabsorption in medullary thick ascending limbs [60]. Furthermore, prostaglandins also appear to inhibit sodium reabsorption in cortical collecting tubules [61] and medullary collecting ducts [62]. The NSAIDs also induce an antinatriuretic effect by virtue of an aldosterone-like action in the distal nephron [63]. Thus, the most frequent effect of NSAIDs on sodium handling is a mild antinatriuresis, which may be transient. More significant antinatriuretic effects would be expected under circumstances in which RBF and GFR were severely reduced. Finally, NSAIDs may blunt the natriuretic and diuretic effects of potent diuretics such as furosemide [64]. This effect probably occurs because of inhibition of renal vasodilatation [65].

Effects of Prostaglandins and NSAIDs on Renal Water Excretion

Prostaglandins oppose the hydro-osmotic effects of arginine vasopressin (AVP) in the kidney both in vitro [66, 67] and in vivo; in addition, vasopressin is known to stimulate prostaglandin synthesis in water-transporting epithelia [68]. Thus, inhibition of endogenous prostaglandin synthesis should enhance the action of arginine vasopressin at the tubular level, thereby promoting a more profound antidiuresis at any given level of AVP. Such an effect of NSAIDs has been documented in vivo under different experimental conditions [69–71]. Prostaglandins of the E series, particularly PGE_2, are most active in antagonizing the hydro-osmotic action of AVP.

Clinical Syndromes Associated with the Use of NSAIDs

Table 3 provides a list of the reported clinical syndromes that may follow the use of NSAID agents. The recognition of adverse renal effects of these drugs has grown remarkably in recent years, reflecting the enormous popula-

Table 3. Clinical syndromes of nephrotoxicity with NSAIDs

Renal insufficiency: Prostaglandin synthesis inhibition results in enhanced renal vasoconstriction, often in the context of diminished basal RBF (congestive heart failure, volume depletion, cirrhosis, nephrotic syndrome, shock states, pre-existent renal disease, or advanced age).

Tubulointerstitial nephritis: Direct nephrotoxicity, often associated with severe proteinuria despite the presence of only foot process fusion in glomeruli.

Hyperkalemia: Prostaglandin synthesis inhibition causes suppression of renin release, leading to hyporeninemic hypoaldosteronism with resultant hyperkalemia.

Sodium and water retention; diuretic resistance: Due to aldosterone-like effect of NSAIDs, as well as antinatriuretic effect of prostaglandin synthesis inhibition; water retention partly secondary to prostaglandin synthesis inhibition and increased effect of arginine vasopressin. Diuretic resistance may be partly a vascular effect.

Anaphylaxis: Often after a second exposure or in aspirin-sensitive patients; anaphylactoid reaction.

tion of patients receiving these drugs and the proliferation of drugs on the market. The following discussion focuses on each of the adverse clinical events described with these drugs.

Renal Insufficiency

This type of adverse effect of NSAIDs is by far the one most commonly reported. In addition, it is the type of nephrotoxicity for which a discrete population of patients at risk has been identified. The greatest number of reported cases of renal insufficiency has occurred with indomethacin use, which probably is partly related to the length of time that the drug has been available for use compared to newer preparations. Several of the most frequent features of indomethacin-induced acute renal failure are listed in Table 4. Several of the most convincing reports have documented depressed urinary prostaglandin levels when renal function deteriorates [16, 30]. However, numerous other persuasive anecdotes exist [72–78]. As shown in Table

Table 4. Clinical features of indomethacin-induced renal failure

Dosage often > 100 mg/day
Oliguria typical
Predisposing factors
    Advanced age
    Volume depletion, shock, and sepsis
    Concomitant diuretic therapy
    Congestive heart failure
    Cirrhosis
    Underlying renal disease
    Postoperative patients with "third space" fluid sequestration
    Any "high-renin" condition
Usually reversible with discontinuation of the drug

4, the population of patients at greatest risk for developing renal failure from indomethacin therapy share several predisposing factors. The greatest risk appears to accompany high-renin states and/or previously impaired renal function. As noted previously, this association is expected in light of the experimental work providing evidence that renal prostaglandins are important protective factors during renal ischemic stress.

The reversible acute renal failure syndrome has been associated with other drugs in the carbo-hetero-cyclic acetic acid class (for example, zomepirac), as well as with drugs in other chemical derivative classes of NSAIDs. For example, zomepirac [77], propionic acid derivatives (such as ibuprofen [79–81] and fenoprofen [82]), and the fenamic acid derivative, meclofenamic acid, all have been associated with acute renal failure syndromes. It is also of interest that salicylic acid (aspirin) and the enolic acid derivative, phenylbutazone, are capable of inducing renal ischemic lesions—particularly in patients with pre-existent renal disease [83–90]. Of current particular interest are recent reports suggesting that sulindac may not induce the renal insufficiency caused by other NSAIDs [91, 92]. The mechanism of this alleged protection is that sulindac sulfide (the active form of the drug) may not inhibit renal prostaglandin synthesis in usual therapeutic doses [92]. However, other recent preliminary communications have questioned this "renal-sparing" effect of sulindac [93, 94]. Clearly, cautious use of sulindac is still warranted until further, more definitive information is available.

Interstitial Nephritis

This type of nephrotoxicity is less common than the usual reversible form of acute renal failure described above. It frequently has a more dramatic onset and is less insidious than the reversible acute renal failure. Eight different NSAIDs have been associated with this reversible clinical syndrome of heavy proteinuria and renal insufficiency [95]. To date, fenoprofen has accounted for 61% of all reported cases. The exact incidence of this syndrome is unknown. Clinical features of this disorder are provided in Table 5. The glomeruli are relatively normal in biopsy specimens in the majority of these cases, despire the heavy proteinuria. Tubules may show mild focal atrophy and dilitation. The interstitium contains edema and minimal focal fibrosis with either a diffuse or focal mononuclear cell infiltrate. An eosinophilic infiltrate

Table 5. Interstitial nephritis associated with NSAIDs; Clinical features

Heavy proteinuria
Tubulointerstitial nephritis on biopsy; glomeruli often have only minimal changes (foot process fusion)
Nonoliguric course common
Flank pain, hematuria, and eosinophilia in some cases
Rapid decline in renal function; steroids have aided resolution in some cases
Variable time to development

has been noted in 30% of all biopsy specimens. Immunofluorescence microscopy is typically normal, although occasional nonspecific immunofluorescent staining of glomeruli and tubules has been noted. Electron microscopy of the glomeruli usually reveals diffuse epithelial foot process fusion. Mesangial electron-dense deposits usually are absent. The value of corticosteroids in the resolution of renal failure and proteinuria is unknown; however, most severe cases have been treated with steroids. Exposure to these drugs has been over a variable length of time in most cases (a mean of 5.7 months in one study [95]); flank pain has been a notable feature in several cases. While the pathogenesis of the lesion is not known, Torres has recently postulated that prostaglandin inhibition may lead to a cycle of immunologic events that culminate in enhanced lymphokine production, thereby allowing a delayed hypersensitivity reaction to proceed unchecked [96]. Alternatively, a direct glomerular or tubular toxicity may be operating in some cases. Also intriguing as a possible cause of the syndrome is the notion that by inhibiting cyclo-oxygenase, arachidonic acid products are stimulated via the lipo-oxygenase pathways to polyenoic acids, including leukotrienes. Thus, the production of a number of synthetic products with known vascular effects actually may be increased by some NSAIDs, at least locally. Finally, the possibility that a delayed hypersensitivity reaction may be present in some cases also has been postulated.

Drugs associated with this type of renal insufficiency include fenoprofen [97–102], indomethacin [103], tolmetin [97, 104], sulindac [105], naproxen [98], benoxaprofen [106], and zomepirac [107, 108].

Hyperkalemia

The inhibition of prostaglandin synthesis results in a decrement in renin release. This decease in renin has led to hypoaldosteronism and hyperkalemia in susceptible patients, particularly those with pre-existent renal insufficiency. Most reports of cases with NSAID-induced hyperkalemia implicate indomethacin [55, 109–111]; however, hyperkalemia remains a potential adverse effect in patients exposed to any of the NSAIDs.

Sodium and Water Retention

Sodium retention as a complication of NSAID therapy is not prominent in most patients. However, in patients with tenuous sodium balance who are susceptible to congestive heart failure, the use of NSAIDs may precipitate symptoms. These effects on sodium excretion may be related to an aldosterone-like effect, to redistribution of renal medullary flood flow, or to a direct antinatriuretic effect of prostaglandin synthesis inhibition. The enhanced end-organ effects of AVP and resultant water retention tendency associations with NSAIDs should be considered in the differential diagnosis of hyponatremia in affected patients. As noted previously, diuretic resistance may occur in patients concomitantly receiving NSAIDs and powerful loop diuretics.

Anaphylaxis

One of the most striking and worrisome reactions associated with these agents has been the growing number of reports of anaphylactoid reactions associated with NSAIDs [112]. Tolmetin, ibuprofen, zomepirac, indomethacin, aspirin, and sulindac have been most frequently associated with this serious adverse reaction. Most of these reactions occur within 1 hr of ingesting the drug. Previous brief exposure to the drug was common in tolmetin cases. Tolmetin and zomepirac are very similar structurally; and, the clustering of anaphylactic reactions with use of these two drugs suggests a common pathogenesis. Aspirin sensitivity may predispose the patient to this reaction with NSAIDs.

Summary

The number of adverse renal effects encountered with the use of NSAIDs can be reduced by recognizing the potential for toxicity and by monitoring renal function in patients known to be at greatest risk for reversible acute renal failure. In this regard, simply by following the serum creatinine in elderly patients and in patients with volume depletion, on diuretics, with heart failure, with liver disease, or with underlying renal disease, many instances of severe acute renal failure can be avoided. Monitoring serum creatinine does not appear to be needed in stable, euvolemic individuals with normal renal function. However, these normal patients should have their renal function checked if an intervening medical event compromises their circulation. If these precautions are taken, NSAIDs may be administered with even greater safety to patients who require them.

References

1. Davis HA, Horton EW: Output of prostaglandins from the rabbit kidney; its increase on renal nerve stimulation and its inhibition by indomethacin. *Br J Pharmacol* 46:658–675, 1972
2. Dunham EW, Zimmerman BG: Release of prostaglandin-like material from dog kidney during nerve stimulation. *Am J Physiol* 219:1279–1286, 1970
3. Morrison AR, Nishikaua K, Needleman P: Thromboxane A_2 biosynthesis in the ureter obstructed isolated perfused kidney of the rabbit. *J Pharmacol Exp Ther* 205:108, 1978
4. McGiff JC, Terragno NA, Molik KU, Lonigro AJ: Release of a prostaglandin E-like substance from canine kidney by bradykinin. *Circ Res* 31:36–48, 1972
5. McGiff JC, Crowshaw K, Terragno NA, Molik KU, Lonigro AJ: Differential effect of nonadrenaline and renal nerve stimulation on vascular resistance in the dog kidney and the release of a prostaglandin E-like substance. *Clin Sci* 42:223–233, 1972
6. Needleman P, Douglas JR, Jarschik G, Steochlein PB, Johnson EM: Release of renal prostaglandins by catecholamines: Relationship to renal endocrine function. *J Pharmacol Exp Ther* 188:453–460, 1974

7. ZUSMAN RM, KEISER HR: Prostaglandin biosynthesis by rabbit renomedullary interstitial cells in tissue culture. Stimulation by vasoactive peptides. *J Clin Invest* 60:215–223, 1977
8. WALKER L, WHORTON A, SMIGEL M, FRANCE R, FROLICH JC: Antidiuretic hormone increases renal prostaglandin synthesis in vivo. *Am J Physiol* 235:F180–F185, 1978
9. HENRICH WL, ANDERSON RJ, BERNS AS, MCDONALD KM, PAULSEN PJ, SCHRIER RW: Role of renal nerves and prostaglandins in control of renal hemodynamics and plasma renin activity during hypotensive hemorrhage in the dog. *J Clin Invest* 61:744–750, 1978
10. HENRICH WL, ANDERSON RJ, BERL T, MCDONALD KM, SCHRIER RW: Role of angiotensin II and prostaglandins in renal response to hypotensive hemorrhage. *Am J Physiol* 235:F46–F51, 1978
11. HENRICH WL, PETTINGER WA, CRONIN RE: The influence of circulating catecholamines and prostaglandins on canine renal hemodynamics during hemorrhage. *Circ Res* 48:424–429, 1981
12. ROTH GJ, STANFORD N, MAJERUS PN: Acetylation of prostaglandin synthetase by aspirin. *Proc Natl Acad Sci USA* 72:3073–3076, 1975
13. HAMBERG M: Inhibition of prostaglandin synthesis in man. *Biochem Biophys Res Comm* 49:720–726, 1972
14. NEWCOMBE DS, THANASSI NM, CIOSEK CP JR: Cartilage cyclic nucleotide phosphodiesterase: Inhibition by anti-inflammatory agents. *Life Sci* 14:505–519, 1974
15. CAMPBELL WB, GRAHAM RM, JACKSON EK: Role of renal prostaglandins in sympathetically mediated renin release. *J Clin Invest* 64:448–456, 1979
16. MUTHER RS, BENNETT W: Effects of aspirin on glomerular filtration rate in normal humans. *Ann Intern Med* 92:386–387, 1980
17. GULLNER HG, GILL JR, BARTER FC: The role of the prostaglandin system in the regulation of renal function in normal women. *Am J Med* 69:718–724, 1980
18. MUTHER RS, BENNETT W: Aspirin-induced depression of glomerular filtration rate in normal humans: Role of sodium balance. *Ann Intern Med* 94:317–321, 1981
19. RICE D, TURNER R, FELTS J, AGUDELLO C, SEMBLE E: Renal failure in patients with rheumatoid arthritis and osteoarthritis on non-steroidal anti-inflammatory drugs (*abstract*). *Fed Proc* 43:1100, 1984
20. JACKSON EK, HEIDERMANN HT, BRANCH RA, GERKENS JF: Low dose intrarenal infusions of PGE$_2$, PGI$_2$ and 6-keto-PGE$_1$ vasodilate in the in vivo rat kidney. *Circ Res* 51:67–72, 1982
21. DUNN M, ZAMBRASKI E: Renal effects of drugs that inhibit prostaglandin synthesis. *Kidney Int* 18:609–622, 1980
22. LEVENSON DJ, SIMMORS CE JR, BRENNER BM: Arachidonic acid metabolism, prostaglandins and the kidney. *Am J Med* 72:354–374, 1982
23. RICE D, TURNER R, FELTS J, AGUDELO C, SEMBLE E: Renal failure in patients with arthritis and osteoarthritis on nonsteroidal antiinflammatory agents (*abstract*). *Fed Proc* 43:1100, 1984
24. OLIVER JA, SCIACCA RR, PINTO J, et al: Participation of the prostaglandins in the control of renal blood flow during acute reductions of cardiac output in the dog. *J Clin Invest* 64:229–237, 1982
25. HENRICH WL, HAMASAKI Y, SAID SI, CAMPBELL WB, CRONIN RE: Dissociation of systemic and renal effects in endotoxemia: Prostaglandin inhibition uncovers an important role of renal nerves. *J Clin Invest* 69:691–699, 1982

26. ZAMBRASKI EJ, DUNN MJ: Prostaglandins and renal function in chronic bile duct-ligated cirrhotic dogs. *Kidney Int* 19:218–224, 1981
27. ZIA P, ZIPSER R, SPECKART R, HORTON R: The measurement of urinary prostaglandin E in normal subjects and high renin states. *J Lab Clin Med* 92:412–416, 1978
28. ZIPSER RD, HOEFS JC, SPECKART PF, ZIA P, HORTON R: Prostaglandins: Modulators of renal function and pressor resistance in chronic liver disease. *J Clin Endocrinol Metab* 48:895–900, 1979
29. BOYER TD, ZIA P, REYNOLDS TB: Effect of indomethacin and prostaglandin A, on renal function and plasma renin activity in alcoholic liver disease. *Gastroenterology* 77:215–222, 1979
30. WALSHE JJ, VENUTO RD: Acute oliguric renal failure induced by indomethacin: Possible mechanism. *Ann Intern Med* 91:47–49, 1979
31. DONKER AJM, ARIOZ L, BRENTJHENS JRH, VANDERHEM GK, HOLLERMAN HJG: The effect of indomethacin on kidney function and plasma renin activity in man. *Nephron* 17:288–296, 1976
32. WHINNERY MA, SHAW JO, BECK N: Thromboxane B_2 and prostaglandin E_2 in the rat kidney with unilateral ureteral obstruction. *Am J Physiol* 242:F220–F225, 1982
33. YARGER WE, SCHOCHEN DD, HARRIS RH: Obstructive nephropathy in the rat: Possible roles for the renin-angiotensin system, prostaglandins, and thromboxanes in renal failure. *J Clin Invest* 65:400–412, 1980
34. CADNAPAPHORNCHOI P, BONDAR NP, MCDONALD FD: Effect of imidazole on the recovery from bilateral ureteral obstruction in dogs. *Am J Physiol* 243:F532–F536, 1982
35. KAWASAKI A, NEEDLEMAN P: Contribution of thromboxane to renal resistance changes in the isolated perfused hydronephrotic rabbit kidney. *Circ Res* 50:486–490, 1982
36. MAUK RH, PATAK RW, FADEM SZ, et al: Effect of prostaglandin E administration in a nephrotoxic vasoconstrictor model of acute renal failure. *Kidney Int* 12:122–130, 1977
37. PATAK RV, FADEM SZ, LIFSCHITZ MD, et al: Study of factors which modify the development of acute renal failure in the dog. *Kidney Int* 15:227–237, 1979
38. WEBB R, CLARK WF, LINDSEY RM, et al: Protective effect of PGE in glycerol induced acute renal failure. *Clin Sci Mol Med* 55:505–507, 1978
39. TORRES VE, STRONG CG, ROMERO JC, et al: Indomethacin enhancement of glycerol acute renal failure in rabbits. *Kidney Int* 7:170–178, 1975
40. LARSSON C, WEBER P, ANGGARD E: Arachidonic acid increases and indomethacin decreases plasma renin activity in the rabbit. *Eur J Pharmacol* 28:391–394, 1974
41. GERBER JC, BRANCH RA, NIES AS, GERKENS JF, SHAND DG, HOLLIFIELD J, OATES JA: Prostaglandins and renin release II. Assessment of renin secretion following infusion of PGI_2, E_2 and D_2 into the renal artery of anesthetized dogs. *Prostaglandins* 15:81–88, 1978
42. BERL T, HENRICH WL, ERICKSON AL, SCHRIER RW: Prostaglandins in the beta-adrenergic and baroreceptor mediated secretion of renin. *Am J Physiol* 236:F472–F477, 1979
43. GERBER JC, NIES AS, OLSEN RD: Control of canine renin release: Macula densa requires prostaglandin synthesis. *J Physiol* 319:419–429, 1981
44. JACKSON EK, HERZER WA, ZIMMERMAN JB, OATES JA, BRANCH RA, GERENS JF: Effects of indomethacin on beta-adrenoreceptor-stimulated renin release in the dog. *J Pharmacol Exp Ther* 222:414–418, 1982

45. SUZUKI S, FRANCO-SAENZ R, MULROW PJ: The role of prostaglandins in the renal response to isoproterenol in the rat in vitro. *Endocrinology* 108:1654–1657, 1981

46. FEURSTEIN G, FEURSTEIN N: The effect of indomethacin on isoprenaline-induced renin secretion in the cat. *Eur J Pharmacol* 61:85–88, 1980

47. ROMERO JC, DUNLAP CL, STRONG GC: The effect of indomethacin and other anti-inflammatory drugs on the renin-angiotensin system. *J Clin Invest* 58:282–288, 1976

48. HENRICH WL: Prostaglandins in renin secretion. *Kidney Int* 19 (Suppl 6):822–830, 1981

49. HENRICH WL, ANDERSON RJ, BERNS AS, McDONALD KM, PAULSEN PJ, SCHRIER RW: Role of renal nerves and prostaglandins in control of renal hemodynamics and plasma renin activity during hypotensive hemorrhage in the dog. *J Clin Invest* 61:744–750, 1978

50. SEYMOUR AA, DAVIS JO, ECHTENKAMP SF, DIETZ JR, FREEMAN RH: Adrenergically induced renin release in conscious indomethacin-treated dogs and rats. *Am J Physiol* 240:F515–F521, 1981

51. SEYMOUR AA, ZEHR JE: Influence of renal prostaglandins on renin control mechanisms in the dog. *Circ Res* 45:13–25, 1979

52. FROLICH JC, HOLLIFIELD JW, VESPER BS, SHAND DG, WILSON JP, SEYBERTH HJ, FROLICH WH, OATES JA: Reduction of plasma renin activity by inhibition of the fatty acid cyclooxygenase: Independence of sodium retention. *Circ Res* 44:781–787, 1979

53. HENRICH WL, CAMPBELL WB: Dissociation of β-adrenergic renin release from the prostaglandin system in the rat (*abstract*). *Clin Res* 31:248A, 1983

54. NORBY LH, WEIDIG J, RAMWILL P, SLOTKOFF L, FLAMENBAUM W: Possible role for impaired renal prostaglandin production in the pathogenesis of hyporeninemic-hypoaldosteronism. *Lancet* I:1118–1121, 1978

55. TAN SY, SHAPIRO R, FRANCO R, STOCKARD H, MULROW PJ: Indomethacin-induced prostaglandin inhibition with hyperkalemia. *Ann Intern Med* 90:783–785, 1979

56. SHEA-DONOHUE PT, BOLGER PM, EISNER GM, SLOTKOFF LM: Effects of PGE_2 on electrolyte and fluid excretion in the canine kidney: Evidence for a direct tubular effect. *Can J Physiol Pharmacol* 57:1448–1452, 1978

57. BRATER DC: Effect of indomethacin on salt and water homeostasis. *Clin Pharmacol Ther* 25:322–330, 1979

58. KAOJAREN S, CHENNAVASIN P, ANDERSON S, BRATER DC: Nephron site of effect of nonsteroidal anti-inflammatory drugs on solute excretion in humans. *Am J Physiol* 244:F134–F139, 1983

59. DUSING R, NICHOLAS V, GLANGER K, KIPHOWSKI J, KRAMER HJ: Prostaglandins participate in the regulation of NaCl absorption in the diluting segments of the nephron in vivo: Effect of furosemide. *Renal Physiol (Basel)* 5:115–123, 1982

60. STOKES JB: Effect of prostaglandin E_2 on chloride transport across the thick ascending limb of Henle. *J Clin Invest* 64:495–502, 1979

61. STOKES JB, KOKKO JP: Inhibition of sodium transport by prostaglandin E_2 across the isolated, perfused rabbit collecting tubule. *J Clin Invest* 59:1099–1104, 1977

62. LINO Y, IMAI M: Effects of prostaglandins on Na transport in isolated collecting tubules. *Pflügers Arch* 373:125–132, 1978

63. FELDMAN D, LOOSE DS, TAN SY: Nonsteroidal anti-inflammatory drugs cause sodium and water retention in the rat. *Am J Physiol* 234:F490–F496, 1978

64. ORLOFF J, HANDLER JS, BERGSTROM S: Effect of prostaglandin (PGE$_2$) on the permeability response of toad bladder to vasopressin, theophylline, and adenosine 3^1, 5^1-monophosphage. *Nature* 205:397–398, 1965
65. NIES AS, GAL J, FADUL S, GERBER JG: Indomethacin furosemide interaction: The importance of renal blood flow. *J Pharmacol Exp Ther* 226:27–32, 1983
66. LIPSON LC, SHARP GWG: Effect of prostaglandin E$_1$ on sodium transport and osmotic water flow in the toad bladder. *Am J Physiol* 220:1046–1052, 1971
67. GRANTHAM JJ, ORLOFF L: Effect of prostaglandin E$_1$ on the permeability response of the isolated collecting tubule to vasopressin, adenosine 3^1, 5^1-monophosphate and theophylline. *J Clin Invest* 47:1154–1161, 1968
68. BURCH RM, HALUSKA PV: Vasopressin stimulates prostaglandin and thromboxane synthesis in toad bladder epithelial cells. *Am J Physiol* 243:F593–F597, 1982
69. ANDERSON RJ, BERL T, MCDONALD KM, SCHRIER RW: Evidence for an in vivo antagonism between vasopressin and prostaglandin in the mammalian kidney. *J Clin Invest* 56:420–426, 1976
70. BERL T, RAZ A, WALD H, HOROWITZ J, CZACKES W: Prostaglandin synthesis inhibition and the action of vasopressin: Studies in man and rat. *Am J Physiol* 232:F529–F537, 1977
71. ZUSMAN RM, VINCI JM, BOWDEN RE, HORWITZ D, KEISER HR: Effect of indomethacin and adrenocorticotrophic hormone on renal function in man: An experimental model of inappropriate diuresis. *Kidney Int* 15:62–70, 1979
72. KOREN JF, BROWN JR, ALISSANDRATOS JK, et al: Indomethacin-induced acute renal failure: Report of a case and review of the literature. *Drug Intell Clin Pharmacy* 14:711–714, 1980
73. FAWAZ-ESTRUP E, HO G JR: Reversible acute renal failure induced by indomethacin. *Arch Intern Med* 141:1670–1671, 1981
74. KLEINKNECHT C, BROYER M, GUBLER MC, PALCOUX JB: Irreversible renal failure after indomethacin in steroid-resistant nephrosis (*letter*). *N Engl J Med* 302:691, 1980
75. TAN SY, SHAPIRO R, KISH MA: Reversible acute renal failure induced by indomethacin. *JAMA* 241:2732–2733, 1979
76. O'MERA ME, EKNOYAN G: Acute renal failure associated with indomethacin administration. *S Med J* 73:587–589, 1980
77. FELLNER SK, ARRAHA HB, WOLFE C: Acute renal failure and zomepirac (*letter*). *Arch Intern Med* 141:1846, 1981
78. GALLER M, FOLKERT VW, SCHLONDORF D: Reversible acute renal insufficiency and hyperkalemia following indomethacin therapy. *JAMA* 246:154–155, 1981
79. FONG HJ, COHEN AH: Ibuprofen-induced acute renal failure with acute tubular necrosis. *Am J Nephrol* 2:28–31, 1982
80. BRANDSETTER RD, MAR DD: Reversible oliguric renal failure associated with ibuprofen treatment. *Br Med J* 2:1149–1155, 1978
81. KIMBERLY RP, SHERMAN RL, MOURADIAN J, et al: Apparent acute renal failure associated with therapeutic aspirin and ibuprofen administration. *Arthr Rheum* 22:281–285, 1979
82. HUSSERL FE, LANGE RK, KANTROW CM: Renal papillary necrosis and pyelonephritis accompanying fenoprofen therapy. *JAMA* 242:1896–1898, 1979
83. KIMBERLY RP, BOWDEN RE, KEISER HR: Reduction of renal function by newer nonsteroidal anti-inflammatory drugs. *Am J Med* 64:804–807, 1978
84. MULHALWAS KK, SHAH GM, WINER RL: Renal papillary necrosis caused by long-term ingestion of pentazocine and aspirin. *JAMA* 246:867–868, 1981

85. EDWARDS KDG, SCHAPEL GJ, JEREMY R, STEELE TW: Possible nephrotoxicity of aspirin in rheumatoid arthritis (*letter*) *Med J Australia* 1:492, 1972
86. NANRA RS, KINCAID-SMITH P: Renal papillary necrosis in rheumatoid arthritis. *Med J Australia* 1:194–197, 1975
87. KIMBERLY RP, GILL JR, BOWDEN RE, et al: Elevated urinary prostaglandins and the effects of aspirin on renal function in lupus erythematosus. *Ann Intern Med* 89:336–341, 1978
88. GOKAL R, MATTHEWS FR: Renal papillary necrosis after aspirin and aclofenac. *Br Med J* 1:1517–1518, 1977
89. MORALES P, STEYN J: Papillary necrosis following phenylbutazone ingestion. *Arch Surg* 103:420–421, 1971
90. WILKINSON EL, BROWN H: The effect of phenylbutazone on water and electrolyte excretion. *Am J Med Sci* 225:153–158, 1953
91. BUNNING RD, BARTH WF: Sulindac: A potentially renal-sparing nonsteroidal anti-inflammatory drug. *JAMA* 248:2864–2867, 1982
92. CIABATTONI G, CINOTTI GA, PIERUCCI A, et al: Effects of sulindac and ibuprofen in patients with chronic glomerular disease. *N Engl J Med* 310:279–283, 1984
93. BRATER DC, ANDERSON S, BAIRD B, CAMPBELL WB: Sulindac does not spare the kidney (abstract). *Clin Res* 31:868A, 1983
94. ROBERTS DG, GERBER JG, NIES AS: Comparative effects of sulindac and indomethacin in humans (abstract). *Clin Res* 32:72A, 1984
95. ABRAHAM PA, KEANE WF: Glomerular and interstitial disease induced by nonsteroidal anti-inflammatory drugs. *Am J Nephrol* 4:1–6, 1984
96. TORES VE: Present and future of the non-steroidal anti-inflammatory drugs in nephrology. *Mayo Clin Proc* 57:389–393, 1982
97. CHATTERJEE GP: Nephrotic syndrome induced by tolmetin (*case report*). *JAMA* 246:1589, 1981
98. BREZIN JH, KATZ SM, SCHWARTZ AB, et al: Reversible renal failure and nephrotic syndrome associated with nonsteroidal anti-inflammatory drugs. *N Engl J Med* 301:1271–1273, 1979
99. FINKELSTEIN A, FRALEY DS, STACHURA I, et al: Fenoprofen nephropathy: Lipoid nephrosis and interstitial nephritis. *Am J Med* 72:81–87, 1982
100. WENDLAND ML, WAGONER RD, HOLLEY KE: Renal failure associated with fenoprofen. *Mayo Clin Proc* 55:103–107, 1980
101. CURT GA, KALDANZ A, WHITLEY LG, et al: Reversible rapidly progressive renal failure with nephrotic syndrome due to fenoprofen calcium. *Ann Intern Med* 92:72–73, 1980
102. HANDA SP: Renal effects of fenoprofen (*letter*). *Ann Intern Med* 93:508, 1980
103. GARY NE, DODELSON R, EISINGER RP: Indomethacin-associated acute renal failure. *Am J Med* 69:135–136, 1980
104. KATZ SM, CAPALDO R, EVERTS EA, et al: Tolmetin: Associated with reversible renal failure and acute interstitial nephritis. *JAMA* 246:253–254, 1981
105. LOMVARDIAS S, PINN VW, WADHWA ML, et al: Nephrotic syndrome associated with sulindac (*letter*). *N Engl J Med* 304:424, 1981
106. FINE W, TALLIS RC, OSMAN KM: Renal failure as a suspected adverse reaction to benoxaprofen. *Postgrad Med J* 58:317–318, 1982
107. RATNER SJ: Zomepirac and renal failure (*letter*). *Ann Intern Med* 96:793, 1982
108. McCARTHY JT, SCHWARTZ GL, PIERIDES AM, et al: Reversible non-oliguric acute renal failure associated with zomepirac therapy. *Mayo Clin Proc* 57:351–354, 1982

109. FINDLING JW, BECKSTROM D, RAWSTHORNE L, et al: Indomethacin-induced hyperkalemia in three patients with gouty arthritis. *JAMA* 244:1127–1128, 1980
110. MACCARTHY EP, FROST GW, STOKES GS: Indomethacin-induced hyperkalemia. *Med J Australia* 1:550, 1979
111. GOLDSZER RC, COUDLEY EL, ROSNER MJ, et al: Hyperkalemia associated with indomethacin. *Arch Intern Med* 141:802–804, 1981
112. ROSSI AC, KNAPP DE: Tolmetin-induced anaphylactoid reactions. *N Engl J Med* 307:499–500, 1982

Renal Damage Induced by Radiologic Contrast Media

Carl M. Kjellstrand, Robert O. Berkseth, and Paul A. Abraham

Contrast administration causes 10% of all cases of acute renal failure and, thus, is a very important entity clinically [1, 2]. Contrast-induced nephropathy was recognized in the 1920s, shortly after the introduction into clinical medicine of examinations with intravascular contrast media [3–5]. Newer contrast media (diatrizoate and iothalamate) were introduced in the 1950s and are used still. They were thought to be safe originally, even in patients with severe renal insufficiency [6–22]. Less than 10 cases per year of contrast media-induced acute renal failure were reported in the 15-year period between 1958 to 1973. In 1978 alone, almost 100 cases were reported in the literature [23]! The explanation for this startling increase probably is due to two factors: first, in the 1960s and 1970s, when these drugs were felt to be safe, renal functional impairment occurring after their use probably was thought to be due to other causes—such as natural history of the renal disease, or other drugs—or it simply was overlooked because of its transient nature; by contrast, patients are currently followed with sequential determinations of the serum creatinine concentration, and contrast media now may be incriminated too often as etiologic in origin. Second, more patients at high risk for this nephropathy now are being exposed to contrast media due to medical advances and increased availability of medical care. Thus, patients with pre-existing renal failure and advanced diabetes mellitus are being aggressively investigated for therapies that were not available for many such patients in the 1960s and early 1970s.

Pharmacology and Physiology

The current contrast agents for intravascular use are 2,4,6-tri-iodinated benzoic acid derivatives. They are distributed in the extracellular space, have

This manuscript was presented as part of a Symposium on *Nephrotoxicity and Drugs.*

insignificant protein-binding, and are excreted by the kidneys as unchanged compounds. The compounds are freely filtered by the glomerulus and are neither secreted nor absorbed by the tubules. Their clearance rate thus approximates that of creatinine. Their half-life is 30 to 60 min when renal function is normal, but it may be delayed to days in severe renal failure [24].

These contrast media have a molecular weight of 600 to 700 daltons, and they are supplied in solutions that are markedly hyperosmolar (1400 to 1800 mOsm/liter). They stimulate the release of antidiuretic hormone (ADH) and may increase urinary oxalate and uric acid excretion two to nine times above baseline values.

Incidence and Risk Factors

The incidence of renal failure after the administration of contrast media is dependent on the presence of a number of risk factors. It may range from well less than 1% in healthy individuals to almost 100% in patients who are at highest risk; for example, the dehydrated patient with diabetes mellitus and underlying severe chronic renal failure [25–28]. Table 1 contains a list of risk factors that have been identified. The only well-documented risk factors are chronic, underlying renal insufficiency and diabetes mellitus. Many of the other factors coexist, and their relative roles have not been delineated. The reported incidence of contrast-induced renal failure is illustrated in Figure 1; the possible summation effect of coexisting risk factors in diabetes mellitus is illustrated in Figure 2. Thus, it is clear that dehydration and the serum creatinine concentration are related, as are chronic renal insufficiency, proteinuria, hypertension, arteriosclerotic peripheral vascular disease, hyperuricemia, and old age. The relative importance and summation effects of these risk factors await larger clinical analysis. A common and dangerous misunderstanding is that the dose of contrast media is important. On the contrary, if a dose-effect relationship should exist, maximum damage has already occurred after the intravascular administration of approximately 30 ml of dye; intravenous urograms and contrast-enhanced computed tomography (CT) thus are no safer than angiography using hundreds of milliliters of contrast media.

Pathogenesis

The pathogenesis of most toxic nephropathies is poorly understood and contrast nephropathy is no exception. Table 2 outlines proposed pathogenetic

Table 1. Proposed risk factors for intravascular contrast media-induced renal damage

Dose of contrast	Specific diagnoses (multiple myeloma or
Repeat exposure to contrast media	postrenal transplant)
Simultaneous use of other nephrotoxic drugs	Hypertension
Pre-existing renal insufficiency	Arteriosclerotic peripheral vascular diseases
Diabetes mellitus	Hyperuricemia, hyperoxalemia
Dehydration	Old age
	Liver disease

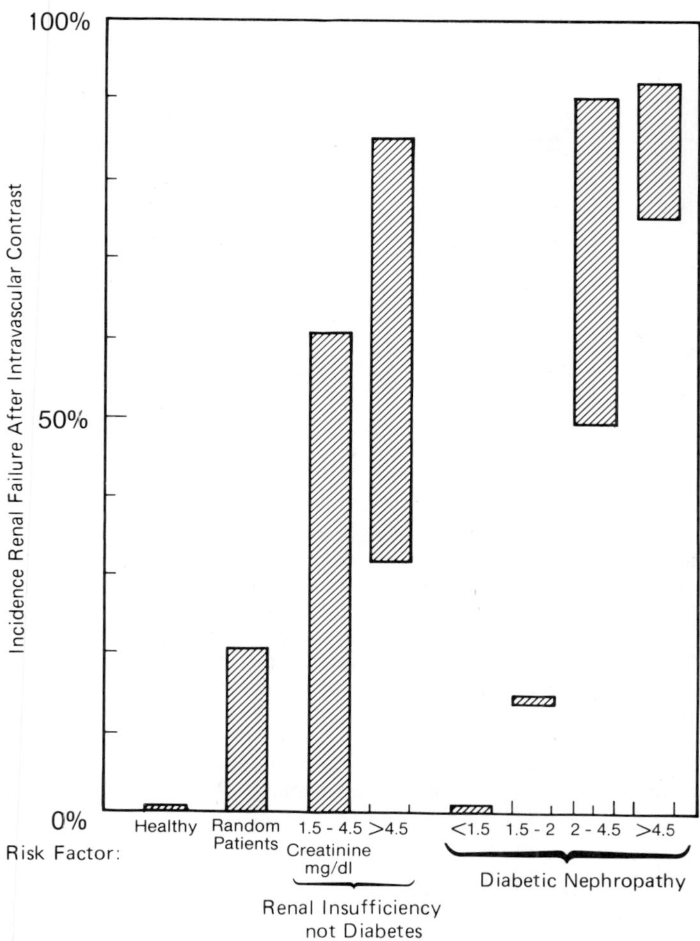

Fig. 1. The incidence of renal failure after intravascular contrast media versus various risk factors. The incidence is much less than 1% in healthy individuals, but it is almost 20% in random patients. There is a direct relationship between the incidence of contrast-induced nephropathy and the severity of pre-existing renal failure. The addition of diabetes mellitus to renal failure markedly increases the risk of contrast nephropathy.

mechanisms. Any pathogenetic theory must acknowledge the clinical observations that contrast nephropathy is transient, rapid in onset, and much more common in patients with underlying renal disease and diabetes mellitus. Contrast media cause sludging of red blood cells and increased blood viscosity [29]; they may also cause prolonged vasoconstriction [30]. Thus, patients are more susceptible to contrast-induced nephropathy if they have underlying damage to the renal microvasculature, such as that observed in association

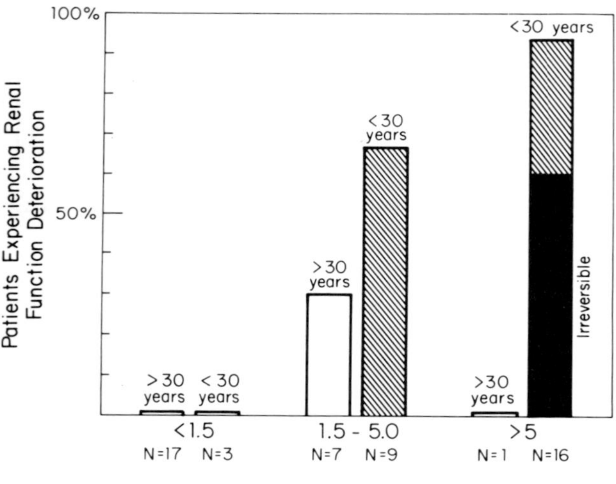

Fig. 2. Graph describing the relationship between contrast nephropathy in diabetes and two risk factors: (1) severity of pre-existing renal failure, and (2) age at onset of diabetes. There is almost no contrast nephropathy in diabetic patients with normal renal function (creatinine < 1.5 mg/dl). With moderate renal failure (creatinine < 1.5 to 5.0 mg/dl), there is a marked increase in the incidence of renal failure. The incidence in patients with juvenile onset diabetes (< 30 yr) is twice that in patients with adult onset diabetes mellitus. Almost all patients with severe renal failure (creatinine > 5 mg/dl) had contrast nephropathy; and, in the juvenile onset group, this was irreversible in more than 50% of the patients. Thus, it seems that advanced pre-existing renal failure and age at onset of diabetes are independent summation risk factors for contrast nephropathy.

with pre-existing renal disease, hypertension, and arteriosclerosis. Studies of renal biopsy specimens in patients with contrast nephropathy have shown acute tubular damage [3, 31, 32]. The presence of renal disease prolongs the exposure to contrast media because of delayed excretion, which may enhance these nephrotoxic mechanisms. The nephrotic syndrome and proteinuria do not seem to be important risk factors for the induction of contrast nephropathy. The clinical course of contrast nephropathy is different from that of oxalate nephropathy. Its sudden onset and rapid resolution is similar to that of acute uric acid nephropathy. Immunologic mechanisms probably

Table 2. Pathogenetic mechanisms in contrast-induced nephropathy

Tubular toxicity	Intratubular uric acid precipitation
Renal ischemia	Intratubular oxalate precipitation
Protein precipitation	Immunologic mechanisms

are operative in only an exceptional patient, but complement activation may play a role in contrast-induced nephropathy in transplanted patients.

Clinical Course and Laboratory Findings

Renal failure occurs shortly after the administration of the contrast media, and it usually resolves within 1 week. Approximately 50% of patients develop oliguria. A few patients develop irreversible renal failure. This risk seems to be related directly to the degree of pre-existent renal failure, particularly if diabetes mellitus is also coexistent. Over 67% of patients with juvenile-onset diabetes mellitus and a serum creatinine concentration greater than 5 mg/dl developed irreversible renal failure after intravenous pyelography [28]. The urinary sediment shows tubular epithelial casts and amorphous urate in most patients and calcium oxalate crystals in a few patients. The fractional excretion of sodium is usually less than 1%. It is common to observe a persistent nephrogram on a 24-hr delayed x-ray film.

Diagnosis

The diagnosis of contrast-induced nephropathy is easy as a rule, but it requires serial determinations of the serum creatinine concentration before and after the contrast study. Changes in the urinary sediment, the appearance of a delayed nephrogram, and a characteristic clinical course with rapid onset and resolution will establish the diagnosis.

Differential diagnoses include cholesterol embolization, catheter-induced trauma of the renal artery, and renal insufficiency due to simultaneous dehydration and other nephrotoxic drugs. In many patients, the diagnosis can only be made retrospectively. Thus, the persistence of renal failure and other manifestations of cholesterol embolization may establish the diagnosis later. Similarly, resolution of renal failure with rehydration or the discontinuation of a nephrotoxic drug may rule out contrast nephropathy in other patients.

Therapy

After nephrotoxicity of contrast media has occurred, no specific therapy is available. Only symptomatic therapy, maintenance of fluid and electrolyte balance, and the use of dialysis can be offered if it should become necessary.

Prophylaxis

To prevent contrast-induced renal insufficiency, one must first identity the patients at risk. A clinical history and measurement of the serum creatinine concentration are sufficient for this purpose. When high-risk patients are identified, one should try to avoid the intravascular use of contrast media. Usually, the necessary information sought by contrast media examination can be obtained by a combination of other procedures. These include radioisotope renography, ultrasonography, tomography, and nonenhanced CT scan. If intravascular dye studies are necessary in patients at risk, then dehydration, acidosis, and hyperuricemia should be corrected first and other nephrotoxic drugs should be discontinued. Although any dose of contrast agent may be sufficient to cause renal failure, it is prudent to plan the examination so that only the smallest amount of contrast necessary is administered.

Several clinical investigators have studied the influence of furosemide and/or mannitol on contrast nephropathy. The results are contradictory, as summarized in Table 3. Shafi and Anto et al [33, 34], using historic control, found the incidence of contrast-induced nephropathy to decline when 250 ml of 20% mannitol was infused intravenously 1 hr after the administration of contrast medium. The incidence fell from 61 to 18% in patients with chronic renal failure secondary to diseases other than diabetes mellitus, and from 92 to 33% in patients with diabetic nephropathy. Old et al [35] in a double-blind prospective randomized study of 24 patients, infused 100 ml of 25% mannitol immediately after contrast study. In the 12 treated patients, the serum creatinine concentration remained stable around 2.4 mg/dl, but it rose from 2.1 to 3.1 mg/dl in the control patients. Also, Oguagha et al [36], using historic control (similar to studies from [33, 34]), observed acute renal failure in only 1 of 17 (18%) patients treated with furosemide given in a 1-mg dosage derived by dividing 4000 by the creatinine clearance (C_{cr}). The serum creatinine concentration in the study patients was approximately 4.0 mg/dl. Beroniade [1] also found that prophylactic furosemide (to maintain a diuresis of 300 ml/hr) prevented acute renal failure after contrast media in seven patients with severe underlying renal disease. He had experienced a high incidence (not specified) in other patients who had received 500 ml of 20% mannitol. His results suggest that furosemide may be more efficient than mannitol. In the largest randomized study by Vosnides et al [37], hypertonic mannitol given in a dose of 100 ml immediately after intravenous pyelography was useless in preventing renal failure. Thus, four patients (13%) developed acute renal failure in each group of 30 treated and 30 control patients.

Our interpretation of these conflicting data is that mannitol and/or loop diuretics reduce the incidence and/or severity of contrast-induced nephropathy. We suggest prophylactic mannitol and furosemide in all patients undergoing intravascular contrast study when the serum creatinine concentration is greater than 2.0 mg/dl. Furosemide in a dose of 100 mg for each 1 mg/dl of serum creatinine is added to 500 ml of 20% mannitol. The infusion is started 1 hr before the administration of contrast medium, at a rate of 20 ml/hr, and is continued throughout the procedure and for 6 hr thereafter. Urine output is replaced with 5% dextrose in one-half normal saline solution with 30 mEq potassium chloride added per liter. We believe this treatment decreases both the risk and the severity of renal failure. As with all treatment, it is not 100% effective; at least one patient with diabetes mellitus and chronic renal insufficiency (serum creatinine, 5 mg/dl) sustained an exacerbation of

Table 3. Summary of results of trials to ameliorate acute contrast-induced nephropathy (ACN)

Reference	Treatment	Baseline creatinine	Result		Study design
			Treated	Control	
33, 34	250 ml 20% mannitol 60 min after contrast	4.0 mg/dl	22% developed ACN	70% developed ACN	Historic control, $N = 77$
37	100 ml hypertonic mannitol immediately after IVP	4.2 mg/dl	13% developed ACN	13% developed ACN	Randomization, $N = 60$
35	100 ml 25% mannitol immediately after contrast study	1.7 to 6.0 mg/dl	Creatinine 2.4 → 2.5 mg/dl	Creatinine 2.1 → 3.1 mg/dl	Double-blind, prospective, randomized, $N = 24$
36	$\frac{400}{C_{cr}}$ mg of furosemide, 60 min after contrast study	4.0 mg/dl	18% developed ACN	70% developed ACN	Historic control, $N = 57$ (same 40 control in study [33, 34])
1	Furosemide	?	Furosemide better than mannitol		Historic control

chronic renal failure after coronary angiography, and this patient needed chronic dialysis.

References

1. BERONIADE VC: Prevention of acute renal failure secondary to radiocontrast agents, in *Abstracts of the Eighth International Congress of Nephrology,* Athens, Greece, University Studio Publishing Company, 1981, p 380
2. HOU SH, BUSHINSKY DA, WISH JB, et al: Hospital-acquired renal insufficiency: A prospective study. *Am J Med* 74:243–248, 1983
3. MILLER GM, WYLIE EJ, HINMAN F: Renal complications from aortography. *Surgery* 35:885–896, 1954
4. CRAWFORD ES, BEAL AC, MOYER JH, DeBAKEY ME: Complications of aortography. *Surg Gynecol Obstet* 104:129–141, 1957
5. ALWALL W, ERLANSON P, TORNBERG A: Clinical course of renal failure occurring after intravenous urography and/or retrograde pyelography. *Acta Med Scand* 152:163–173, 1955
6. SCHWARTZ WB, HURWIT A, ETTINGER A: Intravenous urography in the patient with renal insufficiency. *N Engl J Med* 269:277–283, 1963
7. SCHENKER B: Drip infusion pyelography. Indications and applications in urologic roentgenologic diagnosis. *Radiology* 83:12–21, 1964
8. BISHOP RC, HEETDERK DR, STEWARD BH: Excretory urography in azotemic patients. Revised technique. *J Urology* 91:441–443, 1964
9. WHITESEL JA, HELLER E: Intensification of excretory urogram by continuous infusion of contrast material. *J Urology* 92:224–229, 1964
10. BENGTSSON U, CEDARBON G, FALKHEDEN T, JAGENBURG R: Clearances of inulin and paraaminohippurate before and after urography using high dosage of contrast medium in patients with renal insufficiency. *Scand J Urol Nephrol* 2:173–176, 1968
11. VOLTZ PW, LOGAN B, WOLFF HL: Adequate dose excretory urography: Experience with 25,000 cases. *South Med J* 64:903–906, 1971
12. BARTLEY O, BENGTSSON U, CEDARBON G: Renal function before and after angiography with large doses of contrast media. *Acta Radiol* 8:9–16, 1969
13. BECKER JA, BERDON, WE: Blood clearance of contrast material in patients with impaired renal function. *Radiology* 93:1301–1304, 1969
14. DANFORD RO, DAVIDSON AJ, GOLDMAN RL: Drip-infusion pyelography. *N Engl J Med* 280:1022, 1969
15. FULTON RE, WITTEN DM, WAGONER RD: Intravenous urography in renal insufficiency. *Am J Roentgenol Rad Ther Nucl Med* 106:623–634, 1969
16. BROWN CB, GLANEY JJ, FRY IK, CAHEL WR: High dose excretion urography in oliguric renal failure. *Lancet* 2:952–955, 1970
17. DAVIDSON AJ, BECKER J, ROTHFIELD N, UNGER G, PLOCH OR: An evaluation of the effect of high dose urography on previously impaired renal and hepatic function in man. *Radiology* 97:249–254, 1970
18. FRY IK, CATTEL WR: Excretion urography in advanced renal failure. *Br J Radiol* 44:198–202, 1971
19. EISENBERG RL, BANK WD, HEDGLOCK MW: Renal failure after major angiography. *Am J Med* 68:43–46, 1980
20. BECKER JA, KINLHABWALA M, ZOLAN S: Urography in renal failure. *Radiology* 105:505–507, 1972
21. BOSNIAK MA, SCHWEIZER RD: Urographic findings in patients with renal failure. *Radiol Clin North Am* 10:433–445, 1972

22. TALNER LB: Urographic contrast media in uremia, physiology and pharmacology. *Radiol Clin North Am* 10:421–432, 1972
23. MUDGE GH: Nephrotoxicity of urographic radiocontrast drugs. *Kidney Int* 18:540–552, 1980
24. BERKSETH RO, KJELLSTRAND CM: Radiological contrast-induced nephropathy. *Medic Clin North Am* 68(Suppl 2):351–370, 1984
25. ABRAHAM P, HARKONEN S, KJELLSTRAND CM: Contrast nephropathy, in *Textbook of Nephrology,* edited by MASSEY SG, GLASSOCH KJ, Baltimore, William & William, 1983, chap 43:5, pp 6.205–209
26. HARKONEN S, KJELLSTRAND CJ: Intravenous pyelography in nonuremic diabetic patients. *Nephron* 24:268–270, 1979
27. HARKONEN S, KJELLSTRAND CM: Contrast nephropathy. *Am J Nephrol* 1:69–77, 1981
28. HARKONEN S, KJELLSTRAND CM: Exacerbation of diabetic renal failure following intravenous pyelography. *Am J Med* 63:939–946, 1977
29. DEAN RE, ANDREW JH, READ RC: The red cell factor in renal damage from angiographic media. *JAMA* 187:27–31, 1964
30. SOBIN SS: Nature of adverse reactions to radioopaque agents. *JAMA* 170:1546–1547, 1959
31. KRUNLOVSKY FA, SIRION N, SANTHANAM S, DEL GREGO P, ROXE D, PONARANC MM: Acute renal failure. Association with administration of radiographic contrast material. *JAMA* 239:125–127, 1978
32. VAN ZEE BE, HOY WE, TALLEY TE, JAENIKE JR: Renal injury associated with intravenous pyelography in nondiabetic and diabetic patients. *Ann Intern Med* 89:51–54, 1978
33. SHAFI T, CHOU S, PORUSH JG, et al: Infusion intravenous pyelography and renal function. *Arch Intern Med* 138:1218–1221, 1978
34. ANTO HR, CHOU SY, PORUSH JG, et al: Infusion intravenous pyelography and renal function: Effects of hypertonic mannitol in patients with chronic renal failure. *Arch Intern Med* 141:1652–1656, 1981
35. OLD CW, DUARTE CM, LEHRNER LM, et al: A prospective evaluation of mannitol in the prevention of radiocontrast acute renal failure (abstract). *Clin Res* 29:472A, 1981
36. OGUAGHA C, PORUSH JG, CHOU SY, et al: Prevention of acute renal failure (ARF) following infusion of intravenous pyelography (IVP) in patients with chronic renal insufficiency (CRI) by furosemide (F), in *Abstracts of the Eighth International Congress of Nephrology,* Athens, Greece, University Studio Publishing Company, 1981, p 290
37. VOSNIDES CR, KALOGEROPOULOUS V, SPANOS H, et al: Radio-contrast-induced deterioration of renal function in patients with chronic renal failure, in *Abstracts of the Eighth International Congress of Nephrology,* Athens, Greece, University Studio Publishing Company, 1981, p 306

Antibiotic-Induced Nephrotoxicity

Carlos A. Vaamonde

Renal dysfunction or disease may result from the clinical use of antibacterial agents. The clinical and morphologic expression of antibacterial nephrotoxicity represents a spectrum of alterations ranging from acute renal failure and tubulointerstitial nephropathy to selected renal tubular disorders.

This chapter will be concerned only with the renal effects of aminoglycoside antibiotics. The choice is not difficult, since aminoglycosides are responsible for the large majority of renal toxicity reported clinically with the use of antibiotics, with beta-lactam antibiotics being a distant second and other antibacterials (such as rifampin and amphotericin B) being more rarely involved [1, 2]. In recent years, many excellent reviews have been published on general and specific aspects of aminoglycoside toxicity [3–9]. Although many aminoglycosides are in use, most of the clinical and experimental studies are based on or compared to gentamicin, which is considered to be the prototypic compound.

Molecular and Pharmacologic Aspects of Aminoglycoside Nephrotoxicity

Aminoglycosides are highly polar cations (average pKa of 8.0 or greater) composed of various sugar molecules in glycosidic linkage with amino-containing side chains. Strictly speaking, however, they are aminoglycosidic aminocyclitols; there are no "pure" aminoglycosides as such in clinical use (that is, with amino groups substituted only in the sugar), with the exception of spectinomycin—a pure aminocyclitol [10]. Most of the semisynthetic derivatives are pure substances (streptomycin, tobramycin, amikacin, dibekacin,

---

This manuscript was presented as part of a Symposium on *Nephrotoxicity and Drugs*.

sisomicin, and netilmicin), but neomycin (A, B, and C), kanamycin (A, B, and C), and gentamicin (C_1, C_{1a}, and C_2) are mixtures of compounds of slightly different pharmacologic and antimicrobial activities [10].

Aminoglycosides act by inhibiting the synthesis of bacterial proteins via interference with the activity of ribosomes. Aminoglycosides are stable in aqueous solution, except in the presence of penicillins. Aminoglycosides have a low lipid solubility and a low capacity for penetrating membranes; all aminoglycosides are poorly absorbed from the gut. When given intramuscularly or intravenously, aminoglycosides are rapidly distributed throughout the extracellular fluid. Because of their polar nature, these antibiotics are largely excluded from most cells. They exhibit very low binding to plasma proteins. In humans, binding is less than 30%; in the rat, which is the principal experimental species, it is less than 15%.

It appears that the potential for aminoglycoside nephrotoxicity depends on the number of ionizable amino groups (NH_2^+) contained on their molecule and on the derived cationicity. The cationic charge of the aminoglycoside is correlated with the degree of aminoglycoside-membrane interaction and interference with mitochondrial function [11]. Addition of cationic, diethylaminoethyl (DEAE) substitution groups to an otherwise nontoxic neutral dextran molecule confers nephrotoxic potential to the synthesized dextran-DEAE [12]. Furthermore, other endogenous polyamines that are strongly cationic at physiologic pH (due to their content in NH_2^+), such as spermine and spermidine, are known to be nephrotoxic [13, 14]. Likewise, poly-L-lysine (a compound of repeated units of lysine) also causes injury to the toad bladder epithelium [15]. The number of NH_2^+ groups contained in the molecular structure of commonly used aminoglycosides is: streptomycin = sisomicin = 3, kanamycin = amikacin = 4, gentamicin = tobramycin = netilmicin = 5, and neomycin = 6.

Although a good correlation exists between this cationicity and specific (renal, oto-, or neurotoxicities) or whole animal toxicity [1, 9], it should be emphasized that aminoglycosides with similar cationic charges may exhibit different clinical or experimental toxicities. For example, Soberon et al [16] have shown that aminoglycosides containing five NH_2^+ groups have different nephrotoxicities when tested in the rat. Netilmicin was less nephrotoxic than tobramycin, which (in turn) was less toxic than gentamicin [16]. Therefore, factors other than the molecular cationic charge are of importance. These may include charge orientation or position and an inherent propensity of the aminoglycoside molecular structure for causing toxic injury to intracellular organelles [6, 16].

Aminoglycosides do not undergo metabolism in the body, and they are rapidly excreted by the kidney in humans and experimental animals. The normal half-life in adults of all aminoglycosides in clinical use is about 2 hr. It is approximately slightly less for gentamicin and tobramycin, and somewhat more for streptomycin, kanamycin, and amikacin [17]. In the rat, the excretion of aminoglycosides is much faster than in humans. For example, we have obtained a plasma half-life value of 32 ± 2 (SEM) min in normal Sprague-Dawley rats after a single intravenous (i.v.) dose of 40 mg/kg of gentamicin (Vaamonde et al, unpublished observations), while a value of 1 hr was obtained after a dose of 100 mg/kg given subcutaneously [16].

Renal Handling of Aminoglycosides

Glomerular filtration has been clearly established in both humans and experimental animals as the major route of aminoglycoside elimination from the body by means of clearance studies [18, 19]. Binding of aminoglycoside to plasma protein plays only a minor role in restricting ultrafiltration. However, the degree of protein binding may explain conflicting reports and interpretations of studies of net tubular transport of aminoglycoside [20, 21]. Because of their low protein binding and molecular weight, which is less than that of inulin, the glomerular ultrafiltration of aminoglycoside may be assumed to be similar to that of inulin. However, recent in vivo studies [22] have shown an ultrafiltration ratio of about 0.87 for gentamicin and netilmicin— a value similar to that of lysozyme (muramidase), which is a cationic protein of a low molecular weight of 14,000 daltons.

Following filtration, aminoglycosides are excreted rapidly in the urine, predominantly within the first 6 hr after intramuscular administration. In the first 24 hr, the total amount eliminated in the urine represents about 80 to 90% of the administered dose [23]. As mentioned, excretion is even more rapid in the rat. Within 2 hr after administration, we have recovered in the urine 93 ± 3% of a dose of gentamicin (40 mg/kg) given intravenously (Vaamonde et al, unpublished observations).

Once in the tubular lumen, aminoglycosides undergo cellular uptake by the proximal convoluted tubule and the pars recta. Uptake has been demonstrated for gentamicin and netilmicin by means of microinjection and micropuncture studies in the rat [21, 24–26], and by radioautographic experiments in the rat and rabbit [27–29]. In addition, uptake of gentamicin also has been demonstrated in isolated rat renal cortical slices [21, 30, 31], rabbit tubule suspensions [29, 32], and perfused rat kidneys [33]. Thus, the overwhelming evidence supports the net reabsorption of gentamicin along the proximal tubule. Because of this small (but substantial) aminoglycoside uptake, accumulation of these antibiotics in the renal cortex—achieving concentration ratios several-fold higher than those in plasma—has been reported in human kidneys [34–36] and on numerous occasions in experimental animals [36–39]. Accumulation in the renal medulla and papilla is considerably less.

There is also evidence supporting some degree of antiluminal transport of aminoglycoside. For example, in one study, urinary fractional excretion of gentamicin exceeded delivery of the drug to the superficial distal tubule of the rat, suggesting secretion beyond this segment of the nephron [24]. Furthermore, the inability to demonstrate basolateral uptake of gentamicin by the proximal tubule during peritubular capillary injection experiments in Sprague-Dawley rats [21] may have been related to the inaccessibility in this rat strain of deep nephrons to micropuncture techniques. Indeed, Sheth et al [25] recently demonstrated secretion of gentamicin in the Munich-Wistar rat by micropuncture of deep nephrons, which suggests heterogeneity for gentamicin transport in the rat kidney. In the superficial nephrons, reabsorption is the predominant direction of net transport, whereas net secretion predominates in the juxtamedullary nephrons [25]. Although, the overall transport favors net luminal reabsorption for most aminoglycosides, recent evidence points to the possibility that tubular secretion may be important under certain circumstances. Pastoriza-Munoz et al [26] reported that in Sprague-Dawley rats, netilmicin undergoes both net secretion along the early proximal convoluted tubule and net reabsorption along the pars recta. Furthermore, in comparison to gentamicin, the absorptive flux of netilmicin along the proximal tubule was lower, whereas the secretory flux was higher. The authors concluded that these differences in transport rates could explain the reduced renal cortical accumulation of netilmicin and its lower nephrotoxic potential, compared with gentamicin [26]. The relevance of these acute experiments to the clinical or experimental nephrotoxicity developing after more prolonged administration of aminoglycoside remains to be established.

Gentamicin uptake is dependent on continued oxidative energy (it is inhibited by 2,4-dinitrophenol and by anoxia [30]). The renal accumulation of gentamicin, on the other hand, is not altered by probenecid or N-methylnicotinamide [21, 36, 40, 41], which suggests independence from the organic acid and organic base transport systems.

The steps leading to cellular uptake and to accumulation of gentamicin in the proximal tubule have been elucidated by means of autoradiographic studies [27–29]. They are schematically depicted in Figure 1, and can be summarized as follows. The first step is binding of the cationic aminoglycoside to anionic sites on the brushborder membranes of the proximal tubular cells [28, 41]. The anionic binding sites appear to be made up of one or more phospholipid components (predominantly phosphatidylinositol) [9, 42, 43]. During reabsorption, the aminoglycosides compete for these binding sites with filtered cationic proteins, polypeptides, polyamines, polylysines, and amino acids [41]. Transport and subsequent accumulation of gentamicin is reduced by concomitant administration of other aminoglycosides (tobramycin, neomycin, kanamycin, and netilmicin) [26, 36, 44]. Glucose or phlorizin do not affect gentamicin uptake by isolated rabbit renal brushborder membrane vesicles [45], which suggests that the glucose tubular transport system is not involved.

The membrane-bound aminoglycosides are then engulfed by absorptive endocytosis (pinocytosis) into small vesicles that fuse with primary lysosomes. These transfer the aminoglycosides to secondary lysosomes, where storage and digestion occurs. The transfer of aminoglycosides from tubular lumen to secondary lysosomes takes between 30 to 60 min. Within 10 min after radiolabeled gentamicin was injected, radioactivity was demonstrated in apical vesicles of rat proximal tubular cells [28, 33]. The uptake and intracellular accumulation of aminoglycosides in lysosomes has been demonstrated by Tulkens et al [46–48] in cultured rat fibroblasts and renal tubular cells. Uptake via the basolateral membrane of the proximal tubular cells, although generally

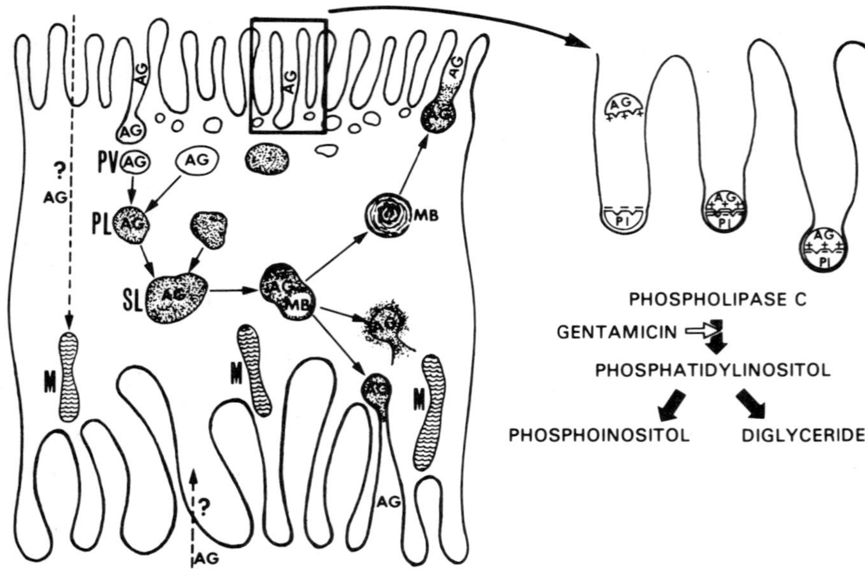

Fig. 1. Possible pathways of aminoglycoside transport and mechanisms of aminoglycoside cellular injury. After binding on brushborder, aminoglycosides (*AG*) are taken up in pinocytotic vesicles (*PV*), which separate from the luminal membrane. These vesicles fuse with primary lysosomes (*PL*), and AG are subsequently transferred to secondary lysosomes (*SL*). The AG may interfere with lysosomal digestion of phospholipids and proteins, inducing formation of myeloid body (*MB*). Later AG labilize lysosomes that may release their lytic content into cytosol or may discharge lysosomal residues outside of the cell via exocytosis. In addition to endocytosis, the existence of other uptake mechanisms at the luminal and contraluminal membrane (*dashed arrows*) may contribute to direct alterations in structure and function of cellular organelles, such as mitochondria (*M*). In the upper right corner, both a schema of the binding of cationic AG with anionic receptors (phosphatidylinositol, *PI*) of the brushborder membrane and subsequent internalization of the AG-membrane receptor complex is shown. On the *lower right corner,* the assumed effect of gentamicin in blocking phospholipase C and in altering the turnover of the membrane-bound receptor is also shown. (Modified from Cojocel and Hook [23] and Feldman, Wang, and Kaloyanides [42])

considered to be a minor route of aminoglycoside cellular penetration, may contribute to the overall renal cortical accumulation of these drugs and to their toxicity [24–26, 31, 36]. Once in the renal tubular cell, it appears that aminoglycosides are in a tightly bound and nonexchangeable pool, which explains the very long half-life in the renal cortex [35, 38] and their ability to bind to homogenates of kidney in vitro [49]. Since these compounds do not undergo metabolism in the renal tubular cells, their elimination is accomplished by exocytosis into the tubular lumen (Fig. 1).

Morphologic Patterns of Aminoglycoside Nephrotoxicity

Aminoglycosides produce acute tubular cell necrosis, largely of the proximal convoluted tubules and pars recta (S_1 and S_2 segments) [35, 50–53]. Although the morphologic changes have been extensively studied in the rat, the findings

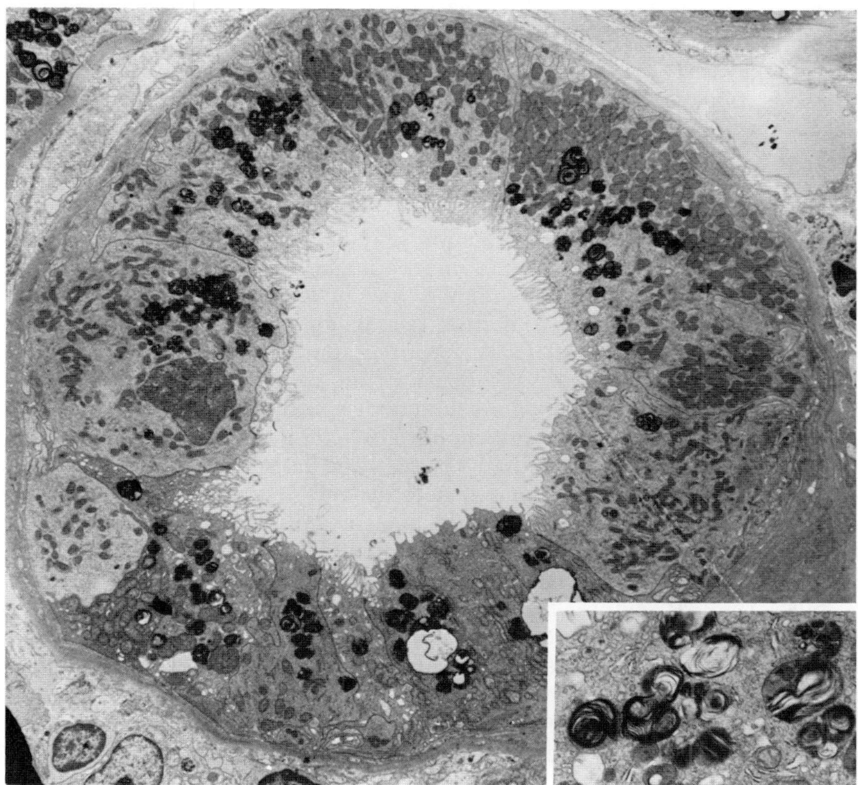

Fig. 2. Electron micrograph obtained from a percutaneous renal biopsy performed in a patient with gentamicin-induced acute renal failure of several days duration. A proximal tubule is shown at low magnification (×6,000). Destruction and disappearance of the brushborder membranes and myeloid bodies are apparent in several cells. Note in the inset (*lower right*), the typical whorled, dark appearance of the myeloid bodies shown at higher magnification (×18,000). (With permission from Victoriano Pardo, M.D., Professor of Pathology, University of Miami School of Medicine)

in human kidneys show the same general pattern (Fig. 2). An increase in the number and size of secondary lysosomes (cytosegrosomes or phagosomes) constitutes the earliest morphologic evidence of toxicity, as shown by electron microscopic studies [50]. In the rat, these changes are seen 48 hr after gentamicin administration; they may extend in late toxicity to the distal tubule [50]. However, they have been shown to be present in human renal biopsy specimens obtained 4 hr after administration of gentamicin in patients with normal renal function [54]. These cytosegrosomes are primary lysosomes that have fused with endocytic or autophagic vacuoles. Many of these secondary lysosomes contain myeloid bodies (Fig. 2), which are characteristic electron-dense lamellar structures of a 5-nm periodic pattern of [54] concentrically arranged and densely packed membranes. These lysosomal alterations, including the formation of myeloid bodies, do not necessarily imply aminoglycoside toxicity; rather, they imply that the person or animal under study has been exposed to these compounds. Furthermore, they are not specific, since many other toxins are capable of inducing their formation [55]. Myeloid bodies probably represent autophagic vacuoles that result from sequestration of membrane and organelle fragments damaged during cellular handling of naturally occurring compounds or potential toxins (aminoglycosides), and that are undergoing lysosomal processing and digestion [55].

Following the initial lysosomal morphologic alterations of the proximal tubular cells, a decrease in the number and height of the microvillae of the brushborder membranes, cytoplasmic vacuolization, and dilatation of the endoplasmic reticulum appear [52]. Depending on the intensity of the lesions, various cellular debris begin to appear in the tubular lumina: brushborder membrane fragments, extruded myeloid bodies, membrane vesicles, and cytoplasmic debris. At this time, mitochondrial swelling becomes prominent; and, as cellular injury evolves, initially patchy and later extensive (particularly in animal experiments) tubular cell necrosis and desquamation with tubular obstruction becomes apparent. By light and transmission electron microscopy, the distal tubules and glomeruli of experimental animals and humans exhibit little change [50, 52, 56].

Since vascular endothelial cells contain negatively charged binding sites and are capable of endocytosis, it is conceivable that glomerular cells may incorporate aminoglycosides [23]. However, the radioautographic studies available [28] do not support this assumption. More recently, with the advent of scanning electron microscopy, considerable interest has been generated by reports suggesting that structural alterations of the glomerular endothelial cells may play a causative role in the development of renal dysfunction in ischemic and nephrotoxic acute renal failure in humans and animals [57–59]. Scanning electron microscopy studies have revealed both decreases in the size and area of endothelial fenestrae and swelling of endothelial cells following experimental aminoglycoside nephrotoxicity [60–62]. However, more recent quantitative investigations [63] have cast some doubt on these earlier findings. Thus, the presumptive role of the glomerular endothelium in the early pathogenesis of gentamicin-induced acute renal failure remains unresolved.

Risk Factors in Aminoglycoside Nephrotoxicity

In assessing the frequency of nephrotoxicity, it is clear that most renal injury tends to cluster around certain patients and specific clinical situations. Because nephrotoxicity may limit the clinical usefulness of aminoglycosides, recognition of factors associated with a greater risk for renal injury is important [1, 64]. These risk factors are listed in Table 1.

Patient-related Factors

Age

Advanced age often has been suggested as a risk factor for aminoglycoside toxicity in retrospective studies [65, 66]. Because muscle mass declines with age and the endogenous creatinine clearance (C_{cr}) depends on creatinine production by muscle, it follows that a normal serum creatinine concentration in an elderly patient may reflect a much lower clearance than in a young patient with an identical serum concentration. Not taking into consideration the patient's age (and body size) will result in a tendency to overdose older

Table 1. Risk factors in aminoglycoside nephrotoxicity

Patient-related factors	
Age[a]	Potassium depletion
Prior renal insufficiency[a]	Magnesium depletion
Dehydration and volume depletion[b]	
Drug-related factors	
Inherent nephrotoxic potential[b]	
Dose[b]	
Duration and frequency of administration[b]	
Drug interactions (drugs with a synergistic effect on aminoglycoside nephrotoxicity)	
Synergism strongly supported[b]	
Cephalothin	
Cyclosporin A	
Probable association (unproven synergism)	
Cis-platin	Methoxyflurane
Other cephalosporins	Loop diuretics[c]
Nonsteroidal anti-inflammatory agents	Amino acids
Unproven factors	
Sex	Prior aminoglycoside exposure
Metabolic acidosis	Renal transplants

[a] Secondary to overdosing.
[b] Most important clinically.
[c] Secondary to volume depletion.

patients. Indeed, two prospective studies using serum aminoglycoside levels as dosage guides have found no significant relationship between nephrotoxicity and age [66, 67]. In addition, because older patients have a lower C_{cr} for each value of serum creatinine, they will be more likely to show an increase in serum creatinine after a renal injury than will younger patients [64]. Therefore, Smith and Smith [64] have concluded that the false assumption that age itself is a risk factor for aminoglycosides is due to: (1) failure to use appropriate control groups, (2) overdosing of elderly patients based on serum creatinine levels, (3) failure to measure serum aminoglycoside levels, and (4) bias in ascribing nephrotoxicity caused by use of serum creatinine increases, rather than percent changes in C_{cr}, as the definition of toxicity.

Prior Renal Insufficiency

The evidence supporting prior renal insufficiency as a risk factor is also flawed by methodologic problems [64]. Since excretion of gentamicin is very closely related to the glomerular filtration rate (GFR), the same considerations discussed above apply to patients with pre-existent renal failure. Thus, unless aminoglycoside serum levels are used to adjust dosage, these patients are prone to overdosage. Although there are studies reporting a greater likelihood of increases in serum creatinine during aminoglycoside treatment in patients with pre-existent renal disease [65, 66], three prospective studies could not find an increased risk with prior renal insufficiency [68–70].

Dehydration and Volume Contraction

Bennett et al [71] demonstrated that a low-sodium diet markedly increased gentamicin nephrotoxicity in the rat. This nephrotoxic potentiation was attributed to a higher renal cortical accumulation of gentamicin [71–73]. Other investigators have found increased renal dysfunction with intravascular volume depletion [74] or diuretic-induced natriuresis [73]; or, they suggested that chloride, rather than sodium, depletion is important [75]. High sodium intake [71], deoxycorticosterone acetate (DOCA)-saline or furosemide-induced sodium chloride diuresis [76], or sodium bicarbonate administration [77, 78] failed to produce a functional or morphologic protective effect. The importance of volume depletion (usually diuretic-induced) was also demonstrated in a prospective clinical study [69]. A 46% incidence of aminoglycoside nephrotoxicity was found in patients with volume depletion, as compared with a 6% incidence in those without volume contraction ($P < 0.005$).

Potassium and Magnesium Depletion

Potassium and magnesium depletion have been suggested as risk factors for experimental aminoglycoside nephrotoxicity [79–81]. Since the clinical counterpart of these findings is not known, it seems prudent to maintain normal body stores of these cations in patients receiving aminoglycosides.

Drug-related Factors

The type of aminoglycoside prescribed, the dose, duration of treatment, and frequency of administration are the most important determinants of aminoglycoside-induced nephrotoxicity.

Inherent Nephrotoxic Potential of Aminoglycosides (Comparative Nephrotoxicity)

The factors determining the different nephrotoxic potential of aminoglycosides are incompletely understood, but they may relate to their intrinsic characteristics, degree of renal cortical accumulation, or other unknown factors. The former include: (1) the number, charge orientation, or position of the NH_2^+ groups [9], (2) an inherent propensity of the aminoglycoside molecule to cause toxic injury to intracellular organelles independent of the renal cortical levels [6, 16], and (3) different transport rates for reabsorption and secretion in different nephron populations [24, 25] or nephronal segments [26].

Comparative Nephrotoxicity

Smith and Lietman [82] have summarized data from 24 prospective, controlled clinical trials reported in the British literature since 1969. The value of the majority of the studies is limited by failure to: (1) use a standard dosage and duration of therapy, (2) evaluate toxicity in an unbiased manner, (3) define nephrotoxicity uniformly, (4) frequently monitor renal function during and after therapy, (5) differentiate patients with other causes of acute renal failure from those with aminoglycoside-induced nephrotoxicity, and (6) enroll sufficient numbers of patients to draw meaningful conclusions.

Clinical comparisons have shown that tobramycin has the same or a lower toxicity than gentamicin [83–85]. Smith et al [85] reported that nephrotoxicity occurred in 26% of patients treated with gentamicin, but in only 13% of patients receiving similar dosages of tobramycin ($P < 0.025$). Sisomicin [82] and amikacin have no greater nephrotoxicity than gentamicin [65, 86], whereas netilmicin appears to have toxicity similar to that of tobramycin [82, 87].

A summary of the relative experimental aminoglycoside nephrotoxicities in rats derived from several studies [16, 53, 61, 88–91] reveals the following rank order (from most to least): neomycin > gentamicin > sisomicin, kamamycin, and amikacin > tobramycin > netilmicin > streptomycin. The different results observed between some clinical and animal studies of comparative nephrotoxicity, such as those of tobramycin versus netilmicin, may be explained by the different species analyzed or by the rat strain used (the Fischer 344 rat being more sensitive to aminoglycoside).

It is apparent that (except for streptomycin) the degree of drug accumulation in the renal cortex does not correlate consistently with the differences in nephrotoxic potential of aminoglycosides. However, it is necessary to consider that in many studies, renal cortical aminoglycoside levels were measured a few or several days after commencing aminoglycoside administration; thus, cellular necrosis and regeneration may have interfered with the measurements. Furthermore, it is conceivable that the very initial cortical aminoglycoside concentration may be of crucial importance in determining cellular injury.

Dose

A strong correlation between the daily and total aminoglycoside dose and toxicity has been easily and consistently demonstrated in animal experiments [16, 88, 92, 93]. Clinical studies using doses lower than 3 mg/kg/d for gentamicin or tobramycin demonstrated a clear relationship between dose and nephrotoxicity [64, 94]. Negative reports have corrected the aminoglycoside dosage according to increased blood levels [68, 86]. At higher dosages (> 4.5 mg/kg/d), such as those used to treat severe sepsis, the correlation has not been as good—perhaps, because the dose-response curve for toxicity is relatively flat in this dosage range or because of other confounding clinical events [64].

Duration and Frequency of Administration

Clinical studies have established that duration of therapy, usually beyond 10 days, is a risk factor for aminoglycoside nephrotoxicity [64, 68]. Although a threshold duration of therapy has not been defined before which aminoglycoside nephrotoxicity does not occur, renal damage is unusual before 5 to 6 days of treatment. Animal studies have clearly established an increased toxicity with frequent administration of aminoglycoside [95, 96]. However, the relationship between frequency of administration and nephrotoxicity has not yet been appropriately evaluated in patients [64]. For any given aminoglycoside, a relationship between dose, serum levels, and renal tissue concentrations has been suggested by Schentag et al [18, 97] and others [94] as accounting for individual patient differences in susceptibility to nephrotoxicity. However, this attractive hypothesis remains to be conclusively proven.

Aminoglycoside Drug Interactions

Many drugs with potential nephrotoxicities of their own are used in combination with aminoglycosides and other antibacterials, particularly in very ill patients (Table 1). These may produce added or increased (synergism) nephrotoxicity. Methoxyflurane [98], cis-platin [99], amphotericin B [100], clindamycin [101], cephalosporins other than cephalotin (for example, methicillin or cephaloridine) [102] all have been reported as adding to the nephrotoxicity of aminoglycoside; but, they appear not to exhibit a synergistic action.

Concomitant use of radiographic contrast agents also should be suspected until proven to be unrelated. Loop diuretics increased nephrotoxicity in animal studies [73, 75, 103]; two clinical studies, however, could not find augmented toxicity [68, 69]. Nevertheless, because of the effect of volume contraction on aminoglycoside nephrotoxicity [71–73], it is necessary to use them carefully. Inhibition of prostaglandin synthesis with indomethacin increased aminoglycoside-induced nephrotoxicity in the rat, which suggests the possibility of a protective role for prostaglandins in this model [104]. The consequences of giving nonsteroidal anti-inflammatory drugs (NSAIDs) to patients treated concomitantly with aminoglycosides are not known.

There is convincing clinical evidence that cephalotin in combination with aminoglycoside causes nephrotoxicity [64, 66, 102]. This was not seen when the combination was used in patients with mild infections [105]. In experimental animals, cephalotin did not influence [106] or protect from aminoglycoside nephrotoxicity [107, 108]. It has recently been reported that significant renal failure can occur when gentamicin and cyclosporin A are used together in patients with bone marrow transplants [109]. When the two drugs were given simultaneously to rats, cyclosporin A induced a synergistic enhancement of gentamicin nephrotoxicity [110].

Unproven Factors

Sex

Gentamicin nephrotoxicity is greater in male rats than in females of the Fischer 344 strain [111]. In the same strain of rat, gentamicin-induced acute tubular necrosis in males and acute tubulointerstitial infiltration in females [112]. We have been unable to confirm these observations in the Sprague-Dawley rat [113]. One prospective clinical study found no sex-related influences [68], while another reported a higher incidence in women [70].

Other

There is no conclusive clinical evidence that metabolic acidosis [114], prior aminoglycoside exposure or nephrotoxicity [64], and renal transplantation per se [64] constitute risk factors. Further work is necessary to confirm the finding that concomitant administration of cationic amino acids to rabbits results in enhanced aminoglycoside nephrotoxicity [115]. The implications for patients receiving hyperalimentation and aminoglycosides are obvious.

Clinical Aspects of Aminoglycoside Nephrotoxicity

The clinical features of aminoglycoside nephrotoxicity have been well characterized in humans and animals, and they are summarized in Table 2. Usually, there is a mild elevation of blood urea nitrogen (BUN) or creatinine accompanied by a normal urine output or frank nonoliguric acute renal failure. The beginning commonly is gradual, and the syndrome may only become apparent at the end of, or after, discontinuation of therapy. The course may be pro-

Table 2. Clinical and renal functional features of aminoglycoside nephrotoxicity

Clinical features
  Normal or high urine output (most common); oliguria is rare
  Gradual onset
  Protracted course
  Reversible
  Blood (↑ BUN, ↑ creatinine, rarely hypokalemia, hypomagnesemia, hypocalcemia)
  Urine (hypo-osmolality, ↑ fractional excretion of Na^+ [not always if polyuria is present], ↑
    cylindruria, ↑ cellular debris, myeloid bodies)

Renal functional abnormalities
  Decreased RBF with preservation of intrarenal flow distribution
  Decreased GFR
    Degree: mild: ↓ GFR without serum abnormalities (most common)
            modest-moderate: ↑ BUN, ↑ creatinine with nonoliguric acute renal failure
              (common)
            severe: oliguric acute renal failure (rare)
  Tubular transport defects
    Enzymuria (brushborder membranes and lysosomal enzymes: early)
    Transport defects
      Low mol wt proteinuria (β-2 microglobulin, muramidase) and aminoaciduria
      Glycosuria, K^+ and Mg^{++} wasting
      Altered uptake of organic acid and bases (renal cortical slices: p-aminohippurate,
        N-methylnicotinamide)
      Decreased concentrating ability (nephrogenic diabetes insipidus)

longed, particularly in the elderly patient. The vast majority of patients do
recover. The presence of risk factors may alter the clinical presentation or
its course, which tends to shorten the time sequence. The earliest urinary
manifestation is the appearance of enzymuria; it is detectable within 24 hr
of a single therapeutic dose of aminoglycoside [116, 117]. The enzymuria
represents fragments of brushborder membrane enzymes (for example, ala-
nine-aminopeptidase or γ-glutamyl transferase) or lysosomal enzymes (for
example, acid phosphatase, N-acetyl-β-D-glucosaminidase [116–118]. The
practical usefulness of measuring enzymuria as an early marker of tubular
damage has not yet been established.

Other evidence of proximal tubular dysfunction may be present in aminoglycoside renal damage. There is urinary wasting of sodium, potassium, magnesium, phosphorus, amino acids, glucose, and low-molecular weight proteins
(β-2 microglobulin, muramidase [lysosymuria]) in some patients [4, 6, 79].
A full Fanconi syndrome can occur rarely [119]. Hypomagnesemia and hypocalcemia may be secondary to depressed parathyroid hormone (PTH) secretion or to skeletal resistance to PTH due to the hypomagnesemia [120,
121].

The gentamicin-induced renal concentrating defect has been the subject
of many studies. The polyuria is associated with urinary hypo-osmolality
[50, 118]; it is vasopressin-resistant [122, 123], with elevated postdehydration
vasopressin levels [124]. A recent micropuncture study in the rat has shown
that the concentrating defect is associated with decreased reabsorption by

the superficial proximal tubule (probably secondary to impaired solute reabsorption) and papillary collecting ducts (secondary to the decreased papillary osmolality) [125]. Another study concluded that the decreased solute reabsorption in the proximal tubule was due to impaired reclamation of bicarbonate, with this anion acting as a poorly reabsorbed solute in the loop of Henle [126]. Urinary excretion of prostaglandin E_2 (PGE_2) has been shown to increase before the appearance of impaired concentrating ability in dogs treated with gentamicin [127]. Indomethacin failed to improve urinary concentration, suggesting that the concentrating defect is PGE_2-independent [124]. In vitro studies have shown gentamicin-induced impairment of water flux in the toad bladder preparation [128].

Pathogenesis of Aminoglycoside Nephrotoxicity

Considerable advancement in the understanding of the pathophysiology of aminoglycoside nephrotoxicity has been made in recent years.

Renal Hemodynamics

Rats that were given gentamicin and were studied with the microsphere technique showed a decreased renal blood flow (RBF), with relatively preserved outer cortical flow [122]. The gentamicin-induced impairment in GFR was primarily mediated by a decrease in the glomerular capillary ultrafiltration coefficient (K_f) of superficial nephrons, rather than by the decreased RBF [56]. The change in K_f was documented 10 days after gentamicin was begun, and it was not accompanied by alterations of glomerular endothelial cells [56]. In the study of Bayliss et al [56], there was an almost complete recovery of inulin microinjected into the tubules, thus minimizing the possibility of a tubular leak of filtrate as a possible cause for the decreased GFR. Intratubular obstruction may be partly responsible for the fall in single-nephron (SNGFR) and total GFR [129] in severe experimental gentamicin nephrotoxicity. Lowering the elevated intratubular pressure improved the depressed SNGFR [129]. Although the histologic evidence of enhanced tubular debris and cast formation favors a pathogenetic role for obstruction, at least at some time along the course of gentamicin nephrotoxicity, it is unclear what role (if any) obstruction may have at the inception of tubular injury.

What causes the decrease of K_f in gentamicin nephrotoxicity is not known. However, it is possible that locally released angiotensin II may mediate—via vasoconstriction—these changes, since administration of the angiotensin-converting enzyme inhibitor, captopril, significantly blunted the decrease of K_f caused by gentamicin [130]. The available evidence suggests that the observed renal hemodynamic changes are not early manifestations of aminoglycoside toxicity, but are events secondary to primary cellular changes occurring in the proximal tubule.

Cellular Mechanisms of Aminoglycoside Toxicity

The final pathway(s) by which aminoglycosides cause tubular cell necrosis remain to be established, but major cellular targets for their action are the plasma membranes, the lysosomes, and the mitochondria. Changes in both the integrity and function of these cellular structures have been described as associated with aminoglycoside treatment, and they undoubtedly are key factors in the pathophysiologic events leading to cellular toxicity.

The luminal binding and transport of aminoglycosides already have been reviewed. Increases in total phospholipid content and in selected phosphoinositides, particularly phosphatidylinositol (PI), have been described in the rat renal cortex after treatment with gentamicin [42, 43, 131]. Similar results were obtained in cultured rat fibroblasts and in rat and human renal tubular cells [46–48, 54, 131]. Subcellular fractionation studies of rat renal cortex have shown that the increase in PI produced by gentamicin involved multiple cell membranes, including mitochondria, brushborder, endoplasmic reticulum, and lysosomes [132]. The mechanism of the increase in PI levels is not entirely elucidated, but it has been attributed to an inhibition of phospholipases A and C [133, 134]. Aminoglycoside inhibited a PI phospholipase C found in the 100,000g supernatant of homogenized renal cortex [133]. Furthermore, Hostetler and Hall [134] demonstrated aminoglycoside inhibition of phospholipases A and C that were obtained from lysosomes isolated from the rat kidney cortex. Indeed, it has recently been shown that gentamicin induces a pH-dependent, Ca^{++}-independent inhibition of the specific phospholipase C for brushborder membrane PI [135]. Comparative inhibition of these phospholipases by other aminoglycosides approximated their known toxicities [133, 135].

Aminoglycosides are typical "lysosomotropic agents" [136]; that is, agents that are taken up in lysosomes either by pinocytosis or by any other mechanism. These agents may stay within the lysosomes and may act either by altering the lysosomal content or the lysosomal ability to degrade engulfed substances, thus inducing lysosomal storage disorders. They also may alter the properties of the lysosomal membrane, thus inducing either an increase or decrease in its permeability toward exogenous substrates or even to lysosomal enzymes, which may cause cell injury by escaping the organelle. Gentamicin inhibits lysosomal enzymes (sphingomyelinase and phospholipases A_1 and C), which are responsible for the early steps in the catabolism of phospholipids and lead to accumulation of all major phosphoinositides [46–48, 131, 133–135]. Morphologically, these changes are translated into the formation of myeloid bodies (Fig. 2). Thus, the concept of gentamicin toxicity has evolved as a lysosomal phospholipidosis or lysosomal overloading phenomena, which is an early manifestation of aminoglycoside cellular damage [42, 46–48]. In addition, as summarized by Feldman et al (Fig. 1) [42], it appears that within the lysosomes, aminoglycosides might interfere with the catabolism of the membrane receptor by directly inhibiting phospholipase C, by modifying substrate-enzyme affinity, or by increasing the intralysosomal pH above the range of the enzyme. The relation of the AG-induced renal phospholipidosis to cellular dysfunction and necrosis remains unresolved. It is possible that labilization or rupture of the lipid-overloaded lysosomes, with release of potent lysosomal hydrolases into the cytosol, or depletion of critical substrates due to suppressed lysosomal catabolism may be responsible for ultimate cellular damage and death [42].

Other mechanisms of injury are also possible, since membrane phospholipids are involved in regulating membrane permeability to calcium [137]. Calcium acts as an effective competitive inhibitor of the gentamicin-membrane receptor interaction [9]. In this context, oral calcium loading significantly decreases gentamicin nephrotoxicity in the intact rat [9, 138]. This finding appears to be specific for aminoglycosides, since calcium loading does not confer protection against mercuric chloride-induced acute renal failure [139]. Furthermore, it is not due to hypercalciuria itself [140, 141]; and, it appears to be independent of PTH suppression [142]. Parathyroidectomy by itself also ameliorates gentamicin renal injury [142]. Likewise, phosphate depletion attenuates gentamicin nephrotoxicity in the rat [141]. The latter effect was independent of alterations in serum calcium, hypercalciuria, and renal cortical gentamicin concentration, but it may have been influenced by low protein intake.

Gentamicin exerts a direct inhibitory effect on renal cortical mitochondrial oxidative phosphorylation in vitro [11, 143]. Mitochondrial dysfunction also occurs during gentamicin nephrotoxicity in vivo before functional or morphologic evidence of severe renal damage appears [144]. Furthermore, gentamicin was found to be a competitive inhibitor of mitochondrial Ca^{++} uptake [145]. This indicates the potential for aminoglycosides to alter membrane function and, thereby, to contribute to toxic cell injury through its interaction with divalent cations.

Studies of renal cortex ion composition in dogs treated with gentamicin showed an early cellular depletion of potassium, magnesium, and phosphorus [146], which may partly explain the potassium and magnesium wasting seen in this animal model [79]. In a latter phase, sodium and calcium content were increased and the activity of Na-K-ATPase fell [146].

We have recently examined the hypothesis that phosphoinositides function as luminal membrane receptors for aminoglycosides in an animal model that was characterized by resistance to gentamicin nephrotoxicity [147]. We have demonstrated that the Sprague-Dawley rat with untreated streptozotocin-induced diabetes mellitus is functionally and morphologically protected from gentamicin-induced acute renal failure [148, 149]. This resistance was associated with a decreased accumulation of gentamicin by the renal cortex [148]; and, it was present as early as 5 days after induction of the experimental diabetes [150]. Furthermore, it was not related to high urine flow or to solute excretion rates, since rats with hereditary diabetes insipidus [148] or with renal glycosuria induced by phlorizin [151] were unprotected from gentamicin. Treatment of the diabetes with insulin resulted in elimination of the protective effect [152]. These studies led us to propose this animal model as being useful for the study of mechanisms of induction and prevention from gentamicin nephrotoxicity [153]. Other investigators have also recently confirmed, in the rat, the protection afforded by untreated diabetes against gentamicin renal injury [154].

The resistant, untreated diabetic rats that were injected with gentamicin at a dose of 100 mg/kg/d for 2 days had renal cortical PI levels that were significantly lower than those of equally injected nondiabetic animals [147]. Moreover, the renal cortex PI content in the diabetic animals was lower even before gentamicin administration [147], which was in accordance with the abnormalities of inositol metabolism described in diabetes [155]. Most importantly, and as predicted from the initial assumption, the nondiabetic glycosuric animals (phlorizin model [151]) and the insulin-treated diabetic rats [152] exhibited normal PI renal cortical levels; and, they were unprotected from the gentamicin nephrotoxic effects. These observations are consistent with the hypothesis that the lower content of phosphoinositides, particularly PI, limits the apical membrane binding and subsequent intracellular transport of gentamicin; this results in lower renal cortical accumulation and prevention of aminoglycoside nephrotoxicity in this animal model.

The intriguing observation that recovery from aminoglycoside nephrotoxicity occurs with continued drug administration remains unexplained [156, 157], but it may be related to the resistance displayed by newly regenerated tubular cells to aminoglycoside toxic effects.

Some of the important questions related to aminoglycoside nephrotoxicity that remain unresolved at this time, and thus require further investigation, are what is: (1) the comparative contribution of apical versus basolateral aminoglycoside uptake to transport and nephrotoxicity? (2) the comparative contribution of dysfunction of the various cellular organelles to the overall aminoglycoside toxicity? (3) the role of calcium and of phosphate depletion? (4) the ultimate cause of cell injury and death? (5) the nature and pathway(s) of the cellular signal(s) that mediate glomerular vasoconstriction, impaired GFR, and acute renal failure? (6) the mechanism(s) of the resistance displayed by newly regenerated tubular cells to toxicity? and (7) the mechanism(s) of the observed differences in nephrotoxicity exhibited by the various aminoglycosides?

Acknowledgments. This work was supported by designated research funds from the Veterans Administration and the Kidney Foundation of South Florida.

References

1. APPEL GB, NEU HC: The nephrotoxicity of antimicrobial agents (three parts). *N Engl J Med* 296:663–670, 722–728, 784–787, 1977
2. PORTER GA, BENNETT WM: Nephrotoxic acute renal failure due to common drugs. *Am J Physiol* 241:F1–F8, 1981
3. FILLASTRE J-P: *Nephrotoxicity. Interactions of Drugs with Membranes Systems: Mitochondria-Lysosomes.* New York and Paris, Masson Pub Inc, USA, 1978
4. APPEL GB, NEU HC: Gentamicin in 1978. *Ann Intern Med* 89:528–538, 1978
5. CRONIN RE: Aminoglycoside nephrotoxicity: pathogenesis and prevention. *Clin Nephrol* 11:251–256, 1979
6. KALOYANIDES GJ, PASTORIZA-MUNOZ E: Aminoglycoside nephrotoxicity. *Kidney Int* 18:571–582, 1980

7. WHELTON A, NEU HC: *The Aminoglycosides. Microbiology, Clinical Use, and Toxicology.* New York, Marcel Dekker, 1982
8. FILLASTRE J-P: *Nephrotoxicity, Ototoxicity of Drugs.* Rouen, Editions Inserm, 1982
9. HUMES HD, WEINBERG JM, KNAUSS TC: Clinical and pathophysiologic aspects of aminoglycoside nephrotoxicity. *Am J Kidney Dis* 2:5–29, 1982
10. PHILLIPS I: Aminoglycosides. *Lancet* 2:311–314, 1982
11. WEINBERG JM, SIMMONS CF JR, HUMES HD: Alterations of mitochondrial respiration induced by aminoglycoside antibiotics. *Res Comm Chem Path Pharmacol* 27:521–531, 1980
12. SIMMONS CF JR, RENNKE HG, HUMES HD: Acute renal failure induced by diethylaminoethyl dextran: Importance of cationic charge. *Kidney Int* 19:424–430, 1981
13. ROSENTHAL SM, FISHER ER, STOHLMAN EF: Nephrotoxic action of spermine. *Proc Soc Exp Biol Med* 80:432–434, 1952
14. TABOR H, TABOR CW: Spermidine, spermine and related amines. *Pharmacol Rev* 16:245–300, 1964
15. MAMELAK M, WISSIG SL, BOGOROCH R, EDELMAN IS: Physiological and morphological effects of poly-L-lysine on the toad bladder. *J Membr Biol* 1:144–176, 1969
16. SOBERON L, BOWMAN RL, PASTORIZA-MUNOZ E, KALOYANIDES GJ: Comparative nephrotoxicities of gentamicin, netilmicin and tobramycin in the rat. *J Pharmacol Exp Ther* 210:334–343, 1979
17. DITTERT IW: Pharmacokinetics of aminoglycosides: general considerations. *Am J Med* 70:77–83, 1977
18. SCHENTAG JJ, JUSKO WJ: Renal clearance and tissue accumulation of gentamicin. *Clin Pharmacol Ther* 22:364–370, 1977
19. CHIU PJ, BROWN A, MILLER G, LONG JF: Renal excretion of gentamicin in anesthetized dogs. *Antimicrob Agents Chemother* 10:277–282, 1976
20. MYERS DR, DEFEHR J, BENNETT WM, PORTER GA, OLSEN GD: Gentamicin binding to serum and plasma proteins. *Clin Pharmacol Ther* 23:356–360, 1978
21. PASTORIZA-MUNOZ E, BOWMAN RL, KALOYANIDES GJ: Renal tubular transport in the rat. *Kidney Int* 16:440–450, 1979
22. PASTORIZA-MUNOZ E, TIMMERMAN D, FELDMAN S, KALOYANIDES GJ: Ultrafilterability of gentamicin and netilmicin *in vivo. J Pharmacol Exp Ther* 220:604–608, 1982
23. COJOCEL C, HOOK JB: Aminoglycoside nephrotoxicity. *Trends Pharmacol Sci* 4:174–179, 1983
24. SENEKJIAN HO, KNIGHT TF, WEINMAN EJ: Micropuncture study of the handling of gentamicin by the rat kidney. *Kidney Int* 19:416–423, 1981
25. SHETH AU, SENEKJIAN HO, BABINO H, KNIGHT TF, WEINMAN EJ: Renal handling of gentamicin by the Munich-Wistar rat. *Am J Physiol* 10:F645–F648, 1981
26. PASTORIZA-MUNOZ E, TIMMERMAN D, KALOYANIDES GJ: Renal transport of netilmicin in the rat. *J Pharmacol Exp Ther* 228:65–72, 1984
27. JUST M, ERDMANN G, HABERMAN E: The renal handling of polybasic drugs. I. gentamicin and aprotinin in intact animals. *Naunyn-Schniedeberg's Arch Pharmacol* 300:57–66, 1977
28. SILVERBLATT FJ, KUEHN C: Autoradiography of gentamicin uptake by the rat proximal tubule cell. *Kidney Int* 15:535–545, 1979
29. VANDEWALLE A, FARMAN N, MORIN J-P, HATT P-Y, BONVALET J-P: Genta-

micin incorporation along the nephron: autoradiographic study on isolated tubules. *Kidney Int* 19:529–539, 1981

30. HSU CH, KURTZ TW, WELLER EJ: In vitro uptake of gentamicin by rat cortical tissue. *Antimicrob Agents Chemother* 12:192–194, 1977
31. KLUWE WM, HOOK JB: Analysis of gentamicin uptake by rat renal cortical slices. *Toxicol Appl Pharmacol* 45:531–539, 1978
32. BARZA M, MURPHY T, HAMBURGER RJ: Uptake of gentamicin by separated viable renal tubules from rabbits. *J Infect Dis* 141:510–517, 1980
33. COLLIER VU, LIETMAN PS, MITCH WE: Evidence for luminal uptake of gentamicin in the perfused rat kidney. *J Pharmacol Exp Ther* 210:247–251, 1979
34. EDWARDS CQ, SMITH CR, BAUGHMAN KL, ROGERS GF, LIETMAN PF: Concentrations of gentamicin and amikacin in human kidneys. *Antimicrob Agents Chemother* 9:925–927, 1976
35. LUFT FC, YUM MN, WALKER PD, KLEIT SA: Gentamicin gradient patterns and morphologic changes in human kidneys. *Nephron* 18:167–174, 1977
36. BENNETT WM, PLAMP CE, ELLIOTT WC, PARKER RA, PORTER GA: Effect of basic amino acids and aminoglycosides of ³H-gentamicin uptake in cortical slices of rat and human kidney. *J Lab Clin Med* 99:156–162, 1982
37. LUFT CF, KLEIT SA: Renal parenchymal accumulation of aminoglycoside antibiotics in rats. *J Infect Dis* 130:656–659, 1974
38. FABRE J, RUDHART M, BLANCHARD P, REGAMEY C: Persistence of sisomicin and gentamicin in renal cortex and medulla compared with other organs and serum in rats. *Kidney Int* 10:444–449, 1976
39. WHELTON A: Renal tubular transport and intrarenal aminoglycoside distribution, in *The Aminoglycosides. Microbiology, Clinical Use, and Toxicology,* edited by WHELTON A, NEU HC, New York, Marcel Dekker, 1982, pp 191–222
40. BERGANT T, WESTLIE L, BRODWALL EK: Influence of probenecid on gentamicin pharmacokinetics. *Acta Med Scand* 191:221–224, 1972
41. JUST M, HABERMANN E: The renal handling of polybasic drugs. 2. In vitro studies with brush border and lysosomal preparations. *Naunyn-Schmiedeberg's Arch Pharmacol* 300:67–76, 1977
42. FELDMAN S, WANG M-Y, KALOYANIDES GJ: Aminoglycosides induce phospholipidosis in the renal cortex of the rat: an early manifestation of nephrotoxicity. *J Pharmacol Exp Ther* 220:514–520, 1982
43. SASTRASINH M, KNAUSS TC, WEINBERG JM, HUMES HD: Identification of the aminoglycoside binding site in rat renal brush border membranes. *J Pharmacol Exp Ther* 222:350–358, 1982
44. KUO C-H, HOOK JB: Specificity of gentamicin accumulation by rat renal cortex. *Life Sci* 25:873–878, 1979
45. LIPSKY JJ, CHENG L, SACKTOR B, LIETMAN PS: Gentamicin uptake by renal tubule brush border membrane vesicles. *J Pharmacol Exp Ther* 215:390–393, 1980
46. TULKENS P, TROUET A: The uptake and intracellular accumulation of aminoglycoside antibiotics in lysosomes of cultured fibroblasts. *Biochem Pharmacol* 27:415–424, 1978
47. TULKENS P: The lysosomal toxicity of gentamicin: a short review, in *Nephrotoxicity, Ototoxicity of Drugs,* edited by FILLASTRE J-P, Rouen, Editions Inserm, 1982, pp 435–443
48. TULKENS P, AUBERT-TULKENS G, VAN HOFF F, TROUET A: The lysosomal toxicity of aminoglycosides, in *Nephrotoxicity: Interaction of Drugs with Membrane Systems: Mitochondria-Lysosomes,* edited by FILLASTRE J-P, New York and Paris, Masson Pub Inc, USA, 1978, pp 231–251

49. KUNIN CM: Binding of antibiotics to tissue homogenates. *J Infect Dis* 121:55–64, 1970
50. KOSEK JC, MAZZE RI, COUSINS MJ: Nephrotoxicity of gentamicin. *Lab Invest* 30:48–57, 1974
51. WELLWOOD JM, LOVELL D, THOMPSON AE, TIGHE JR: Renal damage caused by gentamicin: A study of the effects on renal morphology and urinary enzyme excretion. *J Pathol* 118:171–182, 1976
52. HOUGHTON DC, HARTNETT M, CAMPBELL-BOSWELL M, PORTER GA, BENNETT WM: A light and electron microscopic analysis of gentamicin nephrotoxicity in rats. *Am J Pathol* 82:589–612, 1976
53. HOUGHTON DC, PLAMP CE, DeFEHR JM, BENNETT WM, PORTER GA, GILBERT D: Gentamicin and tobramycin nephrotoxicity. *Am J Pathol* 93:137–152, 1978
54. DeBROE ME, PAULUS GJ, VERPOOTEN GA, ROELS, F, DePREST B, VANHOFF F, TULKENS P, BUYSSENS N: Nephrotoxicity of gentamicin in humans, in *Nephrotoxicity, Ototoxicity of Drugs,* edited by FILLASTRE J-P, Rouen, Editions Inserm, 1982, pp 147–165
55. HRUBAN Z, SLESSERS A, HOPKINS E: Drug induced and naturally occurring myeloid bodies. *Lab Invest* 27:62–70, 1972
56. BAYLIS C, RENNKE HR, BRENNER BM: Mechanisms of the defect in glomerular ultrafiltration associated with gentamicin administration. *Kidney Int* 12:344–353, 1977
57. SOLEZ KL, RACUSEN LC, WHELTON A: Glomerular epithelial cell changes in early postischemic acute renal failure in rabbits and man. *Am J Pathol* 103:163–173, 1981
58. WILLIAMS RH, THOMAS CE, NAVAR LG, EVAN AP: Hemodynamic and single nephron function during the maintenance phase of ischemic acute renal failure in the dog. *Kidney Int* 19:503–513, 1981
59. AVASTHI PS, EVAN AP, HAY D: Glomerular endothelial cells in uranyl nitrate-induced acute renal failure in rats. *J Clin Invest* 65:121–127, 1980
60. AVASTHI PS, EVAN AP, HUSER JW, LUFT FC: Effect of gentamicin on glomerular ultrastructure. *J Lab Clin Med* 98:444–454, 1981
61. LUFT FC, ARONOFF GA, EVAN AP, CONNERS BA: The effect of aminoglycosides on glomerular endothelium: A comparative study. *Res Commun Chem Pathol Pharmacol* 34:89–95, 1981
62. VAAMONDE CA, TEIXEIRA RB, MORALES J, LUFT FC, EVAN AP: Absence of glomerular endothelial cell changes in the diabetic rat protected against gentamicin-induced acute renal failure (*abstract*). *Clin Res* 29:874A, 1981
63. BULGER RE, EKNOYAN G, PURCELL DJ III, DOBYAN DC: Endothelial characteristics of glomerular capillaries in normal, mercuric chloride-induced, and gentamicin-induced acute renal failure in the rat. *J Clin Invest* 72:128–141, 1983
64. SMITH TR, SMITH CR: Risk factors for aminoglycoside nephrotoxicity, in *The Aminoglycosides. Microbiology, Clinical Use, and Toxicology,* edited by WHELTON A, NEU HC, New York, Marcel Dekker, 1982, pp 401–415
65. LANE AZ, WRIGHT GE, BLAIR DC: Ototoxicity and nephrotoxicity of amikacin. *Am J Med* 62:911–918, 1977
66. THE EORTC INTERNATIONAL ANTIMICROBIAL THERAPY PROJECT GROUP: Three antibiotic regimens in the treatment of infection in febrile granulocytopenic patients with cancer. *J Infect Dis* 137:14–29, 1978
67. LAU WK, YOUNG LS, BLACK RE, WINSTON DJ, LINNE SR, WEINSTEIN RJ, HEWITT WL: Comparative efficacy and toxicity of amikacin/carbenicillin versus gentamicin/carbenicillin in leukopenic patients. *Am J Med* 62:959–966, 1977

68. SMITH CR, MAXWELL RR, EDWARDS CG, ROGERS JF, LIETMAN PS: Nephrotoxicity induced by gentamicin and amikacin. *Johns Hopkins Med J* 142:85–90, 1978

69. REYMAN MT, BRADAC JA, COBBS CG, DISMUKES WE: Correlation of aminoglycoside dosage with serum concentration during therapy of serious gram-negative bacillary disease. *Antimicrob Agents Chemother* 16:353–361, 1979

70. MOORE RD, SMITH CR, LIPSKY JJ, MELLITS ED, LIETMAN PS: Risk factors for nephrotoxicity in patients treated with aminoglycosides. *Ann Intern Med* 100:352–357, 1984

71. BENNETT WM, HARTNETT MN, GILBERT DN, HOUGHTON D, PORTER GA: Effect of sodium intake on gentamicin nephrotoxicity in the rat. *Proc Soc Exp Biol Med* 151:736–738, 1976

72. LECOMPTE J, DUMONT L, HILL J, SOUICHI PD, LELORIER J: Effect of water deprivation and rehydration on gentamicin disposition in the rat. *J Pharmacol Exp Ther* 218:231–236, 1981

73. ADELMAN RD: Sodium depletion and diuretics in relation to aminoglycoside nephrotoxicity, in *Nephrotoxicity, Ototoxicity of Drugs,* edited by FILLASTRE J-P, Rouen, Editions Inserm, 1982, pp 213–224

74. FINN WF, FERNANDEZ-REPOLLET E: Contribution of intravascular volume concentration to gentamicin nephrotoxicity (*abstract*). *Kidney Int* 21:217, 1982

75. KAHN T: Effect of furosemide on gentamicin and netilmicin nephrotoxicity (*abstract*). *Kidney Int* 12:527, 1977

76. DEROUGEMONT D, OESCHGER A, KONRAD L, THEIL G, TORHORST J, WENK M, WUNDERLICH P, BRUNNER FP: Gentamicin-induced acute renal failure in the rat: Effect of dehydration, DOCA-saline and furosemide. *Nephron* 29:176–184, 1981

77. CHIU PJS, MILLER GH, LONG JF, WAITZ JA: Renal uptake and nephrotoxicity of gentamicin during urinary alkalinization in rats. *Clin Exp Pharmacol Physiol* 6:317–326, 1979

78. ELLIOTT WC, PARKER RA, HOUGHTON DC, GILBERT DN, PORTER GA, DE-FEHR J, BENNETT WM: Effect of sodium bicarbonate and ammonium chloride ingestion in experimental gentamicin nephrotoxicity in rats. *Res Comm Chem Pathol Pharmacol* 28:483–495, 1980

79. BRINKER KR, BULGER RE, DOBYAN DC, STACEY TR, SOUTHERN PM, HENRICH WL, CRONIN RE: Effect of potassium depletion on gentamicin nephrotoxicity. *J Lab Clin Med* 98:292–301, 1981

80. YARGER WE: Effect of potassium depletion on gentamicin-induced acute renal failure (*abstract*). *Clin Res* 26:806A, 1978

81. RANKIN LI, KROUS H, FRYER AW, WHANG R: Enhancement of gentamicin nephrotoxicity by magnesium depletion in the rat. *Min Electr Metab* 10:199–203, 1984

82. SMITH CR, LIETMAN PS: Comparative clinical trials of aminoglycosides, in *The Aminoglycosides. Microbiology, Clinical Use, and Toxicology,* edited by WHELTON A, NEU HC, New York, Marcel Dekker, 1982, pp 497–509

83. WALKER BD, GENTRY LO: A randomized, comparative study of tobramycin and gentamicin in treatment of acute urinary infections. *J Infect Dis* 134(Suppl):S146–S149, 1976

84. SCHENTAG JJ, PLAUT ME, CERRA FB, WELS PB, WALCZAK P, BUCKLEY RJ: Aminoglycoside nephrotoxicity in critically ill surgical patients. *J Surg Res* 26:270–279, 1979

85. SMITH CR, LIPSKY JJ, LASKIN OL, HELLMAN DB, MELLITS ED, LONGSTRETH J, LIETMAN PS: Double-blind comparison of the nephrotoxicity and auditory toxicity of gentamicin and tobramycin. *N Engl J Med* 302:1106–1109, 1980

86. LERNER SA, SELIGSOHN R, MATZ GJ: Comparative clinical studies of ototoxicity and nephrotoxicity of amikacin and gentamicin. *Am J Med* 62:959–966, 1977

87. LERNER AM, CONE LA, JANSEN W, REYES MP, BLAIR DC, WRIGHT GE, LORBER RR: Randomized, controlled trial of the comparative efficacy, auditory toxicity, and nephrotoxicity of tobramycin and netilmicin. *Lancet* 1:1123–1126, 1983

88. LUFT FC, BLOCH R, SLOAN RS, YUM MN, MAXWELL DR: Comparative nephrotoxicity of aminoglycoside antibiotics in rats. *J Infect Dis* 138:541–545, 1978

89. GILBERT DN, PLAMP CE, STARR P, BENNETT WM, HOUGHTON DC, PORTER GA: Comparative nephrotoxicity of gentamicin and tobramycin in rats. *Antimicrob Agents Chemother* 13:34–40, 1978

90. ORMSBY AM, PARKER RA, PLAMP CE, STEVENS P, HOUGHTON DC, GILBERT DN, BENNETT WM: Comparison of the nephrotoxic potential of gentamicin, tobramycin and netilmicin in the rat. *Curr Therap Res* 25:335–342, 1979

91. HOUGHTON DC, PLAMP CE, GILBERT DN, KOLHEPP S, BENNETT WM, PORTER GA, DeFEHR J, WEBB R: Amikacin nephrotoxicity in the rat. *J Environ Pathol Toxicol* 4:227–291, 1980

92. LUFT FC, YUM MN, KLEIT SA: Comparative nephrotoxicity of netilmicin and gentamicin in rats. *Antimicrob Agents Chemother* 10:845–849, 1976

93. LUFT FC, RANKIN LI, SLOAN RS, FINEBERG NS, YUN MN, WONG L: Comparative low-dose nephrotoxicity of dibekacin, gentamicin and tobramycin. *J Antimicrob Chemother* 9:297–301, 1982

94. DALHGREN JC, ANDERSON ET, HEWITT WL: Gentamicin blood levels: a guide to nephrotoxicity. *Antimicrob Agents Chemother* 8:58–62, 1975

95. FRAME PT, PHAIR JP, WATANAKUNAKORN C, BANNISTER TWP: Pharmacologic factors associated with gentamicin nephrotoxicity in rabbits. *J Infect Dis* 135:952–956, 1977

96. BENNETT WM, PLAMP CE, GILBERT DN, PARKER RA, PORTER GA: The influence of dosage regimen on experimental gentamicin nephrotoxicity: dissociation of peak serum levels from renal failure. *J Infect Dis* 140:576–579, 1979

97. SCHENTAG JJ, CUMBO TJ, JUSKO WJ, PLAUT ME: Gentamicin tissue accumulation and nephrotoxic reactions. *JAMA* 240:2067–2069, 1978

98. MAZZE RI, COUSSINS M: Combined nephrotoxicity of gentamicin and methoxyflurane anesthesia in man. *Br J Anaesth* 45:394–397, 1973

99. GONZALEZ-VITALE JC, HAYES DM, CVITKOVIC E, STERNBERG SS: Acute renal failure after Cis-Dichlorodiamineplatinum (II) and gentamicin-cephalothin therapies. *Cancer Treat Rep* 62:693–698, 1978

100. CHURCHILL DN, SEELEY J: Nephrotoxicity associated with combined gentamicin-amphotericin B therapy. *Nephron* 19:176–181, 1977

101. BUTKUS DE, DeTORRENTE A, TERMAN DS: Renal failure following gentamicin in combination with clindamycin. *Nephron* 17:307–313, 1976

102. WADE JC, SMITH CR, PETTY BG, LIPSKY JJ, CONRAD G, ELLNER J, LIETMAN PS: Cephalothin plus an aminoglycoside is more nephrotoxic than methicillin plus an aminoglycoside. *Lancet* 2:604–606, 1978

103. LAWSON DH, MACADAM RF, SINGH H, GARRAS H, HARTZ S, TURNBULL D, LINTON AL: Effect of furosemide on antibiotic-induced renal damage in rats. *J Infect Dis* 126:593–599, 1972

104. HIGA EMS, SCHOR N, BOIM MA, AJZEN H, RAMOS OL: Prostaglandin inhibition in gentamicin and tobramycin nephrotoxicity (*abstract*). *Clin Res* 30:450A, 1982

105. GIAMARELLOU H, METZIKOFF C, PAPACHRISTOPHOROU AS, DONTAS AS, DAI-

kos GK: Prospective comparative evaluation of gentamicin or gentamicin-plus cephalothin in the production of nephrotoxicity in man. *J Antimicrob Chemother* 5:581–590, 1979

106. HARRISON WO, SILVERBLATT FJ, TURCK M: Gentamicin nephrotoxicity: failure of three cephalosporins to potentiate injury in rats. *Antimicrob Agents Chemother* 8:209–215, 1975

107. BLOCH R, LUFT FC, RANKIN LI, SLOAN RS, YUM MN, MAXWELL DR: Protection from gentamicin nephrotoxicity by cephalothin and carbenicillin. *Antimicrob Agents Chemother* 15:46–49, 1979

108. BARZA M, PINN V, TANGUAY P, MURRAY T: Nephrotoxicity of newer cephalosporins and aminoglycosides alone and in combination in a rat model. *J Antimicrob Chemother* 4(Suppl A):59–68, 1978

109. HOWS JM, PALMER S, WANT S, DEARDEN C, GORDON-SMITH EC: Serum levels of cyclosporin A and nephrotoxicity in bone marrow transplant patients. *Lancet* 2:145–146, 1981

110. WHITING PH, SIMPSON JG: The enhancement of cyclosporin A-induced nephrotoxicity of gentamicin. *Biochem Pharmacol* 32:2025–2028, 1983

111. BENNETT WM, PARKER RA, ELLIOTT WC, GILBERT DN, HOUGHTON DC: Sex-related differences in the susceptibility of rats to gentamicin nephrotoxicity. *J Infect Dis* 145:370–373, 1982

112. KOURILSKY O, SOLEZ K, MOREL-MAROGER L, WHELTON A, DUHOUX P, SRAER J-D: The pathology of acute renal failure due to interstitial nephritis in man with comments on the role of interstitial inflammation and sex in gentamicin nephrotoxicity. *Medicine (Baltimore)* 61:258–268, 1982

113. VAAMONDE CA, GOUVEA W, OWENS B, ALPERT HC: Sex does not influence the protection against gentamicin nephrotoxicity in the diabetic rat (*abstract*). *Kidney Int* 25:238, 1984

114. HSU CH, KURTZ TW, EASTERLING RE, WELLER JM: Potentiation of gentamicin nephrotoxicity by metabolic acidosis. *Proc Soc Exp Biol Med* 146:894–897, 1974

115. SOLEZ K, SILVIA CB, CRAIG T, STOUT R, WHELTON A: Adverse effect of amino acid mixtures in experimental aminoglycoside toxicity (*abstract*). *Clin Res* 28:462A, 1980

116. BECK PR, THOMSON RB, CHAUDHURI AKR: Aminoglycoside antibiotics and renal function: Changes in urinary gamma-glutamyl transferase excretion. *J Clin Pathol* 30:432–437, 1977

117. MONDORF AW, BREIER J, HANDUS J, SCHERBERICH JE, MACKENROOT G, SHAH PM, STILLE W, SCHOEPPE W: Effect of aminoglycosides on proximal tubular membranes of the human kidney. *Eur J Clin Pharmacol* 13:133–142, 1978

118. LUFT FC, PATEL V, YUM MN, PATEL G, KLEIT SA: Experimental aminoglycoside nephrotoxicity. *J Lab Clin Med* 86:213–220, 1975

119. RUSSO JC, ADELMAN RD: Gentamicin-induced Fanconi syndrome. *J Pediatrics* 96:151–153, 1980

120. KELMAR CJH, TAOR WS, REYNOLDS DJ, SMITH DR, SLAVIN BM, BROOK CGD: Hypomagnesemia, hypocalcemia with hypokalemia caused by treatment with high dose gentamicin. *Arch Dis Child* 53:817–820, 1978

121. PATEL R, SAVAGE A: Symptomatic hypomagnesemia associated with gentamicin therapy. *Nephron* 23:50–52, 1979

122. APPEL GB, SIEGEL NJ, APPEL AS, HAYSLETT JP: Hemodynamic and tubular functional alterations in gentamicin induced experimental acute renal failure (*abstract*). *Kidney Int* 14:721, 1978

123. PLAMP CE, REGER K, BENNETT WM, MCCLUNG MR, PORTER GA: Vasopressin resistant polyuria in gentamicin nephrotoxicity (*abstract*). *Clin Res* 26:151A, 1978

124. GORDON JA, DILLINGHAM MA, GUGGENHEIM SJ, GROSSFIELD PD, ANDERSON RJ: The renal concentrating defect after gentamicin administration in the rat. *J Lab Clin Med* 101:903–910, 1983

125. SAFIRSTEIN R, MILLER P, KAHN T: Cortical and papillary absorptive defects in gentamicin nephrotoxicity. *Kidney Int* 24:526–533, 1983

126. KLOTMAN PE, YARGER WE: Reduction of renal blood flow and proximal bicarbonate reabsorption in rats by gentamicin. *Kidney Int* 24:638–643, 1983

127. MCNEIL JS, JACKSON B, NELSON L, BUTKUS DE: The role of prostaglandins in gentamicin-induced nephrotoxicity in the dog. *Nephron* 33:202–207, 1983

128. SOULIERE CR, GOODMAN DBP, APPEL GB, FORREST JN: Gentamicin selectively inhibits antidiuretic hormone induced water flow in the toad urinary bladder (*abstract*). *Kidney Int* 14:733, 1978

129. NEUGARTEN F, AYNEDJIAN HS, BANK N: Role of tubular obstruction in acute renal failure due to gentamicin. *Kidney Int* 24:330–335, 1983

130. SCHOR N, ICHIKAWA I, RENNKE HG, TROY JL, BRENNER BJ: Pathophysiology of altered glomerular function in aminoglycoside-treated rats. *Kidney Int* 19:288–296, 1981

131. MORIN JP, VIOTTE G, VAN HOFF F, TULKENS P, FILLASTRE J-P: Gentamicin-induced nephrotoxicity: a cell biology approach. *Kidney Int* 18:583–590, 1980

132. KNAUSS TC, WEINBERG JM, HUMES HD: Alterations in renal cortical phospholipid content induced by gentamicin: time course, specificity, and subcellular localization. *Am J Physiol* 244:F535–F546, 1983

133. LIPSKY J, LIETMAN PS: Aminoglycoside inhibition of a renal phosphatidylinositol phospholipase C. *J Pharmacol Exp Ther* 220:287–292, 1982

134. HOSTETLER KY, HALL LB: Inhibition of kidney lysosomal phospholipases A and C by aminoglycoside antibiotics: Possible mechanisms of aminoglycoside toxicity. *Proc Natl Acad Sci USA* 79:1663–1667, 1983

135. SCHWERTZ DW, KREISBERG FI, VENKATACHALAM MA: Effects of gentamicin on proximal tubule brush border membrane phosphatidylinositol-specific phospholipase C (*abstract*). *Kidney Int* 25:238, 1984

136. DE DUVE C, DE BARSY T, POOLE B, TROUET A, TULKENS P, VAN HOOF F: Lysosomotropic agents. *Biochem Pharmacol* 23:2495–2531, 1974

137. MITCHELL RH, JAFFERJI SS, JONES HF: The possible involvement of phosphatidylinositol breakdown in the mechanism of stimulus-response coupling at receptors which control calcium gates. *Adv Exp Biol* 83:447–465, 1977

138. ELLIOTT WC, GILBERT DN, DEFEHR J, BENNETT WM, MCCARRON DA: Protection from experimental gentamicin toxicity by dietary calcium loading (*abstract*). *Am Soc Nephrol* 14:89A, 1981

139. PULLIAM JP, HOUGHTON DC, BENNETT WM: High calcium intake does not protect against mercuric chloride-induced acute renal failure (*abstract*). *Kidney Int* 25:236, 1984

140. MCCARRON DA, GILBERT DN, HOUGHTON DC, BENNETT WM: Hypercalciuria per se does not protect from experimental gentamicin nephrotoxicity (*abstract*). *Kidney Int* 25:234, 1984

141. EKNOYAN G, GENTRY L, BULGER R, DOBYAN D: Attenuation of gentamicin induced acute renal failure by phosphate depletion (*abstract*). *Kidney Int* 25:229, 1984

142. PULLIAM JP, HOUGHTON DC, BENNETT WM: Modification of gentamicin

nephrotoxicity in rats following selective parathyroidectomy (*abstract*). *Clin Res* 32:455A, 1984
143. BENDIRDJIAN JP, FOUCHER B, FILLASTRE J-P: Influence de la gentamicine sur le metabolisme energetique de mitochondries de foie et de reins de rats, in *Nephrotoxicity: Interactions of Drugs with Membrane Systems of Mytochondria-Lysosomes,* edited by FILLASTRE J-P, Paris and New York, Masson, 1978, pp 315–332
144. SIMMONS CF JR, BOGUSKY RT, HUMES HD: Inhibitory effects of gentamicin on renal mitochondrial oxidative phosphorylation. *J Pharmacol Exp Ther* 214:709–715, 1980
145. SASTRASINH M, WEINBERG JM, HUMES HD: The effect of gentamicin on calcium uptake by renal mitochondria. *Life Sci* 30:2309–2315, 1982
146. CRONIN RE, NIX KL, FERGUSON ER, SOUTHERN PM, HEINRICH WL: Renal cortex ion composition and Na-K-ATPase activity in gentamicin nephrotoxicity. *Am J Physiol* 242:F477–F483, 1982
147. KALOYANIDES GJ, WANG M, GOUVEA W, KELLEY J, ALPERT H, VAAMONDE CA: Altered phosphatidylinositol metabolism in diabetic rats confers resistance to gentamicin-induced acute renal failure (*abstract*). *Kidney Int* 21:219, 1982
148. TEIXEIRA RB, KELLEY J, ALPERT H, PARDO V, VAAMONDE CA: Complete protection from gentamicin-induced acute renal failure in the diabetes mellitus rat. *Kidney Int* 21:600–612, 1982
149. GOUVEA W, OWENS B, VAAMONDE CM, ALPERT H, VAAMONDE CA: Creatinine and inulin clearances in the evaluation of gentamicin nephrotoxicity in control and streptozotocin-induced diabetic rats (*abstract*). *Kidney Int* 25:230, 1984
150. VAAMONDE CA, BIER RT, GOUVEA W, ALPERT H, KELLEY J, PARDO V: Effect of duration of diabetes on the protection observed in the diabetic rat against gentamicin-induced acute renal failure. *Min Electr Metab* 10:209–216, 1984
151. GOUVEA W, KELLEY J, ALPERT H, PARDO V, VAAMONDE CA: Enhanced solute excretion fails to protect against gentamicin acute renal failure in the phlorizin treated rat (*abstract*). *Kidney Int* 21:217, 1982
152. VAAMONDE CA, ROTH D, KELLEY J, ALPERT H, PARDO V, KALOYANIDES GJ: Insulin reverses the protection afforded by diabetes against gentamicin-induced acute renal failure (*abstract*). *Clin Res* 30:465A, 1982
153. VAAMONDE CA, TEIXEIRA RB, MORALES J, ROTH D, KELLEY J, ALPERT H, PARDO V: A new model for studying drug-induced acute renal failure: the rat with untreated diabetes mellitus, in *Acute Renal Failure,* edited by ELIAHOU EH, London, John Libbey & Co, 1982, pp 96–101
154. CRONIN RE, SPLINTER KL, FERGUSON ER, HEINRICH WL: Gentamicin nephrotoxicity: Protective effect of diabetes on cell injury. *Min Electr Metab* 9:38–44, 1983
155. CLEMENTS RS, REYNERTSON R: Myoinositol metabolism in diabetes mellitus. *Diabetes* 26:215–221, 1977
156. LUFT FC, RANKIN LI, SLOAN RS, YUM MN: Recovery from aminoglycoside nephrotoxicity with continuous drug administration. *Antimicrob Agents Chemother* 3:284–287, 1978
157. GILBERT DN, HOUGHTON DC, BENNETT WM, PLAMP CE, REGER K, PORTER GA: Reversibility of gentamicin nephrotoxicity in rats: recovery during continuous drug administration. *Proc Soc Exp Biol Med* 160:99–103, 1979

Nephrotoxicity Caused
by Cancer Chemotherapy

Richard E. Rieselbach

Complications of cancer and its therapy have a major impact upon the kidney, causing a broad spectrum of abnormalities. Neoplastic processes may damage the kidney via immunologically mediated disease, tumor products, or tumor metabolites. Furthermore, tumor may directly invade the renal parenchyma, ureters, or bladder, resulting in obstruction to urine flow and decreased kidney function. One of the most frequent causes of renal failure in the cancer patient at the present time is nephrotoxicity from cancer chemotherapy agents [1]. The resulting impairment of renal function may impose a particularly difficult burden upon the patient with cancer. If renal failure is not effectively managed, uremia may supervene with its infectious, hemorrhagic, and metabolic complications. Furthermore, the pharmacokinetics of cancer chemotherapeutic agents may be altered substantially when renal function is reduced, thereby limiting the potential for optimal therapy of the underlying cancer. The nephrotoxicity from cancer chemotherapy may be either direct (caused by specific agents) or endogenously produced (caused by chemotherapy-induced tumor lysis).

Direct Nephrotoxicity Caused by
Cancer Chemotherapy Agents

Since nephrotoxicity relating to cancer chemotherapy most often occurs following the administration of cis-platinum, nitrosoureas, or high-dose methotrexate, these agents will be discussed in some detail. Significant nephrotoxicity has been noted on occasion following administration of mitomycin C, mithramycin, and 5-azacytidine; thus, these agents also will be discussed.

This manuscript was presented as part of a Symposium on *The Kidney and Malignant Disease.*

Cis-Platinum

Cis-platinum (cis-diamminedichloroplatinum II) is a recently developed anti-neoplastic agent that has a remarkably broad spectrum of clinical activity in the treatment of solid tumors [1, 2]. Use of this drug has significantly improved the response rate in patients treated for metastatic testicular and ovarian carcinomas [3]. Additionally, cis-platinum is an important component of many treatment programs for the management of bladder carcinoma, squamous cell carcinoma of the head and neck, bronchogenic carcinoma of the lung, cervical, and endometrial cancer [1]. In addition to nephrotoxicity, side effects of the drug include myelosuppression, severe nausea and vomiting, peripheral neuropathy, ototoxicity, and acute anaphylaxis [1]. Early preclinical toxicologic evaluation of cis-platinum revealed that nephrotoxicity was a major side effect [4]; nephrotoxicity also was a prominent side effect with initial clinical trials [5]. A dose of 50 mg/m^2 of body surface area (BSA), administered either as a single dose or in divided doses over a 5-day period, produced nephrotoxicity in a significant percentage of the patients. With higher doses and repeated courses of therapy, nephrotoxicity was noted to be severe, frequently irreversible, and was a major dose-limiting factor [1].

Histopathology and Pathogenesis

The primary site of cis-platinum nephrotoxicity is the tubule. Distal tubules and collecting ducts are affected to a greater degree than proximal tubules [6]. Coagulative necrosis, interstitial edema, and tubular dilatation were the most prominent findings; glomerular changes were not observed [6]. The cytotoxic effect of cis-platinum appears to occur through its interaction with nucleophilic sites in DNA in a manner similar to that of alkylating agents [7]. In biologic fluids that contain a low chloride concentration (that is, intracellular water in which the chloride concentration is 4 mM), the drug's chloride ligands in the *cis* position are replaced by water molecules, thus forming an aquated compound. This positively charged, aquated species then reacts with nucleophilic sites. In plasma, which has an ambient chloride concentration of 103 mM, cis-platinum remains electrically neutral, with the chloride ligands remaining intact on the molecule. Thus, the drug becomes activated only when present within the cell. Cis-platinum is predominantly excreted via the kidney, with recovery of up to 90% of administered platinum in the urine in animal studies [8]. The drug is excreted via glomerular filtration; a recent study demonstrating that free platinum clearance exceeded the glomerular filtration rate (GFR) suggests that tubular secretion of cis-platinum or a metabolite also occurs [9]. Thus, the drug may gain access to renal tubular cells via secretion or reabsorption.

Clinical Manifestations

The initial manifestation of cis-platinum nephrotoxicity is a decrease in GFR with an associated increase in the BUN and serum creatinine concentrations.

Since glomerular injury is not associated with the nephrotoxic process, glomerular proteinuria does not occur; tubular proteinuria may be observed as an early indication of toxicity [10]. Cylindruria is a prominent feature only when severe nephrotoxicity is present [11]. An additional nephrotoxic effect of cis-platinum is renal magnesium wasting [12]. The magnesium loss may, on occasion, be accompanied by hypocalcemia and tetany. In one series of 44 patients, hypomagnesemia was induced by cis-platinum in 52%, including 2 patients who required hospitalization because of symptoms. The median nadir of magnesium concentration in these patients was 0.92 mEq/liter. It usually occurred 21 days following drug administration, after completion of one or two courses of cis-platinum. This complication is readily managed with administration of oral magnesium chloride solution (magnesium, 1 mEq/ml) and usually does not require parenteral magnesium sulfate administration. This tubular defect usually remits spontaneously over a period of weeks if cis-platinum therapy is not reinstituted. However, on occasion it may persist for a longer duration [1].

Prophylactic Measures

The initial clinical studies with cis-platinum were indicative of its prominent antitumor activity. However, the frequent occurrence of severe nephrotoxicity discouraged interest in the drug. Development of cis-platinum to its present level of clinical usefulness was greatly facilitated by studies in which hydration-diuresis maneuvers were used in dogs [13] and subsequently in humans [14]; these maneuvers were extremely effective in preventing or minimizing nephrotoxicity if the dosage did not exceed 120 mg/m² BSA.

Recent studies from the National Cancer Institute indicate that even higher doses of the drug may be tolerated without nephrotoxicity if each dose of cis-platinum is administered in 250 ml of 3% saline (over 30 minutes) in association with i.v. infusion of 250 ml/hr of normal saline with potassium chloride added (20 mEq/liter). This infusion is initiated 12 hr before the first dose of cis-platinum and continued until 12 hr after the last dose on day 5 of chemotherapy. This regimen allowed an administration of 200 mg/m² BSA in five divided daily doses without evidence of a decrease in GFR [15]. These studies are of particular importance because previous studies of cis-platinum administration in both ovarian and testicular cancer have not used cis-platinum doses greater than 100 to 120 mg/m² BSA. When used with moderate hydration (3 liters/d) and mannitol or furosemide diuresis, these or lower doses of cis-platinum have produced an acceptable degree of nephrotoxicity. However, previous experience with higher doses of cis-platinum has shown that an unacceptable incidence of nephrotoxicity occurs at doses greater than 120 mg/m² BSA even with furosemide or mannitol diuresis [16]. The National Cancer Institute study revealed that use of this higher dose of cis-platinum resulted in a markedly increased antitumor effect in patients with testicular and ovarian cancer. Although the mechanism for the apparent protective effect of hypertonic saline from cis-platinum nephrotoxicity is unclear, these findings may relate to the degree of intracellular aquation of cis-platinum. A low intracellular concentration of chloride ion favors the formation of the aquated species of cis-platinum within renal tubular cells, as opposed to a high chloride concentration, which may decrease the concentration of the toxic aquated species.

Another promising approach to limiting cis-platinum nephrotoxicity is pharmacologic inhibition of cis-platinum tubular secretion. Administration of drugs such as probenecid may be effective in decreasing the intracellular concentration of drug by inhibiting its uptake by the contraluminal cell membrane [17].

Methotrexate

Methotrexate (MTX) was one of the earliest cancer chemotherapy agents used. When it is administered in conventional oral or i.v. doses, nephrotoxicity is only an occasional problem. However, renal toxicity occurs with increasing frequency as the MTX dose is increased. Renal failure has been implicated in 20% of the deaths associated with high-dose MTX administration [18]. This drug is excreted primarily by the kidneys. Thus, any change in renal function has an effect on plasma MTX levels and the rate of MTX clearance. If MTX levels are elevated for prolonged periods of time, the organ systems most affected, which are thereby limiting with respect to toxicity, are the bone marrow and gastrointestinal tract [19]. Both of these organ systems contain a substantial proportion of actively proliferating cells. Proliferating or cycling cells are susceptible to the toxic effects of MTX, whereas noncycling (resting) cells are not. Although the ultimate role of MTX in the management of cancer patients is unclear, it has proven to be an extremely effective agent when used as a component of combination chemotherapy regimens for trophoblastic choriocarcinoma, acute lymphocytic leukemia, breast carcinoma, squamous cell carcinoma of the head and neck, osteogenic sarcoma, and nonHodgkin's lymphoma [20]. The major extrarenal toxicities caused by MTX include myelosuppression, mucositis, diarrhea, dermatitis, and hepatitis. This analog of folic acid exerts its cytotoxic activity as a consequence of tight binding to dihydrofolate reductase, with subsequent inhibition and depletion of intracellular reduced folate pools.

Pathogenesis and Histopathology

Presently, there are three hypotheses for the pathogenesis of MTX nephrotoxicity. The most widely accepted one is that MTX or a metabolite precipitates within the distal nephron and causes an intrarenal obstructive nephropathy similar to that observed with acute uric acid nephropathy. MTX is excreted rapidly in the urine, with 54 to 88% of conventional doses undergoing urinary excretion during the first 24 hr after administration [21]. With high doses administered i.v. over a period of 6 hr, urinary excretion has been noted to range from 35 to 53% during the infusion, with 90% of the parent compound excreted by 30 hr [22]. With the use of high doses, a MTX metabolite (7-hydroxymethotrexate) is also excreted in the urine [23]. MTX undergoes urinary excretion via both glomerular filtration and active tubular secretion [24]. At physiologic system pH, the drug is fully ionized; however, its solubility is markedly reduced at the more acid pH usually encountered within the distal nephron [25]. Thus, patients receiving high doses of MTX therapy are extremely prone to nephrotoxicity if they are dehydrated and excreting an acid urine; the nephrotoxicity may occur as a result of MTX precipitation in the distal nephron. Urinary 7-hydroxymethotrexate may also contribute to the precipitate, because its solubility is only 25% of that observed for methotrexate [23]. Figure 1 shows a renal biopsy sample from a patient treated with MTX (3 g/m² BSA) followed by leukovorin rescue therapy

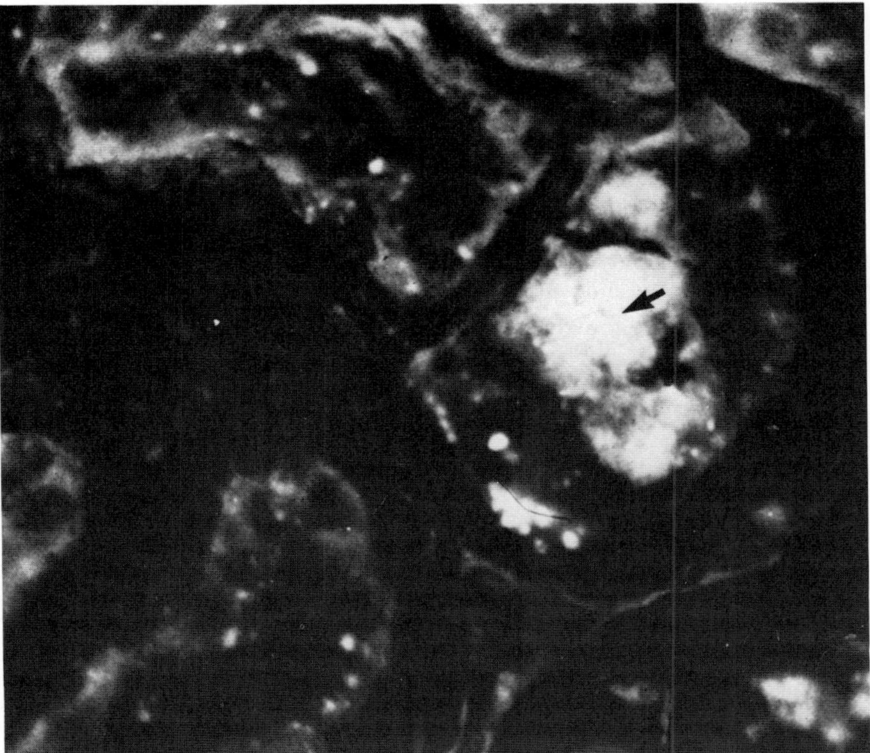

Fig. 1. Renal biopsy sample from a patient who became dehydrated and developed acute renal failure after being treated with methotrexate (MTX; 3 g/m² body surface area) followed by leukovorin rescue. The precipitated material in the renal tubules (*arrow*) strongly reacted with a fluorosceinated rabbit anti-MTX antibody. (Reprinted with permission from [26])

[26]. The patient became dehydrated and developed acute renal failure. The precipitated material in the renal tubules was demonstrated to be MTX. Following the institution of prophylactic urinary alkalinization and hydration as part of the treatment regimen associated with high-dose MTX therapy, the incidence of nephrotoxicity has markedly decreased [27, 28]. This observation would appear to support the importance of intrarenal MTX precipitation as a significant factor in the pathogenesis of nephrotoxicity.

Since the majority of patients with MTX nephrotoxicity present with non-oliguric acute renal failure, this has raised the question of direct tubular toxicity as a second possible pathogenic mechanism. In one report of a patient who developed MTX-induced renal failure following high-dose treatment, post-mortem examination revealed evidence of proximal tubular necrosis without demonstration of intraluminal precipitated material [1]. Furthermore, the nephrotoxicity that occurs following high-dose aminopterin therapy is of great interest with respect to direct tubular toxicity of folic acid antagonists. Aminopterin is 10 times more potent as a folic acid antagonist than equimolar doses of MTX. Thus, high-dose aminopterin protocols call for a dosage that is approximately 10% of the methotrexate dosage in similar protocols. The solubility of MTX and aminopterin in urine at 37°C is equivalent. Therefore, intratubular folic acid antagonist precipitation should be minimized with these protocols. Two patients receiving a high-dose aminopterin protocol who died with nephrotoxicity were not found to have renal tubular precipitates [1].

A third possible pathogenic mechanism involves the direct effect of MTX on glomerular hemodynamics. The administration of high-dose MTX has uniformly resulted in a decrease in GFR, both in pediatric and adult patients [29, 30]. The consistent and reversible decrease in GFR observed after high-dose MTX administration would suggest that constriction of the afferent arteriole may be a mechanism of toxicity, with a resultant decrease in renal perfusion. In this regard, it is interesting to note that pediatric patients receiving high-dose MTX for treatment of osteogenic sarcoma have been observed to develop hypertension during therapy [20].

Clinical Manifestations

In most cases, the clinical course of MTX nephrotoxicity closely resembles the nonoliguric acute renal failure induced by aminoglycosides. Although serum creatinine may progressively increase, urine output characteristically remains high. Flank pain during MTX infusion has been reported in two patients who subsequently developed nephrotoxicity [1]. Since renal function changes rapidly when nephrotoxicity occurs, alterations in serum creatinine may not accurately reflect the decrease in GFR. Thus, serial creatinine clearances are necessary to accurately assess the level of renal function. Alternatively, monitoring serum MTX levels provides a sensitive means of identifying patients who have a delayed MTX excretion pattern owing to a decrease in renal function. Patients who develop severe renal toxicity usually have elevated serum MTX levels as early as 24 hr after treatment. Parameters for monitoring serum MTX levels and the strategy for both prophylaxis of MTX-induced nephrotoxicity and its management recently have been reviewed in detail [1].

Nitrosoureas

The nitrosoureas are a group of cell-cycle nonspecific agents that have proved effective in the treatment of a large number of human cancers [31]. Nephrotoxicity has been observed in patients treated with two of the nitrosourea compounds: streptozotocin and methyl-CCNU. The nephrotoxicity induced by these agents will be discussed separately, since the mechanism and form of nephrotoxicity differs for each agent.

Streptozotocin

This drug has well-established roles in the management of patients with metastatic islet cell carcinoma of the pancreas and carcinoid tumors. Furthermore, additional clinical activity has been reported in Hodgkin's and non-Hodgkin's lymphoma [1]. Toxic effects in humans, in addition to nephrotoxicity, include gastrointestinal symptoms, transient elevations of hepatic enzymes, mild myelosuppression, neurologic deficits, and hypoglycemia [1]. The drug acts through inhibition of DNA synthesis. Functional and morphologic derangements within the kidney are the most significant toxic effects of the drug.

The first sign of nephrotoxicity is proteinuria. This may be followed by a variety of tubular defects that are manifested by hypophosphatemia, renal glycosuria, renal tubular acidosis, and hypokalemia. Acute renal failure has been reported in some patients [32]. Although there are no unequivocal data relating a cumulative dose to the development of nephrotoxicity, renal damage often occurs following a total dose of 4 g/m² BSA [1]. To minimize the possibility of nephrotoxicity, the optimal dosage schedule would appear to be 1.5 g/m² BSA per week or 0.5 g/m² BSA daily for 5 days, with repeated courses every 3 to 4 weeks [1]. The use of hydration and diuretic regimens or a continuous infusion schedule may possibly reduce nephrotoxicity; however, definitive data in this regard are not yet available.

Methyl-CCNU

Methyl-CCNU is a lipid-soluble nitrosourea having antitumor activity in the treatment of malignant gliomas, gastrointestinal adenocarcinomas, malignant melanoma, and other neoplasms [31]. The drug may produce nausea and vomiting and delayed, severe bone marrow toxicity. Nephrotoxicity was not apparent with the early uses of methyl-CCNU. However, long-term observation in patients receiving the drug following the total or partial resection of brain tumors revealed that high-dose therapy may lead to irreversible renal failure [33]. Proteinuria, hypertension, and alterations in urine sediment were absent. The degree of toxicity appears to be dose-dependent. Evidence of renal damage often was not apparent until 18 to 24 months following the completion of nitrosourea therapy. Histologic examination of renal tissue disclosed glomerulosclerosis, focal tubular atrophy, and marked interstitial fibrosis with moderate lymphocyte infiltration. The earliest indication of nephrotoxicity appeared to be a decrease in kidney size. Since the majority of reported patients received a cumulative dose greater than 1500 mg/m² BSA, it is now recommended that methyl-CCNU therapy be limited to a total dose of 1000 to 1250 mg/m² BSA [20].

Mithramycin

Mithramycin has been shown to be an active agent in the treatment of testicular carcinomas and glioblastomas. A variety of metabolic and toxic side effects involving the bone marrow, central nervous system, gastrointestinal tract, and kidneys have limited its widespread use [1]. Use of the drug is associated with a particularly high incidence of nephrotoxicity. Renal histopathologic changes have consisted of renal tubular swelling with hydropic degeneration, proximal and distal tubular necrosis, and eventual tubular atrophy, with sparing of glomeruli. Currently, the major use of this drug is in the management of hypercalcemia, for which a dose of 25 μg/kg is infused either rapidly or over 4 to 24 hr [34]. The desired hypocalcemic effect usually occurs within 24 to 48 hr. Administration of the drug can be repeated if hypercalcemia reoccurs. Nephrotoxicity has been observed when the drug was used in this manner; thus, constant renal monitoring is essential even when the smaller doses of this agent required for treatment of hypercalcemia are used [1].

Mitomycin-C

Mitomycin-C is an antitumor antibiotic that has clinical activity in adenocarcinoma of various origins, as well as various squamous cell, gynecologic neoplasms, and genitourinary cancers [1]. Its major dose-limiting toxicities include cumulative myelosuppression, as well as gastrointestinal, dermatologic, and pulmonary toxicity [1]. The various available studies to date are not in agreement in terms of the actual incidence of nephrotoxicity [1]. However, it would appear that nephrotoxicity is related to a cumulative dose of the drug, and its low incidence in some reports may be a reflection of the comparatively short survival time observed in the patients with the neoplasms for which the drug has been used. Recently, combination chemotherapy programs containing mitomycin-C have been associated with intravascular hemolysis and renal impairment resembling the hemolytic-uremic syndrome [35].

5-Azacytidine

This drug has been used in the treatment of acute myelocytic leukemia. Acute renal failure and renal tubular dysfunction have been associated with its use [1]. Aminoaciduria, phosphaturia, glycosuria, polyuria, and sodium wasting have been observed; renal tubular acidosis has developed in 73% of treatment courses [36]. These tubular abnormalities resolve shortly following the completion of therapy.

As is the case when evaluating the nephrotoxicity observed with any cancer chemotherapy agent, the associated administration of other potential nephrotoxins, such as antibiotics, introduces difficulty in evaluating data relating to the nephrotoxicity of a specific drug. Furthermore, it is possible that some drugs act synergetically to cause nephrotoxicity in the presence of other renal insults. Thus, determining that a given cancer chemotherapy agent is the sole cause of nephrotoxicity may be difficult because of its use in a clinical setting where there are many possible reasons for renal dysfunction.

Endogenous Nephrotoxicity Associated with Cancer Chemotherapy

Treatment of cancer may result in the rapid generation of endogenous nephrotoxins such as uric acid, xanthine, and phosphorus. This complication is of particular concern in patients with rapidly growing tumors that are extremely sensitive to cancer chemotherapy. As a consequence of massive cytolysis, intracellular products of malignant cells are released into the circulation and may produce hyperuricemia, hyperxanthinemia (especially when patients are being treated with allopurinol), hyperphosphatemia, and hyperkalemia. The magnitude of biochemical alterations in this setting is related to tumor burden and is magnified greatly by prior renal insufficiency, since renal excretion is necessary for phosphate, potassium, and uric acid homeostasis. The foregoing metabolic abberations have been described as part of the "acute tumor lysis syndrome" observed in patients with acute leukemia and malignant lymphoma [37]. Nephrotoxicity from hyperphosphatemia or hyperxanthinemia are limited essentially to this setting and, thus, are a rare occurrence. On the other hand, acute uric acid nephropathy (AUAN) is encountered more frequently and must be considered prior to initiating chemotherapy for a variety of malignancies [38].

Acute Uric Acid Nephropathy (AUAN)

Marked overproduction of uric acid may occur spontaneously in the cancer patient, but most often it is precipitated or exacerbated by chemotherapy. A failure to recognize impending AUAN, or a delay in pursuing vigorous therapy, may result in rapidly progressive acute renal failure leading to total cessation of renal function. Any significant degree of renal failure unnecessarily complicates the care of the cancer patient. Thus, prevention or prompt therapy of AUAN is an essential component of effective cancer chemotherapy.

Pathogenesis

The first comprehensive study investigating the pathogenesis of acute uric acid nephropathy in humans was published in 1964 [39]. Data correlating hyperuricosuria with a decrease in GFR, the relatively greater decrease in GFR than renal plasma flow, and the rapid and complete reversibility of renal insufficiency following appropriate therapy were all noted to be compatible with an intrarenal obstructive process caused by precipitation of uric acid in the distal nephron. This postulate was supported by the knowledge that concentration of uric acid increases progressively along the distal nephron as a result of water reabsorption and that uric acid is much less soluble at the acid pH that is often characteristic of tubular fluid within the distal tubule and collecting duct. The postmortem observation of both internal hydronephrosis and uric acid crystals within the collecting ducts of patients with the clinical diagnosis of AUAN at the time of death supported the hypothesis that uric acid precipitation is the cause of the intrarenal obstructive lesion [40]; subsequent studies in animal models have provided further support [41–43].

Diagnosis

AUAN occurs in a rather characteristic clinical setting. Recognition of this setting should serve to alert the physician to this diagnosis as a possible cause of acute renal failure. AUAN is most frequently associated with leukemias [44] or lymphomas [45], although it has been reported in a patient with disseminated carcinoma [46]. AUAN may occur spontaneously in the cancer patient, but it is most often precipitated or exacerbated by chemotherapy, resulting in increased uric acid production via the accelerated degradation of nucleoprotein. Early diagnosis is important because prompt and vigorous therapy of AUAN is an essential component of effective cancer chemotherapy and acute renal failure greatly complicates the care of the cancer patient. Patients with AUAN often have sustained contraction of extracellular fluid volume because of lack of oral intake, gastrointestinal fluid losses, or high fever. All of the foregoing may be associated with adverse reactions to cancer chemotherapy. The presence of a metabolic acidosis and, thus, a markedly acid urine (as a result of complications such as gastrointestinal bicarbonate losses, respiratory insufficiency, or lactic acidosis) is of additional concern, especially when associated with extracellular fluid volume contraction. The most prominent laboratory finding in AUAN is usually severe hyperuricemia associated with evidence of renal failure. However, hyperuricemia alone does not reliably differentiate patients with AUAN from those with other types of acute renal failure. The key to diagnosis of AUAN is hyperuricosuria, which is the basic pathogenic factor. This abnormality is reflected by the detection of urinary uric acid crystals or the documentation of a urinary uric acid-to-creatinine ratio of greater than 1.0 [47]. One of the foregoing observations is necessary to establish this diagnosis. These findings are not observed in acute renal failure of other etiologies or in chronic renal failure, since marked hyperuricosuria is not observed in these settings.

Prophylaxis and Therapy

Prophylaxis and therapy of AUAN is based on minimizing the concentration of uric acid in the urine and enhancing its solubility. Since uric acid is a weak acid, urinary pH plays a predominant role in determining whether a given urine becomes supersaturated. In the physiologic pH range of 4.5 to 7.5, urinary uric acid varies from nearly 100% undissociated to the opposite extreme in alkaline urine. Table 1 indicates the uric acid solubility at a pH of 5.0 and 7.0, as well as that for hypoxanthine and xanthine [48]. Sodium urate tends to remain in a supersaturated state when solubility limits are exceeded, as opposed to free uric acid, which readily undergoes precipitation. At a urinary pH of 5.0, 85% of uric acid is present in the undissociated form; whereas at a pH 7.2, well in excess of 90% is present in the highly soluble ionized form. Any further increase in urinary pH has essentially no effect on solubility. Successful prophylaxis also is based on controlling the load of uric acid presented to the kidney. Hyperuricosuria may be minimized by initiating xanthine oxidase inhibitor with allopurinol therapy at least 48 hr prior to definitive therapy of neoplasms. It has been noted that up to 5 days are required for allopurinol to exert its maximum hypouricemic effect [49]. If the tumor is large and considered to be particularly sensitive to therapy, the dosage of chemotherapy should be modified to avoid an abrupt, marked increase in synthesis of uric acid or oxypurines. Also, drugs that might inhibit tubular absorption of uric acid should be avoided. Vigorous hydration is desirable so that a urine volume of at least 3 liters/d may be achieved prior to induction of cancer chemotherapy. Furthermore, urinary alkalinization should be achieved through an administration of sodium bicarbonate, with the addition of diamox if necessary. In patients who have significant extracellular fluid volume depletion, high fever, vomiting, or diarrhea, hospitalization is recommended prior to instituting cancer chemotherapy so that in addition to allopurinol therapy, an intensive regimen of hydration and urinary alkalinization may be carried out.

With regard to therapy, the same considerations are appropriate for those patients who have renal insufficiency from AUAN but who are not oliguric at the time of presentation. In the presence of oliguria, therapy is more difficult, thus emphasizing the importance of early diagnosis. A detailed regimen for management of AUAN at various stages of presentation has been published recently [50].

Table 1. Solubility of purines in urine[a]

	At pH 5.0	At pH 7.0
Uric acid (mg/liter)	150	2000
Hypoxanthine (mg/liter)	1400	1500
Xanthine (mg/liter)	50	130

[a] Data from [48].

Xanthine Nephropathy

Xanthine nephropathy is rarely encountered. Nevertheless, this complication must be considered when patients with the acute tumor lysis syndrome are treated with allopurinol. Although the normal daily excretion of xanthine is approximately 6 mg, patients who are undergoing rapid tumor lysis and are receiving allopurinol therapy may manifest an increase in urinary xanthine excretion to a level as high as 750 mg/d [51]. The solubility of xanthine in urine at a pH of 5.0 is 50 mg/liter, whereas it is 130 mg/liter at a pH of 7.0 (Table 1). Hypoxanthine is much more soluble (Table 1). In one study, purine excretion was determined following chemotherapy in 7 patients with rapidly growing lymphomas who were receiving 300 to 600 mg/d of allopurinol. The peak urinary xanthine excretion postchemotherapy exceeded the solubility of xanthine at pH 7.0 in 4 of 7 patients [51]. Despite intensive hydration, 2 of these 4 patients developed transient renal failure, with creatinine clearances of 28 and 12 ml/min. The pathogenesis of xanthine nephropathy appears to be similar to that of acute uric acid nephropathy; similar prophylactic and therapeutic principles apply to the enhancement of xanthine solubility as were discussed previously with reference to uric acid solubility.

A recent report concerning the administration of polyethyleneglycol-modified uricase to five patients with advanced cancer raises an interesting possibility for dealing with xanthine nephropathy in patients who have a particularly high urinary purine excretion [52]. The described modification of the uricase molecule produces a preparation retaining some of the enzyme's activity in converting uric acid to highly soluble allantoin, but eliminating its ability to induce an immune response. In all five patients treated, the plasma urate concentration fell to undetectable levels within 60 min of injection and remained undetectable for at least 32 hr, in association with a marked increase in urinary allantoin excretion. Repeated administration 30 days later resulted in similar findings. No toxic effects were observed. Although widespread clinical application of uricase awaits further studies in humans, the foregoing data suggest a potentially valuable therapeutic approach in patients who have marked overproduction of uric acid. Uricase could be used as an alternative to allopurinol, or in combination with a reduced allopurinol dosage.

Hyperphosphatemic Nephropathy

The acute onset of extreme hyperphosphatemia following cancer chemotherapy may result in acute renal failure [53, 54]. Marked hyperphosphatemia, sometimes in excess of 20 mg/dl, may be anticipated after therapy in patients with a large tumor burden who have a reduction in GFR prior to therapy. Intrarenal precipitation of calcium phosphate salts has been suggested as the cause of acute renal failure in this setting [54]. Acute renal failure in response to this "infusion" of phosphate derived from tumor cells undergoing rapid lysis is analogous to reports of acute renal failure observed following the administration of large doses of phosphate [55]. Excessive urinary alkalinization may promote phosphate precipitation in renal tubules, and thus should be avoided in the presence of a high urinary phosphate concentration. If the GFR is already substantially reduced in the presence of marked hyperphosphatemia, dialysis may be necessary to prevent further renal damage. Recovery of renal function usually occurs following reduction of the serum phosphate level [53, 54].

Conclusion

Nephrotoxicity from cancer chemotherapy is a frequent cause of acute renal failure and other renal abnormalities in the cancer patient. A decreased incidence of this complication can be attained with an increased awareness for: (1) the nephrotoxic potential of offending chemotherapy agents, (2) the nephrotoxic dosage of these agents, (3) appropriate prophylactic measures, and (4) the clinical settings that predispose to nephrotoxicity (whether from specific chemotherapy agents or from the generation of endogenous nephrotoxins). Additionally, early diagnosis of nephrotoxicity allowing prompt therapy may minimize adverse effects. The foregoing principles have been reviewed and provide an important consideration in the care of the cancer patient.

References

1. ABELSON HT, GARNICK MB: Renal failure induced by cancer chemotherapy, in *Cancer and the Kidney,* edited by RIESELBACH RE, GARNICK MB, Philadelphia, Lea and Febiger, 1982, p 769
2. ROZENCWEIG M, VON HOFF DD, SLAVIK M, MUGGIA FM: Cis-diamminedichloroplatinum (II), a new anticancer drug. *Ann Intern Med* 86:803–812, 1977
3. EINHORN LH, WILLIAMS SD: The role of cis-platinum in solid tumor therapy. *N Engl J Med* 300:289–291, 1979
4. SCHAEPPI U, HEYMAN IA, FLEISCHMAN RW, ROSENKRANTZ H, ILIEVSKI V, PHELAN R, COONEY DA, DAVIS RD: Cis-dichlorodiammine-platinum (II) (NSC-119875): Preclinical toxicologic evaluation of intravenous injection in dogs, monkeys and mice. *Toxicol Appl Pharmacol* 25:230–241, 1973
5. TALLEY RW, O'BRYAN RM, GUTTERMAN JU, BROWNLEE RW, MCCREDIE KB: Clinical evaluation of toxic effects of cis-diamminedichloroplatinum (NSC-119875): Phase I clinical study. *Cancer Chemother Rep* 57:465–471, 1973
6. GONZALEZ-VITALE JC, HAYES DM, CVITKOVIC E, STERNBERG SS: The renal pathology in clinical trials of cis-platinum (II) diamminedichloride. *Cancer* 39:1362–1371, 1977
7. ROSENBERG B: Cisplatin: Its history and possible mechanisms of action, in *Cisplatin-Current Status and New Developments,* edited by PRESTAYKO AW, CROOKE ST, CARTER SK, New York, Academic Press, 1980, p 9
8. LITTERST CL, LEROY AF, GUARINO AM: Disposition and distribution of platinum following parenteral administration of cis-dichlorodiammineplatinum (II) to animals. *Cancer Treat Rep* 63:1485–1492, 1980
9. JACOBS C, KALMAN SM, TRETTON M, WEINER MW: Renal handling of cis-diamminedichloroplatinum (II). *Cancer Treat Rep* 64:1223–1226, 1980
10. JONES BR, BHALLA RB, MLADEK J, KALEYA RN, GRALLA RJ, ALCOCK NW,

Schwartz MK, Young CW, Reidenberg MM: Comparison of methods of evaluating nephrotoxicity of cis-platinum. *Clin Pharmacol Ther* 24:557–562, 1980

11. HARDAKER WT, STONE RA, McCoy R: Platinum nephrotoxicity. *Cancer* 34:1030–1032, 1974

12. SCHILSKY RL, ANDERSON T: Hypomagnesemia and renal magnesium wasting in patients receiving cisplatin. *Ann Intern Med* 90:929–931, 1979

13. CVITKOVIC E, SPAULDING J, BETHUNE V, MARTIN J, WHITMORE WF: Improvement of cis-dichlorodiammineplatinum (NSC-119875) therapeutic index in an animal model. *Cancer* 39:1357–1361, 1977

14. HAYES DM, CVITKOVIC E, GOLBEY RB, SCHREINER E, HELSON L, KRAKOFF IH: High dose cis-platinum diammine dichloride: Amelioration of renal toxicity by mannitol diuresis. *Cancer* 39:1372–1381, 1977

15. OZOLS RF, CORDEN BJ, JACOB J, WESLEY MN, OSTCHEGA Y, YOUNG RC: High-dose cisplatin in hypertonic saline. *Ann Intern Med* 100:19–24, 1984

16. BHUCHAR VK, LANZOTTI VJ: High-dose cisplatin for lung cancer. *Cancer Treat Rep* 66:375–376, 1982

17. ROSS DA, GALE GR: Reduction of the renal toxicity of cis-dichlorodiammineplatinum (II) by probenecid. *Cancer Treat Rep* 63:781–787, 1979

18. VON HOFF DD, PENTA JS, HELMAN LJ: Incidence of drug-related deaths secondary to high-dose methotrexate and citrovorum factor administration. *Cancer Treat Rep* 61:745–748, 1977

19. BLEYER WA: The clinical pharmacology of methotrexate: New applications of an old drug. *Cancer* 41:36–51, 1978

20. GARNICK MB, MAYER RJ, ABELSON HT: Acute renal failure associated with cancer treatment, in *Acute Renal Failure,* edited by BRENNER BM, LAZARUS JM, Philadelphia, WB Saunders, 1982, p 527

21. HENDERSEN ES, ADAMSON RH, OLIVERIO VT: The metabolic fate of tritiated methotrexate: II. Absorption and excretion in man. *Cancer Res* 25:1018–1024, 1965

22. PRATT CB, ROBERTS D, SHANKS EC, WARMATH EL: Clinical trials and pharmacokinetics of intermittent high-dose methotrexate- "leucovorin rescue" for children with malignant tumors. *Cancer Res* 34:3326–3331, 1974

23. JACOBS SA, STOLLER RG, CHABNER BA, JOHNS DG: 7-Hydroxymethotrexate as a urinary metabolite in human subjects and rhesus monkeys receiving high dose methotrexate. *J Clin Invest* 57:534–538, 1976

24. LIEGLER DG, HENDERSEN ES, HAHN MA, OLIVERIO VT: The effect of organic acids on renal clearance of methotrexate in man. *Clin Pharmacol Ther* 10:849–857, 1969

25. PITMAN SW, PARKER LM, TATTERSALL MHN, JAFFE N, FREI E III: Clinical trial of high-dose methotrexate (NSC-740) with citrovorum factor (NSC-3590)-toxicologic and therapeutic observations. *Cancer Chemother Rep* 6:43–49, 1975

26. GARNICK MB, MAYER RJ: Management of acute renal failure associated with neoplastic disease, in *Oncologic Emergencies,* edited by YARBORO J, BORNSTEIN R, New York, Grune and Stratton, 1981

27. PITMAN SW, FREI E III: Weekly methotrexate calcium leukovorin rescue: Effect of alkalinization on nephrotoxicity; pharmacokinetics in the CNS, and use in CNS non-Hodgkin's lymphoma. *Cancer Treat Rep* 61:695–701, 1977

28. FREI E: Methotrexate revisited. *Med Pediatr Oncol* 2:227–241, 1976

29. LINK DA, FOSBURG MT, INGELFINGER JR: Renal toxicity of high dose methotrexate. *Pediatr Res* 10:455–459, 1976

30. HOWELL SB, CARMODY J: Changes in glomerular filtration rate associated with high dose methotrexate therapy in adults. *Cancer Treat Rep* 61:1389–1391, 1977

31. KATZ ME, GLICK HJ: Nitrosoureas: A reappraisal of clinical trials. *Cancer Clin Trials* 2:297–316, 1979
32. SCHEIN PS, O'CONNELL MJ, BLOM J, ET AL: Clinical antitumor activity and toxicity of streptozotocin (NSC-85998). *Cancer* 34:993–1000, 1974
33. HARMON WE, COHEN HJ, SCHNEEBERGER EE, GRUPE WE: Chronic renal failure in children treated with methyl-CCNU. *N Engl J Med* 300:1200–1203, 1979
34. MAZZAFERRI EL, O'DORISIO TM, LOBUGLIO AF: Treatment of hypercalcemia associated with malignancy. *Semin Oncol* 5:141–153, 1978
35. PAVEY MD, WILEY EL, ABELOFF MD: Hemolytic-uremic syndrome associated with mitomycin therapy. *Cancer Treat Rep* 66:457–461, 1982
36. PETERSON BA, COLLINS AJ, VOGELZANG NJ, BLOOMFIELD CD: 5-Azacytidine and renal tubular dysfunction. *Blood* 57:182–185, 1981
37. COHEN LF, BALOW JE, MAGRATH IT, PAPLOCK DG, ZIEGLER JL: Acute tumor lysis syndrome. A review of 37 patients with Burkitt's lymphoma. *Am J Med* 68:486–491, 1980
38. RIESELBACH RE, SORENSEN LB: Uric acid metabolism in cancer: Hyperuricemic nephropathy, in *Cancer and the Kidney,* edited by RIESELBACH RE, GARNICK MB, Philadelphia, Lea and Febiger, 1982, p 485
39. RIESELBACH RE, BENTZEL CJ: Uric acid excretion and renal function in the acute hyperuricemia of leukemia. *Am J Med* 37:872–883, 1964
40. FREI E III, BENTZEL CJ, RIESELBACH RE: Renal complications of neoplastic disease. *J Chronic Dis* 16:757–776, 1963
41. SPENCER HW, YARGER WE, ROBINSON RR: Alterations of renal function during dietary induced hyperuricemia in the rat. *Kidney Int* 9:489–500, 1976
42. CONGER JD, FALK SA, GUGGENHEIM SJ, et al: A micropuncture study of the early phase of acute urate nephropathy. *J Clin Invest* 58:681–689, 1976
43. CONGER JD, FALK SA: Intrarenal dynamics in the pathogenesis and prevention of acute urate nephropathy. *J Clin Invest* 59:786–793, 1977
44. GREENBAUM D, STONE H: Dangers of uric acid excretion during treatment of leukemia and lymphosarcoma. *Lancet* 1:73–75, 1959
45. WEISBERGER AS, PERSKY L: Renal calculi and uremia as a complication of lymphoma. *Am J Med Sci* 225:669–673, 1953
46. CRITTENDEN DR, ACKERMANN GL: Hyperuricemic acute renal failure in disseminated carcinoma. *Arch Intern Med* 137:97–99, 1977
47. KELTON J, KELLEY WH, HOLMES EW: A rapid method for the diagnosis of acute uric acid nephropathy. *Arch Intern Med* 138:612–615, 1978
48. KLINENBERG JR, GOLDFINGER SE, SEEGMILLER JE: The effectiveness of the xanthine oxidase inhibitor allopurinol in the treatment of gout. *Ann Intern Med* 62:639, 1965
49. DE CONTI RC, CALABRESI P: Use of allopurinol for prevention and control of hyperuricemia in patients with neoplastic disease. *N Engl J Med* 274:481–486, 1966
50. RIESELBACH RE, SORENSEN L: Acute and chronic hyperuricemic nephropathy, in *Current Therapy in Nephrology and Hypertension,* edited by GLASSOCK RJ, Philadelphia, B.C. Decker (in press, 1984)
51. HANDE KR, PERINI F, HIXSON C, MEGARTH I, CHABNER B: Post-chemotherapy hyperxanthinuria in lymphoma patients on allopurinol: A potential cause of nephropathy (*abstract*). *Clin Res* 27:386, 1979
52. DAVIS S, PARK YK, ABUCHOWSKI A, DAVIS FF: Hypouricaemic effect of polyethyleneglycol modified urate oxidase. *Lancet* 1:281–283, 1981
53. ETTINGER DS, HARKER WG, GERRY HW, SANDERS RC, SARAL R: Hyperphosphatemia, hypocalcemia, and transient renal failure. *JAMA* 239:2472–2474, 1978

54. KANFER A, RICHET G, ROLAND J, CHATELET F: Extreme hyperphosphatemia causing acute anuric nephrocalcinosis in lymphosarcoma. *Br Med J* 1:1320–1321, 1979
55. AYALA G, CHERTOW BS, SHAH JH, WILLIAMS GA, KUKREJA SC: Acute hyperphosphatemia and acute persistent renal insufficiency induced by oral phosphate therapy. *Ann Intern Med* 83:520–521, 1975